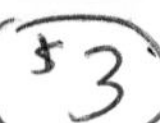

NSCA's Essentials of Personal Training

National Strength and Conditioning Association

Roger W. Earle, MA; CSCS,*D; NSCA-CPT,*D
NSCA Certification Commission

Thomas R. Baechle, EdD; CSCS,*D; NSCA-CPT,*D
Creighton University, Omaha, Nebraska
NSCA Certification Commission

Editors

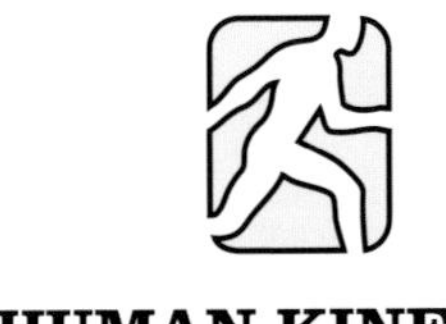

HUMAN KINETICS

Library of Congress Cataloging-in-Publication Data

NSCA's essentials of personal training / Roger W. Earle, Thomas R. Baechle, editors.
p. cm.
Includes bibliographical references and index.
ISBN 0-7360-0015-1 (Hard Cover)
1. Personal trainers. 2. Physical education and training. 3. Muscle strength. 4. Physical fitness--Physiological aspects. I. Earle, Roger W., 1967- II. Baechle, Thomas R., 1943- III. National Strength & Conditioning Association (U.S.)
GV428.7.N73 2003
613.7'1--dc22

2003019033

ISBN-10: 0-7360-0015-1

ISBN-13: 978-0-7360-0015-4

Portions of text in chapters 1-4, 7, 8, 10, 11, 13, 15-18, 21, and 24 are adapted or reprinted, by permission, from chapters 1-5, 7, 9, 10, 12, 14, 15, 17-21, 23, 24, and 26 of T.R. Baechle and R.W. Earle, 2000, *Essentials of Strength Training and Conditioning, Second Edition* (Champaign, IL: Human Kinetics), courtesy of the National Strength and Conditioning Association. We gratefully acknowledge the NSCA and the contributors to *Essentials of Strength Training and Conditioning, Second Edition.*

The Web addresses cited in this text were current as of September 15, 2003 unless otherwise noted.

Acquisitions Editor: Michael S. Bahrke, PhD; **Developmental Editor:** Christine M. Drews; **Assistant Editors:** Sandra Merz Bott and Maggie Schwarzentraub; **Copyeditor:** Joyce Sexton; **Proofreader:** Red Inc.; **Indexer:** Marie Rizzo; **Permission Manager:** Dalene Reeder; **Graphic Designer:** Robert Reuther; **Graphic Artist:** Dawn Sills; **Photo Manager:** Kareema McLendon; **Cover Designer:** Keith Blomberg; **Photographer (cover):** Kelly J. Huff; **Photographer (interior):** Tom Roberts, unless otherwise noted; **Art Manager:** Kelly Hendren; **Illustrator:** Argosy; **Printer:** Creative Printing USA

We thank the Mettler Center in Urbana, Illinois, and FitTek in Mahomet, Illinois, for providing the locations for the photo shoot for this book.

Printed in China 15

Human Kinetics
Web site: www.HumanKinetics.com

United States: Human Kinetics
P.O. Box 5076
Champaign, IL 61825-5076
800-747-4457
e-mail: humank@hkusa.com

Canada: Human Kinetics
475 Devonshire Road, Unit 100
Windsor, ON N8Y 2L5
800-465-7301 (in Canada only)
e-mail: info@hkcanada.com

Europe: Human Kinetics
107 Bradford Road
Stanningley
Leeds LS28 6AT, United Kingdom
+44 (0)113 255 5665
e-mail: hk@hkeurope.com

Australia: Human Kinetics
57A Price Avenue
Lower Mitcham, South Australia 5062
08 8372 0999
e-mail: info@hkaustralia.com

New Zealand: Human Kinetics
P.O. Box 80
Torrens Park, South Australia 5062
0800 222 062
e-mail: info@hknewzealand.com

Contents

Contributors

Anthony A. Abbott, EdD; CSCS,*D; NSCA-CPT,*D; FACSM
Fitness Institute International, Inc., Lighthouse Point, FL

Thomas R. Baechle, EdD; CSCS,*D; NSCA-CPT,*D
Creighton University, Omaha, NE

Lee E. Brown, EdD; CSCS,*D; FACSM
California State University, Fullerton

Jared W. Coburn, MS, CSCS
University of Nebraska, Lincoln

Matthew J. Comeau, PhD, ATC, LAT, CSCS
Arkansas State University

Joel T. Cramer, PhD; CSCS,*D; NSCA-CPT,*D
The University of Texas at Arlington

J. Henry "Hank" Drought, MS; CSCS,*D; NSCA-CPT,*D
Personal Trainers Strength & Conditioning Consulting, Boston, MA

Roger W. Earle, MA; CSCS,*D; NSCA-CPT,*D
NSCA Certification Commission

JoAnn Eickhoff-Shemek, PhD, FACSM, FAWHP
University of South Florida

Todd Ellenbecker, PT, MS, SCS, OCS, CSCS
Physiotherapy Associates, Scottsdale Sports Clinic, Scottsdale, AZ

Avery D. Faigenbaum, EdD; CSCS,*D; FACSM
University of Massachusetts-Boston

John F. Graham, MS, CSCS,*D
Orthopaedic Associates of Allentown, Allentown, PA

Mike Greenwood, PhD, CSCS,*D
Baylor University, Waco, TX

Patrick S. Hagerman, EdD; CSCS,*D; NSCA-CPT,*D
University of Tulsa, Oklahoma

Everett Harman, PhD, CSCS, NSCA-CPT
U.S. Army Research Institute of Environmental Medicine, Natick, MA

Bradley D. Hatfield, PhD, FACSM
University of Maryland, College Park

Allen Hedrick, MA, CSCS,*D
U.S. Air Force Academy, Colorado

Susan L. Heinrich, MS, NSCA-CPT
Pima Community College–West Campus, Tucson, AZ

Carlos E. Jiménez, MD, NSCA-CPT
Ashford Presbyterian Community Hospital, Condado, PR

Phil Kaplan, NSCA-CPT
Phil Kaplan's Fitness, Sunrise, FL

John A.C. Kordich, MEd; CSCS,*D; NSCA-CPT,*D
Pima Community College–West Campus, Tucson, AZ

Len Kravitz, PhD
University of New Mexico, Albuquerque

Tom LaFontaine, PhD, CSCS, NSCA-CPT, FAACVPR, FACSM
PREVENT Consulting Services, Columbia, MO

David Pearson, PhD, CSCS,*D
Ball State University, Muncie, IN

David H. Potach, PT; MS; CSCS,*D; NSCA-CPT,*D
Omaha Sports Physical Therapy, Omaha, NE

Kristin J. Reimers, MS, RD
The Center for Human Nutrition, Omaha, NE

Torrey Smith, CSCS, NSCA-CPT
NSCA Certification Commission

Travis Triplett-McBride, PhD, CSCS,*D
Appalachian State University, Boone, NC

Christine L. Vega, MPH; RD; CSCS,*D; NSCA-CPT,*D
Antilles Consolidated School System, Puerto Rico

Robert Watine, MD, CSCS, NSCA-CPT
Diplomate, American Board of Internal Medicine

Joseph P. Weir, PhD, EPC, FACSM
Des Moines University Osteopathic Medicine, Des Moines, IA

Wayne L. Westcott, PhD, CSCS
South Shore YMCA, Quincy, MA

Mark A. Williams, PhD, FACSM, FAACVPR
The Cardiac Center of Creighton University, Omaha, NE

Reviewers

David H. Potach, PT; MS; CSCS,*D; NSCA-CPT,*D
Omaha Sports Physical Therapy, Omaha, NE

Dan Connaughton, EdD, CSCS
University of Florida, Gainesville

Joel T. Cramer, PhD; CSCS,*D; NSCA-CPT,*D
The University of Texas at Arlington

J. Henry "Hank" Drought, MS; CSCS,*D; NSCA-CPT,*D
Personal Trainers Strength & Conditioning Consulting, Boston, MA

Dick Hannula, BA
Tacoma Swim Club, retired

John A.C. Kordich, MEd; CSCS,*D; NSCA-CPT,*D
Pima Community College–West Campus, Tucson, AZ

June M. Lindle, MA, AEA, ISCA, AAAI/ISMA
Fitness Learning Systems and Harrison Health & Fitness Center, Cincinnati, OH

Terry L. Nicola, MD, MS
University of Illinois Medical Center, Chicago

Steven Plisk, MS, CSCS,*D
Velocity Sports Performance, Norwalk, CT

Mark Rosenberg, MD, NSCA-CPT
Bethesda Memorial Hospital, Boynton Beach, FL

Jaime Ruud, MS, RD
Nutrition Link Consulting, Inc., Lincoln, NE

Darren C. Treasure, PhD
Arizona State University

Gib Willett, PT, MS, CSCS
University of Nebraska Medical Center, Omaha

Preface

You are holding a truly unique book. It is the most complete and authoritative book on personal training, and it is the primary resource for those preparing for the only nationally accredited personal training certification: the NSCA Certification Commission's NSCA-Certified Personal Trainer® (NSCA-CPT®) examination.

This book is written by leading authorities in anatomy, exercise physiology, biomechanics, medicine, psychology, testing and evaluation, nutrition, and exercise science research. In addition, respected professional personal trainers provide in-depth coverage of the academic and practical knowledge, skills, and abilities (KSAs) required of a competent personal trainer. To determine the KSAs, the NSCA Certification Commission and its independent examination service conducted a national survey of personal trainers. The resulting 13 content areas were grouped into six divisions that make up the content of *NSCA's Essentials of Personal Training*:

- **Part 1: The scientific basis of personal training.** The first part of the book contains foundational exercise science–related information about anatomy, physiology, bioenergetics, biomechanics, training adaptations, exercise psychology, motivation and goal setting, and general nutrition guidelines.
- **Part 2: Initial consultation and evaluation.** This section includes detailed guidelines about assessing a client, selecting and administering fitness tests, and interpreting the results based on descriptive and normative data.
- **Part 3: Safe and effective exercise technique.** The chapters in this part of the book describe proper exercise technique and instructional approaches for flexibility; body-weight, free weight, and machine resistance exercises; and cardiovascular activities. Also, targeted muscles and common performance errors are identified.
- **Part 4: Program design.** The focus of this section is the complex process of designing safe, effective, and goal-specific resistance, aerobic, plyometric, and speed training programs.
- **Part 5: Training specialized clients or populations.** This part of the book describes a variety of clients who have special needs and limitations (e.g., prepubescents, pregnant women, the elderly, and athletes) or physical conditions (e.g., obesity, hyperlipidemia, diabetes, hypertension, low back pain, heart disease, epilepsy). This section details how to modify an exercise program; identify exercise contraindications; and when, how, and to whom to refer a client with a condition beyond the personal trainer's scope of practice.
- **Part 6: Safety and legal issues.** The last section provides guidelines on the design and layout of commercial and home fitness facilities, basic exercise equipment maintenance, and important legal issues a personal trainer should understand and be aware of.

NSCA's Essentials of Personal Training contains features and elements that personal trainers will find helpful:

- More than 240 full-color photographs that clearly illustrate and accurately depict proper exercise technique
- Chapter objectives and key points
- Sidebars with practical explanations and applications
- Testing protocols and norms for assessing clients of all ages
- Over 120 chapter questions that can be used to help prepare for the NSCA-Certified Personal Trainer exam
- An appendix covering common personal training business management issues
- A comprehensive glossary of over 300 frequently used terms and concepts that are bolded red in the text
- Many other key terms that are bolded black at their first mention in the text

NSCA's Essentials of Personal Training is the most comprehensive reference available for personal trainers and other fitness professionals. As an exam preparation tool, it is unmatched in its scope and relevance to the NSCA-Certified Personal Trainer examination.

From the Editors

One would think that writing and editing another textbook so soon after completing the second edition of *Essentials of Strength Training and Conditioning* would be too big a task. At times it seemed so; however, this project was manageable because of the tremendous support and expertise of the staff at Human Kinetics Publishers. Thankfully, Chris Drews, the developmental editor, and Dr. Mike Bahrke, the acquisitions editor, both agreed to work with us a third time! Also, we are grateful for the dedication of Maggie Schwarzentraub and Sandra Merz Bott, assistant editors; the consistency of Joyce Sexton, the copyeditor; the vision of Bob Reuther, the graphic designer, and Dawn Sills, the graphic artist; and the patience and eye of Tom Roberts, the photographer. It simply is impossible to create a textbook of almost 700 pages without an effective and complementary system of checks and balances made possible by these people and the dozens of other staff members at Human Kinetics.

We also want to thank Dr. Rainer Martens, president of Human Kinetics, who supported the requests of the editors to create this book in full color.

Special recognition goes to the invaluable and significant content reviews and feedback of a long-time friend and colleague, David H. Potach, PT; MS; CSCS,*D; NSCA-CPT,*D, and to model clients Larry Nesbitt and Gary Rakestraw, whose life changes from regular exercise and healthy eating were truly inspirational.

Most important, the editors dedicate this book to the Earle family—Tonya, Kelsey, Allison, Natalia, and Cassandra—who understood the importance of this project and were willing to make sacrifices to ensure that it was completed. It is because of their patience, devotion, encouragement, and patience (yes, again!) that we were able to imagine, begin, persevere with, and complete this book.

PART I

Exercise Sciences

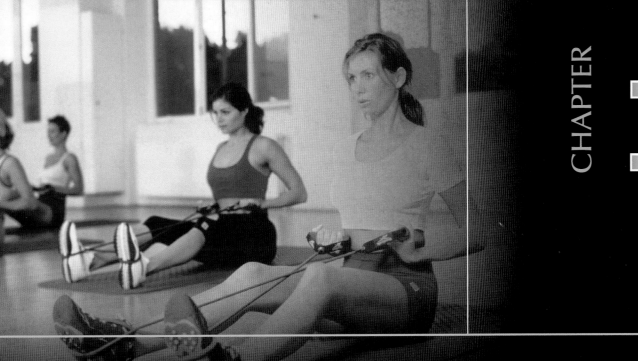

CHAPTER 1

Structure and Function of the Muscular, Nervous, and Skeletal Systems

Len Kravitz

After completing this chapter, you will be able to

- describe the structure, role, and function of skeletal muscle;
- explain the sliding-filament theory of muscular contraction;
- describe the structure and function of the motor unit;
- explain the electrical conduction system of motor nerves;
- describe the structure and role of bone of the skeletal system;
- discuss the composition of all connective tissue; and
- discuss the interrelation of muscle, bone, and connective tissue in force production.

Knowledge of and ability to apply the basic principles of anatomy and physiology of the body in effective resistance training and aerobic endurance training programs is essential for optimal assessment and prescription for clients. This chapter presents and discusses the fundamental concepts of muscle, nerve, bone, and connective tissue.

Muscular System

The muscular system delivers the forces that enable the human body to do work and perform physical activity. This section describes the foundational anatomy and physiology of the gross and microscopic composition of muscle and provides a detailed explanation of the theory of muscle contraction. In addition, we consider the various types and functions of muscle fibers.

There are three types of muscle tissue:

- Cardiac muscle, which composes the walls of the heart, is involuntary muscle and therefore is not subject to conscious control.
- Smooth muscle, which lines the internal organs such as the intestines and stomach, is also involuntary.
- Skeletal muscle is muscle that attaches to the skeleton via tendons to produce bodily movement.

Introduction to Skeletal Muscle

Skeletal muscle is under voluntary control of the nervous system and thus can be stimulated to contract and relax by conscious effort. Accounting for 36% to 45% of the total body weight and composing over 600 different muscles, skeletal muscle tissue is the most plentiful tissue in the human body. To enable the body to move, the muscles usually work together in muscle groups. Furthermore, most of the muscle groups of the trunk and extremities work in opposing pairs, so that when one muscle, referred to as the **agonist,** is initiating a desired movement, the opposite muscle, or the **antagonist,** is being stretched. For example, when one is doing a biceps curl exercise in an upright position, the biceps are the agonists while the triceps are the antagonists.

The muscle that is most directly involved in causing movement is the agonist. The opposing muscle, which can stop or slow down a movement (caused by an agonist), is the antagonist.

The properties of skeletal muscle are elasticity, extensibility, and contractility. The first two properties permit a muscle to be stretched similarly to an elastic band and—when the stretching is discontinued—to return again to its normal resting length. Contractility is the unique ability of a muscle to shorten, produce tension at its endpoints, or do both. Most skeletal muscles can shorten to nearly one-half their resting length. On the other hand, skeletal muscles can be stretched up to 150% of their resting length.

Neural stimulation can lead to three primary types of muscle actions: **concentric action, eccentric action,** and **isometric action.** A concentric action occurs when a muscle overcomes a load and shortens, as in the upward phase of the biceps curl exercise. An eccentric action occurs when a muscle cannot develop sufficient tension and is overcome by an external load, and thus progressively lengthens. Eccentric actions are commonly involved in the deceleration of joint motion. For example, walking down stairs involves an eccentric action of the quadriceps muscle group as it decelerates the flexion action of the knee. Concentric and eccentric muscle actions involve dynamic work, in which the muscle is either moving a joint or controlling its motion. In an isometric action, the muscle generates force against a resistance but does not overcome it and therefore does not shorten, lengthen, or cause joint motion. Many of the body's posture muscles work isometrically to hold or restrain the skeleton in the upright posture in opposition to the force of gravity. It should be noted that certain exercise devices elicit an **isokinetic** muscle action, which is a dynamic muscle action kept at a constant velocity independent of the amount of muscular force generated by the involved muscles. Thus with isokinetic actions, the speed of shortening and lengthening is constant.

Gross Muscle Structure and Organization

The structural component of skeletal muscle is the **muscle fiber,** which is also known as the muscle cell. The muscle fiber is a cylindrical cell that contains hundreds of nuclei. Its length varies from a few millimeters, as in muscles of the eye, to up to 30 centimeters (12 inches), with the longest fibers in the sartorius muscle of the leg. Surrounding the individual muscle fiber and thus separating the fibers from one another is a layer of connective tissue known as the **endomysium** (figure 1.1). The fibers are grouped into different-sized bundles, or

fascicles, which contain up to 150 fibers. Each fasciculus is surrounded by another connective tissue, the **perimysium.** Encasing the entire muscle is an outer **fascia** of connective tissue called the **epimysium.** This dense, protective sheath joins with the other intramuscular tissues to form the strong connective tissue of tendons. The tendons attach to the **periosteum,** which is the outermost covering of the bone. Unlike muscles, tendons have no active contractile properties.

The structural constituent of skeletal muscle is the multinucleated muscle fiber, which is also known as the muscle cell.

Beneath the endomysium and surrounding each muscle fiber is the **sarcolemma,** which is a thin plasma membrane (figure 1.2). The primary function of the sarcolemma is to conduct an electrochemical wave of depolarization along the surface of the muscle fiber. In addition, the sarcolemma serves to insulate muscle fibers from one another during a depolarization occurrence. The sarcolemma also fuses with the endomysium. Within the sarcolemma's basement membrane are **satellite cells,** which have important regulatory functions for cellular growth. The spaces within the muscle fiber hold **sarcoplasm,** a fluid resembling gelatin that contains lipids (fat), glycogen, enzymes, nuclei, mitochondria, and other cellular organelles. The sarcoplasm in muscle cells is analogous to the cytoplasm in other cells of the body; but the sarcoplasm, in contrast to cytoplasm, is a storage site for large amounts of glycogen (for energy utilization) and myoglobin (for oxygen binding). Also within the sarcoplasm are a large number of interconnecting **transverse tubules** (or T tubules) that pass through the muscle fiber. The T tubules are extensions of the sarcolemma that carry impulses through the fiber and serve as transport vesicles for certain substances, such as ions, oxygen, and glucose. Within the muscle fiber as well is a longitudinal system of tubules known as the **sarcoplasmic reticulum.** The sarcoplasmic reticulum is a highly specialized complex that stores calcium ions (Ca^{2+}). The function of this system is described in the theory of muscle contraction.

Microscopic Muscle Structure and Order

Within a muscle fiber, lying parallel to one another, are up to thousands of **myofibrils**—the elements of skeletal muscle that allow the muscle to contract. The myofibrils consist primarily of two proteins, **actin** and **myosin,** which are referred to as **myofilaments.** Close examination of the myofilaments reveals a thinner actin protein compared to a thicker myosin protein. Other proteins present in the myofibrillar complex include troponin, tropomyosin, alpha-actinin, beta-actinin, M protein, C protein, and titin. As seen when the surface of a muscle fiber is viewed with a light microscope, the arrangement of the actin and myosin myofilaments creates distinctive light and dark striations. These striation patterns exist throughout the muscle fiber and explain why skeletal muscle is also called striated muscle. The darker zone is termed the **A band,** and the lighter region is referred to as the **I band.** Protein actin attaches to the **Z line** (or Z disk),

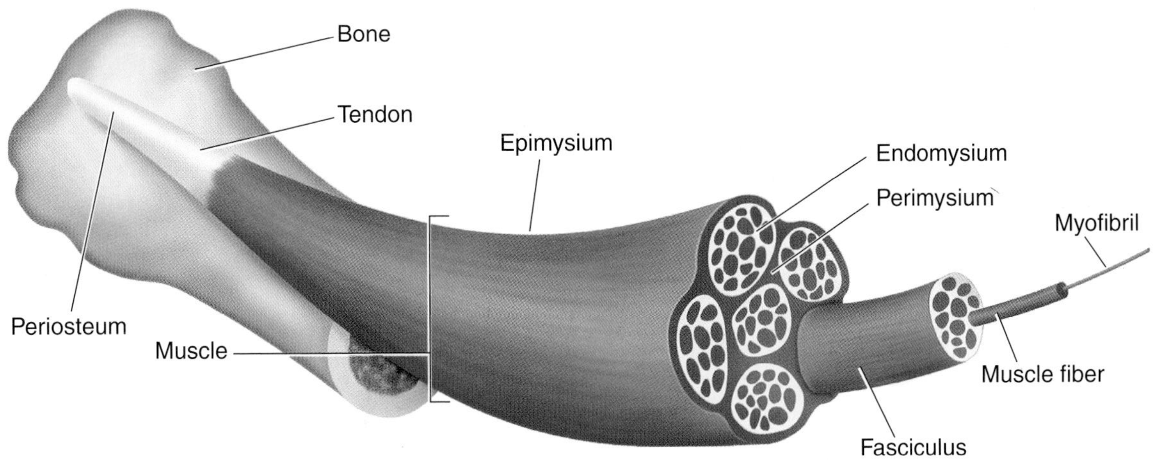

Figure 1.1 The basic structure of muscle.
Reprinted from Wilmore and Costill 1999.

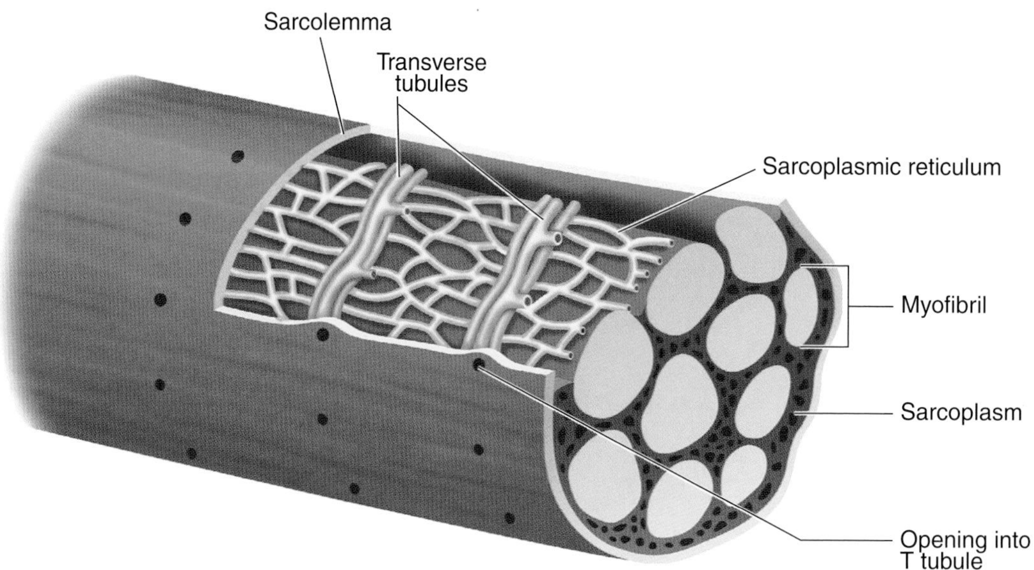

Figure 1.2 Single muscle fiber morphology.
Reprinted from Wilmore and Costill 1999.

which bisects the I band. The Z line attaches to the sarcolemma to bring stability to this ultrastructure of muscle tissue. The repeating sequence from Z line to Z line delineates the functional unit of skeletal muscle, the **sarcomere** (figure 1.3). The myofibrils are composed of numerous sarcomeres, which are joined end to end at the Z line [5]. On either side of the Z line is a lighter I band region, which contains only the actin protein. The darker A band contains myosin and actin proteins. However, in the center of the A band, a gap exists where only myosin is present. This region is the **H zone,** and within its center is a darker area known as the **M line** (the center of the sarcomere), which is produced by proteins that link adjacent myosin filaments.

The functional and contractile unit of skeletal muscle is the sarcomere.

Actin-Myosin Alignment

To understand how muscles contract to create forces for movement, one must examine actin and myosin more closely. Actin is composed of two thin filaments shaped in a double helix, which means that it appears as two strands twisting around each other. Attached are two other important protein constituents, **tropomyosin** and **troponin,** which help with actin's function in muscle contraction (see figure 1.3). Tropomyosin is a long, rope-like protein that spirals around the actin double helix, lies in a groove formed by the actin strands, and blocks the binding sites for actin-myosin interaction or coupling. Troponin is a globular molecule that attaches at regular intervals to the tropomyosin. It has a strong affinity to calcium ions and thus has a crucial function in muscle action and fatigue.

Myosin is a thicker filament with distinct components. The molecule has two globular heads—called myosin heads, S1 units, or cross-bridges—that are attached to protein strands (see figure 1.3). The components containing the cross-bridges are sometimes referred to as the "heavy chains." The protein strands intertwine to form long shafts, "tails," or "light chains." Hundreds of myosin molecules are packed tail to tail in a sheaf, with the globular heads pointed in one direction along half of the filament and in the opposite direction along the other half. In the middle, where no globular heads are present, is the M line. Myosin is secured along its longitudinal axis partly by thin filaments of the protein titin (figure 1.4). Six actin filaments surround each myosin filament. In muscle contraction, the myosin globular heads extend as cross-bridges and bind to specific sites on the actin filament, forming the structural and functional link between the two filaments.

The Sliding-Filament Theory: How Muscle Contracts

The sliding-filament theory of muscle contraction suggests that changes in muscle length occur as the

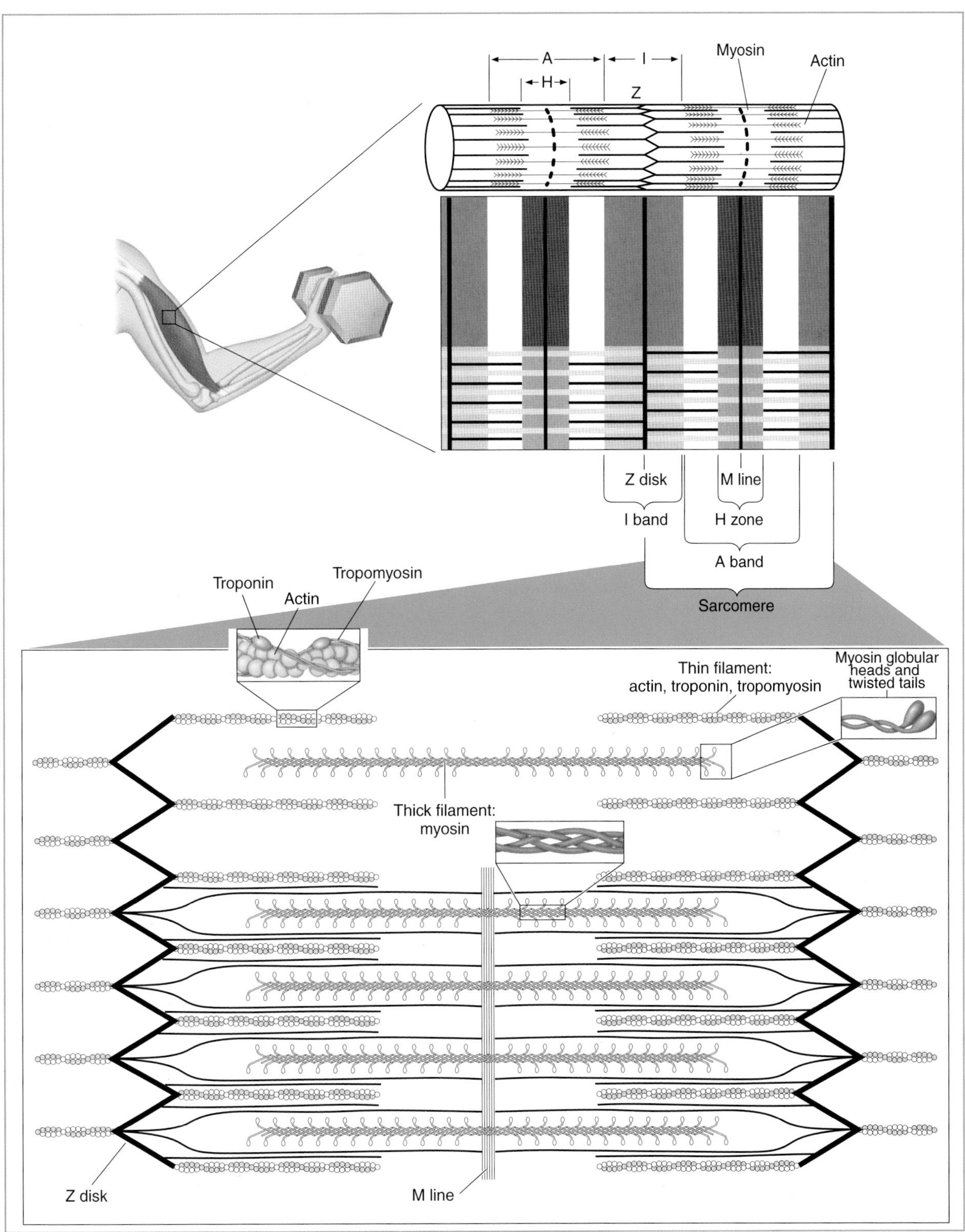

Figure 1.3 The sarcomere: the basic functional unit of the myofibril and the specialized order of actin and myosin filaments.
Reprinted from Wilmore and Costill 1999.

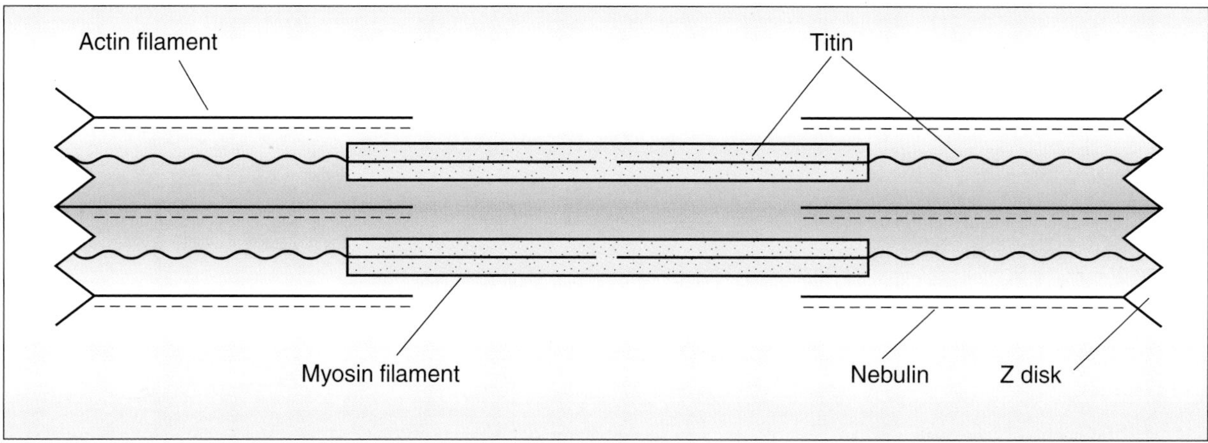

Figure 1.4 Filaments made of titin maintain the spacing of the myosin filaments between the actin filaments.
Reprinted from Wilmore and Costill 1999.

myosin and actin myofilaments slide past each other. The myofilaments do not actually change in their length; it is the sarcomere that is shortening (concentric action) or lengthening (eccentric action), with a resultant production of force. The change of length occurs as the myosin cross-bridges bind to sites on the actin and then rotate, causing the filament sliding. The actin filaments slide over the myosin filaments, with the force of the contraction coming from the myosin cross-bridges. The myosin cross-bridges swivel in an arc around their fixed position, similarly to oars on a boat. As the Z lines of the sarcomere are pulled together (concentric action), the regions of the I band and H zone decrease. There is no change in the length of the myosin, depicted by the A band. During an isometric contraction, the spacing of the I band and H zone remains unchanged. The energy for this molecular motion comes from the splitting of **adenosine triphosphate (ATP).** The following steps highlight the complex sequence of the sliding-filament theory.

The myofilaments (actin and myosin) do not actually change in their length during a muscle action; it is the sarcomere that is shortening (concentric action) or lengthening (eccentric action), with a resultant production of force.

Initiation of a Muscle Action

Before a muscle cell can act, it must receive an **action potential** from a motor neuron, as explained in the neurological section later in this chapter. After the sarcolemma of the muscle cell receives the action potential, the electrical impulse travels inward through the transverse tubules and sarcoplasmic reticulum. This electrical charge causes the sarcoplasmic reticulum to quickly release calcium ions into the sarcoplasm (figure 1.5). While in a resting state, the tropomyosin protein strands are covering the binding sites on the actin filaments, thus preventing any actin-myosin interaction. However, once the calcium ions are released from the sarcoplasmic reticulum they bind with troponin, which has a strong affinity for calcium ions. Troponin, which lies on top of the tropomyosin, then initiates a molecular process of shifting the tropomyosin molecules off the binding sites (on the actin). The myosin cross-bridges can now attach to the binding sites on the actin filaments.

When the myosin cross-bridges are activated, they bind with actin, leading to the conformational change at the cross-bridges where they swivel in an arc around their fixed position, in an action called the **power stroke.** This causes the actin filaments to slide over (or be pulled over) the myosin protein and muscle shortening to occur (figure 1.6). Present on the globular heads of the myosin cross-bridges is the enzyme ATPase, which speeds up the splitting of ATP to yield adenosine diphosphate (ADP), inorganic phosphate (P_i), and energy. Adenosine triphosphate is the energy molecule for all muscle actions. Immediately after the power stroke, the myosin cross-bridges detach from their receptor site and rotate back to their original positions. Adenosine triphosphate provides the energy required for the dissociation of actin and myosin. Following this detachment of the cross-bridges, **hydrolysis** (or splitting) of ATP can reoccur, and the myosin cross-bridges then reattach to a new bind-

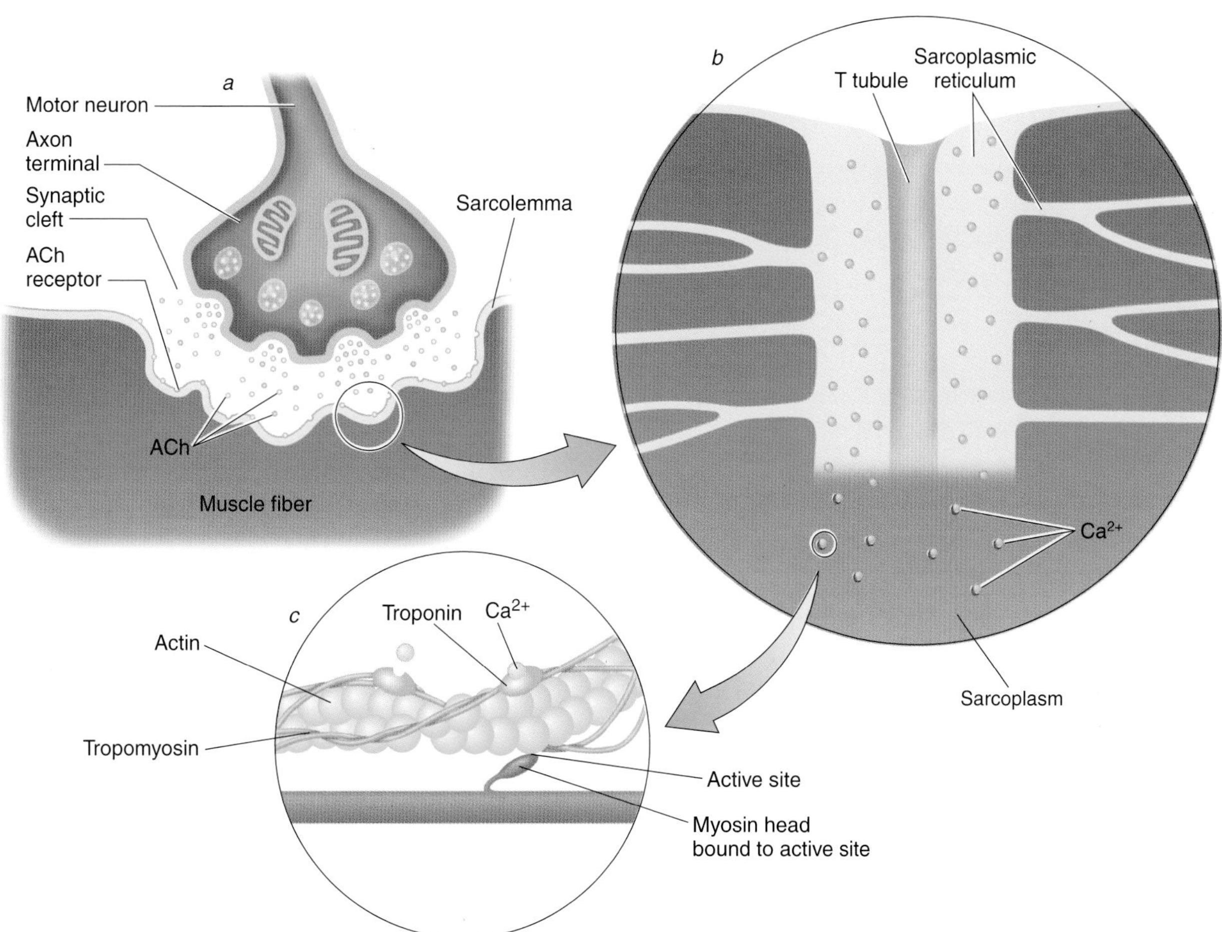

Figure 1.5 The sequence of events leading to a muscle action. ACh = acetylcholine; Ca^{2+} = calcium ions.
Reprinted from Wilmore and Costill 1999.

ing site on the actin filaments farther along, undergo another power stroke, and cause actin sliding over myosin. In an isometric action, the myosin cross-bridges continue to bind, swivel, and detach; but they reattach at the same sites, as no movement is occurring in the sarcomere. In an eccentric muscle action, the myosin cross-bridges are undergoing the attaching, power stroke, detaching, and recombining movements, only the Z lines are now moving apart due to the lengthening occurrence in an eccentric muscle action.

In all muscle actions, the cross-bridges do not act in a synchronized manner. Each pair of cross-bridges acts independently. If the cross-bridges responded simultaneously, human movement would be very jerky. Therefore, at any given moment during a muscle action, some of the cross-bridges are actively generating force via their power strokes, while other cross-bridges are attaching or detaching from their receptor sites on the actin filaments.

In all muscle actions, the cross-bridges do not act in a synchronized manner. Each pair of cross-bridges acts independently. If they responded simultaneously, human movement would be very jerky.

End of Muscle Action

The muscle actions continue until the muscle is no longer stimulated, thus preventing further release of calcium ions from the sarcoplasmic reticulum. During this recovery, calcium ions in the sarcoplasm are returned to the sarcoplasmic reticulum for storage by an ATP-mediated calcium-pumping system. With the removal of calcium, troponin becomes deactivated; this leads to a shift of tropomyosin to its resting position, covering the receptor sites for the myosin cross-bridges (on the actin filaments). The hydrolysis of ATP ceases and the muscle fiber returns to a relaxed state.

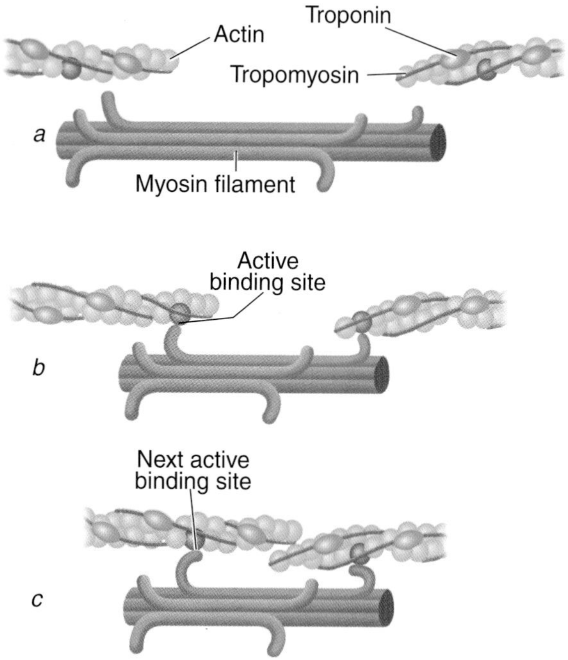

Figure 1.6 Muscle fiber myofilaments illustrating the sliding-filament theory: *(a)* relaxed, *(b)* contracting, and *(c)* fully contracted.
Reprinted from Wilmore and Costill 1999.

Muscle Fiber Types

Skeletal muscle has traditionally been classified according to the myosin heavy-chain protein it possesses. There are two distinct fiber types: **fast-twitch** (or **Type II**) and **slow-twitch** (or **Type I**). Fiber types are differentiated by their metabolic and contractile properties. Fast-twitch fibers have the ability to generate rapid, powerful muscle actions. This is due to a number of metabolic factors such as a speedy level of calcium ion release, a high level of myosin ATPase, and a highly developed sarcoplasmic reticulum. The fast-twitch fiber's speed of shortening and force development is three to five times faster than that of slow-twitch fibers [2]. The fast-twitch fibers use predominantly a blood glucose and muscle glycogen fuel source and thus are predominantly recruited in anaerobic-type activities such as a volleyball spike, a tennis serve, or a weight training workout. Fast-twitch muscle fibers can be further subdivided into two primary groups: Type IIa and Type IIb [1]. Fast-twitch and slow-twitch fibers can exist as "pure fibers," containing only one type of myosin heavy chain, or as hybrids, containing multiple forms [1]. The Type IIa fibers are considered intermediate fibers, having a moderate capacity for anaerobic and aerobic energy production. They are referred to as fast-oxidative-glycolytic or FOG fibers. The Type IIb fibers exhibit the most extensive anaerobic potential and are referred to as fast-glycolytic or FG fibers.

Slow-twitch or Type I fibers are characteristically involved in energy production for prolonged aerobic activities, such as step aerobics, aquatic exercise, long-distance running, and stationary cycling. They are described as fatigue resistant, whereas fast-twitch fibers fatigue easily. The slow-twitch fibers have a less developed sarcoplasmic reticulum, which leads to a slower calcium ion-handling capability and a low activity level of myosin ATPase; this in turn inhibits the speed of hydrolysis of ATP. In addition, the glucose and glycolytic control capacity is less developed than in the fast-twitch fibers. However, Type I fibers contain a large number of **mitochondria** and mitochondrial enzymes, which enhances their aerobic metabolism capacity. The Type I fibers are often described as slow-oxidative or SO fibers, with reference to their high involvement in aerobic metabolism and their slower rate of shortening. The SO fibers also have a greater capacity for blood flow, a structural and functional adaptation due to their greater need for oxygen delivery.

Distribution of Fiber Types in Various Populations

It is interesting to note that a person's arm and leg muscles generally have similar proportions of slow-twitch and fast-twitch fibers. One exception is the soleus muscle, an ankle plantar flexor involved in walking and weight-bearing activities, which is predominantly a slow-twitch muscle [5]. Most men, women, and children possess 45% to 55% slow-twitch muscle fibers in their limbs [2]. Type IIa and IIb fibers are fairly evenly distributed. There does not appear to be a gender difference in muscle fiber distribution, just a difference in absolute muscle size. With world-caliber athletes, a distinction in fiber type is often apparent. Sprinters tend to have more fast-twitch fibers in their legs, whereas aerobic endurance athletes demonstrate predominance in slow-twitch fibers. Middle-distance-event athletes frequently have an equal distribution of fast-twitch and slow-twitch fibers. Notwithstanding, fiber type is only one component of athletic success and is not a universally accepted predictor of athletic performance [2]. The fast-twitch and slow-twitch characteristics of muscle fibers appear to be determined within the first few years of life—thus genetically determined—and change very little until late in life. As people grow older they tend to lose fast-twitch fibers as a result of age-related changes and physical inactivity. Fortunately, the intervention of progressive resistance exercise to mature adult clients' exercise programs can delay the loss of muscle mass while enhancing muscle strength, function, and performance in everyday life activities.

Muscle fiber recruitment involves the interaction of the nerve and the muscle fibers innervated by that motor nerve, known as the **motor unit.** This necessitates a further review of the structure and function of the nervous system.

Nervous System

The nervous system is the communication and command system of the body. Its main functions are to sense changes in and around the body, interpret these changes, and then respond with some form of muscle contraction or gland secretion. The nervous system is divided into two parts: the **central nervous system,** which includes the brain and spinal cord, and the **peripheral nervous system,** which consists of the nerves extending from the brain and spinal cord. The skin, joints, tendons, muscles, internal organs, and sense organs send sensory input, via the **afferent neurons** (of the peripheral nervous system), to the central nervous system; and **efferent neurons** (of the peripheral nervous system) send output from the central nervous system to the muscles and glands. The efferent neurons can be further divided into a **somatic** and an **autonomic nervous system.** The somatic nervous system, consisting of motor neurons, innervates skeletal muscle whereas the autonomic nerves excite involuntary organ muscles, such as in the stomach, blood vessels, heart, and intestines. Nerves can be either excitatory or inhibitory. This section focuses primarily on the structure and function of the peripheral nervous system as it relates to physical activity and exercise.

Nerve Fibers: Structure and Function

All movements and exercise are regulated by the body's neural control system. The three main divisions of the neuron are the **cell body, dendrites,** and **axon** (see figure 1.7). The cell body contains the nucleus, nucleolus, various substances, and other organelles. Attached to the cell body are numerous dendrites that transmit sensory messages (relating to heat, cold, pressure, touch, kinesthetic sense, etc.) to the cell body from other neurons. On one side of the cell body is a cone-shaped region known as the **axon hillock.** Extending from the axon hillock is the axon, which transmits messages from the cell body to its end organs. A cell body normally has many dendrites but only one axon.

A multilayered covering known as the **myelin sheath** encircles most of the axons of the peripheral nervous system. The myelin sheath provides insulation and maintenance for the axon. A fiber not covered with this sheath is called unmyelinated, whereas with the sheath it is myelinated. The constituents of the myelin sheath are **Schwann cells,** which wind around the axon many times. Along the myelin sheath are gaps approximately every one to two millimeters, which are called the **nodes of Ranvier.** Electrical impulses are propagated much faster on myelinated axons, as the messages "jump" from one node of Ranvier to the next, in a process called a **saltatory conduction.** The axon splits into numerous branches at its **axon terminals.** On the tips of the axon terminals are synaptic knobs that house vesicles containing communication chemicals known as **neurotransmitters** (e.g., acetylcholine).

The functional unit of the neuromuscular system is the **motor unit,** which consists of the motor nerve and the muscles fibers it innervates. Each motor nerve innervates several muscle fibers, with the ratio of muscle fibers to motor neuron dependent on the muscle's particular function. For instance, precise movements of the eye may have as few as 10 muscle fibers per motor neuron, whereas with large muscle groups a motor neuron may innervate as many as 2,000 or 3,000 muscle fibers [2].

> The functional unit of the neuromuscular system is the motor unit, which consists of the motor nerve and the muscles fibers it innervates.

Nerve Impulses, Depolarization, and Action Potentials

The cell membrane of a nerve and muscle fiber is polarized, which means there is a difference in charges. On the inside of a cell is a high concentration of potassium ions (K^+), and on the outside is a high concentration of sodium ions (Na^+) (see figure 1.8). At rest the internal cell membrane's charge is –70 millivolts in relation to the charge on the outside of the cell. This is the cell's **resting membrane potential,** and the negative charge on the inside means that the cell's outside environment is relatively much more positive. The stability of the resting membrane potential is sustained by the **sodium-potassium pump,** which

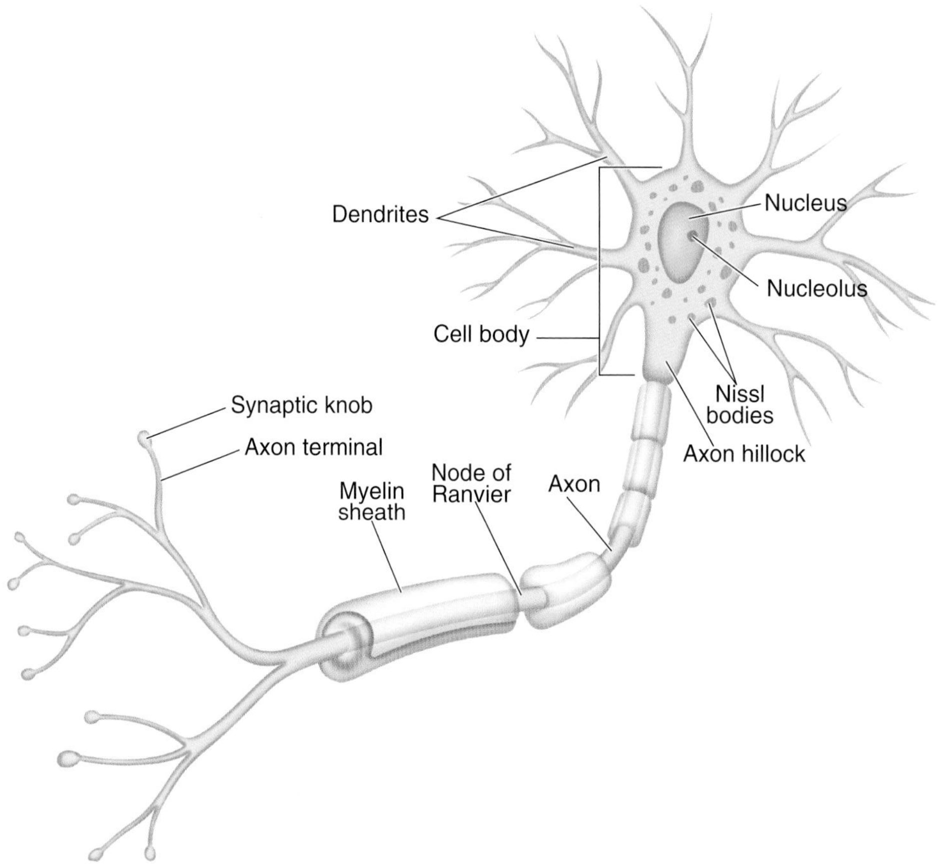

Figure 1.7 Structure of a nerve cell body and axon.
Reprinted from Wilmore and Costill 1999.

helps to regulate the balance of potassium and sodium ions on the inside and outside of the cell, respectively.

At any given moment, the nerve cell membrane undergoes minor changes in electrical charge due to small changes in the cell membrane's external environment. These are referred to as **graded potentials.** If the cell membrane's charge becomes less negative, a **depolarization** is occurring, and if it becomes more negative a **hyperpolarization** is occurring. If the cell membrane's electrical potential changes to a value of –50 to –55 millivolts, it reaches its electrical **threshold** and will conduct an action potential along the axon to the target muscle or organ. The membrane potential will change from the –70 millivolts to a value of +30 millivolts in an action potential. This dramatic voltage change occurs because many sodium ions are rushing into the cell (figure 1.8). When a cell membrane reaches or exceeds its electrical threshold, the entire message becomes an action potential. The principle at work is referred to as the **all-or-none principle** because if threshold is not met, the action potential will not be propagated, and when it is reached the action potential is completely conducted. As the action potential travels along a myelinated nerve, it commences into a saltatory conduction, jumping from node of Ranvier to node of Ranvier toward its end organ. The speed of a nerve transmission along a myelinated axon may be as fast as 100 meters per second (220 miles per hour) [5]. Upon reaching the axon terminals, the action potential will have reached its target organ or a synapse.

When a cell membrane reaches or exceeds its electrical threshold, the entire message becomes an action potential. The principle involved is called the all-or-none principle.

Immediately following the action potential, the motor nerve restores itself to its resting membrane potential. This is called **repolarization** (see figure 1.8). Repolarization initially involves potassium ions moving to the outside of the cell to regain the –70 millivolt resting membrane potential. Upon

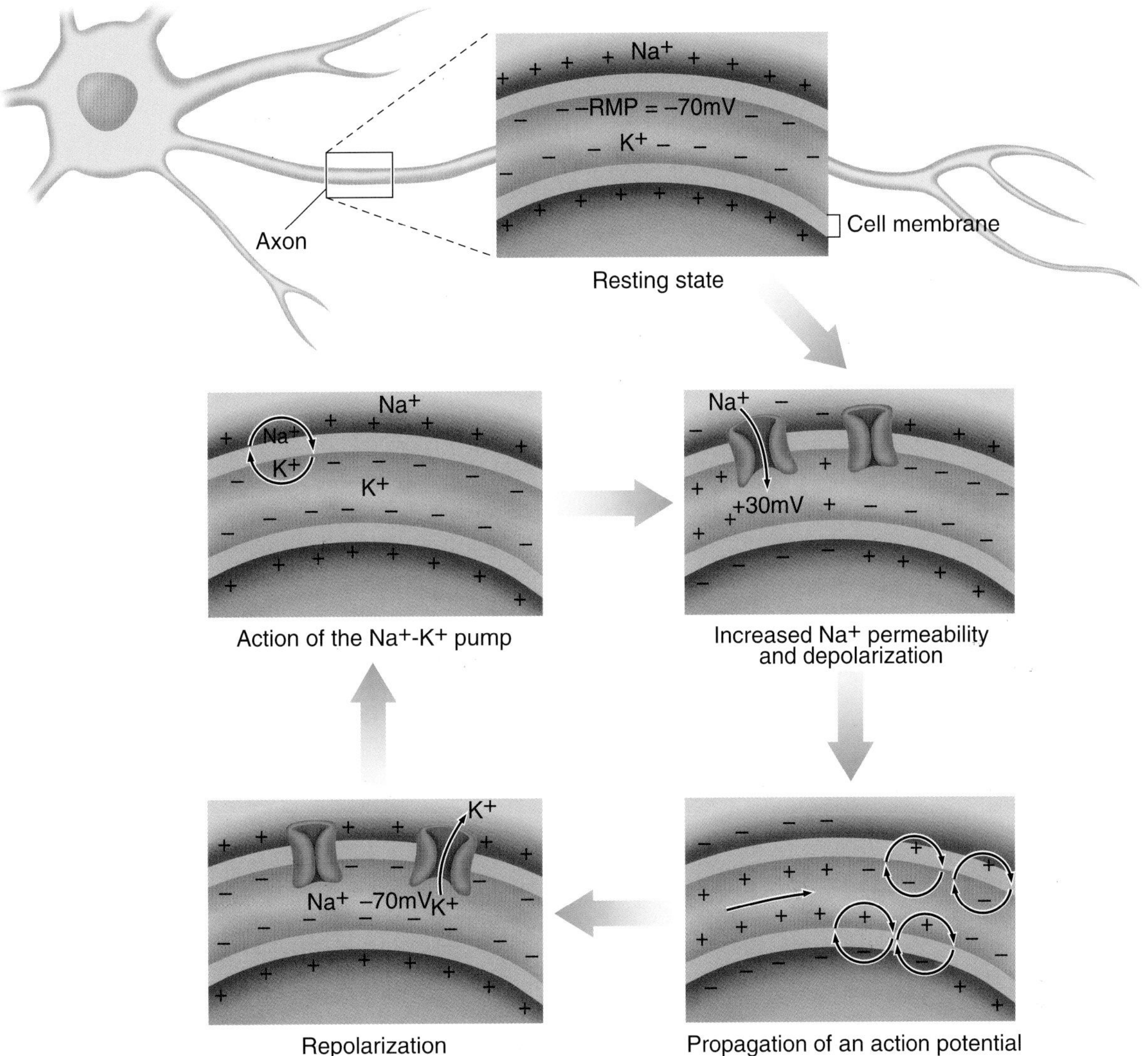

Figure 1.8 The sequence of events during an action potential: the resting state, increased sodium permeability and depolarization, propagation of an action potential, repolarization, and the action of the sodium-potassium pump. K^+ = potassium ions; mV = millivolts; Na^+ = sodium ions; RMP = resting membrane potential.
Reprinted from Wilmore and Costill 1999.

reaching resting membrane potential, the cell has one final process to complete. During the action potential, sodium ions rushed into the cell, while during repolarization potassium ions exited the cell. This created a concentration of sodium ions on the inside and potassium ions on the outside of the cell, a situation opposite to that of the normal cell resting membrane potential. To return the ions to their proper locations, inside or outside of the cell, the sodium-potassium pump is activated, which restores the ion concentration to the correct side of the cell membrane.

The **synapse** is the junction between two nerves where a neurotransmitter will diffuse from the axon terminal of the initial axon to receptor sites on the second nerve, to continue an action potential. Nerves communicate with one another via synapses, whereas nerves communicate to muscles via a **neuromuscular junction.**

Neuromuscular Junction

The function of the neuromuscular junction is to transmit the electrical impulse from the nerve to the muscle (figure 1.9). The action potential reaches the axon terminals of the motor neuron. In the synaptic knobs, vesicles fuse with the terminal membrane and release the neurotransmitters in the space, or cleft, between the neuron and the muscle fiber.

The impulse is received in a specialized segment of the muscle fiber known as the **motor endplate.** The motor endplate visually looks like sarcolemma membrane folded into small cavities that contain the neurotransmitter receptor sites. The binding of the neurotransmitter to the motor endplate leads to a depolarization of the muscle cell membrane. If threshold is met, which is the same electrical threshold in muscle as in nerves, the action potential will spread throughout the sarcolemma, transverse tubules, and sarcoplasmic reticulum (as described earlier in "Muscular System"). Immediately following the action potential, the muscle cell membrane repolarizes and restores itself to resting membrane potential. After the action potential is complete, the neurotransmitters are either destroyed by enzymes or are actively returned to their synaptic vesicles and readied for the next impulse to arrive [5].

The function of the neuromuscular junction is to transmit the electrical impulse from the nerve to the muscle.

The Proprioceptors

Specialized receptors in muscles, joints, and tendons, known as **proprioceptors,** are of particular interest to the personal trainer. It is the proprioceptors that, for example, help clients subconsciously maintain posture and balance when performing a lunge or that inhibit the stretch should the lunge be too deep. These organs relay messages to the central nervous system about muscular changes in the body and limb movement. **Muscle spindles,** which lie parallel to muscle fibers, provide sensory feedback (to the central nervous system) concerning the length change and speed of length change of muscle fibers. Their input may lead to a reflex response, known as the **stretch reflex,** of the central nervous system to inhibit the stretch in a muscle or cause it to contract. Therefore, the muscle spindle protects the muscle from extreme ranges of stretch or from stretches that are performed too fast. For example, one of the reasons personal trainers are encouraged not to do rapid stretching with their untrained clients is that the accelerated movement toward the endpoint of motion may cause muscle damage from the muscle spindle responding with the stretch reflex (i.e., a contracting response while the muscle is lengthening).

Golgi tendon organs lie within the tendons of the musculotendinous region and recognize changes in tension in the muscle. In response to this muscle tension, the central nervous system may reflexively send a message to suppress the muscular force. If a client lifts a barbell that is too heavy for that individual, the Golgi tendon organs elicit an inhibiting message that goes to the muscle, not allowing further movement and thus sparing the muscle from excessive or dangerous tension. Thus the protective role of Golgi tendon organs is to safeguard the muscle from excessive loads that the client may not be properly prepared to execute. **Pacinian corpuscles** are sensory organs located near the musculotendinous junction. Their functional role is to provide sensory information about bodily movement or pressure.

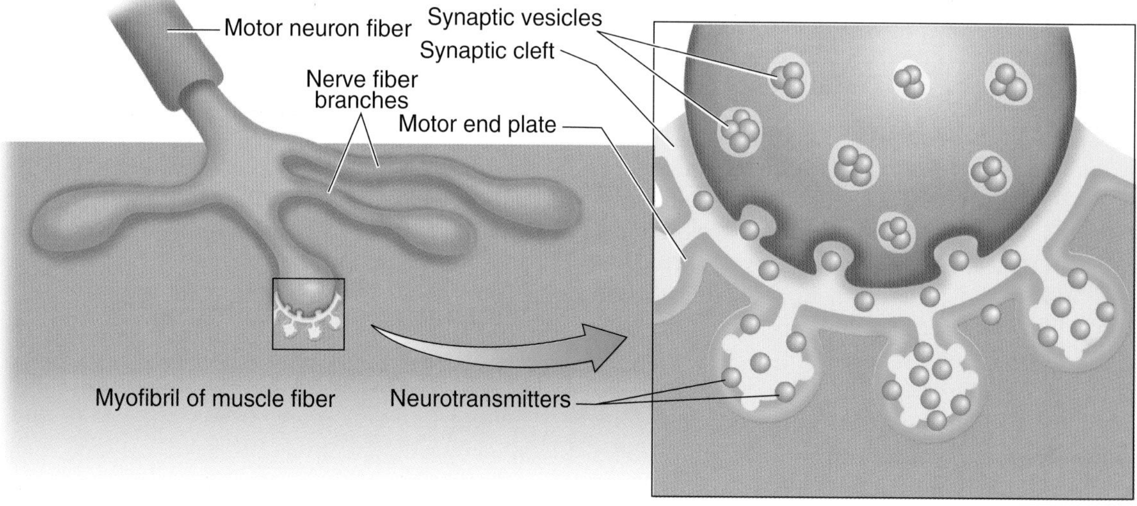

Figure 1.9 Neuromuscular junction.
Reprinted from Wilmore and Costill 1999.

Proprioceptors relay messages to the central nervous system about muscular changes in the body and about limb movement.

Skeletal System

The skeletal system is composed of over 200 bones, linked together by joints that provide the support and foundation for the muscles and organs of the body. It is divided into the **axial skeleton** and **appendicular skeleton.** The axial skeleton, or central skeleton, consists of the skull, vertebral column, sternum, and ribs. The appendicular skeleton consists of the shoulder girdles, arms, legs, and hips. The different shapes of bone (e.g., short, long, flat, and irregular bones) are associated with their function and the loads placed upon them. This section provides an overview of the structure and function of bone and bone growth.

Types of Bone Tissue

Bone tissue or **osseous** tissue is an active, living tissue that consists of two types: **compact bone** and **cancellous bone** (see figure 1.10). Compact bone, or cortical bone, is dense bone distinguished by the arrangement of minerals and cells into the **Haversian system,** which is composed of bone cells, nerves, and blood and lymph vessels. The Haversian system accounts for 80% of the skeletal mass and is situated toward the outer layers of a given bone [4]. The cancellous, spongy, or trabecular bone has no Haversian system and accounts for 20% of the skeletal mass. Cancellous bone is quite porous, with branching struts, called **trabeculae,** that form a latticelike arrangement. This spongy-looking bone tissue allows for marrow and fat storage and yet provides a microstructure for bone strength [4]. The relative percentage of compact and cancellous bone varies in different bones.

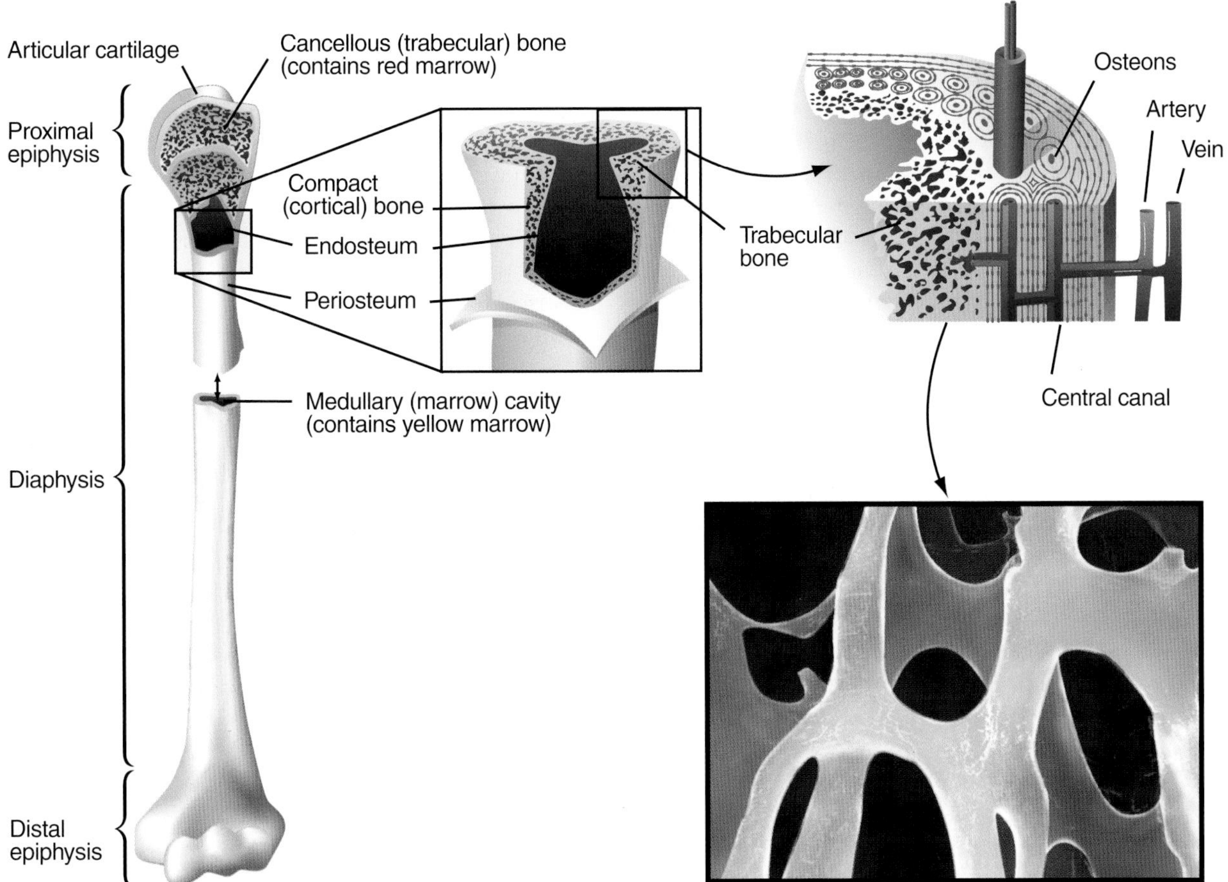

Figure 1.10 Structure of bone and view of bone in cross section.
Reprinted from Plowman and Smith 1997.

Major Functions of Bone Tissue

The functions of bone tissue can be grouped into structural and physiological categories. Structurally, the skeletal system serves as the basis for physical movement and internal organ protection. Physiologically, bone tissue is the region for red blood cell formation and white blood cell formation, called **hematopoiesis.** In addition, bone is a storage area for calcium and phosphate, which are essential for nerve conduction, muscle actions, heart contraction, blood clotting, and energy formation [3]. Because of their different constituencies, compact bone is best adapted for structural support, whereas cancellous bone is best matched for the bone's physiological functions.

Bone Growth and Remodeling

Bone growth, or **ossification,** is the increase in size of bone due to an increase in bone cells. The bone may increase in its thickness or grow longitudinally. Longitudinal growth occurs at the epiphyseal plate (cartilage at the end of the long bone) initially with replacement of the cartilage growth by bone. Although bone is one of the body's hardest structures, it is important to realize that bone growth is a very dynamic and metabolically active tissue process of the body that occurs throughout the life span. A distinguishing aspect of bone is its high content of minerals, such as calcium and phosphate (which give bone its hardness) and organic components (which give bone its resilience). Bone has unique capabilities for growth and self-repair. It adapts to the mechanical loads placed upon it through a process referred to as bone remodeling.

Bone remodeling describes the bone tissue's capability to modify its shape, size, and structure in response to demands imposed upon it. It is a physiological process involving bone **resorption** and formation. Resorption means loss of a substance, in this case bone tissue. Remodeling is an ongoing process of bone turnover, replacement, maintenance, and repair [3]. It is a balanced process of bone resorption and bone formation. In elderly populations or in persons with some diseases, the bone resorption is greater than bone formation, resulting in a reduction in bone mineral density.

The bone matrix consists of three types of bone cells: **osteoclasts, osteoblasts,** and **osteocytes.** The osteoclasts are bone-destroying cells that cause the resorption of bone tissue. Osteoblasts are bone-forming cells that lead to the deposition of bone tissue. Osteocytes are mature osteoblasts that help regulate bone remodeling.

Bone Health

1. A loss of bone mineral density results in weak bones that are susceptible to fracture.
2. The most common sites for fracture are the hip, spine, and wrist.
3. Bone mineral density is highly related to long-term physical activity.
4. Exercise may be beneficial in preventing fractures by increasing strength.

Connective Tissue

The human body consists of numerous tissues. The connective tissue structures of great interest to the personal trainer are the tendons, ligaments, and fascia. Whether the personal trainer is leading group exercise classes, where forces and stretches are involved, or collaborating on a client's rehabilitation program, he or she will need a working knowledge of connective tissues. This section deals with the function and structure of these connective tissues.

Tendons

Muscles attach to bone via strong tissues called **tendons.** The tendons transfer the tension created by the muscle to the bones, causing movement. The main constituent of tendon is the protein **collagen,** arranged in bundles in a somewhat wavy manner. Collagen, an inelastic tissue with great tensile strength, is the most abundant protein in the body and a structural component of all living tissue. Collagen fibers provide a negligible amount of extensibility. The collagen molecule consists of three amino acids that wind together as a triple helix. The collagen bundles are oriented along the long axis of the tendon, which is the direction of the physiological loads placed on tendons. This facilitates the tendon's ability to withstand great loads without overextending or deforming. The collagen fibrils have intermolecular cross-links that fortify the rope-like, unyielding characteristic of tendon. In addition, the tendon's multiple layers of connective tissue contribute to its rigid framework and robust strength.

The main constituent of tendon is the protein collagen, which is an inelastic tissue with great tensile strength. It is the most abundant protein in the body and a structural component of all living tissue.

Another constituent contributing to the tensile strength of tendon connective tissue is **ground substance.** Ground substances are nonfibrous materials composed of several different molecules, which when combined create a more stable and rigid structure.

Ligaments

The **ligaments** bind bone to bone, providing support to the joint. Therefore, unlike tendons, the ligaments attach to bones at both ends. The composition of ligaments is similar to that of tendons, with collagen bundles located parallel to one another. Depending on the bone shapes to which they are attached, the ligaments exhibit various shapes, such as thin sheets, thick cords, or band structures. Ligaments also have a concentration of the protein **elastin.** Elastin has a very complex biochemical composition that allows ligaments some extensibility with return to their undeformed length once a stretch or force is removed. This characteristic provides a balance of support and resilience to the joint.

Elastin has a very complex biochemical composition that allows ligaments some extensibility and an ability to return to their undeformed length.

Fascia

Fascia is a Latin word that means bandage or band. From an anatomical viewpoint, fascia is a broad term used to designate all connective tissues that do not have a specific name. Fascia varies in shape and thickness relative to the functional demands placed upon it. There are three types of fascia. The outermost fascia, or superficial fascia, lies directly below the skin. This bilayered tissue has varying amounts of fat within it. The characteristic ability of skin to move is furnished by this outermost fascia. Directly below the superficial fascia is the deep fascia. This is much more compact and tough than the superficial fascia. The deep fascia fuses with muscles and bones. It also serves to separate internal organs and muscles from one another. The innermost fascia is the subserous fascia. It is a **serous,** or fluid-containing, membrane that directly covers the internal viscera. The pericardium, which surrounds the heart, is also a subserous type of fascia. All of the connective tissues of muscle (discussed earlier in "Muscular System"), including the sarcolemma, endomysium, perimysium, and epimysium, are forms of fascia that have specific names according to where they are found.

Fascia has three major functions. First, it provides the intramuscular framework that binds muscle, safeguarding its stability. Second, it permits forces developed by the muscle to be transmitted securely and efficiently. Lastly, it offers a necessary insulation between various organs and tissues of the body, permitting their proficient function without inhibition to adjacent structures.

CONCLUSION

The known benefits of exercise include improvements in muscular strength and endurance, body composition, glucose metabolism, coronary risk factors, bone mineral density, and psychological well-being. For the personal trainer, the foundation of program design is an appreciation of the anatomy and physiology of the human body. Understanding the structural concepts presented in this chapter will help ensure the personal trainer's ability to provide a safe, effective, and successful training environment for all clients.

STUDY QUESTIONS

1. Which of the following is the correct sequence of components from smallest muscle structure to largest muscle structure?
   - A. fascia, perimysium, epimysium, endomysium
   - B. myofilament, myofibril, fiber, fasciculus
   - C. endomysium, epimysium, perimysium, fascia
   - D. muscle cell, fasciculus, myofibril, fiber

2. Which of the following describes the properties of Type I and Type II muscle fibers?

	Type I	Type II
A.	high force	slow speed
B.	fast speed	high endurance
C.	high endurance	high force
D.	slow speed	low force

3. Which of the following changes in muscle length and tension are associated with a muscle spindle and a Golgi tendon?

	Muscle spindle	Golgi tendon organ
A.	rapid muscle length change	increase in muscle tension
B.	decrease in muscle tension	slow muscle length change
C.	slow muscle length change	decrease in muscle tension
D.	increase in muscle tension	fast muscle length change

4. Which of the following is true regarding bone health?
   - I. Decreased bone mineral density is related to an increased risk of fracture.
   - II. The most common sites for fracture are the humerus, tibia, and femur.
   - III. Bone mineral density is promoted by chronic participation in a physically-active lifestyle.
   - IV. Exercise may be beneficial in preventing fractures by decreasing the concentration of osteocytes.

   A. I and III only
   B. II and IV only
   C. I, II, and III only
   D. II, III, and IV only

APPLIED KNOWLEDGE QUESTION

Complete the following chart to describe the role each of the following structures or substances has during a muscle action.

Structure/Substance	Role during a muscle action
Myosin cross-bridges	
ATP	
Calcium	
Troponin	
Tropomyosin	
Acetylcholine	

REFERENCES

1. Gardiner, P.F. 2001. *Neuromuscular Aspects of Physical Activity.* Champaign, IL: Human Kinetics.
2. McArdle, W.D., F.I. Katch, and V.L. Katch. 1996. *Exercise Physiology: Energy, Nutrition, and Human Performance,* 4th ed. Baltimore: Williams & Wilkins.
3. Plowman, S.A., and D.L. Smith. 1997. *Exercise Physiology for Health, Fitness and Performance.* Boston: Allyn & Bacon.
4. Robergs, R.A., and S.O. Roberts. 1997. *Exercise Physiology: Exercise, Performance, and Clinical Applications.* St. Louis: Mosby.
5. Wilmore, J.H., and D.L. Costill. 1999. *Physiology of Sport and Exercise,* 2nd ed. Champaign, IL: Human Kinetics.

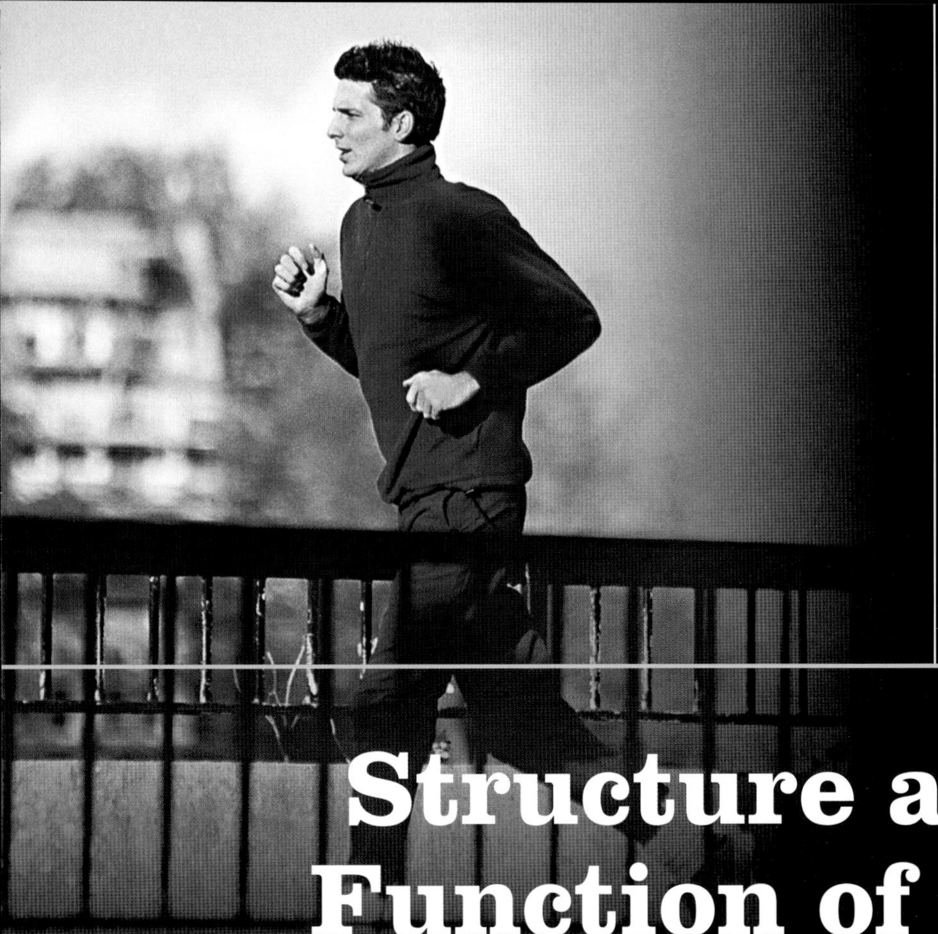

CHAPTER 2

Structure and Function of the Cardiovascular and Respiratory Systems

Mark A. Williams

After completing this chapter, you will be able to

- describe the anatomical and physiological characteristics of the cardiovascular system;
- describe the electrical conduction system of the heart and the basic electrocardiogram;
- describe the mechanisms that control the circulation of blood throughout the body;
- describe the anatomical and physiological characteristics of the respiratory system;
- explain the exchange of gases between the lungs and the blood; and
- understand the mechanisms that control respiration.

This chapter summarizes cardiovascular and respiratory anatomy and physiology so that the personal trainer can design appropriate and effective exercise programs. It is critical for the personal trainer to have a clear understanding of this material in order to offer appropriate recommendations for programs of aerobic conditioning and muscular strength and endurance. Within this chapter are anatomical and physiological descriptions of the heart, blood vessels, and lungs.

Cardiovascular Anatomy and Physiology

The primary roles of the cardiovascular system are transport of nutrients, removal of waste products, and assistance with maintenance of the environment for all the body's functions. This section describes the anatomy and physiology of the heart and the blood vessels.

The Heart

The heart is a muscular organ that is two interconnected but separate pumps; the right side of the heart pumps blood through the lungs, and the left side pumps blood through the rest of the body. Each pump has two chambers: an **atrium** and a **ventricle** (figure 2.1). The right and left atria function primarily as blood reservoirs, delivering blood into the right and left ventricles. The right and left ventricles supply the main force for moving blood through the pulmonary and peripheral circulations, respectively [4, 8].

Heart Rate

Heart rate (HR; the number of heartbeats per minute) can be assessed at various pulse sites (e.g., radi-

THE CARDIOVASCULAR SYSTEM TRANSPORTS OXYGEN FROM THE LUNGS TO THE TISSUES FOR USE IN CELLULAR METABOLISM AND THE REMOVAL OF CARBON DIOXIDE, THE MOST ABUNDANT BY-PRODUCT OF METABOLISM, FROM THE TISSUES AND LUNGS.

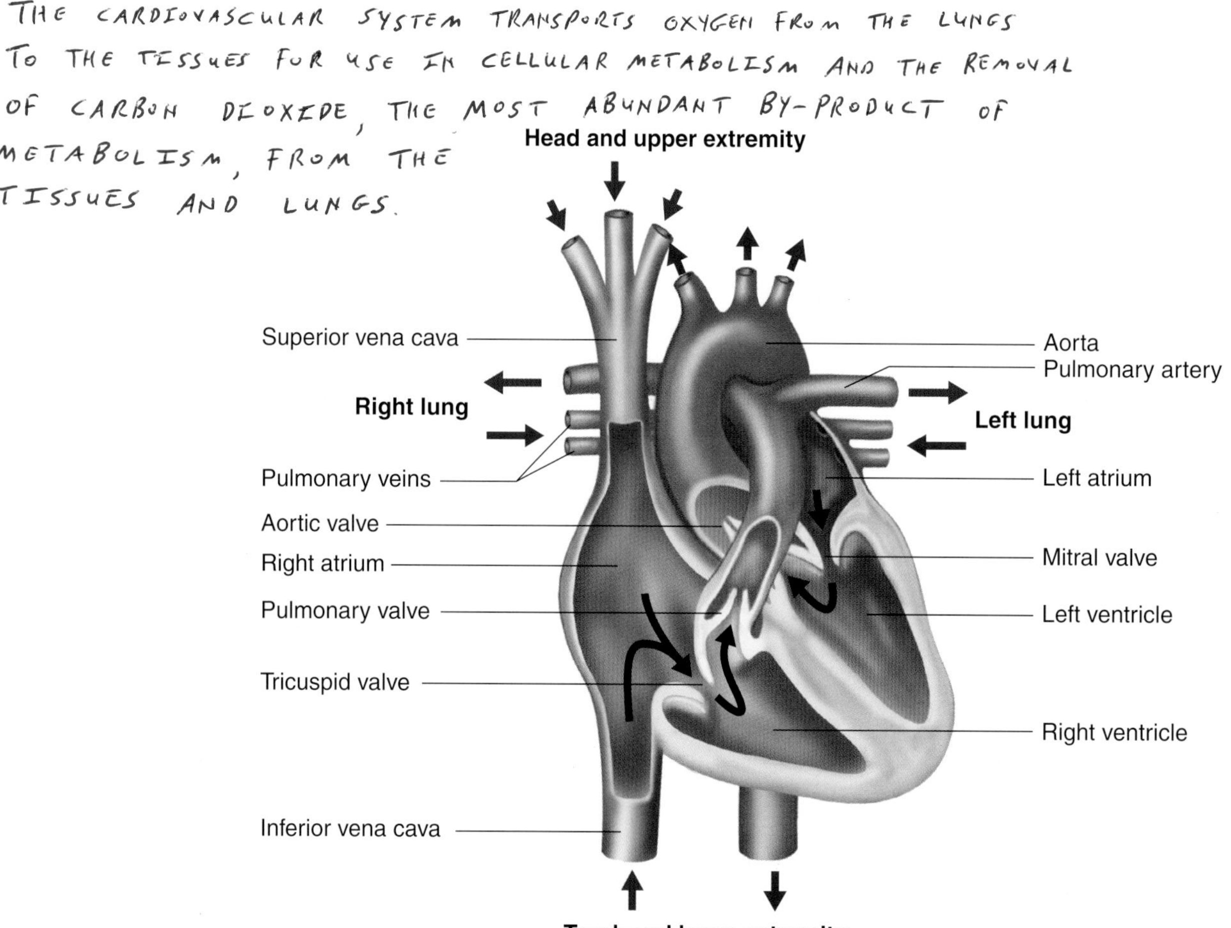

Figure 2.1 Structure of the human heart and course of blood flow through its chambers.
Reprinted from Baechle and Earle 2000.

al, carotid), through use of a stethoscope to listen to the heart, or by recording the electrocardiogram.

The **pulse** is the beat that can be felt against the wall of an artery when the heart beats and pushes blood through the artery. The pulse rate is usually the same as the heart rate. It is easier to feel the pulse in arteries that come close to the skin. Although there are several arteries that can be used to feel a pulse, the radial or carotid arteries are commonly used (figure 2.2).

The radial artery is an easy artery to use when one is checking the heart rate during or after exercise. Clients can usually be easily taught the correct technique. The steps listed in "Locating the Pulse and Determining the Heart Rate" may help the client take the radial or carotid pulse.

Locating the Pulse and Determining the Heart Rate

Radial Pulse

- Bend the elbow with the arm at the side. The palm of the hand should be up.
- The radial artery is located on the inside of the wrist near the base of the thumb.
- Using the middle (long) and index (pointer) fingers, gently feel for the radial artery.

Carotid Pulse

- Using the middle (long) and index (pointer) fingers, gently feel the carotid artery on either side of the neck, in the space between the windpipe (trachea) and muscle (right or left sternocleidomastoid), beneath the lower jawbone.
- *Caution:* Some pressure needs to be applied to allow one to feel the pulse, but too much pressure may cause reduced blood flow to the head. Therefore the client should be careful not to press too hard on the artery and should not press on both arteries at the same time.

Determining the Heart Rate

- Count either the radial or the carotid pulse rate for 10 seconds and multiply by 6 to get the heart rate for one minute.

The resting heart rate normally ranges from 60 to 100 beats per minute; fewer than 60 beats per minute is called **bradycardia,** and more than 100 beats per minute is referred to as **tachycardia** [9]. Chapter 16 includes complete guidelines for estimating maximal heart rate and establishing target heart rates in order to meet fitness goals.

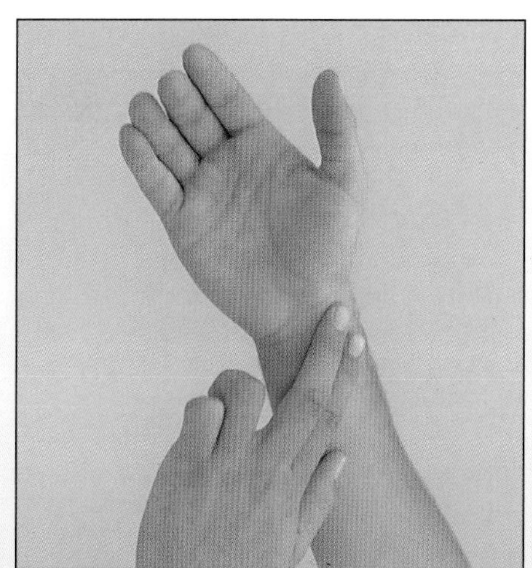

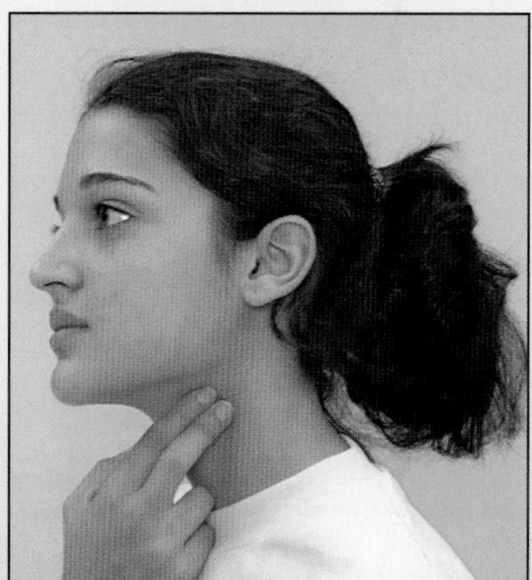

Figure 2.2 Radial pulse and carotid pulse determination.

Stroke Volume

Although both the right and left ventricles eject blood with each contraction and thus each ventricle has a stroke volume (SV), generally it is the left ventricle that is referred to in discussions of **stroke volume.** Stroke volume is the amount of blood ejected by the left ventricle, measured in milliliters. Two physiological mechanisms are responsible for the regulation of stroke volume. The first is a consequence of the **end-diastolic volume** (the volume of blood available to be pumped by the left ventricle at the end of the filling phase, or diastole). As end-diastolic blood volume increases, myocardial muscle fibers are stretched; in the normal heart, this results in a more forceful contraction. The second means is through the action of **catecholamines,** hormones of the sympathetic nervous system, which when secreted into the bloodstream produce a more forceful ventricular contraction and greater systolic emptying of the heart [9].

Cardiac Output

The amount of blood pumped by the heart, **cardiac output,** is determined by the stroke volume and the heart rate and can be ascertained using the following equation:

$$\text{cardiac output} = \text{SV} \times \text{HR} \quad \textbf{(2.1)}$$

Cardiac output ($\dot{Q}$) is usually expressed as the volume of blood, either in liters or in milliliters, ejected per minute [4, 7].

The Heart's Electrical Conduction System

A specialized electrical conduction system (figure 2.3) provides the electrical stimulus for the mechanical contraction of the heart. The conduction system is composed of

- the **sinoatrial (SA) node,** the intrinsic pacemaker, where rhythmic electrical impulses are normally initiated;
- the **internodal pathways** that conduct the impulse from the SA node to the **atrioventricular (AV) node;**
- the AV node, where the impulse is delayed slightly before passing into the ventricles;
- the **atrioventricular (AV) bundle,** which conducts the impulse to the ventricles; and
- the **left** and **right bundle branches,** which transmit the electrical impulse to the ventricles and further divide into the **Purkinje fibers,** which in turn conduct the impulse to all parts of the ventricles.

The SA node is a small area of specialized muscle tissue located in the upper lateral wall of the right atrium. The fibers of the node are continuous with the muscle fibers of the atrium, with the result that each electrical impulse that begins in the SA node normally spreads immediately into the atria. The conduction system is organized so that the impulse does not travel into the ventricles too rapidly; this allows time for the atria to contract and empty blood into the ventricles before ventricular contraction begins. It is primarily the AV node and its associated conductive fibers that delay each impulse entering into the ventricles [4, 8].

The left and right bundle branches lead from the AV bundle into the ventricles. These conduction fibers generally have characteristics quite opposite to those of the AV nodal fibers; that is, they are large and transmit impulses at a much higher velocity. As the bundle branches give way to the Purkinje fibers, which more completely penetrate the ventricles, the impulse travels quickly throughout the entire ventricular system and causes both ventricles to contract at approximately the same time [4, 8].

The SA node normally controls the rhythm of electrical stimulation of the heart and ultimately the heart's contraction patterns. Its discharge rate generally ranges between 60 and 80 times per minute. The inherent rhythm and conduction of electrical signals through the heart muscle are influenced by the brain's cardiovascular center (medulla); this center transmits signals to the heart through the **sympathetic nervous system** and **parasympathetic nervous system,** both of which are components of the autonomic nervous system. Stimulation of the sympathetic nerves accelerates firing of the SA node, causing the heart to beat faster. Stimulation of the parasympathetic nervous system slows the rate of SA node discharge, which slows the heart rate.

Electrocardiogram

The electrical activity of the heart can be recorded at the surface of the body; a graphic representation of this activity is called an **electrocardiogram (ECG).** A normal electrocardiogram, seen in figure 2.4, is composed of a P wave, a QRS complex (the QRS complex is often three separate waves: a Q wave, an R wave, and an S wave), and a T wave. The P wave and the QRS complex are recordings of the electrical stimulus as it moves through atrial and then ventricular myocardial tissue. The P wave rep-

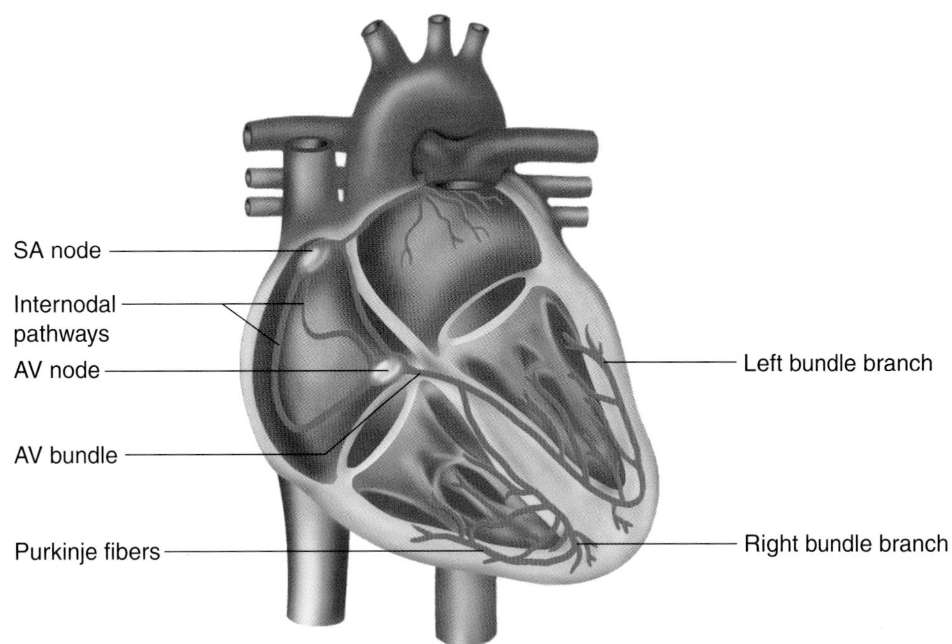

Figure 2.3 The electrical conduction system of the heart. SA = sinoatrial; AV = atrioventricular.
Reprinted from Baechle and Earle 2000.

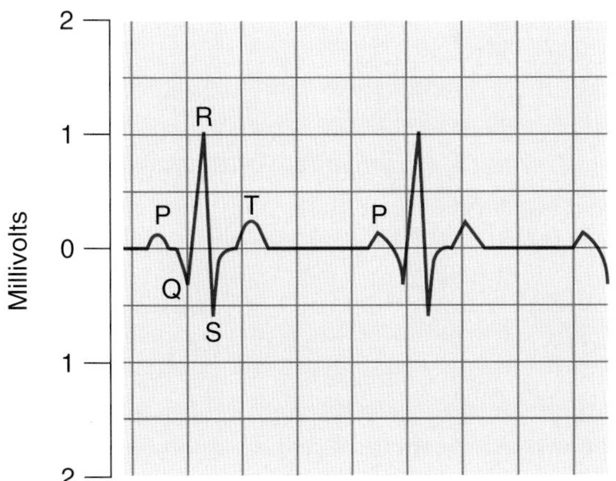

Figure 2.4 Normal electrocardiogram.

resents **atrial depolarization,** which initiates atrial contraction. The QRS complex is the recording of **ventricular depolarization,** which initiates ventricular contraction. In contrast, the T wave reflects the electrical recovery following ventricular depolarization and is referred to as **ventricular repolarization.** Although **atrial repolarization** occurs as well, its wave formation usually occurs during the time of ventricular depolarization and is thus masked by the QRS complex [4, 5].

The Blood Vessels and Circulation

The circulation of the heart and lungs (central circulation) and that of the rest of the body (peripheral circulation) form a single closed-circuit system with two components: an arterial system, which carries blood away from the heart, and a venous system, which returns blood toward the heart (figure 2.5). As blood returns to the heart from the peripheral circulation **(venous return)**, it enters the heart from inferior and superior vena cavae and into the right atrium. From the right atrium, blood passes into the right ventricle, through the pulmonary arteries, entering the lungs. With the exchange of oxygen and carbon dioxide in the lungs, blood returns to the heart through the pulmonary veins into the left atrium, where it is delivered to the left ventricle, and then to the body's arterial circulation. The distribution of the blood volume throughout the circulatory system at rest is also seen in figure 2.5. The blood vessels of each system are identified in the figure as well [9].

The circulation of the heart and lungs (central circulation) and that of the rest of the body (peripheral circulation) form a single closed-circuit system with two components: an arterial system, which carries blood away from the heart, and a venous system, which returns blood toward the heart.

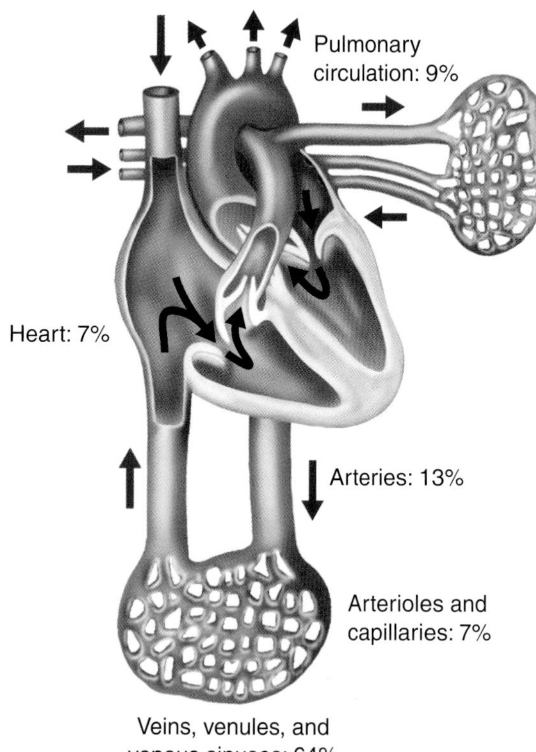

Figure 2.5 The arterial *(right)* and venous *(left)* components of the circulatory system. The percent values indicate the distribution of blood volume throughout the circulatory system at rest.
Reprinted from Baechle and Earle 2000.

Arteries

The function of **arteries** is to transport blood pumped from the heart. Because blood pumped from the heart is under relatively high pressure, arteries have strong, muscular walls. Small branches of arteries called **arterioles** act as control vessels through which blood enters the capillaries. Arterioles play a major role in the regulation of blood flow to the capillaries. Arterioles have strong, muscular walls that are capable of closing the arteriole completely or allowing it to be dilated severalfold, thus vastly altering blood flow to the capillaries in response to the needs of the tissues [4, 8].

Capillaries

The function of **capillaries** is to exchange oxygen, fluid, nutrients, electrolytes, hormones, and other substances between the blood and the various tissues of the body. The capillary walls are very thin and allow for movement of these substances into and out of these tissues [4].

Venules and Veins

As blood begins the process of moving back toward the heart through the venous portion of the circulation, **venules** collect blood from the capillaries and gradually converge blood into the progressively larger **veins.** Because the pressure in the venous system is very low, venous walls are thin. However, they are surrounded by muscle tissue, which allows them to constrict **(vasoconstriction)** or dilate **(vasodilation)** greatly, thereby allowing the venous circulation to act as a reservoir for blood, in either small or large amounts [4, 8]. In addition, some veins, such as those in the legs, contain one-way valves that help maintain venous return by preventing blood flow away from the heart, which is particularly helpful when the body is in the upright position.

Control of Circulation

The movement of blood (blood flow) throughout the body is a function of resistance in the body. As resistance is reduced, blood flow is increased; and as resistance increases, blood flow is reduced. The amount of resistance to blood flow is primarily a function of the diameter of the systemic arterial vessels. The resistance of the entire systemic circulation is called the **total peripheral resistance.** As blood vessels throughout the body become constricted, total peripheral resistance increases; with dilation, peripheral resistance decreases [4].

Blood vessel dilation and constriction, and therefore peripheral resistance, are affected by a variety of factors including type of exercise, sympathetic nervous system stimulation, local muscle tissue metabolism, and responses to environmental stressors, particularly heat stress. During aerobic exercise (as well as prior to activity in anticipation of exercise), sympathethic nervous system stimulation causes arterial vasodilation leading to increased blood flow. However, the greatest increase in blood flow to active muscles is primarily the result of local factors related to muscle tissue metabolism during exercise, including increased temperature, carbon dioxide, and acidity—all of which lead to vasodilation [8]. At the same time, blood flow to other organ systems that are less essential during activity is reduced by constriction of arterioles **(shunting)**. Together with vasoconstriction of the large vessels of the venous system, these latter two responses provide for more blood to move into the central circulation, ultimately increasing blood supply to working muscles. Similarly, with resistance exercise involving low resistance over many repetitions, responses are comparable to those for aerobic work. However, heavy resistance exercise increases resistance to blood flow to the working muscle.

In the case of activity during heat stress, the body adjusts to exercise with peripheral dilation to enhance the body's cooling mechanism. This may, however, limit the return of blood to the heart (venous return) as blood pools in the periphery. The decrease in venous return would reduce cardiac output if the heart rate did not increase adequately to offset reduced venous return. This explains why heart rate is frequently more elevated during activity in the heat than under more normal temperatures. If heart rate is unable to adequately compensate for reduced venous return, cardiac output will diminish and blood supply to the working muscles could actually become limited.

The movement of blood throughout the body is a function of resistance in the body. As resistance is reduced, blood flow is increased; as resistance increases, blood flow is reduced. Constriction and dilation of blood vessels, which influence resistance, are primarily affected by type of exercise, responses to exercise of the sympathetic nervous system, and local metabolic factors.

Blood Pressure Defined

Systolic blood pressure (SBp) is the pressure exerted against the arterial walls as blood is forcefully ejected during ventricular contraction **(systole)**. When systolic blood pressure and heart rate are measured simultaneously, they are also useful in describing the work of the heart and can provide an indirect estimation of myocardial oxygen uptake [9]. This estimate of the work of the heart, referred to as the **rate-pressure product**, or double product, is obtained according to the following equation:

$$\text{rate-pressure product} = \text{HR} \times \text{SBp} \qquad \textbf{(2.2)}$$

Conversely, **diastolic blood pressure** (DBp) is the pressure exerted against the arterial walls when no blood is being forcefully ejected through the vessels **(diastole)**. It provides an indication of peripheral resistance or vascular stiffness, tending to decrease with vasodilation and increase with vasoconstriction.

Systemic Pressure Patterns

In systemic circulation, pressure is highest in the aorta and arteries and rapidly falls off within the venous circulation (figure 2.6). Because pumping by the heart is pulsatile, arterial pressure fluctuates between a systolic level and a diastolic level. As the blood flow continues through the systemic circulation, its pressure falls progressively to nearly 0 mmHg (millimeters of mercury; venous pressure) by the time it reaches the termination of the vena

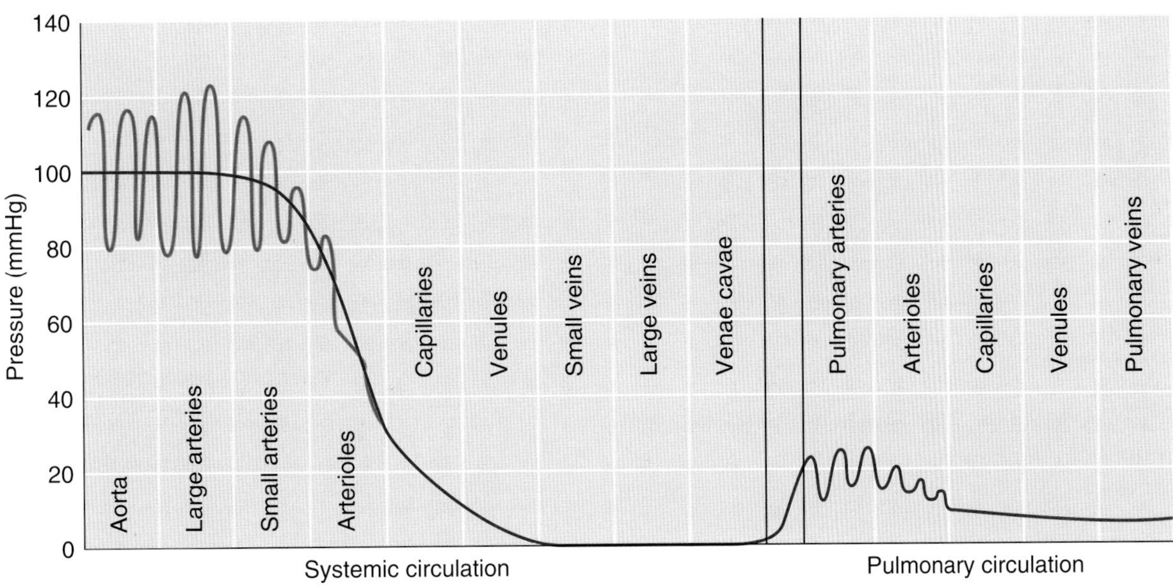

Figure 2.6 Blood pressures in the various portions of the circulatory system.
Reprinted from Guyton and Hall 1996.

cava in the right atrium [4]. With use of a blood pressure cuff (sphygmomanometer) on the arm and a stethoscope, blood pressure at rest normally ranges from 100 to 139 systolic and 60 to 89 diastolic. **Hypertension** (high blood pressure) at rest is commonly defined as ≥140/90 mmHg (either or both numbers) [9]. With aerobic exercise, systolic pressure can normally rise to as much as 220 to 260 mmHg, while diastolic pressure remains at the resting level or decreases slightly [4, 7]. In comparison, extremely high blood pressure values have been observed during heavy resistance exercise (>300/180 mmHg) especially when the Valsalva maneuver is used. Ordinarily, however, blood pressure values rarely reach these levels, particularly as work is reduced [1, 2].

The **mean arterial pressure** is the average blood pressure throughout the cardiac cycle. However, it is not the average of systolic and diastolic pressures. Rather, because the arterial pressure usually remains nearer to the diastolic level than to the systolic level during the greater portion of the cardiac cycle, the mean arterial pressure is usually less than the average of the systolic and diastolic pressures.

$$\text{mean arterial blood pressure} = [(\text{SBp} - \text{DBp}) \div 3] + \text{DBp} \tag{2.3}$$

Oxygen and Carbon Dioxide Transport and Exchange

Two major functions of the cardiovascular system are the transport of oxygen from the lungs to the tissues for use in cellular metabolism and the removal of carbon dioxide, the most abundant by-product of metabolism, from the tissues to the lungs.

> The cardiovascular system transports nutrients and removes waste products while helping to maintain the environment for all the body's functions. The blood transports oxygen from the lungs to the tissues for use in cellular metabolism and transports carbon dioxide—the most abundant by-product of metabolism—from the tissues to the lungs, where it is removed from the body.

Oxygen

Although oxygen can be transported in very small amounts in the fluid portion of blood, and when transported in this manner is important in many physiologic functions, it is the combination of oxygen and an important component of the blood, hemoglobin, that is primarily responsible for transporting oxygen to meet the body's oxygen demands. Men have about 15 to 16 grams of hemoglobin per 100 milliliters of blood, and women have about 14 grams of hemoglobin per 100 milliliters of blood. One gram of hemoglobin can carry 1.34 milliliters of oxygen; thus the oxygen capacity of 100 milliliters of blood is about 20 milliliters of oxygen in men and a little less in women [7].

The movement of a gas—in this case oxygen—across a cell membrane is called **diffusion.** It is a function of the concentration of the gas and the resulting partial pressure exerted by the molecular motion of the gas. Diffusion occurs when there is a **concentration gradient** (a greater concentration of a gas on one side of the cell membrane compared to that on the other side of the membrane), the result being the movement of the gas from high concentration to low concentration. At the tissue level, where oxygen is utilized and carbon dioxide produced, their partial pressures at times differ considerably from those in arterial blood. As oxygen is utilized by the tissue cells, the partial pressure of oxygen within the cells becomes considerably less than that immediately outside the muscle cell. This difference in concentration facilitates the rapid diffusion of oxygen from blood across the cell membrane and into the cell. In addition, an increase in acidity, temperature, or concentration of carbon dioxide (all of which occur with exercise, for example) reduces the effectiveness of hemoglobin to hold oxygen, allowing more oxygen to become available. This phenomenon is illustrated in figure 2.7 by the **oxyhemoglobin dissociation curve,** which describes the impact of increased metabolism on oxygen dissociation, in this case, the curve shifting downward and to the right [7, 9].

> As blood temperature, concentration of carbon dioxide, and acidity increase with exercise, oxygen more readily dissociates from hemoglobin, and its availability to active cells increases.

Carbon Dioxide

The way in which carbon dioxide is removed from the system has some similarities to oxygen transport, but the vast amount of carbon dioxide is removed by a more complex process. Only a limited quantity of carbon dioxide (about 5%) produced during metabolism is transported out of the cell by diffusion and subsequently transported by the plasma to the lungs. Importantly, however, just as with oxygen, this limited amount of carbon dioxide

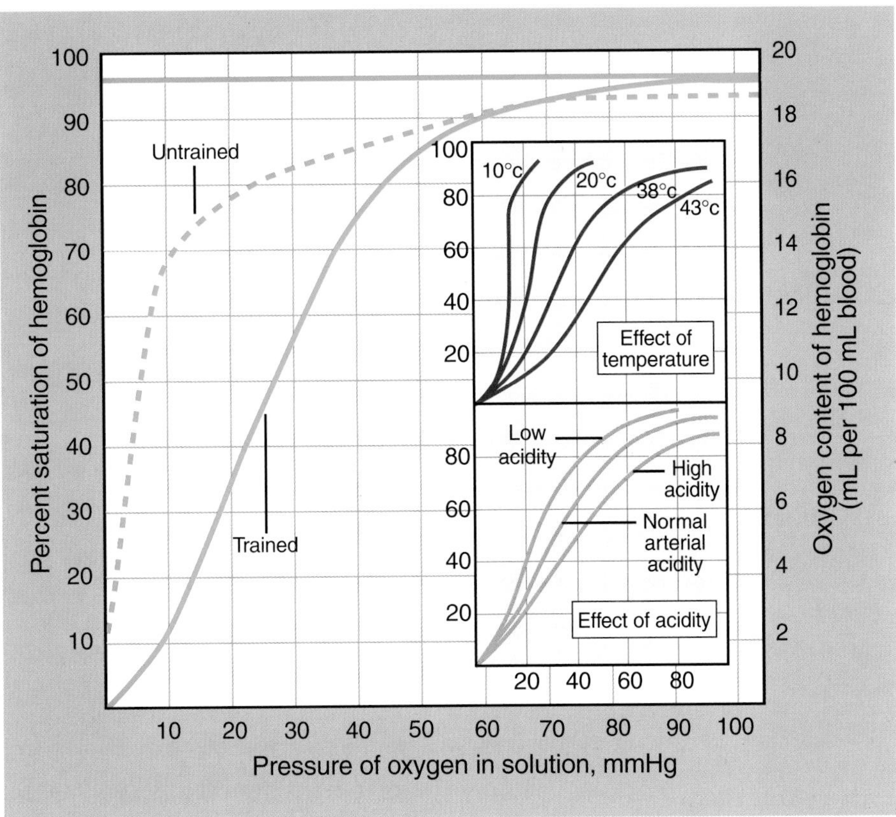

Figure 2.7 The oxyhemoglobin dissociation curve.
Reprinted from McArdle, Katch, and Katch 1996.

contributes to various other physiologic processes establishing the partial pressure of carbon dioxide in the blood. Some carbon dioxide is also transported via hemoglobin, but this too is a limited amount [7]. The greatest amount of carbon dioxide removal, approximately 70%, results from a process involving its combination with water in the red blood cells and subsequent delivery to the lungs in the form of bicarbonate (HCO_3^-) [4, 7].

Oxygen Uptake

Oxygen uptake is the amount of oxygen utilized by the tissues of the body. The capacity to utilize oxygen is primarily related to the ability of the heart and circulatory system to transport blood (and oxygen) and to the ability of body tissues to extract (utilize) oxygen from the blood. Cardiac output describes the volume of blood transported, and **arteriovenous oxygen difference** (a-$\bar{v}O_2$ difference) is used to determine the amount of oxygen extracted from the transported blood. Arteriovenous oxygen difference is the difference in the oxygen content of arterial blood versus venous blood and is expressed in milliliters of oxygen per 100 milliliters of blood.

The capacity to utilize oxygen is primarily related to the ability of the heart and circulatory system to transport blood (and oxygen) and the ability of body tissues to extract (utilize) oxygen from the blood.

Oxygen uptake ($\dot{V}O_2$) may be calculated as follows:

$$\dot{V}O_2 = \dot{Q} \times \text{a-}\bar{v}O_2 \text{ difference} \quad \textbf{(2.4)}$$

where $\dot{Q}$ is the cardiac output (heart rate × stroke volume) in milliliters per minute.

For example,

$$\dot{V}O_2\text{rest} = (80 \text{ beats/min} \times 65 \text{ ml blood/beat}) \times 6 \text{ ml } O_2/100 \text{ ml blood} = 312 \text{ ml } O_2/\text{min}$$

or

$$\dot{V}O_2\text{rest} = (\text{HR} \times \text{SV}) \times \text{a-}\bar{v}O_2 \text{ difference}$$

To get the usual units for oxygen uptake (i.e., ml · kg^{-1} · min^{-1}), one then divides the result by the person's weight in kilograms.

$$312 \text{ ml } O_2/\text{min} \div 75 \text{ kg} = 4.2 \text{ ml } O_2 \cdot \text{kg}^{-1} \cdot \text{min}^{-1}$$

Equation 2.4 is a manipulation of the **Fick equation,** which expresses the relationship of cardiac output, oxygen uptake, and arteriovenous oxygen difference:

$$\dot{Q} = \dot{V}O_2 \div a\text{-}\bar{v}O_2 \text{ difference} \quad (2.5)$$

For example,

$$\dot{Q} = 312 \text{ ml } O_2/\text{min} \div 6 \text{ ml } O_2/100 \text{ ml blood}$$
$$= 5{,}200 \text{ ml blood/min}$$
$$= 5.2 \text{ L blood/min}$$

This equation is helpful for understanding the relationship of each parameter to the others and for developing a clearer picture of how exercise may affect each [9].

The oxygen demand of working muscles during aerobic exercise is directly related to their mass, metabolic efficiency, and level of work. **Maximal oxygen uptake ($\dot{V}O_2max$)** is described as the greatest amount of oxygen that can be utilized at the cellular level for the entire body. Maximal oxygen uptake has been found to correlate well with the degree of physical conditioning and is recognized as the most accepted measure of cardiopulmonary fitness [3]. However, maximal oxygen uptake has more recently been differentiated from **peak oxygen uptake,** in that maximal oxygen uptake is more often a theoretical or potential value (a value achieved when each component is at its maximal attainable level) and peak oxygen uptake describes an actual measured value that is subject to change based on various factors including fitness level, level of health or illness, and subject motivation. By changing values for HR, SV, and a-$\bar{v}O_2$ difference in equation 2.4, one is able to recognize the impact of exercise on oxygen uptake [9].

For example,

$$\dot{V}O_2 = (185 \text{ beats/min} \times 110 \text{ ml blood/beat})$$
$$(\text{HR}) \quad \times \quad (\text{SV})$$
$$\times\ 13 \text{ ml } O_2/100 \text{ ml blood}$$
$$a\text{-}vO_2 \text{ difference}$$
$$\dot{V}O_2 = 2{,}646 \text{ ml } O_2/\text{min}$$
$$2{,}646 \text{ ml } O_2/\text{min} \div 75 \text{ kg} = 35.3 \text{ ml} \cdot \text{kg}^{-1} \cdot \text{min}^{-1}$$

Resting oxygen uptake is generally estimated at 3.5 ml $O_2 \cdot kg^{-1} \cdot min^{-1}$, the actual value for a given individual being dependent upon the metabolic rate and those parameters that affect it. The value 3.5 ml $O_2 \cdot kg^{-1} \cdot min^{-1}$ is also described as one **metabolic equivalent,** or one **MET.** Peak oxygen uptake values generally range from 35 to 80 ml $\cdot kg^{-1} \cdot min^{-1}$, or 10 to 22.9 METs, in normal, healthy individuals and depend upon a variety of physiological parameters including age as well as conditioning level [4, 7].

Respiratory Anatomy and Physiology

The primary function of the respiratory system is the basic exchange of oxygen and carbon dioxide. This section deals with the anatomy and physiology of the lungs and the control of respiration.

> The primary function of the respiratory system is the basic exchange of oxygen and carbon dioxide.

The Lungs

The anatomy of the human respiratory system is depicted in figure 2.8. As air passes through the nose, the nasal cavities perform three distinct functions: warming, humidifying, and purifying the air [4]. Air is then distributed to the lungs by way of the trachea, bronchi, and bronchioles. The **trachea** is called the first-generation respiratory passage, and the right and left main **bronchi** are the second-generation passages; each division thereafter is an additional generation **(bronchioles)**. There are approximately 23 generations before the air finally reaches the **alveoli,** where gases are exchanged in respiration [4].

Minute ventilation (the volume of air breathed per minute) provides for appropriate levels of alveolar gas concentrations [6]. It is a function of **tidal volume** (the amount of air moved during inhalation or exhalation, with each breath) and the **respiratory rate** (frequency of breathing). **Inspiratory reserve volume** represents the maximal volume of air that may be inspired beyond normal resting inspired tidal volume. Conversely, **expiratory reserve volume** is the maximal volume of air that may be exhaled beyond normal resting expired tidal volume. The volume of air moved that results from maximal inspiration and maximal expiration is the **forced vital capacity.** However, even with maximal exhalation, there remains a volume of air in the lungs **(residual lung volume)** that prevents the lungs from collapsing upon themselves. The combination of forced vital capacity and the residual lung volume is **total lung capacity.**

With inspiration, air enters the gas exchange area (the alveoli). However, air also enters and occupies other areas of the respiratory passages: the nose, mouth, trachea, bronchi, and bronchioles. This area as a whole is not useful for gas exchange and is called the **anatomical dead space** (figure 2.9). The normal volume of this air space is approximately

150 milliliters in young adults, and the volume increases with age. Because the respiratory passages stretch with deep breathing, it should be recognized that anatomical dead space increases as tidal volume increases. Nevertheless, tidal volume increases relatively more than the volume of the anatomical dead space does, resulting in a lesser percentage of tidal volume as a component of the anatomical dead space. Thus, increasing tidal volume (deeper breathing) provides for more efficient ventilation than simply increasing frequency of breathing alone [4, 6].

Physiological dead space refers to alveoli in which poor blood flow, poor ventilation, or other problems with the alveolar surface impair gas exchange (figure 2.9). The physiological dead space in

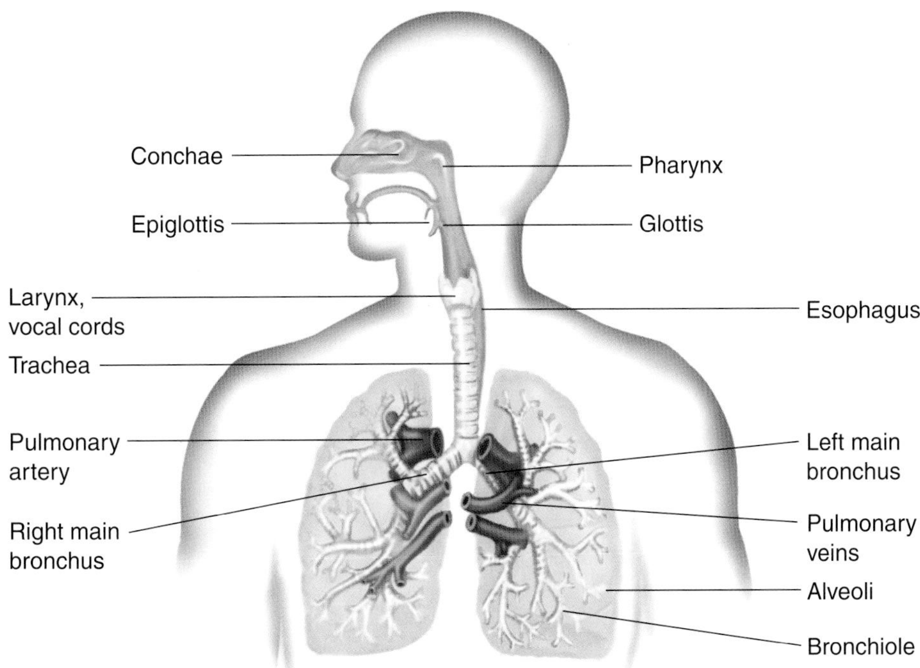

Figure 2.8 Gross anatomy of the human respiratory system.
Reprinted from Baechle and Earle 2000.

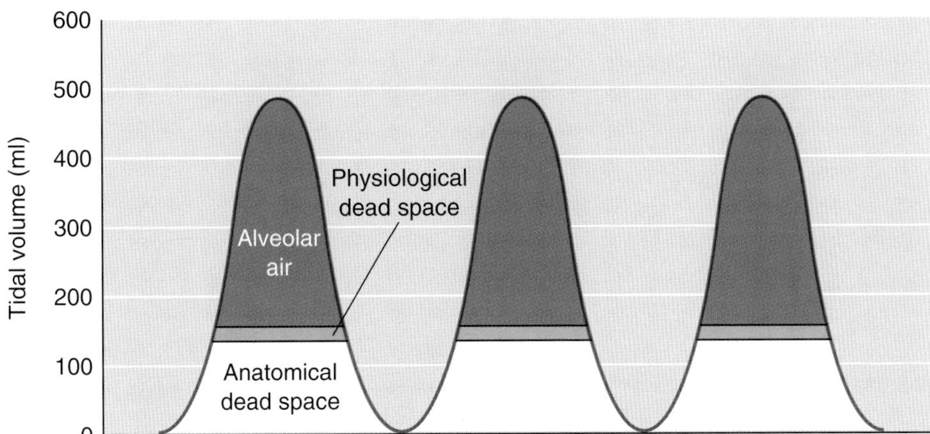

Figure 2.9 Distribution of tidal volume in a healthy client at rest. The tidal volume comprises about 350 milliliters of ambient air that mixes with alveolar air, about 150 milliliters of air in the larger passages (anatomical dead space), and a small portion of air distributed to either poorly ventilated or underperfused alveoli (physiological dead space).
Reprinted from McArdle, Katch, and Katch 1996.

the lungs of healthy people is usually negligible because all or nearly all alveoli are functional. Certain types of lung disease (e.g., chronic obstructive lung disease, pneumonia), however, can significantly reduce alveolar function, increasing physiological dead space by as much as 10 times the volume of anatomical dead space [4, 6].

Exchange of Air

The amount and movement of air and expired gases in and out of the lungs are controlled by expansion and recoil of the lungs. The lungs do not actively expand and recoil themselves. Rather they are acted upon to do so in two ways: (1) by downward and upward movement of the diaphragm to lengthen and shorten the chest cavity and (2) by elevation and depression of the ribs to increase and decrease the back-to-front diameter of the chest cavity (figure 2.10).

Normal, quiet breathing is accomplished almost entirely by movement of the diaphragm. During inspiration, contraction of the diaphragm creates a negative pressure (vacuum) in the chest cavity, and air is drawn into the lungs. During expiration, the diaphragm simply relaxes; the elastic recoil of the lungs, chest wall, and abdominal structures compresses the lungs, and air is expelled. During heavy breathing, the elastic forces alone are not powerful enough to provide the necessary respiratory response. The required extra force is achieved mainly by contraction of the abdominal muscles, which push the abdomen upward against the bottom of the diaphragm [4, 7].

The second method for expanding the lungs is to raise the rib cage. Because the chest cavity is small and the ribs are slanted downward while in the resting position, elevating the rib cage allows the ribs to project almost directly forward so that the sternum can move forward and away from the spine. The muscles that elevate the rib cage are called muscles of inspiration; they include the external intercostals, the sternocleidomastoids, the anterior serrati, and the scaleni. The muscles that depress the chest are muscles of expiration and include the abdominal muscles (rectus abdominis, external and internal obliques, and transversus abdominis) and the internal intercostals [4, 6, 9].

Pleural pressure is the pressure in the narrow space between the lung pleura and the chest wall **pleura** (membranes enveloping the lungs and lining the chest walls). This pressure is normally slightly negative. Because the lung is an elastic structure, during normal inspiration as the chest cage expands it pulls on the surface of the lungs and creates a more negative pressure, thus enhancing inspiration. During expiration, the events are essentially reversed [4, 9].

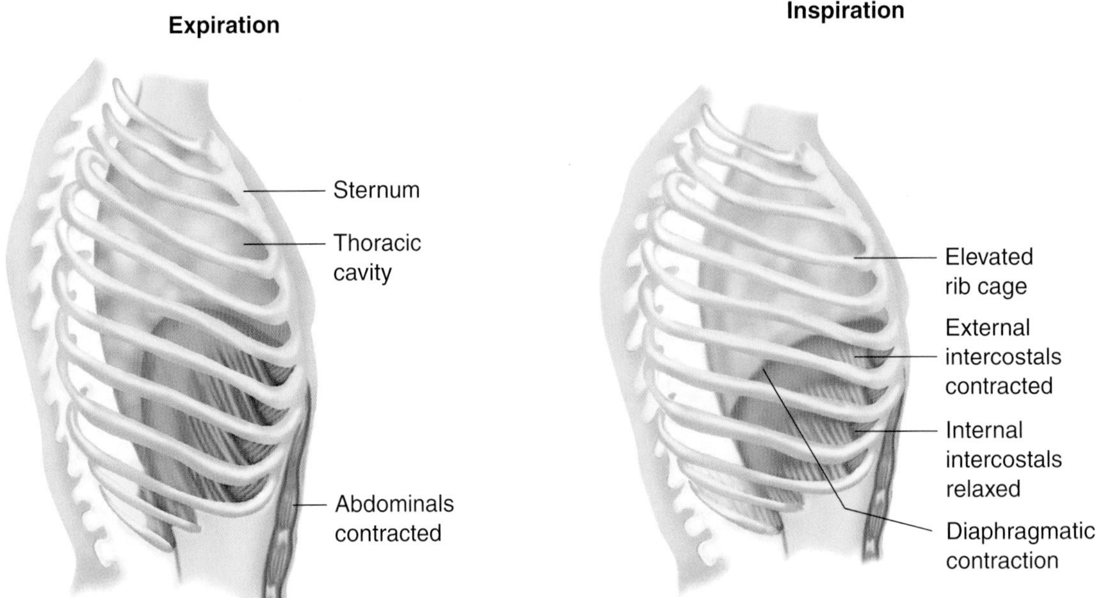

Figure 2.10 Contraction and expansion of the thoracic cage during expiration and inspiration, illustrating diaphragmatic contraction, elevation of the rib cage, and function of the intercostals. The vertical and anteroposterior diameters increase during inspiration.
Reprinted from Baechle and Earle 2000.

Alveolar pressure is the pressure inside the alveoli when the **glottis** is open and no air is flowing into or out of the lungs. The glottis is the narrowest part of the larynx where air passes through the trachea. A fibrocartilage cover opens and closes, thus allowing for movement of air and at the same time protecting the trachea from foreign bodies. When the glottis is open and no air is flowing into or out of the lungs, the pressure in all parts of the respiratory tree is the same all the way to the alveoli and is equal to the atmospheric pressure. To cause inward flow of air during inspiration, the pressure in the alveoli must fall to a value slightly below atmospheric pressure. During expiration, alveolar pressure must rise above atmospheric pressure [4, 9].

Exchange of Respiratory Gases

With ventilation, oxygen diffuses from the alveoli into the pulmonary blood, and carbon dioxide diffuses from the blood into the alveoli. The process of diffusion allows for the movement of oxygen and carbon dioxide through the alveolar capillary membrane. At rest, the partial pressure of oxygen in the alveoli is about 60 mmHg greater than that in the pulmonary capillaries. Thus, oxygen diffuses into the pulmonary capillary blood. Similarly, carbon dioxide diffuses in the opposite direction. This process of gas exchange is so rapid as to be thought of as instantaneous [4, 7].

With ventilation, oxygen diffuses from the alveoli into the pulmonary blood, and carbon dioxide diffuses from the blood into the alveoli.

Control of Respiration

The nervous system controls the rate of ventilation by adjusting the rate and depth of breathing in order to meet the demands of the body. Thus, arterial blood oxygen concentration and carbon dioxide concentration are hardly altered, even during strenuous exercise [4] such as spinning and heavy resistance training.

The body's **respiratory center** is composed of several widely dispersed groups of neurons located bilaterally in the lower portion of the brain stem (the pons and medulla oblongata). The respiratory center is divided into three major collections of neurons [4] (figure 2.11):

- The *dorsal respiratory group* plays the fundamental role in the initiation of respiration. It is also the primary generator of the rhythm of respiration, serving to maintain regularity of breathing frequency.
- The *ventral respiratory group* of neurons has several important functions. First, respiratory signals from these neurons contribute to the respiratory drive for increased pulmonary ventilation. Second, stimulation of some of the neurons in the ventral group causes inspiration or expiration, depending on where the stimulus is located. These neurons are especially important in providing the expiratory signals to the powerful abdominal muscles during more forceful expiration.
- The *pneumotaxic center* helps to control both the rate and pattern of breathing. The primary effect of this center is to control the duration of the filling

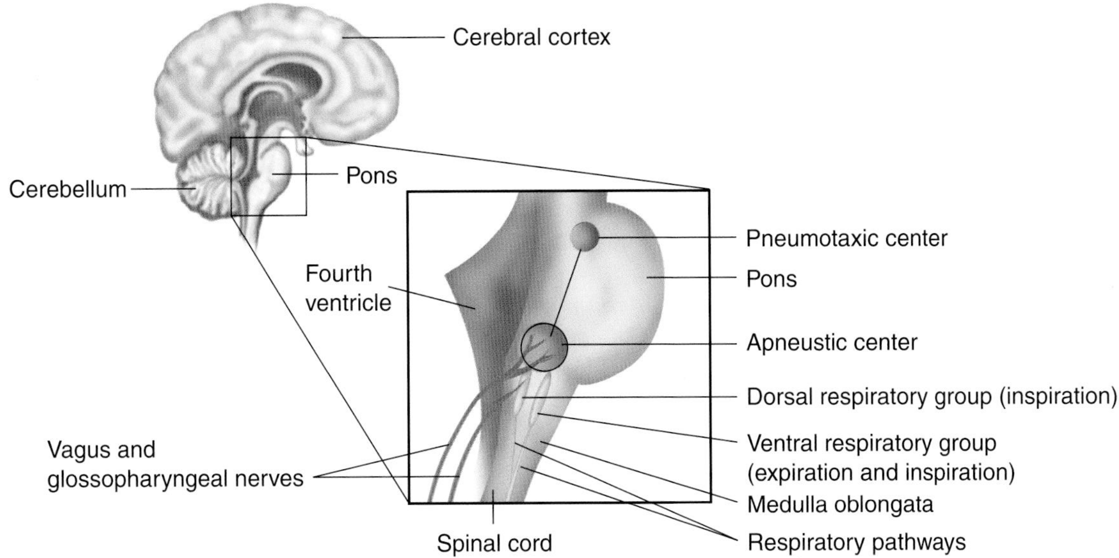

Figure 2.11 The brain's respiratory center.
Reprinted from Baechle and Earle 2000.

cycle of the lungs, the limiting factor in inspiration volume. A secondary effect of this control is its impact on the rate of breathing. As inspiration shortens, expiration is also shortened, thus increasing the rate of respiration. Conversely as inspiration is increased, expiration is also increased, and the rate of respiration is decreased [4].

The nervous system controls the rate of ventilation by adjusting the rate and depth of breathing so that arterial blood oxygen concentration and carbon dioxide concentration are hardly altered, even during strenuous exercise.

CONCLUSION

Knowledge of cardiovascular and respiratory anatomy and physiology can help the personal trainer understand the scientific basis for aerobic conditioning and muscular strength and endurance programming, as well as the expected adaptations to both aerobic and resistance exercise. This information can be of particular value when one is developing the goals of a conditioning program and can provide a basis for clinical evaluation and the selection parameters included in such an evaluation process.

STUDY QUESTIONS

1. Which of the following is the correct sequence of structures that the blood passes through after it leaves the left ventricle?
   A. arteries, capillaries, veins, right atrium
   B. pulmonary vein, lungs, right atrium, right ventricle
   C. left atrium, pulmonary artery, lung, right ventricle
   D. vein, right atrium, right ventricle, pulmonary artery
2. Which of the following are components of oxygen uptake ($\dot{V}O_2$)?
   I. heart rate
   II. body weight
   III. stroke volume
   IV. a-$\bar{v}O_2$ difference

   A. I, II, and III only
   B. II, III, and IV only
   C. I, III, and IV only
   D. I, II, and IV only
3. Which of the following compose total lung capacity?
   I. minute ventilation
   II. residual lung volume
   III. forced vital capacity
   IV. tidal volume

   A. I and II only
   B. II and IV only
   C. I and III only
   D. II and III only
4. Which of the following control the expansion and recoil of the lungs to create air exchange during heavy breathing?
   I. abdominal muscle activity
   II. ribcage movement
   III. diaphragm movement
   IV. pectoral muscle activity

A. I and III only
B. II and IV only
C. I, II, and III only
D. I, II, III, and IV

APPLIED KNOWLEDGE QUESTION

A 38-year-old, 132-lb female has been using an elliptical trainer for her aerobic workouts. Her exercise heart rate is 140 bpm, her stroke volume is 100 ml/beat, and her a-$\bar{v}O_2$ difference is 11 ml O_2/100 ml blood. At what MET level is she exercising?

REFERENCES

1. Fleck, S.J. 1988. Cardiovascular adaptations to resistance training. *Medicine and Science in Sports and Exercise* 20: S146-S151.
2. Fleck, S.J., and W.J. Kraemer. 1998. Resistance training: Physiologic responses and adaptations. Part 2. *Physician and Sportsmedicine* 16: 63-73.
3. Franklin, B.A., and J.L. Roitman. 2001. Cardiorespiratory adaptations to exercise. In: *ACSM's Resource Manual for Guidelines for Exercise Testing and Prescription,* 4th ed., J.L. Roitman, ed. Baltimore: Lippincott Williams & Wilkins, pp. 160-166.
4. Guyton, A.C., and J.E. Hall. 1996. *Textbook of Medical Physiology,* 9th ed. Philadelphia: Saunders.
5. Larry, J.A., and S.F. Schaal. 2001. Normal electrocardiograms. In: *ACSM's Resource Manual for Guidelines for Exercise Testing and Prescription,* 4th ed., J.L. Roitman, ed. Baltimore: Lippincott Williams & Wilkins, pp. 411-414.
6. Mahler, D.A. 2001. Respiratory anatomy. In: *ACSM's Resource Manual for Guidelines for Exercise Testing and Prescription,* 4th ed., J.L. Roitman, ed. Baltimore: Lippincott Williams & Wilkins, pp. 74-81.
7. McArdle, W.D., F.I. Katch, and V.L. Katch. 1996. *Exercise Physiology: Energy, Nutrition, and Human Performance,* 4th ed. Baltimore: Williams & Wilkins.
8. Murray, T.D., and J.M. Murray. 2001. Cardiovascular anatomy. In: *ACSM's Resource Manual for Guidelines for Exercise Testing and Prescription,* 4th ed., J.L. Roitman, ed. Baltimore: Lippincott Williams & Wilkins, pp. 65-73.
9. Williams, M.A. 2000. Cardiovascular and respiratory anatomy and physiology: Response to exercise. In: *Essentials of Strength Training and Conditioning,* 2nd ed., T.R. Baechle and R.W. Earle, eds. Champaign, IL: Human Kinetics, pp. 115-136.

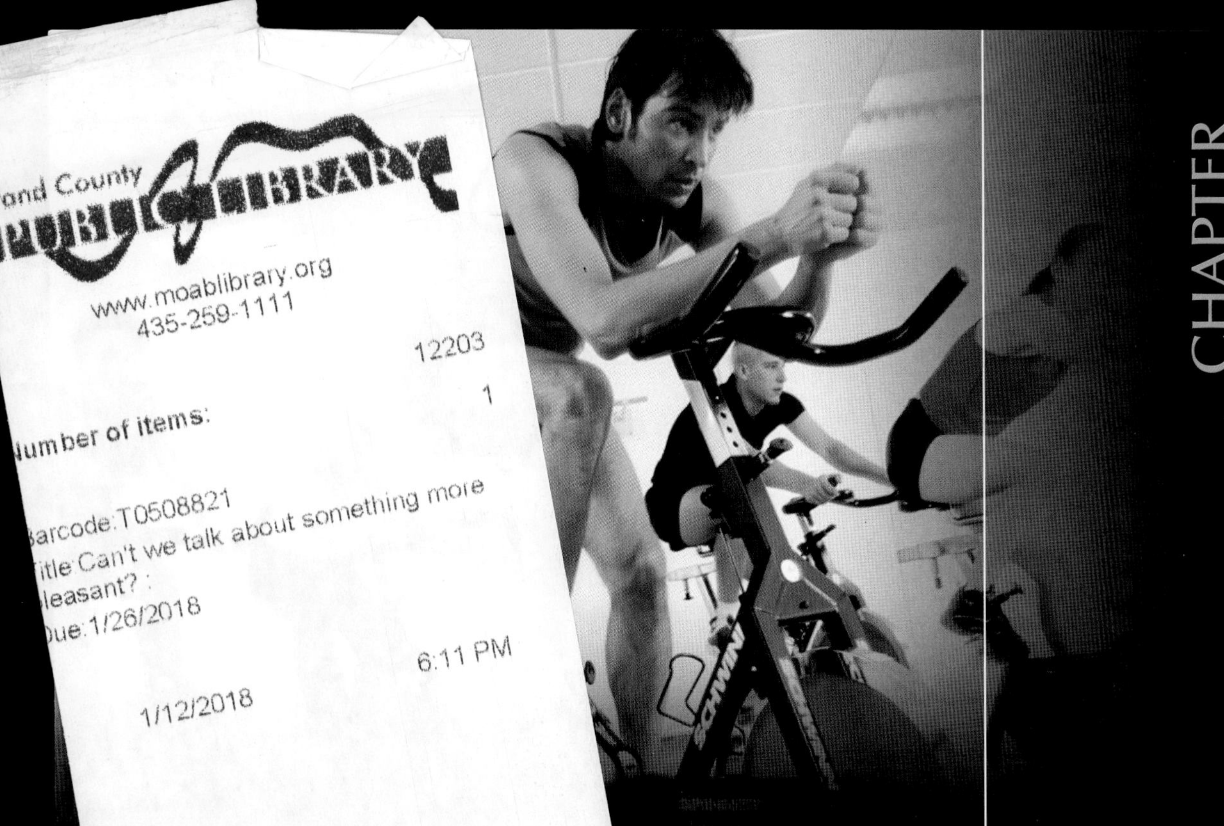

CHAPTER 3

energetics

avis Triplett-McBride

After completing this chapter, you will be able to

- understand the basic terminology of bioenergetics and metabolism related to exercise and training;
- discuss the central role of adenosine triphosphate in muscular activity;
- explain the basic energy systems present in the human body and the ability of each to supply energy for various activities;
- discuss the effects of training on the bioenergetics of skeletal muscle;
- recognize the substrates used by each energy system and discuss patterns of substrate use with various types of activities; and
- develop training programs that demonstrate an understanding of human bioenergetics and metabolism, especially the metabolic specificity of training.

To properly and effectively design exercise and training programs, a personal trainer must have knowledge of the production and use of energy in biological systems. After defining essential bioenergetics terminology, including the role of adenosine triphosphate, this chapter deals with the three basic energy systems that are utilized to replenish adenosine triphosphate in human skeletal muscle. Then we look at how substrates are used for various types of activities, including specifics on how each type of substrate is broken down for energy production, and how the main substrate, muscle glycogen, is replenished. Finally we discuss the metabolic specificity of training, which refers to the limitations of each energy system and the contribution of each energy system to physical activity.

Essential Terminology

The ability or capacity to perform physical work requires **energy.** In the human body, the conversion of chemical energy to mechanical energy is necessary for movement to occur. **Bioenergetics,** or the flow of energy in a biological system, primarily concerns the conversion of food—or large carbohydrate, protein, and fat molecules that contain chemical energy—into biologically usable forms of energy. The breakdown of chemical bonds in these molecules releases the energy necessary to perform physical activity.

The process of breaking down large molecules into smaller molecules, such as the breakdown of carbohydrates into glucose, is generally accompanied by the release of energy and is termed **catabolic.** The synthesis of larger molecules from smaller molecules can be accomplished using the energy released from catabolic reactions. This building-up process is termed **anabolic,** and an example of this process is the formation of proteins from amino acids. The human body is in a constant state of anabolism and catabolism, which is defined as **metabolism,** or the total of all the catabolic and anabolic reactions in the body. Energy obtained from catabolic reactions is used to drive anabolic reactions, through an intermediate molecule, **adenosine triphosphate (ATP).** Without an adequate supply of ATP, muscular activity and muscle growth would not be possible. Thus, when designing training programs, personal trainers should have a basic understanding of how exercise affects ATP use and resynthesis.

Adenosine triphosphate is composed of adenine, a nitrogen-containing base; ribose, a five-carbon sugar (adenine and ribose together are called adenosine); and three phosphate groups (figure 3.1). The removal of one phosphate group yields **adenosine diphosphate (ADP);** removal of a second phosphate group yields **adenosine monophosphate (AMP).** Adenosine triphosphate is classified as a high-energy molecule because it stores large amounts of energy in the chemical bonds of the two terminal phosphate groups. The breaking of these chemical bonds releases energy to power various reactions in the body. Because muscle cells store ATP only in limited amounts and activity requires a constant supply of ATP to provide the energy needed for contraction, ATP-producing processes must also occur in the cell.

Composition of Adenosine Triphosphate

- Adenine (a nitrogen-containing base) ⟩ Together called *adenosine*
- Ribose (a five-carbon or pentose sugar) ⟩
- Three phosphate groups — Together called *triphosphate*

The author would like to acknowledge the contributions of Drs. Michael Conley and Michael Stone to this chapter. Much of the content is directly attributed to Dr. Conley's work in the second edition and Dr. Stone's work in the first edition of *Essentials of Strength Training and Conditioning,* published by Human Kinetics.

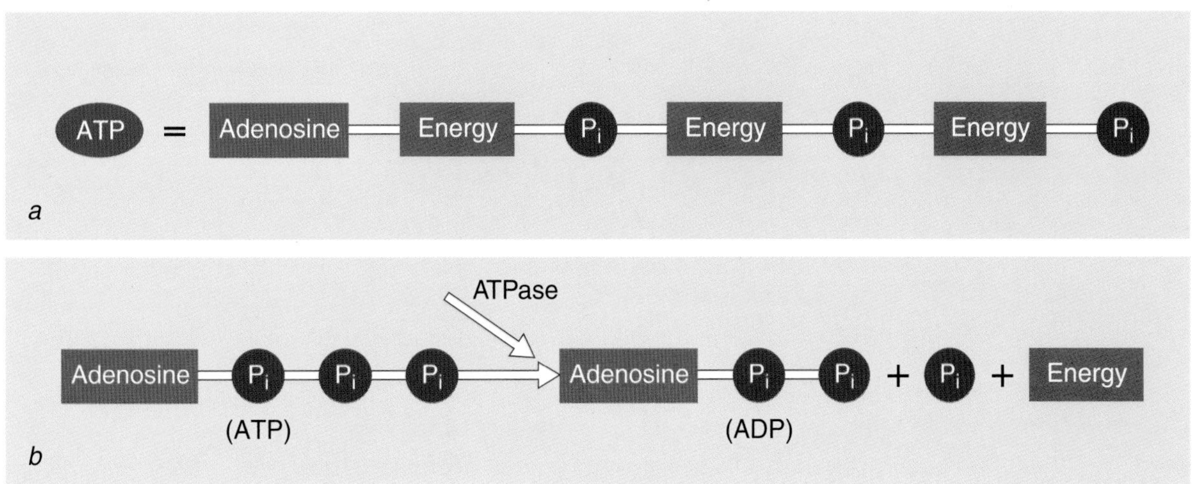

Figure 3.1 *(a)* The structure of an ATP (adenosine triphosphate) molecule, showing the high-energy phosphate bonds. *(b)* When the third phosphate on the ATP molecule is separated from adenosine by the action of adenosine triphosphatase (ATPase), energy is released.
Reprinted from Baechle and Earle 2000.

Energy Systems

Three energy systems exist in the human body to replenish ATP [66, 77]:

- Phosphagen system (an anaerobic process, i.e., one that occurs in the absence of oxygen)
- Glycolysis (two types: fast glycolysis and slow glycolysis)
- Oxidative system (an aerobic process, i.e., one that requires oxygen)

Of the three main food components (carbohydrates, fats, and proteins), only carbohydrates can be metabolized for energy without the direct involvement of oxygen [9].

> Energy stored in the chemical bonds of ATP is used to power muscular activity. The replenishment of ATP in human skeletal muscle is accomplished by three basic energy systems: (1) phosphagen, (2) glycolytic, and (3) oxidative.

Phosphagen System

The **phosphagen system** is the primary source of ATP for short-term, high-intensity activities (e.g., jumping and sprinting) but is active at the start of all types of exercise regardless of intensity [11]. For instance, even during the first few seconds of an easy 5K jog or a moderate-intensity spinning class, the energy for the muscular activity is derived primarily from the phosphagen system. This energy system relies on the chemical reactions of ATP and creatine phosphate, both phosphagens, which involve the enzymes myosin adenosine triphosphatase (ATPase) and creatine kinase. **Myosin ATPase** catalyzes the breakdown of ATP to form ADP and inorganic phosphate (P_i) and release energy. **Creatine kinase** catalyzes the synthesis of ATP from creatine phosphate and ADP; creatine phosphate supplies a phosphate group that combines with ADP to form ATP.

These reactions provide energy at a high rate; however, because ATP and creatine phosphate are stored in the muscle in small amounts, the phosphagen system cannot supply enough energy for continuous, long-duration activities [13]. Generally, Type II (fast-twitch) muscle fibers contain greater concentrations of phosphagens than Type I (slow-twitch) fibers [45].

Creatine kinase activity primarily regulates the breakdown of creatine phosphate. An increase in the muscle cell concentration of ADP promotes creatine kinase activity; an increase in ATP concentration inhibits it [66]. At the beginning of exercise, ATP is broken down to ADP, releasing energy for muscular contraction. This increase in ADP concentration activates creatine kinase to catalyze the formation of ATP from the breakdown of creatine phosphate. Creatine kinase activity remains elevated if exercise continues at a high intensity. If exercise is discontinued, or continues at an intensity low enough to allow glycolysis or the oxidative system to supply an adequate amount of ATP for the muscle cells' energy demands, the muscle cell concentration of ATP will likely increase. This increase in ATP then results in a decrease in creatine kinase activity.

Glycolysis

Glycolysis is the breakdown of carbohydrates, either **glycogen** stored in the muscle or glucose delivered in the blood, to produce ATP [10, 54]. The ATP provided by glycolysis supplements the phosphagen system initially and then becomes the primary source of ATP for high-intensity muscular activity that lasts up to about two minutes, such as keeping a good volley going in a rigorous game of racquetball [77]. The process of glycolysis involves many enzymes catalyzing a series of chemical reactions (figure 3.2). The enzymes for glycolysis are located in the cytoplasm of the cells (the sarcoplasm in muscle cells).

As seen in figure 3.2, the process of glycolysis may occur in one of two ways, termed **fast glycolysis** and **slow glycolysis.** During fast glycolysis, the end-product, **pyruvate,** is converted to lactic acid, providing energy (ATP) at a faster rate than with slow glycolysis, in which pyruvate is transported to the mitochondria for energy production through the oxidative system. (Fast glycolysis has commonly been called *anaerobic glycolysis,* and slow glycolysis has been termed *aerobic glycolysis,* as a result of the ultimate fate of the pyruvate. However, because glycolysis itself does not depend on oxygen, *these terms are not practical for describing the process* [10].) The fate of the end-products is controlled by the energy demands within the cell. If energy must be supplied at a high rate, such as during resistance training, fast glycolysis is primarily used. If the energy demand is not as high and oxygen is present in sufficient quantities in the cell, for example at the beginning of a low-intensity dance aerobics class, slow glycolysis is activated. Another by-product of interest is reduced nicotinamide adenine dinucleotide (NADH), which goes to the electron transport system for further ATP production ("reduced" refers to the added hydrogen).

The net reaction for fast glycolysis may be summarized as follows:

$$\text{glucose} + 2P_i + 2\text{ADP} \ \square\ 2\text{lactate} + 2\text{ATP} + H_2O \quad \textbf{(3.1)}$$

The net reaction for slow glycolysis may be summarized as follows:

$$\text{glucose} + 2P_i + 2\text{ADP} + 2\text{NAD}^+ \ \square\ 2\text{pyruvate} + 2\text{ATP} + 2\text{NADH} + 2H_2O$$

Energy Yield of Glycolysis

Glycolysis produces a net of two molecules of ATP from one molecule of glucose. However, if glycogen (the stored form of glucose) is used, there is a net production of three ATPs because the reaction of **phosphorylating** (adding a phosphate group to) glucose, which requires one ATP, is bypassed [54] (see figure 3.2).

Glycolysis Regulation

Glycolysis is stimulated during intense muscular activity by ADP, P_i, ammonia, and a slight decrease in pH and is strongly stimulated by AMP [10, 54, 78]. It is inhibited by the markedly lowered pH that may be observed during periods of inadequate oxygen supply and by increased levels of ATP, creatine phosphate, citrate, and free fatty acids [10, 37, 54] that are usually present at rest. The phosphorylation of glucose by hexokinase (see figure 3.2) primarily controls glycolysis [10, 51, 54]; but we must also consider the rate of glycogen breakdown to glucose, which is catalyzed by phosphorylase (figure 3.2), in the regulation of glycolysis [10, 65, 67]. In other words, if glycogen is not being broken down into glucose quickly enough and the supply of free glucose has already been depleted, glycolysis will be slowed.

Another important consideration in the regulation of any series of reactions is the **rate-limiting step,** that is, the slowest reaction in the series. The rate-limiting step in glycolysis is the conversion of fructose-6-phosphate to fructose-1,6-biphosphate (see figure 3.2), a reaction catalyzed by the enzyme phosphofructokinase (PFK). Thus, the activity of PFK is the primary factor in the regulation of the rate of glycolysis. Activation of the phosphagen

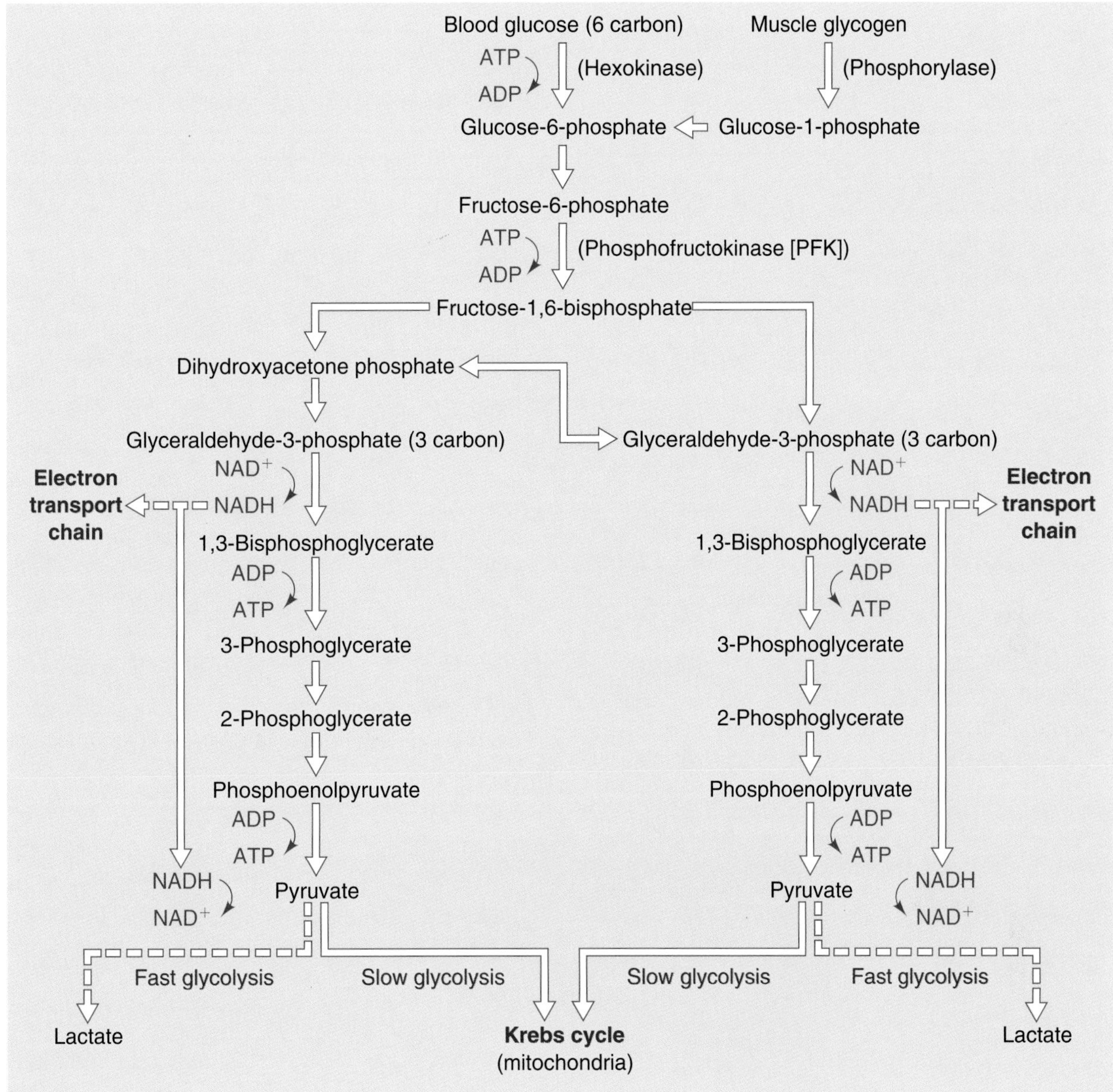

Figure 3.2 Glycolysis. ATP = adenosine triphosphate; ADP = adenosine diphosphate; NAD^+, NADH = nicotinamide adenine dinucleotide.
Reprinted from Baechle and Earle 2000.

energy system stimulates glycolysis (by stimulating PFK) to contribute to the energy production of high-intensity exercise [10, 81]. Ammonia produced during high-intensity exercise as a result of increased AMP or amino acid deamination (removing the amino group of the amino acid molecule) can also stimulate PFK.

Lactic Acid and Blood Lactate

Fast glycolysis occurs during periods of reduced oxygen availability in the muscle cells and results in the formation of the end-product **lactic acid.** Muscular fatigue experienced during exercise is often associated with high muscle tissue concentrations of lactic acid [34]. Lactic acid accumulation in tissue is the result of an imbalance between production and utilization or breakdown [52]. As lactic acid accumulates, there is a corresponding increase in hydrogen ion concentration, which is believed to inhibit glycolytic reactions and directly interfere with muscle contraction, possibly by inhibiting calcium binding to troponin [27, 62] or by interfering with actin-myosin cross-bridge formation [23, 27, 37, 62, 80]. Also, the decrease in pH levels (to more acidic) from the increased hydrogen ion concentration inhibits the enzyme activity of the cell's energy systems [2, 37]. The overall effect is a decrease in available energy and muscle contraction force during exercise [34, 37].

Lactic acid is converted to its salt, **lactate,** by buffering systems in the muscle and blood [7, 10]. Unlike lactic acid in the muscle, lactate is not believed to be a fatigue-producing substance [10]. Instead, lactate is often used as an energy substrate, especially in Type I and cardiac muscle fibers [3, 57, 87]. It is also used in **gluconeogenesis,** the formation of glucose from lactate and non-carbohydrate sources, during extended exercise and recovery [7, 57]. Blood lactate concentrations reflect lactic acid production and clearance. The clearance of lactate from the blood indicates a person's ability to recover. Lactate can be cleared by oxidation within the muscle fiber in which it was produced, or it can be transported in the blood to other muscle fibers to be oxidized [57]. Lactate can also be transported in the blood to the liver, where it is converted to glucose. This process is referred to as the **Cori cycle** and is depicted in figure 3.3.

Normally there is a low concentration of lactate in blood and muscle. The reported normal range of lactate concentration in blood is 0.5 to 2.2 mmol · L^{-1} at rest [31, 60]. Lactic acid production increases with increasing exercise intensity [31, 69] and appears to depend on muscle fiber type. The higher rate of lactic acid production by Type II muscle fibers may reflect a concentration or activity of glycolytic enzymes that is higher than that of Type I muscle fibers [3, 19, 63].

Gollnick, Bayly, and Hodgson [31] have reported that blood lactate concentrations normally return to pre-exercise values within an hour after activity. Light activity during the postexercise period has been shown to increase lactate clearance rates [25, 31, 38], and aerobically trained [31] and anaerobically trained [61, 64] individuals have faster lactate

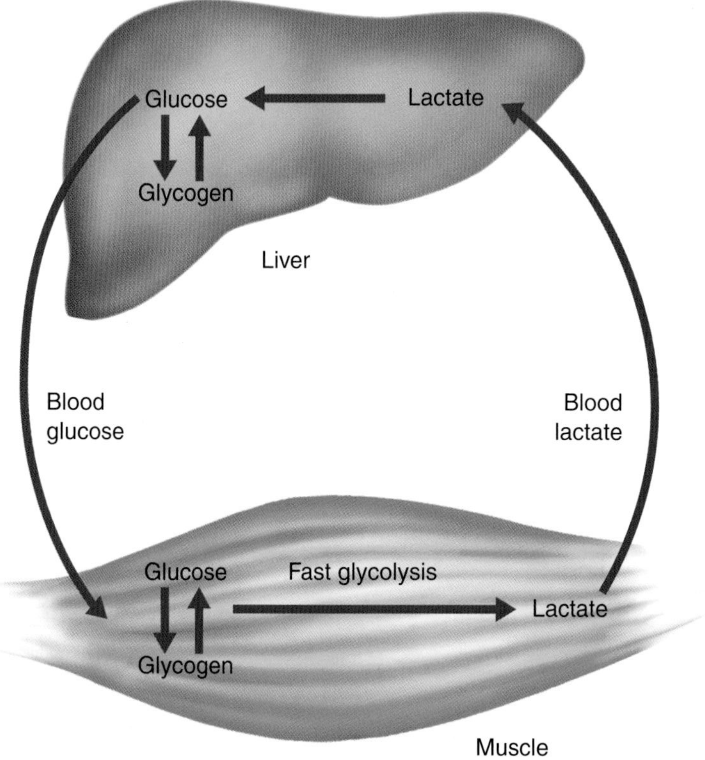

Figure 3.3 The Cori cycle.
Reprinted from Baechle and Earle 2000.

clearance rates than untrained people. Peak blood lactate concentrations occur approximately five minutes after the cessation of exercise [31], a delay frequently attributed to the time required to buffer and transport lactic acid from the tissue to the blood [47].

Recent evidence suggests that there are specific inflection points in the lactate accumulation curve (figure 3.4) as exercise intensity increases [14, 49]. The exercise intensity or relative intensity at which blood lactate begins an abrupt increase above the baseline concentration has been termed the **lactate threshold (LT)** [88]. The LT represents an increasing reliance on anaerobic mechanisms. The LT typically begins at 50% to 60% of maximal oxygen uptake in untrained subjects and at 70% to 80% in trained subjects [12, 24]. A second increase in the rate of lactate accumulation has been noted at higher relative intensities of exercise. This second point of inflection, termed the **onset of blood lactate accumulation (OBLA)**, generally occurs when the concentration of blood lactate is near 4 mmol · L^{-1} [39, 74, 79]. The breaks in the lactate accumulation curve may correspond to the points at which intermediate and large motor units are recruited during increasing exercise intensities [46]. The muscle cells associated with large motor units are typically Type II fibers, which are particularly suited for anaerobic metabolism and lactic acid production.

Some studies suggest that training at intensities near or above the LT or OBLA changes the LT and OBLA so that lactate accumulation occurs later at a higher exercise intensity [14, 17]. This shift probably occurs as a result of several factors but, in particular, because of the increased mitochondrial content that allows for greater production of ATP through aerobic mechanisms. The shift allows the individual to perform at higher percentages of maximal oxygen uptake without as much lactate accumulation in the blood [10, 14].

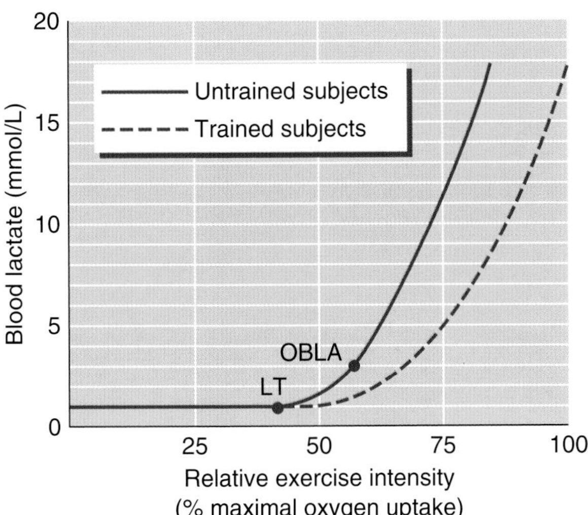

Figure 3.4 Lactate threshold (LT) and onset of blood lactate accumulation (OBLA).
Reprinted from Baechle and Earle 2000.

The Oxidative (Aerobic) System

The **oxidative system** is the primary source of ATP at rest and during aerobic activities and uses primarily carbohydrates and fats as substrates [77]. Clients who are walking on a treadmill, doing water aerobics, or participating in a yoga class are relying primarily on the oxidative system. Protein is normally not metabolized significantly, except during long-term starvation and long bouts (>90 minutes) of exercise [16, 55]. At rest, approximately 70% of the ATP produced is derived from fats and 30% from carbohydrates. Following the onset of activity, as the intensity of the exercise increases, there is a shift in substrate preference from fats to carbohydrates. During high-intensity aerobic exercise, almost 100% of the energy is derived from carbohydrates, if an adequate supply is available. However, during prolonged, submaximal, steady-state work there is a gradual shift from carbohydrates back to fats and protein as energy substrates [10].

Glucose and Glycogen Oxidation

The oxidative metabolism of blood glucose and muscle glycogen begins with glycolysis. If oxygen is present in sufficient quantities, then the end-product of glycolysis, pyruvate, is not converted to lactic acid but is transported to the **mitochondria** (specialized cellular organelles where the reactions of aerobic metabolism occur). When pyruvate enters the mitochondria, it is converted to acetyl CoA (CoA stands for coenzyme A) and can then enter the **Krebs cycle** for further ATP production. Also transported there are two molecules of NADH produced during glycolytic reactions. The Krebs cycle, a series of reactions that continues the oxidation of the substrate begun in glycolysis, produces two ATPs indirectly from guanine triphosphate (GTP) for each molecule of glucose (figure 3.5). Also produced in the Krebs cycle from one molecule of glucose are an additional six molecules of NADH and two molecules of reduced flavin adenine dinucleotide ($FADH_2$).

These molecules transport hydrogen atoms to the **electron transport chain (ETC)** to be used to produce ATP from ADP [10, 58]. The ETC uses the

NADH and $FADH_2$ molecules to rephosphorylate ADP to ATP (figure 3.6). The hydrogen atoms are passed down the chain, a series of electron carriers known as **cytochromes,** to form a concentration gradient of protons to provide energy for ATP production, with oxygen serving as the final electron acceptor (resulting in the formation of water). Because NADH and $FADH_2$ enter the ETC at different sites, they differ in their ability to produce ATP. One molecule of NADH can produce three molecules of ATP, whereas one molecule of $FADH_2$ can produce only two molecules of ATP. The production of ATP during this process is referred to as **oxidative phosphorylation.** The oxidative system, beginning with glycolysis, results in the production of approximately 38 ATPs from the degradation of one glucose molecule [10, 77]. Table 3.1 summarizes the ATP yield of these processes.

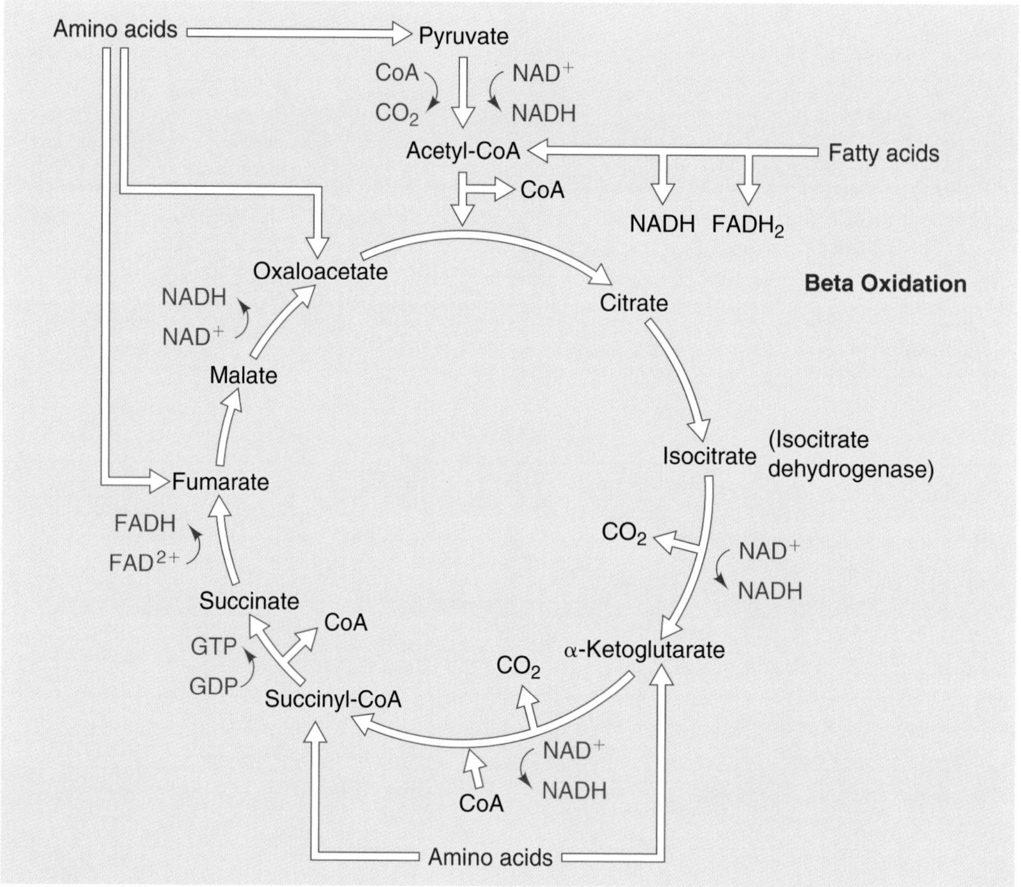

Figure 3.5 The Krebs cycle. CoA = coenzyme A; FAD^{2+}, $FADH_2$ = flavin adenine dinucleotide; GDP = guanine diphosphate; GTP = guanine triphosphate; NAD^+, NADH = nicotinamide adenine dinucleotide.
Reprinted from Baechle and Earle 2000.

ADP+P_i ADP+P_i ADP+P_i

NADH / NAD^+ → FAD^{2+} / $FADH_2$ → CoQ / CoQ → Cyt *b* / Cyt *b* → Cyt c_1 / Cyt c_1 → Cyt *c* / Cyt *c* → Cyt *a* / Cyt *a* → Cyt a_3 / Cyt a_3 → H_2O / $½O_2$

ATP ATP ATP

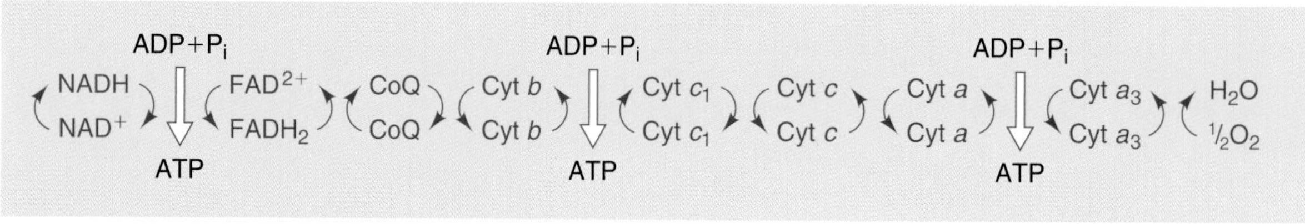

Figure 3.6 The electron transport chain. CoQ = coenzyme Q; Cyt = cytochrome; ATP = adenosine triphosphate; ADP = adenosine diphosphate; P_i = inorganic phosphate; NADH, NAD^+ = nicotinamide adenine dinucleotide; $FADH_2$, FAD^{2+} = flavin adenine dinucleotide; H_2O = water; O_2 = oxygen.
Reprinted from Baechle and Earle 2000.

Fat Oxidation

Fats can also be used by the oxidative energy system. Triglycerides stored in fat cells can be broken down by an enzyme known as hormone-sensitive lipase. This enzyme releases free fatty acids from the fat cells into the blood, where they can circulate and enter muscle fibers [10, 42, 54, 65]. Additionally, limited quantities of triglycerides are stored within the muscle, along with a form of hormone-sensitive lipase, to serve as a source of free fatty acids within the muscle [10, 20]. Free fatty acids enter the mitochondria, where they undergo **beta oxidation,** a series of reactions in which the free fatty acids are broken down, resulting in the formation of acetyl CoA and hydrogen atoms (figure 3.5). The acetyl CoA enters the Krebs cycle directly, and the hydrogen atoms are carried by NADH and $FADH_2$ to the ETC [10, 54]. An example of the ATP produced from a typical triglyceride molecule is shown in table 3.2.

TABLE 3.1

Total Energy Yield From the Oxidation of One Glucose Molecule

Process	ATP production
Slow glycolysis	
Substrate-level phosphorylation	4
Oxidative phosphorylation: 2 NADH (3 ATP each)	6
Krebs cycle (2 rotations through the Krebs cycle per glucose)	
Substrate-level phosphorylation	2
Oxidative phosphorylation: 8 NADH (3 ATP each)	24
Via GTP; 2 $FADH_2$ (2 ATP each)	4
Total	40*

Note: Glycolysis consumes 2 ATP (if starting with glucose), so net ATP production is 40 – 2 = 38. This figure may also be reported as 36 ATP depending on which shuttle system is used to transport the NADH to the mitochondria. ATP = adenosine triphosphate; NADH = nicotinamide adenine dinucleotide; GTP = guanine triphosphate; $FADH_2$ = flavin adenine dinucleotide.

TABLE 3.2

Total Energy Yield From the Oxidation of One (18-Carbon) Triglyceride Molecule

Process	ATP production
1 molecule of glycerol	22
18-carbon fatty acid metabolism*	
147 ATP per fatty acid × 3 fatty acids/triglyceride molecule	441
Total	463

*Other triglycerides that contain different amounts of carbons will yield more or less ATP. ATP = adenosine triphosphate.

Protein Oxidation

Although not a significant source of energy for most activities, protein can be broken down into its constituent amino acids by various metabolic processes. These amino acids can then be converted into glucose (in a process known as gluconeogenesis), pyruvate, or various Krebs cycle intermediates to produce ATP (figure 3.5). The contribution of amino acids to the production of ATP has been estimated to be minimal during short-term exercise but may contribute 3% to 18% of the energy requirements during prolonged activity [8, 75]. The major amino acids that are oxidized in skeletal muscle appear to be the **branched-chain amino acids** (leucine, isoleucine, and valine), although alanine, aspartate, and glutamate may also be used [33]. The nitrogen-containing waste products of amino acid breakdown are eliminated through the formation of urea and small amounts of ammonia, which end up in the urine [10]. The elimination of ammonia is important because ammonia is toxic and is associated with fatigue [54, 77].

Oxidative (Aerobic) System Regulation

The rate-limiting step in the Krebs cycle (see figure 3.5) is the conversion of isocitrate to α-ketoglutarate, a reaction catalyzed by the enzyme isocitrate dehydrogenase. Isocitrate dehydrogenase is stimulated by ADP and normally inhibited by ATP. The reactions that produce NADH or $FADH_2$ also influence the regulation of the Krebs cycle. If NAD^+ and FAD^{2+} are not available in sufficient quantities to accept hydrogen, the rate of the Krebs cycle is reduced. Also, when GTP accumulates, the concentration of succinyl CoA increases, which inhibits the initial reaction (oxaloacetate + acetyl CoA □ citrate + CoA) of the Krebs cycle. The ETC is inhibited by ATP and stimulated by ADP [10, 54]. Figure 3.7 presents a simplified overview of the metabolism of fat, carbohydrate, and protein.

All three energy systems are active at a given time; however, the extent to which each is used depends primarily on the intensity of the activity and secondarily on its duration [18, 77].

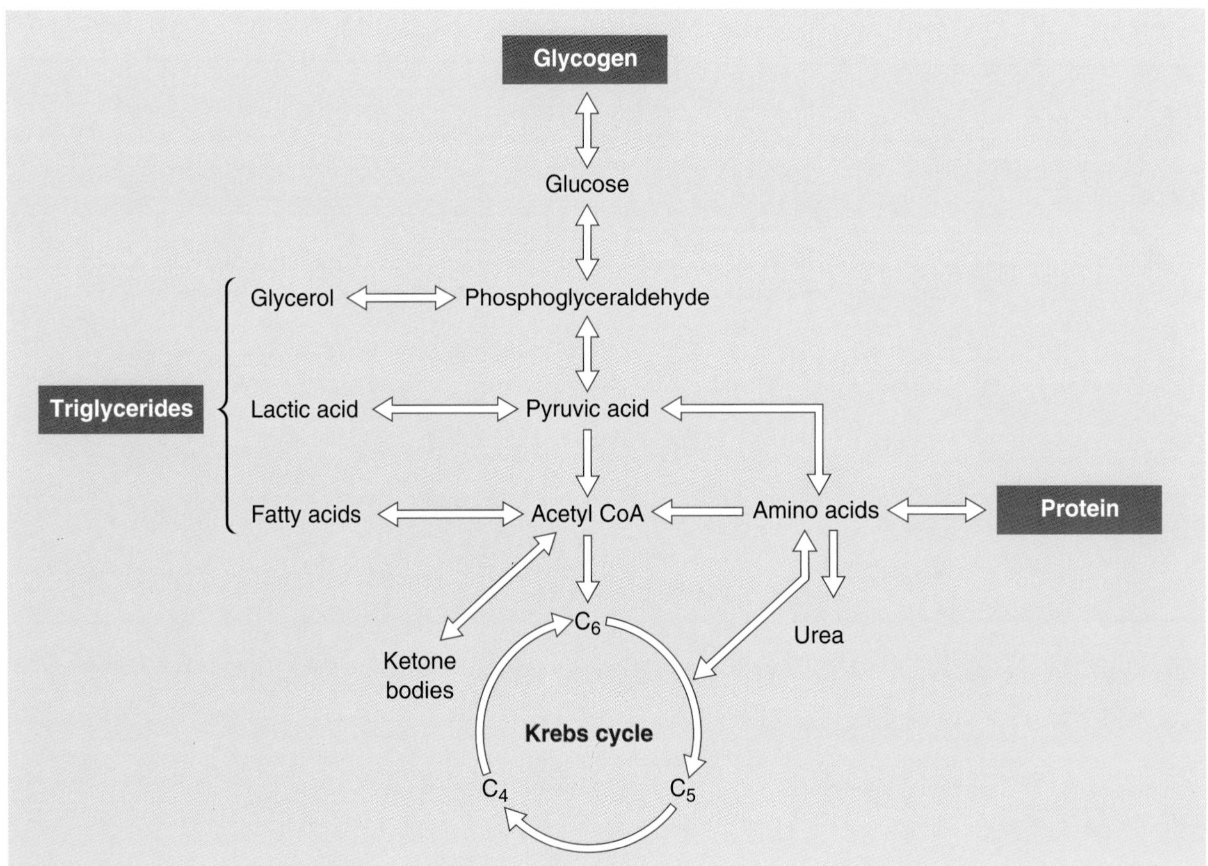

Figure 3.7 The metabolism of fat, carbohydrate, and protein share some common pathways. Note that all three are reduced to acetyl CoA and enter the Krebs cycle.
Reprinted from Baechle and Earle 2000.

Energy Production and Capacity

The phosphagen, glycolytic, and oxidative energy systems differ in their ability to supply energy for activities of various intensities and durations (tables 3.3 and 3.4). **Exercise intensity** is defined as a level of muscular activity that can be quantified in terms of **power** output, with power defined as the amount of physical work performed for a particular duration of time [50].

Activities such as performing resistance training and performing a serve in tennis that are high in intensity and thus have a high power output, require rapidly supplied energy and rely almost entirely on the energy supplied by the phosphagen system. Activities that are of lower intensity but longer duration, such as a 10-mile (16-kilometer) bike ride or swimming laps in the pool, require a large energy supply and rely on the energy supplied by the oxidative energy system (table 3.3). The primary source of energy for activities between these two extremes differs depending on the intensity and duration of the event (table 3.4). In general, short, high-intensity activities (e.g., jumping or kicking and punching moves in cardio kickboxing) rely on the phosphagen energy system and fast glycolysis. As the intensity decreases and the duration increases, the emphasis gradually shifts to slow glycolysis and the oxidative energy system [10, 18, 70].

The duration of the activity also influences which energy system is used. Specific exercises within a prescribed program can range in duration from approximately five seconds (e.g., one set of bench press at 90% of the 1RM [1-repetition maximum]) to more than an hour (e.g., low-intensity, extended-duration treadmill walking). If an individual makes a best effort (an effort that results in the best possible performance for a given activity), the time considerations shown in table 3.4 are reasonable [10, 21, 37, 68, 80, 82].

TABLE 3.3

Rankings of Rate and Capacity of Adenosine Triphosphate (ATP) Production

System	Rate of ATP production	Capacity of ATP production
Phosphagen	1	5
Fast glycolysis	2	4
Slow glycolysis	3	3
Oxidation of carbohydrates	4	2
Oxidation of fats and proteins	5	1

Note: 1 = fastest/greatest; 5 = slowest/least; ATP = adenosine triphosphate.

TABLE 3.4

Effect of Event Duration on Primary Energy System Used

Duration of event	Intensity of event	Primary energy system(s)
0-6 sec	Very intense	Phosphagen
6-30 sec	Intense	Phosphagen and fast glycolysis
30 sec to 2 min	Heavy	Fast glycolysis
2-3 min	Moderate	Fast glycolysis and oxidative system
>3 min	Light	Oxidative system

At no time, during either exercise or rest, does any single energy system provide the complete supply of energy. During exercise, the degree to which anaerobic and oxidative systems contribute to the energy being produced is determined primarily by the exercise intensity and secondarily by exercise duration [10, 18, 21].

In general, there is an inverse relationship between the relative rate and total amount of ATP that a given energy system can produce. As a result, the phosphagen energy system primarily supplies ATP for high-intensity activities of short duration (e.g., sprint across a football field), the glycolytic system for moderate- to high-intensity activities of short to medium duration (e.g., running once around a track), and the oxidative system for low-intensity activities of long duration (e.g., 20-mile [32-kilometer] bike ride).

Metabolic Specificity of Training

Appropriate exercise intensities and rest intervals can permit the "selection" of specific energy systems during training for specific athletic events or training goals (e.g., to improve short-term endurance) [10, 58, 77]. Few sports or physical activities require maximal sustained-effort exercise to exhaustion or near exhaustion. Most sports and training activities (such as football, cardio kickboxing, spinning, and resistance training) are intermittent in nature and therefore produce metabolic profiles that are very similar to that for a series of high-intensity, constant- or near-constant-effort exercise bouts interspersed with rest periods. In this type of exercise, the power output (a measure of exercise intensity) produced during each exercise bout is much greater than the maximal power output that can be sustained using aerobic energy sources. Chapters 15, 16, and 17 discuss training methods that allow appropriate metabolic systems to be stressed.

Substrate Depletion and Repletion

Energy substrates—molecules that provide starting materials for bioenergetic reactions, including phosphagens (ATP and creatine phosphate), glucose, glycogen, lactate, free fatty acids, and amino acids—can be selectively depleted during the performance of activities of various intensities and durations. Subsequently, the amount of energy that can be produced by the bioenergetic systems decreases. Fatigue experienced during many activities is frequently associated with the depletion of phosphagens [30, 41] and glycogen [9, 10, 37, 43, 72]; the depletion of substrates such as free fatty acids, lactate, and amino acids typically does not occur to the extent that performance is limited. Consequently, the depletion and repletion pattern of phosphagens and glycogen following physical activity is important in exercise bioenergetics.

Phosphagens

Fatigue during exercise appears to be at least partially related to the decrease in phosphagens. Phosphagen concentrations in muscle are more rapidly depleted as a result of high-intensity anaerobic exercise than of aerobic exercise [30, 41]. Creatine phosphate can decrease markedly (50% to 70%) during the first stage (5-30 seconds) of high-intensity exercise and can be almost eliminated as a result of very intense exercise to exhaustion [40, 44, 48, 59]. Muscle ATP concentrations do not decrease by more than about 60% from initial values, however, even during very intense exercise [40, 48]. It is also important to note that dynamic muscle actions, such as a complete repetition of a weight training exercise, use more metabolic energy and typically deplete phosphagens to a greater extent than do isometric muscle actions, such as arm wrestling, in which there is no visible shortening of the muscle [6].

Postexercise phosphagen repletion can occur in a relatively short period; complete resynthesis of ATP appears to occur within three to five minutes, and complete creatine phosphate resynthesis can occur within eight minutes [35, 41, 56]. Repletion of phosphagens occurs largely as a result of aerobic metabolism [35], although fast glycolysis can contribute to ATP resynthesis after high-intensity exercise [12, 15].

Glycogen

Limited stores of glycogen are available for exercise. Approximately 300 to 400 grams of glycogen is stored in the body's total muscle, and about 70 to 100 grams is stored in the liver [73]. Resting concentrations of liver and muscle glycogen can be influenced by training and dietary manipulations [26, 73]. Research suggests that both anaerobic training, including sprinting and resistance training [5], and typical aerobic training [28, 29] can increase resting muscle glycogen concentration (figure 3.8).

The rate of glycogen depletion is related to exercise intensity [73]. Muscle glycogen is a more important energy source than is liver glycogen during moderate- and high-intensity exercise; liver glyco-

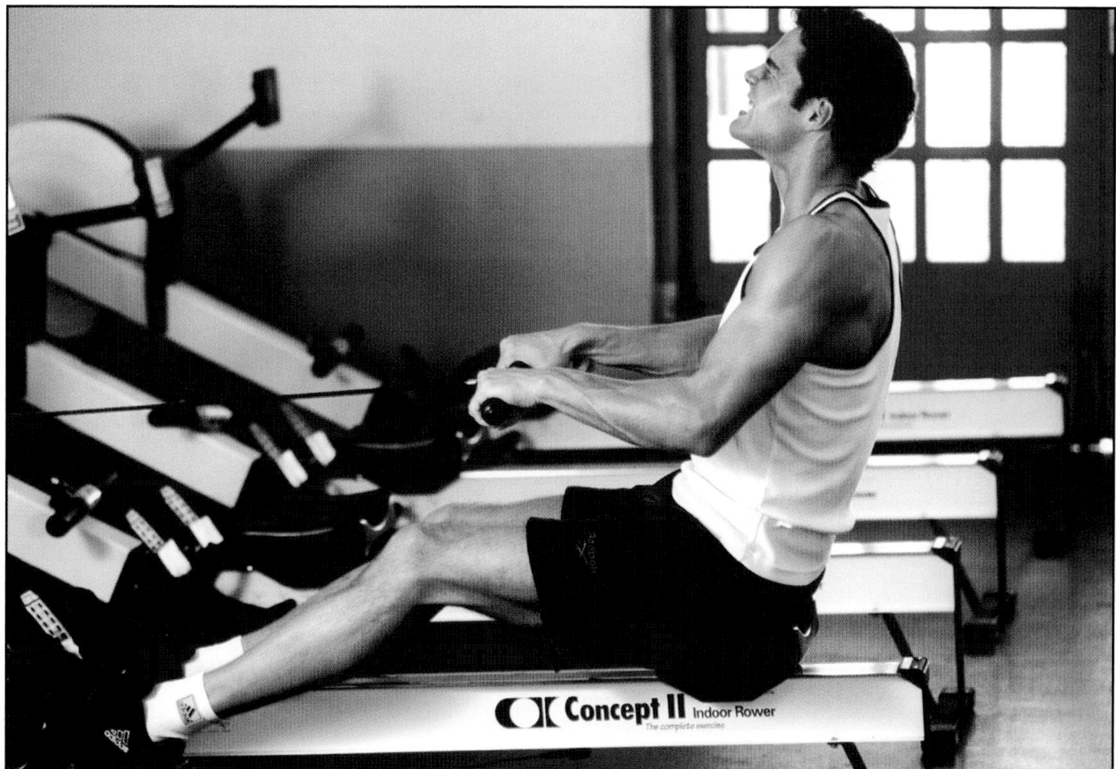

Figure 3.8 Both resistance and aerobic training can increase resting muscle glycogen concentration.

gen appears to be more important during low-intensity exercise, and its contribution to metabolic processes increases with duration of exercise. Increases in relative exercise intensity of 50%, 75%, and 100% of maximal oxygen uptake result in increases in the rate of muscle **glycogenolysis** (the breakdown of glycogen) [72]. At relative intensities of exercise above 60% of maximal oxygen uptake, muscle glycogen becomes an increasingly important energy substrate; and the entire glycogen content of some muscle cells can become depleted during exercise [71].

Very high intensity, intermittent exercise, such as resistance training or half-court basketball, can cause substantial depletion of muscle glycogen (decreases of 20% to 60%) with relatively few sets of exercise (low total workloads) [53, 68, 80, 83]. Although phosphagens may be the primary limiting factor during resistance exercise with few repetitions or few sets, muscle glycogen may become the limiting factor for resistance training with many total sets and larger total amounts of work [68, 77]. This type of exercise could cause selective muscle fiber glycogen depletion (more depletion in Type II fibers) that can also limit performance [22, 68]. As with other types of dynamic exercise, the rate of muscle glycogenolysis during resistance exercise depends on intensity. However, it appears that equal amounts of total work produce equal amounts of glycogen depletion, regardless of relative exercise intensity [68].

Repletion of muscle glycogen during recovery is related to postexercise carbohydrate ingestion. Repletion appears to be optimal if 0.7 to 3.0 grams of carbohydrate per kilogram of body weight is ingested every two hours following exercise [26, 73]. Muscle glycogen may be completely replenished within 24 hours, provided sufficient carbohydrate is ingested [26, 73]. However, if the exercise has a high eccentric component (associated with exercise-induced muscle damage), more time may be required to completely replenish muscle glycogen.

Oxygen Uptake and the Aerobic and Anaerobic Contributions to Exercise

Oxygen uptake (or consumption) is a measure of a person's ability to take in and use oxygen. The higher the oxygen uptake, the more fit the person is thought to be. During low-intensity exercise with a constant power output, oxygen uptake increases for the first few minutes until a steady state of uptake (oxygen demand equals oxygen consumption) is reached (figure 3.9) [1, 39]. At the start of the exercise bout, however, some of the energy must be supplied through anaerobic mechanisms [84]. This anaerobic contribution to the total energy cost of exercise is termed the **oxygen deficit** [39, 58]. After exercise, oxygen uptake remains above pre-exercise levels for a period of time that varies according to the intensity and length of the exercise. Postexercise oxygen uptake has been termed the **oxygen debt** [39, 58], or the **excess postexercise oxygen consumption (EPOC)** [10]. The EPOC is the oxygen uptake above resting values used to restore the body to the pre-exercise condition [76]. Researchers have observed only small to moderate relationships between the oxygen deficit and the EPOC [4, 36]; the oxygen deficit may influence the size of the EPOC, but the two are not equal.

Anaerobic mechanisms provide much of the energy for work if the exercise intensity is above the maximal oxygen uptake that a person can attain (figure 3.10). For instance, if a client who was not used to that type of activity jumped right into an advanced spinning class, most of the energy would be supplied by anaerobic mechanisms. Generally, as the contribution of anaerobic mechanisms supporting the exercise increases, the exercise duration decreases [1, 32, 85, 86].

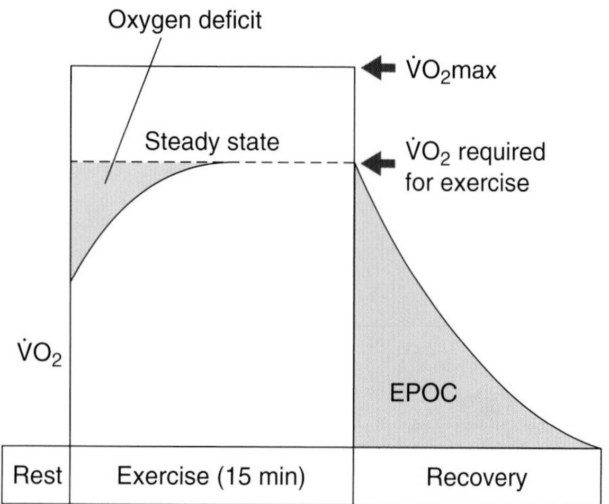

Figure 3.9 Low-intensity, steady-state exercise metabolism: 75% of maximal oxygen uptake ($\dot{V}O_2$max). EPOC = excess postexercise oxygen consumption; $\dot{V}O_2$ = oxygen uptake.
Reprinted from Baechle and Earle 2000.

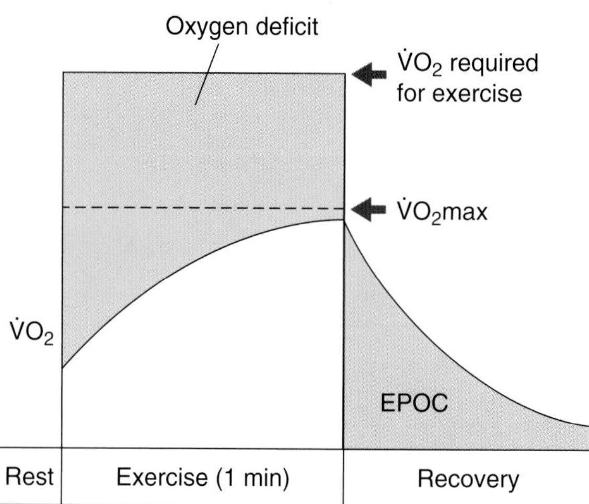

Figure 3.10 High-intensity, non-steady-state exercise metabolism (80% of maximum power output). The required $\dot{V}O_2$ here is the oxygen uptake that would be required to sustain the exercise if such an uptake were possible to attain. Because it is not, the oxygen deficit lasts for the duration of the exercise. EPOC = excess postexercise oxygen consumption; $\dot{V}O_2$max = maximal oxygen uptake.
Reprinted from Baechle and Earle 2000.

CONCLUSION

One can design more productive training programs through an understanding of how energy is produced during various types of exercise and how energy production can be modified by specific training regimens. Which energy system is used to supply energy for muscular contraction is determined primarily by the intensity of exercise and secondarily by the duration of exercise. Metabolic responses and the subsequent training adaptations are largely regulated by those characteristics (e.g., intensity and duration) and form the basis of metabolic specificity of exercise and training. This principle of specificity allows for enhanced physical adaptation and program results through the implementation of precise training programs.

STUDY QUESTIONS

1. Which of the following describes the process of fast glycolysis?

   I. a breakdown of glycogen
   II. its end product is converted to lactic acid
   III. a breakdown of glucose
   IV. its end product is sent to the Krebs Cycle

   A. I and II only
   B. III and IV only
   C. I, II, and III only
   D. II, III, and IV only

2. Which of the following describes what a client would be doing to allow the oxidative system to contribute the greatest *percentage* toward total ATP production?

   A. sitting quietly
   B. walking
   C. jogging
   D. sprinting

3. Which of the following energy systems is capable of producing the greatest amount (capacity) of ATP?

   A. phosphagen
   B. fast glycolysis
   C. slow glycolysis
   D. oxidative

4. Which of the following energy systems is capable of producing ATP at the greatest rate?

   A. phosphagen
   B. fast glycolysis
   C. slow glycolysis
   D. oxidative

APPLIED KNOWLEDGE QUESTION

Fill in the chart to describe the changes in the sources of energy to produce ATP as a client participates in a maximum treadmill test. Write *Most* if it is the primary source of energy during the activity. Write *Least* if it is the least used source of energy during the activity.

Activity	Carbohydrate	Fat
While client is sitting in a chair listening to the personal trainer		
The first few seconds of the treadmill test		
During a stage that the client reached steady-state		
At the end of the test as the client reaches maximum		

REFERENCES

1. Åstrand, P.O., and K. Rodahl. 1970. *Textbook of Work Physiology,* 2nd ed. New York: McGraw-Hill.
2. Barany, M., and C. Arus. 1990. Lactic acid production in intact muscle, as followed by ^{13}C and ^{1}H nuclear magnetic resonance. In: *Human Muscle Power,* N.L. Jones, N. McCartney, and A.J. McComas, eds. Champaign, IL: Human Kinetics, pp. 153-164.
3. Barnard, R.J., V.R. Edgerton, T. Furakawa, and J.B. Peter. 1971. Histochemical, biochemical and contractile properties of red, white and intermediate fibers. *American Journal of Physiology* 220: 410-441.
4. Berg, W.E. 1947. Individual differences in respiratory gas exchange during recovery from moderate exercise. *American Journal of Physiology* 149: 507-530.
5. Boobis, I., C. Williams, and S.N. Wooten. 1983. Influence of sprint training on muscle metabolism during brief maximal exercise in man. *Journal of Physiology* 342: 36-37P.
6. Bridges, C.R., B.J. Clark III, R.L. Hammond, and L.W. Stephenson. 1991. Skeletal muscle bioenergetics during frequency-dependent fatigue. *American Journal of Physiology* 29: C643-C651.
7. Brooks, G.A. 1986. The lactate shuttle during exercise and recovery. *Medicine and Science in Sports and Exercise* 18: 360-368.
8. Brooks, G.A. 1987. Amino acid and protein metabolism during exercise and recovery. *Medicine and Science in Sports and Exercise* 19: S150-S156.
9. Brooks, G.A., K.E. Brauner, and R.G. Cassens. 1973. Glycogen synthesis and metabolism of lactic acid after exercise. *American Journal of Physiology* 224: 1162-1186.
10. Brooks, G.A., and T.D. Fahey. 1984. *Exercise Physiology: Human Bioenergetics and Its Applications.* New York: Wiley.
11. Brooks, G.A., K.J. Hittelman, J.A. Faulkner, and R.E. Beyer. 1971. Temperature, skeletal muscle mitochondrial functions and oxygen debt. *American Journal of Physiology* 220: 1053-1068.
12. Cerretelli, P., G. Ambrosoli, and M. Fumagalli. 1975. Anaerobic recovery in man. *European Journal of Applied Physiology* 34: 141-148.
13. Cerretelli, P., D. Rennie, and D. Pendergast. 1980. Kinetics of metabolic transients during exercise. *International Journal of Sports Medicine* 55: 178-180.
14. Davis, J.A., M.H. Frank, B.J. Whipp, and K. Wasserman. 1979. Anaerobic threshold alterations caused by endurance training in middle-aged men. *Journal of Applied Physiology* 46: 1039-1046.
15. diPrampero, P.E., L. Peeters, and R. Margaria. 1973. Alactic O_2 debt and lactic acid production after exhausting exercise in man. *Journal of Applied Physiology* 34: 628-632.
16. Dohm, G.L., R.T. Williams, G.J. Kasperek, and R.J. VanRij. 1982. Increased excretion of urea and N-methylhistidine by rats and humans after a bout of exercise. *Journal of Applied Physiology* 52: 27-33.
17. Donovan, C.M., and G.A. Brooks. 1983. Endurance training affects lactate clearance, not lactate production. *American Journal of Physiology* 244: E83-E92.
18. Dudley, G.A., and T.F. Murray. 1982. Energy for sport. *NSCA Journal* 3 (3): 14-15.
19. Dudley, G.A., and R. Terjung. 1985. Influence of aerobic metabolism on IMP accumulation in fast-twitch muscle. *American Journal of Physiology* 248: C37-C42.
20. DuFax, B., G. Assmann, and W. Hollman. 1982. Plasma lipoproteins and physical activity: A review. *International Journal of Sports Medicine* 3: 123-136.
21. Edington, D.E., and V.R. Edgerton. 1976. *The Biology of Physical Activity.* Boston: Houghton Mifflin.
22. Essen, B. 1978. Glycogen depletion of different fiber types in man during intermittent and continuous exercise. *Acta Physiologica Scandinavica* 103: 446-455.
23. Fabiato, A., and F. Fabiato. 1978. Effects of pH on the myofilaments and sarcoplasmic reticulum of skinned cells from cardiac and skeletal muscle. *Journal of Physiology* 276: 233-255.
24. Farrel, P.A., J.H. Wilmore, E.F. Coyle, J.E. Billing, and D.L. Costill. 1979. Plasma lactate accumulation and distance running performance. *Medicine and Science in Sports* 11 (4): 338-344.
25. Freund, H., and P. Gendry. 1978. Lactate kinetics after short strenuous exercise in man. *European Journal of Applied Physiology* 39: 123-135.
26. Friedman, J.E., P.D. Neufer, and L.G. Dohm. 1991. Regulation of glycogen synthesis following exercise. *Sports Medicine* 11 (4): 232-243.
27. Fuchs, F., Y. Reddy, and F.N. Briggs. 1970. The interaction of cations with calcium binding site of troponin. *Biochimica et Biophysica Acta* 221: 407-409.
28. Gollnick, P.D., R.B. Armstrong, B. Saltin, W. Saubert, and W.L. Sembrowich. 1973. Effect of training on enzyme activity and fiber composition of human muscle. *Journal of Applied Physiology* 34: 107-111.
29. Gollnick, P.D., R.B. Armstrong, W. Saubert, K. Piel, and B. Saltin. 1972. Enzyme activity and fibre composition in skeletal muscle of untrained and trained men. *Journal of Applied Physiology* 33: 312-319.
30. Gollnick, P.D., and W.M. Bayly. 1986. Biochemical training adaptations and maximal power. In: *Human Muscle Power,* N.L. Jones, N. McCartney, and A.J. McComas, eds. Champaign, IL: Human Kinetics, pp. 255-267.
31. Gollnick, P.D., W.M. Bayly, and D.R. Hodgson. 1986. Exercise intensity, training diet and lactate concentration in muscle and blood. *Medicine and Science in Sports and Exercise* 18: 334-340.
32. Gollnick, P.D., and L. Hermansen. 1982. Significance of skeletal muscle oxidative enzyme enhancement with endurance training. *Clinical Physiology* 2: 1-12.
33. Graham, T.E., J.W.E. Rush, and D.A. Maclean. 1995. Skeletal muscle amino acid metabolism and ammonia production during exercise. In: *Exercise Metabolism,* M. Hargreaves, ed. Champaign, IL: Human Kinetics, pp. 41-72.
34. Häkkinen, K. 1992. Effects of fatiguing heavy resistance loading on voluntary neural activation and force production in males and females. In: *Proceedings of the Second North American Congress on Biomechanics.* Chicago: North American Congress on Biomechanics, pp. 567-568.
35. Harris, R.C., R.H.T. Edwards, E. Hultman, L.O. Nordesjo, B. Nylind, and K. Sahlin. 1976. The time course of phosphocreatinine resynthesis during recovery of the quadriceps muscle in man. *Pfluegers Archives* 97: 392-397.
36. Henry, F.M. 1957. Aerobic oxygen consumption and alactic debt in muscular work. *Journal of Applied Physiology* 3: 427-450.
37. Hermansen, L. 1981. Effect of metabolic changes on force generation in skeletal muscle during maximal exercise. In: *Human Muscle Fatigue,* R. Porter and J. Whelan, eds. London: Pittman Medical.

38. Hermansen, L., and I. Stenvold. 1972. Production and removal of lactate in man. *Acta Physiologica Scandinavica* 86: 191-201.

39. Hill, A.V. 1924. Muscular exercise, lactic acid and the supply and utilization of oxygen. *Proceedings of the Royal Society of London [Biological Sciences]* 96: 438.

40. Hirvonen, J., S. Ruhunen, H. Rusko, and M. Harkonen. 1987. Breakdown of high-energy phosphate compounds and lactate accumulation during short submaximal exercise. *European Journal of Applied Physiology* 56: 253-259.

41. Hultman, E., and H. Sjoholm. 1986. Biochemical causes of fatigue. In: *Human Muscle Power,* N.L. Jones, N. McCartney, and A.J. McComas, eds. Champaign, IL: Human Kinetics, pp. 215-235.

42. Hurley, B.F., D.R. Seals, J.M. Hagberg, A.C. Goldberg, S.M. Ostrove, J.O. Holloszy, W.G. Wiest, and A.P. Goldberg. 1984. Strength training and lipoprotein lipid profiles: Increased HDL cholesterol in body builders versus powerlifters and effects of androgen use. *Journal of the American Medical Association* 252: 507-513.

43. Jacobs, I., P. Kaiser, and P. Tesch. 1981. Muscle strength and fatigue after selective glycogen depletion in human skeletal muscle fibers. *European Journal of Applied Physiology* 46: 47-53.

44. Jacobs, I., P.A. Tesch, O. Bar-Or, J. Karlsson, and R. Dotow. 1983. Lactate in human skeletal muscle after 10 and 30 s of supramaximal exercise. *Journal of Applied Physiology* 55: 365-367.

45. Jansson, E., C. Sylven, and E. Nordevang. 1982. Myoglobin in the quadriceps femoris muscle of competitive cyclists and in untrained men. *Acta Physiologica Scandinavica* 114: 627-629.

46. Jones, N., and R. Ehrsam. 1982. The anaerobic threshold. In: *Exercise and Sport Sciences Review,* vol. 10, R.L. Terjung, ed. Philadelphia: Franklin Press, pp. 49-83.

47. Juel, C. 1988. Intracellular pH recovery and lactate efflux in mouse soleus muscles stimulated in vitro: The involvement of sodium/proton exchange and a lactate carrier. *Acta Physiologica Scandinavica* 132: 363-371.

48. Karlsson, J. 1971. Lactate and phosphagen concentrations in working muscle of man. *Acta Physiologica Scandinavica* 485: 358-365.

49. Kindermann, W., G. Simon, and J. Jeul. 1979. The significance of the aerobic-anaerobic transition for the determination of work load intensities during endurance training. *European Journal of Applied Physiology* 42: 25-34.

50. Knuttgen, H.G., and P.V. Komi. 1992. Basic definitions for exercise. In: *Strength and Power in Sport: The Encyclopedia of Sports Medicine,* P.V. Komi, ed. Oxford, England: Blackwell Scientific, pp. 3-8.

51. Krebs, H.A. 1972. The Pasteur effect and the relation between respiration and fermentation. *Essays in Biochemistry* 8: 2-34.

52. Kreisberg, R.A. 1980. Lactate homeostasis and lactic acidosis. *Annals of Internal Medicine* 92 (2): 227-237.

53. Lambert, C.P., M.G. Flynn, J.B. Boone, T.J. Michaud, and J. Rodriguez-Zayas. 1991. Effects of carbohydrate feeding on multiple-bout resistance exercise. *Journal of Applied Sports Science Research* 5 (4): 192-197.

54. Lehninger, A.L. 1973. *Bioenergetics.* Menlo Park, CA: W.A. Benjamin. 1973.

55. Lemon, P.W., and J.P. Mullin. 1980. Effect of initial muscle glycogen levels on protein catabolism during exercise. *Journal of Applied Physiology: Respiration in Environmental Exercise Physiology* 48: 624-629.

56. MacDougall, J.D., G.R. Ward, D.G. Sale, and J.R. Sutton. 1977. Biochemical adaptations of human skeletal muscle to heavy resistance training and immobilization. *Journal of Applied Physiology* 43: 700-703.

57. Mazzeo, R.S., G.A. Brooks, D.A. Schoeller, and T.F. Budinger. 1986. Disposal of blood [1-13C] lactate in humans during rest and exercise. *Journal of Applied Physiology* 60 (10): 232-241.

58. McArdle, W.D., F.I. Katch, and V.L. Katch. 1986. *Exercise Physiology: Energy, Nutrition, and Human Performance,* 2nd ed. Philadelphia: Lea & Febiger.

59. McCartney, N., L.L. Spriet, G.J.F. Heigenhauser, J.M. Kowalchuk, J.R. Sutton, and N.L. Jones. 1986. Muscle power and metabolism in maximal intermittent exercise. *Journal of Applied Physiology* 60: 1164-1169.

60. McGee, D.S., T.C. Jesse, M.H. Stone, and D. Blessing. 1992. Leg and hip endurance adaptations to three different weight-training programs. *Journal of Applied Sports Science Research* 6 (2): 92-95.

61. McMillan, J.L., M.H. Stone, J. Sartin, R. Keith, D. Marple, C. Brown, and R.D. Lewis. 1993. 20-hour physiological responses to a single weight-training session. *Journal of Strength and Conditioning Research* 7 (1): 9-21.

62. Nakamura, Y., and A. Schwartz. 1972. The influence of hydrogen ion concentration on calcium binding and release by skeletal muscle sarcoplasmic reticulum. *Journal of General Physiology* 59: 22-32.

63. Opie, L.J., and E.A. Newsholme. 1967. The activities of fructose-1,6-diphosphate, phosphofructokinase, and phosphoenolpyruvate carboxykinase in white and red muscle. *Biochemical Journal* 103: 391-399.

64. Pierce, K., R. Rozenek, M. Stone, and D. Blessing. 1987. The effects of weight training on plasma cortisol, lactate, heart rate, anxiety and perceived exertion (abstract). *Journal of Applied Sports Science Research* 1 (3): 58.

65. Pike, R.L., and M. Brown. 1975. *Nutrition: An Integrated Approach,* 2nd ed. New York: Wiley.

66. Poortmans, J.R. 1984. Protein turnover and amino acid oxidation during and after exercise. *Medicine and Science in Sports and Exercise* 17: 130-147.

67. Richter, E.A., H. Galbo, and N.J. Christensen. 1981. Control of exercise-induced muscular glycogenolysis by adrenal medullary hormones in rats. *Journal of Applied Physiology* 50: 21-26.

68. Robergs, R.A., D.R. Pearson, D.L. Costill, W.J. Fink, D.D. Pascoe, M.A. Benedict, C.P. Lambert, and J.J. Zachweija. 1992. Muscle glycogenolysis during differing intensities of weight-resistance exercise. *Journal of Applied Physiology* 70 (4): 1700-1706.

69. Rozenek, R., L. Rosenau, P. Rosenau, and M.H. Stone. 1993. The effect of intensity on heart rate and blood lactate response to resistance exercise. *Journal of Strength and Conditioning Research* 7 (1): 51-54.

70. Sahlin, K., M. Tonkonogi, and K. Soderlund. 1998. Energy supply and muscle fatigue in humans. *Acta Physiologica Scandinavica* 162 (3): 261-266.

71. Saltin, B., and P.D. Gollnick. 1983. Skeletal muscle adaptability: Significance for metabolism and performance. In: *Handbook of Physiology,* L.D. Peachey, R.H. Adrian, and S.R. Geiger, eds. Baltimore: Williams & Wilkins, pp. 540-555.

72. Saltin, B., and J. Karlsson. 1971. Muscle glycogen utilization during work of different intensities. In: *Muscle Metabolism During Exercise,* B. Pernow and B. Saltin, eds. New York: Plenum Press, pp. 289-300.

73. Sherman, W.M., and G.S. Wimer. 1991. Insufficient carbohydrate during training: Does it impair performance? *International Journal of Sports Nutrition* 1 (1): 28-44.

74. Sjodin, B., and I. Jacobs. 1981. Onset of blood lactate accumulation and marathon running performance. *International Journal of Sports Medicine* 2: 23-26.
75. Smith, S.A., S.J. Montain, R.P. Matott, G.P. Zientara, F.A. Jolesz, and R.A. Fielding. 1998. Creatine supplementation and age influence muscle metabolism during exercise. *Journal of Applied Physiology* 85: 1349-1356.
76. Stainsby, W.M., and J.K. Barclay. 1970. Exercise metabolism: O_2 deficit, steady level O_2 uptake and O_2 uptake in recovery. *Medicine and Science in Sports* 2: 177-195.
77. Stone, M.H., and H.S. O'Bryant. 1987. *Weight Training: A Scientific Approach.* Minneapolis: Burgess International.
78. Sugden, P.H., and E.A. Newsholme. 1975. The effects of ammonium, inorganic phosphate and potassium ions on the activity of phosphofructokinase from muscle and nervous tissues of vertebrates and invertebrates. *Biochemical Journal* 150: 113-122.
79. Tanaka, K., Y. Matsuura, S. Kumagai, A. Matsuzuka, K. Hirakoba, and K. Asano. 1983. Relationships of anaerobic threshold and onset of blood lactate accumulation with endurance performance. *European Journal of Applied Physiology* 52: 51-56.
80. Tesch, P. 1980. Muscle fatigue in man, with special reference to lactate accumulation during short intense exercise. *Acta Physiologica Scandinavica* 480: 1-40.
81. Tesch, P.A., B. Colliander, and P. Kaiser. 1986. Muscle metabolism during intense, heavy resistance exercise. *European Journal of Applied Physiology* 55: 362-366.
82. Tesch, P.A., L.L. Plouz-Snyder, L. Ystrom, M.J. Castro, and G.A. Dudley. 1998. Skeletal muscle glycogen loss evoked by resistance exercise. *Journal of Strength and Conditioning Research* 12: 67-73.
83. Thorstensson, P. 1976. Muscle strength, fiber types and enzymes in man. *Acta Physiologica Scandinavica* 102: 443.
84. Warren, B.J., M.H. Stone, J.T. Kearney, S.J. Fleck, G.D. Wilson, and W.J. Kraemer. 1992. The effects of short-term overwork on performance measures and blood metabolites in elite junior weightlifters. *International Journal of Sports Medicine* 13 (5): 372-376.
85. Wells, J., B. Balke, and D. Van Fossan. 1957. Lactic acid accumulation during work. A suggested standardization of work classification. *Journal of Applied Physiology* 10: 51-55.
86. Whipp, B.J., C. Scard, and K. Wasserman. 1970. O_2deficit-O_2debt relationship and efficiency of aerobic work. *Journal of Applied Physiology* 28: 452-458.
87. York, J., L.B. Oscai, and D.G. Penny. 1974. Alterations in skeletal muscle lactate dehydrogenase isozymes following exercise training. *Biochemical and Biophysical Research Communications* 61: 1387-1393.
88. Yoshida, I. 1984. Effect of dietary modifications on lactate threshold and onset of blood lactate accumulation during incremental exercise. *European Journal of Applied Physiology* 53: 200-205.

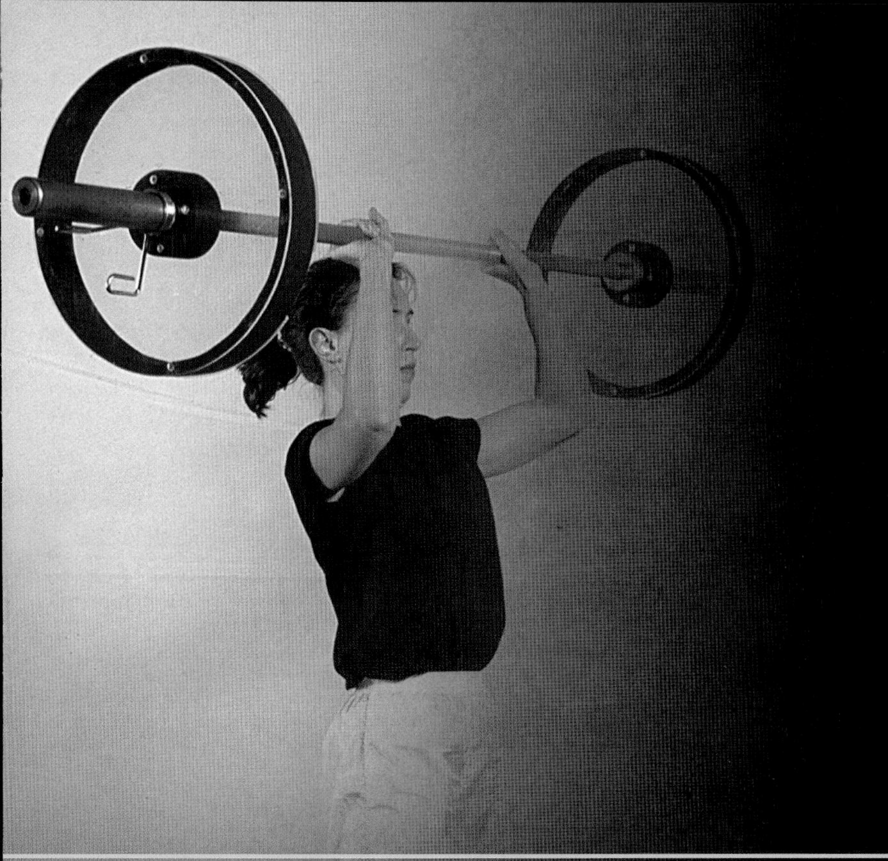

CHAPTER 4

Biomechanics

Everett Harman

After completing this chapter, you will be able to

- recognize the various types of levers of the musculoskeletal system;
- quantify linear and rotational work and power;
- understand the factors contributing to human strength and power;
- evaluate the resistive force and power patterns of exercise devices based on their sources of resistance; and
- analyze movements in sport, work, and daily life and make movement-oriented exercise prescriptions.

In order to understand human movements, including those involved in sport, exercise, and daily activities, a personal trainer must have a working knowledge of basic **biomechanics** of the musculoskeletal system. In contrast to **anatomy,** which is the study of the various physical components that make up the body, biomechanics is the science of how those components work together to create movement. Knowledge of both disciplines is useful for understanding how the human "machine" carries out body movements and the stresses and strains it undergoes in doing so. This enhances the personal trainer's ability to design safe and effective exercise programs.

The principles of biomechanics underlie almost every movement in sport, exercise, and activities of daily living. Knowledge of biomechanics is essential to personal trainers because it enhances their ability to select exercises to meet clients' goals and minimizes the likelihood of injury in almost any exercise setting.

This chapter begins with a description of the various types of levers in the musculoskeletal system. It then explains how basic principles of biomechanics relate to physical training and the manifestation of human strength and power. We next turn to the various sources of resistance to the muscles, including gravity, inertia, friction, fluid resistance, and elasticity, as well as the exercise devices that employ these sources of resistance. The final section of the chapter deals with the application of biomechanics to movement analysis and exercise prescription for the attainment of specific training goals.

Levers of the Musculoskeletal System

Levers involving bones, joints, and skeletal muscles bring about most movements of the limbs and the whole body. Muscles not acting through bony levers include those of the face, tongue, heart, arteries, and sphincters. However, body movements that are characteristic of sport, exercise, and most daily life activities act primarily through the levers of the skeleton in order to exert forces on the ground, objects, and other people. A basic knowledge of leverage enables an understanding of how the body is able to carry out such movements. The following are some basic definitions:

lever—A rigid or partially rigid structure that can rotate about a pivot point. (The term "about" is used in biomechanics literature to describe movement around a certain position or joint.) When a force is exerted on the lever in a direction not in line with the pivot point, then the lever tends to rotate about the pivot point. The lever will exert force on any object impeding its rotation (figure 4.1).

fulcrum—The point about which the lever pivots.

line of action of a force—The line along which the force acts, passing through the force's point of application.

moment arm (also called **lever arm, force arm,** or **torque arm**)—A line starting from and perpendicular to the line of action of the force, extending to the fulcrum.

torque (or **moment**)—The tendency of a force to rotate an object about a fulcrum. Quantitatively, torque is the magnitude of the force multiplied by the length of its moment arm.

muscle force—The force exerted by a muscle at either of its ends when it is electrochemically stimulated to shorten.

resistive force—Force due to such factors as gravity, inertia, or friction that tends to prevent a muscle from shortening.

mechanical advantage—The ratio of the output force to the applied force in a particular leverage system. This is the same as the ratio of the length of the moment arm through which the muscle force acts to the length of the moment arm though which the resistive force acts (figure 4.2). A mechanical advantage greater than 1.0 means that the force exerted on the resisting object by the lever is greater than the applied force. When the mechanical advantage is less than 1.0, the lever exerts a smaller force on the resisting object than the force applied to the lever. The latter situation represents a disadvantage in common terms. However, there are advantages as to movement range and speed that are described more fully later in the chapter.

first-class lever—A lever for which the applied and resistive forces act on opposite sides of the fulcrum (figure 4.2).

second-class lever—A lever for which the applied and resistive forces act on the same side of the fulcrum, with the resistive force acting through a moment arm shorter than that of the applied force, thus providing a mechani-

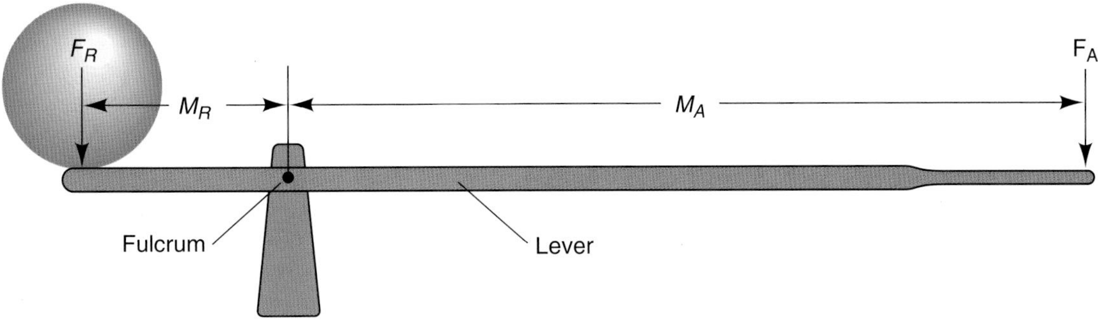

Figure 4.1 A lever. Force exerted perpendicular to the lever at one contact point is resisted by another force at a different contact point. F_A = force applied to the lever; M_A = moment arm of the applied force; F_R = force resisting the lever's rotation; M_R = moment arm of the resistive force.
Reprinted from Baechle and Earle 2000.

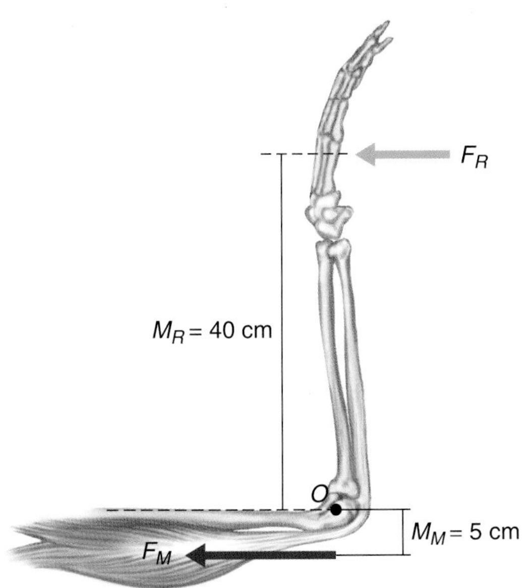

Figure 4.2 A first-class lever (the forearm). Extending the elbow against resistance. O = fulcrum; F_M = muscle force; F_R = resistive force; M_M = moment arm of the muscle force; M_R = moment arm of the resistive force. Mechanical advantage = $M_M \div M_R$ = 5 cm ÷ 40 cm = 0.125, and, being less than 1.0, is a disadvantage in common terms. This is a first-class lever, because muscle force and resistive force act on opposite sides of the fulcrum. During isometric exertion or constant-speed joint rotation, $F_M \times M_M = F_R \times M_R$. Because M_M is much smaller than M_R, F_M must be much greater than F_R; this is disadvantageous in that a large muscle force is required to push against a small external resistance.
Reprinted from Baechle and Earle 2000.

cal advantage greater than 1.0. An example of this is seen when the soleus and gastrocnemius muscles contract so that a standing person rises up on the balls of the feet (figure 4.3). Because of the mechanical advantage, when the body is stationary or moving upward at a constant speed, the force applied by the muscles is less than the resistive force (body weight).

third-class lever—A lever for which the applied and resistive forces act on the same side of the fulcrum (figure 4.4), but with the resistive force acting through a longer moment arm than that of the applied force, thus providing a mechanical advantage of less than 1.0. Because of the low mechanical advantage, the force applied by the muscles has to be greater than the resistive force.

Anatomical Planes of the Human Body

Figure 4.5 shows a person in the standard **anatomical position,** standing erect with arms down at the sides and palms forward. The standard anatomical views of the body are in the **sagittal, frontal,** and **transverse** planes; these are views from the side, front, and top of the body, respectively, in the anatomical position. These three anatomical planes, which are perpendicular to each other, are useful for describing the major body movements. Some examples of exercises within these planes are sit-up (sagittal plane), side bend (frontal plane), and seated hip adduction (transverse plane).

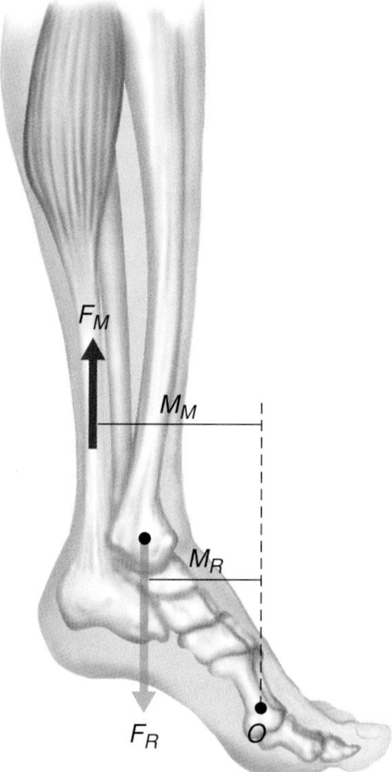

Figure 4.3 A second-class lever—the foot during plantar flexion against resistance, as when one is standing up on the toes. F_M = muscle force; F_R = resistive force; M_M = moment arm of the muscle force; M_R = moment arm of the resistive force. When the body is raised, the ball of the foot, being the point about which the foot rotates, is the fulcrum (O). Because M_M is greater than M_R, F_M is less than F_R.
Reprinted from Baechle and Earle 2000.

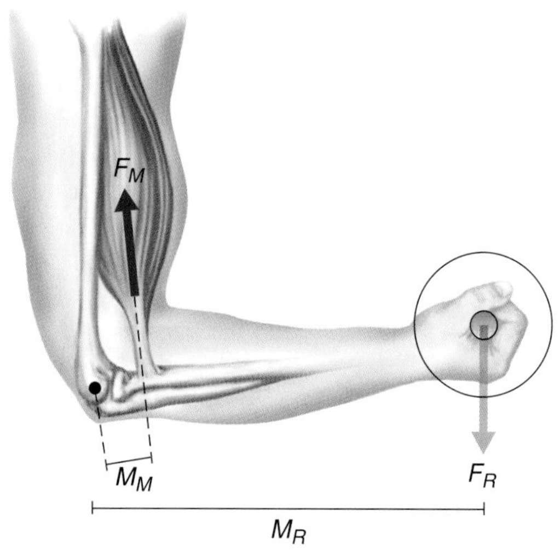

Figure 4.4 A third-class lever—the forearm during the arm curl exercise. F_M = muscle force; F_R = resistive force; M_M = moment arm of the muscle force; M_R = moment arm of the resistive force. Because M_M is much smaller than M_R, F_M must be much greater than F_R.
Reprinted from Baechle and Earle 2000.

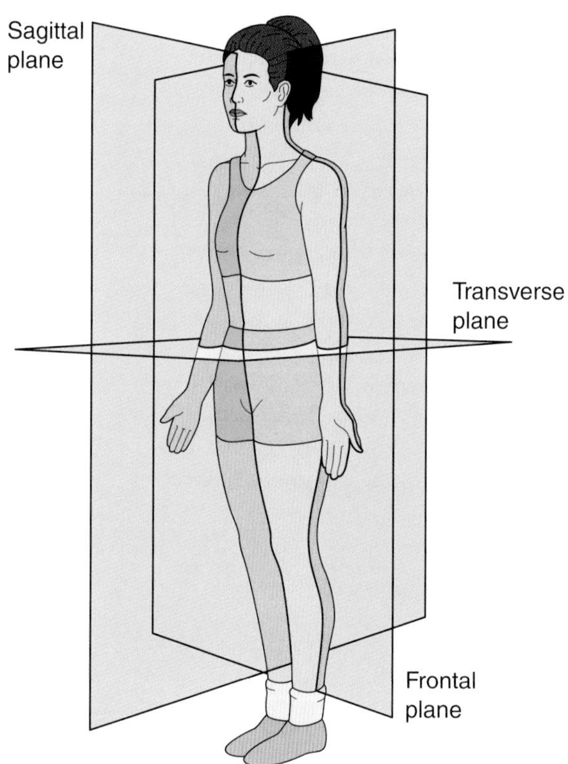

Figure 4.5 The three major planes of the human body in the anatomical position.
Reprinted from Baechle and Earle 2000.

Human Strength and Power

The differences between the common and scientific definitions of power can be confusing. As the term is commonly used, power refers to "vigor, energy, the capacity for exerting mechanical force or doing work" [1]. Thus, frequently the terms "strength" and "power" are used interchangeably to describe the ability to exert force in sport or other life activities. However, in both science and engineering, "strength" and "power" have distinctly different meanings. Personal trainers should be aware of the more precise definition of power and the way it relates to various human activities. This section provides scientific definitions of both strength and power and shows how various factors contribute to their manifestation.

Defining Strength, Power, and Work

In general, the term **strength** is recognized as referring to the ability to exert force [33]. However, there are many ways in which strength can be measured. The most obvious, and likely the oldest, method of quantitatively measuring strength is to see how much weight a person can lift. Other, more qualitative, measures include contests in which people directly pit their strength against each other, as in arm wrestling or tug-of-war. Recent advances in technology, such as electronic force transducers, have greatly expanded the ways in which strength can be measured.

Virtually all physical activities in life involve the **acceleration** (increase in velocity) or **deceleration** (decrease in velocity, also termed negative acceleration) of body segments, the whole body, or external objects (e.g., lifting and/or accelerating grocery bags, trash cans, hammers, axes, or sport implements). According to the force-velocity relationship, the force that a muscle can exert decreases as movement speed increases [29]. However, individuals differ in the degree to which their ability to exert force declines with increasing speed of movement [20]. Thus, measurement of strength with an isometric or low-speed test may not tell much about how an individual might perform in activities requiring acceleration at high speed, such as Ping-Pong, kickboxing, chopping wood, or swatting a fly. For that reason, Knuttgen and Kraemer [21] suggested a more specific definition of strength: the amount of force that can be exerted at a particular speed of movement. The direct measurement of force at various speeds requires sophisticated equipment; but indirect tests—such as one test measuring the distance that balls of different weights can be thrown—can provide similar information relevant to individual strength patterns. Whether simple or sophisticated, direct or indirect, such testing provides much more information than do isometric or maximal lift tests.

Some physical training professionals like to use the term "power" to specify the ability to exert force at relatively high speed and the term "strength" to indicate the ability to lift a weight slowly or exert isometric force [28]. In everyday speech, physical power usually refers to the ability to exert force. The limited meaning of isometric and low-speed strength scores has led to a heightened interest in power as a measurement of the ability to exert force at higher speeds. Yet, as precisely defined in science and engineering, **power** means "the time rate of doing work" [26], where **work** is quantitatively defined as the product of the force exerted on an object and the distance the object moves in the direction in which the force is exerted:

$$\text{work} = \text{force} \times \text{distance} \tag{4.1}$$

$$\text{power} = \text{force} \times \text{distance} \div \text{time} = \text{work} \div \text{time} \tag{4.2}$$

Rearranging the variables, it can also be shown that

$$\text{power} = \text{force} \times \text{velocity} \tag{4.3}$$

For example, if a work crew uses a pulley to hoist an 800-pound piano off the ground 20 feet into a second-story window, the amount of work done against gravity is 20 feet times 800 pounds, equaling 16,000 foot-pounds of work, regardless of any horizontal movement of the piano during its ascent or any variation in the speed at which it is lifted. If it took the crew 40 seconds to hoist the piano, the average power would be 16,000 foot-pounds divided by 40 seconds, equaling 400 foot-pounds per second. One **horsepower** is equal to 550 foot-pounds per second, so the crew would be generating 400 ÷ 550 = 0.73 horsepower. Because the crew pulls on the pulley rope intermittently (i.e., they pull on the rope, pause and regrasp the rope farther up, then pull on the rope again), in order to average a power output of 400 foot-pounds per second, the power exerted during the actual pull phases is considerably higher. For that reason, during most human activities, peak power is much higher than average power.

Work and Power in SI Units

In the **International System of Units** (abbreviated SI from the French) [23], the unit of force is the newton (N), and the unit of distance is the meter (m). Thus, work is quantified in newton-meters (N · m), also called joules, and power in joules per second, also called watts (W). In the United States, we use a combination of traditional and international units. The rate of power consumption of many electrical devices, such as microwave ovens and some exercise machines, is generally given in watts, while the power output of gasoline engines is usually provided in horsepower. One horsepower is equivalent to 746 watts. One can also multiply by 1.36 to convert from foot-pounds of work to joules or from foot-pounds per second of power to watts.

These conversions may be useful for comparing equipment that is rated using the different systems. Unfortunately, one must be careful to distinguish between power consumption and power output. Since motors are not completely efficient, the power consumption of an electric motor is greater than its output power. Thus, it is most relevant to compare the output power of different machines, rather than power consumption. Table 4.1 provides additional factors to convert from traditional U.S. units to SI units.

Work and Power During Physical Activity

Power output is relevant to both short and long human activities. Aerobic activities like running,

TABLE 4.1

Conversion Between Various Units

pounds × 4.448 = newtons
newtons × 0.2248 = pounds
kilograms force × 2.205 = pounds
pounds × 0.4536 = kilograms force
kilograms force × 9.807 = newtons
newtons × 0.1020 = kilograms force
feet × 0.3048 = meters
inches × 0.02540 = meters
miles × 1,609 = meters
foot-pounds × 1.356 = joules
foot-pounds per second × 1.356 = watts
horsepower × 745.7 = watts
miles per hour × 1.467 = feet per second
miles per hour × 0.4470 = meters per second
degrees × 0.01745 = radians

swimming, and cycling are all activities whose performance depends on the ability to sustain power output through the oxidation of fuel. During running, most of the mechanical work is done in raising the body with each stride, and a smaller proportion is used for horizontal acceleration. The net vertical work done by the muscles per stride equals body weight times the vertical distance the body's center of mass is raised. Average power output during a time period is body weight times vertical distance traveled per stride times the number of strides during the time interval divided by the time interval in seconds.

The limiting factor in power output when activities last for several minutes or more is the ability of the circulatory system to supply oxygen to the working muscles. The energy-generating mechanisms within the mitochondria must also be able to utilize the oxygen that is brought to the muscle tissue. The body is not extremely efficient, so that much of the energy generated during physical activity is dissipated as heat. Typically, the efficiency of muscular activity is only in the 20% to 30% range [24]. Therefore, the energy consumed is about four times the mechanical work produced.

Power output is also crucial to very short physical exertions. Many sports require the athlete to exert maximal force in a short period of time—for example, when jumping, throwing a ball, serving in tennis, hitting a softball, or driving a golf ball (figure 4.6). Similarly, performing self-defense movements, swatting a fly, shaking down a thermometer, hammering a nail, and running up a flight of stairs require short, very fast exertions. Obviously, the power that can be generated during very short time intervals is much greater than the power that can be generated during sustained activity. A person who can maintain a power output of 200 watts for several minutes while running or cycling may be able to average 1,500 watts during a vertical jump.

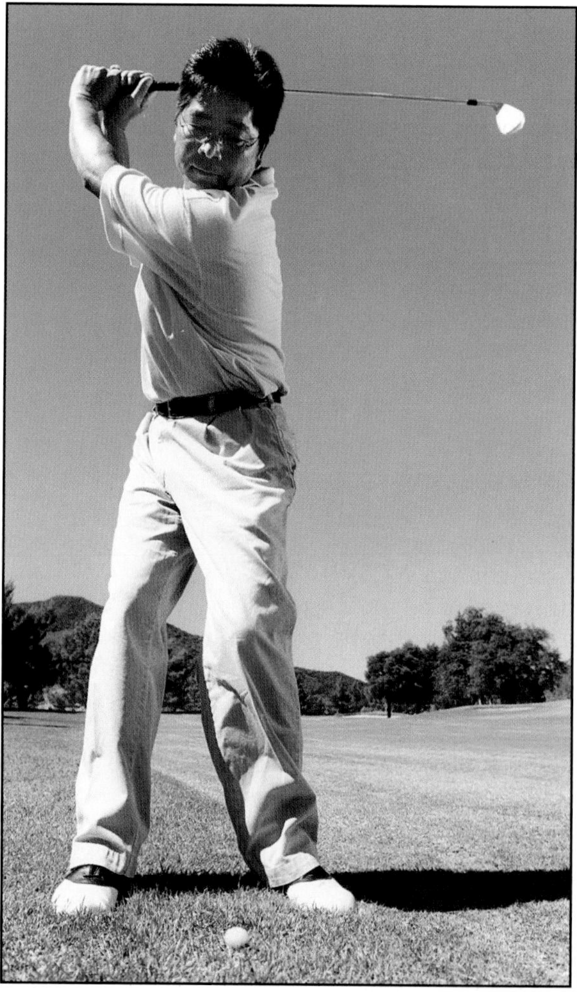

Figure 4.6 Power output is crucial to a golf swing because force must be exerted at high speed.

Most general fitness exercises, such as calisthenics, weight training, swimming, and yoga, are performed relatively slowly. For that reason, such exercises have limited application for improving speed and power. Exercises more appropriate for improving power output include sprinting, jumping, "explosive" weight training exercises such as power cleans and snatches, cardio kickboxing, and martial arts training. "Power lifting" is a misnomer because although it requires high force, it does not require fast movement. Several other sports (e.g., high jump, shot put, baseball hitting) are more dependent on power than is power lifting [8].

Knowledge of the scientific definitions of strength and power has prompted use of the term "power" to refer to the ability to exert force at high speed and "strength" actually to refer to the ability to exert force at low speed. However, "strength" refers to the ability to exert force at whatever the speed of movement. Thus, the terms "high-speed strength" and "low-speed strength" more accurately describe what is generally meant by "power" and "strength," respectively.

A full picture of a person's strength in a particular body movement requires more than one test to produce a set of scores representing the force that could be exerted over a range of movement speeds. Such testing can provide a relatively comprehensive picture of an individual's strength. It can distinguish between individuals excelling at low-speed strength and those excelling at high-speed strength. Such measures can be useful for identifying strengths, weaknesses, and potential aptitudes for various physical activities. For example, a dancer who excels at high-speed strength has the basic ability to do high leaps. An ice-skater excelling at high-speed strength may be training to do multiple jumping spins. Low-speed strength is useful for many activities such as lifting and moving heavy objects, hiking with a heavy backpack, or withstanding g-forces in a fighter plane.

Strength cannot be described by a single score. Not only do individuals differ in the relative strength of different parts of their body, but they differ in relative strength at different speeds of movement.

Calculating Resistance Training Work

Customarily, a weightlifting exercise session is sometimes quantified by summing the product of weight lifted and number of repetitions for all exercise sets performed. To accurately assess the work involved in a lifting session, it would be necessary to measure the vertical distance the weight moves per repetition. The work for each set of exercise is then:

$$\text{work} = \text{weight} \times \text{vertical distance} \times \text{reps} \qquad \textbf{(4.4)}$$

For free weight exercise, one may measure the vertical distance from the floor to the bar at the bar's low point and high point during the exercise movement. The vertical distance traveled by the weight would be the difference between those two measurements. For a weight stack machine, the low and high points of the stack weights during an exercise repetition can be measured (figure 4.7). These measurements can be made with the lowest-weight plate on the stack because the vertical distance traveled by the weight during a given exercise for an individual should be about the same regardless of the weight used. It is important to use consistent units. With use of the traditional U.S. system, the weight should be in pounds and the distance in feet. In the SI system, the weight should be in newtons (kilograms multiplied by 9.8) and the distance in meters.

In addition, the weight of the body should be considered. For example, when dumbbells are lifted in the lateral raise exercise, the weight of the arms is raised in addition to the weight of the dumbbells. Thus, the total work includes both the work of lifting the dumbbells and the work in lifting the arms. Such considerations are important for exercises in which a significant portion of the body moves vertically. For example, in the squat exercise, most of the body weight is lifted with each repetition, while in the leg press, only the legs move and, depending on the particular machine, the legs may not move vertically at all. Thus, to compare the difficulty of the squat lift and the leg press, one must know something about the geometry of the machine. A fair approximation is to add body weight to the weight of the squat, since most of the body is lifted on each repetition. If the leg press machine involves lifting a stack of weights, then the resistance can be taken as the weight of the stack of weights and the part of the machine holding the weight plates. However, on a sled-type leg press machine, in which the sled travels at an angle instead of vertically, an adjustment must be made to determine the true resistance. For example, if the weight is being pushed up along tracks angled at 45 degrees, the actual resistance is only about 70% of the weight of the sled plus added plates. For angles of the sled tracks relative to the ground of 30 and 60 degrees, the actual resistances are 50% and 87%, respectively, of the weight of the sled plus added plates. Anyone interested in the

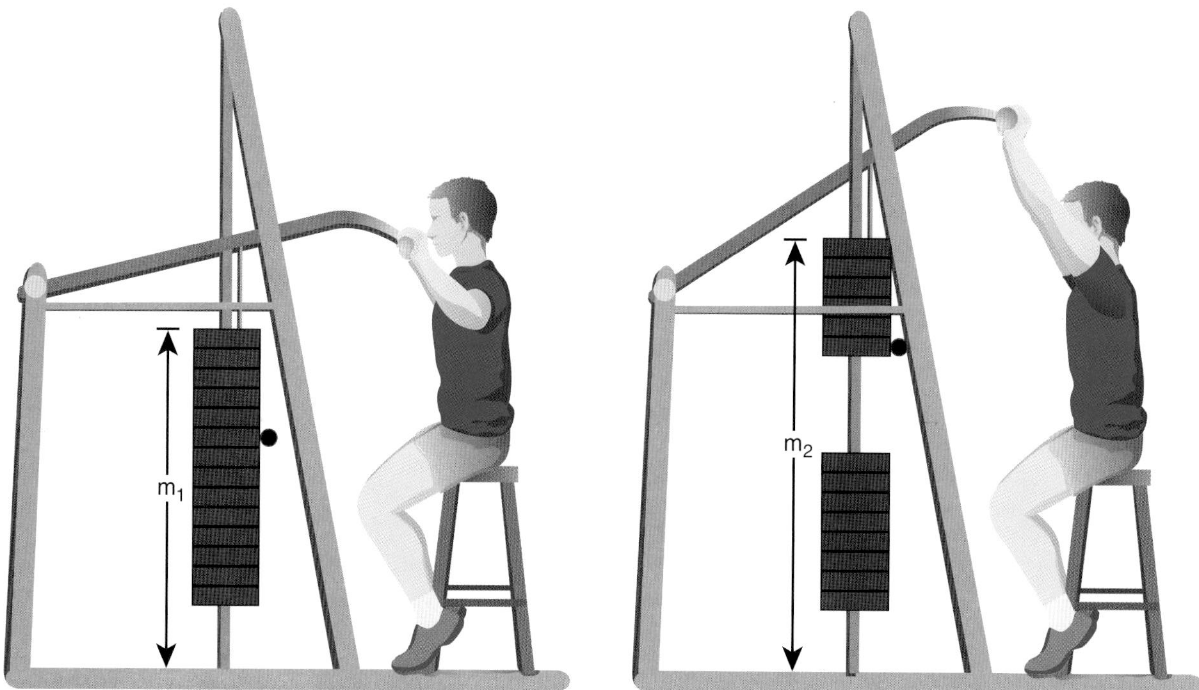

Figure 4.7 Calculation of work during resistance exercise. If the pin is set at 90 pounds, m_1 = 31 inches, and m_2 = 52 inches, the distance lifted in feet is first calculated as (52 in. – 31 in.) ÷ 12 = 1.75 ft. The work done in 10 repetitions can then be calculated, using equation 4.4, as (90 lb) × (1.75 ft) × (10 reps) = 1,575 ft · lb. In the SI system, the weight lifted would be (40.9 kg) × (9.807 N/kg) = 401 N; the distance would be (132 cm – 79 cm) × (0.01 m/cm) = 0.53 m. The work would then be (401 N) × (0.53 m) × (10 reps) = 2,125 joules.

precise calculations can use the following equation, in which the angle is that between the floor and the track along which the sled moves:

$$\text{actual resistance} = \text{sine of the floor-to-track angle} \times (\text{weight of the sled plus added plates}) \quad (4.5)$$

The sine function is available on most calculators, and the angle of the track relative to the ground can be measured with a protractor. If the weight is pushed vertically, the track angle is 90 degrees, the sine of which is 1. Thus, for pushing vertically, no adjustment is needed.

Work and Power in Rotational Movements

The preceding discussion of work and power relates to situations in which force is exerted on an object that moves from one location to another in space. Work and power are also involved when an object is rotated, even if it does not move through space at all. **Angular displacement** is the angle through which an object rotates, commonly measured in degrees. The SI unit for angle is the **radian** (rad), which equals 57.3 degrees. An object's rotational speed is called its **angular velocity.** Although this can be measured in degrees per second, it is necessary to convert to radians per second (rad/sec) in order to calculate **rotational power** as described in the following paragraph (degrees ÷ 57.3 = radians).

Torque should be expressed in newton-meters (N · m). The latter unit of measurement appears the same as the unit used to quantify work. However, in relation to torque, the newtons quantify the magnitude of a force—whose line of action does not pass through the pivot point—that acts to rotate an object about the pivot point. In contrast, for work, the newtons quantify a force acting to move an object through space. Also, for torque, the meters quantify the length of the moment arm (that is perpendicular to the line of action of the force). For work, the meters quantify the distance the object moves in the direction in which the force is applied. Just as for linear work and power, **rotational work** and power are respectively quantified in joules (J) and watts (W) [23]. Equation 4.6 is used to calculate rotational work. Equation 4.2 can then be used to calculate rotational power.

$$\text{work}_J = \text{torque}_{N \cdot m} \times \text{angular displacement}_{rad} \quad (4.6)$$

The velocities at which force must be exerted vary considerably among daily life activities and sport. Some body movements are kept to relatively low speeds by high resistance. For example, when a person pushes a disabled automobile, the vehicle's mass provides resistance to acceleration. When a football lineman pushes against an opponent, both the mass and strength of the opponent provide resistance. In both of these examples, low-speed strength is critical.

On the other hand, in many body movements there is little resistance and the movement gets to high speed in a short time, making high-speed strength most important. For example, when one is blocking or striking to defend oneself, only the mass of the arm provides resistance to acceleration, so that it reaches a high speed in a very short time. This is also true when relatively light implements are held in the hand, such as a Ping-Pong paddle, badminton racket, or flyswatter. Offering little inertial resistance, these light implements reach high speed quickly. Thus, the user's ability to exert force while moving at relatively high speed becomes very important [33].

Biomechanical Factors in Human Strength

Several biomechanical factors relate to physical strength, including neural control, muscle cross-sectional area, arrangement of muscle fibers, muscle length, joint angle, muscle contraction velocity, joint angular velocity, and body mass.

Neural Control

The force output of a muscle is determined by neural signals sent from the brain that specify how many and which motor units are involved in a muscular contraction (recruitment) and the firing rate of the motor units (rate coding) [6]. Muscle force is increased through (a) involvement of more motor units in a contraction, (b) recruitment of larger motor units, or (c) increase in the rate at which the motor units are fired. During the first few weeks of resistance training, much of the improvement in strength can be attributed to **neural adaptations,** by which the brain learns how to produce more force from a given amount of muscle tissue [27]. Thus, percentage gains in strength achieved early in resistance training programs usually greatly exceed percentage increases in muscle fiber size [32].

Often, those embarking on resistance training programs are greatly encouraged by the rapid initial gains they achieve but are then disappointed or discouraged by the slower rate of improvement that follows. This is a critical point at which the personal trainer must be encouraging in order to maintain the client's motivation. It is important to note that although initial gains due to neural adaptations are more rapid, the slower gains due to increases in muscle mass (hypertrophy) continue over a long period of time, resulting in greater strength and improved physical appearance.

Muscle Cross-Sectional Area

In general, the force capability of a muscle relates more closely to its cross-sectional area than to its volume [18, 32]. Consider the case of two muscles that have the same cross-sectional area but different lengths. The longer muscle will have a greater volume and weight, but the same force capability. Also consider the case of two muscles of equal weight and volume, with one longer than the other. With equal volume, the longer muscle will have a smaller cross-sectional area and therefore less force capability. On the basis of these considerations, two people who have different heights but the same body weight and percent body fat will not have the same ability to manipulate their own body weight. The taller individual has smaller muscle cross-sectional area and thus less strength in proportion to body mass. This will make it more difficult for the taller person to do exercises such as push-ups, pull-ups, and sprints.

The strength of a muscle is related primarily to its cross-sectional area rather than its volume. Therefore, all else being equal, a taller person has a smaller muscle cross-sectional area and correspondingly greater difficulty doing body weight resisted exercises than a shorter person with the same muscle mass.

Arrangement of Muscle Fibers

In tests, muscle tissues have been shown capable of producing 23.2 to 145 pounds per square inch (16-100 N/cm^2) of muscle cross-sectional area during maximal contractions [2, 12, 13, 25]. Some of this fairly sizeable variation can be accounted for by the arrangement of fibers within a muscle (figure 4.8) [9, 13]. **Pennate muscles** show featherlike arrangements of the muscle fibers in which the fibers lie at some angle relative to the overall direction of muscle contraction. The **pennation angle** is the angle between the muscle fibers and an imaginary line extending from the muscle's origin to its

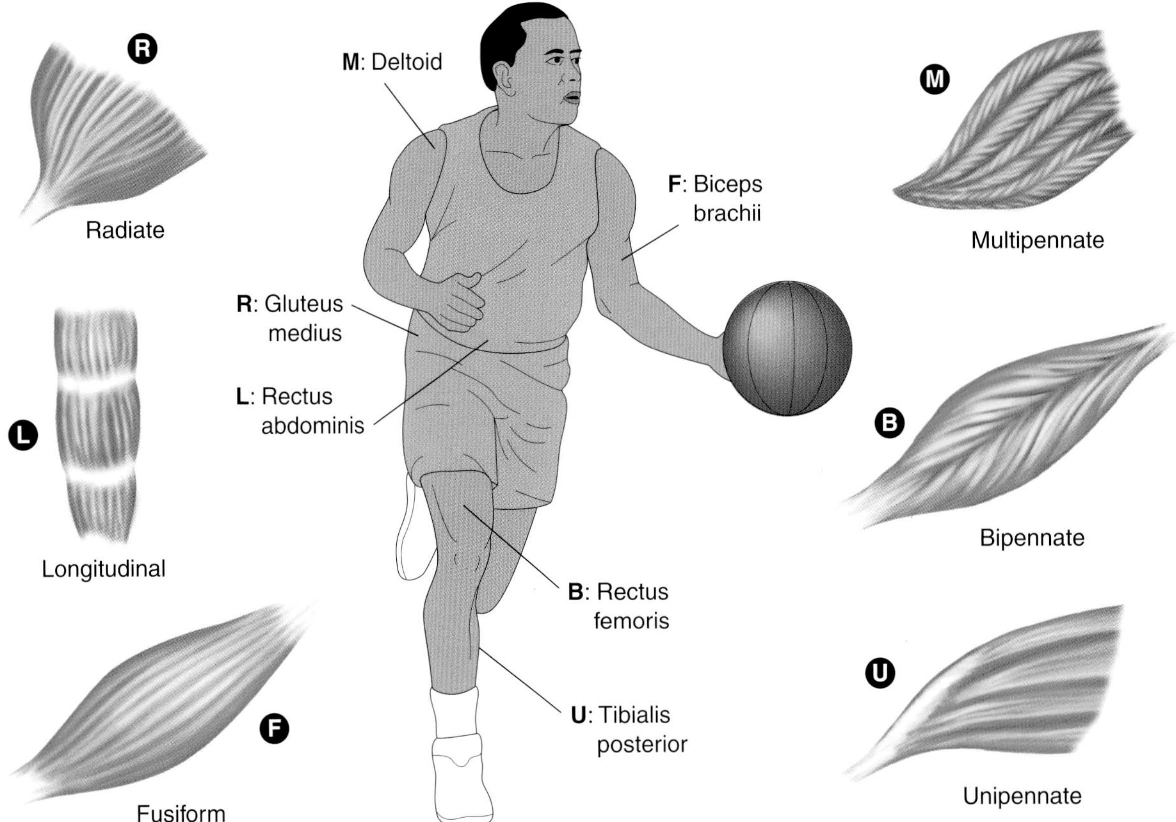

Figure 4.8 The fiber arrangements of various muscles.
Reprinted from Baechle and Earle 2000.

insertion; a pennation angle of 0 degrees indicates no pennation.

Several human muscles are pennate [9]; most often the pennation angle is 15 degrees or less. One advantage of pennation is that more of a muscle's mass can be distributed close to the joint, thereby reducing the rotational inertia that impedes acceleration of the limb [5]. For example, pennation allows much of the calf muscle to be close to the knee, minimizing inertial resistance during running. As a muscle contracts, the pennation angle may actually change, usually increasing as the muscle shortens. In comparison with non-pennate muscles, pennate muscles seem to have more force capability at higher speeds of muscular contraction, particularly near the extremes of the muscle range of motion. Yet a pennate muscle may be less capable of generating isometric, eccentric, or low-speed concentric force [31]. Despite the trade-off related to pennation, this fiber arrangement provides enough advantage for most muscles that many skeletal muscles exhibit the pennate structure [9].

Muscle Length

The maximal possible number of cross-bridge sites is available when a muscle is at its resting length, because in this situation the greatest proportion of the actin and myosin filaments are adjacent to each other (figure 4.9). As a result, the greatest force can be generated by a muscle when it is at its resting length [14]. A smaller proportion of the actin and myosin filaments are next to each other when the muscle is stretched beyond its resting length. The muscle cannot generate as much force as it can at its resting length because there are fewer potential cross-bridge sites. And when the muscle contracts below its resting length, the actin filaments tend to overlap, again diminishing the number of cross-bridge sites.

Thus, force capability is reduced when the muscle is either longer or shorter than its resting length. A personal trainer providing manual resistance to a client should vary the resistance applied throughout the movement in keeping with the changes in force capability of the muscle. Generally, a client

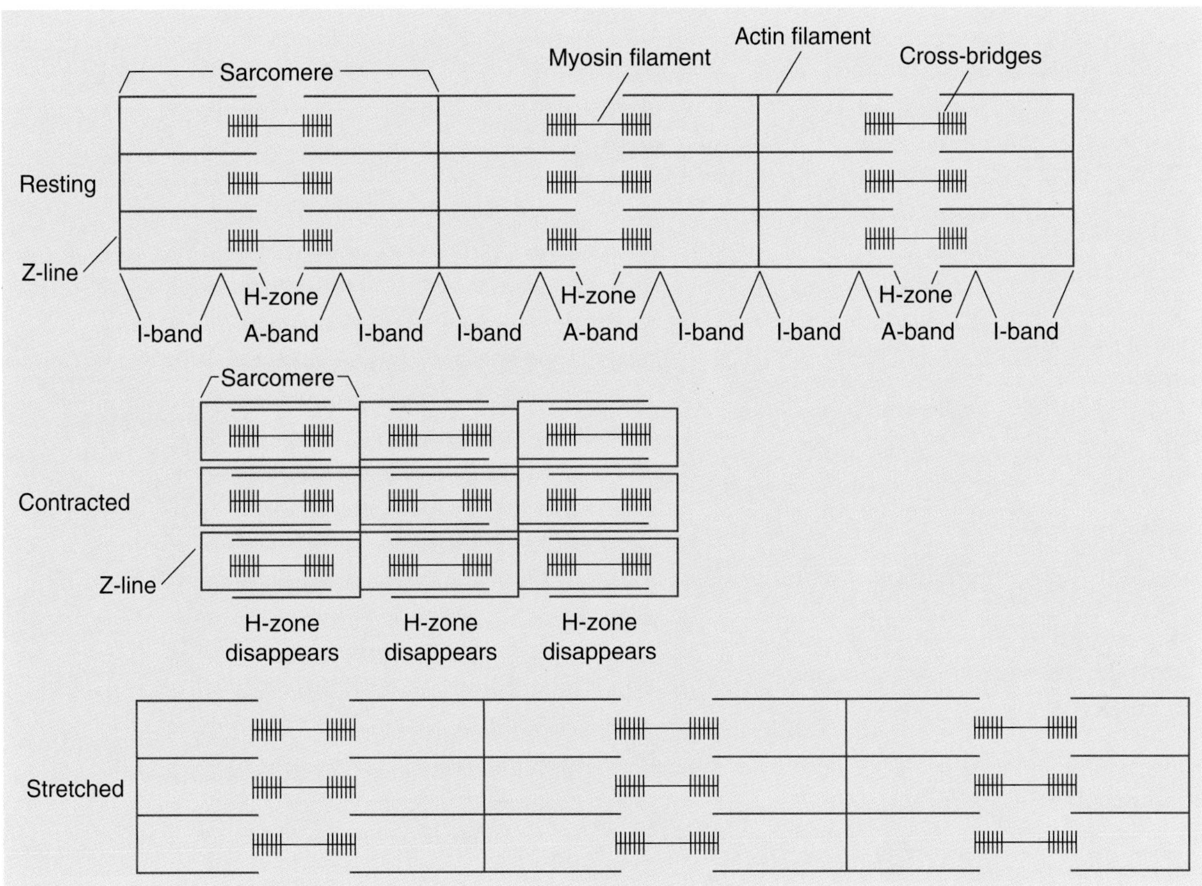

Figure 4.9 The interaction between actin and myosin filaments when the muscle is at its resting length and when it is contracted or stretched. Muscle force capability is greatest when the muscle is at its resting length because of the increased number of potential actin-myosin cross-bridges.
Reprinted from Baechle and Earle 2000.

can exert greater force in the midrange than at the extremes of a body segment range of motion. This is not true for all body segments, however. Thus, it is best to provide enough manual resistance to a movement to keep the speed within a desired range, and allow the force to vary according to the client's ability.

Joint Angle

Virtually all body movements take place by means of rotations about joints. These rotations may be difficult to notice when the hand or foot moves in a straight line. However, careful observation reveals that straight-line movement of the hand or foot is the product of rotations about the shoulder and elbow or hip and knee, respectively. Since rotation requires torque, one can see that muscle forces have their effect by generating torques. For a given muscle, higher force results in higher torque, which means a greater ability to rotate the limb or body part about a joint against resistive torque.

An understanding of the capabilities of muscles that contract across a body joint—to bring about rotational movement of the bones that meet at the joint—requires knowledge of maximal torque capability over the full range of joint motion. The variation in the magnitude of torque that can be generated about a given body joint is due to both (a) the force versus muscle length relationship; and (b) the variation in leverage over the joint range of motion attributable to the geometry of the muscles, tendons, and internal joint structures. Other factors affecting torque capability about a particular body joint include the type of exercise (isotonic, isometric, etc.), the direction of movement (extension or flexion), and the angular velocity. For movement about a particular joint, higher speeds of movement are associated with lower torque capability.

The pattern of maximal muscle torque as a function of joint angle may deviate considerably from the pattern of maximal muscle force as a function of muscle length, for several reasons. First, the muscle's moment arm varies throughout the movement as the axis of rotation and tendon position change. For example, near the beginning and end of the range of elbow motion, the force that the elbow flexor muscles exert must be much greater than at the midrange of motion to generate the same torque. Looking at this another way, a given force by the elbow flexors results in less torque at the extremes of the range of motion than it does in the midrange.

Another reason for the disparity between the pattern of maximal muscle torque as a function of joint angle and the pattern of maximal muscle force is that a group of muscles often act together around a body joint to cause movement. Because of their different configurations, at any particular point in the range of motion the muscles are at different percentages of their resting lengths. This affects the amount of force they can contribute. For example, both the gastrocnemius and soleus muscles are plantar flexors of the foot. The gastrocnemius is a **two-joint muscle,** crossing both the ankle and knee joints. Therefore it is relatively taut when the knee is straight and relatively slack when the knee is bent. In comparison, the soleus crosses only one joint, the ankle, so that soleus tension is unaffected by knee angle. Based on these considerations, the seated calf machine was designed to work the soleus more than the gastrocnemius. When one sits in a bent knee position, the gastrocnemius is slackened to the extent that it cannot exert much force. Thus the soleus becomes primarily responsible for plantar flexion of the foot. Similarly, if one places the ball of the foot onto a relatively high stepping bench and steps up, the soleus does most of the work of plantar flexing the foot because the gastrocnemius muscle is relatively slack.

A final reason for the difference between the pattern of maximal muscle torque as a function of joint angle and the pattern of maximal muscle force is that, when a muscle crosses two body joints (e.g., gastrocnemius, hamstrings, rectus femoris, biceps, and triceps), the muscle's length is affected by both joint angles. For example, when someone who is standing bends forward at the waist, the hamstrings are put under tension. Thus these muscles can generate more knee flexion torque in this body position than when the trunk is upright. The added tension in the hamstrings affects not only the magnitude, but also the pattern, of maximal flexion torque capability about the knee as a function of knee angle [35].

Muscle Contraction Velocity

The force capability of muscle decreases as the velocity of contraction increases, as shown in classic experiments by A.V. Hill on isolated animal muscles [16]. The decline is steepest when speed is increasing from slow to moderate, and less steep when speed is increasing from moderate to fast. Thus the speed-force relationship is not linear. Specific movement techniques can be used to take advantage of this relationship, for example, swinging the arms forward and upward during the vertical jump. This results in a downward force on the trunk at the shoulders, which tends to reduce the upward acceleration of the body. Knee and hip extension are thus slowed down, allowing the muscles that carry out these movements to contract at a slower velocity, at which they can exert greater force for a longer period.

Training with faster movement speeds can modify the shape of the force-velocity curve so that there is less decline in force capability at higher speeds [36]. In order to develop a client's speed-strength, the personal trainer can add sprint interval training to a running program, cardio kickboxing to an aerobics program, and faster movements with light weights to a resistance training program. Some dance styles, such as hip-hop, can involve very fast movements as well.

Joint Angular Velocity

The torque generated by muscle contraction force varies with joint angular velocity in a way specific to the type of muscular action. During isokinetic (constant joint angular velocity) concentric exercise, maximal torque declines as angular velocity increases. However, during eccentric exercise, as joint angular velocity increases, maximal torque increases until joint angular velocity reaches about 90 degrees per second (1.57 rad/sec), then declines gradually [20]. As a result, the greatest muscle force can be obtained during eccentric muscle action. That is why some clients may want to use eccentric movements to train. They usually do this by lowering a weight heavier than they can lift, and getting help from one or two spotters to raise the weight on each repetition. Non-weight exercises have eccentric components as well, during which very high forces can be generated. For example, if a person is stepping down from large rocks while hiking downhill and carrying a relatively heavy backpack, the quadriceps muscles are stretched while exerting high force to decelerate the body's descent. Landing on one leg from a high dance leap is another example.

Strength-to-Mass Ratio

The **strength-to-mass ratio** equals the force the person can exert during a particular movement divided by the mass of the body. This reflects the ability to lift and accelerate one's body, and is especially important for activities involving total body movement, such as sprinting and jumping.

Strength training can improve the strength-to-mass ratio, but only if strength increases by a greater percentage than does body weight. For example, if an individual weighing 150 pounds can leg press 200 pounds, the leg press strength-to-mass ratio is $200 \div 150 = 1.33$. If, after training, the individual weighs 155 pounds and can leg press 220 pounds, the strength-to-mass ratio has increased to $220 \div 155 = 1.42$. However, if the same strength gain is accompanied by a body-weight increase to 170 pounds, the strength-to-mass ratio has actually decreased to 1.29. Such a decrease is not unusual, especially for bodybuilders, whose primary concern is to build up muscle bulk without necessarily improving physical performance. However, for people interested in improving the ability to move their bodies, as in rock climbing, soccer, gymnastics, or even activities of daily living for older people, it is important to increase strength to a greater extent than the body mass. Most sedentary people needn't be concerned about that because most exercise programs will increase their strength while maintaining or decreasing their body mass. However, highly fit athletes must consider whether the exercises they select will likely add body mass to a greater extent than they will increase the strength of muscles key to the given sport.

> Greater strength-to-mass ratio generally means improved physical performance, whether in work, sport, or daily life. Not all exercise programs improve strength-to-mass ratio. If a training regimen increases body mass to a greater extent than it increases strength, then strength-to-mass ratio declines.

Sources of Resistance to Muscle Contraction

The most common sources of resistance experienced by the body during exercise are gravity, inertia, friction, fluid resistance, and elasticity. This section focuses on how these forms of resistance work and how their resistance patterns may differ. We consider resistance training primarily, though these sources of resistance have applications in many types of exercise.

Gravity

All objects have mass and thus exert **gravitational force** on other objects. The force of attraction between any two objects is proportional to the product of the objects' masses and inversely proportional to the square of the distance between them. This means that as the distance between two objects increases, gravitational force decreases more and more markedly. Since the earth is so massive and much closer to us than any other celestial object, its gravitational pull on us far outweighs that of any other object. Because distances from the center of the earth at various points on its surface don't vary much, objects weigh about the same all over the globe. Nevertheless, weight variations are measurable and can affect physical performance.

Weight and mass should not be confused. An object has the same mass (i.e., same number of protons, neutrons, and electrons) wherever it is. However, its weight is the gravitational force that the mass exerts, which is the object's mass times the local acceleration due to gravity. This effect is most noticeable when we compare the weight of an object on earth and on another celestial body, or in space. For example, on the moon, an object of a given mass weighs only one-sixth of its earth weight. Only a balance scale can measure mass rather than weight, because the local acceleration of gravity results in proportional forces on the masses of the object on the scale and the metal blocks that are slid horizontally to determine the object's mass. However, spring or electronic scales can detect only weight, not mass.

The labeling on weight plates can be misleading. A plate has a specific mass, but its weight depends on the local **acceleration of gravity.** Therefore, since the pound is a unit of force, it cannot correctly be applied to a weight plate. Plates labeled in kilograms correctly quantify the plate's mass. However, it is not correct to say that an object weighs a certain number of kilograms, since weight refers to force, not mass. To be correct, one could say "She lifted 35 kilograms" or "The mass of the dumbbell is 5 kilograms."

Applications to Free Weight Training

The force exerted by gravity on an object always acts downward. The moment arm of a weight is always horizontal because the moment arm that produces a torque is, by definition, perpendicular to the line of action of the force. The torque about a given body joint when a weight is held is the product of the weight and the horizontal distance from the weight to that body joint. Although the weight does not change during a lift, its horizontal distance from a given body joint almost always changes throughout the movement. When the weight is horizontally farther from the joint, it exerts more resistive torque; and when it is horizontally closer to the joint, it exerts less resistive torque.

As an example, during a barbell curl the horizontal distance from the barbell to the elbow is greatest when the forearm is horizontal (figure 4.10). In that position the lifter must exert the greatest muscle torque to raise the weight. As the forearm rotates away from the horizontal, in an upward or downward direction, the moment arm decreases and so does the resistive torque due to the weight. There is no resistive torque at all from the weight when it is positioned directly above or below the elbow because the horizontal moment arm has length zero in those positions.

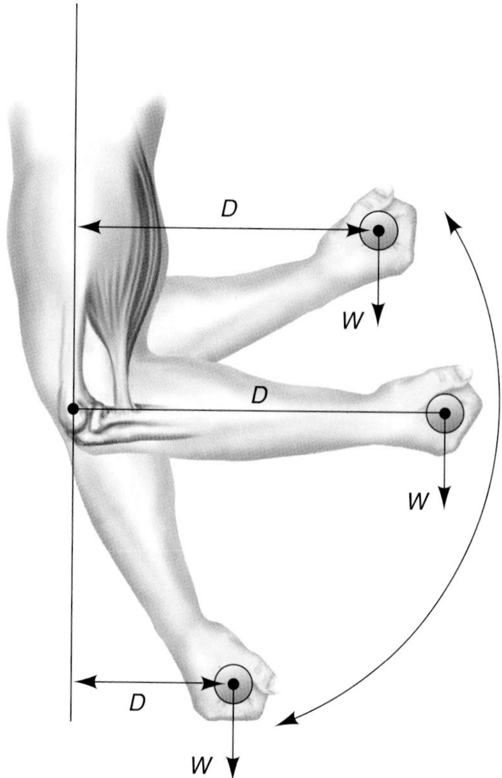

Figure 4.10 The horizontal distance (D) from the weight to the elbow changes throughout the curl movement, causing the torque exerted by the weight (W) of the object to change as well.
Reprinted from Baechle and Earle 2000.

The way in which an exercise is performed can affect the resistive torque pattern and shift the work among muscle groups. For example, during the squat, greater forward trunk inclination positions the weight horizontally farther from the hip, increasing the resistive torque about the hip that the gluteus and hamstring muscles (hip extensors) must work to counteract. Yet the weight is horizontally closer to the knees, reducing the resistive torque about the knees counteracted by the quadriceps (knee extensors).

During any exercise, the combined center of mass of the body and barbell must be positioned above the foot so that the lifter does not fall. Placing the bar in different positions causes the lifter to instinctively adjust body posture to keep the center of mass over the feet and avoid falling. For example, when the barbell is positioned as low as possible on the upper back, the trunk must be inclined relatively far forward to keep the total center of mass over the feet. That brings the bar horizontally far from the hip and close to the knee. As a result, the hip extensors must work harder, while the knee extensors work less. Holding the bar high on the back brings about less trunk inclination and thus shifts some of the lifting work from the hip extensors to the knee extensors. By the same token, holding the bar in front of the shoulders (e.g., the front squat) requires less forward lean than any of the other squat positions, so trunk lean is minimized and the greatest possible load is placed on the knee extensors.

Because individuals differ in body proportions and in the relative strength of different muscle groups, the optimal technique for performing lifts and other physical activities varies from individual to individual. Postural modifications can shift resistance from muscles that are relatively weak to those that are relatively strong. People naturally follow the path of least resistance and generally make such modifications instinctively. However, it often takes the eye of a good personal trainer to find a technique most suitable to the individual.

Modifications in exercise technique can be used to reduce stress on an injured area. The Smith machine is a multipurpose exercise device in which a barbell is restricted to movement along tracks. This device can be useful for technique modifications because it has the advantage of allowing the feet to be positioned behind or in front of the center of mass of the body-plus-barbell without causing a fall. If a back injury necessitates removing some of the stress from the back, the feet can be positioned a foot (30 centimeters) or more forward of their normal position. A lifter in the same body position with a free weight would fall, but the Smith machine prevents that because the tracks restrict horizontal movement. With the feet farther forward, the trunk stays more upright. That decreases the horizontal moment arm about the lower back, thus reducing the torque the back muscles must generate. At the same time, the length of the horizontal moment arm about the knee is increased, making the quadriceps do more work. If a Smith machine is not available, the front squat can be used for a similar, though less pronounced, effect.

Applications to Weight-Resisted Machine Training

Gravity is the source of resistance for weight stack and plate-loaded machines, just as it is for free weights. However, with free weights, the direction of movement is relatively unrestricted, and the pattern of resistance about each body joint depends on how the movement pattern affects the horizontal distance from the weight to the joint. In contrast, the direction and pattern of resistance in weight-resisted machines are manipulated by levers, gears, cams, pulleys, and cables. That makes it difficult to determine the actual level and pattern of resistance. The resistive force cannot usually be determined by numbers inscribed on the plates unless one weighs the plates and analyzes the leverage system.

If the handle of a weight-resisted machine is connected to the weights via a cable that passes over a single round pulley, as on most pulldown machines, then the resistance is equal to the weight lifted and is constant throughout the exercise movement. If there is a cam of variable radius in the system, then the resistance is variable and cannot be readily determined. If the handle is connected to the weights via a lever, the actual resistance is again variable and cannot be determined without a quantitative analysis of the leverage system.

During the 1970s, Nautilus Sports/Medical Industries® popularized an exercise machine that used a cam of variable radius to vary the length of the moment arm through which a weight stack acted over the range of joint motion. This was said to provide a desired pattern of resistance intended to match the individual's pattern of torque capability (figure 4.11). The idea was to provide less resistance at segments of the range of motion where the muscles could not provide much torque and greater resistance where the muscles could apply more torque. The underlying assumptions were that everyone had basically the same torque capability pattern for a given body movement, and that the lifting movement had to be at a slow steady speed. Studies have shown that cam-based machines succeed to only a limited degree in matching typical human torque capability patterns, and sometimes do not do so at all [10, 19].

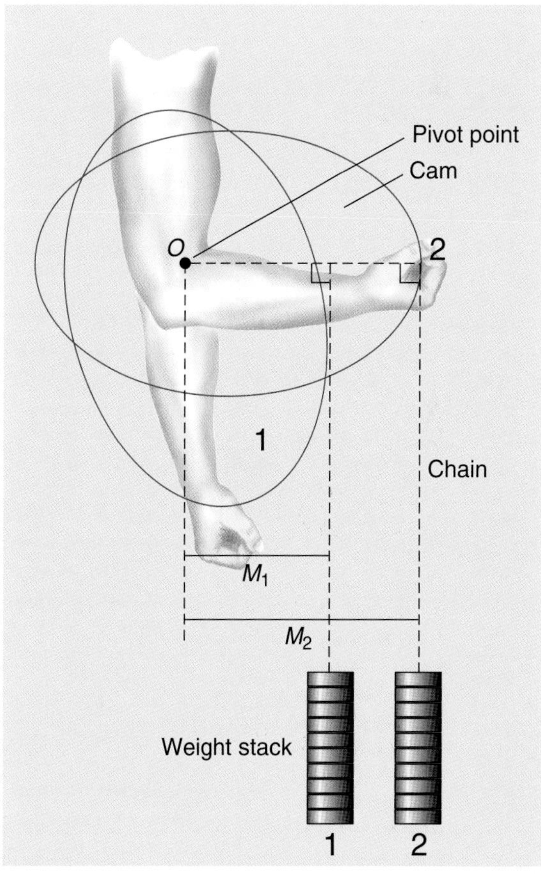

Figure 4.11 In cam-based weight-resisted machines, the moment arm (M) through which the weight acts (horizontal distance from chain to pivot point) varies during the exercise movement. When the cam is rotated from position 1 to position 2, the moment arm of the weight, and thus the resistive torque, increases.
Reprinted from Baechle and Earle 2000.

Applications to Other Physical Activities

Any form of calisthenics is basically gravity-resisted exercise, although additional resistance can come from inertia and the elastic properties of muscles and tendons. Each body segment of an individual has a given mass and center-of-mass location. The farther horizontally the center of mass of a body segment is from a joint, the greater the resistive moment arm and the greater the muscle force must be to provide the torque needed to support the body segment. Thus, it is much more difficult to support a fully abducted straight leg than a slightly abducted straight leg. The deltoid muscles tire much more rapidly when the arms are held out horizontally in a dance or aerobics class than when they are held in a lower position.

Knowledge of the relationship of body position to resistive torque allows the personal trainer to control the difficulty level of an exercise. For example, the resistance that the hip flexors and abdominals encounter in the leg raise exercise can be reduced by bending the knees, thus bringing the center of mass of the legs closer to the hips. Conversely, the resistance can be increased by straightening the knees, bringing the leg center of mass farther from the hips.

One can also control the difficulty level of aerobic exercise by applying the principle that the work done against gravity is proportional to the vertical distance a weight is lifted. This applies to limb and total body weight in addition to the weight of objects lifted. Different people can work at different levels of difficulty in the same aerobics class by lifting their limbs to a greater or lesser extent. In a step class, one can also control the difficulty level by choosing the step height. Selecting a step that is 25% higher will increase the work of stepping up on it by 25%, assuming the same body position at the low and high points of the movements. It is important to note that in order to get the full benefit of using a higher step, the client should step fully up onto the step and straighten the knees, thereby lifting the body center of mass as high as possible.

Any exercise in which the whole body or body segments are lifted involves work against gravity. During running, the body is repeatedly lofted into the air by the action of the leg and hip muscles. Most of the muscular work in running serves to raise the body vertically rather than to propel it forward, because gravity pulls downward while the only horizontal resistance is from the air and from the braking force of the ground against the foot when it lands.

Obviously, the work done in repeatedly raising the body during running is proportional to the weight of the client, all else being equal. A client's body weight is roughly proportional to body volume, while the ability to provide oxygen to working muscles is dependent on the cross-sectional area of blood vessels [3]. Because volume is a cubic measure (x^3) and area is a square measure (x^2), as body size increases there is generally a reduced maximal rate at which oxygen can be supplied to working muscle. The reason is that increases in body size are accompanied by increases in body weight that are proportionally larger than the increases in blood vessel cross-sectional area. Therefore, a smaller physically fit client of a given age and gender is generally expected to have a higher maximal oxygen uptake per unit body mass ($ml \cdot min^{-1} \cdot kg^{-1}$) than a larger physically fit client, even though individual differences in factors such as heart volume and mitochondrial density can come into play. This effect is magnified during uphill running because of the increased vertical component of body movement. One can see why competitive distance runners are typically small and slim. The same principles apply to aerobic dance.

The effects of gravity are less during exercise in which the whole body is not lifted. In stationary cycling, large people can generally sustain a higher power output than smaller people because their muscles and circulatory systems are larger. Because they have to lift only their legs rather than their whole body during cycling, their body size does not hurt their performance. In outdoor bicycling, body size does not provide as much advantage because a larger body creates greater wind resistance and rolling resistance due to increased deformation of the tires. In addition, when cycling in hilly terrain, the larger client encounters the same impediments in raising the body uphill that the runner encounters.

The least effect of gravity is seen in swimming and water aerobics because of the **buoyant force** pushing up on the body, which is equal to the weight of the water displaced by the body. Therefore, clients' underwater weights are only a small fraction of their weights on dry land. For example, without considering air in the lungs, a 154-pound (70-kilogram) client of 10% body fat would weigh only 10.9 pounds (4.9 kilograms) underwater, whereas a client of the same weight but 30% body fat would weigh only 4.7 pounds (2.1 kilograms) underwater. Air in the lungs serves to decrease weight even more. Thus, the work against gravity is minimally involved in water exercise, and fluid resistance becomes much more important.

Inertia

Inertia is the resistance to acceleration, and acceleration is quantitatively defined as the change in velocity divided by the change in time [26]. According to Isaac **Newton's second law,** force equals mass times acceleration. Thus, for a given force, a smaller mass will show greater acceleration. Also, more force is required for greater acceleration of a given mass. These considerations apply directly to any exercise in which the speed of movement of the body or of an implement changes.

Virtually all body movements involve acceleration and deceleration. During running, for example, the arms and legs are repeatedly accelerated and decelerated. Throwing a ball, swinging a tennis racket, and even getting out of a chair or picking up a bag of groceries all involve acceleration rather than constant-rate movement. Any body movement starting from a standstill or involving a change in speed or direction is accelerative in nature and encounters inertial resistance.

Effects of Inertia on Resistance

Only when a mass is supported in a static position or lifted or lowered at a constant rate is the resistive force equal to the force of gravity on the mass, and the direction of the resistance is only downward. However, if there is any acceleration at all, it is accompanied by **inertial resistance** in addition to the gravitational resistance. The magnitude of the inertial resistance equals mass times acceleration, and the direction of the inertial resistance is opposite to the direction of the acceleration. The inertial resistance may coincide with the direction of the gravitational resistance, or may act in any other direction. When an object is lifted off the ground it must be accelerated vertically to get from a stationary position to an upward velocity. Therefore, both gravity and inertia resist the lifter. That is why the force on the object to get it moving vertically is always greater than the object's weight. However, once the object starts moving, vertical acceleration or deceleration can add to or subtract from the resistance, respectively.

Ballet dancers frequently have to leap into the air, sometimes staying aloft long enough to do one or more complete turns. To provide more time in the air for performing turns or other maneuvers, greater jump height is required, which in turn is dependent on the vertical takeoff velocity. The greater the takeoff velocity, the higher the dancer will leap and the longer the dancer will be in the air to accomplish the desired movements. The attainment of takeoff velocity necessitates vertical acceleration of the body. To merely stand still, the dancer must exert a force on the ground equal to body weight. But to reach a high takeoff velocity, the dancer must exert force on the ground much greater than body weight. During vertical leaps, it is not unusual for the force exerted on the ground to exceed two to three times body weight [11].

In a typical step class, most of the work done is against gravity; such work is accomplished when the whole body or body segments are raised. In exercise classes in which the body movements are much faster, as in cardio kickboxing and hip-hop, inertial resistance becomes significant. The muscles must exert considerable force to accelerate the limbs to high speed and decelerate them toward the end of the range of motion. The many rapid changes in direction require much acceleration and deceleration. Thus, even though the limbs themselves may be relatively light, such exercise can require high forces.

Javelin throwing provides an example of how the resistance encountered during acceleration of an object can far exceed the object's weight. A javelin, whose mass is in the vicinity of 2 pounds (1 kilogram), can provide more than 100 pounds (450 newtons) of resistive force to a world-class thrower. The throwing motion is accomplished within a tenth of a second, with an average power exceeding 3,000 watts [4].

Effects of Varying Acceleration During Resistance Training

Acceleration and deceleration are used in **"cheat" lifting movements.** Sometimes a lifter becomes so determined to increase the weight lifted that lifting technique deteriorates to permit completion of the lift. For example, if there is a point in the movement **("sticking point")** at which the resistive force is too great to overcome when lifting at a relatively constant rate, the lifter may accelerate the bar before that point so that the bar has enough momentum to carry it past the sticking point. Accomplishing the lift by means of this technique does not mean that the lifter has become stronger. Such techniques are generally discouraged except during "explosive" lifting exercises like the power clean, power snatch, and high pull.

When a weight is lowered during a repetition, the muscle acts eccentrically because it is stretched while active. If the lifter exerts less upward force on the bar than the bar's weight, the bar will accelerate downward and its velocity will increase. The less upward force the lifter exerts, the more the downward bar velocity is accelerated by gravity. If the upward force on the bar drops to zero, the bar is in free fall, with its downward velocity increasing every second by 32 feet (9.8 meters) per second. If the lifter desires to slow the downward velocity of the bar, then the lifter must exert upward force on the bar that is greater than the bar weight. If the lifter waits until the bar is close to its low point before slowing down its descent, and the bar must be brought to a stop in a very short time, the force of deceleration can greatly exceed bar weight. That is why this type of movement can cause injury. Thus, it is safer to lower the weight in a controlled manner during each repetition rather than to let it come down quickly and have to decelerate it at the bottom of the movement.

All lifts involve some acceleration at the beginning to bring the bar from a zero to an upward velocity and some deceleration near the top of the lift to bring the bar's velocity back to zero. With this acceleration pattern, the agonist muscles receive resistance in excess of bar weight early in the range of motion but resistance less than bar weight toward the end of the range of motion [22]. The lifter decelerates the bar by either (a) reducing upward force on the bar to less than bar weight to let some or all of the bar's weight decelerate it; or (b) pushing down against the bar using the antagonist muscles, which work eccentrically as they bring the bar to a halt. In either case, the deceleration has the effect of providing less resistance to the agonist muscles late in the range of motion.

Compared to a slow lift with minimal acceleration of a given weight, a lift involving higher acceleration (an **"explosive" lift**) provides greater resistance to the muscles involved early in the lift and less resistance to the muscles involved toward the end of the lift. During a power clean with a heavy weight, for example, the strong leg, hip, and back muscles accelerate the bar vertically to a high enough velocity that, even though the weaker upper body muscles cannot exert vertical force equal to the bar's weight, the bar continues to travel upward until the force of gravity decelerates the bar to zero velocity at the top of the lift.

Effects of Varying Acceleration During Exercise Other Than Resistance Training

Acceleration can have a great effect on exercises other than weight training. Generally, doing a given exercise faster increases acceleration forces. Power output increases as well because (1) more work against gravity per unit time is done in lifting the body or body segments at a faster cadence, and (2) more work against inertia (resistance to acceleration) is performed per unit time both because the forces of acceleration are higher and because the cadence is faster.

These principles apply to many physical activities, such as dancing, aerobics, running, and martial arts. For example, dancing a slow waltz or other slow dance involves little acceleration and thus involves relatively low forces and low power output. In contrast, a vigorous polka, samba, or hip-hop dance is characterized by considerably higher forces and power output. Tai chi is a form of martial arts exercise that is performed extremely slowly and deliberately. Therefore, the forces of acceleration are virtually nil and the power output is low. In contrast, taekwondo, a Korean martial art, involves very fast kicks and hand strikes, as well as leaps into the air. Thus, the forces on the musculoskeletal system are much higher than in tai chi, and the power output is greater.

Sprint running involves much higher forces and power output than does long-distance running because of the faster cadence and greater accelerative forces. Thus, sprint interval training on a track is an excellent means of improving strength of the leg and hip muscles. Even the torso and arm musculature is worked because of the high accelerative forces and pumping action involved. In addition, the greater range of motion in sprinting as compared to long-distance running provides another training benefit.

When an object in the hands is held still or moved at a constant velocity, it exerts constant resistance due to gravity, and only in the downward direction. However, vertical or horizontal acceleration of the object requires additional force in the direction of the acceleration according to Newton's second law.

Bracketing

Bracketing is a type of training in which an exercise or sport movement is performed with lighter-than-normal and heavier-than-normal resistance [4]. Inertial resistance can be used along with other modalities in such training. For example, if an athlete sprints while wearing a weight vest, the resistance to acceleration is increased according to Newton's law equating force to mass times acceleration. A baseball player can train with a lighter-than-usual bat in order to practice high-speed movement. The lower inertia of the lighter bat allows the bat to achieve higher speed. In contrast, a heavier-than-usual bat provides greater inertial resistance, which slows down the speed of the swing and provides higher inertial resistance. This training method allows the athlete to train the neuromuscular system over a wider range of the force-velocity curve than does training with only the normal bat.

Bracketing may be used to improve ability in nonsport activities as well. For example, a client who wishes to get in shape to hike in the mountains may engage in a bracket training program on smaller hills closer to home two to six weeks before the planned mountain hiking. After establishing a base with a few hikes using a relatively light backpack at a leisurely-to-moderate pace, the client could add hikes with a backpack heavier than planned for mountain use, but at a slower pace than planned for the mountains. Also included would be hikes using a backpack lighter than planned for mountain use, but at a faster pace than planned for the mountains.

Friction

When two surfaces pressed together rub against each other, there is resistance due to **friction.** Various exercise devices use friction for resistance, such as belt- or brake pad-resisted cycle ergometers and frictional wrist curl devices. For each such device, the resistive force is roughly proportional to the force pressing the two surfaces together. However, for a given set of surfaces in contact and compressive force, it takes more force to get the movement started than to keep it moving. Once the movement starts, the resistance does not change much even as the speed changes. Friction-resisted devices sometimes have an adjustment knob that alters the force compressing the two contacting surfaces together, thus changing the resistance.

Several exercise devices utilize friction for resistance. For example, various companies make devices used to simulate skating movements. A smooth board or flexible sheet is placed on the ground; and the client, wearing a soft bootie, slides side to side on the board in a skating movement. Friction provides resistance to sliding. The work required of the push-off leg depends on the weight of the client, the level of friction between the board and booties, and the distance between the ends of the board. Such devices, which are relatively inexpensive and compact, provide an alternative to running. Both aerobic and anaerobic interval training can be performed on these devices, depending on the speed of movement. The virtual absence of impact with such exercise makes it advantageous for clients recovering from injuries, and the specificity of the movement provides excellent training for ice-skaters or in-line skaters when weather or access to facilities is problematic.

Another friction-based device consists of a cord passing through a braking element that is attached to a door, a piece of furniture, or other stationary object. Braking friction can be adjusted to provide a wide range of resistance. This type of device has been used by NASA (National Aeronautics and Space Administration) and has been popular among swimmers. Its main limitation is that it provides concentric, but not eccentric, resistance. However, its portability and relatively low price are advantageous, particularly for clients who travel frequently.

Fluid Resistance

When pushing an object through a fluid (a liquid or gas) or pushing fluid past or around an object or through an opening, one encounters resistive force. **Fluid resistance** is a major factor in sports such as swimming, cycling, speed skating, skydiving, baseball, golf, and javelin throwing. In swimming the fluid is water, and in the other sports the fluid is air. There are also exercise machines that use fluid to provide resistance. In hydraulic machines, the fluid is a liquid, while in pneumatic machines, the fluid is a gas.

Fluid resistance comes from **surface drag,** caused by the friction of fluid molecules passing along the surface of an object, and **form drag,** caused by the force of the molecules pressing against the front or rear of an object that is passing through the fluid.

There is also resistance due to the creation of waves. Generally, the cross-sectional (frontal) area has the greatest effect on form drag; the larger the area, the more drag [34].

Applications to Swimming

Swimming is the most fundamental of **aquatic exercises.** The body encounters fluid resistance as it is propelled through the water. The swimmer tries to minimize form drag of the body by offering the least amount of cross-sectional area in the direction of travel. Obviously, the shape of the individual's body itself does not offer much room for change, unless a considerable amount of body girth can be lost. However, the position of the body in the water can affect form drag even more than body shape does. Maintaining a horizontal body position by keeping the feet up reduces form drag. Because the lower legs and feet usually have a low percentage of body fat and a high percentage of bone, the legs tend to drop in the water. The swimmer must counter this by kicking, which is the primary means of keeping the feet up. The "angle of attack" is the angle of the swimmer's body relative to the horizontal. The smaller the angle of attack, the less the form drag. Among the various swim strokes, the angle of attack, and thus the resistance, are lowest for the front crawl and progressively higher for the back crawl, butterfly, and breaststroke [34].

While attempting to minimize form drag, the swimmer tries to maximize the drag of the hand pushing rearward through the water so as to exert as much pushing force against the water as possible. This is accomplished by the position of the hands and fingers as well as the movement path of the hand through the water. If the swimmer pushes backward against the water in a straight line, the desired drag of the water against the hand is reduced because of the momentum and turbulence of the water. Therefore, to increase the drag of the hand in the water, good freestyle swimmers seek relatively immobile water while they stroke, by pushing backward in relatively complex curved patterns. This enables a harder push against the water through a greater portion of the swim stroke. Also, sideward movement of the hand through the water can generate propulsive force through a "lift" effect as for an airplane wing. Synchronized swimmers use this "sculling" action very effectively [34].

Body fat is not as much of an impediment during swimming as it is during land-based exercise such as running or aerobic dance. This is so because of the buoyant force exerted by the water. Fat is less dense than water. Because buoyant force is equal to the weight of the water displaced, the buoyant force on fat is greater than its weight. Therefore, fat helps the body float. Bone and muscle are denser than water; thus they tend to pull the body down. A person who is obese may be able to float without any muscular effort, whereas a lean person must work to stay afloat. The longer the swimming distance, the more advantageous it is to have a layer of body fat because of its insulating value in addition to its buoyancy. For long-distance open-water swims such as across the English Channel, the advantages of moderate body fat outweigh the disadvantage of increased form drag.

Applications to Non-Swimming Aquatic Exercise

Although swimming is generally considered the preferred fluid-resisted exercise, alternative aquatic exercises are usually a better choice for people who cannot swim well and do not have the inclination to take swimming lessons. Non-swimming aquatic exercise, sometimes called water aerobics, can take various forms. The client may stand in the shallow end of the pool and march, run, or kick against the resistance of the water. Alternatively, the client may wear paddles on the hands or other devices to increase the fluid drag encountered when moving through the water. The more of the body that is submerged, the greater the buoyant force countering body weight. For example, in water up to the neck, the client supports only about 10% of body weight, whereas in water at waist level, the client must support about 50% of body weight [17]. People can perform exercise in the deep end of the pool using flotation devices to keep the head above water. Such exercise is widely used by physical therapists and athletic trainers and in health clubs for physical conditioning and rehabilitation.

Applications to Exercise Machines

Some exercise machines use fluid to provide resistance. This is accomplished with cylinders in which a piston forces fluid through an opening during the exercise movement. The resistance is roughly proportional to the velocity of piston movement [15]. Thus, when the piston is pushed faster the resistive force increases; and when the piston is pushed more slowly, the resistive force decreases. Because of this relationship, fluid cylinders allow rapid acceleration early in the exercise movement and little acceleration after higher speeds are reached. The increasing resistance with increasing speed places an effective limit on how rapid the movement can get. Some machines of this type have adjustment knobs or buttons to change the size of the orifice through which the fluid flows. When the orifice is larger, the resistance increases to a lesser degree as velocity of the piston increases. Thus, a higher movement speed can be reached when the orifice is larger. The orifice adjustment allows exercise at different movement speeds.

Fluid-resisted machines do not provide an eccentric exercise phase unless specifically designed to do so through the use of pumps. This contrasts to standard resistance exercise, in which a muscle group acts concentrically while raising the weight and the same muscle group acts eccentrically while lowering the weight. Thus, weight-resisted exercise can be called concentric-eccentric. With most fluid-resisted machines that do not provide eccentric resistance, a muscle group acts concentrically for movement in one direction (e.g., flexion), and the antagonist muscle group acts concentrically for movement in the opposite direction (e.g., extension). Fluid-resisted exercise can then be called concentric-concentric.

In summary, while free weights or weight machines involve alternate concentric and eccentric actions of the same muscle with little or no rest in between, fluid-resisted machines generally involve alternate concentric actions of antagonistic muscle groups, with each muscle group resting while its antagonist works. The absence of eccentric muscle action during fluid-resisted exercise suggests that such training is unlikely to provide optimal benefits for activities in daily life or sport that rely upon eccentric muscle actions (e.g., walking downstairs, lowering a box to the floor) or the stretch-shortening cycle (e.g., running, jumping, throwing).

Applications to Other Fluid-Resisted Exercise

Kayaking, canoeing, and rowing are all forms of fluid-resisted exercise. One propels the boat by pulling the blade of the paddle or oar through the water. Fluid resistance is encountered both by the hull of the boat traveling through the water and by the blade of the paddle as it is pressed against the water. The more streamlined the boat, the faster it travels through the water. That affects the speed of movement of the paddler or rower. If the boat travels faster, the paddler has to pull faster to exert force against the water, thereby increasing the speed of muscle contraction. Thus, all else equal, a rower in a wide, less streamlined boat will likely exert higher forces at lower muscle contraction speeds, while a rower in a more narrow, streamlined boat will exert lower muscle forces but at higher muscle contraction speeds.

A standard dryland rowing machine is fluid resisted as well. When the client pulls on a handle, a cable spins a fan. Resistance is provided by the air pressing against the fan blades. The degree of resistance can be changed by opening a sliding door in the housing around the fan. The larger the opening, the more the resistance because more air is available to press against the fan blades. Such machines provide a good simulation of the work involved in rowing a boat. Because both racing shells and better rowing machines have sliding seats, the exercise is mainly for the legs, with some involvement of the back and arms.

Elasticity

Several commercial exercise devices, particularly those seen on television infomercials, use elastic components such as springs or bands for resistance. One such device consists of an elastic band, both ends of which are attached to a bar. With the bar in the hands, the client stands with one or both feet on the middle of the elastic band and performs various exercise movements that stretch the band. Another device consists of a pair of elastic bands attached at one end. The bands can be affixed to a stationary object so that the free ends can be pulled on via handles or cuffs. A third such device provides resistance to a push-up movement via elastic bands that extend from a handle in one hand, around the back and over a pad, to a handle in the other hand. All these devices are relatively inexpensive and can enable convenient exercise in hotel rooms during travel. However, they are limited as to the movements for which they can provide resistance and the variability of the resistance.

The primary characteristic of **elastic resistance** is that tension increases with the degree of stretching. Thus, exercise movements using elastic resistance always begin with low resistance and end with high resistance. This pattern is not in keeping with the force capability patterns of most human muscle groups, which generally exhibit considerable decline in force capability toward the end of an exercise movement. Also, the degree to which resistance can be adjusted may be limited by the number of elastic elements provided. If the standard resistance training progression is to be followed, resistance should be adjustable enough to allow the number of exercise repetitions within the prescribed range. It would not be desirable for one level of resistance to allow more than the prescribed range of repetitions and the next higher level of resistance to permit less than the prescribed range of repetitions. See chapter 13 for descriptions of proper technique for performing exercises with resistance bands.

Electronically Controlled Devices

The resistance of some training devices, including some strength training equipment, step-mills, elliptical trainers, and rowing machines, is electronically controlled. The resistance itself may be provided by any of the means described previously, or via electromagnetism or a motorized pump. Whatever the form of resistance, such devices are electronically regulated. The distinguishing characteristic of these machines is that they use feedback and control technology to regulate the degree of resistance during an exercise movement. For example, the isokinetic dynamometers frequently used by physical therapists maintain constant joint angular velocity by matching resistive force to muscle force. Some models permit only concentric exercise, while others allow both concentric and eccentric exercise. More complex machines even allow the client to specify acceleration patterns. Some machines permit the user to specify the resistive force, resistive power, or velocity of movement. The potential exists to simulate or design any type of resistance modality via electronic and computer-controlled machines.

"Negative" Work and Power

Because power is the product of force and velocity, exerting upward (positive) force on a weight that is moving in a downward ("negative") direction (as in the lowering phase of weightlifting exercise) results in negative calculated work and power. Such "negative" work and power reflect eccentric muscle action [30]. Other types of eccentric muscle action also result in negative work and power. For example, when a tennis player suddenly changes direction to go after a ball, active muscles are stretched before they contract. If we arbitrarily call muscle shortening positive and lengthening negative, we can see that muscle power (which is the product of muscle force and muscle velocity) during eccentric muscle action is negative. Lowering of the body or a weight and deceleration of the body or an object are very common human movements. These all result in negative calculated work and power.

For negative work and power to occur, there must be potential or kinetic energy in the body or object being lowered or decelerated. **Gravitational potential energy** is the product of an object's weight and the distance it can fall, while **kinetic energy** is one-half the product of the object's mass and the square of its velocity. The amount of negative work performed in lowering an object is equal in magnitude to that object's weight times the distance it is lowered. The amount of **negative work** performed in decelerating a moving object to zero velocity is equal in magnitude to the object's kinetic energy before it is decelerated. The total negative work is the sum of the work of lowering and of decelerating. Because power equals work divided by time, negative work results in **negative power.** If an object is decelerated in a very short time, the peak negative force and power are very great. It is not surprising, then, that injuries such as anterior cruciate ligament (ACL) tears frequently occur when an athlete moving at high speed suddenly comes to a stop or changes direction.

Movement Analysis and Exercise Prescription

The **specificity principle** is widely recognized [7, 32]. It states that training is most effective when it is similar in key ways to the physical activity in which improvement is sought **(target activity)**, such as the type of muscle contraction and the pattern, range, and velocity of movement [33]. For an athlete, the target activity is a sport movement, like hitting a baseball or a sprint start. Similarly, nonathletes frequently wish to improve their ability to perform specific body movements in addition to improving their overall physical fitness. A worker, for instance, may want to be able to lift equipment onto a worktable without asking for help. A person who is elderly may want to be able to walk upstairs without difficulty. Physical fitness refers to the ability to perform important physical activities. Clearly, what physical activities are important depends very much on the individual's age, medical status, and personal goals. Whatever these are, the principle of specificity can facilitate the attainment of physical fitness goals.

In practice, specificity means that there should be similarity between the training and target activities with respect to the muscle groups involved, as well as the direction and range of movement. That is not to say that the training program should include only exercises similar to the target activity. A balanced whole-body training program is important for general health and physical performance. However, exercises selected according to the specificity principle can give a decided advantage in improving performance. Thus a whole-body training program supplemented with specific exercises is most beneficial for improvement of performance and avoidance of injury.

Ideally, one can quantitatively analyze a target activity using high-speed video and other tools of biomechanics. However, such equipment is not widely available. Alternatively, the personal trainer can use home video or simple visual observation to identify the characteristics of a target activity for the purpose of selecting appropriately specific exercises. The key is to identify the joints about which resisted body movements occur during the target activity and the directions of movement. Exercises that involve similar movement around the same joints are then selected. Videotape that can be played back in slow motion is particularly useful for identifying the component body movements of the target activity. For example, observation of a worker lifting a toolbox may show that the movement mainly involves knee and hip extension as well as lateral trunk movement.

A basic set of body movements, providing a manageable framework for movement-oriented exercise prescription, is illustrated in figure 4.12. The set of all possible body movements is simplified to only those in the frontal, sagittal, and transverse planes (see figure 4.5). Despite this, the training effect overlaps enough so that training muscles using exercises within the planes also strengthens them for movements between the planes.

An exercise program that included exercise for all the movements in figure 4.12 would be both comprehensive and balanced. However, some of the movements are usually not included in typical exercise programs while others account for a disproportionate share of the workout. Some important movements not usually exercised in typical resistance training programs (and examples of activities in which the movements are used) include shoulder internal and external rotation (throwing, pulling weeds), knee flexion (hiking, sprinting), hip flexion (kicking, sprinting, getting out of bed), ankle dorsiflexion (walking, running), hip internal and external rotation (dancing, tennis), hip adduction and abduction (horseback riding, lateral movement), torso rotation (truck loading, throwing), and all the neck movements (impact absorption, wearing a hard hat or helmet). However, it is important to include exercises specific to the target activities in an exercise program in order to both improve performance and reduce the likelihood of injury.

A personal trainer can use figure 4.12 to design comprehensive and balanced training programs, determine deficiencies in existing programs, and identify exercises that could improve performance in work, sport, and routine as well as occasional physical activities of daily life. Visually observing a sport, work, or daily life activity, with or without the assistance of high-speed video, enables identification of the movements particularly important to that physical activity. Specific training exercises can be selected to provide resistance to those movements over the characteristic ranges of motion.

As an example of analyzing a target movement for the purpose of prescribing exercises, we can use figure 4.12 to qualitatively analyze the physical work task of loading boxes onto a truck. Observation indicates that the following movements are key components of truck loading: knee extension, hip extension, lower back extension, shoulder flexion, and elbow flexion. If the worker must lift the box and then turn 90 degrees to load the truck, lower back transverse plane rotation is also involved. Thus, a possible list of specific exercises can include the squat, the forward dumbbell raise, the barbell curl, and stack-machine trunk rotation. The power clean may be added as a more ballistic and specific exercise movement. If free weights are not available, similar exercises can be performed using loaded boxes.

The specificity principle is a major consideration when the personal trainer is designing an exercise program to improve target activity performance in work, sport, or daily life. It is necessary to analyze the target activity qualitatively and/or quantitatively to determine the specific movements involved. Exercises that utilize similar movements around the same body joints receive special emphasis in the exercise program.

Wrist—sagittal
Flexion
Exercise: wrist roller
Activity: opening jar

Extension
Exercise: reverse wrist curl
Activity: tennis backhand

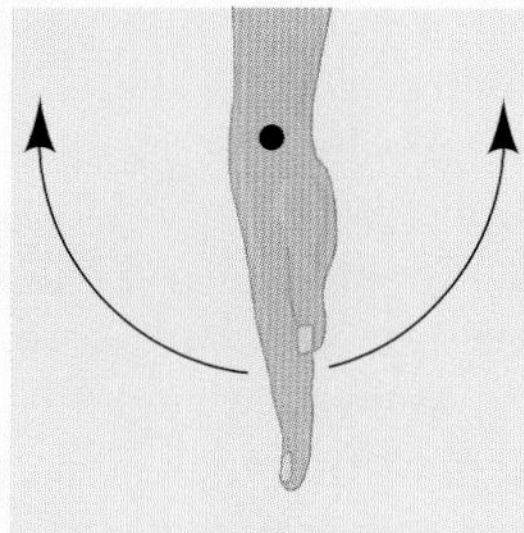

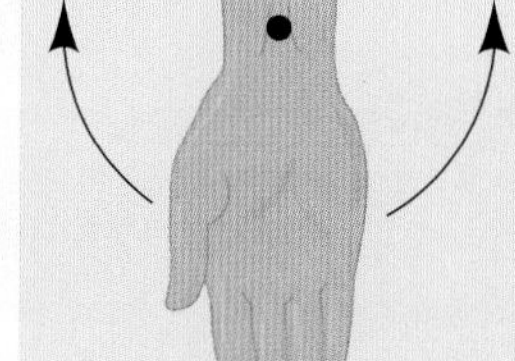

Wrist—frontal
Ulnar deviation
Exercise: aquatic hand paddles
Activity: golf swing

Radial deviation
Exercise: Indian club work
Activity: lifting a child

Elbow—sagittal
Flexion
Exercise: dumbbell curl
Activity: bowling

Extension
Exercise: narrow-grip pushup
Activity: pushing a cart

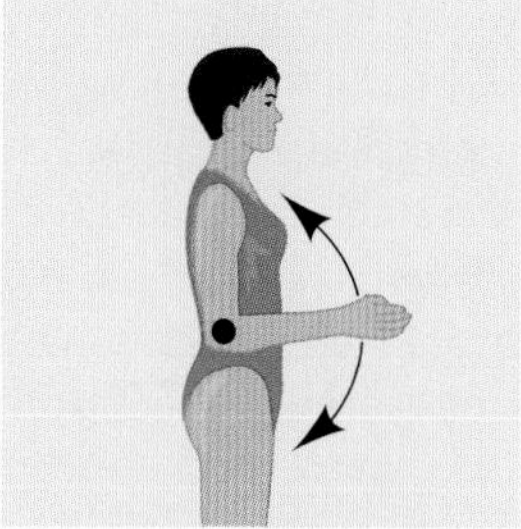

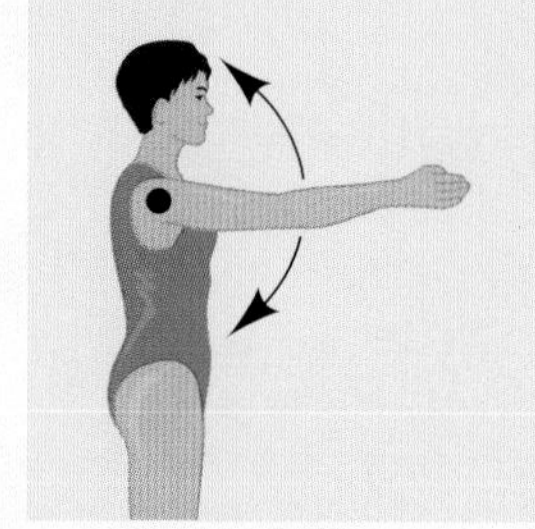

Shoulder—sagittal
Flexion
Exercise: swimming backstroke
Activity: placing books on a shelf

Extension
Exercise: rowing
Activity: tamping soil

Shoulder—frontal
Adduction
Exercise: wide-grip pullup
Activity: swimming

Abduction
Exercise: lateral arm raise
Activity: reach for climbing handhold

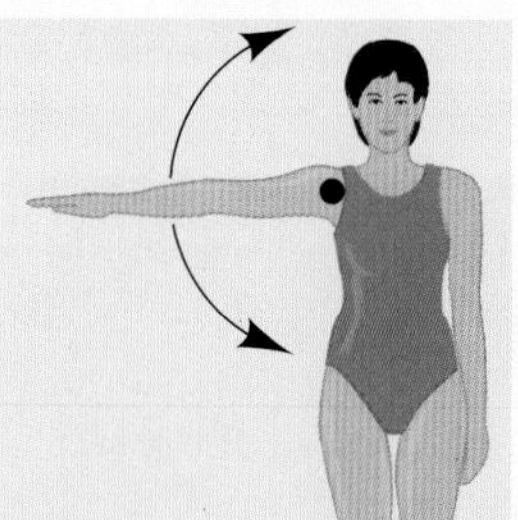

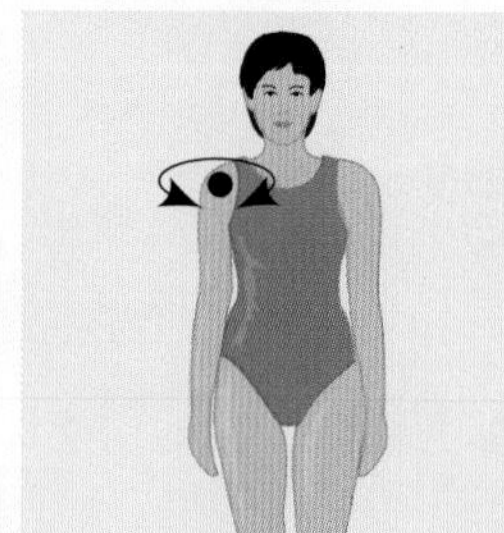

Shoulder—transverse
Internal rotation
Exercise: aquatic hand paddle
Activity: baton twirling

External rotation
Exercise: aquatic hand paddle
Activity: using a screwdriver

Shoulder—transverse
Adduction
Exercise: fly stack machine
Activity: tennis forehand

Abduction
Exercise: elastic band row
Activity: opening a door

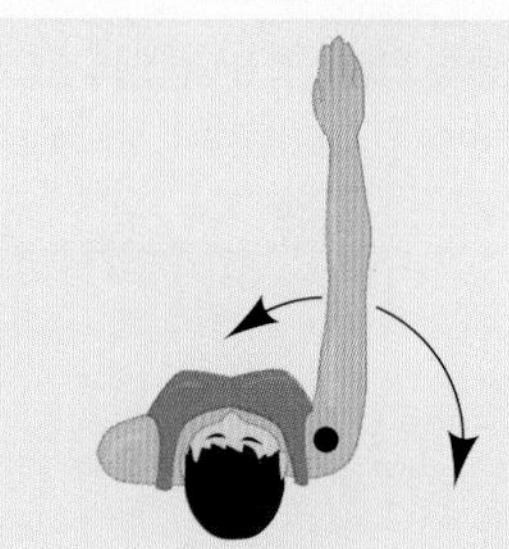

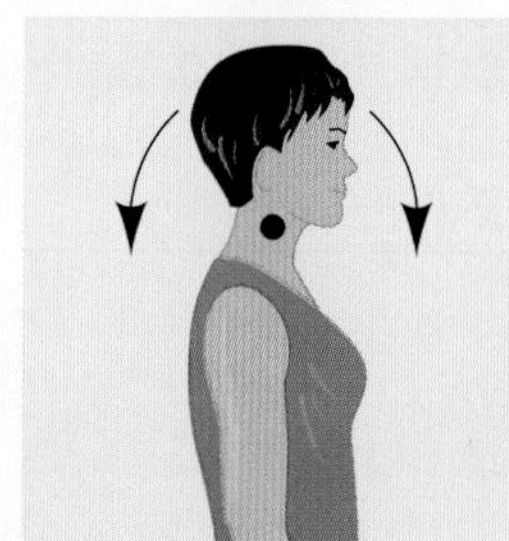

Neck—sagittal
Flexion
Exercise: self-resisted neck flexion
Activity: tolerate motorcycle acceleration forces

Extension
Exercise: neck machine exercise
Activity: hold up head while cycling

Neck—transverse
Left rotation
Exercise: self resistance
Activity: catching a baseball in the outfield

Right rotation
Exercise: self resistance
Activity: backing up automobile

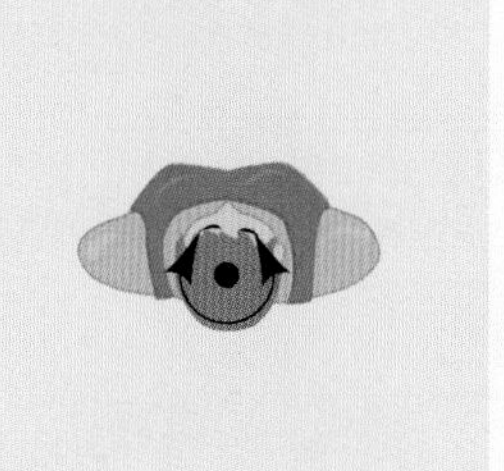

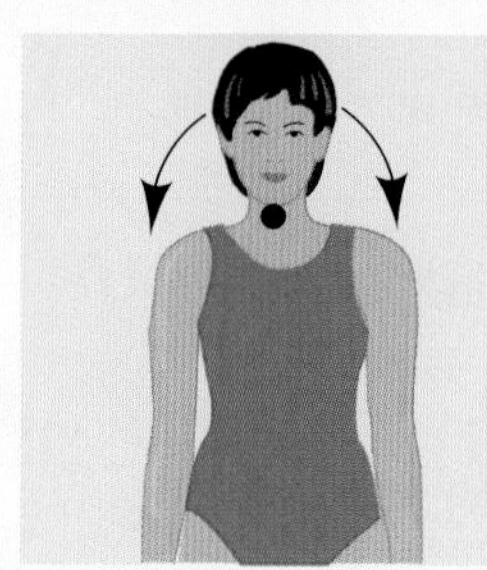

Neck—frontal
Left tilt
Exercise: self-resisted head tilt
Activity: tolerate g-forces in fighter plane

Right tilt
Exercise: neck machine exercise
Activity: escape from wrestling hold

Figure 4.12 Major body movements. Planes of movement are relative to the body in the anatomical position. The list includes common exercises that provide resistance to the movements and related physical activities.
Adapted from Harman, Johnson, and Frykman 1992.

Lower back—sagittal
Flexion
Exercise: sit-up
Activity: get out of bed

Extension
Exercise: back machine
Activity: lift boxes of supplies

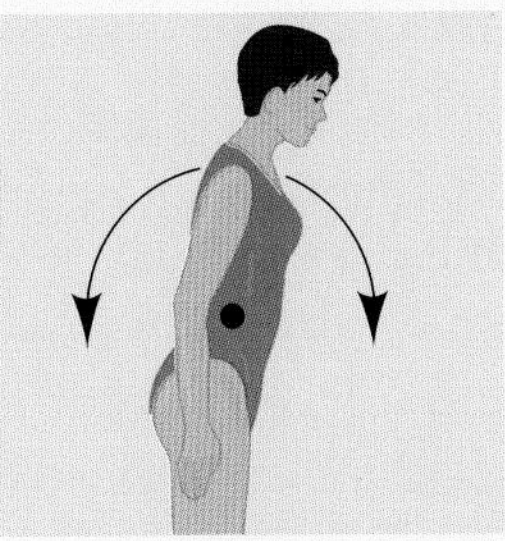

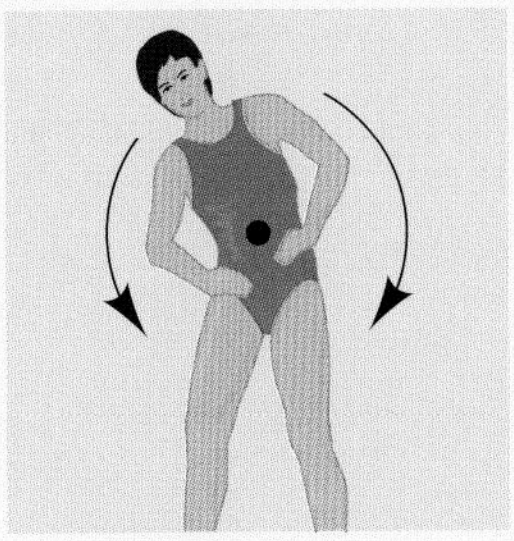

Lower back—frontal
Left tilt
Exercise: side tilt with bar on shoulders
Activity: walking with a suitcase in the right hand

Right tilt
Exercise: side bend with dumbbell in one hand
Activity: carrying a toolbox in left hand

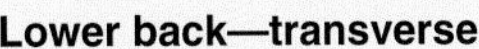

Lower back—transverse
Left rotation
Exercise: medicine ball side toss
Activity: baseball swing

Right rotation
Exercise: torso stack machine
Activity: chopping wood

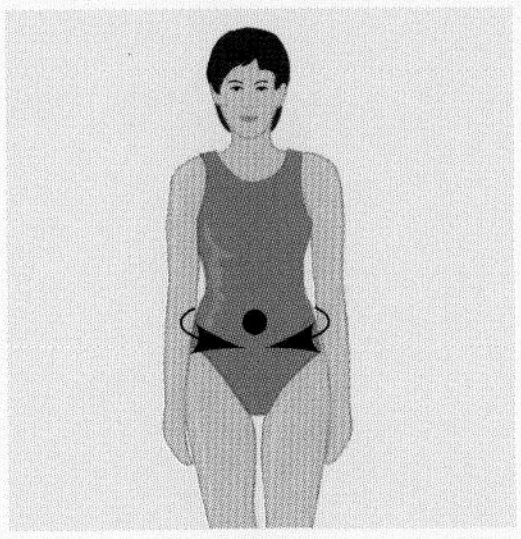

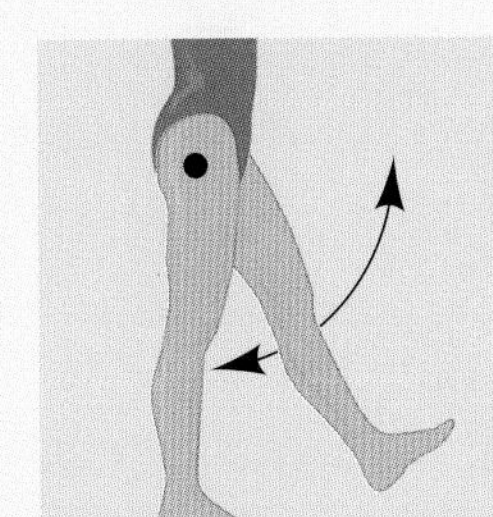

Hip—sagittal
Flexion
Exercise: high stepping
Activity: self-defense kick

Extension
Exercise: cross-country ski machine
Activity: walking uphill

Hip—frontal
Adduction
Exercise: sideward shuffle
Activity: riding a horse

Abduction
Exercise: skating slide board
Activity: sidestepping an obstacle

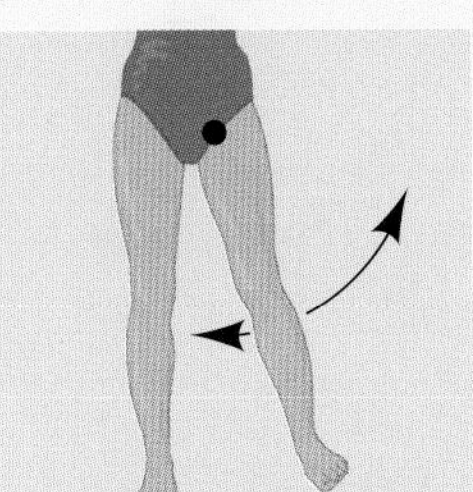

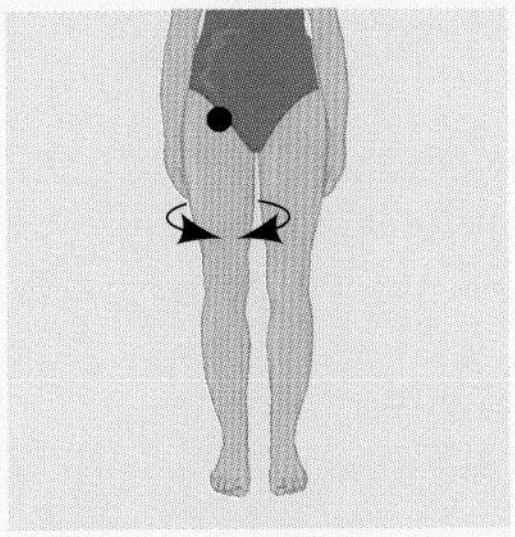

Hip—transverse
Internal rotation
Exercise: sand box
Activity: swing dancing

External rotation
Exercise: sand box
Activity: ice skating turn

Hip—transverse
Adduction
Exercise: cardio-kickbox inward sweep kick
Activity: soccer kick

Abduction
Exercise: cardio-kickbox outward sweep kick
Activity: stepping over a fence

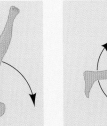

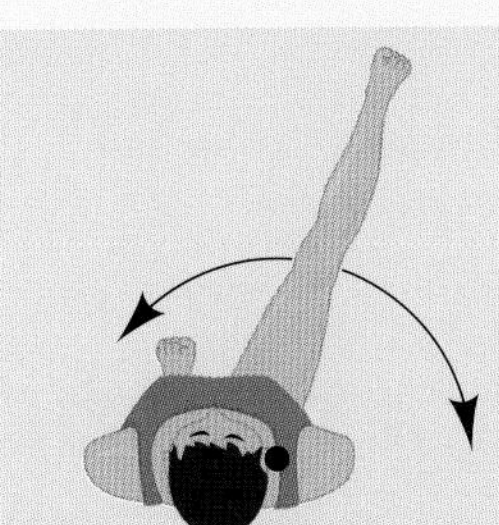

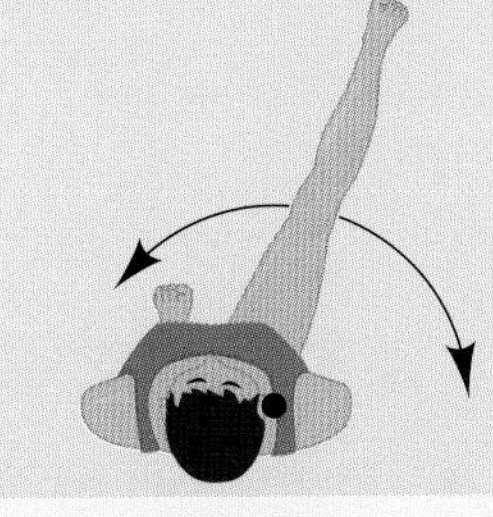

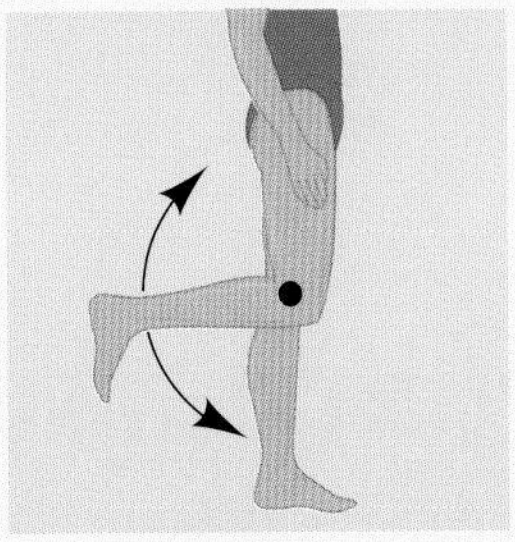

Knee—sagittal
Flexion
Exercise: interval sprints
Activity: rock climbing

Extension
Exercise: step class
Activity: walking upstairs

Ankle—sagittal
Dorsiflexion
Exercise: pushup with insteps on a large ball
Activity: SCUBA diving

Plantarflexion
Exercise: walking
Activity: standing on tiptoes

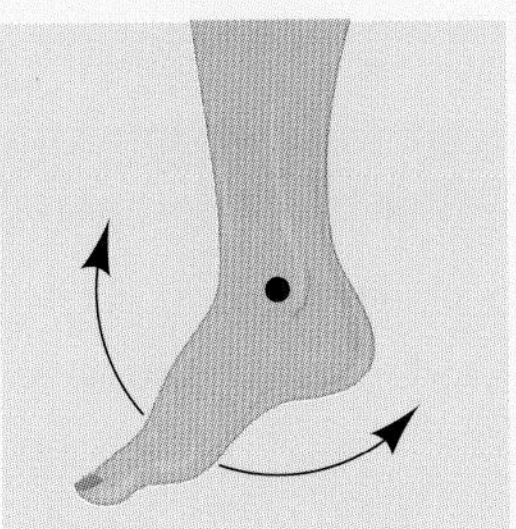

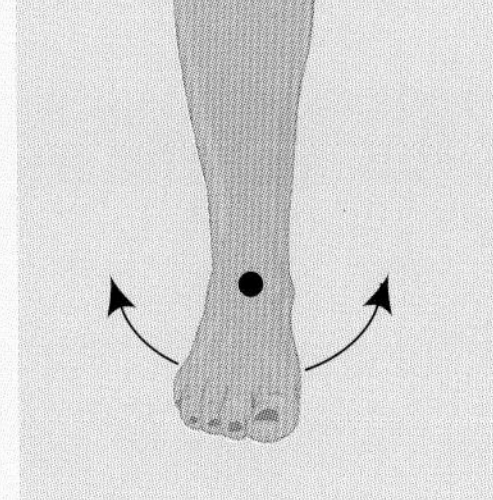

Ankle—frontal
Inversion
Exercise: medicine ball catch with feet
Activity: walking across a hillside (downhill foot)

Eversion
Exercise: walking in sand
Activity: walking across a hillside (uphill foot)

Figure 4.12 *(continued)*

CONCLUSION

The understanding of basic biomechanical principles is important for understanding how exercises bring about the desired training effect while minimizing the likelihood of injury. A personal trainer with a solid foundation in biomechanics is better prepared to help establish training goals, as well as to prescribe an exercise program that is effective in improving the physical capabilities of the client both efficiently and safely.

STUDY QUESTIONS

1. Which of the following exercise modes requires the client to produce the most power?
   A. 1RM squat
   B. 1RM leg press
   C. 3RM bench press
   D. 3RM hang clean
2. Using 220 lb (100 kg) for each and allowing 90 degrees of knee flexion at the bottom of each movement, which of the following exercises produces the most work?
   A. back squat
   B. horizontal leg press
   C. 15 degree leg press
   D. 60 degree leg press
3. Which of the following changes will increase concentric force production?
   A. decreased rate coding
   B. increased pennation
   C. increased contraction velocity
   D. decreased leverage over the joint range of motion
4. At what point during the upward movement phase of the standing barbell curl exercise can the biceps brachii muscles produce the greatest torque?
   A. At the beginning, because the muscle is at its longest length.
   B. At 45 degrees of flexion, because the moment arm is at its shortest length.
   C. At 90 degrees of flexion, because the moment arm is at its longest length.
   D. At the end, because the muscle is at its shortest length.

APPLIED KNOWLEDGE QUESTION

Fill in the chart with examples of resistance training exercises for each source of external resistance that can be applied to the body.

Source of external resistance	Resistance training exercises
Gravity	
Inertia	
Fluid	
Elasticity	
Electronically-controlled	

REFERENCES

1. Abate, F., ed. 1996. *The Oxford Dictionary and Thesaurus,* American ed. New York: Oxford University Press.
2. Alexander, R., and A. Vernon. 1975. The dimensions of the knee and ankle muscles and the forces they exert. *Journal of Human Movement Studies* 1: 115-123.
3. Åstrand, P., and K. Rodahl. 1986. *Textbook of Work Physiology,* 3rd ed. New York: McGraw-Hill.
4. Bartonietz, K. 2000. Hammer throwing: Problems and prospects. In: *Biomechanics in Sport: Performance Enhancement and Injury Prevention,* V.M. Zatsiorsky, ed. London: Blackwell Science, pp. 458-486.
5. Challis, J.H. 2000. Muscle-tendon architecture and athletic performance. In: *Biomechanics in Sport: Performance Enhancement and Injury Prevention,* V.M. Zatsiorsky, ed. London: Blackwell Science, pp. 33-55.
6. Enoka, R.M. 2001. *Neuromechanics of Human Movement.* Champaign, IL: Human Kinetics.
7. Fleck, S.J., and W.J. Kraemer. 1997. *Designing Resistance Training Programs,* 2nd ed. Champaign, IL: Human Kinetics.
8. Garhammer, J. 1989. Weight lifting and training. In: *Biomechanics of Sport,* C. Vaughn, ed. Boca Raton, FL: CRC Press, pp. 169-211.
9. Gregor, R.J. 1989. The structure and function of skeletal muscle. In: *Kinesiology and Applied Anatomy,* 7th ed., P.J. Rasch, ed. Philadelphia: Lea & Febiger, pp. 34-35.
10. Harman, E. 1983. Resistive torque analysis of 5 Nautilus exercise machines. *Medicine and Science in Sports and Exercise* 15 (2): 113.
11. Harman, E.A., M.T. Rosenstein, P.N. Frykman, and R.M. Rosenstein. 1990. The effects of arms and countermovement of vertical jumping. *Medicine and Science in Sports and Exercise* 22 (6): 825-833.
12. Haxton, H.A. 1944. Absolute muscle force in the ankle flexors of man. *Journal of Physiology* 103: 267-273.
13. Hay, J.G., and J.G. Reid. 1982. *The Anatomical and Mechanical Bases of Human Motion.* Englewood Cliffs, NJ: Prentice Hall.
14. Herzog, W. 2000. Mechanical properties and performance in skeletal muscles. In: *Biomechanics in Sport: Performance Enhancement and Injury Prevention,* V.M. Zatsiorsky, ed. London: Blackwell Science, pp. 21-32.
15. Higdon, A., W.B. Stiles, A.W. Davis, and C.R. Evces. 1976. *Engineering Mechanics.* Englewood Cliffs, NJ: Prentice Hall.
16. Hill, A.V. 1970. *First and Last Experiments in Muscle Mechanics.* London: Cambridge University Press.
17. Humphrey, J. 2002. Treating the athlete: Aquatic advantages. *Training and Conditioning* 12 (5): 28-34.
18. Ikai, M., and T. Fukunaga. 1968. Calculation of muscle strength per unit cross-sectional area of human muscle by means of ultrasonic measurement. *Internationale Zeitschrift fur angewandte Physiologie, einschliesslich Arbeitphysiologie* 26: 26-32.
19. Johnson, J.H., S. Colodny, and D. Jackson. 1990. Human torque capability versus machine resistive torque for four Eagle resistance machines. *Journal of Applied Sport Science Research* 4 (3): 83-87.
20. Jorgensen, K. 1976. Force-velocity relationship in human elbow flexors and extensors. In: *Biomechanics V-A,* P.V. Komi, ed. Baltimore: University Park Press.
21. Knuttgen, H., and W. Kraemer. 1987. Terminology and measurement in exercise performance. *Journal of Applied Sport Science Research* 1 (1): 1-10.
22. Lander, J.E., B.T. Bates, J.A. Sawhill, and J. Hamill. 1985. A comparison between free-weight and isokinetic bench pressing. *Medicine and Science in Sports and Exercise* 17 (3): 344-353.
23. *Le Système International d'Unites (SI),* 6th ed. 1991. Sevres, France: Bureau International des Poids et Mesures.
24. McArdle, W.D., F.I. Katch, and V.L. Katch. 2001. *Exercise physiology: Energy, nutrition, and human performance,* 5th ed. Baltimore: Lippincott Williams & Wilkins.
25. McDonagh, M.J.N., and C.T.M. Davies. 1984. Adaptive response of mammalian skeletal muscle to exercise with high loads. *European Journal of Applied Physiology* 52: 139-155.
26. Meriam, J.L., and L.G. Kraige. 2002. *Engineering Mechanics: Dynamics,* 5th ed. New York: Wiley.
27. Moritani, T., and H.A. deVries. 1979. Neural factors versus hypertrophy in the time course of muscle strength gain. *American Journal of Physical Medicine* 58 (3): 115-130.
28. Neumann, G. 1988. Special performance capacity. In: *The Olympic Book of Sports Medicine,* A. Dirix, H.G. Knuttgen, and K. Tittel, eds. London: Blackwell Scientific.
29. Perrine, J.J., and V.R. Edgerton. 1978. Muscle force-velocity and power-velocity relationships under isokinetic loading. *Medicine and Science in Sports* 10 (3): 159-166.
30. Prilutsky, B.I. 2000. Eccentric muscle action in sport and exercise. In: *Biomechanics in Sport: Performance Enhancement and Injury Prevention,* V.M. Zatsiorsky, ed. London: Blackwell Science, pp. 56-85.
31. Scott, S.H., and D.A. Winter. 1991. A comparison of three muscle pennation assumptions and their effect on isometric and isotonic force. *Journal of Biomechanics* 24 (2): 163-167.
32. Semmler, J.G., and R.M. Enoka. 2000. Neural contributions to changes in muscle strength. In: *Biomechanics in Sport: Performance Enhancement and Injury Prevention,* V.M. Zatsiorsky, ed. London: Blackwell Science, pp. 3-20.
33. Siff, M. 2000. Biomechanical foundations of strength and power training. In: *Biomechanics in Sport: Performance Enhancement and Injury Prevention,* V.M. Zatsiorsky, ed. London: Blackwell Science, pp. 103-139.
34. Vorontsov, A.R., and V.A. Rumyantsev. 2000. Resistive forces in swimming. In: *Biomechanics in Sport: Performance Enhancement and Injury Prevention,* V.M. Zatsiorsky, ed. London: Blackwell Science, pp. 184-231.
35. Williams, M., and L. Stutzman. 1959. Strength variation through the range of joint motion. *Physical Therapy Review* 39 (3): 145-152.
36. Zatsiorsky, V.M. 1995. *Science and Practice of Strength Training.* Champaign, IL: Human Kinetics.

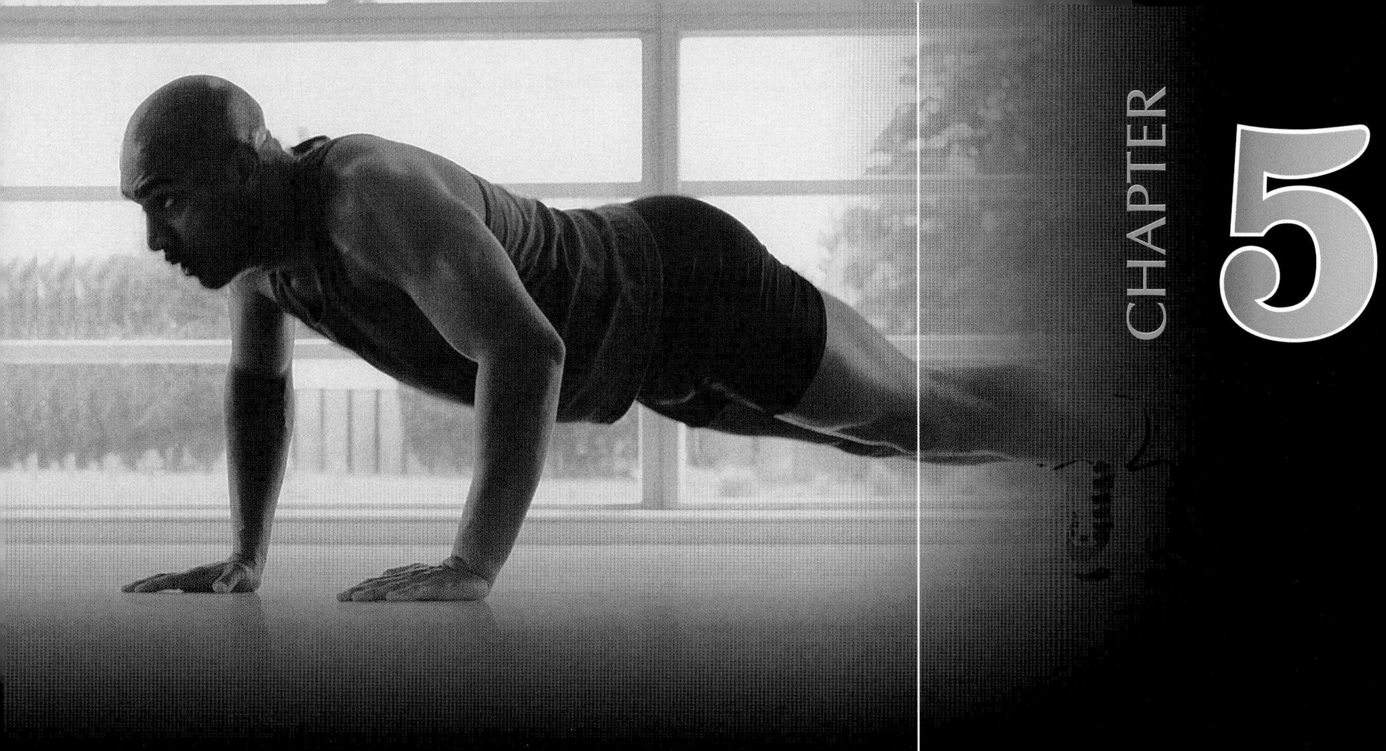

Resistance Training Adaptations

Lee E. Brown | Joseph P. Weir

After completing this chapter, you will be able to

- describe the acute and chronic adaptations to resistance exercise;
- identify factors that affect the magnitude or rate of adaptations to resistance training;
- design resistance training programs that maximize the specific adaptations of interest;
- design resistance training programs that avoid overtraining; and
- understand the effects of detraining and how to reduce them.

As clients embark on a resistance training program, their bodies respond in several notable ways. This chapter examines the physiological adaptations that occur with resistance training, both during acute bouts of training and over time. Personal trainers who understand these adaptations can design resistance training programs that will best meet clients' individual needs. Such personal trainers have a keen sense of how to train each physiological system with the client's personal goals in mind.

This chapter explains general adaptations that result from progressive overload. These include neurological, muscle and connective tissue, skeletal, metabolic, hormonal, cardiovascular, and body composition changes. As with all types of exercise training, resistance training is highly specific, so particular areas of resistance training specificity will be examined. The impact of gender, age, and genetics on physiological adaptations will then be explained. Finally, overtraining as an unwanted physiological response that must be prevented in the personal training setting will be discussed, and the effects of detraining and how to avoid them will be explained.

Basic Adaptations to Resistance Training

In studying the adaptations to resistance training, it is useful to distinguish between acute and chronic adaptations. Acute adaptations, which are often referred to as "responses" to exercise, are the changes that occur in the body during and shortly after an exercise bout. As an example, fuel substrates in muscle such as creatine phosphate (CP) can become depleted during an exercise bout. In contrast, chronic adaptations refer to changes in the body that occur after repeated training bouts and persist long after a training session is over. For example, long-term resistance training results in increases in muscle mass, which largely drive the increase in force production capability of the muscle. Two subsequent sections of this chapter address the acute and chronic adaptations that typically occur with resistance training.

> Acute adaptations are changes that occur in the body during and shortly after an exercise bout. Chronic adaptations are changes in the body that occur after repeated training bouts and that persist long after a training session is over.

The key to inducing increases in muscle size and strength is to place the system under **overload;** that is, the neuromuscular system must experience a training stress that it is not accustomed to experiencing. The same holds true if one is considering adaptations in bone and connective tissue. Progressive overload results in the muscle's ability to handle heavier loads, and this indicates that a variety of physiological adaptations have occurred.

A large volume of literature describes the adaptations to resistance training overload. The rapidity with which overload increases the capacity for muscle to handle heavier loads at the start of a training program suggests that there is a dramatic increase in the activation of motor units during the initial phases of resistance training. Scientific studies have indicated that such improvements in strength associated with the early stages of resistance training are primarily due to neurological adaptations. In addition, during this time the quality of muscle protein (e.g., myosin heavy chains and myosin ATPase) also changes to allow for more rapid and forceful contractile capabilities.

Although the ultimate magnitude of morphological size of a muscle is primarily determined by genetic factors, numerous studies have established that resistance training leads to muscle hypertrophy. Hypertrophy of muscle fibers is usually not measurable until approximately 8 to 12 weeks after the initiation of the training program. The continued interplay of hypertrophic and neurological adaptations to resistance training continues with long-term training. The impact of long-term training on muscle hypertrophy remains less well studied, but the absolute magnitude of gains in muscle size and strength is lower as clients approach their genetic limits. Nevertheless, continued training over a client's lifetime helps to improve quality of life and minimize the consequences of aging.

A variety of cellular adaptations occur with resistance training programs. These include changes in anaerobic enzyme quantity, changes in stored energy substrates (e.g., glycogen and phosphagens), increased myofibrillar protein content (i.e., increased actin and myosin proteins), and increased noncontractile muscle proteins. In addition, important changes occur within the central and peripheral nervous system to help in the activation of motor units to produce specific force and power requirements. Furthermore, a variety of changes occur in other physiological systems (e.g., endocrine, immune, and cardiovascular systems) that support the neuromuscular adaptations to a resistance training program. All these adaptations support the neuromuscular improvements in force, velocity, and power capabilities in the body consequent to resistance training.

Acute Adaptations

The short-term changes that occur in the neuromuscular system during and immediately after a training session drive the chronic adaptations. This section presents an overview of the major acute responses to resistance exercise, specifically exploring responses involving the neurological, muscular, and endocrine systems. These acute responses are summarized in table 5.1.

Neurological Changes

Performance of resistance training, as of all physical activity, requires activation of skeletal muscle. The process of skeletal muscle activation involves action potential generation on the muscle cell membrane (sarcolemma) via acetylcholine release from the alpha motor neuron that **innervates** (stimulates) a particular muscle cell. The action potential is manifested as a voltage change on the sarcolemma that can be recorded with either surface or intramuscular electrodes. The technique of recording these electrical events is referred to as **electromyography** (EMG). The size of an EMG signal varies as a function of muscle force output, but is also affected by

TABLE 5.1

Acute Responses to Resistance Training

Variable	Acute response
Neurological responses	
EMG amplitude	Increases
Number of motor units recruited	Increases
Muscular changes	
Hydrogen ion concentration	Increases
Inorganic phosphate concentration	Increases
Ammonia levels	Increases
ATP concentration	No change or slight decrease
CP concentration	Decreases
Glycogen concentration	Decreases
Endocrine changes	
Epinephrine concentration	Increases
Cortisol concentration	Increases
Testosterone concentration	Increases
Growth hormone concentration	Increases

EMG = electromyogram; ATP = adenosine triphosphate; CP = creatine phosphate.

other factors such as fatigue and muscle fiber composition [20]. Much of what we know about neurological responses and adaptations to resistance training comes from studies using EMG.

Control of muscle force is accomplished by the interplay of two control factors: motor unit recruitment and rate coding [21]. Motor unit **recruitment** simply refers to the process in which tasks that require more force involve the activation of more motor units. An individual performing a 100-pound (45-kilogram) bench press would need to turn on more motor units than would be required to perform a 50-pound (23-kilogram) bench press. **Rate coding** refers to control of motor unit firing rate (number of action potentials per unit of time). Within certain limits, the faster the firing rate, the more force is produced. Therefore, a motor unit that was activated at a rate of, say, 20 times per second during the 50-pound bench press may be firing at 30 times per second during the 100-pound bench press. As a general rule, small muscles (like those in the hands) that require very precise motor control achieve full recruitment at relatively low percentages of maximum force output (e.g., 50% of maximum), and after this point depend entirely on firing rate to increase force production. In contrast, large muscles like those in the quadriceps employ recruitment up to 90% of maximum or more, and maximum firing rates tend to be lower than for the small muscles [5]. Therefore, one can generalize that small muscles depend more heavily on firing to control force output while large muscles tend to depend more heavily on recruitment.

During a typical set of resistance exercise using weights, a pool of motor units in the involved muscle is activated and each motor unit is firing at some rate. As the person progresses from one repetition to the next, the muscle begins to fatigue, and changes in recruitment and firing rate occur. It is likely that motor unit recruitment increases over time to compensate for the loss in force production capability of the previously activated motor units [78]. In addition, motor units that were firing at low rates at the start of the set may have to fire at higher rates (rate coding) as the set progresses in response to the fatigue associated with the task. These changes are manifested in changes in the surface EMG signal. Specifically, the size of the surface EMG signal gets larger during a set of resistance training exercise [73]. This reflects changes in motor unit recruitment and firing rate.

Motor unit recruitment is based on the **size principle** [23] (figure 5.1). In general, motor units that innervate slow-twitch motor units innervate fewer fibers than motor units that innervate fast-twitch fibers. In addition, both the muscle fiber size and alpha motor neuron diameters of slow-twitch motor units are smaller than those of their fast-twitch counterparts. The smaller neuron size of slow-twitch motor units results in a lower threshold for activation for these motor neurons. Therefore, they are recruited at low force levels. In contrast, large motor neurons, such as those that typically innervate fast-twitch muscle fibers, have higher recruitment thresholds and are recruited at higher force levels. As the force requirements of a task increase and more motor units are recruited, the nervous system recruits larger motor units [23].

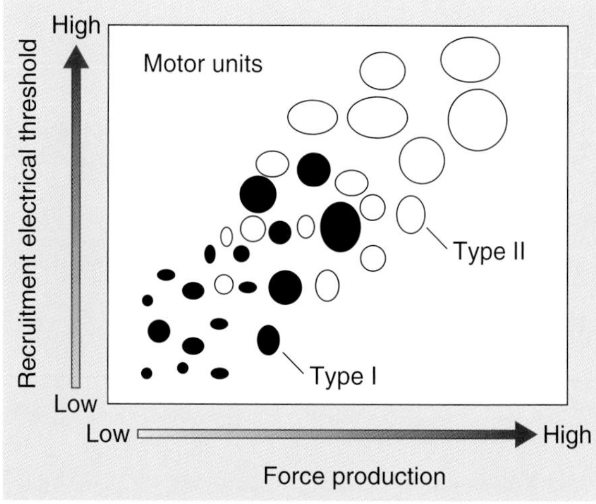

Figure 5.1 Graphic representation of the size principle.
Reprinted from Baechle and Earle 2000.

One implication of the size principle is that to recruit high-threshold (fast-twitch) motor units, one must engage in tasks that require high force outputs. In addition, the terms slow-twitch and fast-twitch do not imply that the nervous system turns on slow-twitch motor units only during slow contractions and fast-twitch motor units only during fast contractions. Rather, motor unit recruitment follows the size principle and is therefore dependent on the force production requirements of a task, so that fast-twitch fibers are recruited even during slow (or isometric) contractions if the force demands are high enough.

Recruitment of motor units for force production follows the size principle, meaning that smaller motor units are recruited at lower force levels and larger motor units are recruited at higher force levels.

Muscular Changes

As already noted, during a set of resistance exercise, muscles experience fatigue. While fatigue is a highly complex phenomenon, it is clear that the acute changes in muscle cells include accumulation of metabolites and depletion of fuel substrates. The factors involved are tied to the metabolic pathways that are primarily stressed during anaerobic activities (like resistance training), specifically the phosphagen system and glycolysis. Metabolites that accumulate include hydrogen ion (H^+, which results in a decrease in muscle pH), inorganic phosphate (P_i), and ammonia [70]. All of these have been studied as potential causes of muscle fatigue.

As noted earlier, CP can become depleted during resistance exercise, reflecting the reliance on the phosphagen system during typical resistance training. Creatine phosphate is important for phosphorylation of adenosine diphosphate (ADP) to adenosine triphosphate (ATP) during high-intensity exercise, and depletion of CP likely leads to decreased power production. Although complete glycogen depletion is unlikely to occur with resistance training, glycogen breakdown is an important factor in the supply of energy for this type of training [68, 86]. In fact, it has been estimated that over 80% of the ATP production during bodybuilding-type resistance training comes from glycolysis [64]. Therefore, glycogen levels decrease in response to high-intensity resistance training. This points to the importance of adequate dietary carbohydrate for those who perform resistance training [38, 66].

During and immediately after resistance exercise, metabolites accumulate and fuel substrates are depleted; thus, clients need to include adequate carbohydrate in their diets.

Endocrine Changes

Hormones are blood-borne molecules that are produced in glands called endocrine glands. There are two primary types of hormones: protein/peptide hormones and steroid hormones. Two examples of protein/peptide hormones are growth hormone and insulin. Steroid hormones are all derived from a common precursor (cholesterol) and include hormones such as testosterone (the primary male sex hormone) and estrogen (the primary female sex hormone).

Many hormones have effects on either the growth or the degradation of tissue such as muscle tissue. **Anabolic** hormones such as testosterone, growth hormone (GH), and insulin tend to stimulate growth processes in tissues, while **catabolic** hormones such as cortisol function to use tissue degradation to help maintain homeostasis of variables such as blood glucose. The concentration of many of these hormones is affected by an acute bout of exercise. Indeed, changes in some hormone concentrations are needed to support the metabolic response to exercise. For example, exercise results in increases in concentrations of epinephrine. Epinephrine increases fat and carbohydrate breakdown by the cell so that more ATP will be available for muscle contraction. Epinephrine also has effects on the central nervous system, which should facilitate motor unit activation. The hormonal response to resistance exercise is dependent on the characteristics of the training bout. As a general rule, bouts that have higher volume and shorter rest periods elicit stronger endocrine responses than do bouts with lower volume and longer rest periods [56]. Similarly, large muscle mass exercises have more of a powerful stimulus than do small muscle mass exercises.

Other hormone concentrations are increased during a bout of resistance training, but they may have little effect on that particular exercise bout. For example, testosterone concentrations are elevated with resistance training [42, 58, 62, 91]. Among its many effects, testosterone increases skeletal muscle protein synthesis. Therefore, it is important for development of muscle mass. The cumulative effect of acute increases in testosterone concentrations with an exercise bout may contribute to the long-term accretion of muscle mass, but the influence of testosterone on the function of the cell during that exercise session is likely negligible.

Chronic Adaptations

Chronic adaptations are long-term changes in the structure and function of the body as a consequence of exercise training. With respect to resistance training, the general adaptations that one sees following prolonged resistance training are increases in strength and muscle mass. Increases in strength are influenced by changes in neurological function as well as changes in muscle mass. In addition, changes in muscle enzyme and substrate concentrations may influence muscle endurance. These chronic adaptations are summarized in table 5.2.

Neurological Changes

It is a common observation that increases in strength occur rapidly during the early stages of a resistance training program and that they are larger than can be accounted for by changes in muscle size (figure

TABLE 5.2

Chronic Adaptations to Resistance Training

Variable	Chronic adaptation
Muscle performance	
Muscle strength	Increases
Muscle endurance	Increases
Muscle power	Increases
Muscle enzymes	
Phosphagen system enzyme concentrations	May increase
Phosphagen system enzyme absolute levels	Increase
Glycolytic enzyme concentrations	May increase
Glycolytic enzyme absolute levels	Increase
Muscle substrates	
ATP concentration	May increase
ATP absolute levels	Increase
CP concentration	May increase
CP absolute levels	Increase
ATP and CP changes during exercise	Decrease
Lactate increase during exercise	Decreases
Muscle fiber characteristics	
Type I CSA	Increases (<Type II)
Type II CSA	Increases (>Type I)
% Type IIa	Increases
% Type IIb	Decreases
% Type I	No change
Body composition	
% Fat	Likely decreases
Fat-free mass	Increases
Metabolic rate	Likely increases

(continued)

TABLE 5.2 *(continued)*

Variable	Chronic adaptation
Neurological changes	
EMG amplitude during MVC	Likely increases
Motor unit recruitment	Likely increases
Motor unit firing rate	Increases
Co-contraction	Decreases
Structural changes	
Connective tissue strength	Likely increases
Bone density/mass	Likely increases

ATP = adenosine triphosphate; CP = creatine phosphate; CSA = cross-sectional area; EMG = electromyogram; MVC = maximal voluntary contraction.

5.2). These early strength gains are often attributed to so-called neural factors [77], and several studies have indicated that strength increases consequent to resistance training are influenced by increases in neural drive [22, 39, 51, 55]. In addition to the discrepancy between hypertrophic and strength increases early in a training program, neural factors have mainly been assumed to exist based on increases in EMG amplitude measured during maximal contractions [39, 55, 77].

The influence of neural factors on strength gains is believed to be dominant in the early phases of a training program (one to two months), and thereafter strength increases are primarily mediated by hypertrophy [43, 88] (figure 5.3). Much of this effect is likely due to improvements in skill in performing the resistance exercises, especially in individuals who are using free weight exercises that require balance and efficiency of movement in order to be performed well. However, some evidence suggests that part of this effect is due to changes in motor unit recruitment and firing rate. With respect to motor unit recruitment, the argument is that many untrained individuals are unable to activate all the motor units that are available, and resistance training may result in an increase in the ability to activate high-threshold motor units, leading to an increase in force production capability that is independent of muscle hypertrophy. We should note, however, that according to some studies, untrained individuals are able to recruit all available motor units [7, 74, 87]. In addition, not all studies show an increase in EMG amplitude following resistance training programs

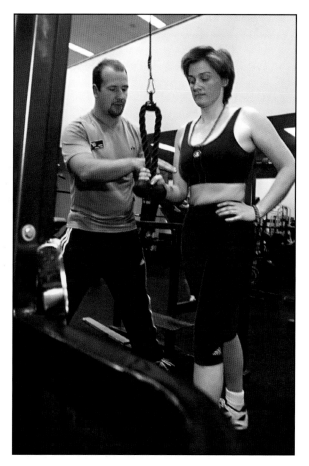

Figure 5.2 In the early stages of a resistance training program, increases in strength often occur rapidly and are larger than can be accounted for by changes in muscle size. These increases are often attributed to neural factors.

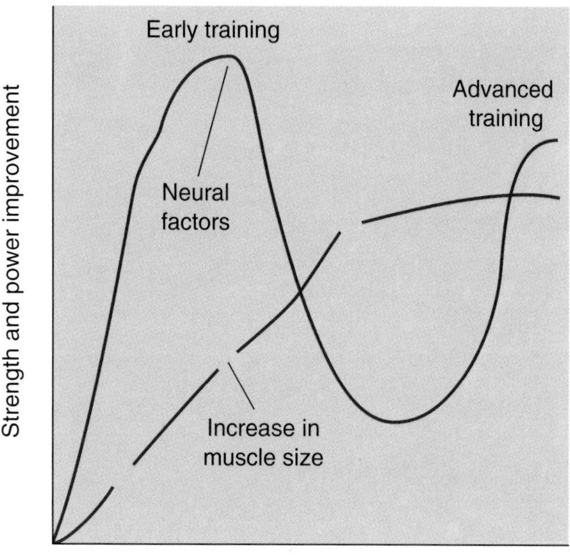

Figure 5.3 The changes in neural and muscular size contributions of improvements in strength.
Reprinted from Baechle and Earle 2000.

[33, 106]. Recent evidence suggests that resistance training can also increase maximal motor unit firing rates [82]. This would also increase muscle force production capability independent of hypertrophy.

During the early phases of a training program, neural factors—including those related to improved skill, motor recruitment, and firing rate—are the primary reason for strength gains; thereafter, strength increases are primarily caused by hypertrophy.

In addition to changes in motor unit recruitment and firing rate, other neurological adaptations have been reported in the literature. **Co-contraction** (or coactivation) refers to the simultaneous activation of an agonist and an antagonist during a motor task. As an example, during knee extension exercise, the quadriceps muscles are the agonists (prime movers) while the hamstrings serve as the antagonist. Several studies have shown significant co-contraction during isometric and isokinetic contractions of the knee joint [80, 85, 107]. Decreased co-contraction would decrease the antagonist torque that must be overcome by the agonist during a contraction, thus enhancing the expression of strength. There appear to be decreases in co-contraction following isometric resistance training [13]. Whether similar changes in co-contraction occur during dynamic exercise, such as with free weights, is unknown but appears likely. Other work has shown changes in motor neuron excitability [89] and increases in motor unit synchronization following resistance training [76]. Neural factors have also been inferred from observations that unilateral resistance training results in increases in strength of the untrained limb [45, 105, 106], as well as from observations that isometric resistance training at one joint angle results in strength increases that are larger at the trained angle than at other joint angles [54, 99, 106].

Muscle Tissue Changes

Resistance training results in adaptations in muscles, tendons, and ligaments. The most obvious adaptation in skeletal muscle is **hypertrophy,** that is, an increase in muscle size (cross-sectional area). Resistance training results in an increase in cross-sectional area of both Type I and Type II muscle fibers. However, Type II fibers show a greater degree of hypertrophy than Type I fibers [99, 94] and also suffer from greater atrophy following detraining [48]. The increase in cross-sectional area is attributed to an increase in both the size and number of myofibrils within a given muscle fiber. Thus resistance training causes an increase in protein synthesis (and/or a decrease in protein degradation) resulting in a greater number of actin and myosin filaments. The increase in myofibril number is possibly the result of "splitting" of existing myofibrils into separate "daughter" myofibrils [34]. **Hyperplasia,** or the increase in number of muscle fibers, has not been definitively shown to occur in humans, but there is evidence for hyperplasia in animal models [3]. The net result of an increase in muscle cross-sectional area, and the associated increase in actin and myosin filaments, is an increase in force and power production capability of the muscle.

The primary adaptation of skeletal muscle to long-term resistance training is hypertrophy, or increased cross-sectional area of the muscle fiber, resulting in increased force and power production capability.

With respect to muscle fiber types, resistance training induces a fiber subtype shift from Type IIb to Type IIa muscle fibers [36, 94]. These subtype shifts are observable after just a few training sessions [92] and likely reflect a change in the myosin heavy-chain composition of the muscle cell. Therefore, resistance training alters not only the quantity of muscle tissue (hypertrophy) but also its quality. However, to date there is little evidence to suggest that resistance training can induce a shift from slow- to fast-twitch fibers or vice versa.

The hypertrophic response to resistance training is the net result of an increase in protein synthesis relative to protein breakdown in the muscle cell [100]. Protein synthesis clearly increases following resistance training [15, 67]. The extent of protein degradation is less clear, but it is improbable that increased degradation does not occur since the hypertrophic response to resistance training is less than would be expected solely on the basis of the magnitude of the increased protein synthesis seen following resistance training bouts [15]. The protein degradation may be a consequence of muscle damage that has occurred during training, and there is some speculation that the damage may be a stimulus for hypertrophy. In support of this notion, researchers have shown that training responses are enhanced when eccentric contractions are included in the training as occurs during typical resistance training [16, 44, 63], and eccentric contractions are primarily implicated in the development of delayed-onset muscle soreness and muscle damage.

Skeletal Changes

It is tempting to think of the skeletal system as an inert framework comprising simply a set of levers that muscles act upon to create movement. However, bone tissue is very much "alive" and is a dynamic tissue. In addition to its role in movement and protection, bone serves as a depot for important minerals, most notably calcium. **Osteoporosis** is the consequence of long-term net demineralization of bone. In recent years, resistance training has been studied for its possible influence on bone mineral density. Bone tissue is significantly affected by strain; that is, deformation of bone rapidly stimulates bone cells to begin activities that stimulate bone formation [2]. Therefore, it seems logical to examine the effects of resistance training on bone formation, especially in the context of osteoporosis. Because osteoporosis is mainly, though not exclusively, a condition associated with postmenopausal women, most research has focused on women. Specifically, research has focused on the effect of resistance training on the accumulation of bone tissue prior to menopause, as well as on the effect of resistance training on the decline in bone mass associated with menopause. Menopause is particularly critical in the development of osteoporosis because hormones like estrogen, which facilitate bone formation, markedly decline after menopause. Accumulation of bone mass prior to menopause is considered important because the greater the bone mass prior to menopause, the less severe the consequences of loss of bone mass.

The research literature has shown quite clearly that, in cross-sectional studies, stronger women tend to have thicker and stronger bones. However, selection bias may influence such studies [2]. Intervention studies are less clear as to whether resistance training programs result in increases in bone mass. Some of these studies show no significant effect of resistance training on bone tissue [8, 84], while others have shown that resistance training programs can positively affect bone tissue [101, 71]. Differences between studies are influenced by factors such as length and characteristics (e.g., intensity, volume, type of exercises) of the training programs, small sample sizes, differences in the extent of bone demineralization prior to training, gender, and age. Nonetheless, there is enough evidence in the literature to suggest that resistance training is very likely to have a positive effect on bone tissue. Therefore, in addition to the obvious effects of resistance training on muscle mass and strength, resistance training may lead to decreased risk for osteoporosis, fractures, and falls in later life.

The greater the bone mass prior to menopause, the less severe are the consequences of loss of bone mass. Resistance training may lead to decreased risk for osteoporosis, fractures, and falls in later life.

Metabolic Changes

Research has shown that chronic resistance training induces a variety of cellular changes that affect the metabolism of skeletal muscle. All studies of metabolic adaptations to resistance training are complicated by the fact that hypertrophy will dilute enzyme and substrate levels, so that changes in absolute levels may result in no change of relative levels (e.g., per unit of muscle mass). In addition, relative decreases in concentrations may simply reflect hypertrophy.

Resistance training primarily stresses anaerobic metabolism, and therefore one should expect that any enzymatic or substrate adaptations would involve anaerobic metabolism. Anaerobic metabolism is typically thought of as having two components: the phosphagen system and glycolysis. Studies conflict regarding increases in substrate and enzyme concentrations in either of these components. With respect to the phosphagen system, some studies have demonstrated that resistance training does not result in increased concentration of ATP or CP [98], while others have shown increases in these variables [69]. Similarly, some data suggest that the enzymes involved in this system, creatine kinase and myokinase, are not found in higher concentrations following resistance training [97]. However, other data do indicate that resistance training results in higher concentrations of these enzymes [18]. Differences between studies likely reflect differences in training mode and volume and indicate the importance of designing programs to meet the specific needs of individual clients.

With respect to glycolytic activity, research has typically shown that key enzymes involved in the glycolytic pathway (e.g., phosphofructokinase, lactate dehydrogenase) are not found in higher concentrations following resistance training [57]. However, these results may be specific to the type of resistance training performed, since bodybuilders who perform higher-volume training with shorter rest periods than power lifters have glycolytic enzyme concentrations similar to those of aerobic endurance athletes such as swimmers [98]. This suggests that high-volume resistance training may induce glycolytic enzymatic adaptations that increase muscle endurance.

For both the phosphagen and glycolytic adaptations to resistance training just described, it is important to note that although some studies indicate no change in the concentrations of key substrates and enzymes, the total volume of these substrates and enzymes in a given muscle will be higher due to the increase in total muscle mass. Therefore, the absolute muscle endurance will likely increase following resistance training. This is evident in an increased ability to perform additional repetitions of a resistance training exercise [10, 96].

Hormone Changes

While resistance training can cause large changes in hormone concentrations during and after a bout of training, the long-term effects of resistance training on resting hormone concentrations are less clear. Also, the understanding of these effects is complicated by the fact that overtraining can cause changes in hormone concentrations that are different from those seen during "normal" training situations. That said, some evidence suggests that prolonged resistance training results in chronically elevated testosterone concentrations [40, 62] that should facilitate an environment conducive to muscle growth. This effect appears blunted in older individuals [41]. There does not appear to be a chronic training effect on resting GH concentrations [40, 42, 62]. However, the cumulative effect of acute increases in GH in response to resistance training likely has a significant influence on long-term muscle hypertrophy.

Chronic resistance training may also affect the magnitude of the endocrine response and the sensitivity of tissues to a hormone. Research has shown that several training sessions are required before an increase in testosterone concentration is elicited by resistance exercise [62]. Similarly, chronic resistance training alters the acute epinephrine response to bouts of exercise [37, 60]. Chronic training may affect sensitivity by increasing the quantity of the receptors for the hormone on the target tissue [53]. Through up-regulation of hormone receptors, the effect of a given concentration of a hormone is amplified.

Cardiovascular Changes

Resistance training places a much different stress on the cardiovascular system than does cardiovascular endurance exercise such as running or cycling, and therefore the effects on the cardiovascular system are quite different. With respect to aerobic endurance performance, resistance training has not been shown to result in an increase in peak $\dot{V}O_2$ [46, 61, 72]. This likely stems from the fact that while heart rate values are elevated during resistance training, the total metabolic demands are lower during resistance training than are those associated with comparable heart rate values elicited during aerobic endurance exercise [17]. Therefore there is little stimulus for increased peak $\dot{V}O_2$. This indicates that it is misleading to use target heart rate zones during resistance exercise as an indicator of cardiovascular fitness training.

Although resistance training programs do not typically improve maximal oxygen consumption to the extent seen with other modes of cardiovascular training (e.g., running, cycling), they augment the development of cardiovascular endurance performance and improve running efficiency while not causing any negative effects on the development of maximal oxygen consumption [46, 47, 80]. Therefore, although resistance training does not directly increase peak $\dot{V}O_2$, it can serve as an important adjunct to cardiovascular training. Nonetheless, to achieve optimal results in increasing the cardiorespiratory endurance capabilities of a client requires aerobic endurance-specific training. Chapter 16 provides the details of such programs for achieving improvements in maximal oxygen consumption and discusses the effects of such training on strength gains.

Increasing cardiorespiratory endurance capabilities requires aerobic endurance-specific training to achieve optimal results; however, resistance training can augment cardiovascular endurance performance and running efficiency by increasing muscle strength and power.

As noted previously, resistance training depends primarily on anaerobic metabolism to generate ATP for muscle contractions. Therefore, it is not surprising that resistance training does not appear to improve skeletal muscle cellular aerobic function as assessed by oxidative enzyme activity and capillary density. However, it does induce increases in capillarization so that capillary supply is maintained in spite of increased muscle size [36]. Both myoglobin [97] and mitochondrial density [69] tend to decrease with resistance training. Both of these changes reflect the effects of hypertrophy and the lack of oxidative stress (and therefore stimulus) that occurs during resistance training.

Despite the lack of improvement in skeletal muscle cellular aerobic function, it is important to note that normal increases in muscle size (i.e., hypertrophy) with resistance training do not reduce muscle endurance. On the contrary, increases in muscle size and strength due to resistance training increase local muscle endurance [10, 96]. That is, a hypertrophied muscle, with the corresponding increases in strength and volume of metabolic enzymes and substrates (but not necessarily a higher density), can do more work over time.

Body Composition Changes

A variety of models have been developed to quantify body composition. For the personal trainer, the model that best relates to the needs of clients is the two-component model, which segregates the body into fat mass and fat-free mass (FFM). The FFM is composed of tissues such as muscle, bone, and connective tissue. As noted previously, resistance training can affect all of these components, so it follows that a resistance training program that induces hypertrophy will directly affect body composition. That is, increases in FFM, independent of changes in fat mass, will decrease body fat percentage. According to several studies, resistance training increases FFM and decreases body fat percentage in men [11], women [19, 83], and persons who are elderly [49].

Resistance training may also affect the amount of fat mass in the body as a consequence of the direct effect of the training on energy consumption. Higher-volume training burns more calories than lower-volume training. In addition, resistance training elevates energy consumption during the recovery period between training sessions, further facilitating fat loss [90].

An added benefit of resistance training is that increases in FFM, especially muscle mass, may increase resting metabolic rate and total daily energy expenditure. This occurs because muscle tissue, unlike fat tissue, has a high metabolic rate. That is, since the normal resting energy requirements of muscle are high, clients with more muscle mass should burn more calories at rest and throughout the day. However, while some studies have shown that resistance exercise can increase resting metabolic rate [49, 83], others have not [11, 19]. It is also unclear whether resistance training significantly increases total daily energy expenditure [83]. Nonetheless, given the clear effect of resistance exercise on FFM and its possible effect on resting metabolic rate, resistance training should be a critical component of any comprehensive program to control body fat.

Factors That Influence Adaptations to Resistance Training

A variety of factors affect the adaptations to resistance training described in the previous sections. These include factors such as **specificity** (i.e., the ability of the body to make adaptations that uniquely enhance performance in activities that are most similar to the exercise stressor), sex, age, and genetics. These factors affect the magnitude and rate of long-term adaptations that occur in the body. The following subsections explore these topics.

Specificity

Exercise training has been shown to be highly specific. That is, the body adapts to exercise in such a way that it can perform optimally in relation to that particular type of exercise stressor, but not necessarily other types of exercise. For instance, distance running has little to no positive effect on bench press performance. However, specificity also influences resistance exercise adaptations. In terms of resistance exercises, the correlations between static and dynamic performance are poor [4]. A variety of studies have examined the effect of one type of resistance training on performance of other types of resistance exercise. In general, strength increases are larger in modes of exercise like those used during training. For example, resistance training with weights results in much larger performance increases on the weights than are seen with isokinetic tests [104]. Isometric exercise training has also been shown to have little to no effect on performance of free weight exercises that involve the same muscle groups. Thus, it appears that the effects of resistance training are specific to the contraction mode with which the exercise was performed.

Resistance training adaptations are also specific with respect to the velocity with which contractions have been performed in training. That is, strength increases tend to be greater when individuals are tested in situations that involve contractions occurring at velocities similar to those experienced during training [6, 104]. Therefore, for people who are performing resistance exercise to improve athletic performance, one should tailor the training program as much as possible to involve types of contractions similar to those seen during the athletic competition. Likewise, although all clients will benefit from a well-rounded resistance training program, an older client desiring the strength and endurance to carry heavy bags of groceries long distances would benefit from walking with handweights, and a client desiring the strength to do home improvement projects such as pounding fence posts or repairing a deck would benefit from pushing and pulling exercises.

Sex

Males and females respond to resistance training in much the same manner. There is no adaptation disparity between the sexes, yet males and females show significant quantitative differences in strength, muscle mass, and hormone levels. With respect to muscle strength, much of the difference between the sexes is attributable to differences in body size and body composition. Specifically, men tend to be larger than women, and the associated differences in muscle mass contribute to strength differences. Similarly, women tend to have a higher percentage of body fat than men; therefore most women have less muscle per pound of body weight. These differences in body size and body composition are largely driven by differences in hormone levels between men and women, most notably differences in testosterone and estrogen levels. Interestingly, sex-related differences in strength are larger in the upper body than in the lower body [9], which likely reflects sex differences in the distribution of muscle mass [75]. That is, women and men tend to exhibit similar lower body strength, whereas men typically have much greater upper body strength than women.

When one looks at sex differences in strength on a per pound of fat-free mass basis, strength differences shrink [9, 108]. When assessed per unit of muscle cross-sectional area, sex differences are negligible [50]. Furthermore, muscle architecture characteristics are similar between males and females [1]. Thus it appears that the force production capability of a given amount of muscle is not affected by whether one is male or female.

The force production capability of a given amount of muscle is not affected by a person's sex.

Age

The process of aging produces a variety of changes in all body systems. The neuromuscular system is no exception. Starting in the 30s, muscle mass appears to decline progressively with time [52]. This loss of muscle mass is referred to as **sarcopenia.** In addition to the loss in muscle mass, some evidence suggests that muscle quality also declines with age [27]. That is, for a given amount of muscle, the amount of force that can be generated by that muscle declines. Aging skeletal muscle experiences muscle loss more severely in the high-threshold fast-twitch motor units [65]. Therefore, as individuals age they not only have diminished ability to produce force; they also have diminished ability to produce force rapidly. These aging effects on skeletal muscle affect performance in physical tasks such as those required for everyday activities, and may be associated with the increased incidence of falls that occurs with age.

As individuals age they not only have diminished ability to produce force; they also have diminished ability to produce force rapidly.

Fortunately, these deleterious effects of aging can be moderated or even reversed (over the short term) with a program of high-intensity resistance training. Numerous studies have shown that resistance training can increase muscle mass and strength in persons who are elderly [14, 24, 26]. In addition, the training can result in significant improvements in muscle function in particular and also general motor performance (e.g., walking, stair climbing) [25]. Strength gains can be dramatic (upward of 200% for knee extension strength), and increases in muscle size may occur in both Type I and Type II muscle fibers [26]. Resistance training in people who are elderly also increases bone density [79]. Chapter 18 presents a more comprehensive overview of resistance training in older adults.

Genetics

Information about the physiological variables mentioned in the previous sections collectively demonstrates that human beings do not pick their successful activities as much as the activities pick them. This is due at least in part to what each individual brings to the table when beginning a resistance training program. Several factors are beyond an individual's capacity to change. That is, people are limited by their genetic potential. Relative percentage of Type I and Type II fibers limits hypertrophy and either explosive or aerobic endurance capabilities. Sex plays a role in hormonal expression, further placing a ceiling on hypertrophy and thereby strength. Age limits the available muscle mass and the propagation of action potentials, which together limit not only strength but also the speed of movement. A personal trainer cannot devise a program that will take a client beyond the client's genetic capabilities. However, the average untrained client can make much improvement within that client's genetic potential.

Overtraining

Although physical adaptations are best brought about by increases in training volume and intensity, at certain points in a training program, more is not better. Inappropriate levels of volume or intensity can lead to a phenomenon known as **overtraining.** As the term suggests, overtraining is a condition in which an individual trains too much, resulting in "staleness" and general fatigue. The overtraining condition does not enhance strength and power levels in the client but leads to decreased performance. A detailed discussion of the many aspects of resistance exercise overtraining (e.g., metabolic, neuromuscular, endocrine) as both a physical and a psychological phenomenon is beyond the scope of this chapter, and the reader is referred to other detailed reviews on the topic [28, 95]. Because of the danger of overtraining, the toleration of and recovery from resistance exercise stress are crucial factors that must be monitored carefully in every resistance training program.

Overtraining in resistance exercise has received much less attention than aerobic overtraining, as significantly fewer studies have been reported. These studies make it clear that what we have found to be markers of overtraining in aerobic endurance exercise are not always representative of overtraining in resistance exercise. It appears that the two primary types of overtraining in resistance exercise are too much intensity and too much volume [28]. Yet each has been difficult to study. However, it is clear that resistance exercise overtraining can lead to decreases in neuromuscular performance [12, 29, 30, 31, 32]. It is interesting to note that, at least in experimental situations, inducing an overtraining state requires a very severe exercise intervention but can be accomplished through repeated bouts of high-intensity exercise (~100% 1RM [1-repetition maximum]) but with relatively low volume [29, 30, 31]. Many overtraining syndromes are a function of the rate of progression—that is, attempting to do too much too soon before the body's physiological adaptations can cope with the stress. This typically results in extreme soreness or injury.

Individuals may fall into either or both of two overtraining scenarios: (1) overtraining of a muscle group or (2) overtraining of the body. Both scenarios are common, and many people may experience both. Overtraining is most often a result of increasing the volume of the program at too rapid a pace. In addition, some people may maintain too many days at high intensity without varying their load or taking a rest. Effective program design includes increasing and decreasing the total volume of the workout and using the concepts of periodization to plan changes in volume, intensity, and recovery [95] (see chapter 23). The difficulty in dealing with real overtraining and the symptoms that may develop is that there is no 100% accurate measurement for the onset of overtraining: Generally, once symptoms develop, overtraining is certain and strength gains have stopped. Once symptoms have developed, the most effective cure is rest [28].

Some programs utilize short periods of overwork followed by rest or reduced training to achieve the benefits of a "rebound" or supercompensation in physical strength and power [28]. This process of "overreaching" is best used only by elite athletes in conjunction with experienced coaches, and most clients would be best served by more moderate training regimens.

Symptoms of Overtraining From Resistance Exercise

- Plateau followed by decrease of strength gains
- Sleep disturbances
- Decrease in lean body mass (when not dieting)
- Decreased appetite
- A cold that just won't go away
- Persistent flu-like symptoms
- Loss of interest in the training program
- Mood changes
- Excessive muscle soreness

Detraining

Detraining refers to the physiological and performance adaptations that occur when an individual ceases an exercise training program. These changes are the exact opposite of what occurs during training programs, and the individual regresses toward his or her condition prior to starting the program. Specifically, muscle tissue loses mass [48, 93], and the changes in neurological function (e.g., recruitment, rate coding, co-contraction) that occurred with training dissipate [39]. Thus the muscle becomes weaker and less powerful. Skeletal muscle atrophy appears to occur faster in the fast-twitch muscle fibers [48].

There is relatively little research on the detraining process with resistance training as compared to the training process, so the rapidity of the detraining process is poorly understood. However, short-term detraining (14 days) appears to have little effect on muscle strength and explosive power in experienced resistance-trained athletes [48] and recreational strength trainers [59], suggesting that the effects are relatively slow. Extended detraining (32 weeks) did result in significant decreases in muscle strength in previously resistance-trained females, but values were still above pretraining levels [93]. Detraining appears to affect different aspects of neuromuscular performance differently. For example, isometric strength performance appears to decay more rapidly than other strength measures [59, 102, 103]. Similarly, performance on anaerobic metabolic tests (i.e., Wingate test) is more severely affected by detraining than performance on strength and explosive power tests [59]. The effects of detraining can be significantly reduced with the incorporation of just one to two training sessions per week [35]; clients with unexpectedly busy or difficult schedules may maintain a certain level of strength by training once or twice a week.

CONCLUSION

Resistance training is a very potent physiological stimulus. It has substantive effects on almost every system in the body, including effects on muscle, bone, nerve, hormones, and connective tissue. Although resistance training is not a panacea, its effects are almost universally positive; and personal trainers should encourage all clients to engage in a vigorous program of resistance training. Benefits include improved appearance, improved body composition, increased muscle strength and power, increased muscle endurance, and stronger bones and connective tissue. These changes can improve quality of life and may have significant health benefits, including the attenuation of the deleterious effects of sarcopenia during aging and possibly attenuation of the effects of osteoporosis. In addition, the increased muscle performance (strength, endurance, power) will likely improve the performance of activities of daily living, so that tasks like carrying groceries and changing a tire are more easily accomplished.

STUDY QUESTIONS

1. Which of the following is most likely to occur during a set of 10 repetitions at 75% of the 1RM for the squat exercise?
   A. motor unit recruitment increases
   B. rate coding decreases
   C. muscle pH increases
   D. ATP stores increase
2. Which of the following is most responsible for the strength gain a client would experience following three weeks of a beginning resistance training program?
   A. muscle hypertrophy
   B. muscle hyperplasia
   C. increased co-contraction
   D. improved skill in performing the exercise
3. Which of the following are the most influential age-related changes that may decrease a client's ability to exhibit muscular strength?
   I. decreased ability to produce force rapidly
   II. decreased bone density
   III. decreased muscle mass
   IV. decreased muscle glycogen stores
   A. I and III only
   B. II and IV only
   C. I and IV only
   D. II and III only
4. All of the following are symptoms of overtraining from resistance exercise EXCEPT:
   A. increased hunger and thirst
   B. inconsistent or interrupted sleep
   C. nonpurposeful decreases in lean body mass
   D. leveled-off improvements or losses in muscular strength

APPLIED KNOWLEDGE QUESTION

Complete the following chart to describe two ways the body's systems adapt to chronic participation in a resistance training program.

System	Two adaptations
Nervous	
Muscular	
Skeletal	
Metabolic	
Hormonal	
Cardiovascular	

REFERENCES

1. Abe, T., W.F. Brechue, S. Fujita, and J.B. Brown. 1998. Gender differences in FFM accumulation and architectural characteristics of muscle. *Medicine and Science in Sports and Exercise* 30 (7): 1066-1070.
2. American College of Sports Medicine. 1995. Position stand: Osteoporosis and exercise. *Medicine and Science in Sports and Exercise* 27: i-vii.
3. Antonio, J., and W.J. Gonyea. 1993. Skeletal muscle hyperplasia. *Medicine and Science in Sports and Exercise* 25 (12): 1333-1345.
4. Baker, D., G. Wilson, and B. Carlyon. 1994. Generality versus specificity: A comparison of dynamic and isometric measures of strength and speed-power. *European Journal of Applied Physiology* 68 (4): 350-355.
5. Basmajian, J.V., and C.J. DeLuca. 1985. *Muscles Alive: Their Functions Revealed by Electromyography,* 5th ed. Baltimore: Williams & Wilkins, p. 164.
6. Behm, D.G., and D.G. Sale. 1993. Intended rather than actual movement velocity determines velocity-specific training response. *Journal of Applied Physiology* 74 (1): 359-368.
7. Bellemare, F., J.J. Woods, R. Johansson, and B. Bigland-Ritchie. 1983. Motor unit discharge rates in maximal voluntary contractions of three human muscles. *Journal of Neurophysiology* 50: 1380-1392.
8. Bemben, D.A., N.L. Fetters, M.G. Bemben, N. Nabavi, and E.T. Koh. 2000. Musculoskeletal responses to high- and low-intensity resistance training in early postmenopausal women. *Medicine and Science in Sports and Exercise* 32 (11): 1949-1957.
9. Bishop, P., K. Cureton, and M. Collins. 1987. Sex difference in muscular strength in equally-trained men and women. *Ergonomics* 30 (4): 675-687.
10. Braith, R.W., J.E. Graves, S.H. Leggett, and M.L. Pollock. 1993. Effect of training on the relationship between maximal and submaximal strength. *Medicine and Science in Sports and Exercise* 25 (1): 132-138.
11. Broeder, C.E., K.A. Burrhus, L.S. Svanevik, and J.H. Wilmore. 1992. The effects of either high-intensity resistance or endurance training on resting metabolic rate. *American Journal of Clinical Nutrition* 55 (4): 802-810.
12. Callister, R., R.J. Callister, S.J. Fleck, and G.A. Dudley. 1990. Physiological and performance responses to overtraining in elite judo athletes. *Medicine and Science in Sports and Exercise* 22 (6): 816-824.
13. Carolan, B., and E. Cafarelli. 1992. Adaptations in coactivation after isometric resistance training. *Journal of Applied Physiology* 73 (3): 911-917.
14. Charette, S.L., L. McEvoy, G. Pyka, C. Snow-Harter, D. Guido, R.A. Wiswell, and R. Marcus. 1991. Muscle hypertrophy response to resistance training in older women. *Journal of Applied Physiology* 70: 1912-1916.
15. Chesley, A., J.D. MacDougall, M.A. Tarnopolsky, S.A. Atkinson, and K. Smith. 1992. Changes in human muscle protein synthesis after resistance exercise. *Journal of Applied Physiology* 73 (4): 1383-1388.
16. Colliander, E.B., and P.A. Tesch. 1990. Effects of eccentric and concentric muscle actions in resistance training. *Acta Physiologica Scandinavica* 140: 31-39.
17. Collins, M.A., K.J. Cureton, D.W. Hill, and C.A. Ray. 1991. Relationship between heart rate to oxygen uptake during weight lifting exercise. *Medicine and Science in Sports and Exercise* 23 (5): 636-640.
18. Costill, D.L., E.F. Coyle, W.F. Fink, G.R. Lesmes, and F.A. Witzman. 1979. Adaptations in skeletal muscle following strength training. *Journal of Applied Physiology* 46: 96-99.
19. Cullinen, K., and M. Caldwell. 1998. Weight training increases fat-free mass and strength in untrained young women. *Journal of the American Dietetic Association* 98 (4): 414-418.
20. DeLuca, C.J. 1997. The use of surface electromyography in biomechanics. *Journal of Applied Biomechanics* 13: 135-163.
21. Deschenes, M. 1989. Short review: Rate coding and motor unit recruitment patterns. *Journal of Applied Sport Science Research* 3 (2): 33-39.
22. Dons, B., K. Bollerup, F. Bonde-Peterson, and S. Hanacke. 1979. The effect of weight-lifting exercise related to muscle fiber composition and muscle cross-sectional area in humans. *European Journal of Applied Physiology* 40: 95-106.
23. Enoka, R.M. 1994. *Neuromechanical Basis of Kinesiology,* 2nd ed. Champaign, IL: Human Kinetics, p. 194.
24. Fiatarone, M.A., E.C. Marks, N.D. Ryan, C.N. Meredith, L.A. Lipsitz, and W.J. Evans. 1990. High-intensity strength training in nonagenarians. Effects on skeletal muscle. *Journal of the American Medical Association* 263: 3029-3034.
25. Fiatarone, M.A., E.R. O'Neill, N.D. Ryan, K.M. Clements, G.R. Solares, M.E. Nelson, S.B. Roberts, J.J. Kehayias, L.A. Lipsitz, and W.J. Evans. 1994. Exercise training and nutritional supplementation for physical frailty in very elderly people. *New England Journal of Medicine* 330 (25): 1769-1775.
26. Frontera, W.R., C.N. Meredith, K.P. O'Reilly, H.G. Knuttgen, and W.J. Evans. 1988. Strength conditioning in older men: Skeletal muscle hypertrophy and improved function. *Journal of Applied Physiology* 64: 1038-1044.
27. Frontera, W.R., D. Suh, L.S. Krivickas, V.A. Hughes, R. Goldstein, and R. Roubenoff. 2000. Skeletal muscle fiber quality in older men and women. *American Journal of Physiology* 279: C611-C616.
28. Fry, A.C., and W.J. Kraemer. 1997. Resistance exercise overtraining and overreaching. *Sports Medicine* 23 (2): 106-129.
29. Fry, A.C., W.J. Kraemer, J.M. Lynch, N.T. Triplett, and L.P. Koziris. 1994. Does short-term near maximal intensity machine resistance training induce overtraining? *Journal of Strength and Conditioning Research* 8 (3): 188-191.
30. Fry, A.C., W.J. Kraemer, F. Van Borselen, J.M. Lynch, J.L. Marsit, E.P. Roy, N.T. Triplett, and H.G. Knuttgen. 1994. Performance decrements with high-intensity resistance exercise overtraining. *Medicine and Science in Sports and Exercise* 26 (9): 1165-1173.
31. Fry, A.C., W.J. Kraemer, F. Van Borselen, J.M. Lynch, N.T. Triplett, L.P. Koziris, and S.J. Fleck. 1994. Catecholamine responses to short-term, high-intensity resistance exercise overtraining. *Journal of Applied Physiology* 77 (2): 941-946.
32. Fry, A.C., J.M. Webber, L.W. Weiss, M.D. Fry, and Y. Li. 2000. Impaired performances with excessive high-intensity free-weight training. *Journal of Strength and Conditioning Research* 14 (1): 54-61.
33. Garfinkel, S., and E. Cafarelli. 1992. Relative changes in maximal force, EMG, and muscle cross-sectional area after isometric training. *Medicine and Science in Sports and Exercise* 24: 1220-1227.
34. Goldspink, G. 1992. Cellular and molecular aspects of adaptation in skeletal muscle. In: *Strength and Power in Sport:*

The Encyclopedia of Sports Medicine, P.V. Komi, ed. Oxford, England: Blackwell Scientific, pp. 211-229.

35. Graves, J.E., M.L. Pollock, S.H. Leggett, R.W. Braith, D.M. Carpenter, and L.E. Bishop. 1988. Effect of reduced training frequency on muscular strength. *International Journal of Sports Medicine* 9 (5): 316-319.
36. Green, H., C. Goreham, J. Ouyang, M. Bull-Burnett, and D. Ranney. 1999. Regulation of fiber size, oxidative potential, and capillarization in human muscle by resistance exercise. *American Journal of Physiology* 276 (2 Pt 2): R591-R596.
37. Guezennec, Y., L. Leger, F. Lhoste, M. Aymonod, and P.C. Pesquies. 1986. Hormone and metabolite response to weight-lifting training sessions. *International Journal of Sports Medicine* 7: 100-105.
38. Haff, G.G., M.H. Stone, B.J. Warren, R. Keith, R.L. Johnson, D.C. Nieman, F. Williams, and K.B. Kirksey. 1999. The effect of carbohydrate supplementation on multiple sessions and bouts of resistance exercise. *Journal of Strength and Conditioning Research* 13(3): 111-117.
39. Häkkinen, K., and P.V. Komi. 1983. Electromyographic changes during strength training and detraining. *Medicine and Science in Sports and Exercise* 15: 455-460.
40. Häkkinen, K., A. Parkarinen, M. Alen, H. Kauhanen, and P.V. Komi. 1988. Neuromuscular and hormonal adaptations in athletes to strength training in two years. *Journal of Applied Physiology* 65: 2406-2412.
41. Häkkinen, K., A. Pakarinen, W.J. Kraemer, A. Häkkinen, H. Valkeinen, and M. Alen. 2001. Selective muscle hypertrophy, changes in EMG and force, and serum hormones during strength training in older women. *Journal of Applied Physiology* 91 (2): 569-580.
42. Häkkinen, K., A. Pakarinen, W.J. Kraemer, R.U. Newton, and M. Alen. 2000. Basal concentrations and acute responses of serum hormones and strength development during heavy resistance training in middle-aged and elderly men and women. *Journal of Gerontology* 55 (2): B95-B105.
43. Harris, R.T., and G.A. Dudley. 2000. Neuromuscular anatomy and adaptations to conditioning. In: *Essentials of Strength Training and Conditioning,* T.R. Baechle and R.W. Earle, eds. Champaign, IL: Human Kinetics, pp. 15-23.
44. Hather, B.M., P.A. Tesch, P. Buchannon, and G.A. Dudley. 1991. Influence of eccentric actions on skeletal muscle adaptation to resistance training. *Acta Physiologica Scandinavica* 143: 177-185.
45. Hellebrandt, F.A., A.M. Parrish, and J.J. Houtz. 1947. Cross education: The influence of unilateral exercise on the contralateral limb. *Archives of Physical Medicine* 28: 76-85.
46. Hickson, R.C., B.A. Dvorak, E.M. Gorostiaga, T.T. Kurowski, and C. Foster. 1988. Potential for strength and endurance training to amplify endurance performance. *Journal of Applied Physiology* 65: 2285-2290.
47. Hoff, J., J. Helgerud, and U. Wisloff. 1999. Maximal strength training improves work economy in trained female cross-country skiers. *Medicine and Science in Sports and Exercise* 31 (6): 870-877.
48. Hortobagyi, T., J.A. Houmard, J.R. Stevenson, D.D. Fraser, R.A. Johns, and R.G. Israel. 1993. The effects of detraining in power athletes. *Medicine and Science in Sports and Exercise* 28 (8): 929-935.
49. Hunter, G.R., C.J. Wetzstein, D.A. Fields, A. Brown, and M.M. Bamman. 2000. Resistance training increases total energy expenditure and free-living physical activity in older adults. *Journal of Applied Physiology* 89 (3): 977-984.
50. Ikai, M., and T. Fukunaga. 1968. Calculation of muscle strength per unit cross-sectional area of human muscle by means of ultrasonic measurement. *Int Z Angew Physiol* 26 (1): 26-32.
51. Ikai, M., and A.H. Steinhaus. 1961. Some factors modifying the expression of human strength. *Journal of Applied Physiology* 16: 157-163.
52. Imamura, K., H. Ashida, T. Ishikawawa, and M. Fujii. 1983. Human major psoas muscle and sacrospinalis muscle in relation to age: a study by computed tomography. *Journal of Gerontology* 38 (6): 678-681.
53. Inoue, K., S. Yamasaki, T. Fushiki, T. Kano, T. Moritani, K. Itoh, and E. Sugimoto. 1993. Rapid increase in the number of androgen receptors following electrical stimulation. *European Journal of Applied Physiology* 66 (2): 134-140.
54. Kitai, T.A., and D.G. Sale. 1989. Specificity of joint angle in isometric testing. *European Journal of Applied Physiology* 58: 744-748.
55. Komi, P.V., J.T. Viitasalo, R. Rauramaa, and V. Vihko. 1978. Effect of isometric strength training on mechanical, electrical, and metabolic aspects of muscle function. *European Journal of Applied Physiology* 40: 45-55.
56. Kraemer, W.J. 1992. Endocrine responses and adaptations to strength training. In: *Strength and Power in Sport: The Encyclopedia of Sports Medicine,* P.V. Komi, ed. Oxford, England: Blackwell Scientific, pp. 291-304.
57. Kraemer W.J., S.J. Fleck, and W.J. Evans. 1996. Strength and power: Physiological mechanisms of adaptation. *Exercise and Sport Science Reviews* 24: 363-397.
58. Kraemer, W.J., K. Häkkinen, R.U. Newton, M. McCormick, B.C. Nindl, J.S. Volek, L.A. Gotshalk, S.J. Fleck, W.W. Campbell, S.E. Gordon, P.A. Farrell, and W.J. Evans. 1998. Acute hormonal responses to heavy resistance exercise in younger and older men. *European Journal of Applied Physiology* 77 (3): 206-211.
59. Kraemer, W.J., L.P. Koziris, N.A. Ratamess, K. Häkkinen, N.T. Triplett-McBride, A.C. Fry, S.E. Gordon, J.S. Volek, D.N. French, M.R. Rubin, A.L. Gomez, M.T. Sharman, J.M. Lynch, M. Izquierdo, R.U. Newton, and S.J. Fleck. 2002. Detraining produces minimal changes in physical performance and hormonal variables in recreationally strength-trained men. *Journal of Strength and Conditioning Research* 16 (3): 373-382.
60. Kraemer, W.J., B.J. Noble, B. Culver, and R.V. Lewis. 1985. Changes in plasma proenkephalin peptide F and catecholamine levels during graded exercise in men. *Proceedings of the National Academy of Sciences* 82: 6349-6351.
61. Kraemer, W.J., J.F. Patton, S.E. Gordon, E.A. Harman, M.R. Deschenes, K. Reynolds, R.U. Newton, N.T. Triplett, and J.E. Dziados. 1995. Compatibility of high intensity strength and endurance training on hormonal and skeletal muscle adaptations. *Journal of Applied Physiology* 78 (3): 976-989.
62. Kraemer, W.J., R.S. Staron, F.C. Hagerman, R.S. Hikida, A.C. Fry, S.E. Gordon, B.C. Nindl, L.A. Gotshalk, J.S. Volek, J.O. Marx, R.U. Newton, and K. Häkkinen. 1998. The effects of short-term resistance training on endocrine function in men and women. *European Journal of Applied Physiology* 78 (1): 69-76.
63. LaCerte, M., B.J. deLateur, A.P. Alquist, and K.A. Questad. 1992. Concentric versus combined concentric-eccentric isokinetic training programs: Effect on peak torque of human quadriceps femoris muscle. *Archives of Physical Medicine and Rehabilitation* 73: 1059-1062.
64. Lambert, C.P., and M.G. Flynn. 2002. Fatigue during high-intensity intermittent exercise. Applications to bodybuilding. *Sports Medicine* 32 (8): 511-522.

65. Larsson, L. 1978. Morphological and functional characteristics of the ageing skeletal muscle in man. *Acta Physiologica Scandinavica* (Suppl) 457: 1-36.
66. Leveritt, M., and P.J. Abernethy. 1999. Effect of carbohydrate restriction on strength performance. *Journal of Strength and Conditioning Research* 13: 52-57.
67. MacDougall, J.D., M.J. Gibala, M.A. Tarnopolsky, J.R. MacDonald, S.A. Interisano, and K.E. Yarasheski. 1995. The time course for elevated muscle protein synthesis following heavy resistance exercise. *Canadian Journal of Applied Physiology* 20 (4): 480-486.
68. MacDougall, J.D., S. Ray, D.G. Sale, N. McCartney, P. Lee, and S. Garner. 1999. Muscle substrate utilization and lactate production during weightlifting. *Canadian Journal of Applied Physiology* 24: 209-215.
69. MacDougall, J.D., G.R. Ward, D.G. Sale, and J.R. Sutton. 1977. Biochemical adaptation of human skeletal muscle to heavy resistance training and immobilization. *Journal of Applied Physiology* 43: 700-703.
70. MacLaren, D.P., H. Gibson, M. Parry-Billings, and R.H.T. Edwards. 1989. A review of metabolic and physiological factors in fatigue. *Exercise and Sport Sciences Reviews* 17: 29-66.
71. Maddalozzo, G.F., and C.M. Snow. 2000. High intensity resistance training: Effects on bone in older men and women. *Calcified Tissue International* 66: 399-404.
72. Marcinik, E.J., J. Potts, G. Schlabach, S. Will, P. Dawson, and B.F. Hurley. 1991. Effects of strength training on lactate threshold and endurance performance. *Medicine and Science in Sports and Exercise* 23: 739-743.
73. Masuda, K., T. Masuda, T. Sadoyama, M. Inaki, and S. Katsuta. 1999. Changes in surface EMG parameters during static and dynamic fatiguing contractions. *Journal of Electromyography and Kinesiology* 9 (1): 39-46.
74. Merton, P.A. 1954. Voluntary strength and fatigue. *Journal of Physiology (London)* 123: 553-564.
75. Miller, A.E.J., J.D. MacDougall, M.A. Tarnopolsky, and D.G. Sale. 1993. Gender differences in strength and muscle fiber characteristics. *European Journal of Applied Physiology* 66: 254-262.
76. Milner-Brown, H.S., R.B. Stein, and R.G. Lee. 1975. Synchronization of human motor units: Possible roles of exercise and supraspinal reflexes. *Electroencephalography and Clinical Neurophysiology* 38: 245-254.
77. Moritani, T., and H.A. deVries. 1979. Neural factors vs. hypertrophy in the time course of muscle strength gain. *American Journal of Physical Medicine* 58: 115-130.
78. Moritani, T., and Y. Yoshitake. 1998. 1998 ISEK Congress Keynote Lecture. The use of surface electromyography in applied physiology. *Journal of Electromyography and Kinesiology* 8: 363-381.
79. Nelson, M.E., M.A. Fiatarone, C.M. Morganti, I. Trice, R.A. Greenberg, and W.J. Evans. 1994. Effects of high-intensity strength training on multiple risk factors for osteoporotic fractures. *Journal of the American Medical Association* 272: 1909-1914.
80. Osternig, L.R., J. Hamill, J.E. Lander, and R. Robertson. 1986. Co-activation of sprinter and distance runner muscles in isokinetic exercise. *Medicine and Science in Sports and Exercise* 18: 431-435.
81. Paavolainen, L., K. Häkkinen, I. Hamalainen, A. Nummela, and H. Rusko. 1999. Explosive-strength training improves 5-km running time by improving running economy and muscle power. *Journal of Applied Physiology* 86: 1527-1533.
82. Patten, C., G. Kamen, and D.M. Rowland. 2001. Adaptations in maximal motor unit discharge rate to strength training in young and older adults. *Muscle and Nerve* 24 (4): 542-550.
83. Poehlman, E.T., W.F. Denino, T. Beckett, K.A. Kinaman, I.J. Dionne, R. Dvorak, and P.A. Ades. 2002. Effects of endurance and resistance training on total daily energy expenditure in young women: A controlled randomized trial. *Journal of Clinical Endocrinology and Metabolism* 87 (3): 1004-1009.
84. Pruitt, L.A., D.R. Taaffe, and R. Marcus. 1995. Effects of a one-year high-intensity versus low-intensity resistance training program on bone mineral density in older women. *Journal of Bone Mineral Research* 10: 1788-1795.
85. Psek, J.A., and E. Cafarelli. 1993. Behavior of coactive muscles during fatigue. *Journal of Applied Physiology* 74: 170-175.
86. Robergs, R.A., D.R. Pearson, D.L. Costill, W.J. Fink, D.D. Pascoe, M.A. Benedict, C.P. Lambert, and J.J. Zachweija. 1991. Muscle glycogenolysis during different intensities of weight-resistance exercise. *Journal of Applied Physiology* 70 (4): 1700-1706.
87. Rutherford, O.M., D.A. Jones, and D.J. Newham. 1986. Clinical and experimental application of percutaneous twitch superimposition technique for the study of human muscle activation. *Journal of Neurology, Neurosurgery, and Psychiatry* 49: 1288-1291.
88. Sale, D.G. 1992. Neural adaptation to strength training. In: *Strength and Power in Sport: The Encyclopedia of Sports Medicine,* P.V. Komi, ed. Oxford, England: Blackwell Scientific, pp. 249-265.
89. Sale, D.G., J.D. MacDougall, A.R.M. Upton, and A.J. McComas. 1983. Effects of strength training upon motoneuron excitability in man. *Medicine and Science in Sports and Exercise* 15: 57-62.
90. Schuenke, M.D., R.P. Mikat, and J.M. McBride. 2002. Effect of an acute period of resistance exercise on excess post-exercise oxygen consumption: Implications for body mass management. *European Journal of Applied Physiology* 86: 411-417.
91. Schwab, R., G.O. Johnson, T.J. Housh, J.E. Kinder, and J.P. Weir. 1993. Acute effects of different intensities of weightlifting on serum testosterone. *Medicine and Science in Sports and Exercise* 25: 1381-1385.
92. Staron, R.S., D.L. Karapondo, W.J. Kraemer, A.C. Fry, S.E. Gordon, J.E. Falkel, F.C. Hagerman, and R.S. Hikida. 1994. Skeletal muscle adaptations during early phase of heavy-resistance training in men and women. *Journal of Applied Physiology* 76: 1247-1255.
93. Staron, R.S., M.J. Leonardi, D.L. Karapondo, E.S. Malicky, J.E. Falkel, F.G. Hagerman, and R.S. Hikida. 1991. Strength and skeletal muscle adaptations in heavy-resistance trained women after detraining and retraining. *Journal of Applied Physiology* 70 (2): 631-640.
94. Staron, R.S., E.S. Malicky, M.J. Leonardi, J.E. Falkel, F.C. Hagerman, and G.A. Dudley. 1990. Muscle hypertrophy and fast fiber type conversions in heavy resistance-trained women. *European Journal of Applied Physiology* 60: 71-79.
95. Stone, M.H., R.E. Keith, J.T. Kearny, S.J. Fleck, G.D. Wilson, and N.T. Triplett. 1991. Overtraining: A review of the signs, symptoms, and possible causes. *Journal of Applied Sport Science Research* 5 (1): 35-50.
96. Stone, W.J., and S.P. Coulter. 1994. Strength/endurance effects from three resistance training protocols with women. *Journal of Strength and Conditioning Research* 8 (4): 231-234.

97. Tesch, P.A. 1992. Short- and long-term histochemical and biochemical adaptations in muscle. In: *Strength and Power in Sport: The Encyclopedia of Sports Medicine,* P. Komi, ed. Oxford, England: Blackwell Scientific, pp. 239-248.

98. Tesch, P.A., A. Thorsson, and E.B. Colliander. 1990. Effects of eccentric and concentric resistance training on skeletal muscle substrates, enzyme activities and capillary supply. *Acta Physiologica Scandinavica* 140: 575-580.

99. Thepaut-Mathieu, C., J. Van Hoecke, and B. Maton. 1988. Myoelectrical and mechanical changes linked to length specificity during isometric training. *Journal of Applied Physiology* 64: 1500-1505.

100. Tipton, K.D., and R.R. Wolfe. 2001. Exercise protein metabolism and muscle growth. *International Journal of Sport Nutrition and Exercise Metabolism* 11 (1): 109-132.

101. Vincent, K.R., and R.W. Braith. 2002. Resistance exercise and bone turnover in elderly men and women. *Medicine and Science in Sports and Exercise* 34: 17-23.

102. Weir, J.P., D.J. Housh, T.J. Housh, and L.L. Weir. 1995. The effect of unilateral eccentric weight training detraining on joint angle specificity, cross-training, and the bilateral deficit. *Journal of Orthopaedic and Sports Physical Therapy* 22 (5): 207-215.

103. Weir, J.P., D.J. Housh, T.J. Housh, and L.L. Weir. 1997. The effect of unilateral concentric weight training and detraining on joint angle specificity, cross-training, and the bilateral deficit. *Journal of Orthopaedic and Sports Physical Therapy* 25: 264-270.

104. Weir, J.P., T.J. Housh, S.A. Evans, and G.O. Johnson. 1993. The effect of dynamic constant external resistance training on the isokinetic torque-velocity curve. *International Journal of Sports Medicine* 14 (3): 124-128.

105. Weir, J.P., T.J. Housh, and L.L. Weir. 1994. Electromyographic evaluation of joint angle specificity and cross-training after isometric training. *Journal of Applied Physiology* 77: 197-201.

106. Weir, J.P., T.J. Housh, L.L. Weir, and G.O. Johnson. 1995. Effects of unilateral isometric strength training on joint angle specificity and cross-training. *European Journal of Applied Physiology* 70: 337-343.

107. Weir, J.P., D.A. Keefe, J.F. Eaton, R.T. Augustine, and D.M. Tobin. 1998. Effect of fatigue on hamstring coactivation during isokinetic knee extensions. *European Journal of Applied Physiology* 78: 555-559.

108. Winter, E.M., and R.J. Maughan. 1991. Strength and cross-sectional area of the quadriceps in men and women. *Journal of Physiology (London)* 438: 175.

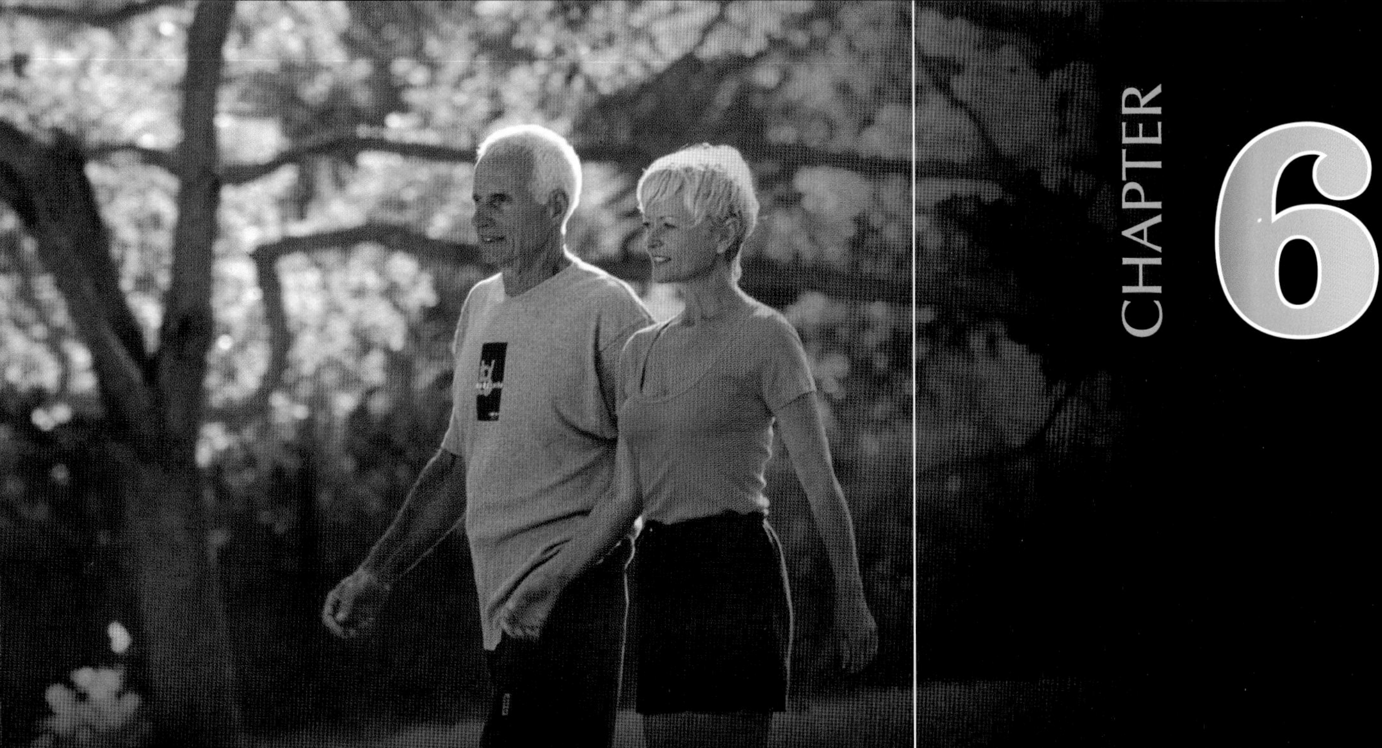

Aerobic Training Adaptations

Lee E. Brown | Matthew J. Comeau

After completing this chapter, you will be able to

- identify acute physiological responses to aerobic training;
- identify chronic physiological adaptations to aerobic training;
- understand the factors that influence adaptations to aerobic training;
- understand and identify the physiological factors associated with overtraining; and
- identify the physiological consequences of detraining.

The primary purpose of this chapter is to discuss the effects of aerobic exercise on the body's physiological processes and to explain the adaptations that occur. The effects of aerobic exercise are regulated by the intensity, frequency, and duration of the activity. Paramount among these is intensity. In other words, the body adapts to a stressor in proportion to that stressor. Generally speaking, then, if one exercises at a greater heart rate during aerobic exercise, the training adaptation will be greater than if one exercises at a lower heart rate. Of course, this assumes that frequency and duration are constant across aerobic training sessions. It is the interplay of these components that results in aerobic physiological changes. A word of caution is relevant, though, in that maximal or extreme exercise often can hinder training adaptation.

Basic Adaptations to Aerobic Training

With aerobic training, the body adapts through alteration of physiological processes or systems as indicated in table 6.1. The sections that follow explain in further detail exactly how these changes occur.

The overall adaptation to recurring aerobic exercise is one that represents a more efficient body, resulting in less effort by all organs at every possible level of exercise.

Cardiovascular Changes

The cardiovascular system consists of two components: (1) the heart and (2) the vasculature (i.e., blood vessels). An understanding of how each component is affected by aerobic training is important for the personal trainer.

Heart

The heart adapts well to the stresses placed on it. In the presence of certain chemicals, such as epinephrine, norepinephrine, and acetylcholine, the heart increases or decreases the rate at which it works. The changes that occur due to aerobic training will occur acutely due to presence of chemicals and will continue to occur with prolonged periods of training. The following sections detail the acute and chronic changes associated with aerobic training. For specific information with regard to the cardiovascular system's structure and function, refer to chapter 2.

TABLE 6.1

Summary of Adaptations to Aerobic Conditioning in Untrained Individuals

Variable	Response
$\dot{V}O_2$max	↑
Resting heart rate	↓
Exercise heart rate (submax)	↓
Maximum heart rate	↔ or slight ↓
a-$\bar{v}O_2$ difference	↑
Stroke volume	↑
Cardiac output	↑
Systolic blood pressure	↔ or slight ↑
Oxidative capacity of the muscle	↑

Reprinted from American College of Sport Medicine 1998.

Acute Reponses

During exercise, an increased stimulation or excitation of the heart occurs in order to supply blood to parts of the body where it is needed, such as skeletal musculature. Although this is not the only reason for an increase in blood flow, a simple explanation is excitation of the heart, or lack thereof, as the sympathetic nervous system or parasympathetic nervous system, respectively, releases neurotransmitters (epinephrine, norepinephrine, acetylcholine). Because of the effect of the nervous system, the heart rate (HR) and stroke volume (SV) increase during exercise. The increase in HR and SV ultimately increases the cardiac output (CO). The following formula helps to identify the relationship between HR and SV in determining cardiac output:

$$CO = HR \times SV \tag{6.1}$$

In order to understand the true effects of aerobic exercise on the heart, however, one must look at each portion of the CO formula more specifically. As just mentioned, direct stimulation of the heart by the central nervous system is responsible for the change in HR. The HR ultimately increases as a result of stimulation from the sympathetic nervous system, but the initial increase in heart rate is due to an inhibition of the parasympathetic nervous system [42].

Stroke volume increases for three reasons: (1) changes in preload, (2) changes in afterload, and (3) changes in myocardial contractility. The change in **preload,** defined as the pressure on the heart at the end of diastole [29], occurs because of an increase in blood flow back to the heart. More blood in the confines of the atrium contributes to the increased pressure. There is also a stretching of the walls of the heart. This affects the **Frank-Starling mechanism,** whereby a stretch placed on the walls of the heart results in a greater contractile force. A greater contractile force allows greater volumes of blood to be pushed from the heart with each beat [33].

Second, the change in **afterload,** which can be defined as the resistance or impedance to ventricular emptying [11], can contribute to a decrease in total peripheral resistance. As aerobic exercise intensity increases from a resting state to maximal exercise, there is a 50% to 60% reduction in peripheral resistance due to the vasodilation that occurs in an effort to supply the working skeletal muscle with blood [42]. However, at intensities near maximal levels, some vasoconstriction occurs because of sympathetic stimulation in an effort to offset the large amount of blood flow to the musculature [11].

Third, myocardial contractility responds to exercise in a positive manner. Because of the increase in venous return to the heart, which leads to an increased filling, the Frank-Starling mechanism causes the contractility of the heart to increase. The cumulative effect is an overall increase in stroke volume above sedentary values, going as high as 184 milliliters in a male marathoner [29].

Tables 6.2 and 6.3 display approximate cardiac changes in males and females [81, 82]. The most distinctive property of SV is that during an aerobic exercise bout it increases to maximal levels at 40% to 60% of $\dot{V}O_2$max and then plateaus long before HR reaches its maximum [80]. Heart rate increases more linearly during aerobic exercise, that is, in direct response to the level of exercise. Figures 6.1 and 6.2 display the changes in both HR and SV during exercise [80]. The overall increase in CO may be as much as four times during maximal aerobic exercise in an untrained individual and as much as six times in a marathoner.

Chronic Adaptations

With regard to cardiovascular changes that are more chronic and attributable exclusively to aerobic endurance-type training, hypertrophy of the heart is a response similar to that occurring in skeletal muscle as a result of resistance training. The size of the chambers of the heart increases approximately 40% overall and is the main reason the SV and subsequently the CO are higher in people who undertake aerobic endurance training. This increase is due to the overload placed on the heart during aerobic exercise. The increase in the overload above resting levels causes an increase in the overall size of the heart, as well as an increase in the thickness of the left ventricular wall [3, 33, 80]. It is worth noting that the changes in the size of the heart resulting from training occur regardless of age or gender [18, 65, 67].

One of the most prominent changes associated with long-term aerobic exercise is a decreased resting and submaximal exercise heart rate. A training-induced reduction in heart rate has been shown to occur with training in as little as two weeks [19], but some studies have shown that the reduction takes 10 weeks [63]. This response is believed to come from an increased parasympathetic influence, decreased sympathetic influence, and lower intrinsic heart rate [80].

TABLE 6.2

Changes in Cardiovascular Variables and a-$\bar{v}O_2$ Difference at 60% of $\dot{V}O_2$max

Variable	Pretraining (mean ± SD)	Posttraining (mean ± SD)
	Exercise heart rate (beats/min)	
Total	140.1 ± 16.3	135.8 ± 14.8*
Men	138.1 ± 15.6	132.8 ± 13.3**
Women	141.7 ± 16.7	138.2 ± 15.5**
	Stroke volume (ml/beat)	
Total	98.6 ± 22.2	109.2 ± 23.6*
Men	114.8 ± 19.8	127.5 ± 19.2**
Women	85.9 ± 14.5	95.0 ± 15.4**
	Cardiac output ($L \cdot min^{-1}$)	
Total	13.7 ± 3.1	14.7 ± 3.1*
Men	15.8 ± 2.9	16.9 ± 2.9*
Women	12.0 ± 2.0	13.0 ± 2.2*
	a-$\bar{v}O_2$ difference (ml/100 ml)	
Total	10.3 ± 1.6	10.9 ± 1.6*
Men	11.4 ± 1.3	12.1 ± 1.3*
Women	9.5 ± 1.2	10.1 ± 1.2*

* Significant difference ($p < 0.05$) pre- to posttraining.

** Significant difference ($p < 0.05$) pre- to posttraining and significant difference ($p < 0.05$) between men and women.

Adapted from Wilmore et al. 2001.

TABLE 6.3

Changes in Blood Pressure at 60% of $\dot{V}O_2$max

Variable	Pretraining (mean ± SD)	Posttraining (mean ± SD)
	Systolic BP (mmHg)	
Total	164.2 ± 21.5	163.4 ± 21.1
Men	177.5 ± 18.7	175.7 ± 18.0
Women	154.5 ± 17.9	154.3 ± 18.6
	Diastolic BP (mmHg)	
Total	75.2 ± 11.7	70.1 ± 10.5*
Men	76.5 ± 11.7	71.5 ± 9.8*
Women	74.4 ± 11.5	69.0 ± 10.9*

* Significant difference ($p < 0.05$) pre- to posttraining.

Adapted from Wilmore et al. 2001.

Another adaptation to aerobic exercise is an increased blood volume. This is due to an increase in the water component of blood (plasma), as well as an increase in hemoglobin, the oxygen-carrying component of blood [56]. A larger blood volume leads to a greater stroke volume during rest. Subsequently, according to the cardiac output formula presented earlier, this results in a lower resting heart rate as displayed in table 6.4 [33].

Heart rate increases linearly with increasing levels of aerobic exercise. However, the adaptation to aerobic exercise is a decreased heart rate at every intensity level including rest, with the exception of maximal heart rate, which is not affected by training.

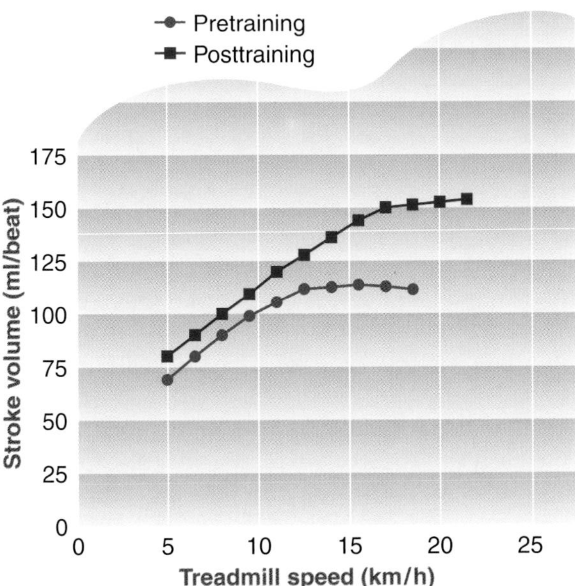

Figure 6.1 Changes in stroke volume with aerobic endurance training during walking, jogging, and running on a treadmill at increasing velocities.
Reprinted from Wilmore and Costill 1999.

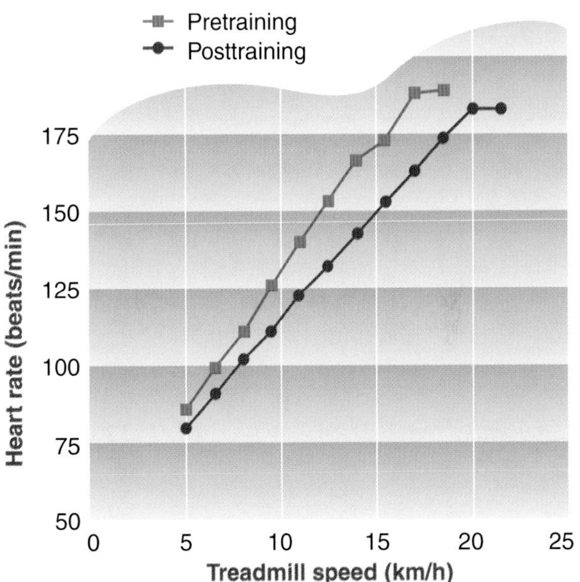

Figure 6.2 Changes in heart rate with endurance training during walking, jogging, and running on a treadmill at increasing velocities.
Reprinted from Wilmore and Costill 1999.

TABLE 6.4

Response of Stroke Volume and Heart Rate to Maximal Exercise

	Stroke volume (ml)	Heart rate (beats/min)
	Resting	
Untrained client	75	75
Marathoner	105	50
	Maximum	
Untrained client	110	195
Marathoner	162	185

Reprinted from Guyton and Hall 2000.

Blood Vessels

The other portion of the cardiovascular system is the vasculature or blood vessels themselves. To aid in understanding the complex response of the vasculature to exercise, it is separated into two distinct sections: (1) coronary vasculature and (2) skeletal or peripheral vasculature.

Acute Coronary Vascular Responses

Coronary vasculature, composed of the right and left coronary arteries, vasodilates during exercise as a result of the increased oxygen demand placed on the heart muscle. The vasodilation response comes about due to changes in arterial pressure, metabolic regulation, and autoregulation [42].

Chronic Coronary Vascular Adaptations

An increase in the cross-sectional area of coronary arteries has been reported [7, 34], with the suggestion that the coronary arteries increased in proportion to the changes in ventricular mass. As to the effect on coronary arterioles, it is commonly believed that density increases due to aerobic endurance training [79]. At the same time, no change in capillary density has been shown to occur with aerobic endurance training [9].

Acute Peripheral Vascular Responses

Several theories have been advanced to explain the changes in peripheral vasculature in response to aerobic exercise. There is no special acute change to blood flow due to aerobic exercise, however. Therefore, the changes that raise blood flow above resting values with an increase in intensity occur through many different mechanisms. An increase in sympathetic stimulation, local metabolism, or a "pumping effect" elicited by rhythmical contraction-relaxation may be the cause of an increase in blood flow to the exercising musculature [35]. At the same time, blood flow to other areas of the body, such as the abdominal region and the skin, is decreased via these same mechanisms.

Chronic Peripheral Vascular Adaptations

Prolonged aerobic training leads to an increase in the density of the capillary beds [47], which allows for better diffusion of oxygen and other metabolites, as well as to structural changes in the already existing vasculature. According to one study [36], the increase may be as great as 15% after long periods of aerobic training. Another study [40] showed an increased capillary density not only around slow-twitch fibers, but also around both subsets of fast-twitch fibers, in cross-country skiers compared to untrained men. The greater capillary density allows for a decrease in the diffusion distance of oxygen at the level of the capillary. This permits better uptake of oxygen at the muscle level. For a more thorough explanation of oxygen diffusion, see the section on respiratory changes later in this chapter.

The adaptation of the vasculature, both coronary and peripheral, to aerobic exercise is, for the most part, one of increased density.

Metabolic Changes

Closely associated with the increase in blood flow and improved function of the cardiovascular system is the need to supply adequate energy. In general, adaptations to aerobic endurance training allow the body to perform for extended periods of time at a given intensity. Therefore, there must be some adaptation of the energy systems of the body to allow for this change. As noted earlier, blood flow increases not only to the heart, but also to the level of the musculature. Now another piece of the puzzle needs to be put in place. Not only do the energy systems of the body become more efficient at producing energy, but the use of substances in the body (e.g., fat) that allow for greater energy production also becomes more efficient.

With this change in substrate utilization, an overall, often visible change occurs in the body. An alteration in body composition is that visible change. Stored energy in the form of fat is more frequently utilized during aerobic training than in any other type of training, leading to this change in body composition. But in order for the transformation to occur, changes in the endocrine system, which is primarily responsible for hormone release, allow the body to become more efficient at energy production. The following section describes adaptations in the energy systems, body composition, and the endocrine system in response to aerobic exercise.

Energy Systems

The production of energy is the most critical part of the ability to exercise. If energy is not present, the ability to exercise will be nonexistent. Energy production for brain function is the body's first priority, but the amount of energy needed to perform muscle contractions is very large in comparison. Therefore, the overall energy need for aerobic exercise is extremely large. The body meets these demands not only by increasing the fuel stores, but also by increasing the efficiency with which it burns fuel.

Acute Responses

Aerobic exercise in an untrained person who is beginning an exercise program is inefficient. Limitations in the cardiovascular and respiratory systems impose a limit on the metabolic processes that take place in order to allow aerobic exercise to occur. Poor performance for a short time period is the ultimate result. Therefore, aerobic exercise has very small acute effects on aerobic energy systems. See chapter 3 for a review of the energy systems as they pertain to aerobic exercise.

Chronic Adaptations

There are two main reasons for the primary changes in the energy systems resulting from aerobic exercise. First, the body adapts by storing more fuel. Second, the body increases its ability to utilize that fuel through enzymatic processes and physiological adaptation at the cellular level. The sections that follow address each component individually.

Substrate Storage Adaptations Adaptations with regard to storage of substrate, primarily glycogen, increase due to aerobic training [24, 80]. There is also an increase in the intramuscular triglyceride concentration as a result of aerobic training [25, 26]. An increased concentration of available substrate for utilization results in an increased time to exhaustion. Depending on the intensity of the exercise, the greater availability of free-fatty acids (FFA) from triglycerides directly affects the stress placed on glycogen stores [28, 38]. Figure 6.3 shows which fuel sources predominate during aerobic exercise at different intensity levels.

Lactate threshold is defined as the point at which the body switches from the use of fat as the predominant fuel source to the use of carbohydrate. This also represents the point at which the body switches from the use of aerobic energy processes to rely more on anaerobic energy sources. Because of this change in the energy systems being utilized, lactate increases. Since aerobic training allows trained individuals to burn fat for longer periods of time at increasing intensity levels compared with those who are untrained, there should be a shift in the lactate threshold similar to the shift shown in figure 6.3. Figure 6.4 displays the shift in lactate threshold that occurs with aerobic training.

Enzymatic and Cellular Adaptations Several key elements associated with the energy systems of the body are of major interest in aerobic research. These

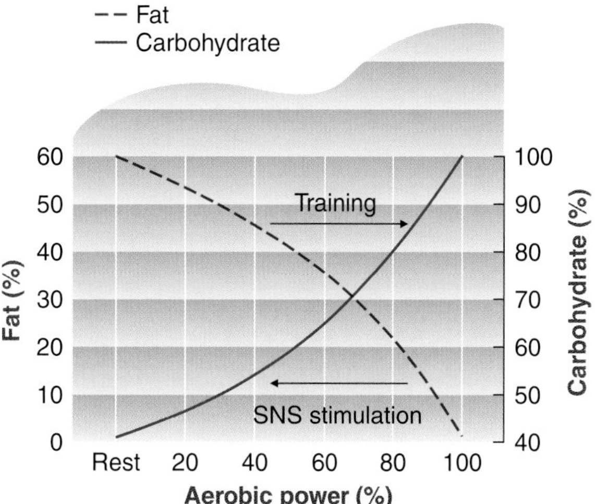

Figure 6.3 The reliance on carbohydrate for energy increases with the intensity (%$\dot{V}O_2$max) of aerobic exercise, whereas the use of fat tends to decline as the exercise intensity increases. Training tends to shift both curves to the right, while the stimulation from the sympathetic nervous system (SNS) declines. As a result, aerobic training tends to decrease the need for carbohydrate as the primary energy source but increases the use of fat.

Reprinted from Wilmore and Costill 1999 with adaptations from Brooks and Mercier 1994.

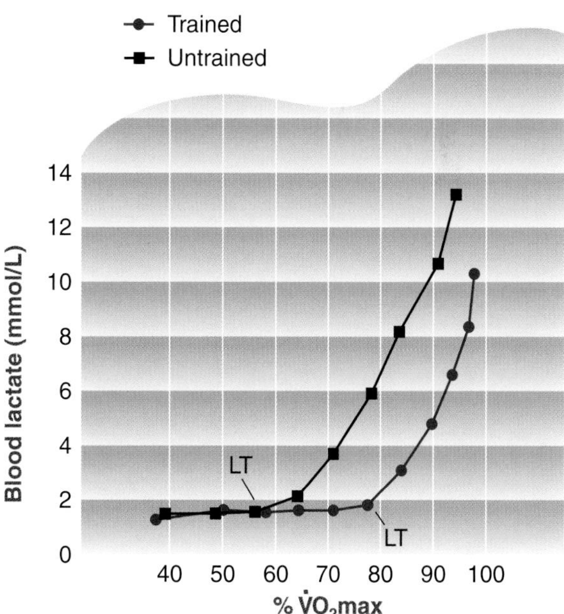

Figure 6.4 Effects of exercise intensity on the accumulation of blood lactate in untrained and aerobic endurance-trained individuals. The point at which blood lactate begins to rise above the resting level is sometimes called the blood lactate threshold (LT).

Reprinted from Wilmore and Costill 1999.

enzymes include hexokinase (HK), phosphofructokinase (PFK), lactate dehydrogenase (LDH), succinate dehydrogenase (SDH), and citrate synthase (CS) and are the focus of this section.

Hexokinase, the enzyme responsible for the phosphorylation of glucose after entry into the cell, has been shown to increase with aerobic training [71]. It is hypothesized that this adaptation facilitates the entry of glucose into the glycolytic pathway and ultimately benefits aerobic activity [11].

Phosphofructokinase, another vital enzyme in the glycolytic pathway, is often referred to as the rate-limiting enzyme of glycolysis. The response of this enzyme to aerobic exercise appears to be much more inconsistent than the response associated with HK. In fact, because the research literature conflicts [5, 30, 43, 73], the general consensus is there is no effect of aerobic exercise on PFK activity or concentration [11].

Lactate dehydrogenase, the enzyme responsible for reversible conversion of pyruvate to lactate, is also affected by aerobic conditioning. Two specific forms of LDH are of interest to exercise scientists. The LDH enzyme found in muscle is called LDH_M. This enzyme has a high affinity for the conversion of pyruvate to lactate. Another LDH enzyme, LDH_H, is found in the heart. This enzyme has a high affinity for the conversion of lactate to pyruvate. The need to discuss both has to do with the alteration in the type of enzyme found after aerobic exercise. Aerobic exercise decreases the concentration of LDH_M while increasing the concentration of LDH_H in the muscle fiber [2]. Therefore, more pyruvate is allowed to proceed into oxidative metabolism (Krebs cycle) with aerobic training.

As noted earlier, aerobic exercise increases levels of the enzymes primarily responsible for increased utilization of glucose or glycogen through oxidative pathways. Succinate dehydrogenase (SDH) is no different. Considering the high demand placed on oxidative metabolism during aerobic exercise, SDH activity increases as a result of aerobic training [14, 30].

Finally, in the present context CS is no different from any of the other enzymes mentioned. Aerobic endurance training improves CS activity [44] regardless of gender [13]. Therefore, CS follows the same adaptations as other enzymes. Figure 6.5 displays the changes associated with aerobic training in two of the key enzymes.

Several cellular adaptations also take place during aerobic exercise, including an increase in the mitochondrial content [38], as well as an increase in the number of glucose transporters ($GLUT_4$) [85].

The mitochondria are often referred to as the "powerhouses" of the cell because of the large amount of adenosine triphosphate (ATP) production that occurs in the mitochondria via the electron transport system (see chapter 3). Because of the utilization of oxygen for energy production during aerobic exercise, the body responds by increasing the mitochondrial content in the muscle fiber [38]. This increase in mitochondrial density makes the production of ATP a much more efficient process.

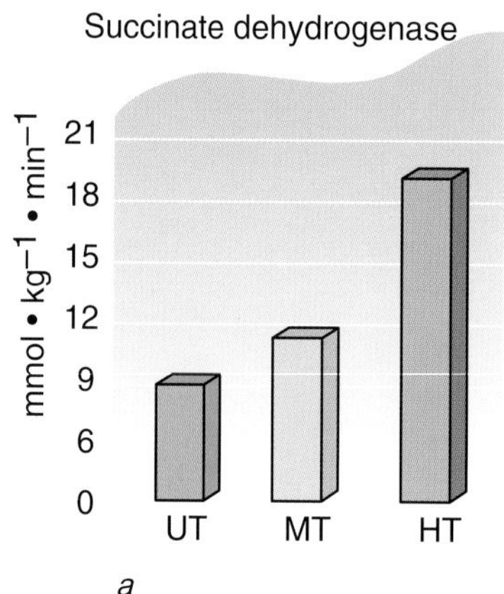

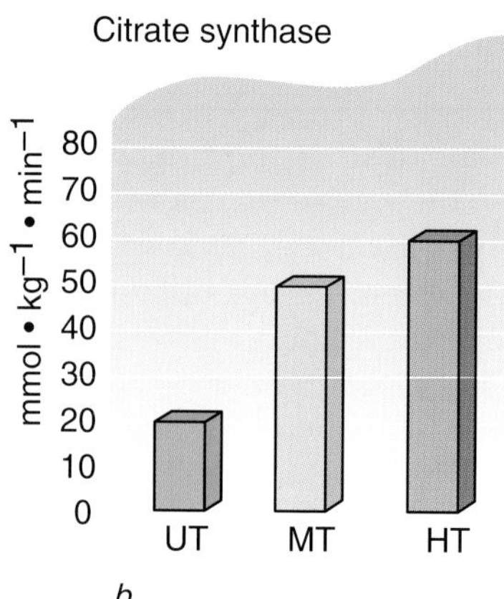

Figure 6.5 Leg muscle (gastrocnemius) enzyme activities of untrained (UT) individuals, moderately trained (MT) joggers, and highly trained (HT) marathon runners. Enzyme levels shown are for *(a)* succinate dehydrogenase and *(b)* citrate synthase, two of many enzymes that participate in the oxidative production of adenosine triphosphate.
Reprinted from Wilmore and Costill 1999.

Glucose enters the cell via facilitated diffusion (see figure 6.6) [61] with the help of a glucose transporter (GLUT), more specifically $GLUT_4$ [39]. These $GLUT_4$ transporters are activated from an intracellular pool to move toward the cell membrane in a process called translocation by way of insulin activity or muscle activation [39, 53]. Understanding glucose transport is important because of the strong relationship between the availability of glucose and aerobic performance at higher intensities [12]. Aerobic exercise training has been shown to increase the concentration of $GLUT_4$, as well as the overall $GLUT_4$ activity [62, 70].

The body responds to the demands of repeated aerobic exercise by increasing the available fuel sources as well as the enzymes responsible for utilizing those fuel sources through respective energy pathways.

Body Composition

One of the positive adaptations to aerobic exercise is a change in body composition. Often, when a reduction of body fat is advised, aerobic exercise is recommended. Currently the recommendation is for sedentary people to get approximately 20 to 30 minutes of moderate exercise a day. This could be a brisk walk. Health issues aside, one of the most noticeable changes with such a regimen is a reduction in fat mass (FM).

Acute Responses

Unfortunately, because of the complex changes that occur in the body over time in response to aerobic exercise, there are no acute changes in body composition. When clients perform aerobic exercise for a period of time, though, observable changes occur.

Chronic Adaptations

The greatest observable change over time with aerobic exercise is a reduction in fat mass. Aerobic exercise for 12 weeks can reduce FM [10]. However, it has also been demonstrated that high-intensity exercise is not necessary in order for the change to occur [32]. Short bouts of exercise may enhance weight loss and produce changes in cardiorespiratory fitness similar to those obtained with long bouts (30 minutes) in sedentary, obese females [41]. Evidence also suggests a greater adherence rate to exercise with short bouts [41]. To preserve fat-free mass, concurrent resistance and aerobic training are needed [60, 77]. Aerobic exercise has also been shown to have a positive effect on body composition due to suppression of appetite [31].

Aerobic exercise has a positive effect on fat mass because fat is the predominant fuel source during aerobic exercise.

Endocrine System

The endocrine system is a very broad system that incorporates the communication between 11 different organs. All of the glands play a specific role in exercise; and through their adaptation to training, performance is enhanced. The glands of primary concern with regard to metabolism are the pancreas, adrenal cortex, and adrenal medulla.

Pancreas

The pancreas is the endocrine gland that plays the largest role in metabolism because of the production and release of insulin and glucagon. Both of these are essential to uptake or release of glucose, which is vital to the survival of the body.

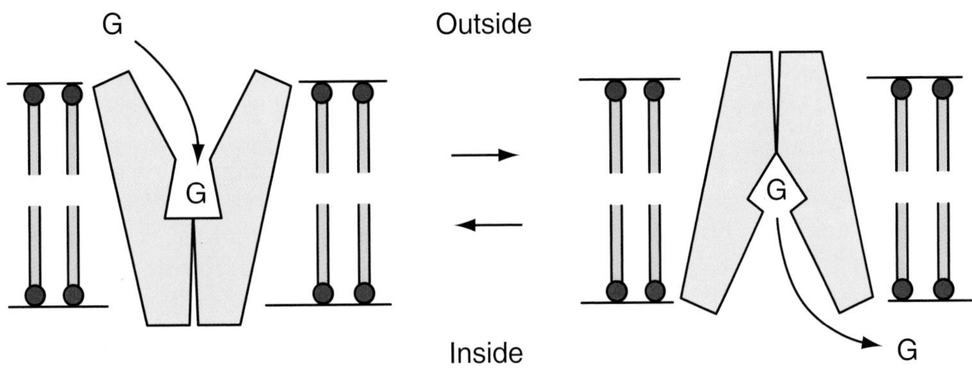

Figure 6.6 Facilitated diffusion of glucose via $GLUT_4$ transporters. G = glucose.
Reprinted from Powell and Shepherd 1996.

Acute Responses A single bout of high-intensity aerobic exercise has been shown to increase the sensitivity of insulin [55] and actually stimulates insulin-mediated glucose uptake in non-insulin-dependent diabetes mellitus (NIDDM) [21, 22]. A single bout of exercise has been shown to increase insulin-stimulated whole-body glucose uptake for up to 48 hours postexercise [55]. Thus, glucose uptake is increased after a single bout of exercise.

Chronic Adaptations Aerobic training has also been shown to have a positive effect on insulin secretion. Trained individuals have an increased sensitivity to insulin and an increase in insulin responsiveness [20]. In fact, the greater sensitivity to insulin counteracts the decline in sensitivity that occurs with aging [66].

Adrenal Cortex

Cortisol is the only substance released from the adrenal cortex that plays a direct role in metabolism. Cortisol is responsible for stimulating the conversion of proteins to be utilized by the aerobic and glycogen systems and for maintenance of normal blood sugar levels, and it also promotes the utilization of fats. All of these factors play a large role in the utilization of energy substrates and consequently in performance of aerobic exercise.

The response of cortisol blood concentration to aerobic exercise follows a similar path whether in relation to an acute bout of activity in an untrained athlete or as a chronic adaptation to repeated bouts of aerobic exercise. The reason is that the cortisol concentration response to aerobic exercise is determined primarily by the intensity of the bout [6] and by duration [6, 8]. This general response is one of increase in cortisol blood concentration followed ultimately by a decrease over time. One study [48] demonstrated that trained individuals had an elevated level of cortisol at rest compared with nontrained individuals. Another observation from this study was that for every level of testing (50%, 70%, and 90% of $\dot{V}O_2$max), aerobically trained individuals responded with less of an increase in cortisol concentration compared to the untrained individuals [48]. However, individuals in the trained group exhibited the general response regardless of their training level. A possible reason is an increased ability to utilize and mobilize FFA in trained compared with nontrained individuals. There appears to be an inverse relationship between cortisol concentration and FFA levels [80]. Also, because of the heightened psychological stress experienced during exercise testing, untrained individuals may have a greater response to exercise [51].

Adrenal Medulla

The term used to describe the response of the adrenal medulla to exercise is the **sympathoadrenal response** [41]. The term reflects the fact that the response of the adrenal medulla to exercise, which corresponds to the release of catecholamines (epinephrine and norephinephrine), is more a reaction from both the sympathetic nervous system and the adrenal medulla than from the adrenal medulla alone. As with many other hormones in the body, there is a training effect on catecholamines. Untrained individuals have a larger rise in catecholamine release than trained individuals. This blunted overall response is one of the rationales for why exercise may help relieve stress.

It is important to note that the catecholamine response to exercise is a very complex issue that is beyond the scope of this text. The response to exercise, whether acute or chronic, may be different depending on the tissue. Gender has also been shown to affect the catecholamine response [75].

Acute Responses Epinephrine and norepinephrine play a large role in the regulation of metabolism. Therefore, one would assume that stresses placed on the body would cause an increased release of epinephrine and norepinephrine. This is not the case. Although the release of norepinephrine and epinephrine increases during exercise, it does not follow the same pattern of response in aerobic endurance-trained versus nonaerobic endurance-trained persons.

In contrast to what occurs with other hormones, the adaptation of the catecholamines to exercise is rather rapid [54, 84]. The main hypothesis for the response observed in epinephrine and norepinephrine is that the exercise session does not feel as difficult (i.e., it causes less stress) than when the program began [50].

Chronic Adaptations As discussed earlier, heart rate decreases as a result of aerobic endurance training, and an increase in parasympathetic stimulation via the vagus nerve occurs as well. Similarly, an adaptation in the sympathoadrenal system is a likely component. The receptors responsible for binding with norepinephrine, which are found in the heart, decrease in number as a result of extended periods of aerobic training [58]; and heart rate thereby decreases. There is also a decrease in the overall release of epinephrine and norepinephrine when measured at a constant workload [83]. However, the response is the opposite during hard- to maximal-intensity aerobic exercise bouts.

Neurological Changes

The neurological changes that result from aerobic training are primarily an adaptation type of change as opposed to an increase in the number of neurons, motor units, and so on. The changes that have been observed occur due to adaptation over time. Therefore this section deals only with chronic adaptations of the nervous system.

Researchers have demonstrated a morphological change in the neuromuscular junction of aerobic endurance-trained mice [1, 27]. However, there was no change in the diameter of the nerve fibers involved [1]. These findings clearly demonstrate a neurological adaptation to aerobic training that can be hypothesized to occur in humans. Likewise, in rats, running influenced basic motor neuron properties, for example leading to a more negative resting membrane potential [4]. The authors of that study speculated that an increased density or localization of membrane ion channels was responsible for the changes.

As with resistance training, neurophysiological changes occur in direct relation to exposure to aerobic exercise.

Skeletal Changes

There are not many skeletal changes associated with aerobic-type exercise. Among the effects most often referred to as positive are the increase in bone mineral density and the alterations that occur in articular cartilage. The effects on bone mineral density are the more important of the two, especially in view of the natural loss of bone mineral content as people age. With age, bone mineral density decreases and consequently more bone injuries such as fractures occur. Figure 6.7 demonstrates the changes in bone mineral density of women throughout life [68].

One troubling fact about aerobic exercise and bone mineral density is that there appears to be little to no increase in bone density in the normal healthy active population as a result of aerobic exercise. If bone mineral density does increase as a result of weight-bearing exercise (e.g., running) the increase is site specific, occurring primarily in the tibia and femoral neck as compared with swimming and biking, which are non-weight bearing aerobic exercises [23, 57, 72]. In nonhealthy or older individuals, bone mineral density has been shown to increase in other areas. A meta-analysis showed that the bone density of the lumbar spine was greater in postmenopausal women who exercised compared to those who did not [46]. However, the difference was not an increase over the value in controls, but rather a reflection of loss of bone density in the control individuals.

It has long been understood that if a sedentary person begins weight-bearing aerobic exercise, running for example, then the bone density of that individual will increase according to **Wolff's law,** which basically states that bone will be laid down

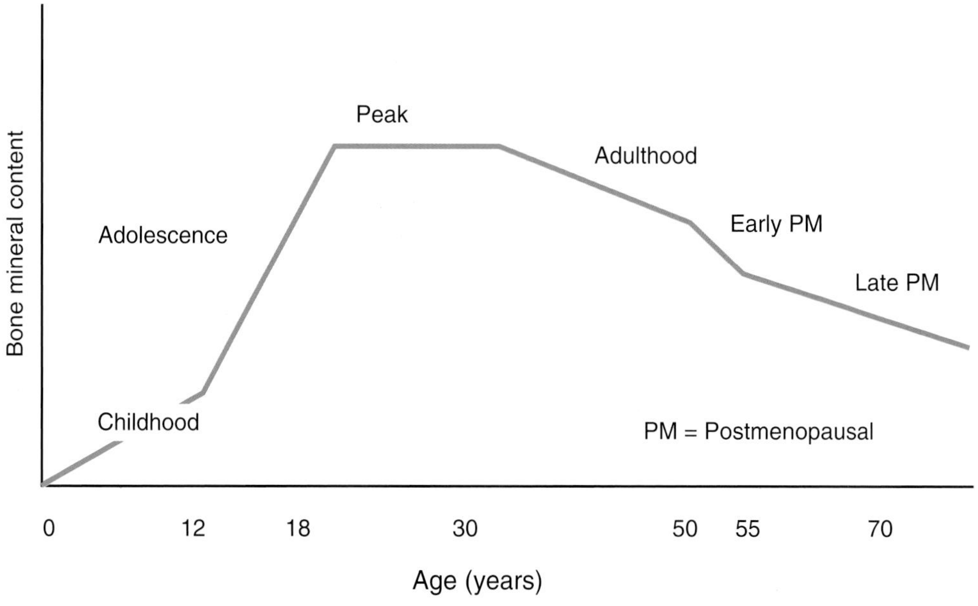

Figure 6.7 Bone mineral content changes throughout female life span.
Reprinted from Snow-Harter 1992.

where needed. Bone, like other organs of the body, adapts according to the applied stresses. However, the available literature deals primarily with postmenopausal women and older men and does not include a great deal of information on normal healthy individuals.

Articular cartilage adapts similarly when stress is applied. Cartilage in joints has three primary functions: (1) to distribute force in the joint, (2) to provide stability, and (3) to provide near-frictionless movement.

Acute Responses

One study showed an increased bone density of the femur in postmenopausal women and in men over 50 due to high-impact aerobic exercise that included stepping and jumping exercise [78]. However, after a period of continued training, the body as usual adapts to the stress of weight-bearing exercise. Therefore, the changes in bone density are acutely displayed, but as the training continues and becomes more chronic, no further adaptation is observed.

Chronic Adaptations

Because of the body's ability to adapt, unless new stresses are imposed on the body, the bone does not change above and beyond what is needed to maintain its integrity. Alterations in the mode of aerobic exercise performed may be one way to continue to place new stresses on the body. In contrast, there are encouraging results with regard to the changes that occur in cartilage due to long-term aerobic exercise. These include an increase in the thickness of the meniscus as well as increases in hydroxyproline and calcium concentrations after 12 weeks of training in comparison to the values in nonexercisers [76]. Although degenerative changes have been shown in animals engaged in long-duration weight-bearing exercise (i.e., running), this has not been the case in humans. The general consensus is that high-impact aerobic exercise (e.g., running) does not predispose the joints to degenerative changes.

> Aerobic training is associated with site-specific increases in bone mineral density. Of all types of aerobic exercise, high-impact weight-bearing activity is the most beneficial for increasing bone mineral density. The overall health of articular cartilage is not jeopardized during high-impact aerobic exercise (e.g., running).

Respiratory Changes

The respiratory system has an extremely close relationship to the cardiovascular changes with aerobic training that were described earlier in the chapter. While blood flow increases during exercise, allowing for more oxygen to be transported to the working muscles, the ability of oxygen to diffuse across the alveolar membrane also increases with aerobic training. The exact mechanism is still unclear, but this increase is seen in people who train aerobically compared to sedentary adults (figure 6.8). Another respiratory change with aerobic training relates to the body's ability to utilize oxygen. As described earlier, the body adapts when necessary, and this is true of the respiratory system as well. The following sections deal with the mechanisms that allow for this more efficient use of oxygen and the ability to meet the body's increased requirement.

Acute Responses

The response of the respiratory system to a bout of aerobic exercise depends on the intensity of the training session (see figure 6.9). Because of the need to supply oxygen, the respiration rate (i.e., pulmonary ventilation) increases as exercise intensity increases.

Chronic Adaptations

Many components of the respiratory system adapt to aerobic exercise. The changes include changes in

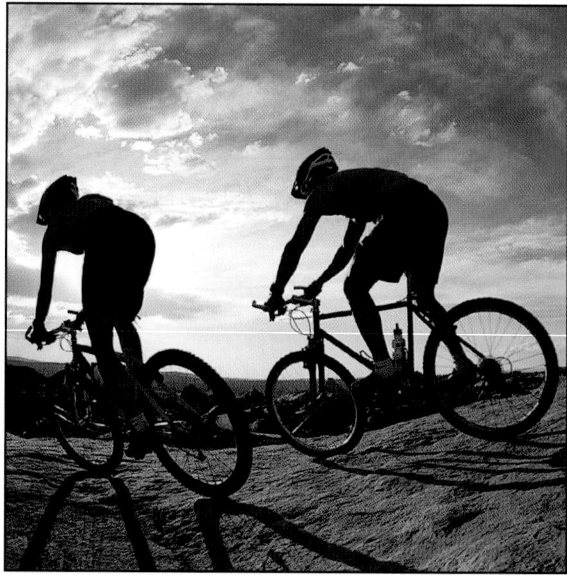

Figure 6.8 Aerobic exercise such as mountain biking increases respiratory adaptations.

lung volumes, carrying capacity of the blood, and diffusion ability of the lungs. All play a vital role in the adaptations of the respiratory system to chronic aerobic exercise.

The lungs adapt to aerobic exercise in much the same way as other tissues of the body. A study of two male marathoners who averaged 45 to 70 miles (64 to 121 kilometers) per week over a three-year period showed increases in total lung capacity and improvement in functional residual capacity [45]. (For an explanation of lung function, see chapter 2.) Other research, however, demonstrated no change in ventilatory performance in healthy male individuals after 19 weeks of training [16].

The diffusion capacity of the lung increases during exercise primarily by increasing the blood flow through the lung. This occurs directly from an increase in pulmonary blood flow particularly to the upper portions of the lungs. This results in greater lung perfusion. So while more blood is being brought into the lungs, there is also an increase in the amount of air exchanged per minute, which allow more alveoli to become involved. This leads to an increase in gas exchange.

The number of oxygen-carrying molecules in the muscle, known as myoglobin, also increases with aerobic training. According to one study [37], the total myoglobin concentration increased 13% to 45% after 14 weeks of training.

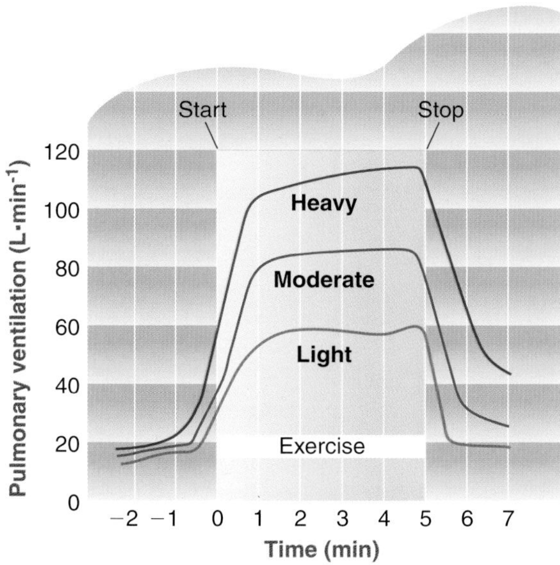

Figure 6.9 The ventilatory response to light, moderate, and heavy aerobic exercise. The individual exercised at each of the three intensities for five minutes. The ventilation volume tended to plateau at a steady-state value at the light and moderate intensities but continued to increase at the heavy intensity.
Reprinted from Wilmore and Costill 1999.

Factors That Influence Adaptations to Aerobic Training

The physiological adaptations to aerobic training that have been addressed in this chapter are influenced by a number of individual factors. These include the types of activity that the person engages in (i.e., specificity), genetics, sex, and age. All these factors play a role in determining the success one may see with aerobic training.

Specificity

The effects of exercise are all subject to the rule of specificity. This means that adaptations occur as a consequence of the training and in a fashion specifically related to the training. In short, if the exercise involves cycling, then the training adaptations will be most closely related to cycling performance. This is true also for running, swimming, or training on an ergometer or treadmill. The body seeks to adapt to the stress it encounters in as specific a manner as possible, a principle that has obvious implications for the design of training programs. While programming is beyond the scope of the chapter, it is important for the personal trainer to bear in mind that any exercise program will produce adaptations very closely related to the specific activities the client engages in.

However, human beings are not lab rats or robotic machines that merely react to the world around them or function like a computer running a series of instructions through a written program. We have the extended capability of modifying our environment and applying the physiological adaptations that we acquire in one area to another area. The body adapts to any stress it experiences so long as the stress is applied in appropriate amounts over a period of time. It is important to remember this concept with regard to specificity. If a client wants to be a good sprinter, the client needs to run sprints; if the client desires to be a good long-distance runner, the client must run long distances. Although the concept is simple, the personal trainer must be creative in order to overcome possible boredom with these types of exercise. Instead, alternative types of exercise or cross-training exercises such as pool running, use of elliptical trainers, and use of stair steppers all lend themselves to the aerobic adaptations that are being sought. It is worth noting here that an "upper limit" with regard to training adaptations exists and is different for each individual.

With aerobic endurance training, adaptations will be aerobic in nature. The key is for the heart rate to be elevated to a submaximal level for an extended period of time.

Genetics

It is safe to say that each of us is born with a theoretical ceiling of human performance that we may attain. This ceiling is not absolute but rather falls within a range of values that is dependent on the training stimulus and motivation levels. However, there appears to be an absolute level that each of us is unable to exceed based on genetic factors we inherited from our ancestors. There is a saying that the best training begins with choosing the right parents. While we obviously do not have control over this factor, it does play a major role in our development.

However, research has shown that the body is not completely unchangeable. For example, people who undertake aerobic-type exercise for an extended period of time see an increase in the number of fast-twitch oxidative fibers that take on more characteristics of slow-twitch muscle fibers, leading to an improved aerobic performance. According to one investigation, the slow-twitch fibers in the legs of people undergoing aerobic endurance training were 7% to 22% larger than the fast-twitch fibers [64]. At the same time, though, it appears that those who perform well in a particular sport requiring predominantly one muscle fiber type over another tend to gravitate to that sport (see table 6.5).

Sex

The physiological changes due to aerobic exercise are similar for males and females. However, some

TABLE 6.5

Percentages of Cross-Sectional Areas of Slow-Twitch (ST) and Fast-Twitch (FT) Fibers in Selected Muscles of Male and Female Athletes

					Cross-sectional area (μm²)	
Athlete	Gender	Muscle	% ST	% FT	ST	FT
Sprint runners	M	Gastrocnemius	24	76	5,878	6,034
	F	Gastrocnemius	27	73	3,752	3,930
Distance runners	M	Gastrocnemius	79	21	8,342	6,485
	F	Gastrocnemius	69	31	4,441	4,128
Cyclists	M	Vastus lateralis	57	43	6,333	6,116
	F	Vastus lateralis	51	49	5,487	5,216
Swimmers	M	Posterior deltoid	67	33	—	—
Weightlifters	M	Gastrocnemius	44	56	5,060	8,910
	M	Deltoid	53	47	5,101	8,450
Triathletes	M	Posterior deltoid	60	40	—	—
	M	Vastus lateralis	63	37	—	—
	M	Gastrocnemius	59	41	—	—
Canoeists	M	Posterior deltoid	71	29	4,920	7,040
Shot-putters	M	Gastrocnemius	38	62	6,367	6,441
Nonathletes	M	Vastus lateralis	47	53	4,722	4,709
	F	Gastrocnemius	52	48	3,501	3,141

Reprinted from Wilmore and Costill 1999.

basic differences affect the absolute amounts of the changes. Women on average have less muscle mass and more body fat than their male counterparts. They also have smaller hearts and lungs, and an overall smaller blood volume. Research has shown that when males and females are matched for age, females typically have a lower cardiac output, stroke volume, and oxygen consumption than a man at 50% of $\dot{V}O_2$max. With that said, the adaptations to exercise for both males and females are approximately the same.

Age

One can think of age in terms of maturational age and old age. With regard to maturational age, in the early stages of life, cardiorespiratory adaptations are attenuated by the child's maturational level. In other words, a child's body is not ready to produce maximum performance levels because it has not fully developed yet. This is in contrast to the situation with old age, which is characterized by a decline in physiological performance. A unique property of the body is that it tends to have the best ability in relation to aerobic performance at the end of puberty. Research has shown that females reach peak $\dot{V}O_2$max between 12 and 15 years of age and that males do not reach peak $\dot{V}O_2$max until 17 to 21 years of age. After this period, there is a plateau and then a gradual decrease as we age.

Once maturity has been reached, the effects of cardiorespiratory training can be fully realized. These effects are well maintained through middle age but then slowly decline. Much of the decline can be negated through continued training regimens. Aerobic endurance-trained athletes who are older exhibit only slight declines during the fifth and sixth decades when they maintain training, whereas those who stop training show declines similar to those in untrained individuals. In five middle-aged men, 100% of the age-related decline in aerobic power that had occurred over 30 years was reversed by six months of aerobic endurance training [52]. Figure 6.10 depicts changes in $\dot{V}O_2$max with age in both trained and untrained men.

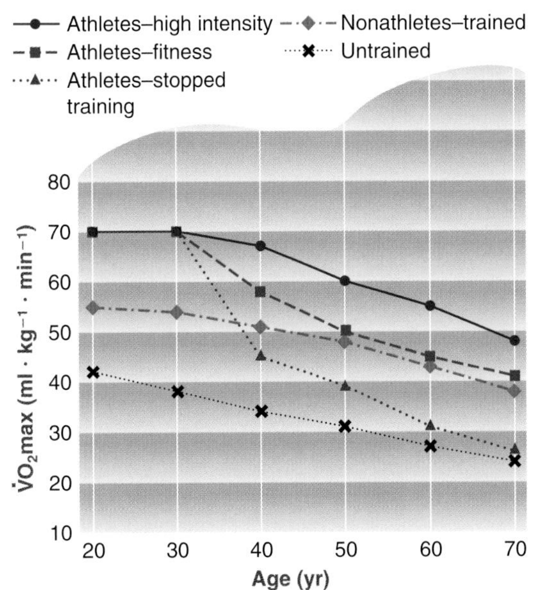

Figure 6.10 Changes in $\dot{V}O_2$max with age for aerobically trained and untrained men.

Reprinted from Wilmore and Costill 1999.

Overtraining

A recognized decline in performance is defined as overtraining. According to Hans Selye's general adaptation syndrome, when the stimulus or stressor becomes too great in relation to the body's ability to adapt, performance will suffer.

This phenomenon is generally preceded by overreaching, which is the precursor to overtraining. Overreaching may be defined as the plateau in performance that precedes a decline. Besides the plateau in performance, critical variables need to be monitored for change, including an altered resting heart rate, altered mood states, sleep pattern disruption, and reduced appetite. "Common Markers of Aerobic Endurance Overtraining" are listed below.

Common Markers of Aerobic Endurance Overtraining

Decreased performance

Decreased percentage of body fat

Decreased maximal oxygen uptake

Altered blood pressure

Increased muscle soreness

Decreased muscle glycogen

Altered resting heart rate

Increased submaximal exercise heart rate

Altered cortisol concentration

Decreased total testosterone concentration

Decreased sympathetic tone (decreased nocturnal and resting catecholamines)

Increased sympathetic stress response

Adapted from Kraemer 2000.

Although measurement of some of the factors listed on page 115 requires invasive techniques, several of the markers can be monitored very noninvasively. Markers of performance (i.e., $\dot{V}O_2max$, changes in blood pressure or resting heart rate, increased muscle soreness) can be measured through meticulous tracking of both objective and subjective information from the client. Being familiar with each client's progression through training is essential to eliminating overtraining. For personal trainers who want a more definitive answer that may require some invasiveness, the exercise physiology department at a nearby college would be a good source of information. With that said, the best way to prevent overtraining is through steady progression, but ultimately adequate rest. The client should be aware that rest is as important as training, if not more so. Without rest, adaptation cannot occur, and this situation can lead to symptoms of overtraining.

Detraining

The ways in which the body responds to detraining are analogous to the ways in which it responds to training. Once exercise is stopped, muscular endurance decreases after only two weeks. One study showed reductions in the muscles' respiratory ability as well as in muscle glycogen over a four-week period, along with an increase in lactate, which demonstrates obvious changes in the muscle metabolism [17]. The training-induced bradycardia that occurs as a consequence of aerobic conditioning is quickly lost with detraining [49, 74]. Another investigation demonstrated that when aerobic endurance-trained rats stopped training, there was a site-specific decrease in the bone mineral density of the tibia [69].

CONCLUSION

Aerobic exercise affects the body in many ways, structurally, metabolically, and physiologically. The acute and chronic effects of aerobic exercise are dependent on the frequency, intensity, and duration of the exercise and the unique characteristics of each client. The key to any training program is a continual yet gradual progression over time. Adaptations to aerobic training do not occur overnight. At the same time, though, the hard work put into developing a good aerobic foundation can be lost in just a few short weeks. Therefore, it is essential that personal trainers educate and guide their clients through a lifestyle change to achieve the longest-lasting results.

STUDY QUESTIONS

1. A 35-year-old female began an exercise program four months ago in which she has been running on the treadmill four days per week. Which of the following describes the adaptations that are most likely to occur with this program?

	Increased	Decreased
A.	maximal exercise HR	capillary density
B.	systolic BP	a-$\bar{v}O_2$ difference
C.	mitochondrial density	submax exercise HR
D.	blood volume	insulin sensitivity

2. Which of the following changes in the body's substrate use and enzyme levels is due to an adaptation to chronic aerobic exercise?

   A. increased reliance on carbohydrates
   B. decreased reliance on free fatty acids
   C. increased concentration of $GLUT_4$
   D. decreased concentration of hexokinase

3. Clients possessing predominantly Type II muscle fibers in their lower body probably would perform well in which of the following activities or events?
   I. Olympic weightlifting
   II. 10-kilometer road race
   III. 100-meter sprint
   IV. triathlon

   A. II and IV only
   B. I and III only
   C. I, II, and III only
   D. II, III, and IV only

4. Which of the following is most likely to occur as a result of aerobic endurance overtraining?
   A. decreased $\dot{V}O_2$ max
   B. increased muscle glycogen
   C. increased body fat percentage
   D. decreased sympathetic stress response

APPLIED KNOWLEDGE QUESTION

Complete the following chart to describe two ways the body adapts to chronic participation in an aerobic training program.

System	Two adaptations
Nervous	
Energy	
Skeletal	
Cardiovascular (blood vessels)	
Endocrine	
Cardiovascular (heart)	

REFERENCES

1. Andonian, M.H., and M.A. Fahim. 1988. Endurance exercise alters the morphology of fast- and slow-twitch rat neuromuscular junctions. *International Journal of Sports Medicine* 9 (3): 218-223.
2. Apple, F.S., and P.A. Tesch. 1989. Ck and Ld isozymes in human single muscle fibers in trained athletes. *Journal of Applied Physiology* 66 (6): 2717-2720.
3. Åstrand, P., and K. Rodahl. 1986. *Textbook of Work Physiology,* 3rd ed. New York: McGraw-Hill.
4. Beaumont, E., and P. Gardiner. 2002. Effects of daily spontaneous running on the electrophysiological properties of hindlimb motoneurones in rats. *Journal of Physiology* 540 (Pt 1): 129-138.
5. Bishop, D., D.G. Jenkins, M. McEniery, and M.F. Carey. 2000. Relationship between plasma lactate parameters and muscle characteristics in female cyclists. *Medicine and Science in Sports and Exercise* 32 (6): 1088-1093.
6. Bonen, A. 1976. Effects of exercise on excretion rates of urinary free cortisol. *Journal of Applied Physiology* 40 (2): 155-158.
7. Bove, A.A., and J.D. Dewey. 1985. Proximal coronary vasomotor reactivity after exercise training in dogs. *Circulation* 71 (3): 620-625.
8. Brandenberger, G., and M. Follenius. 1975. Influence of timing and intensity of muscular exercise on temporal patterns of plasma cortisol levels. *Journal of Clinical Endocrinology and Metabolism* 40 (5): 845-849.

9. Breisch, E.A., F.C. White, L.E. Nimmo, M.D. McKirnan, and C.M. Bloor. 1986. Exercise-induced cardiac hypertrophy: A correlation of blood flow and microvasculature. *Journal of Applied Physiology* 60 (4): 1259-1267.
10. Broeder, C.E., K.A. Burrhus, L.S. Svanevik, J. Volpe, and J.H. Wilmore. 1997. Assessing body composition before and after resistance or endurance training. *Medicine and Science in Sports and Exercise* 29 (5): 705-712.
11. Brooks, G.A., T.D. Fahey, T.P. White, and K.M. Baldwin. 2000. *Exercise Physiology: Human Bioenergetics and Its Applications*, 3rd ed. Mountain View, CA: Mayfield.
12. Brooks, G.A., and J. Mercier. 1994. Balance of carbohydrate and lipid utilization during exercise: The crossover concept. *Journal of Applied Physiology* 76 (6): 2253-2261.
13. Carter, S.L., C.D. Rennie, S.J. Hamilton, and M. Tarnopolsky. 2001. Changes in skeletal muscle in males and females following endurance training. *Canadian Journal of Physiology and Pharmacology* 79 (5): 386-392.
14. Chilibeck, P.D., G.J. Bell, T. Socha, and T. Martin. 1998. The effect of aerobic exercise training on the distribution of succinate dehydrogenase activity throughout muscle fibres. *Canadian Journal of Applied Physiology* 23 (1): 74-86.
15. Clark, A.L., I. Skypala, and A.J. Coats. 1994. Ventilatory efficiency is unchanged after physical training in healthy persons despite an increased exercise tolerance. *Journal of Cardiovascular Risk* 1 (4): 347-351.
16. Coast, J.R., P.S. Clifford, T.W. Henrich, J. Stray-Gundersen, and R.L. Johnson Jr. 1990. Maximal inspiratory pressure following maximal exercise in trained and untrained subjects. *Medicine and Science in Sports and Exercise* 22 (6): 811-815.
17. Costill, D.L., W.J. Fink, M. Hargreaves, D.S. King, R. Thomas, and R. Fielding. 1985. Metabolic characteristics of skeletal muscle during detraining from competitive swimming. *Medicine and Science in Sports and Exercise* 17 (3): 339-343.
18. Crouse, S.F., J.J. Rohack, and D.J. Jacobsen. 1992. Cardiac structure and function in women basketball athletes: Seasonal variation and comparisons with nonathletic controls. *Research Quarterly for Exercise and Sport* 63 (4): 393-401.
19. Dart, A.M., I.T. Meredith, and G.L. Jennings. 1992. Effects of 4 weeks endurance training on cardiac left ventricular structure and function. *Clinical and Experimental Pharmacology and Physiology* 19 (11): 777-783.
20. Dela, F., K.J. Mikines, M. von Linstow, N.H. Secher, and H. Galbo. 1992. Effect of training on insulin-mediated glucose uptake in human muscle. *American Journal of Physiology* 263 (6 Pt 1): E1134-E1143.
21. Devlin, J.T., M. Hirshman, E.D. Horton, and E.S. Horton. 1987. Enhanced peripheral and splanchnic insulin sensitivity in NIDDM men after single bout of exercise. *Diabetes* 36 (4): 434-439.
22. Devlin, J.T., and E.S. Horton. 1985. Effects of prior high-intensity exercise on glucose metabolism in normal and insulin-resistant men. *Diabetes* 34 (10): 973-979.
23. Duncan, C.S., C.J. Blimkie, C.T. Cowell, S.T. Burke, J.N. Briody, and R. Howman-Giles. 2002. Bone mineral density in adolescent female athletes: Relationship to exercise type and muscle strength. *Medicine and Science in Sports and Exercise* 34 (2): 286-294.
24. Ebeling, P., R. Bourey, L. Koranyi, J.A. Tuominen, L.C. Groop, J. Henriksson, M. Mueckler, A. Sovijarvi, and V.A. Koivisto. 1993. Mechanism of enhanced insulin sensitivity in athletes: Increased blood flow, muscle glucose transport protein (GLUT-4) concentration, and glycogen synthase activity. *Journal of Clinical Investigation* 92 (4): 1623-1631.
25. Essen, B. 1977. Intramuscular substrate utilization during prolonged exercise. *Annals of the New York Academy of Sciences* 301: 30-44.
26. Essen, B., L. Hagenfeldt, and L. Kaijser. 1977. Utilization of blood-borne and intramuscular substrates during continuous and intermittent exercise in man. *Journal of Physiology* 265 (2): 489-506.
27. Fahim, M.A. 1997. Endurance exercise modulates neuromuscular junction of C57BL/6NNia aging mice. *Journal of Applied Physiology* 83 (1): 59-66.
28. Fink, W.J., D.L. Costill, and M.L. Pollock. 1977. Submaximal and maximal working capacity of elite distance runners. Part II. Muscle fiber composition and enzyme activities. *Annals of the New York Academy of Sciences* 301: 323-327.
29. Franklin, B.A. 2001. Normal cardiorespiratory responses to acute aerobic exercise. In: *ACSM's Resource Manual for Guidelines for Exercise Testing and Prescription*, J.L. Roitman, ed. Philadelphia: Lippincott Williams & Wilkins, pp. 141-149.
30. Green, H.J., S. Jones, M. Ball-Burnett, B. Farrance, and D. Ranney. 1995. Adaptations in muscle metabolism to prolonged voluntary exercise and training. *Journal of Applied Physiology* 78 (1): 138-145.
31. Grilo, C.M., and K.D. Grownell. 2001. Interventions for weight management. In: *ACSM's Resource Manual for Guidelines for Exercise Testing and Prescription*, J.L. Roitman, ed. Philadelphia: Lippincott Williams & Wilkins, pp. 584-591.
32. Gutin, B., P. Barbeau, S. Owens, C.R. Lemmon, M. Bauman, J. Allison, H.S. Kang, and M.S. Litaker. 2002. Effects of exercise intensity on cardiovascular fitness, total body composition, and visceral adiposity of obese adolescents. *American Journal of Clinical Nutrition* 75 (5): 818-826.
33. Guyton, A.C., and J.E. Hall. 2000. *Textbook of Medical Physiology*, 10th ed. Philadelphia: Saunders.
34. Haskell, W.L., C. Sims, J. Myll, W.M. Bortz, F.G. St Goar, and E.L. Alderman. 1993. Coronary artery size and dilating capacity in ultradistance runners. *Circulation* 87 (4): 1076-1082.
35. Haughlin, M.H., R.J. Korthuis, D.J. Duncker, and R.J. Bache. 1996. Control of blood flow to cardiac and skeletal muscle during exercise. In: *Section 12: Exercise: Regulation and Integration of Multiple Systems*, L.B. Rowell and J.T. Shepherd, eds. New York: Oxford University Press, pp. 705-769.
36. Hermansen, L., and M. Wachtlova. 1971. Capillary density of skeletal muscle in well-trained and untrained men. *Journal of Applied Physiology* 30 (6): 860-863.
37. Hickson, R.C. 1981. Skeletal muscle cytochrome C and myoglobin, endurance, and frequency of training. *Journal of Applied Physiology* 51 (3): 746-749.
38. Holloszy, J.O., and E.F. Coyle. 1984. Adaptations of skeletal muscle to endurance exercise and their metabolic consequences. *Journal of Applied Physiology* 56 (4): 831-838.
39. Hoppeler, H., and R. Billeter. 1991. Conditions for oxygen and substrate transport in muscles in exercising mammals. *Journal of Experimental Biology* 160: 263-283.
40. Ingjer, F. 1979. Capillary supply and mitochondrial content of different skeletal muscle fiber types in untrained and endurance-trained men: A histochemical and ultrastructural study. *European Journal of Applied Physiology and Occupational Physiology* 40 (3): 197-209.
41. Jakicic, J.M., R.R. Wing, B.A. Butler, and R.J. Robertson. 1995. Prescribing exercise in multiple short bouts versus one continuous bout: Effects on adherence, cardiorespiratory fitness, and weight loss in overweight women. *International Journal of Obesity and Related Metabolic Disorders* 19 (12): 893-901.

42. Janicki, J.S., D.D. Sheriff, J.L. Robotham, and R.A Wise. 1996. Cardiac output during exercise: Contribution of the cardiac, circulatory, and respiratory systems. In *Section 12: Exercise: Regulation and Integration of Multiple Systems,* L.B. Rowell and J.T. Shepherd, eds. New York: Oxford University Press, pp. 651-704.

43. Jansson, E., and C. Sylven. 1986. Activities of key enzymes in the energy metabolism of human myocardial and skeletal muscle. *Clinical Physiology* 6 (5): 465-471.

44. Jong-Yeon, K., R.C. Hickner, G.L. Dohm, and J.A. Houmard. 2002. Long- and medium-chain fatty acid oxidation is increased in exercise-trained human skeletal muscle. *Metabolism* 51 (4): 460-464.

45. Kaufmann, D.A., and E.W. Swenson. 1981. Pulmonary changes during marathon training: A longitudinal study. *Respiration* 41 (4): 217-223.

46. Kelley, G. 1998. Aerobic exercise and lumbar spine bone mineral density in postmenopausal women: A meta-analysis. *Journal of the American Geriatrics Society* 46 (2): 143-152.

47. Kiens, B., B. Essen-Gustavsson, N.J. Christensen, and B. Saltin. 1993. Skeletal muscle substrate utilization during submaximal exercise in man: Effect of endurance training. *Journal of Physiology* 469: 459-478.

48. Luger, A., P.A. Deuster, S.B. Kyle, W.T. Gallucci, L.C. Montgomery, P.W. Gold, D.L. Loriaux, and G.P. Chrousos. 1987. Acute hypothalamic-pituitary-adrenal responses to the stress of treadmill exercise: Physiologic adaptations to physical training. *New England Journal of Medicine* 316 (21): 1309-1315.

49. Martin, W.H. 3rd, E.F. Coyle, S.A. Bloomfield, and A.A. Ehsani. 1986. Effects of physical deconditioning after intense endurance training on left ventricular dimensions and stroke volume. *Journal of the American College of Cardiology* 7 (5): 982-989.

50. Mazzeo, R.S. 1991. Catecholamine responses to acute and chronic exercise. *Medicine and Science in Sports and Exercise* 23 (7): 839-845.

51. McArdle, W.D., F.I. Katch, and V.L. Katch. 2000. *Essentials of Exercise Physiology,* 2nd ed. Philadelphia: Lippincott Williams & Wilkins.

52. McGuire, D.K., B.D. Levine, J.W. Williamson, P.G. Snell, C.G. Blomqvist, B. Saltin, and J.H. Mitchell. 2001. A 30-year follow-up of the Dallas Bedrest and Training Study: II. Effect of age on cardiovascular adaptation to exercise training. *Circulation* 104 (12): 1358-1366.

53. Megeney, L.A., P.D. Neufer, G.L. Dohm, M.H. Tan, C.A. Blewett, G.C. Elder, and A. Bonen. 1993. Effects of muscle activity and fiber composition on glucose transport and GLUT-4. *American Journal of Physiology* 264 (4 Pt 1): E583-E593.

54. Mendenhall, L.A., S.C. Swanson, D.L. Habash, and A.R. Coggan. 1994. Ten days of exercise training reduces glucose production and utilization during moderate-intensity exercise. *American Journal of Physiology* 266 (1 Pt 1): E136-E143.

55. Mikines, K.J., B. Sonne, P.A. Farrell, B. Tronier, and H. Galbo. 1988. Effect of physical exercise on sensitivity and responsiveness to insulin in humans. *American Journal of Physiology* 254 (3 Pt 1): E248-E259.

56. Morganroth, J., B.J. Maron, W.L. Henry, and S.E. Epstein. 1975. Comparative left ventricular dimensions in trained athletes. *Annals of Internal Medicine* 82 (4): 521-524.

57. Mussolino, M.E., A.C. Looker, and E.S. Orwoll. 2001. Jogging and bone mineral density in men: Results from Nhanes III. *American Journal of Public Health* 91 (7): 1056-1059.

58. Ohman, E.M., J. Butler, J. Kelly, J. Horgan, and K. O'Malley. 1987. Beta-adrenoceptor adaptation to endurance training. *Journal of Cardiovascular Pharmacology* 10 (6): 728-731.

59. O'Toole, M.L. 1998. Overreaching and overtraining in endurance athletes. In: *Overtraining in Sport,* R.B. Kreider, A.C. Fry, and M.L. O'Toole, eds. Champaign, IL: Human Kinetics, pp. 3-17.

60. Pierson, L.M., W.G. Herbert, H.J. Norton, G.M. Kiebzak, P. Griffith, J.M. Fedor, W.K. Ramp, and J.W. Cook. 2001. Effects of combined aerobic and resistance training versus aerobic training alone in cardiac rehabilitation. *Journal of Cardiopulmonary Rehabilitation* 21 (2): 101-110.

61. Richter, E.A. 1996. Glucose utilization. In *Section 12: Exercise: Regulation and Integration of Multiple Systems,* L.B. Rowell and J.T. Shepherd, eds. New York: Oxford University Press, pp. 912-951.

62. Rodnick, K.J., E.J. Henriksen, D.E. James, and J.O. Holloszy. 1992. Exercise training, glucose transporters, and glucose transport in rat skeletal muscles. *American Journal of Physiology* 262 (1 Pt 1): C9-C14.

63. Rubal, B.J., A.R. Al-Muhailani, and J. Rosentswieg. 1987. Effects of physical conditioning on the heart size and wall thickness of college women. *Medicine and Science in Sports and Exercise* 19 (5): 423-429.

64. Saltin, B., K. Nazar, D.L. Costill, E. Stein, E. Jansson, B. Essen, and D. Gollnick. 1976. The nature of the training response; peripheral and central adaptations of one-legged exercise. *Acta Physiologica Scandinavica* 96 (3): 289-305.

65. Schairer, J.R., S. Keteyian, J.W. Henry, and P.D. Stein. 1993. Left ventricular wall tension and stress during exercise in athletes and sedentary men. *American Journal of Cardiology* 71 (12): 1095-1098.

66. Seals, D.R., J.M. Hagberg, W.K. Allen, B.F. Hurley, G.P. Dalsky, A.A. Ehsani, and J.O. Holloszy. 1984. Glucose tolerance in young and older athletes and sedentary men. *Journal of Applied Physiology* 56 (6): 1521-1255.

67. Seals, D.R., J.M. Hagberg, R.J. Spina, M.A. Rogers, K.B. Schechtman, and A.A. Ehsani. 1994. Enhanced left ventricular performance in endurance trained older men. *Circulation* 89 (1): 198-205.

68. Shaw, J.M., K.A. Witzke, and K.M. Winters. 2001. Exercise for skeletal health and osteoporosis prevention. In: *ACSM's Resource Manual for Guidelines for Exercise Testing and Prescription,* J.L. Roitman, ed. Philadelphia: Lippincott Williams & Wilkins, pp. 299-307.

69. Shimamura, C., J. Iwamoto, T. Takeda, S. Ichimura, H. Abe, and Y. Toyama. 2002. Effect of decreased physical activity on bone mass in exercise-trained young rats. *Journal of Orthopaedic Science* 7 (3): 358-363.

70. Slentz, C.A., E.A. Gulve, K.J. Rodnick, E.J. Henriksen, J.H. Youn, and J.O. Holloszy. 1992. Glucose transporters and maximal transport are increased in endurance-trained rat soleus. *Journal of Applied Physiology* 73 (2): 486-492.

71. Soar, P.K., C.T. Davies, P.H. Fentem, and E.A. Newsholme. 1983. The effect of endurance-training on the maximum activities of hexokinase, 6-phosphofructokinase, citrate synthase, and oxoglutarate dehydrogenase in red and white muscles of the rat. *Bioscience Reports* 3 (9): 831-835.

72. Stewart, A.D., and J. Hannan. 2000. Total and regional bone density in male runners, cyclists, and controls. *Medicine and Science in Sports and Exercise* 32 (8): 1373-1377.

73. Takekura, H., and T. Yoshioka. 1990. Different metabolic responses to exercise training programmes in single rat muscle fibres. *Journal of Muscle Research and Cell Motility* 11 (2): 105-113.

74. Takenaka, K., Y. Suzuki, K. Kawakubo, Y. Haruna, R. Yanagibori, H. Kashihara, T. Igarashi, F. Watanabe, M. Omata, F. Bonde-Petersen, and A. Gunji. 1994. Cardiovascular effects of 20 days bed rest in healthy young subjects. *Acta Physiologica Scandinavica* (Suppl) 616: 59-63.

75 Tarnopolsky, L.J., J.D. MacDougall, S.A. Atkinson, M.A. Tarnopolsky, and J.R. Sutton. 1990. Gender differences in substrate for endurance exercise. *Journal of Applied Physiology* 68 (1): 302-308.

76. Vailas, A.C., R.F. Zernicke, J. Matsuda, S. Curwin, and J. Durivage. 1986. Adaptation of rat knee meniscus to prolonged exercise. *Journal of Applied Physiology* 60 (3): 1031-1034.

77. Walberg, J.L. 1989. Aerobic exercise and resistance weight-training during weight reduction: Implications for obese persons and athletes. *Sports Medicine* 7 (6): 343-356.

78. Welsh, L., and O.M. Rutherford. 1996. Hip bone mineral density is improved by high-impact aerobic exercise in postmenopausal women and men over 50 years. *European Journal of Applied Physiology and Occupational Physiology* 74 (6): 511-517.

79. White, F.C., M.D. McKirnan, E.A. Breisch, B.D. Guth, Y.M. Liu, and C.M. Bloor. 1987. Adaptation of the left ventricle to exercise-induced hypertrophy. *Journal of Applied Physiology* 62 (3): 1097-1110.

80. Wilmore, J.H., and D.L. Costill. 1999. *Physiology of Sport and Exercise*, 2nd ed. Champaign, IL: Human Kinetics, pp. 206-242.

81. Wilmore, J.H., P.R. Stanforth, J. Gagnon, T. Rice, S. Mandel, A.S. Leon, D.C. Rao, J.S. Skinner, and C. Bouchard. 2001. Cardiac output and stroke volume changes with endurance training: The Heritage Family Study. *Medicine and Science in Sports and Exercise* 33 (1): 99-106.

82. Wilmore, J.H., P.R. Stanforth, J. Gagnon, T. Rice, S. Mandel, A.S. Leon, D.C. Rao, J.S. Skinner, and C. Bouchard. 2001. Heart rate and blood pressure changes with endurance training: The Heritage Family Study. *Medicine and Science in Sports and Exercise* 33 (1): 107-116.

83. Winder, W.W., J.M. Hagberg, R.C. Hickson, A.A. Ehsani, and J.A. McLane. 1978. Time course of sympathoadrenal adaptation to endurance exercise training in man. *Journal of Applied Physiology* 45 (3): 370-374.

84. Winder, W.W., R.C. Hickson, J.M. Hagberg, A.A. Ehsani, and J.A. McLane. 1979. Training-induced changes in hormonal and metabolic responses to submaximal exercise. *Journal of Applied Physiology* 46 (4): 766-771.

85. Wojtaszewski, J.F., and E.A. Richter. 1998. Glucose utilization during exercise: Influence of endurance training. *Acta Physiologica Scandinavica* 162 (3): 351-358.

CHAPTER 7

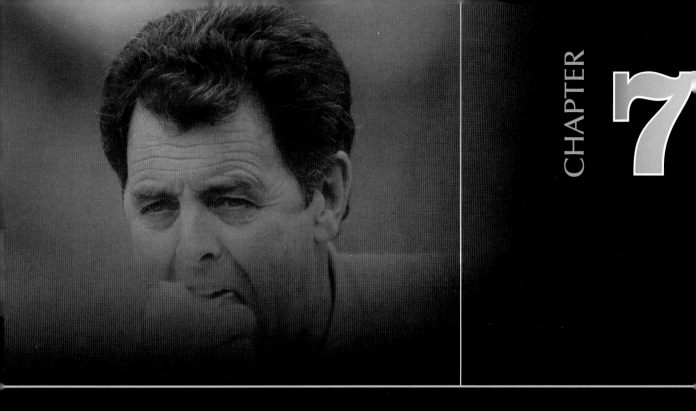

Nutrition in the Personal Training Setting

Kristin J. Reimers

After completing this chapter, you will be able to

- be aware of a personal trainer's scope of practice to know when to refer clients to a nutrition professional;
- review a client's diet and estimate his or her energy expenditure and requirement;
- understand the changes in a client's nutritional and fluid requirements due to exercise;
- advise clients on guidelines for weight gain and weight loss; and
- recognize the role and appropriateness of dietary supplementation

Nutrition and physical activity are two pieces of the same pie. Focusing on one at the exclusion of the other will yield less than optimal results for clients. Personal trainers can enhance their overall effectiveness by maintaining a core knowledge base in nutrition and by individualizing their nutrition advice. Nutrition assessment and recommendations should match the needs and goals of the client and will vary accordingly. And lastly, the personal trainer's guidance is enhanced by knowledge of "when to say when"—that is, when referral to a nutrition expert will benefit the client.

Role of the Personal Trainer Regarding Nutrition

Television, newspapers, magazines, and Web sites are the major sources of nutrition information for most Americans. Nutrition information communicated as sound bites and advertisements makes for much confusion. Personal trainers have the opportunity to help clear the confusion by being a source of credible, individualized nutrition information.

It is well within the scope of practice of the personal trainer who possesses fundamental nutrition knowledge to address misinformation and to give advice as it relates to general nutrition for physical performance, disease prevention, weight loss, and weight gain. An important part of the core knowledge, from the standpoint of both ethics and safety, is the ability to recognize more complicated nutrition issues and know how and to whom to refer clients.

Referral to a nutrition professional is indicated when the client has a disease state (i.e., diabetes, heart disease, gastrointestinal disease, eating disorder, elevated cholesterol, etc.) that is affected by nutrition. This type of nutrition information is called medical nutrition therapy and falls under the scope of practice of a licensed nutritionist, registered dietitian, or both. Referral is also indicated when the complexity of the nutrition issue is beyond the competence of the personal trainer, which will vary. Identifying nutrition professionals to whom the personal trainer is comfortable referring clients, and with whom the personal trainer can communicate about clients, will create a smooth referral process. Registered dietitians can be located through the local dietetic group or through the American Dietetic Association's Web site, www.eatright.org. To facilitate communication, the client should sign a release of information form so that the personal trainer and the nutrition professional can communicate about the client's needs.

Personal trainers should refer clients to a nutrition professional when the client has a disease state that is affected by nutrition or when the complexity of the nutrition issue is beyond the competence of the personal trainer.

Dietary Assessment

Should a client seek nutrition information that is within the scope of the personal trainer's practice, the personal trainer may want to assess the client's diet. A complete nutrition assessment includes dietary data, anthropometric data, biochemical data (lab tests), and clinical examination (condition of skin, teeth, etc.) Although a personal trainer is usually not involved in the comprehensive assessment, the ability to assess the diet of clients is beneficial. (*Note:* The term "diet" as used throughout this chapter refers to the usual eating pattern of the individual, not a restrictive weight loss plan.)

Dietary Intake Data

Before the personal trainer can give valid nutrition advice, gleaning some information about the client's current diet is imperative. How balanced is the client's current diet? Is the client allergic to certain foods? Is the client vegetarian? Is he or she restricting food groups? Dieting to lose weight? Is he or she a sporadic eater? Has the individual just adopted a new way of eating? The answers to all of these questions and others may influence the personal trainer's advice to the client.

Gathering dietary intake data is a simple concept, but it is extremely complex to do. Most people have difficulty recalling fully and accurately what they ate. Research shows that there is a tendency to underestimate or underreport actual intake, especially in persons who are overweight.

Keeping in mind these general shortcomings, the personal trainer has three methods for gathering dietary intake data to choose from:

- Dietary recall
- Diet history
- Diet records

The diet recall has clients report what they have eaten in the past 24 hours. The diet history has clients answering questions about usual eating habits, likes and dislikes, eating schedule, medical history, weight history, and so forth. The diet record is typically a log, filled out for three days, in which the client records everything consumed (foods, beverages, and supplements).

The three-day diet record is considered the most valid of the three methods for assessing the diet of an individual. However, a valid record requires scrupulous recording as well as scrupulous analysis. The pitfall of this method is that recording food intake usually inhibits eating, and recorded intake thus underestimates true intake. To get useful data, the personal trainer should ask only the most motivated clients to complete this process. The diet recall or diet history is more appropriate for many clients.

The personal trainer should never make assumptions about a client's eating habits. Assessing the client's diet is essential before one makes dietary recommendations.

Evaluating the Diet

When the personal trainer has successfully gathered what he or she feels is valid dietary intake data, several options exist for evaluating the information. One way to evaluate the client's diet is to compare the number of servings from each food group to the recommended guidelines given in the **Food Guide Pyramid,** developed by the U.S. Department of Agriculture (USDA) [41]. For clients who are keenly interested in nutrition, a more detailed analysis of the diet using diet analysis software may be indicated. Both methods are reviewed here.

Food Guide Pyramid

The USDA Food Guide Pyramid (figure 7.1) displays recommended types and amounts of food to eat daily. The pyramid classifies foods into five groups:

1. Bread, cereal, rice, and pasta
2. Fruit
3. Vegetables
4. Milk, yogurt, and cheese
5. Meat, poultry, fish, dry beans, eggs, and nuts

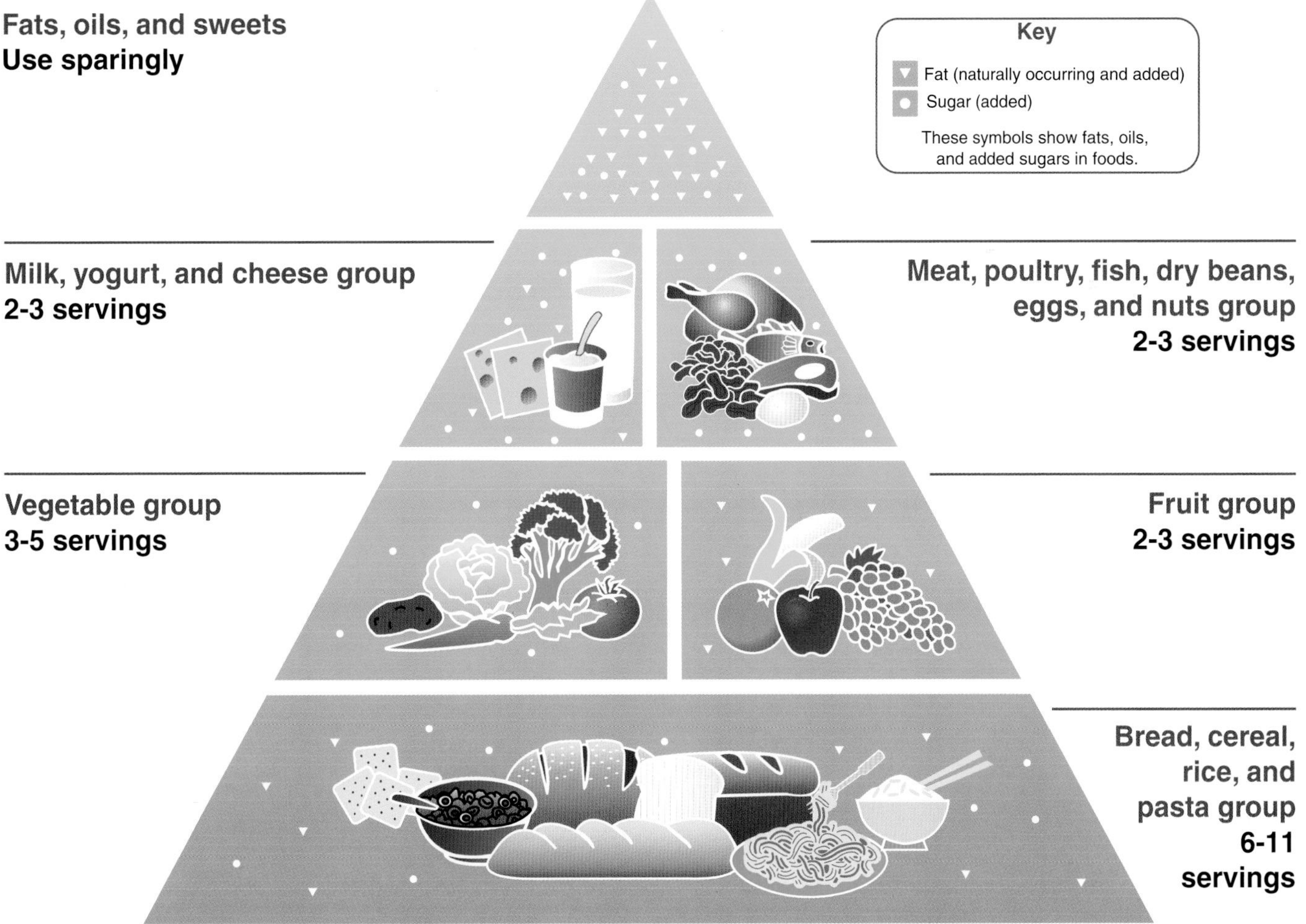

Figure 7.1 Food Guide Pyramid.
SOURCE: U.S. Department of Agriculture/U.S. Department of Health and Human Services.

Foods within each group have similar nutrient compositions and are considered interchangeable; however, balance and variety within each food group is encouraged. For example, the combination of an orange, an apple, and a pear provides more essential nutrients than do three apples, although either example provides the recommended two to four servings. In general, breads, cereal, rice, and pasta provide carbohydrates (sugar and starch), as do fruits and vegetables. These foods are also the primary sources of dietary fiber, riboflavin, thiamin, niacin, folate, vitamin C, and beta-carotene. Meat, poultry, fish, dry beans, eggs, and nuts are major contributors of protein, iron, zinc, and vitamin B_{12} in the diet. Dairy products are excellent sources of dietary protein, calcium, and riboflavin.

The tip of the pyramid is labeled fats, oils, and sweets. Consumers are urged to "use sparingly." This recommendation is based in part on concerns about excess caloric intake for the general population. However, fats, oils, and sweets have a place in clients' diets. When added to a balanced, varied diet, fats and sweets can serve as affordable, convenient sources of calories for those with high caloric needs. Clients with lower caloric requirements should eat these foods in moderation but not completely omit them from the diet.

The USDA Food Guide Pyramid is an excellent starting point from which to evaluate the adequacy of a client's diet. As a rule of thumb, if a diet provides the minimum number of servings from each group, it is adequate for vitamins and minerals. However, if the diet excludes an entire food group, specific nutrients may be lacking. For example, exclusion of meat from the diet increases the risk of inadequate protein, iron, zinc, and vitamin B_6 intake. Exclusion of milk and dairy products increases the risk of inadequate calcium and riboflavin intake. Exclusion of all animal foods means that the diet lacks vitamin B_{12}. Exclusion of fruits and vegetables increases the risk of inadequate vitamin C and beta-carotene intake; and exclusion of breads and cereals increases the risk of inadequate riboflavin, thiamin, and niacin.

Although the pyramid may give the impression that one food group is more important than another, each group provides key nutrients that are more difficult to acquire in the diet if that group is omitted.

The guidelines may need to be adjusted to meet the dietary requirements specific to a client's training program [32]. For example, consuming the maximum number of servings from the Food Guide Pyramid provides about 2,800 kilocalories (kcal), while the minimum number of servings provides about 1,600 calories. Table 7.1 shows examples of

TABLE 7.1

Servings at Various Calorie Levels

	Minimum servings			
	1,600 calories	2,800 calories	3,600 calories	5,000 calories*
Bread, cereal, rice, pasta	6	11	14	18
Vegetable	3	5	7	10
Fruit	2	4	5	7
Milk, yogurt, cheese	2	3	4	6
Meat, poultry, fish, eggs, dry beans, nuts	5 oz (140 g)	7 oz (196 g)	9 oz (252 g)	14 oz (392 g)
Added fats and oils	25 g (5 tsp)	32 g (6 1/2 tsp)	42 g (8 1/2 tsp)	49 g (10 tsp)
Added sugar	11 tsp	18 tsp	24 tsp	28 tsp

*This chart represents a high-carbohydrate, low-fat diet. Obviously the servings become unreasonable at 5,000 calories; it is hard for even the biggest eater to consume 17 servings of vegetables and fruits in a day. Usually individuals who require higher-calorie diets eat more fats, oils, and sugars to get the extra calories.

What's a Serving?

A serving is not necessarily a helping. A helping is the amount a person eats. A helping is much bigger than a serving in many cases. The following are the defined servings of each of the food groups:

- Bread: one slice bread, one small muffin, or dinner roll
- Cereal: 1 ounce (28 grams) ready-to-eat cereal or 1/2 cup cooked cereal
- Pasta and rice: 1/2 cup cooked
- Raw leafy vegetables (lettuce): 1 cup
- Other vegetables: 1/2 cup
- Fruit: one medium apple, orange, or banana, or 1/2 cup canned fruit
- Juices: 3/4 cup
- Milk: 1 cup
- Yogurt: 1 cup
- Cheese: 1 1/2 to 2 ounces (42-56 grams)
- Meat: 2 to 3 ounces cooked (56-85 grams)
- Equivalent to 1 ounce of meat: one egg; 1/2 cup dried beans, cooked; 2 tablespoons peanut butter

the number of servings from each group that would be needed at varying calorie levels, and "What's a Serving?" defines serving sizes.

Computerized Diet Analysis

Computerized analysis is worth it only if the client accurately and completely records usual intake for three consecutive days. Even if the diet is recorded perfectly, the analysis will not be completely accurate because all software programs have shortcomings. Many foods listed in the database have missing values for some vitamins and minerals, meaning that analysis for that nutrient is missing for that food, resulting in an erroneously low intake. Additionally, without fail, some foods that the client eats are not in the database, so it is necessary to make substitutions and best guesses. At best, dietary analysis gives a general idea of nutrient intake, and at worst it does not reflect usual intake at all.

Computerized analysis of the diet is only as good as the recorded information (i.e., "garbage in/garbage out").

Before asking clients to assess their diet, it is helpful for personal trainers to complete a computerized diet analysis on themselves to recognize the bias that recording can impose on true habits. Additionally, analyzing one's own diet makes one aware of the level of detail needed to accurately assess a diet.

In many cases, the personal trainer does not have the training, time, or resources to complete a computerized dietary analysis. This is an area where many personal trainers turn to dietitians for assistance. Another option for motivated clients is to refer them to Web sites where they can enter their own diet and receive feedback (see the list below). These websites are excellent resources to use in that they put the responsibility and ownership on the client. Additionally, some clients feel more comfortable asking questions and reporting intake in private situations.

Analysis of a client's diet is a detailed, time-consuming process that requires expertise. The personal trainer should consider referral of the analysis to a dietitian or refer the client to self-directed diet analysis.

Web Sites Offering Diet Analysis

- www.cyberdiet.com. Users can obtain answers to their personal diet questions, weight loss information, and nutrition and exercise monitoring. E-counseling service is also available.
- www.usda.gov/cnpp. The USDA Web site allows users to enter their food intake; the program then compares intake to the Healthy Eating Index.
- www.shapeup.org. This site was designed as a one-stop for weight loss. It provides access to personalized menus, support groups, and other aids.

Energy

Energy is commonly measured in kilocalories (kcal). A kilocalorie is a measure of energy that equates to the heat required to raise the temperature of 1 kilogram of water 1 degree Celsius (or 2.2 pounds of water 1.8 degrees Fahrenheit). The general public refers to this as a calorie. (The terms "calorie" and "energy" are used interchangeably in this chapter.)

Factors Influencing Energy Requirements

Three factors make up the energy requirement of adults: resting metabolic rate, physical activity, and thermic effect of food. Each of these factors can be affected directly or indirectly by age, genetics, body size, body composition, environmental temperature, training conditions, nontraining physical activity, and caloric intake. For youth, growth is another variable that increases the energy requirement.

Resting metabolic rate (RMR) is the largest contributor to total energy requirement, accounting for approximately 60% to 75% of daily energy expenditure. It is a measure of the calories required for maintaining normal body functions such as respiration, cardiac function, and thermoregulation. One way to think of this is to think of the energy a person would expend by simply lying in bed all day and doing nothing. Factors that increase RMR include gaining lean body tissue, young age, growth, abnormal body temperature, menstrual cycle, and hyperthyroidism. Factors that decrease RMR include low caloric intake, loss of lean tissue, and hypothyroidism. All things equal, RMR can vary up to 20% between individuals due to normal genetic variations in metabolism.

The second largest component of energy requirement is physical activity. Of all the components, this one is the most variable. The amount of energy needed for physical activity depends on the intensity, duration, and frequency of training. It also depends on the environmental conditions; that is, extreme heat or cold increases calorie expenditure. When estimating how physically active a client is, the personal trainer needs to remember to ascertain how physically active the client is aside from structured exercise. Even if they have an exercise routine, those with the sedentary lifestyle of a desk job and sedentary leisure activities would be considered only lightly active.

The **thermic effect of food** is the increase in energy expenditure above the RMR that can be measured for several hours following a meal. The thermic effect of food is the energy needed to digest and assimilate foods, approximately 7% to 10% of the total energy requirement.

Estimating Energy Requirements

A true estimation of **energy requirement** (i.e., energy expended in a day) is difficult to obtain directly. Therefore surrogate methods are used. One such method is to measure calorie intake. This method is valid if the client is maintaining a stable body weight, because stable body weight indicates that energy intake equals energy expenditure. For the motivated client who accurately records intake, the best way to determine energy requirement by this method is to assess the calorie intake from the three-day food log. If that is not possible, there are mathematical equations that roughly estimate caloric expenditure. However, it is difficult to calculate energy needs because of the many variables affecting caloric requirements and the significant inter- and intra-individual variation. It is essential to stress that these equations are only estimates and are meant to serve as a frame of reference. Actual energy expenditure of individuals will vary widely. Table 7.2 provides factors that can be used for energy requirement estimation. For example, for a male who weighs 170 pounds (77 kilograms) and is highly physically active, the requirement would be roughly 3,900 kcal (23×170).

Another method for calculating energy expenditure is to first calculate **resting energy expenditure** (REE), then multiply it by a factor based on activity level. Several equations for estimating REE exist. One set of the REE equations, developed by the World Health Organization [28], is shown in table 7.3.

The result is the number of calories that are likely expended by the person in one day. Clients wishing to maintain current body weight would then need to consume the same number of calories that they expend per day.

It is difficult, if not impossible, to obtain an accurate estimate of a client's energy expenditure. Basing the estimation on intake is one method. Another method is to use an equation such as those provided in this chapter. Regardless of the method, these are rough estimates of the actual expenditure.

TABLE 7.2

Estimated Daily Calorie Needs of Males and Females by Activity Level

	Male		Female	
Activity level	kcal/lb	kcal/kg	kcal/lb	kcal/kg
Light	17	38	16	35
Moderate	19	41	17	37
Heavy	23	50	20	44

Light activity level: Walking on a level surface at 2.5 to 3.0 mph, garage work, electrical trades, carpentry, restaurant trades, housecleaning, child care, golf, sailing, table tennis.

Moderate activity level: Walking 3.5 to 4.0 mph, weeding and hoeing, carrying a load, cycling, skiing, tennis, dancing.

Heavy activity level: Walking with load uphill, tree felling, heavy manual digging, basketball, climbing, football, soccer.

TABLE 7.3

Estimated Daily Calorie Needs Based on Resting Energy Expenditure (REE) and Activity Level

1. To calculate the REE, choose one of these 6 formulas [28]:

Males 18-30 years	(15.3 × weight in kg) + 679
Males 30-60 years	(11.6 × weight in kg) + 879
Males >60 years	(13.5 × weight in kg) + 487
Females, 18-30 years	(14.7 × weight in kg) + 496
Females, 30-60 years	(8.7 × weight in kg) + 829
Females >60 years	(10.5 × weight in kg) + 596

2. Then, multiply the REE by a factor to account for activity level to estimate daily calorie needs:

Level of activity	Activity factor (× REE)
Very light	1.3
Light	1.5-1.6
Moderate	1.6-1.7
Heavy	1.9-2.1
Exceptional	2.2-2.4

Adapted from National Research Council 1989.

Nutrients

Once the personal trainer knows a client's diet habits and energy requirements, he or she can assess general nutritional needs. To understand the relationship between the body and food, as well as to provide nutrition guidance, it is important to have an understanding of the nutrients that compose foods. This section reviews the six nutrients: protein, carbohydrate, fat, vitamins, minerals, and water.

Protein

For centuries, protein was considered the staple of the diet and the source of speed and strength for athletic endeavors. Although we now know that carbohydrates are the main energy source for humans, even today, protein remains the main nutrient of interest, especially among bodybuilders, weightlifters, and others who resistance train.

General Requirements

When answering the question, "How much protein does my client need?" the personal trainer must consider two key factors, energy intake and source of the protein. Protein is burned for energy when fewer calories are consumed than are expended, so protein cannot be used for the intended purpose of building and replacing lean tissue. Thus, when caloric intake goes down, protein requirement goes up. Dietary protein requirements were derived from research on subjects who were consuming adequate calories. Requirements for clients who are dieting for weight loss are higher than standard requirements.

Additionally, protein requirements are based on "reference proteins" such as meat, fish, poultry, dairy products, and eggs, which are considered high-quality proteins. If protein in the diet comes mostly from plants, the requirement is higher. Assuming that a client's energy intake is adequate and that most of his or her protein is from animal sources, the client's needs may be met by the Recommended Dietary Allowance (RDA) for protein for healthy, sedentary adults: 0.8 grams per kilogram of body weight for both adult men and women [28].

Increased Requirements for Intense Training

Intense physical training increases protein requirements. The protein requirement of aerobic endurance athletes can reach 1.4 grams per kilogram of body weight, due in part to increased use of protein as a fuel source during exercise [21]. Resistance training can increase requirements to 1.8 grams per kilogram of body weight [21]. Because most athletes do not fall neatly into one category (aerobic endurance- or resistance-trained athletes), a general recommendation is 1.5 to 2.0 protein grams per kilogram of body weight. Athletes consuming a vegan diet or a low-calorie diet may require more than 2.0 grams per kilogram of body weight.

The personal trainer should be aware that excessively high protein intakes (e.g., greater than 4 grams per kilogram of body weight per day) are not indicated for clients with impaired renal function, those with low calcium intake, or those who are restricting fluid intake. These situations could be exacerbated by a high protein intake. For the most part, however, concerns about potential negative effects of high protein intakes are unfounded, especially in healthy individuals. Proteins consumed in excess of amounts needed for the synthesis of tissue are used for energy or stored.

Carbohydrate

Carbohydrate is required for the complete metabolism of fatty acids. Roughly 50 to 100 grams of carbohydrate (the equivalent of three to five pieces of bread) per day prevents **ketosis** (high levels of ketones in the bloodstream), which results from incomplete breakdown of fatty acids [45]. Beyond that basal requirement, the role of carbohydrate is to provide fuel for energy, and thus the amount of carbohydrate needed by clients depends on their total energy requirement. Carbohydrate recommendations are also based on clients' mode of training.

Because dietary carbohydrate replaces muscle and liver glycogen used during high-intensity physical activity, a high-carbohydrate diet (up to 60-70% of total calories) is commonly recommended for physically active individuals. However, it is important to note that a variety of diets, with various carbohydrate, protein, and fat mixtures, have been shown to be equally effective in supporting training and performance [7, 29, 30]. Not all clients need or want to consume a high-carbohydrate diet. Some physically active individuals certainly benefit from a high-carbohydrate diet, but others do not benefit; and in the worst case, some experience negative effects, such as an increase in serum triglycerides, from consuming a high-carbohydrate diet. Individualizing carbohydrate intake based on the training program and diet history is imperative.

One important factor to consider in determining recommendations for carbohydrate intake is the training program. If a client is an aerobic endurance athlete, for example a distance runner, road cyclist, triathlete, or cross-country skier, who trains aerobically for long durations (90 minutes or more daily), he or she should replenish glycogen levels by consuming maximal levels of carbohydrate. A common recommendation is 8 to 10 grams per kilogram of body weight [17, 35, 37]. This is equivalent to 600 to 750 grams of carbohydrate (2,400-3,000 kcal from carbohydrate) per day for an individual weighing 165 pounds (75 kilograms). This level has been shown to adequately restore skeletal glycogen within 24 hours [1, 9, 18, 22, 31]. More recently, research has shown that athletes engaged in high-intensity, intermittent activities, such as soccer players, also benefit from high-carbohydrate diets [4, 39].

However, the majority of physically active individuals do not train *aerobically* for more than an hour each day. Research on the carbohydrate needs of these individuals is sparse. Moderately low carbohydrate intake and muscle glycogen levels seem to have a minor impact, if any, on resistance training performance [26, 40, 42, 47]. Intake of approximately half of that recommended for aerobic endurance exercise appears adequate to support training and performance of strength, sprint, and skill exercise; thus an intake of 5 to 6 grams per kilogram of body weight per day is reasonable [8, 36].

Dietary Fat

The human body has a low requirement of dietary fat. It is estimated that individuals should consume at least 3% of energy from omega-6 (linoleic) fatty acids and 0.5% to 1% from omega-3 (linolenic) fatty acids to prevent true deficiency [10]. Even though the requirement is low, inadequate fat intake is a potential problem for otherwise healthy individuals who overly restrict dietary fat. Very low–fat diets, such as those sometimes prescribed for patients with severe heart disease, are not recommended for healthy, active individuals. In fact, reducing dietary fat to 10% or less of total calories may worsen blood lipid profiles [11]. Additionally, diets with less than 15% fat may decrease testosterone production, thus decreasing metabolism and muscle development [43]. Recognizing the risk of inadequate fat intake, both the American Heart Association and the Subcommittee on Nutrition of the United Nations recommend that fat provide at least 15% of the total calories in the diets of adults and at least 20% of total calories in the diets of women of reproductive age.

Personal trainers need to be aware of their clients' perception toward dietary fat. "Fat phobia" can lead to diets void of meat and dairy products, which in turn increases the risk of protein, calcium, iron, and zinc deficiency. A moderate- or lower-fat diet should be encouraged; a no-fat diet is dangerous.

It is, of course, the overconsumption rather than the underconsumption of fat that has held the attention of scientists, health care providers, and the general public for the past several decades, specifically with respect to the relationship between dietary fat and cardiovascular disease. High levels of cholesterol or unfavorable ratios of lipoproteins are associated with increased risk of heart disease. A low-fat diet, specifically one low in saturated fat, can decrease total cholesterol in individuals who respond to such a diet. It is from this premise that public health recommendations for fat are made.

Approximately 34% of calories in the typical American diet are from fat [12]. The recommendation for the general public from most health organizations is that fat contributes 30% or less of the total calories consumed. It is recommended that 20% of the total calories (or two-thirds of the total fat intake) come from monounsaturated or polyunsaturated sources and 10% from saturated fats (one-third of total fat intake).

Fat guidelines for physically active individuals are higher than standard "heart healthy" guidelines. Research shows that during periods of heavy aerobic endurance training, increasing dietary fat to a level as high as 50% of calories does not negatively affect plasma lipids [7, 19]. Consumption of high fat diets (38% of calories from fat) in the presence of adequate calorie intake has been shown to enhance performance in trained runners [27]. Indeed, fat intakes greater than 30% are common in elite athletes [15]. In light of the differing metabolism of fats in individuals, the Subcommittee on Nutrition of the United Nations recommends an upper limit for fat intake of 35% of total calories for physically active people.

Personal trainers typically find that many of their clients already consume a diet lower in fat than the goal. It is advisable for a personal trainer to consider the following before making recommendations about decreasing dietary fat.

When Should the Client Decrease Dietary Fat?

In general, there are three reasons for individuals to reduce dietary fat:

1. *Need to increase carbohydrate intake to support training* (see the earlier section on carbohydrate). In this case, to ensure adequate protein provision, fat is the nutrient to decrease so that caloric intake can remain similar while the person is increasing carbohydrate.
2. *Need to reduce total caloric intake to achieve weight loss.* Achieving a negative calorie balance is the only way to reduce body fat. Fat can be a source of excess calories because fat is dense in calories (fat has 9 kcal/gram vs. 4 kcal/gram in carbohydrate and protein). Studies have also suggested that the good flavor of high-fat foods increases the likelihood of overeating these foods. Thus, decreasing excess dietary fat can help reduce caloric intake. (The recommendation to reduce dietary fat should not be made before assessment of dietary intake. The individual may already have a low-fat diet.)
3. *Need to decrease elevated blood cholesterol.* Manipulation of fat and carbohydrate may be necessary if medically indicated for clients who have high blood cholesterol levels or a family history of heart disease. This diet therapy should be provided by a registered dietitian.

Protein, carbohydrates, and fats are all essential nutrients. Excess or deficiency of any one will be problematic. With so many media messages targeting single nutrients, sometimes in a positive light, sometimes negative, it is important for the personal trainer to help clients stay focused on the total diet, not an individual nutrient.

Vitamins and Minerals

Dietary Reference Intakes (DRIs) are recommendations of the Food and Nutrition Board of the National Academy of Sciences for the intake of vitamins and minerals, to be used for planning and assessing diets for healthy people (table 7.4). A personal trainer who has the computerized analysis of a client's diet can assess actual vitamin and mineral intake compared to the DRIs. Starting in 1997 the DRIs replaced the *Recommended Dietary Allowances* that had been published since 1941. Dietary Reference Intakes represent a new approach, with the emphasis on long-term health instead of deficiency diseases. The DRIs are split into four categories:

1. *Recommended dietary allowance* is the intake that meets the nutrient needs of almost all healthy individuals in a specific age and sex group. The RDA reflects the population mean plus two standard deviations, so it is not a minimum number as it is sometimes assumed to be.
2. *Adequate intake* is a goal intake when sufficient scientific information is unavailable to estimate the RDA.
3. *Estimated average requirement* is the intake that meets the estimated nutrient need of half the individuals in a specific group.
4. *Tolerable upper intake level* is the maximum intake that is unlikely to pose risks of adverse health effects in almost all healthy individuals in a group.

Instead of being published in one volume as were the RDAs, the DRIs have been published as separate nutrient groups, each group having its own volume. The first book was published in 1997; several more have followed. The reader is referred to the Web site www.nap.edu, where full texts of the reports are posted. It is important to remember that the recommendations for nutrient intakes represent the state of the science at the time, and as such, continue to evolve.

Historically, focus has been on inadequate nutrient intake. However, both inadequate intakes and excessive intakes are problematic. Accordingly the new DRIs include an upper limit, or the amount of a nutrient that may cause negative side effects. Personal trainers should watch for excessively high vitamin and mineral intakes in clients who are taking a number of supplements that may overlap in their ingredients.

TABLE 7.4

Recommended Dietary Allowances and Upper Limits of Select Vitamins and Minerals

Specific vitamin or mineral	RDA or AI		Upper limit
	Male	Female	
Vitamin A (μg/day)	**900**	**700**	3,000
Vitamin C (mg/day)	**90**	**75**	2,000
Vitamin E (mg/day)	**15**	**15**	1,000
Vitamin K (μg/day)	120	90	ND
Thiamin (mg/day)	**1.2**	**1.1**	ND
Riboflavin (mg/day)	**1.3**	**1.1**	ND
Niacin (mg/day)	**16**	**14**	35
Vitamin B_6 (mg/day)	**1.3**	**1.3**	100
Folate (μg/day)	**400**	**400**	1,000
Vitamin B_{12} (μg/day)	2.4	2.4	ND
Pantothenic acid (mg/day)	5	5	ND
Biotin (μg/day)	30	30	ND
Calcium (mg/day)	1,000	1,000	2,500
Chromium (μg/day)	35	25	ND
Iron (mg/day)	**8**	**18**	45
Magnesium (mg/day)	**400-420**	**310-320**	350
Phosphorus (mg/day)	**700**	**700**	4,000
Selenium (μg/day)	**55**	**55**	400
Zinc (mg/day)	**11**	**8**	40

Note: This table (taken from the Dietary Reference Intake reports, see www.nap.edu) presents Recommended Dietary Allowances (RDAs) in **bold type** and adequate intakes (AIs) in ordinary type. RDAs are set to meet the needs of almost all (97-98%) individuals in a group. The AI for adults and gender groups is believed to cover needs of all individuals in the group, but lack of data does not allow specifying of the percentage of individuals covered by this intake. ND = not determined.

From www.nap.edu

Dietary intake of vitamins and minerals includes intake from food as well as from dietary supplements. Personal trainers can assess a client's intake on the basis of the Dietary Reference Intakes.

Water

Fluid intake is a nonissue for some and an obsession for others. Some carry water with them and quaff so much that frequent trips to the bathroom are in order. Others seem to shun water almost entirely, leaving to question how they can remain upright. A variety of issues have set the stage for confusion about how much and what to drink. Surprisingly little research exists on the water requirements of humans. Research that does exist is primarily limited to hospitalized patients, soldiers, or serious athletes in hot environments. Assumptions that thirst will drive adequate water intake, and taking comfort in the fact that kidneys will do their job, have largely led scientists to overlook the issue of hydration in healthy individuals.

General Fluid Intake Guidelines

Unlike the situation with many other nutrients, it is impossible to set a general requirement for water. Common knowledge and folklore have put the requirement at anywhere from 64 ounces (1.9 liters) per day to 2 gallons (7.5 liters). Both could be right, depending on the situation. The reality is that water requirements change based on environment, sweating, body surface area, calorie intake, body size, lean muscle tissue, and so on, leading to tremendous inter- and intra-individual variation. Instead of looking at prescriptive amounts to be consumed each day, it is important for personal trainers to assess each client's situation and to individualize recommendations.

It is impossible to set a generic water recommendation, such as eight glasses of water a day. Each individual's water requirement varies over time, as do requirements among various people.

The basic goal of fluid intake is avoid dehydration, that is, maintain fluid balance. The state of fluid balance exists when the water that is lost from the body through urine, through insensible loss from skin and lungs, and through feces, is replaced. The kidneys dilute or concentrate urine to keep the body's internal milieu unchanged regardless of significant changes in intake. Thirst is triggered at about 1% dehydration. Thus, "Just drink when you are thirsty" is a recommendation that probably works quite well to maintain fluid balance for individuals in temperature-controlled environments who are sedentary and who have plenty of fluid readily available.

The average fluid intake needed to offset fluid losses in sedentary adults may range from 1.5 to 2.7 quarts (1.4-2.6 liters) per day. The question is often asked if higher fluid intakes are healthful. The answer is unclear, but an emerging area of study examining the relationship between disease prevention and fluid intake indicates that high fluid intakes may be preventive against bladder cancer, kidney stones, gallstones, and colon cancer [6, 20, 25, 34].

While most individuals who are not under physical or environmental stress maintain hydration status with normal intake, the relationship between consuming higher amounts of fluid and disease prevention is being examined.

Fluid Intake and Exercise

Although the answers regarding general fluid intake during sedentary conditions are unclear, more is known about fluid intake and exercise. Guidelines have been developed for individuals before, during, and after exercise.

Before Exercise Consuming at least 1 pint (0.5 liters) of fluid two hours before activity provides the fluid needed to achieve optimal hydration and allows enough time for urination of excess fluid [2].

During Exercise Preventing dehydration is difficult for physically active people exercising in a warm environment. Continuous sweating during prolonged exercise can exceed 1.9 quarts (1.8 liters) per hour, increasing water requirements significantly. Unless sweat losses are replaced, body temperature rises, leading to heat exhaustion, heat stroke, and even death. Paradoxically, during exercise, humans do not adequately replace sweat losses when fluids are consumed at will. In fact, most individuals replace only about two-thirds of the water they sweat off during exercise. Personal trainers must be aware of this tendency and make their clients aware of it as well. During times of high sweat loss under physical stress, a systematic approach to water replacement is necessary because thirst is not a reliable indicator of fluid needs.

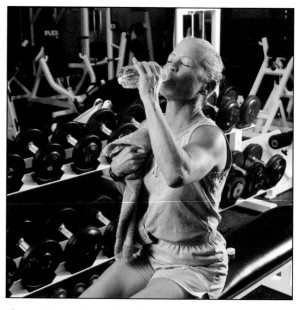

Figure 7.2 Clients should start drinking water before they are thirsty and continue to drink throughout their workout.

When heat or intensity of exercise lead to profuse sweating, a client should drink early and frequently, for example, at 10- to 30-minute intervals. The amount to be consumed depends on how much that client is losing via sweat. In ambient conditions, sweat rate loss may be less than 250 milliliters per hour, whereas in hot environments, sweat rates can exceed 2 liters per hour. Monitor sweat loss by checking body weight before and after the activity.

After fluids enter the stomach, they empty to the small intestine, and then nutrients are absorbed into the bloodstream for distribution throughout the body. Larger volumes (e.g., 8 fluid ounces, or 237 milliliters) tend to empty from the stomach more rapidly than small volumes, so chugging is preferred over sipping as long as it does not cause stomach discomfort. Concern about feeling waterlogged is common. However, research suggests that the cause of stomach discomfort is usually a result of dehydration, not the result of too much water. The amount consumed will vary based on the temperature and humidity. Some clients make the mistake of drinking the same amount on cool days as on hot days, which in a few cases has led to water overload.

After Exercise Slight dehydration is common in almost all physical endeavors, and therefore rehydration is necessary. However, "preventive maintenance" is also important. Starting hydrated, as well as consuming fluids during activity, is commonly overlooked but is a very important part of the systematic approach to hydration.

A systematic approach to ensuring adequate rehydration is to record body weight immediately before and after a workout. (For accuracy, clients should remove sweaty clothes before weighing.) Each pound (0.45 kilograms) lost during a workout represents 1 pint (0.5 liters) of fluid loss. Thus, for each pound lost, 1 pint of fluid needs to be consumed. During the rehydration process, urine is produced before full rehydration occurs. Thus, consuming 20% more than the amount of sweat loss is an adequate guideline for fluid intake [38]. Ideally, the amount of fluid clients need to replace should be measured into water bottles, pitchers, and so forth so that rehydration is not left to chance.

Clients who have a goal of weight loss may misperceive acute weight loss during a workout as loss of fat and therefore see it as positive. It is important for personal trainers to clarify with clients that the acute weight loss during a workout is water, not fat, and must be replaced.

Monitoring Hydration Status

Although not as sensitive as weight change, other indicators of hydration status can be useful monitoring tools. Signs of dehydration include dark yellow, strong-smelling urine; decreased frequency of urination; rapid resting heart rate; and prolonged muscle soreness [3]. Normal urine production for adults is about 1.2 quarts (1.1 liters) per day, or 8 to 10 fluid ounces (237-296 milliliters) per urination four times per day. Normal urine is the color of lemon juice, except in clients who are taking supplemental vitamins, which tend to make the urine bright yellow.

What to Drink Before and After Activity

All fluids, from beverages and from food, contribute to the body's fluid requirement. Juice and soft drinks are 89% water; milk is 90% water, and even pizza is 50% water. Before and after physical activity, water or other beverages such as milk, juice, carbonated or uncarbonated soft drinks, and sport drinks, are suitable choices for fluid replacement. For clients who eat many fruits, vegetables, and soups, much of their water requirement may be coming from foods.

Whether consuming caffeine-containing beverages causes dehydration is a frequently asked question. Data show that tolerance to caffeine occurs in one to four days and that persons who are tolerant do not experience increased urine output. Thus, caffeine-containing beverages contribute to hydration [14].

When significant sweating has occurred, consumption of sodium chloride (salt) in the form of beverages or food minimizes urine output and hastens recovery of water and electrolyte balance [23, 24]. In practical terms, this means that consuming a wide variety of beverages and foods after training is important. In fact, most fluid consumption occurs during and around mealtimes.

All foods and fluids contribute to hydration, including foods like pizza and beverages like coffee.

What to Drink During Activity

The goal of fluid replacement during exercise is to move the fluid from the mouth, through the gut, and into circulation rapidly and to provide a volume that matches sweat losses. The way to achieve this is to provide fluids that are absorbed rapidly and that the client finds palatable. A variety of fluids can serve as effective fluid replacements during exercise [16]. Cool water is an ideal fluid replacement. Other options include commercial sport drinks or homemade sport drinks, such as diluted juice or diluted soft drinks. Although plain water can meet fluid requirements in most cases, some people find flavored drinks more palatable than water and consequently drink more [46]. During aerobic endurance training, carbohydrate along with water intake can be helpful if activities last more than an hour [5].

Commercial sport drinks contain water, sugars, and electrolytes (usually sodium, chloride, and potassium). The sugar content of sport drinks is slightly less than the amount in most soft drinks and juices. Carbohydrate concentration of commercial sport drinks ranges from 6% to 8%, a solution that tends to be absorbed rapidly. People can make their own sport drinks by diluting two parts soft drink to one part water and adding salt (1/8 teaspoon, or 0.7 milligrams, per quart). Another option is to ingest solid food (fruit, sport bars, cereal bars, cookies, etc.) or sport gel as a carbohydrate source along with plain water.

Clients who are monitoring calorie intake in an effort to maintain or lose weight may be averse to consuming the extra calories in sport drinks. In this case, the cost:benefit of consuming carbohydrate must be examined. It is worth remembering that the benefits of carbohydrate during aerobic endurance training are important for competitive clients wanting to increase speed and aerobic endurance, but might be less so for a client who is training primarily for health and fitness.

Weight Gain

There are two basic reasons clients may attempt to gain weight: to improve physical appearance or to enhance athletic performance. For weight gain in the form of muscle mass, a combination of diet and progressive resistance training is essential. However, genetic predisposition, body type, and compliance determine the client's progress. Muscle tissue is approximately 70% water, 22% protein, and 8% fatty acids and glycogen. If all the extra calories consumed are used for muscle growth during resistance training, then about 2,500 extra kilocalories are required for each 1-pound (0.45-kilogram) increase in lean tissue. This includes the energy needed for tissue assimilation as well as the energy expended during resistance training. Thus, 350 to 700 kcal above daily requirements would supply the calories needed to support a 1- to 2-pound (0.45- to 0.9-kilogram) weekly gain in lean tissue as well as the energy requirements of the resistance training program.

To accomplish increased caloric intake, it is recommended that clients eat larger portions of foods at mealtime, eat more items at each meal, eat frequently, or choose higher-calorie foods. Practical experience shows that it is difficult for clients to gain weight if they are eating less than five times per day. To accommodate frequent eating, some use meal replacement drinks.

Gaining muscle increases protein requirements. Protein needs are estimated to be 1.5 to 2.0 grams per kilogram of body weight per day and may be higher if the client's primary source of protein is plant based. Plant proteins have a lower biological value than animal proteins.

The two primary nutrition principles for weight gain are to increase calorie intake and to increase (or maintain at an adequate level) protein intake.

Weight Loss

People who have weight loss, specifically fat loss, as a goal can be split into two general groups: those who are normal weight but want to lose body fat for aesthetic reasons, and those who are overweight or obese, that is, have a body mass index greater than 25 or 30, respectively. Chapter 19 provides detailed information on weight loss. The following are general principles to be considered when a client embarks on a weight loss regimen:

- The ability to achieve and maintain minimal body fat is largely genetic. Some individuals are able to do so while maintaining health and performance. Others experience health and performance problems.
- Whether clients can gain muscle and lose body fat simultaneously depends primarily on their level of training. Previously untrained clients can both lose body fat and gain lean body mass as a result of caloric restriction and training; however, it is unlikely that trained persons who already possess a relatively low percentage of body fat can achieve body mass reduction without losing some lean body mass.
- An average of 1 to 2 pounds (about 0.5-1.0 kilograms) per week represents a daily caloric deficit of approximately 500 to 1,000 kcal. Faster rates of weight loss can lead to dehydration

and decrease vitamin and mineral status [13]. Substantial weight loss by caloric restriction will result in loss of marked amounts of lean body mass [44]. Fat loss rates vary depending on body size. The rate of loss of 1% total body weight per week is a common guideline. For example, losing at a rate of 1%, a 110-pound (50-kilogram) client would strive for about a 1-pound (0.45-kilograms) weight loss per week, while a 331-pound (150-kilogram) client would aim to lose about 3 pounds (1.5 kilograms) per week.

- The diet should be composed of food low in energy density. **Energy density** refers to the calories per weight or volume of food. Examples of foods with low energy density are broth-based soup, salad greens, vegetables, and fruits. In general, foods with low energy density contain a high proportion of water and fiber. These are foods that people can eat in large portions without consuming excess calories. This can help control hunger and lower caloric intake [33].
- The diet should be nutritionally balanced and should provide a variety of foods. See the first section of this chapter on the Food Guide Pyramid.

The guiding principle for weight loss is to help clients achieve a negative energy balance. Many clients think the issue is more complex than that, so the personal trainer should keep them focused on this principle.

Evaluating Weight Loss Diets

Weight loss diet plans are endless—high protein, low fat, low carbohydrate, this shake, that bar, fat burners, don't eat at night, eat six times a day, eat one time a day—and the list goes on. What makes things confusing is that every client can name at least one person for whom at least one of these methods has worked. In addition, each client can think of many people for whom nothing seems to work. The truth is, *any* method will lead to fat loss if, and only if, the person achieves a negative calorie balance. Input has to be less than output, period. As personal trainers answer their clients' questions about diets they read about or see on TV, it is essential to keep in mind that calories-in have to be less than calories-out for fat loss to occur.

Clearly, it is impossible to keep up with every new diet, and a personal trainer does not need to. Instead, one evaluates a diet not on the claims it makes, but by the foods (and therefore nutrients) that are included and excluded. Exclusion of one or more groups of foods is an indicator that the diet may be deficient in certain nutrients, or that it is too restrictive for clients to stay on for the long term. It is also important to evaluate the calorie intake that the diet implicitly or explicitly recommends. Very low calorie diets can lead to higher loss of lean tissue, are limited in nutrients, and may decrease compliance. Last but not least, personal trainers need to talk to clients about what they are really doing, not what the diet plan says. Often, the two are different.

In addition to foods, the personal trainer should examine whether a diet plan includes dietary supplements. Stimulants such as ephedrine or caffeine are commonly added to weight loss supplements. These types of supplements are generally contraindicated in individuals with high blood pressure or other medical conditions. Use of stimulants for weight loss should be implemented only under the supervision of a physician. In many cases, clients are not aware of all the ingredients in the supplement they ingest. The personal trainer can ask the client to bring in the container so they can review the contents together. At this time the personal trainer can gather information on any questionable ingredients.

Dietary Supplements

Dietary supplements cover the spectrum from traditional vitamin-mineral tablets to prehormones such as androstenedione. Because of the diversity of dietary supplements, it is difficult to give blanket recommendations or guidelines about them. The following information provides a general overview of the science and regulation of dietary supplements.

Dietary Supplement Regulation

Dietary supplements are under the same safety and purity regulations as foods, as well as by truth-in-labeling laws. However, supplements do not fit perfectly under food regulation. Thus regulations continue to be defined under the Dietary Supplement Health and Education Act of 1994 (DSHEA). This act was a landmark law for supplements, affirming the status of dietary supplements as a category of food, not drugs, and defining dietary supplements as products "intended to supplement the diet." The ingredients of a supplement include vitamins, minerals, herbs/botanicals, amino acids, a substance that increases the total dietary intake, or variations and combinations thereof.

In January of 2000, the Food and Drug Administration ruled that supplement manufacturers can make claims on the label about the body's structure or function that the supplement affects but cannot claim to diagnose, prevent, cure, or treat disease. In other words, it is permissible to say that a calcium supplement will "help maintain bone health" but not permissible to say that calcium will "help prevent osteoporosis."

Although the Food and Drug Administration does not have the resources to monitor and test individual supplements, a few independent organizations offer quality testing and approval. One independent company, ConsumerLab.com, tests supplements for quality and purity and provides the results on their Web site. Supplements that pass the test can carry the ConsumerLab seal of approved quality on the label. An independent, voluntary organization called United States Pharmacopoeia (USP) is developing a pilot Dietary Supplement Certification Program. The acronym USP on the label is meant to assure the consumer that the label information is accurate and that the company follows good manufacturing practices.

Evaluating Supplement Regimens

It is estimated that 48% of U.S. adults take some kind of dietary supplement. Vitamin and mineral supplements remain the types of supplements most commonly used. Although vitamin-mineral supplements are perceived to be without risk, this is not the case. The personal trainer must decide whether to recommend a vitamin-mineral supplement to a client based on the client's food intake. The content of the supplement should round out, that is, supplement, the individual's diet. There are common scenarios of appropriate use of supplements: for example, people who do not consume dairy products take a calcium supplement, or people who travel a great deal use vitamin-mineral supplements to ensure that they are getting needed nutrients. It is not uncommon to observe among dietary supplement users that their diet is quite adequate without supplements. Likewise, it is often the client who does not use dietary supplements who has an inadequate diet that may benefit from supplementation.

Excesses are just as dangerous as inadequate intakes. For example, excess iron can be dangerous for those with a silent genetic disorder called hemochomotasis, whereby the body absorbs and stores excess iron in tissues, leading to multisystem failure. Excess zinc can decrease high-density lipoprotein cholesterol, and excess calcium is a risk for kidney stones. When evaluating a client's supplement regimen, it is important to evaluate all sources of the nutrient. Because vitamins and minerals are often added to a variety of supplements (shakes, powders, etc.) as well as breakfast cereal, sport bars, and energy drinks, there is increasing likelihood of excessive intakes. Excessive intakes, especially of iron, calcium, zinc, magnesium, niacin, B_6, and vitamin A, should be corrected by changing the supplement regimen.

A common finding is that the individual's supplementation choices do not match the inadequacies of the diet, causing excess intakes of some nutrients and not correcting the low intakes. Helping a client adjust food choices and supplement choices to optimize the vitamin and mineral intake is a useful function of diet analysis.

Besides questions about vitamins and minerals, clients may have questions about other types of supplements such as creatine or amino acids. One way to make sense of the wide array of supplements is to categorize them. Most supplements fit into the categories shown in table 7.5. Evaluation of the particular supplement for a client depends on the individual's goals and situation. For example, meal replacement drinks and bars can be an excellent snack for busy people. Protein supplements can round out protein needs in those who don't eat enough dietary protein, and so on. If a client participates in National Collegiate Athletic Association, United States Olympic Committee, or other competitions where drug testing occurs, it is important to know that some supplements contain banned substances that could lead to a positive drug test. These individuals need to check with their sponsoring organizations for guidelines.

For more specific information on the science and regulation of dietary supplements, check http://dietary-supplements.info.nih.gov/, the Web site of the government office on dietary supplements.

The "Art" of Making Dietary Recommendations

When a personal trainer is evaluating a client's eating habits and giving advice, it is important to keep a few concepts in mind. First, nutritional

TABLE 7.5

Selected Dietary Supplement Categories

Category	Examples
Meal replacements	Drinks and bars
Protein sources	Drinks, powder, tablets
Amino acids	Glutamine, tyrosine
Carbohydrate sources	Sport drinks, energy drinks, bars, gels
Pre- and prohormones*	Androstenedione, DHEA
Biochemicals/Energy metabolites	Creatine, HMB, pyruvate, CLA
Herbs	Ginseng, St. John's wort, guarana

* Pre- and prohormone refers to substances that are precursors to or enhancers of hormone production.

CLA = conjugated linoleic acid; DHEA = dehydroepiandrosterone; HMB = hydroxy metylbutyrate.

status is influenced by intake over a relatively long period. Short-term dietary inadequacies or excesses will minimally influence long-term status. Additionally, the body can accumulate the nutrients it needs through countless combinations of foods consumed over time. There is no "right way to eat" that applies to everyone. Generally speaking, an adequate diet provides nutrients the body needs, provides other components from food that promote health or prevent disease, provides calories at the level needed to achieve desired body weight, and does so in a manner that matches the individual's preferences, lifestyle, training goals, and budget. The beauty of working one-on-one is that this format does not tie the personal trainer to generalized one-size-fits-all dietary recommendations so often communicated by the media, but allows individualization of recommendations. This is one of the keys to effectiveness.

CONCLUSION

The personal trainer can benefit from three fundamental tools when discussing nutrition with their clients. One is factual information, such as that provided in this book, on which to base assessments and recommendations. The second tool is the individualized approach. Personal trainers are likely to find themselves recommending something to one client and advising the next client against it. The ability to match the recommendations to the individual's situation enhances the personal trainer's effectiveness exponentially. The third tool is a network of knowledgeable persons to consult or refer to when clients have nutrition issues outside the scope of the personal trainer's expertise. With these three tools, the personal trainer can help nutrition work for, not against, clients' health and fitness goals.

STUDY QUESTIONS

1. How many servings of the "bread, cereal, rice, and pasta" group does this meal provide?

   1.5 cups cooked oatmeal
   1 cup 1% milk
   ¾ cup apple juice
   2 slices wheat toast with 2 tablespoons peanut butter

A. 8
B. 5
C. 4
D. 3

2. Taking into consideration REE, which of the following is the approximate daily caloric need of a 45-year-old, 176-pound (80-kilogram) male client who has a very light activity level?
   A. 3797 kilocalories
   B. 1983 kilocalories
   C. 2349 kilocalories
   D. 4156 kilocalories
3. Which of the following guidelines should the personal trainer recommend to a client to promote proper fluid intake?

	Before exercise	After exercise
A.	1 gallon (3.8 liters) 30 minutes before	1 pint (0.5 liters) for each lost kilogram
B.	1 cup (237 milliliters) 15 minutes before	1 gallon (3.8 liters) for each lost pound
C.	1 quart (0.9 liters) 1 hour before	1 gallon (3.8 liters) for each lost kilogram
D.	1 pint (0.5 liters) 2 hours before	1 pint (0.5 liters) for each lost pound

4. Assuming no other changes except body fat loss and the same weekly rate of fat loss (1% of the starting weight), approximately how many weeks will it take a 220-pound (100-kilogram) client to reach a goal weight of 200 pounds (91 kilograms)?
   A. 20 weeks
   B. 9 weeks
   C. 5 weeks
   D. 3 weeks

APPLIED KNOWLEDGE QUESTION

Assuming no deficiencies, special requirements, or additional needs, describe the general daily nutrient requirements for a 50-year-old, 154-pound (70-kilogram) female client who has a light activity level.

Nutrient	General daily requirements
Kilocalories	
Protein (grams)	
Carbohydrate (grams)	
Fat (percent of total kilocalories)	
Monounsaturated fat (percent of total fat intake)	
Polyunsaturated fat (percent of total fat intake)	
Saturated fat (percent of total fat intake)	
Vitamin A	
Vitamin E	
Calcium	
Iron	
Fluid	

REFERENCES

1. Ahlborg, B., J. Bergstrom, J. Brohult, L. Ekelund, E. Hultman, and G. Maschio. 1967. Human muscle glycogen content and capacity for prolonged exercise after different diets. *Foersvarsmedicine* 3: 85-99.
2. American College of Sports Medicine. 1996. Position stand. Exercise and fluid replacement. *Medicine and Science in Sports and Exercise* 28: i-vii.
3. Armstrong, L.W., C.M. Maresh, J.W. Castellani, M.F. Bergeron, R.W. Kenefick, K.E. LaGasse, and D. Riebe. 1994. Urinary indices of hydration status. *International Journal of Sports Nutrition* 4: 265-279.
4. Balsom, P.D., K. Wood, P. Olsson, and B. Ekblom. 1999. Carbohydrate intake and multiple sprint sports: With special reference to football (soccer). *International Journal of Sports Medicine* 20: 48-52.
5. Below, P.R., R. Mora-Rodriguez, J. Gonzalez-Alonso, and E.F. Coyle. 1995. Fluid and carbohydrate ingestion independently improve performance during 1 h of intense exercise. *Medicine and Science in Sports and Exercise* 27: 200-210.
6. Borghi, L., T. Meschi, F. Amato, A. Briganti, A. Novarini, and A. Giannini. 1996. Urinary volume, water, and recurrences in idiopathic calcium nephrolithiasis: A 5-year randomized prospective study. *Journal of Urology* 155: 839-843.
7. Brown, R.C., and C.M. Cox. 1998. Effects of high fat versus high carbohydrate diets on plasma lipids and lipoproteins in endurance athletes. *Medicine and Science in Sports and Exercise* 30: 1677-1683.
8. Burke, L.M., G.R. Collier, S.K. Beasley, P.G. Davis, P.A. Fricker, P. Heeley, K. Walder, and M. Hargreaves. 1995. Effect of coingestion of fat and protein with carbohydrate feedings on muscle glycogen storage. *Journal of Applied Physiology* 78: 2187-2192.
9. Costill, D.L., W.M. Sherman, W.J Fink, C. Maresh, M. Witten, and J.M. Miller. 1981. The role of dietary carbohydrates in muscle glycogen resynthesis after strenuous running. *American Journal of Clinical Nutrition* 34: 1831-1836.
10. Davis, B. 1998. Essential fatty acids in vegetarian nutrition. *Vegetarian Diet* 7: 5-7.
11. Dreon, D.M., H.A. Fernstrom, P.T. Williams, and R.M. Krauss. 1999. A very-low-fat diet is not associated with improved lipoprotein profiles in men with a predominance of large, low-density lipoproteins. *American Journal of Clinical Nutrition* 69: 411-418.
12. Ernst, N.D., C.T. Sempos, R.R. Briefel, and M.B. Clark. 1997. Consistency between US dietary fat intake and serum total cholesterol concentrations: The National Health and Nutrition Examination Surveys. *American Journal of Clinical Nutrition* 66 (Suppl): 965S-972S.
13. Fogelholm, G.M., R. Koskinen, J. Laakso, T. Rankinen, and I. Ruokonen. 1993. Gradual and rapid weight loss: Effects on nutrition and performance in male athletes. *Medicine and Science in Sports and Exercise* 25: 371-373.
14. Grandjean, A.C., K.J. Reimers, K.E. Bannick, and M.C. Haven. 2000. The effect of caffeinated, non-caffeinated, caloric and non-caloric beverages on hydration. *Journal of the American College of Nutrition* 19: 591-600.
15. Grandjean, A.C., K.J. Reimers, and J.S. Ruud. 1998. Dietary habits of Olympic athletes. In: *Nutrition in Exercise and Sport*, I. Wolinsky, ed. Boca Raton, FL: CRC Press, pp. 421-430.
16. Horswill, C.A. 1998. Effective fluid replacement. *International Journal of Sport Nutrition* 8: 175-195.
17. Jacobs, K.A., and W.M. Sherman. 1999. The efficacy of carbohydrate supplementation and chronic high-carbohydrate diets for improving endurance performance. *International Journal of Sport Nutrition* 9: 92-115.
18. Kochan, R.G., D.R. Lamb, S.A. Lutz, C.V. Perrill, E.M. Reimann, and K.K. Schlende. 1979. Glycogen synthase activation in human skeletal muscle: Effects of diet and exercise. *American Journal of Physiology* 236: E660-E666.
19. Leddy, J., P. Horvath, J. Rowland, and D. Pendergast. 1997. Effect of a high or a low fat diet on cardiovascular risk factors in male and female runners. *Medicine and Science in Sports and Exercise* 29: 17-25.
20. Leitzmann, M.F., W.C. Willett, E.B. Rimm, M.J. Stampfer, D. Spiegelman, G.A. Colditz, and E. Giovannucci. 1999. A prospective study of coffee consumption and the risk of symptomatic gallstone disease in men. *Journal of the American Medical Association* 281: 2106-2112.
21. Lemon, P.W.R. 1998. Effects of exercise on dietary protein requirements. *International Journal of Sport Nutrition* 8: 426-447.
22. MacDougall, G.R., D.G. Ward, D.G. Sale, and J.R. Sutton. 1977. Muscle glycogen repletion after high intensity intermittent exercise. *Journal of Applied Physiology* 42: 129-132.
23. Maughan, R.J., J.B. Leiper, and S.M. Shirreffs. 1996. Restoration of fluid balance after exercise-induced dehydration: Effects of food and fluid intake. *European Journal of Applied Physiology* 73: 317-325.
24. Maughan, R.J., J.H. Owen, S.M. Shirreffs, and J.B. Leiper. 1994. Post-exercise rehydration in man: Effects of electrolyte addition to ingested fluids. *European Journal of Applied Physiology* 69: 209-215.
25. Michaud, D.S., D. Spiegelman, S.K. Clinton, E.B. Rimm, G.C. Curhan, W.C. Willett, and E.L. Giovannucci. 1999. Fluid intake and the risk of bladder cancer in men. *New England Journal of Medicine* 340: 1390-1397.
26. Mitchell, J.B., P.C. DiLauro, F.X. Pizza, and D.L. Cavender. 1997. The effect of pre-exercise carbohydrate status on resistance exercise performance. *International Journal of Sport Nutrition* 7: 185-196.
27. Muoio, D.M., J.J. Leddy, P.J. Horvath, A.B. Awad, and D.R. Pendergast. 1994. Effect of dietary fat on metabolic adjustments to maximal VO_2 and endurance in runners. *Medicine and Science in Sports and Exercise* 26: 81-88.
28. National Research Council. 1989. *Recommended Dietary Allowances*, 10th ed. Washington, DC: National Academy Press.
29. Pendergast, D.R., P.J. Horvath, J.J. Leddy, and J.T. Venkatraman. 1996. The role of dietary fat on performance, metabolism, and health. *American Journal of Sports Medicine* 24: S53-S58.
30. Phinney, S.D., B.R. Bistrian, W.J. Evans, E. Gervino, and G.L. Blackburn. 1983. The human metabolic response to chronic ketosis without caloric restriction: Preservation of submaximal exercise capability with reduced carbohydrate oxidation. *Metabolism* 32: 769-776.
31. Piehl, K.S., S. Adolfsson, and K. Nazar. 1974. Glycogen storage and glycogen synthase activity in trained and untrained muscle of man. *Acta Physiologica Scandinavica* 90: 779-788.
32. Reimers, K.J. 1994. Evaluating a healthy, high performance diet. *Strength and Conditioning* 16: 28-30.

33. Rolls, B.J., V.H. Castellanos, J.C. Halford, A. Kilara, D. Panyam, C.L. Pelkman, G.P. Smith, and M.L. Thorwart. 1998. Volume of food consumed affects satiety in men. *American Journal of Clinical Nutrition* 67: 1170-1177.
34. Shannon, J., E. White, A.L. Shattuck, and J.D. Potter. 1996. Relationship of food groups and water intake to colon cancer risk. *Cancer Epidemiology, Biomarkers and Prevention* 5: 495-502.
35. Sherman, W.M. 1995. Metabolism of sugars and physical performance. *American Journal of Clinical Nutrition* 62 (Suppl): 228S-241S.
36. Sherman, W.M., J.A. Doyle, D.R. Lamb, and R.H. Strauss. 1993. Dietary carbohydrate, muscle glycogen, and exercise performance during 7 d of training. *American Journal of Clinical Nutrition* 57: 27-31.
37. Sherman, W.M., and G.S. Wimer. 1991. Insufficient carbohydrate during training: Does it impair performance? *Sports Nutrition* 1(1): 28-44.
38. Shirreffs, S.M., A.J. Taylor, J.B. Leiper, and R.J. Maughan. 1996. Post-exercise rehydration in man: Effects of volume consumed and drink sodium content. *Medicine and Science in Sports and Exercise* 28: 1260-1271.
39. Sugiura, K., and K. Kobayashi. 1998. Effect of carbohydrate ingestion on sprint performance following continuous and intermittent exercise. *Medicine and Science in Sports and Exercise* 30: 1624-1630.
40. Symons, J.D., and I. Jacobs. 1989. High-intensity exercise performance is not impaired by low intramuscular glycogen. *Medicine and Science in Sports and Exercise* 21: 550-557.
41. U.S. Department of Agriculture and U.S. Department of Health and Human Services. 1992. *The Food Guide Pyramid.* Home and Garden Bulletin No. 252. Washington, DC: U.S. Government Printing Office.
42. Vandenberghe, K., P. Hespel, B.V. Eynde, R. Lysens, and E.A. Richter. 1995. No effect of glycogen level on glycogen metabolism during high intensity exercise. *Medicine and Science in Sports and Exercise* 27: 1278-1283.
43. Volek, J.S., W.J. Kraemer, J.A. Bush, T. Incledon, and M. Boetes. 1997. Testosterone and cortisol in relationship to dietary nutrients and resistance exercise. *Journal of Applied Physiology* 82: 49-54.
44. Walberg, J.L., M.K. Leidy, D.J. Sturgill, D.E. Hinkle, S.J. Ritchey, and D.R. Sebolt. 1987. Macronutrient needs in weight lifters during caloric restriction. *Medicine and Science in Sports and Exercise* 19: S70.
45. Wardlaw, G.M., and P.M. Insel. 1996. *Perspectives in Nutrition.* St. Louis: Mosby Year Book, p. 76.
46. Wilmore, J.H., A.R. Morton, H.J. Gilbey, and R.J. Wood. 1998. Role of taste preference on fluid intake during and after 90 min of running at 60% of VO_2max in the heat. *Medicine and Science in Sports and Exercise* 30: 587-595.
47. Young, K., and C.T.M. Davies. 1984. Effect of diet on human muscle weakness following prolonged exercise. *European Journal of Applied Physiology* 53: 81-85.

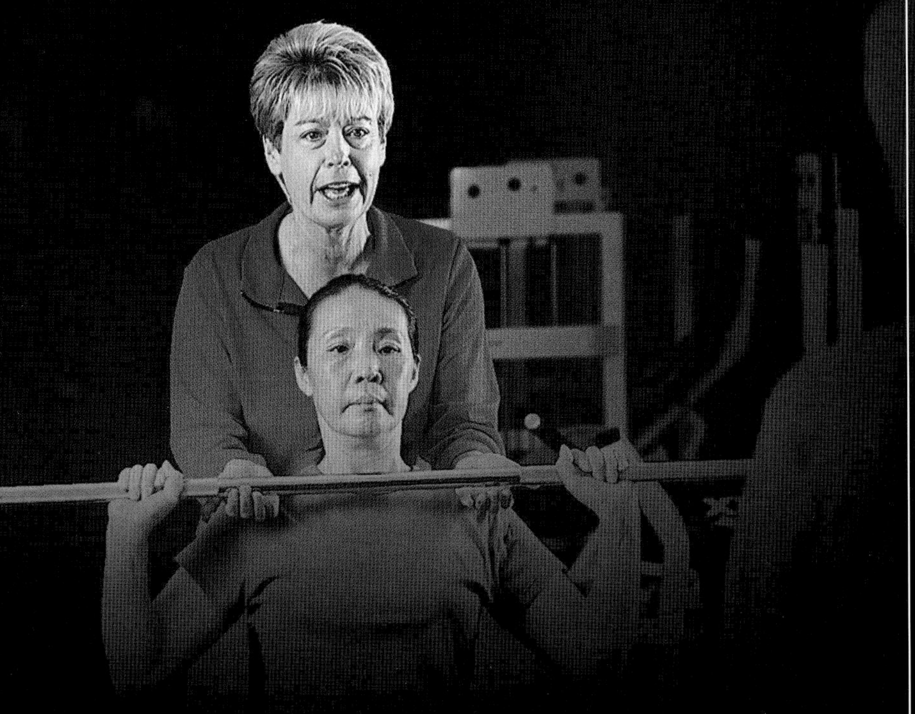

CHAPTER 8

Exercise Psychology for the Personal Trainer

Bradley D. Hatfield | Phil Kaplan

After completing this chapter, you will be able to

- understand the psychological benefits of exercise;
- work with a client to set effective exercise goals;
- recognize the value of motivation; and
- implement methods to motivate a client.

Participation in physical activity can result in desirable health consequences in terms of both acute responses and chronic adaptations in the physiological and psychological domains [62]. Despite the well-known benefits of exercise, current estimates from the National Center for Health Statistics indicate that approximately 40% of American men and women are sedentary during their leisure time [8]. According to one study, fewer than 50% of those who begin a program of regular physical activity will continue their involvement after six months [9]. For those who do adhere, the level of improvement in muscular strength and cardiovascular fitness is probably compromised by a lack of intensity and effort.

Thus for many people, the benefits of exercise remain elusive, and lack of compliance with programs offered by personal trainers results in a less-than-satisfactory experience for both the personal trainer and the client. Although human behavior is challenging to understand and change, understanding and implementing fundamental motivational principles can improve the situation. Although it might appear that some people are naturally more motivated toward achievement than others, in actuality those motivated individuals are employing their own mental strategies. If personal trainers can elicit a client's specific strategy for summoning motivation, and can learn to stimulate a client to employ that strategy, it is possible to turn on motivation in much the same way a switch on the wall can illuminate a room.

The first section of this chapter considers the anxiety-reducing and antidepressive effects of exercise as well as the cognitive benefits, especially for persons who are older; it also outlines some of the scientific evidence for the role of genetic factors in the relationship between exercise and mental health. The second section deals with goals, goal orientations, and effective goal setting. The final sections cover motivation, reinforcement, the development of self-efficacy or confidence, and practical instructions for motivational techniques. Here the personal trainer will find specific steps to use to help clients minimize procrastination, overcome false beliefs, identify and modify self-talk, and employ mental imagery.

Mental Health Aspects of Exercise

In addition to the desirable physiological consequences of physical activity, there is ample scientific evidence that participation in physical activity has significant mental health benefits. Further, people who are aware of such benefits may be encouraged to increase commitment to regular exercise. Notable among the mental health benefits are a reduction of anxiety and depression, decreased reactivity to psychological stress, and enhanced cognition. In this section we discuss the psychological impact of exercise in order to help the personal trainer communicate such benefits to the client for educational and motivational purposes.

Stress Reduction Effects of Exercise: Evidence and Mechanisms

It is estimated that approximately 7.3% of the American population have anxiety-related disorders to the extent that treatment is warranted [35]. In addition, most people experience episodic, and sometimes extended, stress-related symptoms during the course of their lives. Regular physical exercise seems to relieve both state and trait anxiety-related symptoms [47], both of which are related to the stress process. For many people, the alleviation of anxiety through physical activity likely provides a strong rationale for maintaining participation.

State anxiety can be defined as the actual experience of anxiety that is characterized by feelings of apprehension or threat and accompanied by increased physiological arousal, particularly as mediated by the autonomic nervous system [29, 59]. On the other hand, **trait anxiety** is a dispositional factor relating to the probability that a given person is likely to perceive situations as threatening [29, 59]. Typically both forms of anxiety are measured by self-report scales such as the State-Trait Anxiety Inventory [59] or in terms of physiological variables such as muscle tension, blood pressure, or brain electrical activity. Clearly, both acute (i.e., state) and chronic (i.e., trait) anxiety represent negative psychological variables that one would want to avoid, and participation in physical activity seems to effectively alleviate the symptoms associated with anxiety.

According to a recent review of the literature [35], there have been well over 100 scientific studies on the anxiety-reducing effects of exercise. Such a volume of research can be overwhelming, especially when some of the client investigations provide contradictory conclusions. Consequently, personal trainers may feel uncertain about their knowledge of the anxiety reduction effects of exercise.

Small to moderate reductions in anxiety with physical activity have been consistently reported in the exercise psychology literature over the last 30 years [10, 32, 36, 38, 41, 47]. These effects are typically observed for aerobic forms of exercise across a wide range of intensities, although low-intensity and higher-volume resistance training appears to be efficacious as well [4]. (As one would expect, higher-intensity exercise [i.e., above ventilatory threshold] does not seem to provide immediate stress reduction benefits, although some people who are extremely well conditioned may derive a cathartic release from this type of activity.)

There are a number of possible explanations for the anxiety-reducing effects of exercise [28]. One possibility is the rhythmic nature of many forms of physical activity and many exercise routines. People find that walking, running, or cycling at a steady pace for some period of time helps to promote relaxation. Stair stepping and aerobic dance routines are often performed to a cadence or in time to music. In essence, many workout routines are rhythmic. The calming effects of rhythmic exercise may be biological: It is possible that cerebral cortical arousal is inhibited, due to a volley of afferent rhythmic impulses from the skeletal muscles to an inhibitory or "relaxation" site in the brain stem of the central nervous system, and that this causes a "quieting" of the cognitive activity associated with anxiety or stress states [7, 28, 42].

One reason for the anxiety-reducing effects of exercise is the rhythmic nature of the exercise stimulus.

Another possible reason for the stress reduction effect of exercise has been termed the **thermogenic effect** [28, 47]. According to this model, based on work with animals [64], the metabolic inefficiency of the human body that results in heat production during exercise causes a cascade of events leading to relaxation. The part of the brain known as the hypothalamus detects the elevation in the body's temperature and consequently promotes a cortical relaxation effect. This results in decreased activation of alpha and gamma motor neurons to the skeletal muscle extrafusal and intrafusal fibers, respectively. In turn, the reduction in muscle efference results in reduced muscle tension and less sensitivity of the muscle spindles to stretch. This "calming down" effect results in less afferent stimulation or feedback to the brain stem arousal center and causes a relaxation state.

The effects from natural release of beta-endorphin during exercise stress are maintained for some time after exercise because of the half-life of hormonal action. Such an effect, in concert with the rhythmic muscle afference and thermic effects of exercise, may explain the altered state of mental and physical tension people experience immediately after working out.

It is important to remember that exercise may also take place either in a social context or in relative independence from others. In both cases, the exercise session may provide a diversion or time-out from daily concerns that occupy the participant's mind and that cause stress [2]. Additionally, a social setting may involve meaningful social interaction that could alleviate stress.

Finally, accomplishing the exercise goal may serve to alter how a person feels after exercise. Overall, the change in psychological state from exercise is referred to as the "feel-better" phenomenon [43] and may result from a complex interaction of social and psychobiological factors that come together to change the overall psychological state.

Antidepressive Effects of Exercise

As with anxiety, research evidence clearly and consistently reveals that physical exercise yields statistically significant and moderate effect sizes (i.e., reductions) both for men and women who are clinically depressed and for those experiencing less severe forms of depression, with the effects being somewhat larger for those with clinical depression [16, 45]. Although depression is commonly treated by physicians with psychiatric intervention, psychotherapy, or electroconvulsive shock, exercise would seem to be a desirable alternative given its relative cost-effectiveness and lack of unwanted side effects. In addition, physical exercise appears to be as effective as medication in men and women experiencing clinical depression [6]. Because many people have episodic bouts of depression over stressful events in their lives, it seems that exercise offers an appropriate and effective means of coping and feeling better.

As in the case of anxiety, exercise alleviates depression through several mechanisms. Two related possibilities center on the release of biogenic amines in the brain. Central levels of serotonin, an important neurotransmitter with antidepressant effects, are elevated during and following physical activity [13]. Levels of norepinephrine, another neurotransmitter that is lowered during bouts of depression, are also increased with exercise [20]. Beyond the biogenic amine hypothesis, it is also likely that some people benefit from the social interaction that occurs in many exercise settings or from the sense of accomplishment or enhanced self-efficacy that stems from greater strength and flexibility in performing daily activities. This effect may be particularly important for people in older age groups, who may gain a sense of independence and may experience decreased feelings of helplessness as a result of being physically fit.

Although serotonin and norepinephrine levels are lowered during bouts of depression, exercise has an antidepressive effect because it naturally elevates these biogenic amines.

Cognitive Benefits

In addition to the emotional or affective benefits, exercise confers cognitive benefits. People who are physically fit seem to function more effectively than less physically active people on tasks involving intellectual demand. Such outcomes are particularly impressive in men and women in older age groups (i.e., 55 and older), who typically show some degree of cognitive decline in specific functions due to the aging process. In an early study demonstrating the advantageous effects of physical activity on the aging brain, the typical age-related increase in reaction time (RT) was moderated in physically active men compared to those who were less physically active [55]. This effect was even more pronounced for complex or choice RT. Sedentary men showed large age-related increases in these RTs whereas physically active men showed little change (figure 8.1).

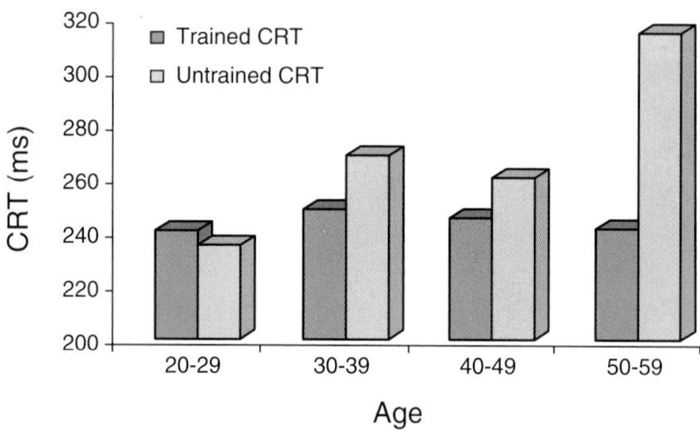

Figure 8.1 Choice reaction time: differences in reaction time at various ages, showing faster times with age in those who are physically active.
Adapted from Sherwood and Selder 1979.

Beyond the basic index of reaction time, mental performance more generally has been shown to be superior in physically fit versus sedentary people. In one study, older men who were physically fit achieved better mental performance on a complex battery of cognitive challenges than sedentary men [23]. The older men who were physically fit performed similarly to a group of younger men on the test battery while also outperforming the sedentary men (figure 8.2).

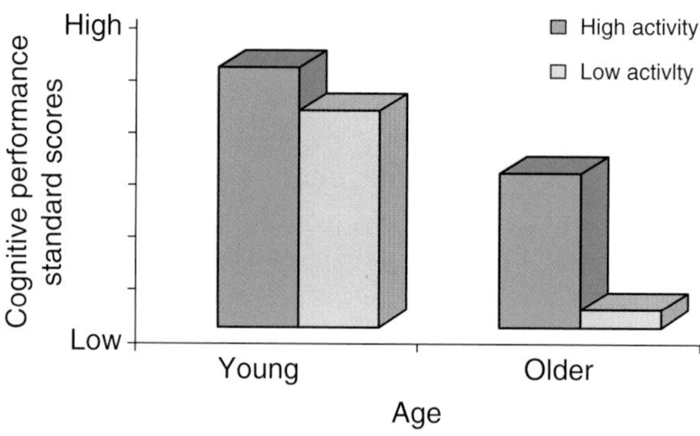

Figure 8.2 Cognitive performance of young and older men with low and high aerobic fitness levels.
Adapted from Dustman et al. 1990.

Vascular Changes

There are a number of possible explanations for the observed cognitive benefits of exercise in elderly persons. One postulate is that physical fitness decreases the decline in cerebral blood flow that normally occurs with aging [23]. Direct evidence for this possibility came from a study of brain blood flow in older retirees who differed in their levels of physical activity [52]. The retirees who were more active showed both superior cognitive functioning and increased perfusion of the cerebral cortex. Such an exercise-induced change would help to deliver oxygen and nutrients to the neural tissue and thereby support the neural processes underlying behavior.

Neurotrophic Factors

In addition to causing such vascular changes, exercise may lead to increases in neurotrophic factors (agents that preserve and nourish brain tissue). An animal study demonstrated that neurotrophic factors increased in rats that engaged in voluntary wheel-running [61]. More specifically, there was an increase in brain-derived neurotrophic factor in the rat hippocampus, a structure in the brain that is integrally involved in memory-related processes. In light of such powerful neurobiological influences in animals, it seems likely that similar changes could occur in humans and contribute to the higher cognitive functioning seen in older fit participants.

There is strong evidence that physical activity is associated with maintenance of levels of dopamine (an essential neurotransmitter involved in motor control processes) in the central nervous system [60]. In addition, research reveals that this neurotransmitter is also related to the learning of new skills as well as mental health (i.e., protection against depression) [60]. The impact of exercise on neurotransmitter function, referred to as the **neurotrophic effect,** likely works in concert with oxygenation to preserve mental functioning.

Neural Efficiency

One of the hallmarks of physically fit men and women is efficiency of musculoskeletal and cardiovascular function. For example, enhanced strength results in recruitment of fewer motor units to accomplish the lifting of a given (i.e., absolute) weight or resistance [19]. Also, lowered heart rate is commonly observed in response to absolute work after exercise training. Such economy of physiological processes also seems to characterize the adaptations in the brain of those who are physically fit.

Specificity and Cognitive Functioning

Just as with peripheral adaptations to exercise training, the psychological benefits seem to be marked by the principle of specificity. The effects have been primarily observed for effortful tasks that involve fluid intelligence, while tasks characterized by crystallized intelligence appear to be relatively unaffected. **Fluid intelligence** refers to reasoning or problem solving, whereas **crystallized intelligence** refers to accumulated knowledge and the ability to recognize words and recall facts. A recent study has indicated that mental tasks involving the frontal lobe executive processes are most affected by physical activity involvement [31].

Interestingly, the frontal lobe in humans is the last region of the brain to mature and the first to show the effects of advanced age. The executive processes housed there function in working memory and in the coordination of complex memory functions, as well as in the inhibition and control of behavior. Because this important area of the brain—serving some of the highest-order cognitive functions—is most susceptible to the deleterious effects of aging, it is reasonable to deduce that it would be most impacted by the positive neurobiological changes that have been discussed. In fact, older adults clearly manifest such specific effects of exercise; one study showed little difference in nonexecutive processes but significant improvement in executive processes in older men and women who engaged in aerobic training versus controls [31]. Because nonexecutive processes, such as speed of word recognition, are less dependent on frontal lobe function and more dependent on other areas of the brain that age less rapidly, it is also reasonable to deduce that the biological benefits of exercise on the brain would be less apparent during the performance of such mental tasks.

Genetic Basis

Finally, a major recent development in exercise science has been work on the genetic basis of physiological adaptations to training. It seems that client differences in the response to exercise are highly dependent on genetic variation. An awareness of genetic factors has much to do with motivational concerns, as some clients will respond favorably to aerobic endurance or resistance training while others may experience frustration in their attempts to improve their level of functioning or change their body composition. Such client variation also relates to the psychological benefits of exercise.

As an example of research on interactions between genes and exercise, one study revealed that cognitive decline in the elderly was particularly related to the presence of the apolipoprotein e4 allele (APOE4) [54]. That is, this particular gene is known to increase the risk for cognitive impairment in the elderly. Carriers of the gene who were less physically active experienced a drop in mental performance over a three-year period compared to those who were more active (i.e., spending more than an hour each day on such activities as walking, bicycling, gardening) and who showed little decline as they aged. This kind of information suggests that the cost of inactivity is particularly high for some individuals and that scientific assessment and understanding of gene-exercise interactions may yield a major motivational impetus for those who are particularly at risk for dementia. Such individuals are ideally suited to achieve benefits from exercise in the form of protection from cognitive decline. Insights into gene-exercise interactions may help people see the importance of a physically active lifestyle. These insights, along with the psychobiological changes discussed previously, substantiate the philosophical belief originating with the ancient Greeks, *mens sana in corpore sano* ("a healthy mind in a healthy body").

Goal Setting

Goal setting is a powerful strategy for increasing the level of participation in exercise programs. This technique can be defined as a strategic approach to behavioral change by which progressive **standards of success** (i.e., goals) are set in an attempt to increasingly approximate a desired **standard of achievement** (i.e., the long-term goal). Importantly, systematic goal setting fosters a sense of mastery and success as people pursue the desired standard or target of achievement. Feelings of success and competency promote commitment and help maintain exercise behavior. Personal trainers can be instrumental in helping clients set goals that prove to be compelling and achievable.

Goal setting is not a one-size-fits-all endeavor. Rather than simply extracting information from an assessment and imposing goals on the client, it is important for the personal trainer to identify the client's true wants and needs and to act as a facilitator in uncovering the goals that the client is most compelled to achieve [26]. Then, together, through directed conversation, the personal trainer and the client should identify goals that are measurable, achievable, and consistent with one another.

Setting Goals for Feedback and Reinforcement

Feedback and reinforcement are critical to the success of a goal-setting program as each progressive goal is sought. For example, a client may want to change body composition by reducing the percentage of fat. The long-term goal could be to shed 60 pounds (27 kilograms) or achieve a target percentage of body fat. This could be accomplished by a series of short-term weight reduction goals to be achieved in specified time frames [15]. **Feedback,** or knowledge of results, is inherent in the completion of or progress toward the short-term goal and leads to the cognitive evaluation of success or failure. Importantly, the realization of success or failure also invokes a corresponding emotional or affective state. Although the client may be far from the ultimate goal of losing 60 pounds, the positive mood or affective state that results from reaching the short-term goal will enhance commitment. Challenging goals that are difficult but within the present ability level of the client are superior to too-easy or very difficult goals in effecting behavior change [33].

> Goal setting is not a one-size-fits-all endeavor. Rather than simply extracting information from an assessment and imposing goals on the client, it is important to identify the client's true wants and needs.

The purpose of a **long-term goal** is to provide a meaningful pursuit for the client. Additionally, a personal trainer can assume that a goal selected by the client has a high level of meaning and purpose because it sets the direction of the short-term goals and provides a destination that the client values. Thus it would seem prudent to conduct initial interviews with clients to assess not just their short-term needs but their core values. Clients are much more likely to pursue and maintain purposeful and meaningful physical activity over a lifetime than they are to maintain activity without purpose or meaning [44]. For example, some people perceive themselves as runners and are so deeply committed to the activity that they are likely to maintain it indefinitely barring injury or chronic health problems.

A **short-term goal** provides a strategy to achieve the long-term goal via attainable steps. Challenging short-term goals are an effective tool to elicit the effort and intensity from the client that will result in a meaningful physiological and psychological change. A challenging goal is one that has about a 50% chance of success. Thus a well-constructed short-term goal represents a compromise between guaranteeing success, as in the case of a goal that is too easy, and requiring too much effort. Short-term goals are meaningless if they are not reasonably difficult; they will lead to going through the motions as opposed to investing real effort. If clients do not achieve a short-term goal initially, they will likely continue to attempt to achieve it or maintain the behavior (e.g., caloric restriction and walking activity in the case of weight reduction) in order to obtain the desired reinforcement. If a short-term goal is not attained in the specified time period, then it needs to be adjusted or replaced with another.

> An effective yet challenging goal is one that has about a 50% chance of success.

The power of **behavioral reinforcement** can be explained on both a psychological and a neurobiological level. Psychologically, the client may experience an increase in **self-esteem** or **self-efficacy** [3]. Reinforcement on a neurobiological level refers to the release of dopamine, which functions to strengthen synaptic pathways involved in learning a behavior. In fact, the two concepts may be inherently linked. Accordingly, feedback and the associated reinforcement are critical to effective goal setting, but feedback cannot reliably occur when short-term goals are vague. Thus it is best to identify objective or highly quantifiable goals so that clients can target effort toward a clear standard resulting in unambiguous knowledge of results. The following sections deal with specific characteristics that enhance the effectiveness of goals.

Types of Goals

The specifics of the long-term and short-term goals vary according to the client. For example, a client's initial fitness level largely determines the number of short-term goals needed to achieve the desired long-term goal. Another general characteristic of goals concerns the amount of control that a client can exert over their attainment. Goals can be categorized as process, performance, and outcome goals depending on the level of personal control that the client has over them. **Process goals** are goals that clients have a high degree of personal control over, whereas **outcome goals** are goals that the client has little control over. **Performance goals** fall in between in relation to personal control.

Process Goals

The amount of effort applied during a workout is an example of a process goal. Other examples are exercise form and technique and positive attitude during an exercise routine. Regardless of the difficulty of the short-term goal, clients can experience success with a high degree of effort if they set a process goal. Such goals may be very important for maintenance of exercise behavior as success or goal accomplishment defined in other ways (i.e., outcome goals) becomes increasingly difficult, a situation that could result in the client dropping out.

Outcome Goals

For some clients, process goals may not be fulfilling. Some need to see progress or accomplishments as gauged by social comparison. For example, they may want to be the fastest walker in the neighborhood walking group or the strongest lifter at the gym. Outcome goals are exemplified by social comparison as in winning or in beating an opponent in a race. Such goals can be highly arousing and can induce great intensity of effort for individuals who like to compare themselves to others. However, outcome goals present less probability of success compared to process goals: Clients can guarantee the effort to achieve an advantage over the "opponent," but they cannot guarantee the outcome itself.

Performance Goals

Performance goals are more difficult to achieve than process goals and are typically stated in terms of a self-referenced personal performance standard for the client rather than in comparison to another client or an opponent. Performance goals are intermediate on the continuum of personal control ranging from low (outcome) to high (process). An example of personalized performance goals that challenge the client to focus on self-improvement in a personally meaningful way is based on the notion of a range or interval goal [46]. For example, during a periodized resistance training program a client may want to improve maximal strength in the squat or bench press exercise. Interval goals are calculated from the client's recent performance history in which a range of success is identified. The limits of the goal are established in the form of a lower (most attainable) and an upper (most challenging) boundary of success. The lower boundary is defined as the client's previous best 1RM performance. To determine the upper boundary, the client "computes" the average of recent performances (three to five) and determines the difference between the average and previous best performance. This difference yields an estimate of the client's performance variability. The difference is then added to the previous best to generate a highly challenging self-referenced level of success.

Overall, it seems appropriate to set a variety of goals or diversify one's goal-setting strategy so as to balance the client's underlying reasons for exercise while maintaining a reasonable probability of success and reinforcement.

Diversified Goal Setting

A successful goal-setting program should involve a diversity of goals, just as financial success entails a diversified financial portfolio [15]. In addition, such diverse goals need to be formed within the context of a sound scientific strategy for long-term goal attainment. Thus the personal trainer needs to incorporate and integrate knowledge from the psychological, biomechanical, physiological, nutritional, and other relevant scientific domains.

A successful goal-setting program should include a diverse combination of short-term and long-term goals.

As an example of a diversified goal-setting approach, think of a middle-aged client who wishes to run a 10K (6.2-mile) race in a time he can feel proud of. The long-term goal may be clearly stated in the form of a desired outcome that will be personally meaningful. Assume that this client has the talent and the ability to achieve the performance goal if he optimizes his effort and trains in a sound strategic manner. However, a number of motivational problems are bound to occur during the training of any client who is striving for a challenging standard of behavior. To overcome the disappointments that can occur if the client focuses on a single performance goal such as "finishing the race in less than an hour," he should also set short-term goals using a goal diversification strategy in the context of a well-designed training program. On some training days the client may set the goal of proper form during foot strike and mechanically sound arm swing and stride length. On other days he may stress resistance training goals to facilitate the efficiency of the lower extremities in an attempt to develop stamina. On still other days, he may concentrate on psychological goals such as positive focus and self-talk during a training run. Positive feedback from the attainment of such process goals can perpetuate the sense of desire and commitment to the long-term goal. Again, the basic principle is that a variety of goals associated with varying levels of personal control may well sustain commitment and adherence to the physical training program.

Goal Orientations

A concept that relates to goal diversification is individual differences—the differing personalities of clients. Consideration of individual differences in clients' perceptions of achievement situations helps to increase the effectiveness of goal setting [22, 49, 51]. For example, clients who gauge their performance improvement on the basis of previous ability level are said to be **task involved.** On the other hand, **ego-involved** or **other-referenced** clients base their sense of improvement on comparison to the performance of one or more others [50]. Such clients are highly aroused by social comparison and put forth greater effort in a situation that permits social comparison, especially if they perceive their own ability or fitness level to be high. A task involvement orientation, on the other hand, may relate to a higher need for personal control; task-involved clients may become discouraged if inappropriate emphasis is placed on comparisons of their achievements to those of others. To be effective in goal setting, the personal trainer must consider these types of individual differences in goal orientation and perceived ability.

During the consultation and assessment session with a new client, the personal trainer should maintain focus on the client's desired goals and expected outcomes, and should develop a sound plan of action.

Tips for Effective Goal Setting

The following suggestions may help the personal trainer develop an effective goal-setting strategy. "Practical Principles of Effective Goal Setting" on page 149 summarizes the primary research-based elements of goal setting.

- Determine the client's perceived needs and desires, and agree on and plan out the long-term goals.
- Figure out the steps and the short-term goals that will lead to long-term achievement. If the goal is to run a marathon and the client has never run even five miles (eight kilometers), the first goal might be to develop the habit of training four times per week; the second might be to run two miles (3.2 kilometers); and the third might be to run in a 10K (6.2-mile) race. The short-term goals should progress from there, ultimately leading up to the point that the client can complete 26.2 miles (42.2 kilometers).
- When starting out with a new client, clarify a preliminary goal based more on achievement than on a measured result. For example, one could set the goal of showing up at the gym three times per week for the first two weeks, or the goal of eating a healthy breakfast every morning. By beginning with goals that are simple to achieve and are free of the pressure of potential impending failure, the personal trainer creates a mind-set of achievement and helps to build a client's self-confidence. Once the client begins accumulating small achievements, the goals should become more challenging.

- Both the personal trainer and client should recognize that absence of required knowledge can often hinder the achievement of long-term goals. Evaluating the client's present level of knowledge will help to set a complementary knowledge-based goal, which might be to learn the names and functions of the major muscle groups or to read a series of recommended nutrition books.
- As time progresses and the client proves committed to the sessions and the result, it is appropriate to set more aggressive goals by identifying specific measures of achievement. These goals might typically include performance and achievement with direct measurement, such as "to bench-press 200 pounds [90 kilograms]," "to walk three miles [4.8 kilometers]," or "to lose 15 pounds [7 kilograms] of fat." These goals should be set in measurable terms so the personal trainer and client can easily discern the moment of achievement.
- Once measurable goals are clarified, attach a time frame to each goal. It is important to recognize that if a goal is not achieved by the assigned date, reevaluation and adjustment of action will move the client closer to the goal. Goals can and should be evaluated and adjusted at regular intervals, perhaps biweekly or monthly.
- Agree on a way to recognize whether or not the program is working. If a goal is to reduce waist girth, some clients may want to use a tape measure whereas others may find it psychologically more helpful to gauge progress by occasionally trying on a pair of pants that they have not worn in years.
- After setting goals, always check to make certain that the client believes they are attainable. If not, work on adjusting the client's belief (i.e., by educating the client) or adjusting the goal.
- Examine the goals to make sure they are compatible with one another. If goals conflict, the client's chance for success may be compromised.
- Goals should be prioritized. If a client comes up with a long list of goals, it is best to first isolate three, for example, that are most important and then to put those three in order of importance.

Attach a time frame to each goal and note if a goal is not achieved by the assigned date. Goals can and should be evaluated and adjusted at regular intervals.

Practical Principles of Effective Goal Setting

1. Make goals specific, measurable, and observable.
2. Clearly identify time constraints.
3. Use moderately difficult goals [33].
4. Record goals and monitor progress.
5. Diversify process, performance, and outcomes.
6. Set short-range goals to achieve long-range goals.
7. Make sure goals are internalized (clients should participate or set their own).

The acronym "SMART" helps to capture these essential points [65]:

Specific
Measurable
Action oriented
Realistic
Time-bound

From Cox 2002 [15].

Motivation

According to its basic definition, **motivation** is a psychological construct that arouses and directs behavior [34]. A **construct** is simply an internal drive or neural process that cannot be directly observed but must be indirectly inferred from observation of outward behavior. For example, a person who rises every day at dawn and works intensely at his or her job is considered to be highly motivated. There are many other examples of constructs in psychology such as personality, ambition, and assertiveness. Although not directly observable, they yield powerful influence on behavior.

The basic definition suggests that motivation has two dimensions: (1) a directional aspect that influences the choices clients make about their time and commitment and (2) the intensity with which they pursue those choices. Such a definition helps clarify the concept of motivation but falls short of offering a strategy or clue regarding how to change behavior. Because regular exercise involvement is such a problem in our society, the following psychological principles are offered as a strategy to increase the level of participation.

The personal trainer and client should together set goals that are specific, measurable, action oriented, realistic, and timely.

Positive and Negative Reinforcement and Punishment

The employment of goal setting is related to the concept of behaviorism, and to clarify the philosophy of motivational practices it is helpful to define the basic concepts used in behavioral or operant conditioning. Formalized by B.F. Skinner [57, 58], **behaviorism** as a view of learning holds that behavior is molded or shaped by its consequences. Accordingly personal trainers can significantly influence exercise adherence by their reactions to a client's behaviors.

A **target behavior** (e.g., completing 45 minutes of a step aerobics class) is termed an **operant,** and the probability that an operant (a behavior) will be repeated in the future increases when the behavior is reinforced. On the other hand, the future likelihood of the behavior's occurring decreases when it is punished. **Reinforcement** is any act, object, or event that *increases* the likelihood of future operant behavior when the reinforcement follows the target behavior; and **punishment** is any act, object, or event that *decreases* the likelihood of future operant behavior when the punishment follows that behavior. Although personal trainers do not engage in purposeful punishment actions, understanding behaviorism can help to clarify their own leadership philosophy and how it relates to enhancing motivation.

Reinforcement *increases* the likelihood that a behavior will be repeated, and punishment *decreases* the likelihood that a behavior will be repeated.

The terms positive and negative reinforcement are often confused. Both terms refer to consequences that increase the probability of occurrence of a desired behavior or operant; but **positive reinforcement** "gives" something to the client in response to his or her behavior, and **negative reinforcement** "takes away" something [40]. An example of positive reinforcement is social approval or congratulations given to a client for completing a workout. An example of negative reinforcement is relieving the client of a disliked chore, such as mopping accumulated sweat from the floor around the exercise equipment, because of successful completion of the workout. In essence, something aversive is "removed" or taken away in order to reward behavior.

Conversely, a personal trainer who focuses on the shortcomings or deficiencies of the client subscribes to a punishing style of motivation since punishment following an event, by definition, decreases the probability of the event's occurring again. **Positive punishment** implies presentation of something aversive such as disapproval, while **negative punishment** implies removal of something in order to decrease the operant. Criticism of a client for poor exercise technique is an example of positive punishment. Removal of a privilege because of poor exercise technique or failure to complete an exercise goal is an example of negative punishment. Although it would seem appropriate for personal trainers to resort to reasonable forms of disapproval or punishment in the case of poor effort, a reinforcing style of leadership focuses on the progress of the client.

Self-Determination Theory

While new routines, new music, or a new piece of equipment can help a client continue to want to exercise, motivation runs deeper in the client's psyche. People are driven to act based on one of two possible stimuli. They either feel a compulsion to move toward a desire (pleasure) or they feel a need to move away from pain. Pain does not mean only physical pain, although sometimes that may be an element to be considered, but more commonly emotional pain. When something becomes increasingly uncomfortable, motivation to move away from the discomfort increases.

Intrinsically motivated behavior is engaged in for the sense of enjoyment derived from it, while extrinsically motivated behavior is engaged to achieve another goal or outcome. In common terms, **intrinsic motivation** implies a true love for the experience of exercise and a sense of fun during its performance. **Extrinsic motivation,** on the other hand, implies a desire to be engaged in behavior to get an external reward. Although originally conceived as independent, the concepts of intrinsic and extrinsic motivation are tied together by the concept of **self-determination** or **internalization** [17, 18]. In essence, self-determination implies that the individual is participating in the activity for his or her own fulfillment as opposed to trying to meet the expectations of others (which would be a "work" orientation). As such, intrinsic and extrinsic motivation represent important landmarks on a motivational continuum or range and are not essentially dichotomous unless one is referring to extremes.

An intrinsically motivated client truly loves to exercise, whereas an extrinsically motivated client typically exercises only to achieve an external reward.

Clients who initially exhibit intrinsic motivation are more likely to maintain their exercise behavior than those who lack intrinsic motivation [53]. Therefore, awareness of a client's location on the motivation continuum holds implications for the type of motivational approach that will be effective in enhancing enjoyment of an exercise program. Major points along the self-determination continuum have been identified [63] and can be summarized [15] as follows:

1. Amotivation: The client has a total lack of intrinsic or extrinsic motivation.
2. External regulation: The client engages in behavior to avoid punishment, not for personal satisfaction.
3. Introjected regulation: The client views exercise and training behavior as a means to a valued end (e.g., getting into correct starting position for resistance training exercise is partly internalized to please the personal trainer).
4. Identified regulation: The client accepts the personal trainer's instructions as beneficial but primarily follows the leadership of the personal trainer instead of initiating exercise behavior.
5. Integrated regulation: The client personally values exercise behavior, internalizes it, and freely engages in it; the client and the personal trainer agree on the goals for the client.

Clients develop greater commitment to their exercise goals if they are intrinsically motivated because they possess the desire to be competent and committed to achieving goals in which they have a personal stake [17]. Although some people may be able to maintain their exercise behavior based solely on extrinsic reinforcement, those who are both intrinsically and extrinsically motivated probably enjoy physical activity and exercise training more, and this makes for a more positive experience for both the client and the personal trainer. Thus clients may have different preferences regarding involvement in goal setting, and the personal trainer can determine whether participation is appropriate. That is, some individuals prefer to have goals formulated by the personal trainer, while others desire to actively participate in the goal setting process. In general, the consideration of client input in the goal-setting process seems well founded.

Effect of Rewards on Intrinsic Motivation

External rewards can play a role in increasing intrinsic motivation and exercise adherence. Although the personal trainer should not count solely on the value of ongoing extrinsic rewards, the promise of a T-shirt, a dinner gift certificate, or a 30-day complimentary health club membership can facilitate early compliance and follow-through. Given this premise, a personal trainer might logically assume that he or she could enhance intrinsically motivated behavior by giving a client even more rewards. For example, if a client derives great satisfaction from running in 10K (6.2-mile) races, it might seem that a trophy or financial reward for each performance would result in even greater satisfaction. In actuality, external rewards or recognition can also reduce intrinsic motivation [17].

A well-known example [56] is the story of a retired psychology professor in need of peace and quiet who was disturbed by the sound of children playing on his lawn. Instead of punishing the playful (i.e., intrinsically motivated) behavior of the children, he gave each child 50 cents and heartily thanked them for the "entertainment" that they had afforded him. The children looked forward to returning the next day. At the end of their next romp on the man's lawn he told them that he was short of money but that he was able to give them 25 cents. A little disappointed, the children returned on a third day and were even more disappointed when they learned that the man had no money to give. Alas, they never returned to play on the man's lawn again! What happened? Exactly what the professor had hoped! If a strong dependency is formed between behavior and reward, removal of the reward is likely to result in a lessening of the behavior. In this manner the reward is perceived in a controlling manner [17]. Rewards can be viewed as "controlling" if the recipient perceives a contingency or connection between the behavior and the reward.

When to Intervene With Motivational Efforts

To be the most effective at motivating a client, the personal trainer needs to be aware of the client's **stage of readiness** for exercise participation. The **transtheoretical model** describes the process a client goes through as he or she "gets ready to start exercise" [5, 48]:

1. Precontemplation: The person does not intend to increase physical activity and is not thinking about becoming physically active.
2. Contemplation: The person intends to increase physical activity and is giving it a thought now and then, but is not yet physically active.
3. Preparation: The person is engaging in some activity, accumulating at least 30 minutes of moderate-intensity physical activity at least one day per week, but not on most days of the week.
4. Action: The person is accumulating at least 30 minutes of moderate-intensity physical activity on five or more days of the week, but has done so for less than six months.
5. Maintenance: The person is accumulating at least 30 minutes of moderate-intensity physical activity on five or more days of the week, and has been doing so for six months or more.

Having identified the client's stage of readiness, the personal trainer can apply the appropriate processes for change or interventions in order to move the client to the next level with the ultimate goals of action and maintenance. The transtheoretical model may appear to be only common sense, but surveying prospective clients to individualize interventions may be helpful. The Stages of Exercise Scale (SES) [11] can be used to conveniently capture the stage of a prospective client. In general, the research has supported the efficacy of this approach [1, 12, 14, 39].

Self-Efficacy: Building Confidence

To have a truly successful experience with a client, it is important to consider the client's motivation in conjunction with his or her confidence about achieving the desired behaviors. For example, there are people who have a poor self-concept or social physique anxiety and therefore lack the confidence to engage in an exercise program [27]. In his social cognitive theory, Bandura [3] described self-efficacy as a person's confidence in his or her own ability to perform specific actions leading to a successful behavioral outcome. Exercise self-efficacy is a powerful predictor of exercise behavior. Self-efficacy is characterized by the degree to which the client is confident of performing the task and by the maintenance of that belief in the face of failure or obstacles. In other words, self-efficacy is related to persistence in striving for goal achievement. Four types of influences affect or build self-efficacy:

1. Performance accomplishments
2. Modeling effects
3. Verbal persuasion
4. Physiological arousal or anxiety

The successful performance of a behavior or of successive approximations of that behavior has the most powerful influence on enhancing self-efficacy for future behavior, and in that sense underscores the relationship of goal accomplishment to building confidence.

Observing others perform a target behavior can also increase self-efficacy by enhancing imitative behavior. For example, some clients may be more confident of effecting a significant behavioral change such as weight loss if they see others similar to themselves in age, gender, and body type reach the same goal.

Another positive influence on self-efficacy is verbal persuasion from a respected source. A person who is respected and who is known to possess expertise in a given area (e.g., strength development or bodybuilding) can significantly influence a client's self-efficacy by offering encouragement and stating, for example, that the client "has potential."

Finally, the client's own interpretation of his or her physiological state before or during exercise also exerts an influence on self-efficacy and can effectively decrease or increase confidence. For example, before performing a maximal repetition to determine 1RM strength in the bench press, the cli-

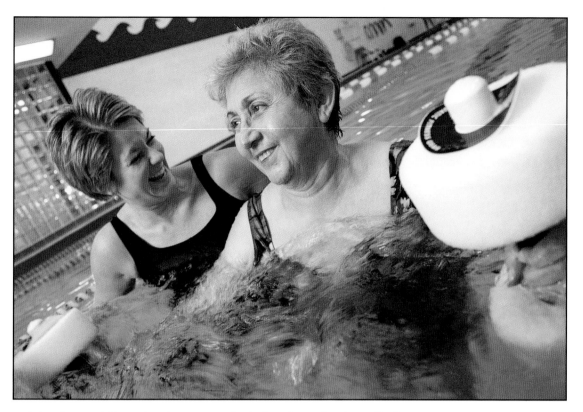

Figure 8.3 Successfully performing an exercise helps clients develop self-efficacy.

ent may judge his or her level of arousal negatively ("I'm too nervous") or positively ("I'm ready").

Achieving success has more impact than anything else on raising a client's self-efficacy.

The next section and "Practical Motivational Techniques" on page 154 outline methods for motivating a client and provide practical motivational techniques to use within the personal training setting.

Methods to Motivate a Client

Sometimes a particular psychological method is helpful in motivating a client. This section offers techniques for minimizing procrastination, overcoming false beliefs, identifying and modifying self-talk, and using mental imagery.

Minimizing Procrastination

The 14th-century philosopher, Jean Buridan, told the story of a mule that starved to death trying to decide between two equidistant bales of hay. The bales of hay were equally desirous, so the mule could not decide which way to go. The fable presents a valuable analogy for human indecision. Health and fitness are attributes desired by everyone, but only a disappointing margin of our population manages to commit to and maintain an exercise lifestyle. If people believe they have too many options that they must decide between—diets, devices, or personal trainers—the decision-making process itself often leads to stagnation. Personal trainers have to think beyond the personal training session and toward influencing clients to exercise not only today, or next week, but for the long haul.

When a client procrastinates, he or she is weighing options, left in a frozen state of indecision, trying to decide if the perceived pain will outweigh the potential benefit.

Identifying False Beliefs

Because quick fixes are so often positioned as solutions, many clients have allowed flawed and misleading information into their belief systems. If, for example, a client believes that weight loss can be achieved only by restricting food intake, he or she

Practical Motivational Techniques

1. Have the client use an exercise log or journal to document baseline measurements and the details of each workout. Teach the client not only to use the journal as a report card for exercise sessions, but also to record emotions, meals, and perspectives on progress.
2. Begin clients with exercise sessions that involve familiar activities. Lack of familiarity with an exercise or exercise mode can frustrate clients and lead to a lack of desire to continue exercising.
3. Whenever possible, offer choices. Keep the client involved in decisions, but offer choices that are equally beneficial. Rather than having the client question whether he or she should exercise at all today, change the decision: "Would you rather do your warm-up on the elliptical climber or the exercise bike today?"
4. Provide feedback often. Look for small achievements. The personal trainer can notice and comment on increases in aerobic capacity, increases in strength, and decreases in body fat while providing exercise assistance. If, for example, the client moves up 5 pounds (2.5 kilograms) in a specific resistance training exercise, make it clear that progress is taking place.
5. One of the best things a personal trainer can do for clients is model the appropriate behavior for a fitness lifestyle; the personal trainer should act as a role model, setting an example of an exercise commitment.
6. Prepare the client for periods during which momentum may be disrupted. If the client understands that even the most dedicated individuals lower the intensity of their training occasionally, those unavoidable or undesired lapses are less likely to result in program abandonment.
7. Utilize social support resources. The personal trainer can check on a client's moods, responses, and adherence by tactful use of telephone contact, e-mail correspondence, and mailing of educational resources or motivational information. If possible, conversations with family members regarding the desired outcome and course of action can all contribute to motivation and adherence by providing a stronger support network at home.
8. Let the past go. If a client feels as if he or she failed to obtain the benefits of an exercise program in the past, focus instead on future goals.
9. Substitute a "be perfect" attitude with a "do your best" outlook. Clients who strive for perfection are guaranteed to hit a point of perceived failure. Teach clients to understand that giving total effort and commitment is the equivalent of excellence.
10. Agree on a motivational affirmation and have the client write it down.

is going to block out the personal trainer's suggestions of a more appropriate caloric intake. Further, many people have been conditioned to believe that exercise is not for them, or that their bodies will not respond to exercise as the bodies of others do. "No pain, no gain" is another flawed belief. This belief increases a person's tendency to overtrain, which can sabotage the potential for results.

Before a personal trainer can attempt to install new empowering beliefs, he or she has to first identify, and then work to change, limiting false beliefs. The first step, therefore, in opening up a clear and effective line of communication between the personal trainer and client must involve a questioning process that includes discussion of the client's present beliefs about fitness and exercise. With education, reasoning, and reinforcement, the personal trainer can then help the client to understand why the false beliefs are in fact deceptive and limiting. With that understanding, the false beliefs are weakened and ultimately dismissed, allowing the client to learn new, correct information.

"No pain, no gain" is a false belief that can encourage overtraining and diminish a client's potential for results.

Questions to Help Identify False Beliefs

To identify false beliefs, personal trainers can ask clients the following questions:

- What is your ideal approach to "getting in shape"?
- What have you tried in the past to achieve the fitness results you want?
- What exercise and nutrition strategies do you feel are important?
- What do you feel you need to do to reshape your body and improve your health and fitness?

Identifying and Modifying Self Talk

Each client has his or her own "internal voice." Sometimes this is a source of motivation, but if this **self-talk** is negative, a person is less likely to accept even the most positively directed affirmations. Over time, strong and repetitive external encouragement can change a client's negative self-talk, but positive affirmations will have more effect if the client changes the negative self-talk first. The following are three simple exercises to identify and modify potentially negative self-talk:

1. Ask the client simply to notice self-talk throughout the day and realize that what they think creates mental pictures, words, and feelings.
2. Once the client has an awareness of the inner voice, direct him or her to identify it at the same point in time each day, ideally just before the scheduled personal training session. For example, if a client has a 5 p.m. personal training appointment each day, ask that client to write down what his or her self-talk is saying at 4:45 p.m. during preparation for the workout.
3. Ask the client to draw a line down the middle of a sheet of paper and on the left-hand side write down precisely what his or her self-talk is saying. Direct the client to write down on the right-hand side what the self-talk *could* say that would be supportive or motivating instead. After the client has done this at a given time each day, encourage him or her to identify self-talk at several pertinent times during each day (such as upon waking or before going to bed), along with what the self-talk could say.
4. After identifying three common self-talk phrases (and three better phrases), the client should write the new phrases (affirmations) down and privately recite the better phrases, at first aloud five or six times each minute at the particular time of day the encouragement is desired, to instill the habit of vocalizing the "better" words. Once the personal trainer helps the client to create this habit, the client can shift to mentally "speaking" the words instead. With practice, the client's positive self-talk will motivate him or her toward success and achievement.

External encouragement will have more effect if the client changes his or her negative self-talk first.

Mental Imagery

At the 1988 Olympic Games in Seoul, track and field athletes who had qualified for the Olympic trials participated in a survey [24]. The survey showed that 83% of the athletes had practiced mental conditioning exercises. Since then, the popularity of mental imagery has grown immensely. The recognized value of mental conditioning for optimal performance is not limited to athletes. Mental conditioning is valuable in music [37], in military training [21], and in rehabilitation [25]—all arenas in which consistency of effort is required for excellence.

Relaxation Exercise for Mental Imagery

Mental imagery should be performed in a relaxed, tension-free state. Sport psychologists use several techniques to facilitate a state of relaxation. **Progressive relaxation,** developed by Jacobson [30], is one of the most commonly practiced techniques for mental imagery. In progressive relaxation the individual is asked to tighten each muscle group, one group at a time, and to follow each contraction with a full relaxation. The first step involves differentiating between the sensations of muscle tension and muscle relaxation. Although one might think the difference to be obvious, even when sitting in a relaxed position a person is probably tensing many muscles. Before asking clients to perform a relaxation or mental imagery exercise, the personal trainer should become familiar with the relaxation process.

Visualization

Visualization involves using the ability of the brain to "draw" and "recall" mental images that can help a client learn how to create positive emotional responses and improve motivation. The following are three simple visualization exercises that can be performed in a relaxed state:

- Witnessing a past success: If a client has "seen" or experienced an achievement or witnessed his or her own excellence, the belief that such a performance is possible becomes concrete. Since the mind and nervous system are closely linked, perception of a remembered event might have the same "belief" power as an actual achievement.
- Witnessing a success yet to be: Even if a client has not yet achieved the desired goal or performance, with developed imagination skills he or she can create a mental movie of success as if it has already happened.
- Witnessing the value: Immediately before, during, or after a workout, the client mentally "sees" the result or valued outcome. This will greatly enhance the client's desire to achieve the outcome.

As a client's imagery becomes more powerful, the sensations the mental images bring about will become more powerful. Each time clients mentally see themselves achieving a goal, lifting the weight, transforming their body, or crossing the finish line, that vision will be accompanied by the feelings of winning and achievement.

CONCLUSION

The mental health aspects of exercise come from its anxiety-reducing and antidepressive benefits, both of which have special applications to new clients and individuals who are older. One method of encouraging regular participation in exercise is for the personal trainer and client to collectively set goals that are specific, measurable, action oriented, realistic, and time-bound. Further, one of the roles of a personal trainer is to motivate clients expediently toward their established goals while minimizing delays, misconceptions, and negative self-talk via methods that include mental imagery and visualization.

STUDY QUESTIONS

1. All of the following describe how exercise provides cognitive benefits EXCEPT:
   A. enhanced oxygen supply to the brain
   B. greater genetic variation
   C. improved neurotransmitter function
   D. heightened neural efficiency
2. Which of the following is an example of an outcome goal?
   A. "I want to do 60 sit-ups in 1 minute."
   B. "I want to do my best not to eat before going to bed tonight."
   C. "I want to be able to bench press more than my friend."
   D. "I want to lose 10 pounds of body fat."
3. Which of the following is an example of negative reinforcement a personal trainer says to a client who just completed a month of consistently walking three times per week?
   A. "Good job! Next month, you do not have to take the time to fill out your own walking workout card—I'll do it for you!"
   B. "Good job! You won the 'Walker of the Month' club!"
   C. "Walking? I thought we talked about you riding the bike instead of walking!"
   D. "Three times per week? It was supposed to be four times per week, so next month you won't be able to keep working out during your lunch hour."

4. Which of the following points along the self-determination or regulation continuum is a client who is highly intrinsically motivated?
   A. introjected
   B. integrated
   C. identified
   D. amotivated

APPLIED KNOWLEDGE QUESTION

Using the seven "Practical Principles of Effective Goal Setting," develop an effective six-month goal setting strategy for a client who says he wants to improve his 1RM leg press from 225 pounds (102 kilograms) to 315 pounds (143 kilograms).

REFERENCES

1. Armstrong, C.A., J.F. Sallis, M.F. Howell, and C.R. Hofstetter. 1993. Stages of change, self-efficacy, and the adoption of vigorous exercise: A prospective analysis. *Journal of Sport and Exercise Psychology* 15: 390-402.
2. Bahrke, M.S., and W.P. Morgan. 1978. Anxiety reduction following exercise and meditation. *Cognitive Therapy and Research* 2: 323-333.
3. Bandura, A. 1997. *Self-Efficacy: The Exercise of Control.* San Francisco: Freeman.
4. Bartholomew, J.B., and D.E. Linder. 1998. State anxiety following resistance exercise: The role of gender and exercise intensity. *Journal of Behavioral Medicine* 21: 205-219.
5. Blair, S.N., A.N. Dunn, B.H. Marcus, R.A. Carpenter, and P. Jaret. 2001. *Active Living Every Day.* Champaign, IL: Human Kinetics.
6. Blumenthal, J.A., M.A. Babyak, K.A. Moore, W.E. Craighead, S. Herman, P. Khatri, R. Waugh, M.A. Napolitano, L.M. Forman, M. Applebaum, M. Doraiswamy, and R. Krishman. 1999. Effects of exercise training on older patients with major depression. *Archives of Internal Medicine* 159: 2349-2356.
7. Bonvallet, M., and V. Bloch. 1961. Bulbar control of cortical arousal. *Science* 133: 1133-1134.
8. Brown, D. 2002. Study says 38 percent of adults are sedentary in leisure time. *Washington Post* (April 8): A2.
9. Buckworth, J., and R.K. Dishman. 2002. *Exercise Psychology.* Champaign, IL: Human Kinetics.
10. Calfas, K.J., and W.C. Taylor. 1994. Effects of physical activity on psychological variables in adolescents. *Pediatric Exercise Science* 6: 406-423.
11. Cardinal, B.J. 1995. The stages of exercise scale and stages of exercise behavior in female adults. *Journal of Sport Medicine and Physical Fitness* 35: 87-92.
12. Cardinal, B.J. 1997. Predicting exercise behavior using components of the transtheoretical model of behavior change. *Journal of Sport Behavior* 20: 272-283.
13. Chaouloff, F. 1997. The serotonin hypothesis. In: *Physical Activity and Mental Health,* W.P. Morgan, ed. Washington, DC: Taylor & Francis, pp. 179-198.
14. Courneya, K.S. 1995. Perceived severity of the consequences of physical inactivity across the stages of change in older adults. *Journal of Sport and Exercise Psychology* 17: 447-457.
15. Cox, R.H. 2002. *Sport Psychology: Concepts and Applications,* 5th ed. Boston: McGraw-Hill.
16. Craft, L.L., and D.M. Landers. 1998. The effect of exercise on clinical depression and depression resulting from mental illness: A meta-analysis. *Journal of Sport and Exercise Psychology* 20: 339-357.
17. Deci, E.L., and R.M. Ryan. 1985. *Intrinsic Motivation and Self-Determination in Human Behavior.* New York: Plenum Press.
18. Deci, E.L., and R.M. Ryan. 1991. A motivational approach to self: Integration in personality. In: *Nebraska Symposium on Motivation 1991: Vol. 38. Perspectives on Motivation: Current Theory and Research in Motivation,* R.A. Dienstbier, ed. Lincoln, NE: University of Nebraska Press, pp. 237-288.
19. deVries, H.A., and T.J. Housh. 1994. *Physiology of Exercise for Physical Education Athletics and Exercise Science.* Madison, WI: Brown and Benchmark.
20. Dishman, R.K. 1997. The norepinephrine hypothesis. In: *Physical Activity and Mental Health,* W.P. Morgan, ed. Washington, DC: Taylor & Francis, pp. 199-212.
21. Druckman, D., and J.A. Swets. 1988. *Enhancing Human Performance: Issues, Theories and Techniques.* Washington, DC: National Academy Press.
22. Duda, J.L. 1989. Relationships between task and ego orientation and the perceived purpose of sport among high school athletes. *Journal of Sport and Exercise Psychology* 11: 318-335.
23. Dustman, R.E., R.Y. Emmerson, R.O. Ruhling, D.E. Shearer, L.A. Steinhaus, S.C. Johnson, H.W. Bonekat, and J.W. Shigeoka. 1990. Age and fitness effects on EEG, ERPs, visual sensitivity, and cognition. *Neurobiology of Aging* 11: 193-200.
24. Golding, J., and S. Ungerleider. 1992. *Beyond Strength: Psychological Profiles of Olympic Athletes.* Madison, WI: Brown and Benchmark.
25. Groden, J., J.R. Cautela, P. LeVasseur, G. Groden, and M. Bausman. 1991. *Imagery Procedures for People With Special Needs: Video Guide.* Champaign, IL: Research Press.
26. Hall, H.K., and A.W. Kerr. 2001. Goal setting in sport and physical activity: Tracing empirical developments and establishing conceptual direction. In: *Advances in Motivation in Sport and Exercise,* G.C. Roberts, ed. Champaign, IL: Human Kinetics, pp. 183-234.
27. Hart, E.A., M.R. Leary, and W.J. Rejeski. 1989. The measurement of social physique anxiety. *Journal of Sport and Exercise Psychology* 11: 94-104.
28. Hatfield, B.D. 1991. Exercise and mental health: The mechanisms of exercise-induced psychological states. In: *Psychology of Sports, Exercise and Fitness,* L. Diamant, ed. Washington, DC: Hemisphere, pp. 17-50.

29. Iso-Ahola, S.E., and B.D. Hatfield. 1986. *Psychology of Sports: A Social Psychological Approach.* Dubuque, IA: Brown.
30. Jacobson, E. 1974. *Progressive Relaxation.* Chicago: University of Chicago Press.
31. Kramer, A.F., S. Hahn, N.J. Cohen, M.T. Banich, E. McAuley, C.R. Harrison, J. Chason, E. Vakil, L. Bardell, R.A. Boileau, and A. Colcombe. 1999. Aging, fitness and neurocognitive function. *Nature* 400: 418-419.
32. Kugler, J., H. Seelback, and G.M. Kruskemper. 1994. Effects of rehabilitation exercise programmes on anxiety and depression in coronary patients: A meta-analysis. *British Journal of Clinical Psychology* 33: 401-410.
33. Kyllo, L.B., and D.M. Landers. 1995. Goal setting in sport and exercise: A research synthesis to resolve the controversy. *Journal of Sport and Exercise Psychology* 17: 117-137.
34. Landers, D.M. 1980. The arousal-performance relationship revisited. *Research Quarterly for Exercise and Sport* 51: 77-90.
35. Landers, D.M., and S.A. Arent. 2001. Physical activity and mental health. In: *Handbook of Sport Psychology,* 2nd ed., R.N. Singer, H.A. Hausenblas, and C.M. Janelle, eds. New York: Wiley, pp. 740-765.
36. Landers, D.M., and S.J. Petruzzello. 1994. Physical activity, fitness, and anxiety. In: *Physical Activity, Fitness, and Health,* C. Bouchard, R.J. Shepard, and T. Stevens, eds. Champaign, IL: Human Kinetics, pp. 868-882.
37. Lim, S., and L. Lipman. 1991. Mental practice and memorization of piano music. *Journal of General Psychology* 118: 21-30.
38. Long, B.C., and R. Van Stavel. 1995. Effects of exercise training on anxiety: A meta-analysis. *Journal of Applied Sport Psychology* 7: 167-189.
39. Marcus, B.H., C.A. Eaton, J.S. Rossi, and L.L. Harlow. 1994. Self-efficacy, decision making, and stages of change: An integrative model of physical exercise. *Journal of Applied Social Psychology* 24: 489-508.
40. Martens, R. 1975. *Social Psychology and Physical Activity.* New York: Harper & Row.
41. McDonald, D.G., and J.A. Hodgdon. 1991. *The Psychological Effects of Aerobic Fitness Training: Research and Theory.* New York: Springer-Verlag.
42. Meijer, E.H., F.T.Y. Smulders, and B.D. Hatfield. 2002. The effects of rhythmic physical activity and the EEG. Paper submitted for presentation at the annual meeting of the Society for Psychophysiological Research, Washington, DC.
43. Morgan, W.P. 1985. Affective beneficence of vigorous physical activity. *Medicine and Science in Sports and Exercise* 17: 94-100.
44. Morgan, W.P. 2001. Prescription of physical activity: A paradigm shift. *Quest* 53: 366-382.
45. North, T.C., P. McCullagh, and Z.V. Tran. 1990. Effects of exercise on depression. *Exercise and Sport Science Reviews* 18: 379-415.
46. O'Block, F.R., and F.H. Evans. 1984. Goal setting as a motivational technique: In: *Psychological Foundations of Sport,* J.M. Silva and R.S. Weinberg, eds. Champaign, IL: Human Kinetics, pp. 188-196.
47. Petruzzello, S.J., D.M. Landers, B.D. Hatfield, K.A. Kubitz, and W. Salazar. 1991. A meta-analysis an the anxiety-reducing effects of acute and chronic exercise. *Sports Medicine* 11: 143-182.
48. Prochaska, J.O., and B.H. Marcus. 1994. The transtheoretical model: The applications to exercise. In: *Advances in Exercise Adherence,* R.K. Dishman, ed. Champaign, IL: Human Kinetics, pp. 161-180.
49. Roberts, G.C. 1993. Motivation in sport: Understanding and enhancing the motivation and achievement of children. In: *Handbook of Research on Sport Psychology,* R.N. Singer, M. Murphy, and L.K. Tennant, eds. New York: Macmillan, pp. 405-420.
50. Roberts, G.C. 2001. Understanding the dynamics of motivation in physical activity: The influence of achievement goals on motivational processes. In: *Advances in Motivation in Sport and Exercise,* G.C. Roberts, ed. Champaign, IL: Human Kinetics, pp. 1-50.
51. Roberts, G.C., and D.C. Treasure. 1995. Achievement goals, motivation climate and achievement strategies and behaviors in sport. *International Journal of Sport Psychology* 26: 64-80.
52. Rogers, R.L., J.A. Meyer, and K.F. Mortel. 1990. After reaching retirement age physical activity sustains cerebral perfusion and cognition. *Journal of American Geriatric Society* 38: 123-128.
53. Ryan, R.M., C.M. Frederick, D. Lepes, N. Rubio, and K.M. Sheldon. 1997. Intrinsic motivation and exercise adherence. *International Journal of Sport Psychology* 28: 335-354.
54. Schuit, A.J., E.J.M. Feskens, L.J. Launer, and D. Kromhout. 2001. Physical activity and cognitive decline, the role of apolipoprotein e4 allele. *Medicine and Science in Sports and Exercise* 33: 772-777.
55. Sherwood, D.E., and D.J. Selder. 1979. Cardiorespiratory health, reaction time and aging. *Medicine and Science in Sports* 11: 186-189.
56. Siedentop, D., and G. Ramey. 1977. Extrinsic rewards and intrinsic motivation. *Motor Skills: Theory Into Practice* 2: 49-62.
57. Skinner, B.F. 1938. *The Behavior of Organisms: An Experimental Analysis.* New York: Appleton Century Crofts.
58. Skinner, B.F. 1953. *Science and Human Behavior.* New York: Macmillan.
59. Spielberger, C.D. 1983. *Manual for the State-Trait Anxiety Inventory (Form Y).* Palo Alto, CA: Consulting Psychologists Press.
60. Spirduso, W.W. 1983. Exercise and the aging brain. *Research Quarterly for Exercise and Sport* 54: 208-218.
61. Tong, L., H. Shen, V.M. Perreau, R. Balazas, and C.W. Cotman. 2001. Effects of exercise on gene-expression profile in the rat hippocampus. *Neurobiology of Disease* 8: 1046-1056.
62. U.S. Department of Health and Human Services. 1996. *Physical Activity and Health: A Report of the Surgeon General.* McLean, VA: International Medical
63. Vallerand, R.J., and G.F. Losier. 1999. An integration analysis of intrinsic and extrinsic motivation in sport. *Journal of Applied Sport Psychology* 11: 142-169.
64. Von Euler, C., and V. Soderberg. 1957. The influence of hypothalamic thermoceptive structures on the electroencephalogram and gamma motor activity. *Electroencephalography and Clinical Neurophysiology* 9: 391-408.
65. Weinberg, R.S., and D. Gould. 1999. *Foundations of Sport and Exercise Psychology.* Champaign, IL: Human Kinetics.

PART II

Initial Consultation and Evaluation

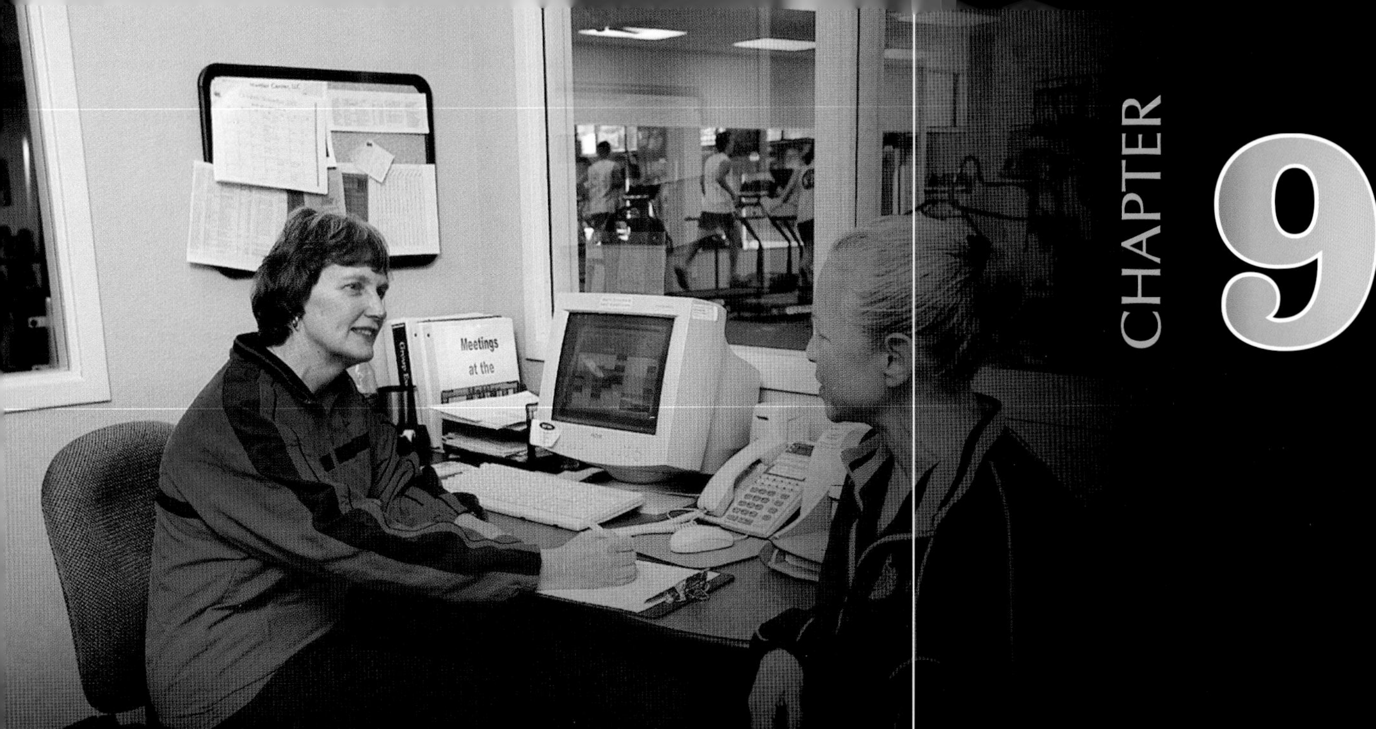

CHAPTER 9

Client Consultation and Health Appraisal

John A.C. Kordich

After completing this chapter, you will be able to

- conduct an initial client interview to assess compatibility, develop goals, and establish a client-trainer agreement;
- understand the process of a preparticipation health appraisal screening;
- identify positive coronary risk factors associated with cardiovascular disease;
- evaluate and stratify the health status of potential clients; and
- recognize individuals requiring referral to health care professionals

The scope of practice of the personal trainer involves the responsibility of interviewing potential clients to gather pertinent information regarding their personal health, lifestyle, and exercise readiness. The consultation process is a vital screening mechanism one can view as instrumental in appraising health status and developing comprehensive programs of exercise to safely and effectively meet the participant's individual objectives. This chapter covers the client consultation; preparticipation health screening; evaluation of coronary risk factors, disease, and lifestyle; interpretation of results; the referral process; and medical clearance.

Purpose of Consultation and Health Appraisal

The NSCA-Certified Personal Trainer® Job (Task) Analysis Committee has defined **scope of practice** for the personal training profession by characterizing personal trainers as "Health/fitness professionals who use an individualized approach to assess, motivate, educate, and train clients regarding their health and fitness needs. They design safe and effective exercise programs and provide the guidance to help clients achieve their personal goals. In addition, they respond appropriately in emergency situations. Recognizing their area of expertise, personal trainers refer clients to other health care professionals when appropriate" [32]. The objective of the client consultation and health appraisal is directly in line with the scope of practice of the personal trainer. Perhaps the best way to describe the role and responsibilities of the personal trainer in the preparticipation screening process is through the acronym MATER.

Personal Trainers MATER

Personal trainers

- **M***otivate* performance and compliance
- **A***ssess* health status
- **T***rain* clients safely and effectively to meet individual objectives
- **E***ducate* clients to be informed consumers
- **R***efer* clients to health care professionals when necessary

The most important principle underlying the client consultation and **health appraisal** process is to screen participants for risk factors and symptoms of chronic cardiovascular, pulmonary, metabolic, and orthopedic diseases in order to optimize safety during exercise testing and participation. Thus this chapter focuses on assessing health status and stratifying risk as a basis for referral to health care professionals.

Delivery Process

Because the health/fitness industry is diverse, there is no specific standardized process for implementing the client consultation and health appraisal mechanism. However, typically, delivery of the process is predicated on four factors that dictate implementation:

1. Credentials of the personal trainer
2. Site of delivery
3. Specific population served
4. Legal statute

As a result of the differences in credentials, delivery sites, populations served, and legal issues, "Steps of the Client Consultation and Health Appraisal" provides an example of the steps that may be involved in the delivery of the consultation and preparticipation health appraisal screening process.

Steps of the Client Consultation and Health Appraisal

- Schedule interview appointment.
- Conduct interview.
- Implement and complete health appraisal forms.
- Evaluate for coronary risk factors, diagnosed disease, and lifestyle.
- Assess and interpret results.
- Refer to an allied health professional when necessary.
- Obtain medical clearance and program recommendations.

Client Consultation

Even though there appears to be no recognized uniform process of administration, there is agreement about the value of an initial interview as the first step in the client consultation to obtain and share essential information associated with the program delivery process [4, 16, 27].

The **initial interview** is a scheduled appointment intended as a mutual sharing of information with the expected outcomes of assessing client-trainer compatibility, discussing goals, and developing a client-trainer agreement.

During the initial interview, the personal trainer and client assess compatibility, develop goals, and establish a client-trainer agreement.

Assessing Client-Trainer Compatibility

As the first step in determining trainer-client compatibility, the personal trainer provides a detailed description of the services available. Important information to convey to the potential client includes an explanation of the personal trainer's formal education, professional experience, certifications, and expertise or specializations, as well as the mission statement, success rate, and unique features of the program delivery system. Other important components that may affect suitability include logistical aspects regarding where and when services are available.

The personal trainer may also need to evaluate the level of exercise readiness by assessing the motivation and commitment of the individual. An attempt to predict compliance may begin with a discussion of past experiences, appreciation for exercise, availability of support, time management and organizational skills, and potential obstacles that may affect exercise adherence. Paper tests are available that are sensitive to predicting levels of exercise readiness and compliance. An attitudinal assessment form is shown on page 179.

It is essential to the decision-making process, as well as to the success of the client, for the personal trainer to provide a detailed description of how the program will be implemented by presenting a road map that informs the potential client of the step-by-step delivery method.

The last step in determining compatibility is to assess suitability and appropriateness. It is important that the personal trainer and potential client agree to boundaries, roles, resources, and expectations and address concerns related to any of the issues or information discussed in the initial interview.

If facts are discovered during the initial interview that would establish incompatibility, it is important for the personal trainer to provide the person with an option to receive services through a referral process.

Discussion of Goals

If compatibility and suitability are established, the next step may be a discussion of goals. The main function of identifying objectives is to provide and define direction as it relates to purpose and motivation. Developing goals that are specific, measurable, action oriented, realistic, and time sensitive is a science and art and a vital element of the training process. Goal setting is discussed in chapter 8.

Establishing the Client-Trainer Agreement

After the personal trainer and client have identified and clarified goals, the next step may be to finalize the trainer-client agreement. Entering into an agreement under the elements of contract law requires a formal process that in most cases is legally driven. Components of a contract include written documentation describing the services, parties involved, expectations of those parties, timeline of delivery, cost structure, and a payment process. Language of the contract should also cover the cancellation policy, termination of contract, and circumstances that would render the document void. An opportunity for discussion regarding the content of the contract should be provided during the consultation. Questions and issues concerning the agreement need to be documented and clarified before receipt of acknowledgment of acceptance. The contract becomes valid when signed by both parties, assuming appropriate legal age and competency [21]. An example of a personal training contract/agreement is provided on page 182.

Preparticipation Health Appraisal Screening

The purpose of the preparticipation health appraisal screening process is to identify known diseases and positive risk factors associated with coronary artery disease, assess lifestyle factors that may require special considerations, and identify individuals who may require medical referral before starting an exercise program.

The preparticipation health appraisal screening process to assess health status begins with the introduction of relevant forms that need to be completed and reviewed before services are provided and any activity occurs. It is essential that the process be cost-effective and time efficient in order to avoid unnecessary barriers to exercise for individuals who do not need a medical clearance to participate [29].

Health appraisal instruments are tools by which information is collected and evaluated to assess appropriateness for various levels of exercise and **referral.** Two instruments are commonly used: (1) **PAR-Q (Physical Activity Readiness Questionnaire)** and (2) **Health/Medical Questionnaire.**

Physical Activity Readiness Questionnaire

The PAR-Q, a tool developed in Canada, consists of a questionnaire that requires self-recall of observations and signs and symptoms experienced by the client, in addition to confirmation of diagnosis by a physician. The PAR-Q form appears on page 183.

The advantages of the PAR-Q are that it is cost-effective, easy to administer, and sensitive in that it identifies individuals who require additional medical screening while not excluding those who would benefit from participation in low-intensity activity [42]. The PAR-Q appears to have limitations in that it was designed essentially to determine the safety of exercise and not necessarily the risk for coronary artery disease. Because of the limitations of the PAR-Q with respect to identifying positive **coronary risk factors,** medications, and contraindications to exercise, it is advisable for personal trainers to use an additional health appraisal instrument for more effective identification of these critical elements.

The Health/Medical Questionnaire is an effective tool to assess the appropriateness of moderate and vigorous levels of exercise in that it can identify positive coronary risk factors associated with coronary artery disease, existing diagnosed pathologies, orthopedic concerns, recent operations, personal history of suggested signs and symptoms, medications, and lifestyle management. A sample health/medical questionnaire appears on page 184.

Information gathered from both health appraisal tools is instrumental in identifying risk factors, stratifying the level of risk, and determining the appropriateness of testing and exercise. Reasons for which clients must seek a physician's clearance before exercise testing or participation are discussed later in this chapter.

Additional Screening

Additional screening forms that provide an opportunity to gather and exchange valuable information include lifestyle inventories, informed consent, and assumption of risk.

Lifestyle Inventories

Lifestyle inventories vary in their format, substance, and depth. However, they usually consist of questions to evaluate personal choices and patterns related to dietary intake, management of stress, level of physical activity, and other practices that may affect the person's health. Although the specific benefits of the inventory results may be unclear, there appears to be some value in qualitatively and quantitatively assessing behaviors that may have a positive or negative impact on facilitating change in an individual's health and fitness. A personal trainer may use a lifestyle inventory to augment previously gathered health- and fitness-related information in an attempt to clarify and confirm personal issues possibly perceived as assets or obstacles to the client's success. In addition, the results of the inventory may provide valuable information for use in developing goals.

The vast majority of the existing standard lifestyle inventory assessments were developed for the average apparently healthy population. Persons with existing health-related conditions who have been previously diagnosed by a physician may not obtain valid and reliable information from the results of the inventories and therefore should rely on diagnostic information from their physician for guidance. The form "Health Risk Analysis" on page 186 is an example of a lifestyle inventory.

Informed Consent

The informed consent form gives clients information about the content and process of the program delivery system. The essential elements of an informed consent include a detailed description of the program, the risks and the benefits associated with participation, a confidentiality clause, responsibilities of the participant, and documentation of acknowledgment and acceptance of the terms described within the form. It has been commonly accepted that the information on this form should be conveyed both verbally and in writing to the client prior to any testing or participation to ensure that the participant knows and understands the risks and circumstances associated with the program. See chapter 25 for a discussion of legal issues regarding informed consent forms. An example of an informed consent form may be found on page 190.

Release/Assumption of Risk Agreement

The legal implications associated with the implementation and execution of the Release/ Assumption of Risk Agreement appear to be unclear at best due to the various legal interpretations associated with waiver documents (see chapter 25). However, in the situation in which a potential client declines to complete the necessary health appraisal and screening forms but wishes to pursue a contractual agreement and participation in an exercise program, there may be another option. It may be appropriate to administer a release/assumption of risk agreement form for people who are apparently healthy and do not appear to be a health risk but may benefit from an exercise program [3]. A release/assumption of risk agreement needs to identify the potential risks associated with participation and establish that the potential client understands those risks and voluntarily chooses to assume the responsibility. The acknowledgment of the content and authorization of this form does not relieve the personal trainer of the duty to perform in a competent and professional manner. An example of a release/assumption of risk agreement form appears on page 191.

Record Keeping

The personal trainer needs to develop a strategy to collect, organize, and store the vital information and materials obtained through the initial interview process. A record-keeping system to verify the completion and receipt of forms, along with other documentation concerning the status of the client, is instrumental in allowing one to move on to the next step of the preparticipation health appraisal screening process.

The scope of practice of the personal trainer involves the responsibility to interview potential clients to gather and assess pertinent information regarding their personal health, medical conditions, and lifestyle in order to safely and effectively meet their individual health/fitness objectives.

Evaluation of Coronary Risk Factors, Disease, and Lifestyle

Once the appropriate forms are completed and the documentation is reviewed, it is necessary to evaluate the content of the information to identify any potential risks associated with the client's present health status. This evaluation helps the personal trainer stratify risk and refer clients to physicians as necessary. The key areas to evaluate include positive risk factors associated with **coronary artery disease (CAD),** medical conditions and diagnosed disease, and current lifestyle.

Coronary Artery Disease Risk Factors

Coronary artery disease is the leading cause of mortality in Western society [6]. **Atherosclerosis** is a progressive degenerative process associated with CAD through which the endothelial lining of the arterial walls becomes hardened and the walls consequently lose elasticity. Over time, deposition of fat and plaque buildup occur and the artery wall narrows, which in turn occludes blood flow through the vascular system to the heart, causing heart tissue to die or leading to a **myocardial infarction.**

Although it is well documented that exercise is a protective preventative mechanism to deter this process, some individuals possess existing factors that put them at greater potential risk for a coronary episode because of the increased demand that exercise imposes on an already compromised system [33].

Identifiable positive risk factors are associated with the potential to acquire CAD. A positive risk factor may be defined as "an aspect of personal behavior or lifestyle, an environmental exposure or inherited characteristic, which, on the basis of epidemiologic evidence, is known to be associated with health related conditions considered important to prevent" [28]. It is necessary to evaluate positive risk factors associated with CAD in order to identify individuals who may be at higher risk during exercise.

Positive Coronary Risk Factors

Epidemiological research suggests that a person's potential risk for developing CAD is associated with the positive coronary risk factors the person possesses. The greater the number and severity of those risk factors, the greater probability of CAD [25]. The seven identifiable positive coronary risk factors that provide a significant correlation to CAD are family history, smoking, hypertension, hypercholesterolemia, impaired fasting glucose levels, obesity, and sedentary lifestyle (see table 9.1, "Coronary Artery Disease Risk Factor Thresholds").

Family History Coronary artery disease appears to have a predisposing genetic connection and a tendency to be familial. Although it is difficult to ascertain whether a genetic code or an environmental influence is involved, it may be safe to speculate that people with a documented family history are more susceptible to CAD [26]. Thus people with a family history possess a risk factor if a myocardial infarction, coronary revascularization, or sudden death

TABLE 9.1

Coronary Artery Disease Risk Factor Thresholds

Positive risk factors	Defining criteria
1. Family history	Myocardial infarction, coronary revascularization, or sudden death before 55 years of age in biological father or other male first-degree relative (i.e., brother or son), or before 65 years of age in biological mother or other female first-degree relative (i.e., sister or daughter)
2. Cigarette smoking	Current cigarette smokers or those who quit within the previous six months
3. Hypertension	Systolic blood pressure ≥140 mmHg or diastolic ≥90 mmHg, confirmed by measurements on at least two separate occasions, or being on antihypertensive medication
4. Hypercholesterolemia	Total serum cholesterol >200 mg/dL (5.2 mmol · L^{-1}) or high-density lipoprotein cholesterol of <35 mg/dL (0.9 mmol · L^{-1}), or on lipid-lowering medication. If low-density lipoprotein cholesterol is available, use >130 mg/dL (3.4 mmol · L^{-1}) rather than total cholesterol of >200 mg/dL.
5. Impaired fasting glucose	Fasting blood glucose of ≥110 mg/dL (6.1 mmol · L^{-1}) confirmed by measurements on at least two separate occasions
6. Obesity[†]	Body mass index of ≥30 kg/m^2 or waist girth of >100 cm (39 in.)
7. Sedentary lifestyle	Persons not participating in a regular exercise program or meeting the minimal physical activity recommendations[‡] from the U.S. Surgeon General's report

Negative risk factor	Defining criteria
High serum high-density lipoprotein cholesterol[§]	>60 mg/dL (1.6 mmol · L^{-1})

Note: For use with American College of Sports Medicine (ACSM) Risk Stratification—*ACSM's Guidelines,* 6th ed.

[†]Professional opinions vary regarding the most appropriate markers and thresholds for obesity; therefore, exercise professionals should use clinical judgment when evaluating this risk factor.

[‡]Accumulating 30 minutes or more of moderate physical activity on most days of the week.

[§]It is common to sum risk factors in making clinical judgments. If high-density lipoprotein (HDL) cholesterol is high, subtract one risk factor from the sum of positive risk factors because high HDL decreases coronary artery disease risk.

Reprinted from ACSM 2000.

occurred before 55 years of age in their biological father or another male first-degree relative (sibling or child), or before 65 years of age in their biological mother or other female first-degree relatives [2].

Cigarette Smoking Overwhelming empirical evidence identifies cigarette smoking as a major positive risk factor for CAD [20]. A linear relationship also appears to exist between the risk for cardiovascular disease and the volume of cigarette smoking and number of years a person smoked [14]. Data suggest that the chemical makeup of cigarettes accentuates risk by elevating myocardial oxygen demand and reducing oxygen transport, causing the cardiovascular system to work harder to obtain a sufficient oxygen supply [15]. In addition, cigarette smoking lowers high-density lipoprotein, which has an impact on the acceleration of the atherosclerotic process [34]. Persons who currently smoke cigarettes, and those who previously smoked but who have quit within the last six months, have a greater potential risk for CAD and have this positive risk factor [2].

Hypertension Hypertension is chronic, persistent sustained elevation of blood pressures. Most individuals who are clinically diagnosed have essential hypertension, which by definition cannot be attributed to any specific cause. Secondary hypertension refers to elevated blood pressures caused by specific factors such as kidney disease and obesity [30].

Regardless of the etiology, hypertension is believed to predispose individuals to CAD through the direct vascular injury caused by high blood pressure and its adverse effects on the myocardium. These include increased wall stress, which dramatically increases the workload of the heart in pumping the extra blood required to overcome peripheral vascular resistance [41]. In general, the higher the blood pressure, the greater the risk for CAD.

Hypercholesterolemia Cholesterol is a fatlike substance found in the tissues of the body that performs specific metabolic functions in the human organism. Cholesterol is carried in the bloodstream by molecular proteins known as high-density lipoproteins (HDLs) and low-density lipoproteins (LDLs). Evidence suggests that the LDL molecules release cholesterol, which penetrates the endothelial lining of the arterial wall and in turn contributes to the atherosclerotic plaque buildup that eventually leads to vascular occlusion and heart attacks [43]. Research has strongly suggested that HDLs act as a protective mechanism by transporting cholesterol through the bloodstream to the liver, where it is metabolized and eliminated.

Epidemiological research has identified a strong relationship between high levels of total cholesterol, high LDL-cholesterol, and low HDL-cholesterol and a higher rate of CAD in both men and women [17]. Individuals who have a total serum cholesterol of >200 mg/dL or an HDL-cholesterol of <35 mg/dL and/or an LDL >130 mg/dL and are on lipid-lowering medication have a greater risk for CAD. It is important to note that the LDL may provide a more predictive value for CAD than the total cholesterol. In any event, people who have these values have a positive risk factor for CAD [2].

Impaired Fasting Glucose Levels Fasting blood glucose levels are markers to assess the body's metabolic function. Elevated levels of circulating glucose in the bloodstream cause a chemical imbalance that impedes the utilization of fats and glucose. As a result, individuals with this metabolic imbalance are more susceptible to atherosclerosis and an increased risk for CAD [5]. Elevated fasting glucose levels may also be early predictive values for the potential onset of diabetes. Individuals who present with fasting glucose values equal to or greater than 110 mg/dL, confirmed by measurements on at least two separate occasions, are considered to be at increased risk for CAD [2].

Obesity Obesity by medical definition is the accumulation and storage of excess body fat. The prevalence of obesity in the United States has reached epidemic proportions. An analysis of the relationship between obesity and CAD is confounded because of the connection between obesity and other risk factors such as physical inactivity, hypertension, hypercholesterolemia, and diabetes. However, most recently, evidence has suggested that obesity in and of itself may be considered an independent risk factor for CAD [23]. In addition to the risk associated with accumulation of excess body fat, there may be an increased risk related to the location and deposition of that stored visceral fat. Persons who store or accumulate excess body fat in the central waist or abdominal area appear to be at greater risk for CAD [18]. The assessments and values associated with obesity as a positive risk factor include a body mass index (BMI) equal to or greater than 30 kilograms bodyweight per height in meters squared (30 kg/m^2) or a waist girth >39 inches (100 centimeters) [2]. Refer to chapter 11 to calculate BMI and measure waist girth.

Sedentary Lifestyle Physical inactivity or a **sedentary** lifestyle is recognized as a leading contributing factor to morbidity and mortality (figure 9.1). Numerous studies have linked a sedentary lifestyle or low fitness to a greater risk of CAD [44]. Substantial evidence suggests that CAD risk for sedentary individuals is significantly greater than for those who are more physically active. Physical activity also has many beneficial effects on other CAD risk factors, for example by decreasing resting systolic and diastolic blood pressures, reducing triglyceride levels, increasing serum HDL-cholesterol levels, and enhancing glucose tolerance and insulin sensitivity [19]. People who do not participate in a regular exercise program or meet the minimal physical activity recommendations (30 minutes or more of accumulated moderate-intensity activity on most, or preferably all, days of the week to expend approximately 200 to 250 calories per day) in the U.S. Surgeon General's report have a positive risk factor for CAD [2].

Negative Coronary Risk Factors

A **negative coronary risk factor** suggests a favorable influence that may contribute to the development of a protective cardiac benefit [31]. High-density lipoproteins appear to provide a protective

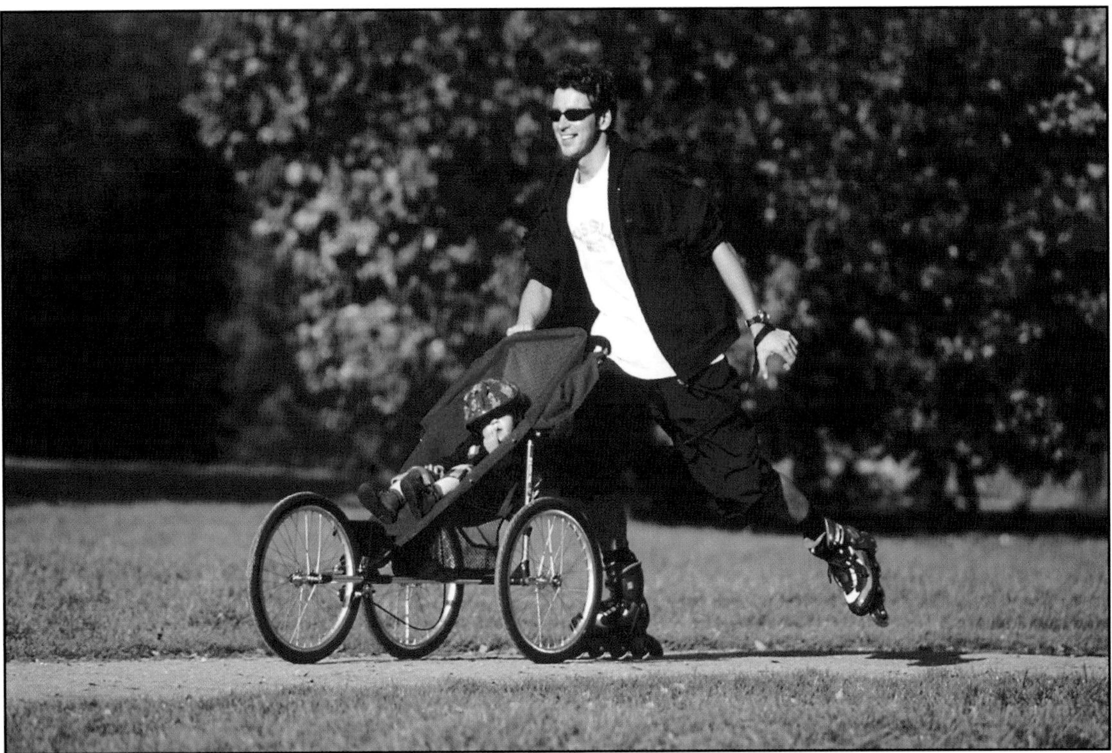

Figure 9.1 Physical activity appears to be a modifiable risk factor associated with CAD in which exercise plays a critical role to deter disease.

mechanism against CAD by removing cholesterol from the body and preventing plaque from forming in the arteries. Research suggests that increases in HDLs are consistent with decreased risk for CAD [12]. Thus, persons who have a serum HDL-cholesterol of >60 mg/dL improve their cholesterol profile and decrease the risk of CAD [2]. If HDL-cholesterol is high (>60 mg/dL), the personal trainer subtracts one risk factor from the sum of positive risk factors shown in table 9.1. The results of this evaluation of CAD risk factors will affect risk stratification and referral, discussed later in this chapter.

The personal trainer must be able to identify and understand positive risk factors and their association with CAD, as well as the potential concerns as they relate to safety.

Identification of Medical Conditions and Diagnosed Disease

Identifying and understanding positive risk factors and their association with CAD, as well as the potential concerns that exist when these risk factors are present, is an important responsibility of the personal trainer in the screening process. However, equally critical is the ability to identify signs and symptoms of various chronic cardiovascular, pulmonary, metabolic, and orthopedic diseases that may contraindicate exercise and could potentially exacerbate an existing condition, thus leading to an adverse impact on the individual's health. Persons who have evidence of a known disease, have symptoms of cardiovascular disease, or are presently on medications to control disease require special attention because of the increased potential risk.

Coronary Artery and Pulmonary Disease

Personal history plays a fundamental and critical role in the process of early detection of CAD. Signs and symptoms suggestive of CAD are important guides in identifying individuals who are at higher risk for the future development of disease. People who exhibit signs and symptoms of a personal history associated with CAD present special safety concerns as to the appropriateness of participating in an exercise program. The health appraisal screening mechanisms mentioned earlier are intended to initially identify those signs and symptoms that have been previously diagnosed or personally detected. However, the personal trainer needs to use enhanced observation throughout the client consultation and health appraisal process to identify and assess signs and symptoms suggestive of cardiovascular and pulmonary disease that the client may exhibit. The major signs or symptoms suggestive of cardiovascular and pulmonary disease are as follows [Reprinted from ACSM 2000; reference 2]:

- Pain, discomfort (or other anginal equivalent) in the chest, neck, jaw, arms, or other areas that may be due to ischemia (lack of blood flow)
- Shortness of breath at rest or with mild exertion
- Dizziness or syncope (fainting)
- Orthopnea (the need to sit up to breathe comfortably) or paroxysmal (sudden, unexpected attack) nocturnal dyspnea (shortness of breath at night)
- Ankle edema (swelling/water retention)
- Palpitations or tachycardia (rapid heart rate)
- Intermittent claudication (calf cramping)
- Known heart murmur
- Unusual fatigue or shortness of breath with usual activities

(These symptoms must be interpreted in the clinical context in which they appear because they are not all specific for cardiovascular, pulmonary, or metabolic disease.)

It is important for personal trainers to understand that these signs and symptoms must be interpreted in a clinical setting for **diagnostic** purposes and that they are not all specific to cardiovascular, pulmonary, and metabolic disease [8]. However, if an individual exhibits these signs or symptoms, it is the role and responsibility of the personal trainer to take appropriate action through the referral process by recommending a medical examination by a physician.

Various pulmonary diseases affect the respiratory system's ability to transport oxygen during exercise to the tissue level via the cardiovascular system. The systematic breakdown that occurs as a result of inadequate oxygen supply creates a greater-than-normal demand on the function of the cardiorespiratory system, in some cases markedly reducing exercise tolerance.

Chronic bronchitis, emphysema, and asthma are considered to be syndromes associated with **chronic obstructive pulmonary disease (COPD)** and are the most common diagnosed diseases related to respiratory dysfunction. Chronic bronchitis is an inflammatory condition caused by persistent production of sputum due to a thickened bronchial wall, which in turn creates a reduction of airflow. Emphysema is a disease of the lung that affects the small airways. An enlargement of air spaces accompanied by the progressive destruction of alveolar-capillary units leads to elevated pulmonary vascular resistance, which in most cases can contribute to heart failure. Asthma is mostly due to a spasmodic contraction of smooth muscle around the bronchi that produces swelling of the mucosal cells lining the bronchi and an excessive secretion of mucous. Constriction of airway paths associated with asthma results in attacks that may be caused by allergic reactions, exercise, air quality factors, and stress [7]. (Chapter 20 provides detailed information.)

Metabolic Disease

As mentioned earlier, an impaired fasting glucose level has been identified as a positive risk factor for CAD and a potential predictor for the development of diabetes. Diabetes mellitus, a metabolic disease, affects the body's ability to metabolize blood glucose properly. The disease is characterized by hyperglycemia resulting from defects in insulin secretion (type 1), insulin action (type 2), or both. Persons with type 1 diabetes are insulin dependent, meaning that they require insulin injections to metabolize glucose. Persons with type 2 diabetes in most cases are able to produce insulin, but the tissue resists it and as a result glycemic control is inadequate. Diabetes is known to be an independent contributing factor in the development of cardiovascular disease. This excessive risk increases the potential for CAD, peripheral vascular disease, and congestive heart failure [11]. Although physical activity and exercise along with dietary modifications and prescribed medications appear to have an impact on the regulation of glucose levels, diabetes still requires ongoing medical attention and warrants precautions [37]. Chapter 19 provides information on working with clients who have diabetes. In addition, diabetes in a client affects risk stratification and referral, which are discussed later in this chapter.

Orthopedic Conditions and Disease

Even though orthopedic limitations and disease do not appear to present the same relative risk as that associated with cardiovascular function, musculoskeletal concerns are an important factor for the personal trainer to consider in assessing an individual's functional capacity and may require a physician's referral before initiation of a program.

Common musculoskeletal concerns related to chronic trauma overuse syndrome, osteoarthritis, and lower back pain present issues and challenges that may need to be assessed on a case-by-case basis. Although these conditions may limit performance and are important to the personal trainer, dealing with individuals who have rheumatoid arthritis, who have had recent surgery, or who have diagnosed degenerative bone disease may involve greater concerns because of the potential implications regarding advanced complications. Issues related to orthopedic replacements, recent surgical procedures, osteoporosis, and rheumatoid arthritis may require communication with a physician and in most cases medical clearance. (Chapter 21 provides detailed information.)

Medications

Individuals being treated by a physician on an ongoing basis may be taking prescribed medications as a therapeutic measure to manage a diagnosed condition or disease. The chemical reactions that occur in the body may influence physiological responses during activity. Various medications may alter heart rate, blood pressures, cardiac function, and exercise capacity. It is important for the personal trainer to understand the classes of commonly used drugs and their effects. For example, beta-blocking medications commonly prescribed for persons with high blood pressure may affect normal increases in heart rates during exercise; as a result, people will have difficulty obtaining, and should not strive to achieve, training heart rates. In addition, monitoring intensity of exercise by using heart rates may be inappropriate because of the masking effect of the medications on heart rates, and therefore ratings of perceived exertion would provide a more effective mechanism to regulate intensity levels of exercise [36].

Lifestyle Evaluation

Identifying an individual's behavioral patterns concerning choices about dietary intake, physical activity, and stress management provides additional information for assessing potential health risks associated with current **lifestyle.** Evidence clearly suggests a strong relationship between lifestyle choices regarding dietary intake, physical activity, and the management of stress on the one hand and the potential risk of CAD and other leading causes of **morbidity** and premature **mortality** on the other hand [39]. The results of this evaluation may influence risk stratification and referral, discussed later in this chapter.

Dietary Intake and Eating Habits

Because of the significant contributory impact of nutritional habits on health and performance, the personal trainer should consider encouraging clients to evaluate their current daily intake. Identifying, quantifying, and assessing a person's daily dietary intake give the personal trainer valuable information for assessing overconsumption, underconsumption, and caloric imbalances that may be contributing factors in the development of disease.

There is a solid link between dietary intake and the development of disease. The most evident connection is between dietary saturated fat and cholesterol and the development of atherosclerosis [13]. Excessive alcohol consumption has also been associated with an increased risk for cardiovascular disease; and diets high in sodium can lead to chronic elevation of systolic blood pressure, or more importantly, can result in worsening of heart failure [24]. Overconsumption of caloric intake may contribute to obesity and diabetes, and underconsumption may lead to degenerative bone diseases and psychological health issues related to disordered eating.

An analysis of a typical dietary intake through documentation of a three-day or seven-day dietary record may be a starting point for assessing the health-related value of the individual's eating habits. A dietary recall or diet history, as discussed in chapter 7, may also be used. The information obtained through these methods may be instrumental as one part of a collective process to identify potential concerns in relation to the risk for disease. See chapter 7 for detailed guidance about seeking information on and evaluating clients' nutrition habits. In addition, strategies and methods have been developed for recognizing and referring individuals who exhibit signs and symptoms related to disordered eating. (Chapter 19 provides details.)

Exercise and Activity Pattern

Identifying patterns of physical activity and exercise helps the personal trainer to recognize individuals with little or no history of physical activity or exercise. As discussed earlier, physical inactivity is a major contributing positive risk factor associated with the development of CAD and requires evaluation to assess potential concerns and level of risk.

An evaluation of physical activity and exercise patterns should include identifying the specific activity and the frequency, volume, and level of intensity (moderate, vigorous) of that activity, as well as documenting signs or symptoms associated with the activity, particularly shortness of breath or chest pains. Any musculoskeletal concerns related to joint discomfort or chronic pain should also be identified.

Stress Management

Epidemiological studies provide evidence that stress is related to the risk for CAD [35]. Several investigations have linked stress with an increase in heart disease. In addition, several prospective studies suggest that **"type A" behavior patterns** may contribute to the overall risk for developing CAD [9].

"Type A" behavior pattern characteristics include hostility, depression, chronic stress produced by situations involving "high demand and low control," and social isolation [1, 38]. These lifestyle stress-related characteristics can be measured psychosocially and physiologically through emotional stress inventories and standard exercise testing [10, 40].

Because of the implications of stress and its impact on developing CAD, it is important for the personal trainer to be able to identify the common signs and symptoms of stress overload and to develop intervention strategies to reduce health risks. The "Health Risk Analysis" on page 186 can be used to assess a client's potential for stress and response to stressors. This inventory will have been completed during the preparticipation health screening.

Once the preparticipation health appraisal screening is complete, the personal trainer should evaluate the client's positive risk factors associated with CAD, medical conditions and diagnosed disease, and current lifestyle. The results of this evaluation will be used for risk stratification.

Interpretation of Results

After the preparticipation health appraisal screening process has taken place and a review and evaluation of coronary risk factors, disease, and lifestyle are complete, the next step in the screening process is to identify individuals who may be at increased risk and to stratify that potential for risk. Stratifying risk for potential health-related concerns is a preliminary step in determining the appropriateness of activity and identifying clients who require referral before beginning an exercise program. In order to meaningfully interpret the results obtained through the screening process, the personal trainer uses the PAR-Q results and the initial risk stratification method to identify people who have a greater potential for risk and may require referral and a clearance from a physician.

PAR-Q

As mentioned earlier, the PAR-Q is easy to administer and is a cost-effective mechanism for initially screening individuals who are apparently healthy and want to engage in regular low-intensity exercise. The PAR-Q has also been shown to be useful in referring individuals who require additional medical screening while not excluding those who may benefit from exercise.

After eliciting objective *yes* or *no* answers to seven questions related to signs and symptoms associated with CAD, orthopedic concerns, and diagnosis by a physician, the self-administered questionnaire form provides direction based on interpretation of the results and specifies recommendations as to the appropriateness of activity and the referral process. Specific recommendations related to this form are discussed later in this chapter in the "Referral Process" section.

Initial Risk Stratification

The intent of the initial **risk stratification** method is to use age, health status, personal symptoms, and coronary risk factor information to initially classify individuals into one of three risk strata for preliminary decision-making purposes [2]. Table 9.2 provides criteria for the risk stratification process.

It is nearly impossible for any set of guidelines or method to address all the potential situations that may arise. However, using a decision-making process to evaluate the information obtained through the initial health appraisal screening process, the personal trainer should be able to classify an individual into one of the three risk categories.

Case Study 9.1 illustrates how the personal trainer might stratify risk using the initial risk stratification process. The personal trainer might obtain the following information during the preparticipation health appraisal screening interview.

Case Study 9.1

Presentation

Ralph D. is a sedentary 36-year-old male tool and die engineer. His father survived a heart attack at age 70. Ralph reports that his blood pressure has been recorded at 136/86 mmHg and that his total cholesterol is 250 mg/dL, with an HDL of 45 mg/dL. His BMI has recently been measured at 30, his hip circumference is 40 inches (102 centimeters), and his waist girth is 47 inches (119 centimeters). Ralph reports no signs or symptoms and indicates that he quit smoking seven months ago.

Analysis

An evaluation of this scenario leads to the conclusion that Ralph presently has three positive coronary risk factors, hypercholesterolemia, sedentary lifestyle, (total cholesterol >200 mg/dL) and obesity (waist girth >39 inches or 100 centimeters; a BMI of 30). Consequently Ralph would be classified according to the stratification as being at moderate risk.

The ability to stratify risk gives the personal trainer the foundation to eventually identify whether it is appropriate to assess and train an individual or refer the individual to a physician for medical clearance.

TABLE 9.2

Risk Stratification

Low risk
Younger individuals[a] who are asymptomatic and meet no more than one risk factor threshold from table 9.1
Moderate risk
Older individuals (men ≥45 years of age; women ≥55 years of age) or those who meet the threshold of two or more risk factors from table 9.1
High risk
Individuals with one or more signs/symptoms listed on page 169 or with known cardiovascular[†], pulmonary[‡], or metabolic[§] disease

[a]Men <45 years of age; women <55 years of age.

[†]Cardiac, peripheral vascular, or cerebrovascular disease.

[‡]Chronic obstructive pulmonary disease, asthma, interstitial lung disease, or cystic fibrosis (see American Association of Cardiovascular and Pulmonary Rehabilitation, 1998, *Guidelines for Pulmonary Rehabilitation Programs,* 2nd ed. Champaign, IL: Human Kinetics, pp. 97-112).

[§]Diabetes mellitus (types 1 and 2), thyroid disorders, renal or liver disease.

Reprinted from ACSM 2000.

Referral Process

The processes described so far (preparticipation health appraisal screening; evaluation of coronary risk factors, disease, and lifestyle; and interpretation of the information obtained through the initial interview and client consultation process) are intended to help identify individuals who will need a referral to a health care professional for **medical clearance** prior to participating in activity. The following referral processes may be implemented to assess readiness and appropriateness for exercise.

Medical Examinations

Regular medical examinations to evaluate health status are normally encouraged for preventative purposes for everyone. It is also reasonable to recommend that persons beginning a new program of activity or exercise consult with a physician prior to participation [22].

PAR-Q Recommendations

After a client has completed the PAR-Q, the personal trainer can derive recommendations from the seven-question form through the following analysis.

If the client gave a *yes* answer *to one or more questions* (which are related to signs and symptoms associated with CAD, orthopedic concerns, and diagnosis by a physician), it is recommended that the individual contact his or her physician and tell the physician which questions elicited *yes* answers before increasing physical activity and taking part in a fitness appraisal or assessment. The client should seek recommendations from the physician regarding the level and progression of activity and restrictions associated with that person's specific needs.

If the client gave *no* answers *to all questions*, there is reasonable assurance that it is suitable for an individual to engage in a graduated exercise program and a fitness appraisal or assessment.

Note also the PAR-Q recommendation that a client who is or may be pregnant talk with her doctor before she starts becoming more active. Chapter 18 provides guidance about conditions in which pregnant women should cease exercising or seek physician advice.

A client must seek physician clearance for exercise testing and participation if he or she answers *yes* to any PAR-Q questions, exhibits any signs or symptoms of cardiovascular or pulmonary disease, is stratified as moderate risk and wants to participate in vigorous exercise, or is stratified as high risk and wants to participate in moderate or vigorous exercise.

Recommendations for Current Medical Examinations and Exercise Testing

Suggested guidelines have been developed for determining when a diagnostic medical examination and submaximal and maximal exercise tests are appropriate before participation in moderate and vigorous exercise, and when a physician's supervision is required to monitor the assessments. Table 9.3 provides the American College of Sports Medicine (ACSM) recommendations for current medical examinations and exercise testing prior to participation and physician supervision of exercise tests [2].

Guidelines and recommendations for medical examinations and exercise testing are interfaced with the initial risk stratification classifications for low, moderate, and high risk. The guidelines are consistent with the notion that as the intensity of the activity increases from moderate (40%-60% maximal oxygen uptake) to vigorous (>60% maximal oxygen uptake), there is an untoward increase in potential risk for the participant. To help users better understand and interpret the recommended guidelines, table 9.3 presents and defines the essential elements associated with medical examinations and exercise testing.

It is important to understand that the guidelines and recommendations for exercise testing clearly distinguish which exercise tests and stratification classifications require a physician's supervision. It is also essential to note the difference between submaximal and maximal exercise tests in order to identify the appropriate recommendation regarding supervision. Submaximal and maximal exercise tests may be defined as follows:

TABLE 9.3

Recommendations for (A) Current Medical Examination* and Exercise Testing Prior to Participation and (B) Physician Supervision of Exercise Tests

	Low risk	Moderate risk	High risk
(A)			
Moderate exercise†	Not necessary‡	Not necessary	Recommended
Vigorous exercise§	Not necessary	Recommended	Recommended
(B)			
Submaximal test	Not necessary	Not necessary	Recommended
Maximal test	Not necessary	Recommended	Recommended

*Within the past year (see G.J. Balady, B. Chaitman, D. Driscoll, et al., 1998, American College of Sports Medicine and American Heart Association joint position statement: Recommendations for cardiovascular screening, staffing, and emergency policies at health/fitness facilities. *Medicine and Science in Sports and Exercise* 30: 1009-1018).

†Absolute moderate exercise is defined as activities that are approximately 3-6 METs (metabolic equivalents) or the equivalent of brisk walking at 3 to 4 mph for most healthy adults. Nevertheless, a pace of 3 to 4 mph might be considered to be "hard" to "very hard" by some sedentary, older persons. Moderate exercise may alternatively be defined as an intensity well within the individual's capacity, one that can be comfortably sustained for a prolonged period of time (~45 min), that has a gradual initiation and progression, and is generally noncompetitive. If an individual's exercise capacity is known, relative moderate exercise may be defined by the range 40%-60% maximal oxygen uptake.

‡The designation "Not necessary" reflects the notion that a medical examination, exercise test, and physician supervision of exercise testing would not be essential in the preparticipation screening; however, they should not be viewed as inappropriate.

§Vigorous exercise is defined as activities of >6 METs. Vigorous exercise may alternatively be defined as exercise intense enough to represent a substantial cardiorespiratory challenge. If an individual's exercise capacity is known, vigorous exercise may be defined as an intensity of >60% maximal oxygen uptake.

When physician supervision of exercise testing is "Recommended," the physician should be in close proximity and readily available should there be an emergent need.

Reprinted from ACSM 2000.

A **submaximal test** is a nondiagnostic practical assessment, typically referred to as a field test, that is inexpensive, is easy to administer, and does not normally require maximal effort. These tests are typically administered by certified personal trainers.

A **maximal test** is commonly performed in a clinical setting with use of specialized diagnostic equipment to assess an individual's functional capacity through maximal effort. Testing is relatively complex, and direct measurements are used to assess physiological responses. Because of the diagnostic capabilities and the high risk of cardiac complications, physicians supervise the administration of these tests.

The following recommendations apply to the levels of stratified risk [2]:

Low risk: It is not necessary to have a current medical examination and an exercise test prior to participation in moderate and vigorous exercise. It is also not necessary for a physician to supervise a submaximal or maximal exercise test.

Moderate risk: It is not necessary to have a current medical examination and exercise test for moderate exercise; however, these are recommended for vigorous exercise. It is not necessary for a physician to supervise a submaximal exercise test, but physician supervision is recommended for a maximal test.

High risk: It is recommended that a current medical examination and exercise test be performed prior to moderate or vigorous exercise, and it is recommended that a physician supervise both submaximal and maximal exercise tests.

The following case studies of information gained during the preparticipation health appraisal screening interview (Case Studies 9.2 and 9.3) provide examples of stratifying risk and making referrals based on recommendations for current medical examinations and exercise testing.

Figure 9.2 provides a flowchart of the referral process.

Case Study 9.2

Presentation

Martha G. is a 56-year-old secretary. Her father died of an MI (myocardial infarction) at the age of 45. Martha reports that her LDL-cholesterol has been recorded at 125 mg/dL. Her BMI is 25. She reports that she has an active lifestyle that includes golf, tennis, and a daily walking routine.

Analysis

On the basis of the information in this scenario, although Martha has only one positive coronary risk factor for family history (father died of an MI before the age of 55), she would be considered at moderate risk also due to her age (over 55). According to the guidelines and recommendations for medical examinations and exercise testing, it would not be necessary for Martha to have a current diagnostic medical examination and exercise test for moderate exercise; but these assessments would be recommended for vigorous exercise. In addition, it would not be necessary for a physician to supervise a submaximal test, but physician supervision would be recommended for a maximal test.

Case Study 9.3

Presentation

Kathleen K. is a 47-year-old sedentary female. Kathleen reports a total cholesterol of 210 mg/dL with an HDL-cholesterol reading of 68 mg/dL. She stands five feet two inches (157 centimeters) tall, and her body weight is 110 pounds (50 kilograms) with a BMI of 20. Her blood pressure taken on two separate occasions is recorded as 120/80 mmHg. She reports that she was diagnosed with type 1 diabetes in early childhood.

Analysis

A review of the scenario shows that Kathleen has two positive coronary risk factors, a sedentary lifestyle and hypercholesterolemia (total cholesterol level >200 mg/dL). However, she presents an HDL-cholesterol level of 68 mg/dL, which gives her a negative risk factor (HDL-cholesterol >60 mg/dL) that cancels one of the positive risk factors—leaving her with one total positive risk factor. It would initially appear that her age (younger than 55) and one risk factor would classify her at low risk. However, the fact that she has been diagnosed with a metabolic disease (type 1 diabetes) places her in the stratification classification of high risk.

Consequently, according to the guidelines and recommendations for medical examination and exercise testing, it would be necessary for Kathleen to have a diagnostic test and medical examination for both moderate and vigorous exercise. In addition, it would be recommended that a physician supervise both submaximal and maximal exercise tests.

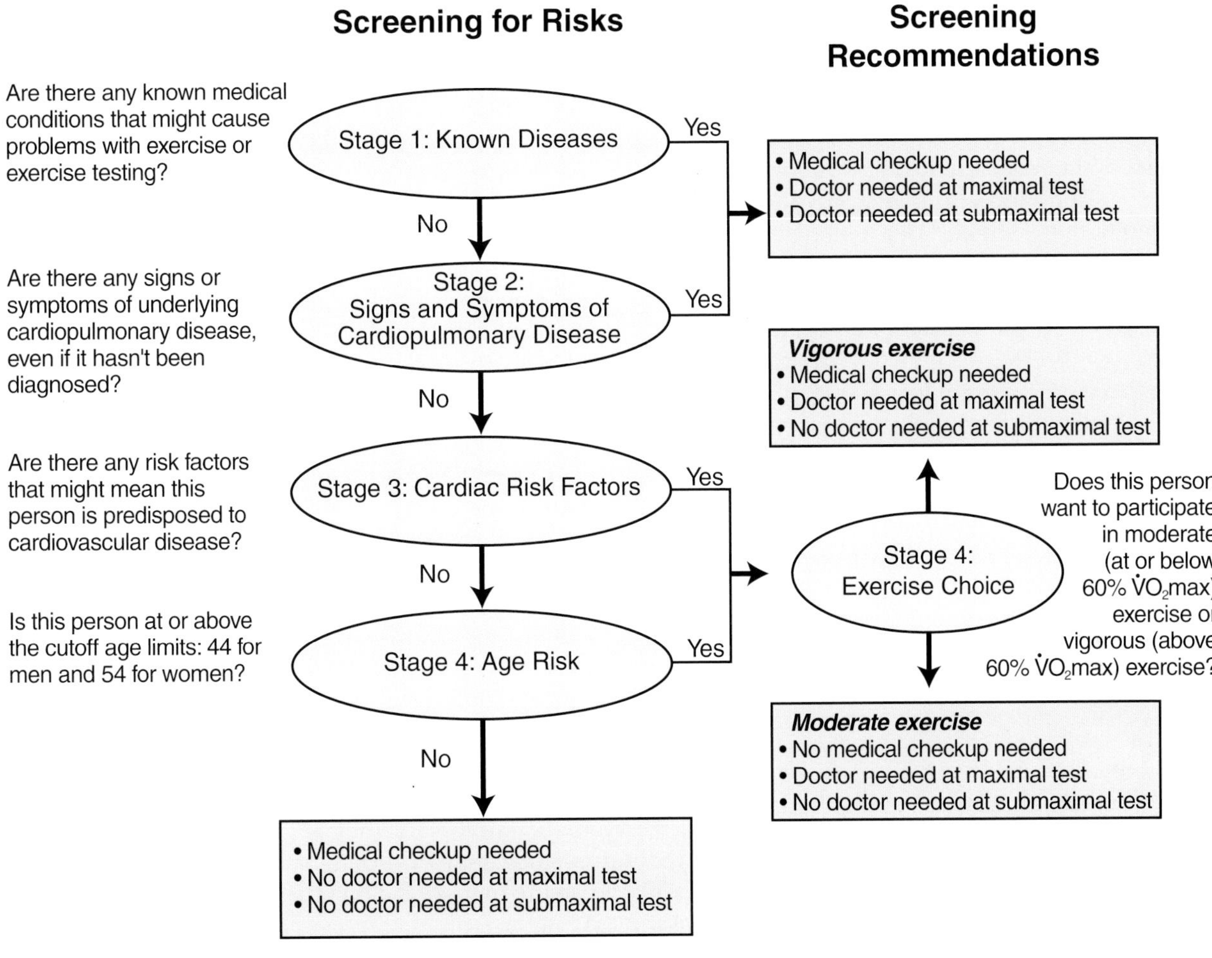
Screening for Risks
Screening Recommendations
Are there any known medical conditions that might cause problems with exercise or exercise testing?
Stage 1: Known Diseases
Yes
No
• Medical checkup needed
• Doctor needed at maximal test
• Doctor needed at submaximal test
Are there any signs or symptoms of underlying cardiopulmonary disease, even if it hasn't been diagnosed?
Stage 2: Signs and Symptoms of Cardiopulmonary Disease
Yes
No
Vigorous exercise
• Medical checkup needed
• Doctor needed at maximal test
• No doctor needed at submaximal test
Are there any risk factors that might mean this person is predisposed to cardiovascular disease?
Stage 3: Cardiac Risk Factors
Yes
No
Does this person want to participate in moderate (at or below 60% $\dot{V}O_2max$) exercise or vigorous (above 60% $\dot{V}O_2max$) exercise?
Stage 4: Exercise Choice
Is this person at or above the cutoff age limits: 44 for men and 54 for women?
Stage 4: Age Risk
Yes
No
Moderate exercise
• No medical checkup needed
• Doctor needed at maximal test
• No doctor needed at submaximal test
• Medical checkup needed
• No doctor needed at maximal test
• No doctor needed at submaximal test

Figure 9.2 The referral process.
Reprinted from Olds and Norton 1999.

Medical Clearance

In the cases in which referral is considered necessary, it is the personal trainer's responsibility to encourage **medical clearance** as a reasonable and safe course of action. A recommendation to consult with a physician prior to participation in an exercise program should not be considered an abdication of responsibility by the personal trainer, but rather a concerted effort to obtain valuable information and professional guidance to assure safety and protection of the individual's health.

Physician Referral

Once medical clearance is recommended, the personal trainer should give the client a physician's referral form in order to obtain the necessary information about health status, physical limitations, and restrictions that would be required to make future fitness program recommendations. An example of a physician's referral form appears on page 192.

The physician's referral form includes an assessment of the individual's functional capacity; a classification of ability to participate based upon the evaluation; identification of preexisting conditions that may be worsened by exercise; prescribed medications; and fitness program recommendations. Chapter 25 includes discussion of the personal trainer's scope of practice as related to referral.

Program Recommendations

The physician recommendations provide the personal trainer with guidance and directions regarding what specific concerns and needs the individual has and which programs are appropriate. On the basis of the results obtained during the diagnostic medical examination and exercise tests, a physician may recommend an unsupervised, supervised, or medically supervised exercise program.

An **unsupervised program** is commonly recommended for people who are apparently healthy or presumably healthy with no apparent risks. This type of program recognizes the positive health-associated benefits that regular activity provides in relation to the relatively low risk involved in participation. These programs may be designed and initiated with the support of a personal trainer, the intended long-term eventual outcome being a combination of consistent weekly training sessions conducted by the personal trainer and other sessions that are self-directed and unsupervised.

A **supervised program** may be recommended for people who have limitations or preexisting conditions that would restrict involvement but not limit participation. These programs are usually directed by a certified fitness professional, such as a certified personal trainer, who monitors intensity and modifies activity to meet the special concerns of the participant.

A **medically supervised program** may be recommended for individuals who present a higher potential risk due to a predisposed condition, multiple risk factors, or an uncontrolled disease. These programs are directed and monitored by allied health professionals in clinical settings with immediately accessible emergency response capabilities.

Although there is no guarantee that the specific initial program recommendation will meet the client's needs, it is important for those involved in the referral and recommendation process to eventually identify the program that will provide the most effective support and safety.

In cases in which referral is considered necessary, it is the personal trainer's responsibility to encourage medical clearance as a reasonable and safe course of action.

CONCLUSION

The client consultation and health appraisal process is directly in line with the scope of practice of the personal trainer to motivate, assess, train, educate, and refer when necessary. In order to develop programs of exercise that will safely and effectively meet the individual's objectives, the personal trainer needs to gather pertinent information and documentation that will be used to assess health status, evaluate potential for risk, and refer for medical clearance when necessary.

STUDY QUESTIONS

1. Which of the following should a personal trainer do during the initial meeting with a new client?

   I. Perform a submaximal bike test to estimate the client's $\dot{V}O_2$ max.
   II. Have the client complete a medical history form.
   III. Evaluate the client's level of exercise readiness.
   IV. Discuss the client's goals for his or her exercise program.

   A. I and II only
   B. III and IV only
   C. I, II, and III only
   D. II, III, and IV only

2. Which of the following should be included in an informed consent?

   I. a summary of the client's testing results
   II. benefits associated with participation
   III. the client's exercise goals
   IV. responsibilities of the client

   A. I and III only
   B. II and IV only
   C. I, II, and III only
   D. II, III, and IV only

3. Which of the following factors discovered at a preparticipation health appraisal screening reveal a client's risk of coronary artery disease?
   I. HDLs: 33 mg/dL
   II. family history: uncle died of stroke at age 42
   III. blood pressure: 128/88 mm Hg; measured twice
   IV. quit smoking 60 days ago
   A. I and III only
   B. II and IV only
   C. I and IV only
   D. II and III only
4. Which of the following clients is in the highest risk stratification for coronary artery disease?
   A. 44-year-old male whose father died of a heart attack at 60 years of age
   B. 46-year-old male with a serum cholesterol reading of 205 mg/dL
   C. 48-year-old female with a BMI of 30
   D. 50-year-old female who has COPD

APPLIED KNOWLEDGE QUESTION

A 45-year-old sedentary male accountant wants to begin working with a personal trainer. After completing the initial interview and preparticipation health appraisal screening, the personal trainer learns the following information about the client:

Family history: both his father and grandmother had heart attacks at age 60

Cigarette smoking: Non-smoker

Resting blood pressure: 122/86 mm Hg

Blood lipids: Serum cholesterol 240 mg/dL; HDLs 35 mg/dL

Fasting glucose: 100 mg/dL

BMI: 25

Evaluate and stratify his health status.

REFERENCES

1. Almada, S.L., A.B. Zonderman, R.B. Shekelle, A.R. Dyer, M.L. Daviglus, P.T. Costa Jr., and J. Stamler. 1991. Neuroticism and cynicism and risk of death in middle-aged men: The Western Electric Study. *Psychosomatic Medicine* 53 (2): 165-175.
2. American College of Sports Medicine. 2000. *ACSM's Guidelines for Exercise Testing and Prescription,* 6th ed. Philadelphia: Lippincott Williams & Williams.
3. American College of Sports Medicine. 1992. *ACSM's Health/Fitness Facility Standards and Guidelines.* Champaign, IL: Human Kinetics.
4. American College of Sports Medicine. 1998. *ACSM's Resource Manual for Guidelines for Exercise Testing and Prescription,* 3rd ed. Baltimore: Williams & Wilkins.
5. American Diabetes Association. 1998. Report of the Expert Committee on the Diagnosis and Classification of Diabetes Mellitus. *Diabetes Care* 21: S5-S19.
6. American Heart Association. 2001. *2001 Heart and Stroke Statistical Update.* Dallas: American Heart Association.
7. American Thoracic Society. 1995. Standards for diagnosis and care of patients with chronic obstructive pulmonary disease. *American Journal of Respiratory and Critical Care Medicine* 152: S77-S120.
8. Brownson, R., P. Remington, and J. Davis, eds. 1998. *Chronic Disease Epidemiology and Control.* Washington, DC: American Public Health Association, pp. 379-382.
9. Burns, J., and E. Katkin. 1993. Psychological, situational, and gender predictors of cardiovascular reactivity to stress: A multi-variate approach. *Journal of Behavioral Medicine* 16: 445-466.
10. Carrol, D., J.R. Turner, and S. Rogers. 1987. Heart rate and oxygen consumption during mental arithmetic, video game, and graded static exercise. *Psychophysiology* 24 (1): 112-121.
11. Caspersen, C.J., and G.W. Heath. 1993. The risk factor concept of coronary heart disease. In: *ACSM's Resource Manual for Guidelines for Exercise Testing and Prescription,* 2nd ed. Philadelphia: Lea & Febiger, pp. 151-167.
12. Cholesterol: Up with the good. 1995. *Harvard Heart Letter* 5 (11): 3-4.
13. Committee on Diet and Health Food and Nutrition Board Co. 1989. *Diet and Health* 7.
14. Doll, R., and R. Peto. 1976. Mortality in relation to smoking: 20 year's observations on male British doctors. *British Medical Journal* 2: 1525-1536.
15. Donatelle, R.J. 2001. *Health—The Basics,* 5th ed. San Francisco: Benjamin Cummings.

16. Drought, H.J. 1990. Personal training: The initial consultation. *Conditioning Instructor* 1 (2): 2-3.
17. Expert Panel on Detection, Evaluation and Treatment of High Blood Cholesterol in Adults. 1993. Summary of the second report of the National Cholesterol Education Program (NCEP) Expert Panel on Detection, Evaluation and Treatment of High Blood Cholesterol in Adults (Adult Treatment Panel II). *Journal of the American Medical Association* 269: 3015-3023.
18. Expert Panel. 1998. Executive summary of the clinical guidelines on the identification, valuation, and treatment of overweight and obesity in adults. *Archives of Internal Medicine* 158: 1855-1867.
19. Fletcher, G.F., G. Balady, S.N. Blair, J. Blumenthal, C. Caspersen, B. Chaitman, S. Epstein, E.S. Sivarajan Froelicher, V.F. Froelicher, I.L. Pina, and M.L. Pollock. 1996. Statement on exercise: Benefits and recommendations for physical activity programs for all Americans. A statement for health professionals by the Committee on Exercise and Cardiac Rehabilitation of the Council on Clinical Cardiology, American Heart Association. *Circulation* 94 (4): 857-862.
20. Glantz, S.A., and W.W. Parmley. 1996. Passive and active smoking. A problem for adults. *Circulation* 94 (4): 596-598.
21. Herbert, D.L., and W.G. Herbert. 1993. *Legal Aspects of Preventative and Rehabilitative Exercise Programs,* 3rd ed. Canton, OH. Professional Reports Corporation.
22. Howley, E.T., and B.D. Franks. 1992. *Health Fitness Instructor's Handbook,* 2nd ed. Champaign, IL: Human Kinetics.
23. Hubert, H.B., M. Feinleib, P.M. McNamara, and W.P. Castelli. 1983. Obesity as an independent risk factor for cardiovascular disease: A 26-year follow-up of participants in the Framingham Heart Study. *Circulation* 67 (5): 968-977.
24. Joint National Committee on Detection, Evaluation, and Treatment of High Blood Pressure. 1993. The fifth report of the Joint National Committee on Detection, Evaluation, and Treatment of High Blood Pressure (JNCV). *Archives of Internal Medicine* 153: 154-183.
25. Kannel, W.B., and T. Gordon. 1974. The Framingham Study: An epidemiological investigation of cardiovascular disease. Section 30. Public Health Service, NIH, DHEW Pub. No. 74-599. Washington, DC: U.S. Government Printing Office.
26. Klieman, C., and K. Osborne. 1991. *If It Runs in Your Family: Heart Disease: Reducing Your Risk.* New York: Bantam Books.
27. Kordich, J.A. 2000. Evaluating your client: Fitness assessment protocols and norms. In: *Essentials of Personal Training Symposium Study Guide.* Lincoln, NE: NSCA Certification Commission.
28. Last, J.M. 1988. *A Dictionary of Epidemiology,* 2nd ed. New York: Oxford University Press.
29. McInnis, K.J., and G.J. Balady. 1999. Higher cardiovascular risk clients in health clubs. *ACSM's Health and Fitness Journal* 3 (1): 19-24.
30. National Heart, Lung, and Blood Institute. 1993. National High Blood Pressure Education Program Working Group report on primary prevention of hypertension. *Archives of Internal Medicine* 153 (2): 186-208.
31. NIH Consensus Development Panel on Triglyceride, High Density Lipoprotein, and Coronary Heart Disease. 1993. Triglyceride, high-density lipoprotein, and coronary heart disease. *Journal of the American Medical Association* 269: 505-510.
32. NSCA-CPT Job Analysis Committee. 2001. *NSCA-CPT Content Description Manual.* Lincoln, NE: NSCA Certification Commission.
33. Olds, T., and K. Norton. 1999. *Pre-Exercise Health Screening Guide.* Champaign, IL: Human Kinetics.
34. Pasternak, R.C., S.M. Grundy, D. Levy, and P.D. Thompson. 1996. 27th Bethesda Conference: Matching the intensity of risk factor management with the hazard for coronary disease events. Task Force 3. Spectrum of risk factors for coronary heart disease. *Journal of the American College of Cardiology* 27 (5): 957-1047.
35. Pieper, C., A. LaCroix, and R. Karasek. 1989. The relation of psychosocial dimensions on work with coronary heart disease risk factors: A meta-analysis of five United States databases. *American Journal of Epidemiology* 129: 483-494.
36. Pollock, M.L., D.T. Lowenthal, C. Foster, et al. 1991. Acute and chronic responses to exercise in patients treated with beta blockers. *Journal of Cardiopulmonary Rehabilitation* 11 (2): 132-144.
37. Report of the Expert Committee on the Diagnosis and Classification of Diabetes Mellitus. 1997. *Diabetes Care* 20 (7): 1183-1197.
38. Russek, L.G., S.H. King, S.J. Russek, and H.I. Russek. 1990. The Harvard Mastery of Stress Study 35-year follow-up: Prognostic significance of patterns of psychophysiological arousal and adaptation. *Psychological Medicine* 52: 271-285.
39. Schuler, G., R. Hambrecht, G. Schlierf, J. Niebauer, K. Hauer, J. Neumann, E. Hoberg, A. Drinkmann, F. Bacher, M. Grunze, et al. 1992. Regular physical exercise and low-fat diet: Effects on progression of coronary artery disease. *Circulation* 86 (1): 1-11.
40. Sims, J., and D. Carrol. 1990. Cardiovascular and metabolic activity at rest and during physical challenge in normal tenses and subjects with mildly elevated blood pressure. *Psychophysiology* 27: 149-160.
41. The sixth report of the Joint National Committee on Prevention, Detection, Evaluation, and Treatment of High Blood Pressure (JNC VI). 1997. *Archives of Internal Medicine* 157: 2413-2446.
42. Thomas, S., J. Reading, and R.J. Shepard. 1992. Revision of the physical activity readiness questionnaire (PAR-Q). *Canadian Journal of Sport Sciences* 17: 338-345.
43. U.S. Department of Health and Human Services. 1989. *Report of the Expert Panel on Detection, Evaluation, and Treatment of High Blood Cholesterol in Adults.* Department of Health and Human Services, Public Health Services, NIH Pub. No. 89-2925. Washington, DC: U.S. Government Printing Office.
44. U.S. Department of Health and Human Services. 1996. *Physical Activity and Health: A Report of the Surgeon General.* Atlanta: U.S. Department of Health and Human Services, Centers for Disease Control and Prevention and Health Promotion.

The Attitudinal Assessment

The assessment should not only be viewed as an assessment of physical condition, but also as a gauge of attitude, outlook, and perspective. For each question, ask the client to rate him or herself on a scale of 1-4. The first time you go through this exercise, your client might want to answer only the first section for each question (denoted with an asterisk (*). You might come back whenever you feel the client is ready and complete the rest of each question. In the first part of each question, the assessment of where the client stands right now, the most motivated and driven athletes would likely have at least seven ratings of a "4" and not a single rating below a "3." Clients with three or more questions for which the answer was a "1" will need extra assistance to develop proper goals and may require frequent rewards, discussion, and education.

1. What would you consider your present attitude toward exercise?

1 - I can't stand the thought of it.
2 - I'll do it because I know I should, but I don't enjoy it.
3 - I don't mind exercise, and I know it is beneficial.
4 - I am motivated to exercise.

*Your answer: _____

How would you like to feel about exercise, if you could change your feelings?

Your Answer: _____

Describe why and any specifics of how you would like to change your feelings about exercise and how those feelings might bring about positive change in your life:

2. What would you consider your present attitude toward goal achievement?

1 - I feel that whatever happens, happens, and I'll roll with the punches.
2 - I set goals and believe it adds clarity and gives me some control over my outcome.
3 - I write down my goals and believe it is a very valuable exercise in determining my future performance and achievement.
4 - I have written goals and I review them often. I believe I have the power to achieve anything I desire and know that setting goals is a vital part of achievement.

*Your answer: _____

How would you like to feel about goal achievement, if you could change your feelings?

Your answer: _____

Describe why and any specifics of how you would like to change your feelings about goal achievement and how those feelings might bring about positive change in your life:

3. How important to you are the concepts of health and well-being?

1 - I don't need to put any effort into bettering my health.
2 - I make certain I devote some time and effort into bettering my physical body.
3 - I am committed to maintaining and working to improve my health and physical well-being.
4 - My health and well being are the foundation of all that I achieve, and they must remain my top priorities.

*Your answer: _____

How would you like to feel about the concepts of health and well-being, if you could change your feelings?

Your answer: _____

Describe why and any specifics of how you would like to change your feelings about the concepts of health and well-being and how those feelings might bring about positive change in your life:

(continued)

4. How strong and driving is your desire for improvement?

1 - I'm really pretty satisfied with the way things are. Striving for improvement might leave me frustrated and disappointed.
2 - I'd like to improve but don't know that it's worth all the work involved.
3 - I love feeling as if I've bettered myself and am open to any suggestions for improvement.
4 - I'm driven to excel and am committed to striving for consistent and ongoing improvement.

*Your answer: _____

How strong and driven would you like to feel about improvement?

Your answer: _____

Describe why and any specifics of how you would like to change your feelings about improvement and how those feelings might bring about positive change in your life:

5. How do you feel about yourself and your abilities (self-esteem)?

1 - I am not comfortable with the way I look, feel, or perform in most situations.
2 - I would love to change many things about myself although I am proud of who I am.
3 - I'm very good at the things I must do, take pride in many of my achievements, and am quite able to handle myself in most situations.
4 - I have great strength, ability, and pride.

*Your answer: _____

How would you like to feel about yourself and your abilities, if you could change your feelings?

Your answer: _____

Describe why and any specifics of how you would like to change your feelings about yourself and your abilities and how those feelings might bring about positive change in your life:

6. How do you feel about your present physical condition in terms of the way you look?

1 - I would like to completely change my body.
2 - There are many things about my reflection in the mirror that I'm not comfortable with.
3 - For the most part I look OK, and I can look really good in the right clothing, but I do feel uncomfortable with a few things about my physical appearance.
4 - I am proud of my body and am comfortable in any manner of dress in appropriate situations.

*Your answer: _____

How would you like to feel about the way you look, if you could change your feelings?

Your answer: _____

Describe why and any specifics of how you would like to change your feelings about the way you look and how those feelings might bring about positive change in your life:

7. How do you feel about your present physical condition in terms of overall health?

1 - I wish I felt healthy.
2 - I feel healthy for my age compared to most people I meet.
3 - I maintain a high level of health.
4 - I am extremely healthy.

*Your answer: _____

How would you like to feel about yourself and your abilities, if you could change your feelings?

Your answer: _____

Describe why and any specifics of how you would like to change your feelings about yourself and your abilities and how those feelings might bring about positive change in your life:

8. **How do you feel about your physical condition in terms of your performance in any chosen physical fields of endeavor (sports, training, etc.)?**

   1 - I feel as if I'm in very poor condition and am uncomfortable when faced with a physical challenge.
   2 - I am not comfortable with my performance abilities; however, I am comfortable training to improve.
   3 - I feel pretty good about my ability to perform physically although I would like to improve.
   4 - I have exceptional physical abilities and enjoy being called upon to display them.

*Your answer: _____

How would you like to feel about your performance, if you could change your feelings?

Your answer: _____

Describe why and any specifics of how you would like to change your feelings about your performance and how those feelings might bring about positive change in your life:

9. **How strongly do you believe that you can improve your body?**

   1 - I believe most of my physical shortcomings are genetic, and most efforts to change would be a waste of time.
   2 - I've seen many people change their bodies for the better and am sure with enough effort I can see some improvement.
   3 - I strongly believe the proper combination of exercise and nutrition can bring about some improvement.
   4 - I know without question that with the proper combination of exercise and nutrition I can bring about dramatic changes in my body.

*Your answer: _____

How would you like to feel about your ability to improve your body, if you could change your feelings?

Your answer: _____

Describe why and any specifics of how you would like to change your feelings about your ability to improve your body and how those feelings might bring about positive change in your life:

10. **When you begin a program or set a goal, how likely are you to follow through to its fruition?**

   1 - I've never been real good at following things through to the end.
   2 - With the right motivation and some evidence of results I think I might stick to a program.
   3 - I have the patience and ability to commit to a program and will give it a chance in order to assess its value.
   4 - Once I set a goal, there's no stopping me.

*Your answer: _____

How would you like to feel about following through on goals, if you could change your feelings?

Your answer: _____

Describe why and any specifics of how you would like to change your feelings about following through on goals and how those feelings might bring about positive change in your life:

From *NSCA's Essentials of Personal Training* by Roger W. Earle and Thomas R. Baechle, 2004, Champaign, IL: Human Kinetics. Courtesy of Phil Kaplan Fitness.

Personal Training Contract/Agreement

Congratulations on your decision to participate in an exercise program! With the help of your personal trainer, you greatly improve your ability to accomplish your training goals faster, safer, and with maximum benefits. The details of these training sessions can be used for a lifetime.

In order to maximize progress, it will be necessary for you to follow program guidelines during supervised and (if applicable) unsupervised training days. Remember, exercise and healthy eating are EQUALLY important!

During your exercise program, every effort will be made to assure your safety. However, as with any exercise program, there are risks, including increased heart stress and the chance of musculoskeletal injuries. In volunteering for this program, you agree to assume responsibility for these risks and waive any possibility for personal damage. You also agree that, to your knowledge, you have no limiting physical conditions or disability that would preclude an exercise program.

A physician's examination is recommended for (1) *all* participants with *any* exercise restrictions; and (2) *all* men ≥45 years old and *all* women ≥55 years old. Personal training participants in either or both of these categories who do NOT have a prior physician examination MUST acknowledge they have been informed of its importance. By signing below, you accept full responsibility for your own health and well-being AND you acknowledge an understanding that no responsibility is assumed by the leaders of the program.

It is recommended that all program participants work with their personal trainer three (3) times per week. However, due to scheduling conflicts and financial considerations, a combination of supervised and unsupervised workouts is possible.

Personal Training Terms and Conditions

1. Personal training sessions that are not rescheduled or cancelled 24 hours in advance will result in forfeiture of the session and a loss of the financial investment at the rate of one session.
2. Clients arriving late will receive the remaining scheduled session time, unless other arrangements have been previously made with the trainer.
3. The expiration policy requires completion of all personal training sessions within 120 days from the date of the contract. Personal training sessions are void after this time period.
4. No personal training refunds will be issued for any reason, including but not limited to relocation, illness, and unused sessions.

Description of program: ____

Total investment: ________________

Method of payment: ________________

WE WISH YOU THE BEST OF LUCK ON YOUR NEW PERSONAL TRAINING PROGRAM!

____
Participant's name (please print clearly)

________________________________ Date: ____________________
Participant's signature

________________________________ Date: ____________________
Parent/guardian's signature (if needed)

________________________________ Date: ____________________
Witness' signature

Physical Activity Readiness
Questionnaire - PAR-Q
(revised 2002)

PAR-Q & YOU

(A Questionnaire for eople Aged 15 to 69)

Regular physical activity is fun and healthy, and increasingly more people are starting to become more active every day. Being more active is very safe for most people. However, some people should check with their doctor before they start becoming much more physically active.

If you are planning to become much more physically active than you are now, start by answering the seven questions in the box below. If you are between the ages of 15 and 69, the PAR-Q will tell you if you should check with your doctor before you start. If you are over 69 years of age, and you are not used to being very active, check with your doctor.

Common sense is your best guide when you answer these questions. Please read the questions carefully and answer each one honestly: check YES or NO.

YES	NO	
❑	❑	**1. Has your doctor ever said that you have a heart condition and that you should only do physical activity recommended by a doctor?**
❑	❑	**2. Do you feel pain in your chest when you do physical activity?**
❑	❑	**3. In the past month, have you had chest pain when you were not doing physical activity?**
❑	❑	**4. Do you lose your balance because of dizziness or do you ever lose consciousness?**
❑	❑	**5. Do you have a bone or joint problem (for example, back, knee or hip) that could be made worse by a change in your physical activity?**
❑	❑	**6. Is your doctor currently prescribing drugs (for example, water pills) for your blood pressure or heart condition?**
❑	❑	**7. Do you know of any other reason why you should not do physical activity?**

If you answered

YES to one or more questions

Talk with your doctor by phone or in person BEFORE you start becoming much more physically active or BEFORE you have a fitness appraisal. Tell your doctor about the PAR-Q and which questions you answered YES.

- You may be able to do any activity you want — as long as you start slowly and build up gradually. Or, you may need to restrict your activities to those which are safe for you. Talk with your doctor about the kinds of activities you wish to participate in and follow his/her advice.
- Find out which community programs are safe and helpful for you.

NO to all questions

If you answered NO honestly to all PAR-Q questions, you can be reasonably sure that you can:

- start becoming much more physically active – begin slowly and build up gradually. This is the safest and easiest way to go.
- take part in a fitness appraisal – this is an excellent way to determine your basic fitness so that you can plan the best way for you to live actively. It is also highly recommended that you have your blood pressure evaluated. If your reading is over 144/94, talk with your doctor before you start becoming much more physically active.

DELAY BECOMING MUCH MORE ACTIVE:

- if you are not feeling well because of a temporary illness such as a cold or a fever – wait until you feel better; or
- if you are or may be pregnant – talk to your doctor before you start becoming more active.

PLEASE NOTE: If your health changes so that you then answer YES to any of the above questions, tell your fitness or health professional. Ask whether you should change your physical activity plan.

Informed Use of the PAR-Q: The Canadian Society for Exercise Physiology, Health Canada, and their agents assume no liability for persons who undertake physical activity, and if in doubt after completing this questionnaire, consult your doctor prior to physical activity.

No changes permitted. You are encouraged to photocopy the PAR-Q but only if you use the entire form.

NOTE: If the PAR-Q is being given to a person before he or she participates in a physical activity program or a fitness appraisal, this section may be used for legal or administrative purposes.

"I have read, understood and completed this questionnaire. Any questions I had were answered to my full satisfaction."

NAME ______________________________

SIGNATURE ______________________________ DATE ______________

SIGNATURE OF PARENT ______________________________ WITNESS ______________
or GUARDIAN (for participants under the age of majority)

Note: This physical activity clearance is valid for a maximum of 12 months from the date it is completed and becomes invalid if your condition changes so that you would answer YES to any of the seven questions.

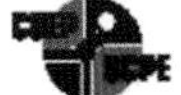

Supported by: 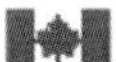 Health Canada Santé Canada

Health/Medical Questionnaire

Date: ____________________

Name: ______________________ Date of birth: ________ Soc. Sec. #: ____________

Address: ____

Street City State Zip

Phone (H): ____________ (W): ____________ E-mail address:______________

In case of emergency, whom may we contact?

Name: ______________________ Relationship: ______________________

Phone (H): ______________________ (W): ______________________

Personal physician

Name: ______________________ Phone: ____________ Fax: ____________

Present/Past History

Have you had OR do you presently have any of the following conditions? (Check if *yes.*)

___ Rheumatic fever
___ Recent operation
___ Edema (swelling of ankles)
___ High blood pressure
___ Injury to back or knees
___ Low blood pressure
___ Seizures
___ Lung disease
___ Heart attack
___ Fainting or dizziness
___ Diabetes
___ High cholesterol
___ Orthopnea (the need to sit up to breathe comfortably) or paroxysmal (sudden, unexpected attack) nocturnal dyspnea (shortness of breath at night)
___ Shortness of breath at rest or with mild exertion
___ Chest pains
___ Palpitations or tachycardia (unusually strong or rapid heartbeat)
___ Intermittent claudication (calf cramping)
___ Pain, discomfort in the chest, neck, jaw, arms, or other areas
___ Known heart murmur
___ Unusual fatigue or shortness of breath with usual activities
___ Temporary loss of visual acuity or speech, or short-term numbness or weakness in one side, arm, or leg of your body
___ Other

Family History

Have any of your first-degree relatives (parent, sibling, or child) experienced the following conditions? (Check if *yes.*) In addition, please identify at what age the condition occurred.

___ Heart attack
___ Heart operation
___ Congenital heart disease
___ High blood pressure
___ High cholesterol

___ Diabetes

___ Other major illness ________________________

Explain checked items: ____

____

____

Activity History

1. How were you referred to this program? (Please be specific.) ____________________

____

____

2. Why are you enrolling in this program? (Please be specific.) ____________________

____

____

3. Are you presently employed? Yes ___ No ___
4. What is your present occupational position? ____________________
5. Name of company: ____________________
6. Have you ever worked with a personal trainer before? Yes ___ No ___
7. Date of your last physical examination performed by a physician: ____________________
8. Do you participate in a regular exercise program at this time? Yes ___ No ___ If yes, briefly describe:

____

____

9. Can you currently walk 4 miles briskly without fatigue? Yes ___ No ___
10. Have you ever performed resistance training exercises in the past? Yes ___ No ___
11. Do you have injuries (bone or muscle disabilities) that may interfere with exercising? Yes ___ No ___ If yes, briefly describe: ____________________

____

12. Do you smoke? Yes ___ No ___ If yes, how much per day and what was your age when you started? Amount per day ______ Age ______
13. What is your body weight now? ____ What was it one year ago? ____ At age 21? ____
14. Do you follow or have you recently followed any specific dietary intake plan, and in general how do you feel about your nutritional habits? ____________________

____

15. List the medications you are presently taking. ____________________

____

____

16. List in order your personal health and fitness objectives.
    a. ____
    b. ____

    ____

    c. ____

    ____

Health Risk Analysis

This form is a learning tool to identify positive and negative aspects of your health behavior. Though many of the effects are based on real findings from large epidemiological investigations, the estimates are generalized and should not be taken too literally. It is impossible to predict with accuracy how long you will live or when you will die.

Plus one (+1) represents a positive effect that could add a year to your life or life to your years, and minus one (-1) indicates a loss in the quantity or quality of life. A zero (0) indicates no shortening or lengthening of your longevity. If none of the categories listed for a factor apply to you, enter 0.

I. Coronary Heart Disease (CHD) Risk Factors

Cholesterol, total cholesterol/HDL ratio

Under 160	160-200	200-220	220-240	Over 240
<3	3-4	4-5	5-6	>6
+2	+1	–1	–2	–4

Blood pressure $\left(\frac{systolic}{diastolic}\right)$

110	110-130	130-150	150-170	170
60-80	60-80	80-90	90-100	>100
+1	0	–1	–2	–4

Smoking

Never	Quit	Smoke cigar or pipe or close family member smokes	1 pack cigarettes daily	2 or more packs daily
+1	0	–1	–3	–5

Heredity

No family history of CHD	1 close relative over 60 with CHD	2 close relatives over 60 with CHD	1 close relative under 60 with CHD	2 or more close relatives under 60 with CHD
+2	0	–1	–2	–4

Body weight (or fat)

5 lb below desirable weight	5 lb below to 4 lb above desirable weight	5-20 lb overweight	20-35 lb overweight	>35 lb overweight
(<10% fat—M; <16% fat—F)	(10-15% fat—M; 16-22% fat—F)	(15-20% fat—M; 22-30% fat—F)	(20-25% fat—M; 30-35% fat—F)	(>25% fat—M; >35% fat—F)
+2	+1	0	–2	–3

Sex

Female under 55 years	Female over 55 years	Male	Stocky male	Bald, stocky male
0	–1	–1	–2	–4

Stress

Phlegmatic, unhurried, generally happy	Ambitious but generally relaxed	Sometimes hard-driving, time-competitive	Hard-driving, time-conscious, competitive (Type A)	Type A with repressed hostility
+1	0	0	–1	–3

Physical activity

High-intensity, over 30 minutes daily	Intermittent, 20-30 minutes 3-5 times/week	Moderate, 10-20 minutes 3-5 times/week	Light, 10-20 minutes 1-2 times/week	Little or none
+2	+2	+1	0	–2

TOTAL: I. CHD Risk Factors ________

Enter on Scoring Summary

II. Health Habits (related to good health and longevity)

Breakfast

Daily	Sometimes	None	Coffee	Coffee and doughnut
+1	0	–1	–2	–3

Regular meals

3 or more	2 daily	Not regular	Fad diets	Starve and stuff
+1	0	–1	–2	–3

Sleep

7-8 hr	8-9 hr	6-7 hr	9 hr	6 hr
+1	0	0	–1	–2

Alcohol

None	Women 3/wk	Men 1-2 daily	2-6 daily	6 daily
+1	+1	+1	–2	–4

TOTAL: II. Health Habits ________

Enter on Scoring Summary

III. Medical Factors

Medical exam and screening tests (blood pressure, diabetes, glaucoma)

Regular tests, see doctor when necessary	Periodic medical exam and selected tests	Periodic medical exam	Sometimes get tests	No tests or medical exams	
+1	+1	0	0	–1	

Heart

No history of problems self or family	Some history	Rheumatic fever as child, no murmur now	Rheumatic fever as child, have murmur	Have ECG abnormality and/or angina pectoris	
+1	0	–1	–2	–3	

Lung (including pneumonia and tuberculosis)

No problem	Some past problem	Mild asthma or bronchitis	Emphysema, severe asthma, or bronchitis	Severe lung problems	
+1	0	–1	–2	–3	

Digestive tract

No problem	Occasional diarrhea, loss of appetite	Frequent diarrhea or stomach upset	Ulcers, colitis, gall bladder, or liver problems	Severe gastrointestinal disorders	
+1	0	–1	–2	–3	

Diabetes

No problem or family history	Controlled hypoglycemia (low blood sugar)	Hypoglycemia and family history	Mild diabetes (diet and exercise)	Diabetes (insulin)	
+1	0	–1	–2	–3	

Drugs

Seldom take	Minimal but regular use of aspirin or other drugs	Heavy use of aspirin or other drugs	Regular use of amphetamines, barbiturates, or psychogenic drugs	Heavy use of amphetamines, barbiturates, or psychogenic drugs	
+1	0	–1	–2	–3	

TOTAL: III. Medical Factors ______

Enter on Scoring Summary

IV. Safety Factors

Driving in car

4,000 mi/year, mostly local	4,000-6,000 mi/year, local and some highway	6,000-8,000 mi/year, local and highway	8,000-10,000 mi/year, highway and some local	10,000 mi/year, mostly highway	
+1	0	0	–1	–2	

Using seat belts

Always	Most of time (75%)	On highway only	Seldom (25%)	Never	
+1	0	–1	–2	–3	

Risk-taking behavior (motorcycle, skydive, mountain climb, fly small plane, etc.)

Some with careful preparation	Never	Occasional	Often	Try anything for thrills	
+1	0	–1	–1	–2	

TOTAL: IV. Safety Factors ______

Enter on Scoring Summary

V. Personal Factors

Diet

Low-fat, high-complex carbohydrates	Balanced, moderate fat	Balanced, typical fat	Fad diets	Starve and stuff	
+2	+1	0	–1	–2	

Longevity

Grandparents lived past 90, parents past 80	Grandparents lived past 80, parents past 70	Grandparents lived past 70, parents past 60	Few relatives lived past 60	Few relatives lived past 50	
+2	+1	0	–1	–3	

Love and marriage

Happily married	Married	Unmarried	Divorced	Extramarital relationship	
+2	+1	0	–1	–3	

(continued)

V. Personal Factors *(continued)*

Education

Postgraduate or master craftsman	College graduate or skilled craftsman	Some college or trade school	High school graduate	Grade school graduate
+1	+1	0	–1	–2

Job satisfaction

Enjoy job, see results, room for advancement	Enjoy job, see some results, able to advance	Job OK, no results, nowhere to go	Dislike job	Hate job
+1	+1	0	–1	–2

Social

Have some close friends	Have some friends	Have no good friends	Stuck with people I don't enjoy	Have no friends at all
+1	0	–1	–2	–3

Race

White or Asian	Black or Hispanic	American Indian
0	–1	–2

TOTAL: V. Personal Factors ______

Enter on Scoring Summary

VI. Psychological Factors

Outlook

Feel good about present and future	Satisfied	Unsure about present or future	Unhappy in present, don't look forward to future	Miserable, rather not get out of bed
+1	0	–1	–2	–3

Depression

No family history of depression	Some family history—I feel OK	Family history and I am mildly depressed	Sometimes feel life isn't worth living	Thoughts of suicide
+1	0	–1	–2	–3

Anxiety

Seldom anxious	Occasionally anxious	Often anxious	Always anxious	Panic attacks
+1	0	–1	–2	–3

Relaxation

Relax meditate daily	Relax often	Seldom relax	Usually tense	Always tense
+1	0	–1	–2	–3

TOTAL: VI. Psychological Factors ______

Enter on Scoring Summary

VII. For Women Only

Health care

Regular breast and Pap exam	Occasional breast and Pap exam	Never have exam	Treated disorder	Untreated cancer
+1	0	–1	–2	–4

Birth control pill

Never used	Quit 5 years ago	Still use, under 30 years	Use pill and smoke	Use pill, smoke, over 35
+1	0	0	–2	–3

TOTAL: VII. For Women Only ______

Enter on Scoring Summary

SCORING SUMMARY

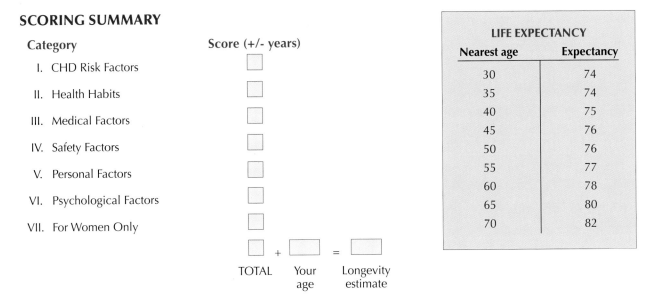

Category	Score (+/- years)
I. CHD Risk Factors	
II. Health Habits	
III. Medical Factors	
IV. Safety Factors	
V. Personal Factors	
VI. Psychological Factors	
VII. For Women Only	

[ ] + [ ] = [ ]

TOTAL + Your age = Longevity estimate

LIFE EXPECTANCY

Nearest age	Expectancy
30	74
35	74
40	75
45	76
50	76
55	77
60	78
65	80
70	82

Now go back and see how you can add years to your life by improving behaviors and lifestyle. Check each category for possible changes you would like to make in your current lifestyle.

From *NSCA's Essentials of Personal Training* by Roger W. Earle and Thomas R. Baechle, 2004, Champaign, IL: Human Kinetics. Adapted from B.J. Sharkey, 2002. *Fitness and Health, Fifth Edition*, (Champaign, IL): Human Kinetics, 63-67,

Informed Consent Form

The tests included in the fitness evaluation will test the following areas of physical fitness: (1) cardiorespiratory endurance, (2) body composition, (3) muscular strength/muscular endurance, and (4) flexibility.

The most physically demanding tests are the cardiorespiratory and muscular strength/muscular endurance tests. The cardiorespiratory test consists of riding a stationary bicycle, walking/running on a treadmill, or stepping up and down from a 12-inch-high bench. The purpose is to examine your heart rate response to submaximal exercise and recovery periods. The muscular strength/endurance tests are either 1-repetition maximum on a bench press machine or the number of curl-ups and/or push-ups performed in one minute.

Muscular fatigue may be experienced during or after these tests. Complications have been few during exercise tests, especially those of a submaximal nature. If the person exercising is not tolerating the test well, it is stopped. Reported complications (1 in 10,000 tests) include faintness and irregularities in heart function. Also, risk of injury getting on or off exercise equipment is possible but rare.

In signing this consent form, you acknowledge that you have read and understood the description of these tests and their complications. In addition, you state that any questions you have about the fitness evaluation have been answered to your satisfaction. Every effort will be made to ensure your health and safety. You enter into the tests willingly and may withdraw at any time.

Information and data obtained from any procedure or within the execution of the program process will be construed as confidential. As such, that information and those data will not be released unless written authorization is provided by the participant named below.

A physician's examination is recommended for (1) *all* participants with *any* exercise restrictions and (2) *all* men ≥45 years old and *all* women ≥55 years old. Personal training participants in either or both of these categories who do NOT have a prior physician examination MUST acknowledge they have been informed of its importance. By signing below, you accept full responsibility for your own health and well-being AND you acknowledge an understanding that no responsibility is assumed by the leaders of the program.

____
Participant's name (please print clearly)

______________________________________ Date: ____________________
Participant's signature

______________________________________ Date: ____________________
Parent/Guardian's signature (if needed)

______________________________________ Date: ____________________
Witness' signature

From *NSCA's Essentials of Personal Training* by Roger W. Earle and Thomas R. Baechle, 2004, Champaign, IL: Human Kinetics.

Release/Assumption of Risk Agreement

In consideration of gaining access to participate in activities associated with ______________________________
Name of program, facility, equipment, and

______________________________, I do hereby waive, release, and forever discharge ______________________
machinery Name of organization/program

______________________________ and its officers, agents, employees, representatives, executors, and all others from any and all responsibilities or liability for injuries or damages resulting from my participation in any activities in said program. __________ (Please initial.)

I understand the policies and procedures set forth by the ______________________ and I have had the opportu-
Name of organization/program

nity to discuss my specific needs in relation to participatory activity; and, as a result, I do voluntarily request the right to participate in this preventive program of exercise. __________ (Please initial.)

Also, in consideration of the above factors, I acknowledge the existence of risks in connection with these activities, assume such risks, and agree to accept the responsibilities for any injuries sustained by my participation in the course via the use of the facilities and/or its equipment. Most specifically, I acknowledge and accept responsibility for injuries arising out of those activities that involve risk in any of the following areas:

- The use of facility equipment
- The performance of fitness-related evaluations to assess functional capacity
- The participation in group activities related to exercise and activity
- Incidents that occur within the institution facility, locker rooms, dressing rooms, showers, and other areas associated with ______________________________
  Name of organization/program

In addition, it was seriously recommended that I consult with a physician before engaging in any activities associated with ______________________________. __________ (Please initial.)
Name of organization/program

Having read the preceding, I acknowledge full understanding of those risks set forth herein and knowingly agree to accept full responsibility for my own exposures to such risks and to waive full responsibility and liability on behalf of ______________________________. __________ (Please initial.)
Name of organization/program

____
Participant's name (please print clearly)

______________________________ Date: ______________________
Participant's signature

______________________________ Date: ______________________
Parent/Guardian's signature (if needed)

______________________________ Date: ______________________
Witness' signature

From *NSCA's Essentials of Personal Training* by Roger W. Earle and Thomas R. Baechle, 2004, Champaign, IL: Human Kinetics.

Physician's Referral Form Pertaining to a Fitness Evaluation and Preventive Program of Exercise

Dear Doctor:

Your patient ______________________________ has contacted us regarding the fitness evaluation conducted by

________________________________. The program is designed to evaluate the individual's fitness status prior to embarking on an exercise program. From this evaluation, an exercise prescription is formulated. In addition, other parameters related to a health improvement program are discussed with the participant. It is important to understand that this program is preventive and is not intended to be rehabilitative in nature.

The fitness testing includes: ____

____

____

A comprehensive consultation will be provided to the participant that serves to review the test results and explain recommendations for an individualized fitness program.

A summary of test results and our recommendations will be kept on file and may be made available to you upon request.

In the interest of your patient and for our information, please complete the following:

A. Has this patient undergone a physical examination within the last year to assess functional capacity to perform exercise? Yes ___ No ___

B. I consider this patient (please check one):

__ Class I: presumably healthy without apparent heart disease eligible to participate in an unsupervised program

__ Class II: presumably healthy with one or more risk factors for heart disease eligible to participate in a supervised program

__ Class III: patient not eligible for this program, and a medically supervised program is recommended

C. Does this patient have any preexisting medical/orthopedic condition(s) requiring continued or long-term medical treatment or follow-up? Yes ___ No ___

Please explain: ____

____

D. Are you aware of any medical condition(s) that this patient may have or may have had that could be worsened by exercise? Yes ___ No ___

E. Please list any currently prescribed medication(s): ______________________________________

____

____

F. Please provide specific recommendations and/or list any restrictions concerning this patient's present health status as it relates to active participation in a fitness program.

____

____

Comments: ____

____

____

Referring physician's signature: ____________________________________

Date: ____________________ Client's name: ____

Phone (H): _______________ Phone (W): _______________

Address: ______________________________ ______________________________

From *NSCA's Essentials of Personal Training* by Roger W. Earle and Thomas R. Baechle, 2004, Champaign, IL: Human Kinetics.

CHAPTER 10

Fitness Assessment Selection and Administration

John A.C. Kordich | Susan L. Heinrich

After completing this chapter, you will be able to

- explain the purposes of performing physical assessments on a client;
- evaluate a test's validity and reliability;
- apply risk stratification criteria to an individual client to determine suitability for specific tests;
- select appropriate tests for individual clients; and
- administer test protocols properly and safely.

After conducting the client consultation and health appraisal, the personal trainer needs to gather more information about the client's current level of fitness and skills before developing a program. There is no "one size fits all" test or battery of assessments that will suit each client and circumstance. Selecting appropriate physical assessments requires thoughtful consideration of the client's health and exercise history, personal goals, and the personal trainer's own experience and training in conducting various assessments. Choosing valid and reliable tests suitable for individual clients and conducting them accurately require practice on the part of the personal trainer. The availability and appropriateness of equipment and facilities, environmental factors, and the client's preassessment preparation influence test selection and implementation.

Having determined the assessment protocols, the personal trainer must conduct them accurately, record and manage the data, and interpret the results. Communicating the results to the client in an individualized program that incorporates his or her goals and interests is the "personal" in personal training. Implementation of the program requires formative and summative evaluation of the program, reassessment of the client's fitness levels and goals, and subsequent adjustments to the program in an ongoing cycle.

Purposes of Assessment

The purposes of **assessment** are to gather **baseline data** and to provide a basis for developing goals and effective exercise programs. Gathering and evaluating the various pieces of information give the personal trainer a broader perspective of the client. The process and the data collected assist the trainer in identifying potential areas of injury and reasonable starting points for recommended intensities and volumes of exercise based on those goals and fitness outcomes.

Gather Baseline Data

There are many valid reasons for administering assessments to clients. The data collected provide

- a baseline for future comparisons of improvement or rate of progress;
- identification of current strengths and weaknesses that may affect program emphasis on specific components;
- assistance in establishing appropriate intensities and volumes of exercise;
- assistance in clarification of short-, intermediate-, and long-term goals;
- identification of areas of potential injury or contraindications prior to program initiation, which may lead to referral to a physician or other health care professional; and
- a record demonstrating prudent judgment and appropriate scope of practice in program design should client injuries develop after a program has begun [12, 22].

The assessment process may fall within the services typically provided to all clients, may constitute an additional revenue stream for the personal trainer, or may do both. However, subjecting clients to a seemingly endless barrage of assessments that have little or no relevance to their program goals is a violation of the trust the client places in the personal trainer to gather necessary information to design a program.

Goal and Program Development

The personal trainer can utilize physical assessment information in conjunction with personal information gathered about the client to plan a time-efficient, specific program that will help the client achieve his or her goals. Understanding personal characteristics and current lifestyle factors about the client helps the personal trainer plan sessions that are reasonable in length, frequency, intensity, and complexity so that the client is more likely to continue adhering to the program. Developing goals with a client is critical for both program design and motivation. (Refer to chapter 8 for more details on motivating clients.)

When possible and appropriate, choosing specific tests that are congruent with a client's goals or preferred mode of exercise may give the client a clearer picture of his or her progress and may be more motivating. For highly trained athletes, choosing an exercise ergometer that most closely matches their mode of exercise (treadmill, cycle, swim flume) leads to a more accurate assessment of their performance [33, 41, 42]. For average or deconditioned clients, the type of test is not as much of a factor in assessing aerobic function; however, a treadmill test will give the average performer his or her highest maximal $\dot{V}O_2$ scores [41]. Clients who seldom if ever ride a bike may experience local muscular fatigue and achieve a lower estimated $\dot{V}O_2max$ value as a result on a bike test compared to a treadmill test [33, 42]. In addition, if clients are tested on a cycle ergometer but will not be riding a bike in their program, they may overlook some of the indicators of their improved performance during the training period.

A timed mile can be easily repeated on occasion during a walking program; if the client can cover the distance more quickly or easily with a lower exercise heart rate or rate of perceived exertion (RPE), the person knows immediately that he or she is making progress. In this instance an appropriate test may match the type of activity the client enjoys doing. However, for clients who are overweight or who have lower body joint issues that make weight-bearing activities painful, the advantages of a non-weight-bearing cycle test may override any concerns about slightly lower estimates of maximal oxygen consumption. Additionally, since cycling tests give results independent of body weight, they are more accurate indicators of progress for a person on a weight loss program than is a treadmill test, whose results are directly related to an individual's body weight [32, 42].

Assessment of health- or skill-related fitness components, or both, provides the personal trainer and client with baseline information that will be used to develop safe, effective, and appropriately challenging goals.

Formative and Summative Evaluations

A primary duty of the personal trainer is to facilitate improvements in the client's physical well-being without causing harm to the client. With the exception of assessing cardiovascular disease risk factors, there is no standardized battery of tests to give each client before designing an appropriate program [8, 15, 27, 38, 39]. The first step in individualizing the personal trainer's approach to each client is determining the specific tests to give to measure various parameters of health- and skill-related fitness. Those decisions are made based on the client's apparent health and level of cardiovascular disease risk, as well as the desired program outcomes expressed by the client.

Formative Evaluation

There are two ways of looking at assessments—as **formative** or **summative evaluations.** Formative evaluations include formal assessment with a specified **test protocol,** as well as the **subjective observations** the personal trainer makes during each interaction with the client. The formal assessments take place before a program begins and periodically throughout the training period. They offer the personal trainer opportunities to "formulate" or plan a program, give the client feedback, and make modifications to the program while it is still in progress.

Although this chapter concerns selecting the specific assessment instruments, it is important to keep in mind that *every* observation of a client provides important data about the client that the personal trainer must consider in designing, implementing, and modifying that client's program. Subjective observations are variable between evaluators and might include, for example, noticing posture, gait, improvements in exercise technique, response to cardiovascular exercise, comments or body language relating to specific exercises or suggestions, and daily energy levels in each exercise session. These provide immediate opportunities for the personal trainer to focus on educating, motivating, and modifying activities for the client.

With the use of a specific test protocol, the data provide **objective** evidence that the personal trainer can compare to relevant standards to interpret the client's performance.

Norm-Referenced Standards

The two reference perspectives for comparison of data involve **norm-referenced standards** and **criterion-referenced standards.** Norm-referenced standards are used to compare the performance of an individual against the performance of others in a like category. Table 10.1 shows percentile values for maximal aerobic power (ml · kg^{-1} · min^{-1}) [15]. These results are reported with **percentile** scores. The results show how the men and women in the study *performed.* In other words, the percentile scores compare the actual "best, worst, and in-between" performance scores of each participant, in this case from a modified Balke treadmill test, against scores of all the other participants of the same gender. The first and last finishers were off the respective ends of this chart, and the rest were statistically divided into percentile rankings. The left side of the chart has descriptive labels to give an "evaluation" to clients that is more familiar than percentile numbers. Some clients may confuse percentile scores with "percent scores" such as those they may have received in school, with 70% generally being a "passing grade." As table 10.1 shows, a score at the 50th percentile (meaning that the person performed better than roughly half of the performers and was outperformed by half) is an average performance. The 70th percentile is above average, and the 90th percentile is well above average, or excellent. Part of interpreting the test results to clients involves educating them on the relative value of their scores.

Many clients are content to know their raw (performance) score and whether they get stronger, faster, or more flexible after training. Clients who are very unfit or who have had negative experiences with fitness testing in the past may have no interest in knowing how poorly they performed compared to others. Other clients feel more motivated with use of the normative data to articulate performance goals and feel a sense of achievement as they "climb the chart."

Criterion-Referenced Standards

What norm-referenced standards do not do is let the client know whether the performance met a **health**

Table 10.1

Percentile Values for Maximal Aerobic Power ($ml \cdot kg^{-1} \cdot min^{-1}$)

Men		Age (years)				
Evaluative description	**Percentiles**	**20-29**	**30-39**	**40-49**	**50-59**	**60+**
Well above average	90	51.4	50.4	48.2	45.3	42.5
	80	48.2	46.8	44.1	41.0	38.1
Above average	70	46.8	44.6	41.8	38.5	35.3
	60	44.2	42.4	39.9	36.7	33.6
Average	50	42.5	41.0	38.1	35.2	31.8
	40	41.0	38.9	36.7	33.8	30.2
Below average	30	39.5	37.4	35.1	32.3	28.7
	20	37.1	35.4	33.0	30.2	26.5
Well below average	10	34.5	32.5	30.9	28.0	23.1

Women		Age (years)				
Evaluative description	**Percentiles**	**20-29**	**30-39**	**40-49**	**50-59**	**60+**
Well above average	90	44.2	41.0	39.5	35.2	35.2
	80	41.0	38.3	36.3	32.3	31.2
Above average	70	38.1	36.7	33.8	30.9	29.4
	60	36.7	34.6	32.3	29.4	27.2
Average	50	35.2	**33.8**	30.9	28.2	25.8
	40	33.8	32.3	29.5	26.9	24.5
Below average	30	32.3	30.5	28.3	25.5	23.8
	20	30.6	28.7	26.5	24.3	22.8
Well below average	10	28.4	26.5	25.1	22.3	20.8

Data provided by Institute for Aerobics Research, Dallas, TX (1994). A modified Balke treadmill test was used with $\dot{V}O_2max$ estimated from the last grade/speed achieved.

Adapted from ACSM 2000.

standard. A health standard could be defined as the lowest performance that would allow an individual to maintain good health and lessen the risk of chronic diseases [25]. Another way of stating this is that a criterion is a specific, minimal standard—one that theoretically each person can strive for, as it is not compared to how other individuals perform. Criterion-referenced standards are set against a combination of normative data and the best judgment of the experts in a given field to identify a specific level of achievement [33]. Criterion-reference standards that have been matched to healthy levels of fitness provide reasonable goals for most people to achieve for improved health.

Unfortunately, there is disagreement on the exact level of performance that accurately reflects a health standard [15, 27, 33, 39]. At least four criterion-referenced health-related fitness batteries of tests are given to school-age children in the United States, but each has a different criterion denoting acceptable performance levels for health [33]. There is no consensus on what determines minimal health standards for adults in all areas, either [33, 39]. For example, despite the normative values for maximal aerobic power presented in table 10.1, there are some data to suggest that, for males between 20 and 39 years of age, a score of 35 ml · kg^{-1} · min^{-1} would represent a health-related criterion standard (about 31.5 ml · kg^{-1} · min^{-1} for women in the same age group) [15, 27, 39, 41]. Does this mean that a client achieving a score higher than the 20th or 30th percentile is healthy? On any fitness test? Not necessarily. The problem is that exact cutoffs for health for each component of fitness for all segments of the adult population have not been identified and universally accepted. For a deconditioned client who scores at or near the bottom of a column on a norm-referenced table, the results may be demoralizing if the client thinks, mistakenly, that he or she must score at or near the top to be *healthy*.

Where they exist, criterion-referenced data provide a reasonable estimate of the level of fitness required for health. In the absence of criterion-referenced data for a test chosen for a particular client, the best way to use the normative tables is to encourage clients with goals related to health to strive for fitness improvements until they reach the "average" or higher levels for a given component, and then to maintain their level of performance [25, 27]. Clients with average or higher levels of performance initially or after training may have already achieved a healthy level of fitness, but may be motivated to improve both health and performance by setting higher performance goals using the norm-referenced tables.

Applying Norm- and Criterion-Referenced Standards

If a 39-year-old woman had a $\dot{V}O_2$max of 34 ml · kg^{-1} · min^{-1}, she scored at the 50th percentile (33.8 is the closest score and she's just barely above that), meaning that 50% of the women her age have a higher $\dot{V}O_2$max and 50% have a lower $\dot{V}O_2$max (see the bolded number in table 10.1). This $\dot{V}O_2$max is average for her age. What the score does not tell her is whether this represents a healthy level of cardiovascular fitness. On the other hand, 31.5 ml · kg^{-1} · min^{-1} is the minimal criterion for health in aerobic power (not noted in this norm-referenced table), and she has achieved a score that exceeds the health standard. The personal trainer and client would need to discuss her interests, performance goals, current program, and time available to determine together how she will maintain (minimal goal) or improve her current level of fitness.

Summative Evaluation

Summative evaluations are final evaluations made when a client completes a specified training period, class, or season. They represent the "sum total" of what has been accomplished in a given period. The same assessments used at the beginning and midpoint of an exercise program can and generally should be used to provide the final evaluation, but how the results are used will differ. For example, if a client has a flexibility goal for a specific joint, the formative evaluation would have included an initial measurement of the range of motion in the joint and a realistic goal for improved flexibility of that joint. The program might include a variety of stretching techniques for that joint with periodic repetitions of the test so the client knows the amount of progress he or she is making toward the goal. At the end of the specified period, the same test is repeated under similar conditions, and the client and personal trainer can determine whether the stated goals were achieved in that time: This evaluation is a "summary" of what was achieved during the specified training period. The formative evaluations are a measure of *progress toward a goal*, and the summative evaluation is a measure of the *degree of attainment of a stated goal*. For most clients, regardless of whether norm- or criterion-referenced standards are used, it is more appropriate to have them compare their own performances over time than to the skills or fitness levels of others.

Assessment Terminology

Assessment is the act of measuring a specific component using a well-constructed, valid, and reliable test. After the assessment is complete, the personal trainer must evaluate the data collected and interpret them meaningfully for the client in relation to his or her program goals. Assessment can be formal, as with specific test protocols that call for consistently followed procedures, or informal, as with all observations of a client performing specific activities and exercises.

Before selecting tests to use with a specific client, the personal trainer must have an understanding of the terminology specific to tests, measurements, and evaluation, and to some extent of the process by which tests are developed. The purpose of this text is not to attempt to list or explain all of the possible choices of assessment instruments available for each health- and skill-related component and each type of client—sedentary, athletic, healthy, or medically compromised. As new research and tests are reported, the personal trainer needs to evaluate new information and decide whether it has a place in the battery of tests used for that personal trainer's particular clientele. A test may be excellent in terms of validity and reliability but still not be appropriate for a specific client—for example, a near-maximal-exertion running test would not be appropriate for a deconditioned adult [25, 27, 33]. Additionally, although some tests may be excellent for measuring a specific component or trait, they may require equipment, facilities, or expertise that the personal trainer does not have (e.g., hydrostatic weighing). Conversely, the fact that a particular piece of equipment or computer-generated test battery is available does not make it appropriate for all clients. The personal trainer must sort through the information and select tests appropriate to each client, while recognizing that some clients will be more interested in personal progress than in multiple formal assessments.

The objective of the personal trainer in selecting assessments for the client is to reduce error and increase the accuracy of the assessment. Questions to answer in attempting to improve the accuracy of a test include the following:

- How reliable and objective was the assessment?
- Was it valid?
- Was the equipment calibrated and did it produce accurate results?
- Was the subject physically or emotionally influenced by anything before or during the test that may have affected the results?
- Was the test protocol followed carefully and were data collected accurately?

When these factors receive adequate attention, the personal trainer may confidently and accurately interpret data and apply the results.

Reliability and Objectivity

Reliability is an expression of the repeatability of a test or the consistency of repeated observations. If a measurement of the same trait under the same conditions yields the same results from one trial to another, the test is reliable (reproducible, consistent, accurate, dependable) [33]. One method of determining the reliability of a test is the **test-retest method.** In this case, a test is repeated with the same individual or group within one to three days unless the test requires near-maximal effort; then a seven-day test period is more appropriate [5]. To determine if the personal trainer is consistent in his or her ability to administer the test, that is, whether **intrarater reliability** exists, there must be a second trial in the same day by the same client and personal trainer [5, 21, 33]. And since a test given by a personal trainer could be consistent without being accurate, scores collected by different personal trainers on the same client are compared in order to determine **interrater reliability** [21, 33]. If more than one personal trainer can consistently get the same result from a client, the test is objective rather than subjective. It is not practical to test a client multiple times per day or per week on the same assessment, so the personal trainer must look for assessments that were proven to have good reliability when they were developed. However, the fact that an assessment had good reliability when developed is meaningless if the personal trainer does not take the time to practice giving the assessment under very strict and standardized conditions.

Validity

Validity means that a test does in fact measure what it claims to measure: that the test score is a "truthful" score. A test that is not reliable cannot be valid, but simply being repeatable does not make a test valid [33]. Does the assessment instrument really test what it claims to be testing? When selecting a test for aerobic capacity, one must choose a test that is long enough and whose intensity is sufficient to require the aerobic system to be the primary energy system. Therefore, a 50-meter (55-yard) or 100-meter (110-yard) sprint test would not give a valid or truthful measure of aerobic capacity. For a test to be valid, it must also be **relevant** [33]. The relevance of a test indicates how well it matches the objectives of the test. In the example just mentioned, a test for assessing speed is not relevant in measuring aerobic capacity. A body mass index (BMI) measurement is a relevant indicator of overweight in a fairly sedentary population, but it is not relevant to a group of athletes with increased lean muscle mass and a low percentage of body fat [9, 24, 32]. **Content validity,** then, means that the test appears to test what it is supposed to test [21, 33]. For example, a 1RM (1-repetition maximum) test is a valid measure of muscular strength, but not muscular flexibility.

Construct validity is a theoretical concept meaning that the test is able to differentiate between performance abilities. In other words, if a test is a sport skill-related test, those with the given sport skills should score better on the test than those who take the test without having previously acquired the skills [21, 33]. For a fitness test, the instrument should be able to truly discern the more highly fit from the unfit.

Criterion-related validity allows personal trainers to use tests in the field or the fitness center, instead of tests that can be done only in laboratory settings or with expensive equipment, because the results of the lab tests and field tests have been statistically compared to each other [33]. A maximal exertion stress test should be given only in a tightly controlled environment, possibly with medical personnel and equipment on hand [8, 15, 25, 41]. Since that is not practical in a fitness center setting, a personal trainer can select a submaximal cardiorespiratory endurance test, such as a treadmill test, step test, or a cycle ergometer test that has been statistically correlated to the **maximal exertion tests** on the basis of certain assumptions: In essence, the more fit the individual, the more work the person should be able to do at a given heart rate and the more total work he or she should be able to perform before reaching maximal heart rate [5, 15, 33, 40]. The results on the **submaximal tests** are not precisely the same as those on the stress test, nor will the estimated $\dot{V}O_2$max score on different types of submaximal tests identically match each other. However, if the margin of error between the submaximal and maximal tests is small, if the test is reliable (can be repeated with the same results), and if it tests what it was supposed to test (has content validity), then it is a good test. Hydrostatic weighing is the standard against which other measures of body fatness have been standardized, but it is an indirect measure of body fatness based on quantitative assumptions of a two-compartment model (fat mass and fat-free mass) [24, 35]. An autopsy is a direct measure, but obviously useless to the personal trainer! Other field measurements, such as skinfold measurements, bioelectrical impedance (BIA), near-infrared interactance (NIR), or anthropometric measures, are doubly indirect [2, 24]. This means that the statistical relationships between each of these methods and the hydrostatic weighing data have been established, and a standard of error has been determined for each method. When a specific test is selected to assess a client, the same test should be used under similar circumstances for posttesting. A skinfold estimate of body fatness cannot reliably be compared to an estimate made by means of BIA or NIR, or vice versa [24]. (See chapter 11 for further discussion.)

A valid test is one that measures what it purports to measure. A reliable test is one that can be repeated with accuracy, by the same tester or another. A good assessment instrument is both valid and reliable.

Factors That Affect Reliability and Validity

All tests have a **standard error of measurement.** This is the difference between a person's observed score—what the result was—and that person's true score, a theoretically errorless score. Empirically any test result consists of a true score and error. All test results contain the true value of the factor being measured as well as the errors associated with the test itself. The error may be constant or random and may be influenced by the client, the personal trainer, the equipment, or the environment [33].

Client Factors

In the process of identifying and selecting appropriate tests it is important to consider factors that may influence client performance and subsequently have an impact on the validity and the reliability of the assessment results. The key client factors to consider when one is selecting tests include health status and functional capacity, age, sex, and pretraining status.

Health Status and Functional Capacity

The health status and functional capacity of a client dictate which assessments are appropriate. Information gathered during the preparticipation screening process (see chapter 9) should be used to identify potential physical limitations. Understanding those limits provides a context for selecting assessments that will reasonably match the capabilities of the individual. As an example, if an individual is sedentary, over the age of 60, and has a functional aerobic capacity of five METs, it may be unreasonable for that person to perform the YMCA Step Test or 1.5-mile (2.4-kilometer) run. Both of these assessments may require a greater metabolic level of performance than 5 METs and in some instances may be considered near-maximal tests for deconditioned individuals [27]. Also, client fatigue, whether a function of recent activities, food and fluid intake, or sleeping patterns or due to the number and physical demands of the assessments being administered in one session, will influence the assessment outcomes [27].

Age

Chronological age and maturity may influence testing performance. For example, the 1.5-mile (2.4-kilometer) run is considered a standard field test to measure aerobic capacity for apparently healthy college-age men and women. However, this same assessment will not appropriately measure aerobic ability of preadolescents, primarily because of the immature physical development of the cardiovascular system and the experiential maturity needed to cover the distance by pacing [10].

Sex

Sex-specific biological factors may influence performances in the chin-up, push-up, and bench press to assess muscular endurance of the upper extremities. Several differences between men and women appear to influence performance: Women tend to have more body fat and less muscle, a smaller shoulder mass that supports less muscle tissue, and as a result less of a mechanical advantage for muscles working at the shoulder [13]. For example, the chin-up test appears to provide reliable results for males; however, it may in some cases fail to differentiate between strength and muscular endurance for females. As a result, the flexed arm hang is sometimes used as an alternative method to assess muscular endurance, through a static rather than a dynamic muscular action, by measuring the length of time the flexed elbow hang position can be sustained. Also, push-up tests to measure dynamic muscular fitness of the upper extremities include a variation to accommodate for the differences in upper body strength; this modification consists of the same standard military push-up position as for men with the exception that the knees are flexed and the ankles are crossed [29]. In addition, the YMCA Fixed-Load Bench Press Test provides different fixed loads for men and women (35 pounds [15.8 kilograms] for women and 80 pounds [36 kilograms] for men), illustrating the sex-specific differences related to client factors that one needs to consider when selecting appropriate tests [17]. (See chapter 11 for the complete procedures for these tests.)

Pretraining Status

The pretraining status of the client may affect test selection when the skills required for the test and the relative level of exertion are considered. Caution should be emphasized in assessment of the untrained, deconditioned individual, even when that client may express a desire to achieve high performance levels. For example, the 1.5-mile (2.4-kilometer) run test and the 12-minute run test are considered near-maximal-exertion tests, as they require the individual to cover distance as quickly as possible [25]. A deconditioned client should have a period of at least four to six weeks of aerobic conditioning before participating in either of these assessments [25]. Clients who are unaccustomed to pacing themselves may do better on subsequent trials of a one-mile (1.6-kilometer) walk test as they learn to adjust their initial pace with a practice trial [8, 33]. Similarly, clients who do not have an opportunity to practice a footwork pattern for an agility test may not get an accurate score. Allowing the client time to practice the movement pattern will yield a better indication of the person's agility [33].

Likewise, a 1RM test in the squat movement may be appropriate for a conditioned individual who has previous experience with that free weight movement pattern. However, for someone with no pretraining experience, the lack of motor skill and the intensity required for the exercise may create an unacceptably high risk for injury [4, 6, 7, 11]. The greater the load, the more stress the joints, muscles, bones, and connective tissues experience [4, 6, 7]. In order to improve safety and reliability, it may be necessary to modify the test to one that estimates maximal strength with a submaximal load, such as a 10RM [7].

One or more practice sessions of the specific exercise with a lighter load to learn the proper technique may be necessary. For the untrained person, adaptations in the coordination of the neuromuscular system may account for most of the initial strength gains in a resistance training program [4, 6, 14]. Even so, a familiarization period may be prudent to acquaint the untrained individual with the new skill involved in the movement and to protect the person from injury. The length of the familiarization period varies by client and the relative intensity required by the strength test chosen.

Also, some muscular endurance tests may involve resistances heavy enough to permit only a limited number of repetitions to be performed by untrained clients. For example, clients with weak or smaller upper body muscles (e.g., younger and older clients, some women, sedentary clients) will not be able to complete very many repetitions (e.g., ≤6) in the push-up test (see page 237) because their body weight—even using the modified body position—is simply too heavy. For these clients, the push-up test becomes one that can be used to assess muscular *strength.*

Personal Trainer Factors

The level of experience and training of the personal trainer has an impact on the selection of assessments. In order to maintain objectivity and reduce intrarater error, testing protocols that require adept technical skills need to match the abilities of the personal trainer. As an example, theoretical prediction errors of ±3.5% or less body fat are considered acceptable on various equations and combinations of skinfold measurements to assess body composition [24], but tester error may account for 3% to 9% variability between raters (interrater reliability) [24]. Errors can be further compounded by failure to follow a protocol, inaccurate identification of measurement sites, improperly calibrated equipment, and the choice of prediction equations [24]. Taking accurate skinfold measurements is a complicated skill that requires about 100 practice opportunities in order for the personal trainer to gain adequate proficiency [24]. To develop intrarater consistency, the personal trainer should do the measurements on different sites and body types [24, 25].

The relative test difficulty and the type of measurement required can affect outcomes. It is not reasonable to expect a personal trainer to read through a protocol, administer an assessment to a client, and get good results without practice. Some tests require quite a bit more skill and practice than others do. For example, relatively little skill on the part of the personal trainer is required to manage a stopwatch and monitor heart rate for a timed one-mile (1.6-kilometer) walk or run test. On the other hand, the skills required to get reliable results on a noncomputerized cycle ergometer test are much more complex and involved (e.g., monitoring and adjusting the workload and pedal cadence on the ergometer; obtaining heart rates every minute of the test) [25, 38].

A personal trainer who is unfamiliar with administration of one assessment may not select it at a given time, but should continue his or her professional development by taking time to practice administration of that assessment for use with future clients.

Equipment Factors

Any mechanism or device used to measure work, performance, or physiological response requires **calibration** in order to accurately measure the specific trait being assessed. Reliability, validity, and objectivity of the assessment are directly affected by the accuracy of the measurement tool. Common mechanisms and devices used in the assessment process that require calibration are cycle, stepping, and treadmill ergometers; blood pressure sphygmomanometers; skinfold calipers and body composition mechanisms; metronomes; and other electronic devices used to measure time, distance, and power. To assure the accuracy of equipment, it is important to institute a scheduled plan for checking and calibrating mechanisms and devices according to manufacturer specification and based on warranty recommendations.

Environmental Factors

Climatic elements and the physical setting of the environment present potential concerns that may influence client performance and safety. Consequently when one is selecting and administering tests, it is necessary to consider environmental planning and quality control assurance related to weather, altitude, and the physical setting of a facility.

Temperature and Humidity

The environment poses challenges and issues related to physiological responses that may have an impact on test administration and performance. High heat and humidity and cold-weather exposure need to be considered in the selection of assessments. High ambient temperatures in combination with high humidity inhibit the body's thermoregulatory system from dissipating heat, which impedes physical endurance performance, poses health risks, and affects test results. Aerobic endurance may be impaired when the temperature approaches 80 degrees Fahrenheit (27 degrees Celsius) and the humidity exceeds 50% [30]. Geographic areas that experience high temperatures along with high humidity may not be suitable for outdoor tests to assess aerobic endurance.

Exposure to cold temperatures, less than 25 degrees Fahrenheit (–4 degrees Celsius), may not have a significant impact on the performance and health of younger apparently healthy individuals; however, older people and those who have cardiovascular and circulatory disorders and respiratory problems may need to use caution. Cold exposure may stimulate the sympathetic nervous system, which can affect total peripheral resistance, arterial pressure, myocardial contraction, and cardiac work [34]. Of particular concern are outdoor performances that require significant effort of the upper extremities. Clients with respiratory conditions, particularly asthma, may also be more prone to problems in cold temperatures as the cold air may trigger a bronchial spasm [15].

Altitude

Altitude can also impair performance of aerobic endurance. Tests to measure aerobic endurance may not correlate with normative performance data when assessment takes place at altitudes higher than 1,900 feet (580 meters) [20]. In addition, individuals not acclimated to altitude changes may require an adaptation period of 10 days before engaging in aerobic endurance assessments [19].

Test Setting

Issues associated with health and environmental control are important factors related to assessment validity and reliability. To minimize external distractions and the potential anxiety related to the assessment process, the testing area should be quiet and private. The personal trainer should project a positive, relaxed, confident demeanor; and the process should be clearly explained and not rushed. The testing room should be well equipped with comfortable furnishings and standardized and calibrated testing devices, and the room temperature should be set at 68 to 72 degrees Fahrenheit (20-22 degrees Celsius), 60% or less humidity, and air circulation of six to eight exchanges per hour [15]. Physical facilities must be inspected for deficiencies, and safety procedures need to be clearly documented and posted. Appropriate emergency equipment must be operable and immediately available in the event that an incident requires an emergency response [15, 23, 27, 38]. (See chapter 24 for more details about recommended facility characteristics.)

The integrity of the assessment process depends on the validity and reliability of the assessments selected and properly administered by a trained fitness professional. Personal trainers should take care to enhance reliability by consistently attending to controllable factors related to the client, personal trainer, equipment, and environment.

Assessment Case Studies

The most important required assessments to initiate and design an exercise program are of the client's cardiovascular disease risk and potential contraindications for specific activities due to known musculoskeletal limitations or diseases. The outcome of the health screening process and risk stratification dictates the selection and administration of all other assessments. Before selecting the assessment instruments for each client, the personal trainer must also consider other factors, including the client's exercise goals, exercise history, attitudes about assessments, the personal trainer's experience and skill in correctly performing the assessments, and the equipment and facilities available. In most cases, more than one assessment instrument may be used to collect the information needed to design a program. The next section further explores these concepts using two case studies. (Refer to table 9.2 on page 172 for details on risk stratification.)

Case Study 10.1: Mrs. G.

Maria G. is a 57-year-old grandmother of four who has been active most of her life. She is 65 inches (165 centimeters) tall and weighs 145 pounds (66 kilograms). She participated in step aerobics and spinning classes three to four times per week at her old club before she moved to be closer to her daughters' families. She is planning on resuming those activities at her new club. She also enjoys occasional games of recreational tennis and golf with her friends. She would like to increase her strength, as she is helping more with the toddlers and finds carrying them and their gear tiring. She has never been a smoker, although her husband still smokes a pack a day. Her father died at age 73 in a car accident, and her 82-year-old mother is still alive. Last month, a local hospital sponsored a health fair, and Mrs. G. took full advantage of the screening opportunities. Her average blood pressure was 129/79 mmHg (millimeters of mercury). Her total cholesterol was 231 mg/dL (milligrams per deciliter) with an LDL count of 150 mg/dL and an HDL score of 65 mg/dL. Her fasting glucose was 93 mg/dL. She also had her body fat tested with a handheld BIA device and was told she was 28% fat. She has no other health problems. See the "Individual Assessment Recording Form for Mrs. G." on the next page for a summary of the assessment findings.

Individual Assessment Recording Form for Mrs. G.

(Pretest) Posttest (circle one)

Client's name: Mrs. G. **Age:** 57

Goals: Increase muscular strength; maintain aerobic capacity and body composition; improve balance and blood lipid profile

Preparticipation screening notes: In 'moderate' risk category; need to receive physician's release prior to prescribing a 'vigorous' activity exercise program

Assessment dates: 8/9/03; 8/11/03

Comments: Will re-evaluate % body fat using skinfold calipers; she previously was active but has not exercised recently; wants to begin aerobic classes again; recently completed a lipid screening (cholesterol: 231 mg/dL; LDLs: 150 mg/dL; HDLs: 65 mg/dL; fasting glucose: 93 mg/dL); husband is a smoker

Vital signs	Score or result	Classification*	Examples and norm- and criterion-referenced standards (chapter 11)
Resting blood pressure	129/79 mmHg	Normal	Example 11.2 (client A) Table 11.4
Resting heart rate	72 bpm	Average	Table 11.2
Body composition measures	**Score or result**	**Classification**	
Height	65 in. (165 cm)	%tile: ~ 80th	Table 11.9
Weight	145 lb (66 kg)	Under "average"	Table 11.11
Body mass index (BMI)	24.1	Normal	Example 11.3 (client A) Table 11.7
Waist circumference	29 in. (74 cm)	Under the "88 cm" cutoff	Table 11.7
Hip circumference	36 in. (91 cm)	—	—
Waist-to-hip ratio	0.81	Moderate risk	Table 11.15
Percent body fat method: BIA	28%	%tile: ~ 60th Criterion: leaner than average	%tile: Table 11.14 Criterion: Table 11.14
Cardiovascular endurance	**Score or result**	**Classification**	
Åstrand-Ryhming cycle test initial work rate: 450 kg·m·min^{-1}	28.64 ml · kg^{-1} · min^{-1}	%tile: ~ 55th Criterion: good	Example 11.5 %tile: Table 11.17 Criterion: Table 11.21
Muscular endurance	**Score or result**	**Classification**	
YMCA bench press test weight: 35 pounds	9 reps @ 35 lb (16 kg)	%tile: 50th	%tile: Table 11.27
Muscular strength	**Score or result**	**Classification**	
Push-up test	3 reps	%tile: 20th	%tile: Table 11.30

(continued)

Individual Assessment Recording Form for Mrs. G. *(continued)*

Flexibility	Score or result	Classification	
YMCA sit and reach test	13 in. (33 cm)	%tile: 30th	%tile: Table 11.31
Other tests	**Score or result**	**Classification**	
**Thomas hip range of motion test	Both tested legs remained on floor	Adequate hip flexor flexibility	
***One-foot stand test, eyes open	Right: 6 sec Left: 9 sec	Low/average	

*Classification refers to either the norm- or criterion-referenced standard, depending on the test and protocol. Refer to the examples and the norm- and criterion-referenced standards provided in chapter 11 for a further explanation of how the classification labels were assigned to Mrs. G.'s test results.

**Protocol and normative data in Howley and Franks [27].

***Protocol and normative data in Hoeger and Hoeger [25].

Risk Factor Analysis

What is Mrs. G.'s risk stratification (see tables 9.1 and 9.2)? Mrs. G. has only one risk factor from the screening, and that is hypercholesterolemia. Both her total and LDL-cholesterol are above the threshold levels for risk (200 mg/dL for total cholesterol and 130 mg/dL for LDL-cholesterol). However, her HDL level at 65 mg/dL is above the 60 mg/dL level, which denotes a positive high number that cancels one of the risk factors. Mrs. G.'s blood pressure and blood glucose are normal, and her BMI score of 24.1 does not indicate an overweight condition. Her percentage of body fat at 28% is in the "leaner than average" category for a woman her age. Mrs. G. does not have a significant family history of cardiovascular disease. She is not a smoker, and although she does have some risk associated with the secondhand smoke from her husband, this is not considered a risk factor for her in determining exercise risk. If she were younger, she would be in the low-risk category, able to participate in a vigorous program without a doctor's release. Because she is over 55 years of age, she is automatically at moderate risk and *should not* participate in *maximal* exercise testing and in a *vigorous* exercise program until she obtains a physician's release (see table 9.3).

Assessment Recommendations

What assessment recommendations would be appropriate for this client? For assessment of cardiovascular endurance, the personal trainer has several choices of activities. Since Mrs. G. used to participate in regular aerobic exercise recently, she would be a candidate for one of the tests that require some preconditioning (e.g., 1.5-mile [2.4-kilometer] run test, 12-minute run test, and the multi-stage YMCA cycle ergometer test) [25, 27, 33]. However, because of her moderate-risk status due to her age, these near-maximal tests must be deemed inappropriate for her at this time without a physician's release. Single-stage or graded treadmill tests, walking tests, cycling tests, and step tests (12-inch [30-centimeter] step or lower) would be acceptable choices since she has no joint complaints and used to participate in two of the three activities.

Since Mrs. G. has not been performing a resistance training program, all maximal (1RM) strength tests are not recommended. Performing a muscular endurance test such as the YMCA fixed-weight bench press test may pose no problem since she has been active; but the activity has not been in a resistance program, and the exercises are unfamiliar. Therefore, an initial familiarization period with various machine or free weight exercises would be the most appropriate starting point for Mrs. G. The personal trainer can use suggested guidelines based on a percentage of the client's body weight to estimate initial loads for a resistance training program [3, 4]. When Mrs. G. is comfortable with the mechanics of performing the exercises and when she becomes better trained, a more standardized strength assessment can be performed. Meanwhile, due to her weak upper body, the personal trainer can use the push-up test to assess Mrs. G.'s relative strength.

If Mrs. G. had expressed concerns related to body weight or body size, it would be prudent to repeat a test for body composition under the prescribed conditions to get the baseline data for future comparisons, since the testing conditions at the health fair are unknown. For measures of body fat it is recommended that the same test be administered under the same conditions by the same tester [24]. Therefore, the personal trainer can re-test Mrs. G. with, for example, skinfold calipers (if the personal trainer is skilled in using this tool). Circumference measures would also provide baseline data for health risks related to excess abdominal fat and also allow Mrs. G. to track changes in her body after participating in an exercise program. (See chapter 11 for further discussion of how to perform these anthropometric measurements.)

Mrs. G. has not expressed a desire to improve athletic performance, and therefore tests for agility, speed, and power are not necessary at this time. Balance, reaction time, and coordination issues related to her activities of daily living may become more apparent and require further investigation and/or programming in the future. If the client continues to participate in tennis and golf, she may welcome some activities related to improved performance after the personal trainer has designed a program to meet her current goal of increased functional strength.

Case Study 10.2: Mr. C.

Paul C. is a 28-year-old accountant in a very busy office. He is six feet (183 centimeters) tall and weighs 260 pounds (118 kilograms) and has never smoked or used tobacco products. Mr. C.'s father had two heart attacks prior to his death at age 47, and Mr. C.'s 34-year-old brother recently underwent triple-bypass surgery after experiencing chest pains. His mother has type 2 diabetes, which is under control. He has not had his fasting blood glucose measured. During the initial interview, Mr. C.'s blood pressure measured 150/96 mmHg; his percentage of body fat was 30, and his waist measurement was 41 inches (104 centimeters) compared to a hip measurement of 44 inches (112 centimeters). His last cholesterol test was over six months ago, and he does not recall the numbers but states "The doctor didn't say anything, so I guess it was okay." Mr. C. has developed asthma, induced by seasonal allergies and exercise. He has an inhaler of albuterol and does find that activity easily winds him and sometimes precipitates an asthma attack. He also reports some intermittent pain in his left knee, probably related to a fall several months ago. He has not had the knee examined by the doctor. Mr. C. has come in at his wife's insistence because she is concerned that he is as much a candidate for a heart attack as his brother was. However, he has never been active or enjoyed exercise and is concerned about how to fit activity into his busy work schedule.

Risk Factor Analysis

What is Mr. C.'s risk stratification (see tables 9.1 and 9.2)? Mr. C. has a number of risk factors at this time. He has a significant family history with both his father and brother having experienced heart attacks or cardiovascular disease prior to age 55. His BMI is 35.3, which classifies him in very high-risk obesity class II (see table 11.7) [9, 15, 24, 25, 36]. The other anthropometric measures support the fact that his excess visceral fat, stored in the abdominal area, puts Mr. C. at high risk of cardiovascular disease, stroke, and diabetes type 2; body fat is ≥30% (see table 11.14); waist circumference is ≥40 inches [102 centimeters] [9, 15]; waist-to-hip ratio is above .94 (see table 11.15) [9, 15, 24, 25, 36]). By his own admission, he is not an active person. His blood pressure is high; two consecutive high blood pressure readings on either systolic (>140 mmHg) or diastolic (>90 mmHG) indicate a referral to a physician for evaluation (see table 11.4). His fasting glucose is unknown at this time. Mr. C. reports no other signs or symptoms of cardiovascular disease, but his blood cholesterol is also unknown at this time. In addition to the four risk factors he presents (family history, obesity, inactivity, high blood pressure), he has a known disease, asthma, and an undiagnosed orthopedic problem (left knee). Mr. C. should be advised not to do any activities until his physician releases him.

Assessment Recommendations

Given Mr. C.'s situation, his physician may designate him as a high-risk client and may choose to perform a diagnostic stress test on this client. If that is the case, and Mr. C. is released for a limited activity program, the personal trainer can use the maximal heart rate and maximal oxygen consumption data from the stress

(continued)

Case Study 10.2: Mr. C. *(continued)*

test in designing the exercise program. If Mr. C. is not stress tested and is released for moderate exercise, the assessment of cardiovascular function will be submaximal, with a bike test as possibly the most appropriate since it is non-weight bearing and may put the least stress on his left knee.

Additional consideration needs to be given to some of the other information provided by this client. He is not an active person, does not particularly enjoy exercise, and is already erecting roadblocks in terms of finding time to exercise. He appears to be in the contemplation, or possibly preparation, stage of readiness for lifestyle change [37]. (See chapter 8, page 152, for more information about the client's psychological readiness for exercise.) Also, the personal trainer could have Mr. C. complete "The Attitudinal Assessment" form (page 179), which gauges attitudes toward exercise.

While awaiting the physician's release, Mr. C. may benefit from sessions to discuss his readiness to change lifestyle behaviors, goal setting, strategies to enhance his adherence to a program, and consultation with a nutrition specialist.

Selecting valid, reliable, and safe assessments that will provide meaningful results requires an understanding of the health status, risk stratification, and goals of the client; level of experience of the personal trainer; availability of equipment; and the specific test characteristics associated with the assessment.

Administration and Organization of Fitness Assessments

Administration of the fitness assessment requires advanced preparation and organization to assure psychometrically sound results and safe outcomes. When organizing and administering the fitness assessment process, one must pay close attention to the details of preparation and the implementation of factors that will have an impact on obtaining safe, accurate, and meaningful results.

Test Preparation

Appropriate and valuable test outcomes are predicated on the ability of the personal trainer to prepare clients by educating them as to the content of the test, pretest requirements, and expectations of the assessment process. Preparation to evaluate someone's level of fitness requires the personal trainer to execute preassessment screening procedures, select appropriate assessments, review safety considerations, verify accuracy of equipment, and perform record-keeping responsibilities. See page 207 for a "Test Preparation and Implementation Checklist."

Verify Appropriateness of Selected Assessments

Selecting valid, reliable, and safe assessments that will provide meaningful results requires an understanding of the goals and health status of the client, level of experience of the personal trainer, and the specific test characteristics associated with the assessment.

Review Safety Considerations

The implementation of a fitness assessment procedure should occur only after a thorough pre-activity screening process that includes an initial interview, execution of a health appraisal tool, completion of appropriate forms, and, when required, recommendations from a physician regarding the management of medical contraindications (see chapter 9). There are documented risks associated with exercise testing; however, evidence suggests that complications are relatively low (.04% or 4 per 10,000) [15, 16].

Select Facilities and Verify Accuracy of Equipment

Ease of administration, cost-effectiveness, availability of equipment, and the facility setting influence the selection and implementation of the assessment process. Two types of assessments, laboratory tests and field tests, may be administered to yield valuable results; but in most situations they are administered under different conditions. **Laboratory tests,** in most cases, are performed in clinical facilities using specialized **diagnostic** equipment to assess an individual's maximal functional capacity. Testing is relatively complex, and direct-measurement tools are used to reduce data error and quantify results based on physiological responses. Because of the diagnostic capabilities of the tests and the high risk of cardiac complications, allied health professionals are responsible for administering the assessment and evaluation process. Table 10.2 provides a list of recommended fitness testing equipment.

Test Preparation and Implementation Checklist

Client's name: ______________________________

Personal trainer's name: ______________________________

	Test preparation	✓	Date/comments
1.	**Verify appropriateness of selected assessments:**		
a.	Identify and evaluate client's specific goals.		
b.	Assess professional expertise associated with the tests to determine appropriateness of current skill level to obtain accurate results.		
c.	Evaluate the characteristics of tests to determine congruency with client's goals and to assess the risk-to-benefit relationship.		
2.	**Review safety considerations:**		
a.	Conduct a preparticipation health appraisal screening.		
b.	Obtain a physician referral and/or medical clearance.		
c.	Distribute and collect completed informed consent and screening forms.		
d.	Review emergency procedures.		
3.	**Select facilities and verify accuracy of equipment:**		
a.	Identify tests that are easy to administer and are cost-effective.		
b.	Select appropriate equipment and confirm availability.		
c.	Calibrate equipment.		
d.	Provide a testing atmosphere that is calm, private, and relaxed.		
e.	Assure the assessment area is safe, clean, set up, and ready for testing.		
f.	Evaluate room temperature and humidity (68-72° F [20-22° C]; 60% humidity).		
4.	**Instruct client on preassessment protocols:**		
a.	Provide clients with pretest instructions. • Adequate rest (6-8 hours the night before testing) • Moderate dietary intake (including adequate hydration) • Abstinence from chemicals that accelerate heart rates (except for presently prescribed medications) • Appropriate attire (loose-fitting clothing and sturdy shoes)		
b.	Explain conditions for starting and stopping procedures of the protocol.		
5.	**Prepare record-keeping system:**		
a.	Create and supply a recording form or system.		
b.	Develop a storage and retrieval system for data that is secure and confidential.		

(continued)

Test Preparation and Implementation Checklist *(continued)*

	Test implementation	✓	Date/comments
1.	**Determine sequence of assessments:**		
a.	Establish an organized and appropriate testing order.		
b.	Develop an appointment schedule for testing.		
2.	**Define and follow test protocols:**		
a.	Provide written test directions and guidelines to client.		
b.	Explain technique, reasons for disqualification, and test scoring.		
c.	Demonstrate test performance and allow time to practice.		
d.	Provide an opportunity for client to ask questions regarding the tests.		
e.	Implement an adequate warm-up and cool-down procedure.		
f.	Spot the clients when appropriate.		

From *NSCA's Essentials of Personal Training* by Roger W. Earle and Thomas R. Baechle, 2004, Champaign, IL: Human Kinetics.

Table 10.2

Fitness Testing Area Equipment

Fitness Testing Area Equipment
Bicycle ergometer
Treadmill or a fixed-step bench
Skinfold calipers or other body composition measuring device
Sit and reach bench or goniometer
Tensiometer or other device for measuring muscular strength and endurance
Perceived exertion chart
Clock
Metronome
Sphygmomanometer (blood pressure cuff)
Stethoscope
Tape measure
Scale
First aid kit

Adapted from ACSM 1998.

Field tests are practical assessments that are inexpensive, are easy to administer, require less equipment, are less time-consuming, can be performed at various venues, and may be more efficient for evaluating large groups. The assessments may be submaximal or maximal and are usually administered by a certified fitness professional. These assessments, which are not diagnostic, use indirect measurements to quantify and extrapolate performance results. The major concerns with the maximal assessments are the potential risks that exist as a result of an individual putting forth a maximal effort without being monitored with diagnostic devices. Because of the cost of laboratory equipment and the consideration of ease of administration, it may not be practical or appropriate for the personal trainer to implement laboratory testing. In any case, one can use field tests effectively and efficiently to obtain the information needed to assess norm or criterion-referenced standards and performance.

Testing equipment must be calibrated; through calibration one checks the accuracy of a measuring device by comparing it with a known standard and making adjustments to provide an accurate reading. Exercise ergometers, which can measure work, need to be calibrated according to the manufacturers' recommendations in order to provide valid and reliable performance-related results. It is important to identify the calibration standards for testing devices and to schedule a routine calibration check to perform adjustments based on manufacturers' recommendations [26].

Instruct Client on Preassessment Protocols

An appointment for the assessment should be scheduled in advance in order for the client to adequately prepare mentally and physically for the event. The client should receive pretest instructions in preparation for the assessment. These include

- adequate rest (e.g., six to eight hours the night before and no vigorous exercise 24 hours preceding the test);
- moderate food intake (e.g., a light meal or snack two to four hours prior to the test);
- adequate hydration (e.g., six to eight glasses of water the day before the test and at least two cups [0.5 liters] of water in the two hours prior to the test);
- abstinence from chemicals that accelerate heart rate (with the exception of prescribed medications);
- proper attire (e.g., loose-fitting clothing, sturdy, tied athletic shoes);
- specific testing procedures and expectations before, during, and after the test; and
- conditions for terminating a test.

It is important for clients to be told that they may terminate a test for any reason at any time. Also, occasionally it may be necessary, for safety reasons, for the personal trainer to terminate a test before its completion. See table 10.3, "General Indications for Stopping an Exercise Test in Low-Risk Adults" [15].

Prepare Record-Keeping System

An organized method to collect, record, and store data is critical in reducing the incidence of error and is instrumental to the evaluation and interpretation of testing results. Creating a systematic method for

Table 10.3

General Indications for Stopping an Exercise Test in Low-Risk Adults

General Indications for Stopping an Exercise Test in Low-Risk Adults
Onset of angina or angina-like symptoms
Significant drop (20 mmHg) in systolic blood pressure or a failure of the systolic blood pressure to rise with an increase in activity
Excessive rise in blood pressure: systolic pressure >260 mmHg or diastolic pressure >115 mmHg
Signs of poor perfusion: light-headedness; confusion; ataxia; pallor; cyanosis; nausea; or cold, clammy skin
Failure of heart rate to increase with increased exercise intensity
Noticeable change in heart rhythm
Client requests to stop
Physical or verbal manifestations of severe fatigue
Failure of the testing equipment

Note: Indications are for nondiagnostic tests performed without direct physician involvement or electrocardiographic monitoring.

Reprinted from ACSM 2000.

collecting and storing data is one of the professional responsibilities associated with the role of the personal trainer. In addition, documentation may provide evidence of reasonable and prudent care in the event that the standard of care is questioned and litigation is pursued [12, 23].

A systematic approach to data collection would include manual recording forms or software programs that allow documentation of raw scores expressed in specific units of measurement. Recording devices should also contain vital client information related to the assessment process and provide space for comments pertaining to the collection of data during the process. In addition, the data collection system should be organized so that testing results can be retrieved from it in a time-efficient manner. This feature is especially important when one is making pretest-to-posttest comparisons during the reassessment process. The system should also have a protective mechanism to assure confidentiality. See the next page for a blank copy of the "Individual Assessment Recording Form" (used in Case Study 10.1) as an example of an assessment recording form that you may use.

Test Implementation

Organizing and implementing an assessment procedure require the personal trainer's detailed attention to a number of tasks: identifying the sequence of the assessments, defining and following testing protocols, collecting and interpreting data, and scheduling a review of the results. Refer to the "Test Preparation and Implementation Checklist" on page 207.

Determine Sequence of Assessments

Organization of a testing procedure demands that the personal trainer identify and determine the proper order of the testing process to assure optimal performance and adequate rest recovery to yield accurate results. Test order is influenced by many factors: number of clients to be tested, components to be evaluated, skill involved, energy system demand, time available, and the specific goal of the client. Many clients do not require a battery of tests as inclusive as the lists that follow. One can use various strategies related to test order; however, the following are examples of logical sequences for clients with general fitness- or athletic performance-related goals [20]:

General Fitness

1. Resting tests (e.g., resting heart rate, blood pressure, height, weight, body composition)
2. Non-fatiguing tests (e.g., flexibility, balance)
3. Muscular strength tests
4. Local muscular endurance tests (e.g., YMCA bench press test, one-minute sit-up test, partial curl-up test)
5. Sub-maximal aerobic capacity tests (e.g., step test, Rockport walking test, Åstrand-Ryhming cycle ergometer test, 1.5-mile [2.4-kilometer] run, 12 minute run/walk)

Athletic Performance

1. Resting tests (e.g., resting heart rate, blood pressure, height, weight, body composition)
2. Non-fatiguing tests (e.g., flexibility, vertical jump)
3. Agility tests (e.g., T-test)
4. Maximum power and strength tests (e.g., 3RM power clean, 1RM bench press)
5. Sprint tests (e.g., 40-yard [37-meter] sprint)
6. Local muscular endurance tests (e.g., one-minute sit-up test, push-up test)
7. Anaerobic capacity tests (e.g., 300-yard [275-meter] shuttle run)
8. Maximal or sub-maximal aerobic capacity tests (e.g., maximum treadmill test, 1.5-mile [2.4-kilometer] run, YMCA cycle ergometer test)

If possible, it is most appropriate to schedule assessments to measure maximum aerobic capacity on a separate day. However, if all assessments are performed on the same day, maximum aerobic tests should be performed last, after a minimum of an hour-long rest recovery period [20].

Define and Follow Test Protocols

Individuals being assessed should receive precise instructions regarding the test prior to the scheduled assessment appointment. The clarity and simplicity of instructions have a direct impact on the reliability and objectivity of a test [28]. Test

Individual Assessment Recording Form

Pretest Posttest (circle one)

Client's name: ______________________ **Age:** ________

Goals: ______________________

____

Preparticipation screening notes: ______________________

____

Assessment dates: ______________________

Comments: ______________________

____

Vital signs	Score or result	Classification
Resting blood pressure		
Resting heart rate		
Body composition measures	**Score or result**	**Classification**
Height		
Weight		
Body mass index (BMI)		
Waist circumference		
Hip circumference		
Waist-to-hip ratio		
Percent body fat method: ________		
Cardiovascular endurance	**Score or result**	**Classification**
Muscular endurance	**Score or result**	**Classification**
Muscular strength	**Score or result**	**Classification**
Flexibility	**Score or result**	**Classification**
Other tests	**Score or result**	**Classification**

instructions should define the protocols, including the purpose of the test, directions on implementation, performance guidelines regarding technique and disqualification, test scoring, and recommendations for maximizing performance. The personal trainer should also provide a demonstration of appropriate test performance and should give the client an opportunity to practice and ask questions concerning the protocol.

It is the responsibility of the personal trainer to assure that testing protocols are followed safely and efficiently. To enhance reliability, strict standardized procedures should be followed with each client, each time the test is administered. Also, the test selected for the pretest should be repeated as the posttest so that a reliable comparison of scores can be made. The personal trainer should institute an adequate warm-up and cool-down procedure when warranted and implement spotting practices when required by the testing protocol.

Administration of the assessments should follow a standardized procedure including mental and physical preparation of the client, verification of the accuracy of the equipment, application of the specific test protocol, ensuring safety throughout the process, and performance of record-keeping responsibilities.

Interpretation and Review of Results

The data collected through the assessment process provide baseline information for the client. The interpretation of the baseline data is dependent on the specific purpose of the assessment and the goals of the client. Common ways to explain data to a client are through norm-referenced and criterion-referenced standards (see chapter 11). The normative approach to data interpretation entails a comparison of test scores with established normative age- and gender-related data to evaluate level of performance with a percentile ranking. This approach tells a client how his or her performance compares to that of others of the same age and sex. Although this may provide positive feedback related to performance, it does not address the health-related status of the individual based on desirable health standards.

Criterion-referenced interpretation uses baseline information as a marker to assess present health risks and to define what changes are necessary to obtain standards that are healthy [33]. A substantial body of research supports the increased risk of mortality with a sedentary lifestyle [15, 18, 25]. Until uniform criterion-referenced health standards are developed and accepted, the best way to use the baseline data is as a reference point for change over time. A client who scores below average, below a criterion-referenced "healthy" score, or at an "increased risk" level will most likely begin a program with moderate intensities of exercise two to three times per week for a relatively short time. As the client shows evidence of motor and physiological adaptations, workloads can progressively increase. This initial stage of training may last four to eight weeks or longer, depending on the client's status and progress. Clients who score in the average or higher categories on the fitness assessments can begin training at higher intensities and with more total volume of exercise per week [31]. (See chapters 15, 16, and 17 for guidelines for developing exercise programs.)

The personal trainer should schedule a review of results immediately or shortly following the assessment process. The client should receive an illustrated summary of the test results, along with an explanation of personal strengths and areas identified that may have room for improvement. It is important to note that testing data are neither good nor bad—they are baseline data to provide a foundation for positive change.

Reassessment

Once the assessments are complete and the personal trainer has reviewed the results with the client, the program is designed and implemented based on the client's goals. The initial assessments, intermediate assessments (repetitions of some or all of the initial assessments), anecdotal records, and exercise logs documenting client progress are all part of the formative evaluation of the client, providing frequent opportunities for feedback and guidance. A time frame for accomplishing goals is set, and posttests are scheduled for that time. This date may be eight or more weeks from program initiation. Some goals may require more or less time for completion. In any case, the summative evaluation should be scheduled just after the posttesting is complete to discuss the client's degree of achievement, review the strengths and weaknesses of the initial program, set new goals, and modify the program where appropriate.

CONCLUSION

If the personal trainer is truly providing individualized programming for his or her clients, the process begins with a thoughtful evaluation of the client's total circumstances—age, health, past experiences with exercise, current training status, exercise readiness, personal interests, and goals. Once these are identified, the personal trainer must consider the appropriateness of various valid and reliable tests that will yield meaningful baseline data from which a program can be developed. The personal trainer must further consider his or her own skills, equipment availability and appropriateness, and environmental factors in selecting the assessment(s) to gather these data. A system of record keeping and storage must be developed to facilitate communication with the client after the initial testing and subsequent follow-up assessments. The entire process is part art and part science. It takes energy and initiative to continually search for assessment protocols relevant to one's clientele and to practice giving them and interpreting them correctly. The personal trainer who does so will increase his or her knowledge, skills, and confidence; and both the personal trainer and the clients will benefit from the effort.

STUDY QUESTIONS

1. A 30-year-old female client is an avid 5-kilometer runner but she would like to improve her time. Which of the following tests is the most appropriate to estimate this client's $\dot{V}O_2max$?
   A. Åstrand-Ryhming cycle ergometer test
   B. YMCA cycle ergometer test
   C. Rockport walking test
   D. 1.5-mile [2.4-kilometer] run
2. A personal trainer performs a skinfold body composition test on a client. If the same test is performed two days later with the same body fat percentage result, this test and the result are said to be
   A. valid.
   B. reliable.
   C. normative.
   D. criterion-referenced.
3. All of the following may increase the standard error of measurement of a push-up test to assess muscular strength EXCEPT:
   A. an inexperienced personal trainer
   B. an injured client
   C. testing a trained client
   D. testing a female client
4. Which of the following is a recommended sequence of tests that promotes the most accurate results when assessing general fitness?
   I. Rockport walking test
   II. sit and reach test
   III. push-up test
   IV. skinfold measurements

   A. I, II, III, IV
   B. IV, III, II, I
   C. I, III, II, IV
   D. IV, II, III, I

APPLIED KNOWLEDGE QUESTION

Four client examples are provided below with a fitness component to be tested. Identify two appropriate fitness assessment tests for each client based upon their background.

Client	Description	Fitness component to be tested	Test one	Test two
27-year-old male	Has been participating in 5-kilometer runs for 3 years	Cardiovascular endurance		
33-year-old female	Has been resistance training consistently for 10 years	Muscular strength		
41-year-old female	Has been diagnosed as obese by her physician	Body composition		
11-year-old male	Has no exercise experience or training	Muscular endurance		

REFERENCES

1. American College of Sports Medicine. 1997. *ACSM's Health/Fitness Facility Standards and Guidelines,* 2nd ed. Champaign, IL: Human Kinetics.
2. Anderson, R.E. 1996. Body composition assessment. In: *Lifestyle and Weight Management Consultant Manual,* R.T. Cotton, ed. San Diego: American Council on Exercise, pp. 70-92.
3. Baechle, T.R., and R.W. Earle. 1995. *Fitness Weight Training.* Champaign, IL: Human Kinetics.
4. Baechle, T.R., and B.R. Groves. 1992. *Weight Training: Steps to Success.* Champaign, IL: Human Kinetics.
5. Baumgartner, T.A., and A.S. Jackson. 1987. *Measurement for Evaluation in Physical Education and Exercise Science,* 3rd ed. Dubuque, IA: Brown.
6. Bompa, T.O., and L.J. Cornacchia. 1998. *Serious Strength Training: Periodization for Building Muscle Power and Mass.* Champaign, IL: Human Kinetics.
7. Brzycki, M. 1993. Strength testing—Predicting a one-rep max from reps-to-fatigue. *Journal of Physical Education, Recreation & Dance* 64 (1): 88-90.
8. Cotton, R.T. 1996. Testing and evaluation. In: *Personal Trainer Manual,* R.T. Cotton, ed. San Diego: American Council on Exercise, pp. 168-205.
9. Dalton, S. 1997. Body weight terminology, definitions, and measurement. In: *Overweight and Weight Management: The Health Professional's Guide to Understanding and Practice,* S. Dalton, ed. Gaithersburg, MD: Aspen, pp. 1-38.
10. Daniels, J., N. Oldridge, F. Nagel, and B. White. 1978. Differences and changes in $\dot{V}O_2$ among young runners 10-18 years of age. *Medicine and Science in Sports* 17: 200-203.
11. Earle, R.W. 2002. Weight training exercise prescription. In: *Essentials of Personal Training Symposium Workbook.* Lincoln, NE: NSCA Certification Commission.
12. Esquerre, R. 2001. Legal liability issues for personal trainers. Presentation at the NSCA's Personal Trainer's Clinic, Fort Lauderdale, FL, May.
13. Faigenbaum, A. 2000. Age and sex-related differences and their implications for resistance training. In: *Essentials of Strength Training and Conditioning,* 2nd ed., T.R. Baechle and R.W. Earle, eds. Champaign, IL: Human Kinetics, pp. 169-186.
14. Fleck, S.J., and W.J. Kramer. 1997. *Designing Resistance Programs.* Champaign, IL: Human Kinetics.
15. Franklin, B.A., M.H. Whaley, and E.T. Howley, eds. 2000. *ACSM's Guidelines for Exercise Testing and Prescription,* 6th ed. Philadelphia: Lippincott Williams & Wilkins.
16. Fuller, T., and A. Movahed. 1987. A current review of exercise testing: Application and interpretation. *Clinical Cardiology* 10 (3): 189-200.
17. Golding, L.A., C.R. Myers, and W.E. Sinning, eds. 1989. *Y's Ways to Physical Fitness: The Complete Guide to Fitness Testing and Instruction.* Champaign, IL: Human Kinetics.
18. Gordon, N.F. 1998. Conceptual basis for coronary artery disease risk factor assessment in clinical practice. In: *ACSM's Resource Manual for Guidelines for Exercise Testing and Prescription,* 3rd ed., J.L. Roitman, ed. Baltimore: Williams & Wilkins, pp. 3-12.
19. Hackney, A.C., D.L. Kelleher, J.T. Coyne, and J.A. Hodgdon. 1992. Military operations at moderate altitude: Effects on physical performance. *Military Medicine* 157 (12): 625-629.

20. Harman, E., J. Garhammer, and C. Pandorf. 2000. Administration, scoring, and interpretation of selected tests. In: *Essentials of Strength Training and Conditioning,* 2nd ed., T.R. Baechle and R.W. Earle, eds. Champaign, IL: Human Kinetics, pp. 287-317.

21. Harman, E., and C. Pandorf. 1994. Principles of test selection and administration. In: *Essentials of Strength Training and Conditioning,* T.R. Baechle, ed. Champaign, IL: Human Kinetics, 275-286.

22. Herbert, D.L. 1996 Legal and professional responsibilities of personal training. In: *The Business of Personal Training,* S.O. Roberts, ed. Champaign, IL: Human Kinetics, pp. 53-63.

23. Herbert, D.L., and W.G. Herbert. 1993. *Legal Aspects of Preventative and Rehabilitative Exercise Programs,* 3rd ed. Canton, OH: Professional Reports Corporation.

24. Heyward, V.H., and L.M. Stolarczyck. 1996. *Applied Body Composition Assessment.* Champaign, IL: Human Kinetics.

25. Hoeger, W.W.K., and S.A. Hoeger. 1999. *Principles and Labs for Physical Fitness,* 2nd ed. Engelwood, CO: Morton.

26. Howley, E.T. 1988. The exercise testing laboratory. In: *Resource Manual for Guidelines for Exercise Testing and Prescription,* S.N. Blair, P. Painter, R.R. Pate, L.K. Smith, and C.B. Taylor, eds. Philadelphia: Lea & Febiger.

27. Howley, E.T., and B.D. Franks. 1997. *Health Fitness Instructor's Handbook,* 3rd ed. Champaign, IL: Human Kinetics.

28. Johnson, B., and J. Nelson. 1974. *Practical Measurements for Evaluation in Physical Education,* 2nd ed. Minneapolis: Burgess.

29. Kordich, J.A. 2002. Evaluating your client: Fitness assessment protocols and norms. In: *Essentials of Personal Training Symposium Workbook.* Lincoln, NE: NSCA Certification Commission.

30. Kraning, K.K., and R.R. Gonzales. 1997. A mechanistic computer simulation of human work in heat that accounts for physical and physiological effects of clothing, aerobic fitness, and progressive dehydration. *Journal of Thermal Biology* 22 (4/5): 331-342.

31. La Forge, R. 1996. Cardiorespiratory fitness and exercise. In: *Personal Trainer Manual,* R.T. Cotton, ed. San Diego: American Council on Exercise.

32. McArdle, W.D., F.I. Katch, and V.L. Katch. 1986. *Exercise Physiology: Energy, Nutrition, and Human Performance.* Philadelphia: Lea & Febiger.

33. Morrow Jr., J.R., A.W. Jackson, J.G. Disch, and D.P. Mood. 2000. *Measurement and Evaluation in Human Performance,* 2nd ed. Champaign, IL: Human Kinetics.

34. Pandolf, K.B., and A.J. Young. 1995. Altitude and cold. In: *Heart Disease and Rehabilitation,* M.L. Pollack and D.H. Schmidt, eds. Champaign, IL: Human Kinetics.

35. Pierson Jr., R.N., J. Wang, and C.N. Boozer. 1997. Body composition and resting metabolic rate. In: *Overweight and Weight Management: The Health Professional's Guide to Understanding and Practice,* S. Dalton, ed. Gaithersburg, MD: Aspen, 39-68.

36. Plombon, M.S., and J.R. Wojcik. 2001. Nutrition and weight management. In: *ACSM's Health and Fitness Certification Review,* J.L. Roitman and K.W. Bibi, eds. Philadelphia: Lippincott Williams & Wilkins.

37. Prochaska, J.O., J.C. Norcross, and C.C. DiClemente. 1994. *Changing for Good: A Revolutionary Six-Stage Program for Overcoming Bad Habits and Moving Your Life Positively Forward.* New York: Avon Books.

38. Rozenek, R., and T.W. Storer. 1997. Client assessment tools for the personal trainer. *Strength and Conditioning* (June): 52-63.

39. Sharkey, B.J. 1991. *New Dimensions in Aerobic Fitness.* Champaign, IL: Human Kinetics.

40. Westcott, W., and T. Baechle. 1999. *Strength Training for Seniors.* Champaign, IL: Human Kinetics.

41. Wilmore, J.H., and D.L. Costill. 1988. *Training for Sport and Activity,* 3rd ed. Dubuque, IA: Brown.

42. Wilmore, J.H., and D.L. Costill. 1999. *Physiology of Sport and Exercise,* 2nd ed. Champaign, IL: Human Kinetics.

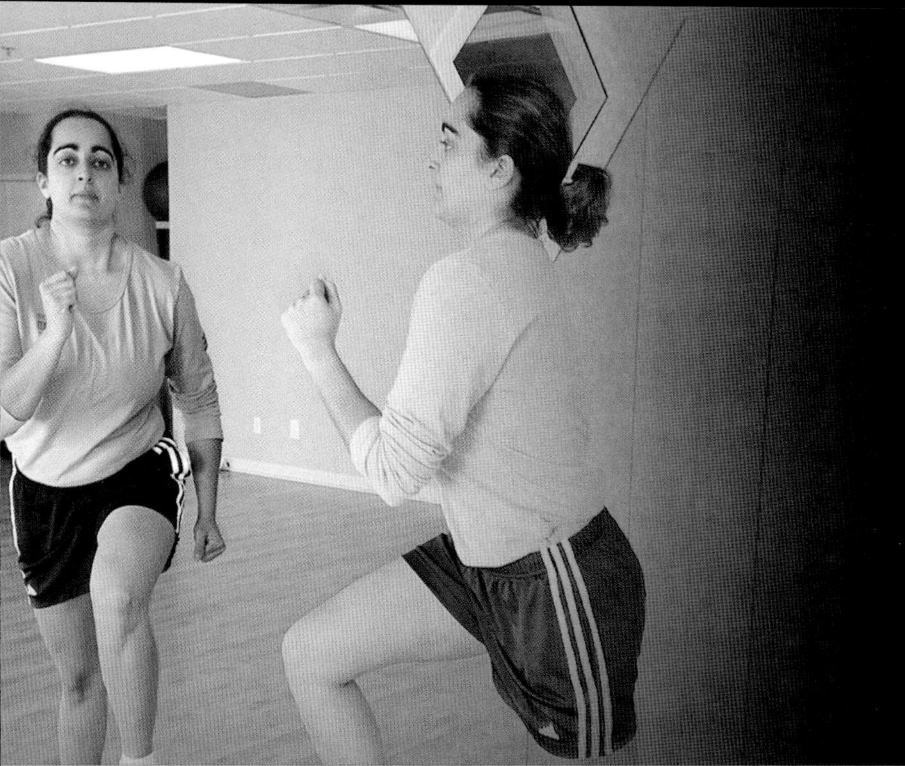

CHAPTER 11

Fitness Testing Protocols and Norms

Joel T. Cramer | Jared W. Coburn

After completing this chapter, you will be able to

- understand the protocols for selected fitness tests;
- correctly administer the selected fitness tests;
- attain valid and reliable measurements of your clients' fitness levels and select appropriate tests for individual clients; and
- compare your clients' results with normative data.

As discussed in chapter 10, personal trainers must choose valid and reliable tests that are suitable for an individual client. To do this effectively, the personal trainer must administer tests accurately and record and interpret the results.

This chapter describes the more frequently used and broadly applied fitness testing protocols for assessing a client's vital signs, body composition, cardiovascular endurance, muscular strength, muscular endurance, and flexibility. Specific descriptive or normative data are also provided for each protocol. More fitness testing protocols are available, but many do not have associated descriptive and normative data and thus are not included here.

Vital Signs

Many of the assessments that a personal trainer performs during a fitness evaluation involve two basic tasks: taking the client's pulse and blood pressure. Sometimes these assessments are performed with the client in a resting state (e.g., measuring resting heart rate); but monitoring heart rate and blood pressure changes with exercise—especially aerobic exercise—is an effective method to determine appropriate exercise intensity (i.e., keeping the client's exercise heart rate in the prescribed target zone).

Heart Rate

Most adults have a resting heart rate (HR) or *pulse* between 60 and 80 beats per minute (beats/min), with the average HR for females 7 to 10 beats/min greater than that for males [11]. Table 11.1 (page 239) provides some general guidelines for resting HR classification, while table 11.2 (page 239) provides resting HR norm values. Three commonly used field techniques for assessing resting HR may be particularly useful for personal trainers: (a) palpation, (b) auscultation, and (c) the use of heart rate monitors.

Equipment

Depending on the specific procedure used to assess HR, any one or a combination of the following devices may be necessary.

- Stopwatch
- Stethoscope
- Heart rate monitor

Palpation Procedure

Palpation is probably the most common and certainly the most cost-effective method for assessing both resting and exercise HR.

1. Use the tips of the index and middle fingers to palpate the pulse. Avoid using the thumb, because its inherent pulse may be confusing and potentially confounding. Any one of the following anatomical landmarks can be used to palpate the pulse:
   - Brachial artery: the anterior-medial aspect of the arm just distal to the belly of the biceps brachii muscle, one inch (two to three centimeters) superior to the antecubital fossa [11].
   - Carotid artery: on the anterior surface of the neck just lateral to the larynx [11]. This position is illustrated in figure 2.2, page 21. *Note:* Avoid applying too much pressure to this location when palpating for HR. Baroreceptors located in the arch of the aorta and the carotid sinuses can sense increases in applied pressure and will feed back to the medulla to decrease HR. Thus, use of the carotid site for measuring HR, if done incorrectly, can result in artificially low HR values.
   - Radial artery: on the anterior-lateral surface of the wrist, in line with the base of the thumb [11]. This position is illustrated in figure 2.2, page 21.
   - Temporal artery: the lateral side of the cranium on the anterior portion of the temporal fossa, usually along the hairline of the head at the level of the eyes.
2. If you are using a stopwatch to keep the time while counting beats, and if you start the stopwatch simultaneously with the first beat, count the first beat as zero (0). If the stopwatch has been running, count the first beat as one (1) [11]. The HR should be counted for 6, 10, 15, 30, or 60 seconds. Use the conversion chart in table 11.3 (page 239) to determine HR in beats per minute for the measurement periods of less than one minute.

Example 11.1

12 heartbeats counted during a 6-second period:

12 beats per 6 sec × 10 = 120 beats/min

18 heartbeats counted during a 10-second period:

18 beats per 10 sec × 6 = 108 beats/min

24 heartbeats counted during a 15-second period:

24 beats per 15 sec × 4 = 96 beats/min

41 heartbeats counted during a 30-second period:

41 beats per 30 sec × 2 = 82 beats/min

Typically, the shorter-duration HR counts (6, 10, and 15 seconds) are used during exercise and postexercise conditions [11]. Not only are short-duration HR counts more time efficient; they may also provide a more accurate representation of momentary HR due to the immediate fluctuations that often occur with changes in exercise intensity. Resting HR, however, is generally assessed with the longer-duration HR counts (30 and 60 seconds) to reduce the risk of miscounts and measurement error.

Auscultation Procedure

Auscultation requires the use of a stethoscope. The bell of the stethoscope should be placed directly on the skin over the third intercostal space just left of the sternum [11]. The sounds heard from the heart beating should be counted for either 30 or 60 seconds [11]. Refer to table 11.3 for the correct conversion factor for the 30-second HR count.

Heart Rate Monitor Procedure

Digital display HR monitors are becoming increasingly popular because of their validity, stability, and functionality [16]. One drawback, however, is the cost of HR monitor equipment. Nevertheless, personal trainers may find that these monitors are a very efficient and convenient way to assess HR at rest and during exercise.

Blood Pressure

Blood pressure (BP) can be defined as the forces of blood acting against vessel walls [1]. The sounds that are emitted as a result of these vibratory forces are called **Korotkoff sounds.** The detection and disappearance of Korotkoff sounds under controlled pressure environments are the basis of most BP measurement methods. Although there are various invasive and noninvasive techniques for determining BP [1], **sphygmomanometry** is the most commonly used field technique and as such provides personal trainers a convenient tool to evaluate their clients' BP. One can also use a mercury or an **aneroid sphygmomanometer.** However, both of these require the use of an inflatable air bladder-containing cuff and a stethoscope to **auscultate** the Korotkoff sounds; thus this procedure is also commonly referred to as the *cuff* or *auscultatory method* [1].

Repeated BP measurements are important for detecting hypertension (table 11.4, page 240, [19]) and for monitoring the antihypertensive effects of an exercise program or dietary changes [1]. When assessing BP, it is imperative to use calibrated equipment that meets certification standards [20] and to follow standardized protocol [19]. It is recommended that BP readings be taken with a mercury sphygmomanometer. However, recently calibrated aneroid sphygmomanometer or validated electronic devices can be used [19].

Factors Affecting Heart Rate Assessment

- Smoking/tobacco products (↑ resting HR; ↑ or ↔ exercise HR)
- Caffeine (↑ or ↔ resting and exercise HR—responses to caffeine consumption are quite variable and depend on previous exposure or consumption; therefore, caffeine consumption should be avoided prior to HR measurements)
- Environmental temperature extremes (↑ resting and exercise HR in hot environmental temperatures; HR responses can be quite variable in cold environmental temperatures and largely dependent on a client's body composition, acclimatization, and metabolism)
- Altitude (↑ HR at altitudes greater than approximately 4,000 feet [1,200 meters])
- Stress (↑ resting and exercise HR)
- Food digestion (↑ resting and exercise HR)
- Body position (↓ HR when supine, ↑ HR from supine to seated position or standing position)
- Time of day (↓ HR first thing in the morning, ↑ or ↔ during afternoon or evening hours)
- Medications (↑, ↔, or ↓ resting and exercise HR—responses to medications are quite variable and contingent on the specific medication)

↑ = increase; ↓ = decrease; ↔ = no significant change.

From Kordich 2002 [14].

Equipment

- Mercury or aneroid sphygmomanometer
- Air bladder-containing cuff
- Stethoscope

Procedure

1. Instruct the client to refrain from smoking or ingesting caffeine at least 30 minutes prior to BP measurements [19].
2. Have the client sit upright in a chair that supports the back with either the right or the left arm and forearm exposed, supinated, and supported at the level of the heart (differences between right and left arm BP measurements are marginal). *Note:* If exposing the arm by rolling or bunching up the sleeves of clothing causes any occlusion of circulation above the cuff site, ask the client to remove the constricting clothing articles [11].
3. Select the appropriate cuff size for the client. See table 11.5 (page 240) for the correct cuff size based on the client's arm circumference. To determine the arm circumference, have the client stand with arms hanging freely at the sides, and take the arm circumference measurements midway between the acromion process of the scapula and the olecranon process of the ulna [11], roughly midway between the shoulder and elbow.
4. Begin BP measurements only after the client has rested for a minimum of five minutes in the position described in step 2 [19].
5. Place the cuff on the arm so that the air bladder is directly over the brachial artery (some cuffs have a line indicating the specific placement over the brachial artery). The bottom edge of the cuff should be one inch (2.5 centimeters) above the antecubital space [1].
6. With the client's palm facing up, place the stethoscope firmly, but not hard enough to indent the skin, over the antecubital space [1]. *Note:* Most personal trainers find it easier to use their dominant hand to control the bladder airflow by placing the air bulb in the palm and using the thumb and forefinger to control the pressure release. The nondominant hand is then used to hold the stethoscope [1].
7. Position the sphygmomanometer so that the center of the mercury column or aneroid dial is at eye level and the air bladder tubing is not overlapping, obstructing, or being allowed to freely contact the stethoscope head or tubing

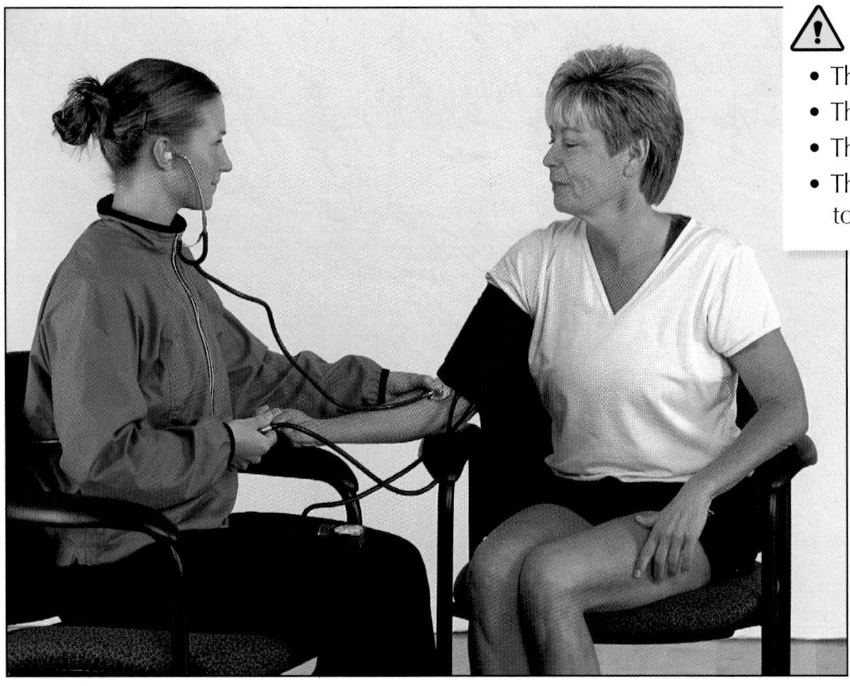

Common Errors

- The stethoscope is on backward.
- The stethoscope bell is under the cuff.
- The dial is not at the tester's eye level.
- The blood pressure cuff is positioned too close to the antecubital space.

Figure 11.1 Common errors when performing a blood pressure assessment.

[11]. See figure 11.1 for common errors when performing a blood pressure assessment.

8. Once the cuff, stethoscope, and sphygmomanometer are in place, quickly inflate the air bladder either (a) to 160 mmHg or (b) to 20 mmHg above the anticipated systolic blood pressure. Upon maximum inflation, turn the air release screw counterclockwise to release the pressure slowly at a rate of 2 to 3 mmHg per second [1].

9. Record both systolic blood pressure (SBP) and diastolic blood pressure (DBP) measurements in even numbers using units of millimeters of mercury (mmHg) to the nearest 2 mmHg on the sphygmomanometer. To do this it is necessary during cuff deflation to make a mental note of the pressure corresponding with the first audible detection of Korotkoff sounds via auscultation, or SBP. The pressure at which the Korotkoff sounds disappear is referred to as the DBP [1]. *Note:* Traditionally, Korotkoff sounds occur as sharp "thud" noises that can be similar to the sounds of gentle finger tapping on the stethoscope head (bell). Consequently, Korotkoff sounds are also similar to the extraneous noises often made when the air bladder tubing is allowed to bump against the stethoscope bell; therefore, it is important to take great care to avoid these erroneous and potentially confusing noises [11].

10. Upon the disappearance of the Korotkoff sounds, carefully observe the manometer for an additional 10 to 20 mmHg of deflation to confirm the absence of sounds. Once the absence of sounds is confirmed, release the remaining pressure rapidly and remove the cuff [1].

11. After a minimum of two minutes rest, measure BP again using the same technique. If the two consecutive measurements of either the SBP or the DBP differ by more than 5 mmHg, take a third BP measurement and record the average of the three SBP and the average of the three DBP measurements as the final scores (i.e., the SBP and the DBP; see example 11.2, Client A). If the consecutive measurements of neither the SBP nor the DBP differ by more than 5 mmHg, average the two SBP scores and average the two DBP scores to determine the final BP (see example 11.2, Client B) [1].

Once a client's BP has been determined, it can be compared to the values in table 11.6 (page 241).

Example 11.2

Client A	*SBP (mmHg)*	*DBP (mmHg)*
Trial 1	132	78
Trial 2	126	80
Difference	*6*	*2*
Trial 3 *(required)*	130	78
Averaged final score	**129**	**79**

Client B	*SBP (mmHg)*	*DBP (mmHg)*
Trial 1	110	68
Trial 2	114	66
Difference	*4*	*2*
Trial 3 *(not required)*	–	–
Averaged final score	**112**	**67**

Factors Affecting Blood Pressure Assessment

- Smoking/tobacco products (↑ resting and exercise)
- Caffeine (BP responses to caffeine consumption are quite variable and depend on previous exposure and consumption; therefore, caffeine consumption should be avoided prior to BP measurements)
- Stress (↑ resting and exercise)
- Body position (↓ when supine, ↑ from supine to seated position or standing position)
- Time of day (↓ first thing in the morning, ↑ or ↔ during afternoon or evening hours)
- Medications (↑, ↔, or ↓ resting and exercise BP—responses to medications are quite variable and contingent on the specific medication)

↑ = increase; ↓ = decrease; ↔ = no significant change.

From Kordich 2002 [14].

Body Composition

The measurement of body composition is of great interest to personal trainers and their clients. A variety of methods are available, each with its own advantages and disadvantages. Regardless of the method chosen, the personal trainer must be meticulous in following the appropriate protocol and must take great care in measuring and evaluating clients.

Body Mass Index

Personal trainers often use the body mass index (BMI) to examine **body mass** related to **stature.** BMI is a somewhat more accurate indicator of body fat than are estimates based simply on height and weight (e.g., height-weight tables).

$$\text{BMI (kg/m}^2\text{)} = \text{body weight (kg)} \div \text{height}^2\ \text{(m}^2\text{)} \quad \textbf{(11.1)}$$

Once a client's BMI has been determined, this value can be compared to those in table 11.7 (page 241).

To calculate BMI, it is necessary to have the client's height and weight. The following instructions describe how to accurately measure height and weight.

Height

Height is a basic anthropometric measurement for which "stature" is a more accurate term [1]. Although stature can be measured in several different ways, the two most common techniques involve (a) using an anthropometer typically located on the upright of a standard platform scale and (b) simply having a client stand with the back against a flat wall. The anthropometer method is convenient but requires access to a standard platform scale. The use of a wall is cost-effective but requires a right-angled device to simultaneously slide against the wall and contact the top of the client's head (crown). Regardless of the specific technique used, the following standard protocol is recommended for assessing a client's stature [1].

Equipment

Depending on the procedure used to assess a client's stature, one of the following devices is necessary.

- Standard platform scale with anthropometer arm
- Flat, ridged, right-angled device (to simultaneously slide against a wall and rest on top of client's crown)

Procedure

1. Ask the client remove all footwear.
2. Instruct the client to stand as erect as possible with feet flat on the floor and heels together.
3. Immediately before taking the measurement, instruct the client to take a deep breath and hold until the measurement has been taken.
4. Rest the anthropometer arm or measurement angle gently on the crown of the client's head.
5. Mark the wall or stabilize the anthropometer, and record the measurement to the nearest centimeter. If only inches are available as a unit of measure, then record the value to the nearest 1/4 to 1/2 inch and convert the measurement in inches to centimeters.

Once a client's height has been measured, the value can be compared to those in tables 11.8 and 11.9 (page 242).

Weight

The term *weight* is defined as the mass of an object under the normal acceleration due to gravity; therefore, a more accurate term to characterize body weight is body mass [1]. An accurate measurement of body mass can be taken only with a calibrated and certified scale. One of the types of scales most commonly used is the platform-beam scale. The personal trainer should adhere to the following standard protocol when assessing a client's body mass [1].

Equipment

- Calibrated and certified scale

Procedure

1. Ask the client to remove as much clothing and jewelry as feasible.
2. Instruct the client to step gently onto the scale and remain as still as possible throughout the measurement.
3. Record the weight to the nearest 1/4 pound or, when a sensitive metric scale is available, to the nearest 0.02 kilograms [1].
4. Convert the measurement in pounds to kilograms using the following equation:

$$\text{pounds (lb)} \div 2.2046 = \text{kilograms (kg)} \quad \textbf{(11.2)}$$

Body weight measurements can be compared to the values in table 11.10 (page 243) for men and to those in table 11.11 (page 243) for women based on age and height. For example, for a 36-year-old female client who is 60 inches (152.4 centimeters) tall and weighs 135 pounds (61.2 kilograms), table 11.11 indicates that she is 2 pounds (1.1 kilograms) below the average weight for women her age based on her height.

Factors Affecting Body Mass Assessment

- Previous meals (↑ after meal consumption)
- Time of day (↓ first thing in the morning, ↑ during afternoon or evening hours)
- Hydration status (↓ when dehydrated; body mass will ↓ postexercise due to sweat loss)

↑ = increase; ↓ = decrease; ↔ = no significant change.

Example 11.3

Client A

A female client is measured with a height of 65 inches and a weight of 145 pounds.

Stature = 65 inches × 0.0254 = 1.651 meters
Mass = 145 pounds ÷ 2.2046 = 65.8 kilograms
BMI = 65.8 ÷ (1.651 × 1.651)
= 65.8 ÷ 2.726
= 24.1

From table 11.7, a BMI of 24.1 is normal.

Client B

A male client is measured with a height of 69 inches and a weight of 214 pounds.

Stature = 69 inches × 0.0254 = 1.753 meters
Mass = 214 pounds ÷ 2.2046 = 97.1 kilograms
BMI = 97.1 ÷ (1.753 × 1.753)
= 97.1 ÷ 3.073
= 31.6

From table 11.7, a BMI of 31.6 is consistent with Class I obesity.

Skinfolds

A skinfold (SKF) indirectly measures the thickness of subcutaneous fat tissue. Skinfold measurements are highly correlated with body density measurements from underwater weighing. Percent body fat estimated from skinfolds is valid and can be reliably measured by properly trained personal trainers.

Equipment

- Skinfold caliper
- Nonelastic (i.e., plastic or metal) tape measure
- Pen or other marking device

General Considerations for Skinfold Testing

- Take all skinfold measurements on the right side of the body.
- Take the skinfold measurements when the client's skin is dry and free of lotion. In addition, skinfold measurements should always be taken before exercise. Exercise-induced changes in the hydration status of different body tissues can significantly affect the thickness of a skinfold.
- Carefully identify, measure, and mark the skinfold site.
- Grasp the skinfold firmly between the thumb and fingers. The placement of the thumb and fingers should be at least one centimeter (0.4 inches) away from the site to be measured.
- Lift the fold by placing the thumb and index finger approximately eight centimeters (three inches) apart on a line that is perpendicular to the long axis of the skinfold. The long axis is parallel to the natural cleavage lines of the skin. The thicker the fat tissue layer, the greater the separation between the thumb and finger in order to lift the fold.
- Keep the fold elevated while taking the measurement.
- Place the jaws of the caliper perpendicular to the fold, one centimeter (0.4 inches) away from the thumb and index finger, and release the jaw pressure slowly.
- Record the skinfold measurement after one to two seconds (but within four seconds) after the jaw pressure has been released.
- If the caliper is not equipped with a digital display (Skyndex II™), read the dial of the caliper to the nearest 0.1 millimeters (Harpenden™), 0.5 millimeters (Lange™ or Lafayette™), or 1

millimeter (Slim Guide™, Fat-O-Meter™, The Body Caliper™, or Accu-measure™). Studies have been conducted to compare skinfold measurements and body composition estimates from different types of calipers [8, 21]. The practical implications, however, regarding any potential variations among skinfold calipers are marginal.

- Take a minimum of two measurements at each site. If the values vary by more than two millimeters or 10%, take an additional measurement.

Harrison et al. 1988 [9].

Procedure for Specific Skinfold Sites

1. Select an appropriate combination of skinfold sites for the client.

Skinfold site	Gender
Chest	Men, women
Midaxilla	Men, women
Triceps	Men, women, boys, girls
Subscapula	Men, women
Abdomen	Men, women
Suprailium	Men, women
Thigh	Men, women
Medial calf	Boys, girls

2. Carefully identify and mark the appropriate skinfold sites:
   - Chest: Take a diagonal fold half the distance between the anterior axillary line (imaginary line extending from the front of the armpit downward) and the nipple for men (figure 11.2a), and one-third of the distance from the anterior axillary line to the nipple for women.
   - Midaxilla: Take a vertical fold on the midaxillary line (imaginary line extending from the middle of the armpit downward; it divides the body into front and back halves) at the level of the xiphoid process (bottom of the sternum) (figure 11.2b).
   - Triceps: Take a vertical fold on the posterior midline of the upper arm (over the triceps muscle), halfway between the acromion (top of shoulder) and olecranon processes (elbow); the elbow should be extended and relaxed (figure 11.2c).
   - Subscapula: Take a fold on a diagonal line coming from the vertebral (medial) border to one to two centimeters (0.8 inches) from the inferior angle (bottommost point) of the scapula (figure 11.2d).
   - Abdomen: Take a vertical fold at a lateral distance of approximately two centimeters (one inch) from the umbilicus (figure 11.2e).
   - Suprailium: Take a diagonal fold above the crest of the ilium (top of the pelvis) at the spot where an imaginary line would come down from the anterior axillary line (figure 11.2f).
   - Thigh: Take a vertical fold on the anterior aspect of the thigh midway between hip and knee joints (figure 11.2g).
   - Medial calf: Have the client place the right leg on a bench with the knee flexed at 90 degrees. On the medial border, mark the level of the greatest calf girth. Raise a vertical skinfold on the medial side of the right calf one centimeter (0.4 inches) above the mark, and measure the fold at the maximal girth (figure 11.2h).
3. Using the appropriate population-specific equation from table 11.12 (page 244), calculate the estimated body density from the skinfold measurements.
4. Enter the body density into the appropriate population-specific equation from table 11.13 (page 245) to calculate the percent body fat.
5. Compare the percent body fat to the normative values in table 11.14 (page 246).

From Baumgartner and Jackson 1999 [5]; Heyward 1988 [10].

Bioelectrical Impedance Analysis and Near-Infrared Interactance Techniques for Measuring Body Composition

Bioelectrical impedance analysis (BIA) has been developed as a potential method for measuring body composition. Bioelectrical impedance analysis works via measurement of the amount of impedance or resistance to a small, painless electrical current passed through the body between two electrodes, which are often placed on the wrist and ankle [7]. The underlying concept is that leaner clients conduct this electrical current with less resistance than those who are carrying more adipose tissue. Some authors have suggested that BIA methods for determining body composition are roughly as accurate as skinfold techniques except for clients who are either very lean or obese, in which cases BIA is not as accurate [6]. Others, however, have questioned the validity and sensitivity of BIA body composition assessments [7, 17] and have stated that BIA measurements can be easily and significantly affected by factors such as hydration status, skin temperature, and racial characteristics [17].

The **near-infrared interactance (NIR)** method of measuring body composition is derived from its use in agriculture to assess the body composition in animals, quality of meats, and lipid concentrations in grains [17]. This method works on the principles of the wavelength changes of light that is absorbed and reflected by different tissues in the

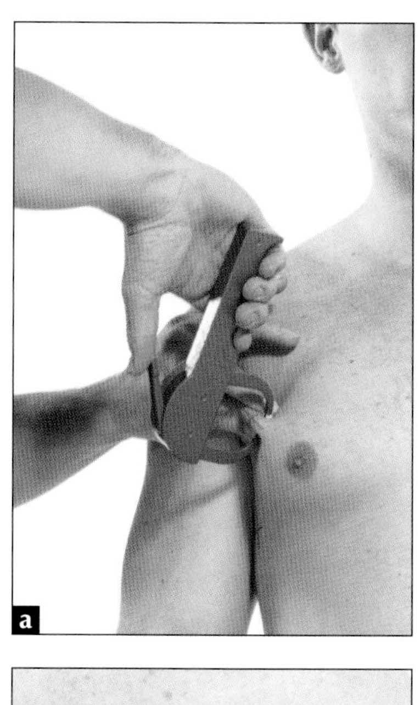

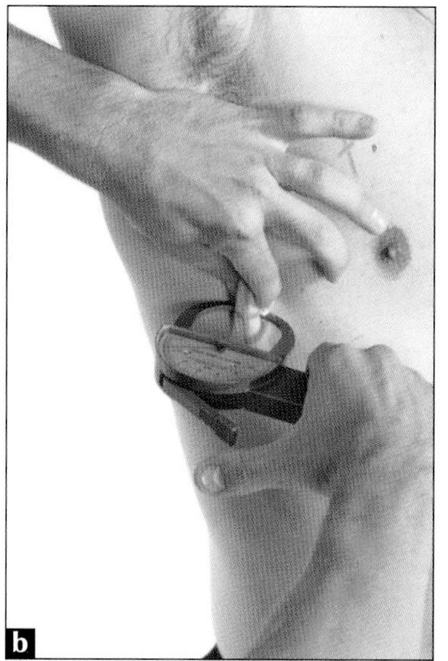

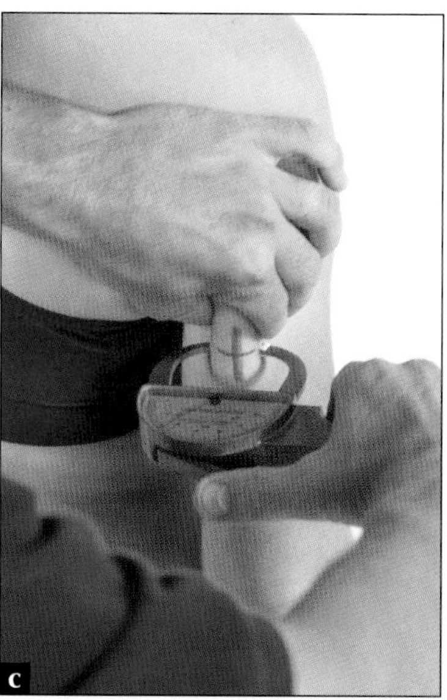

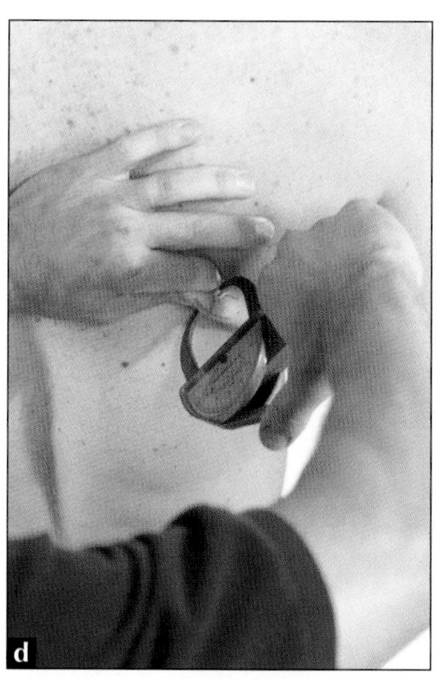

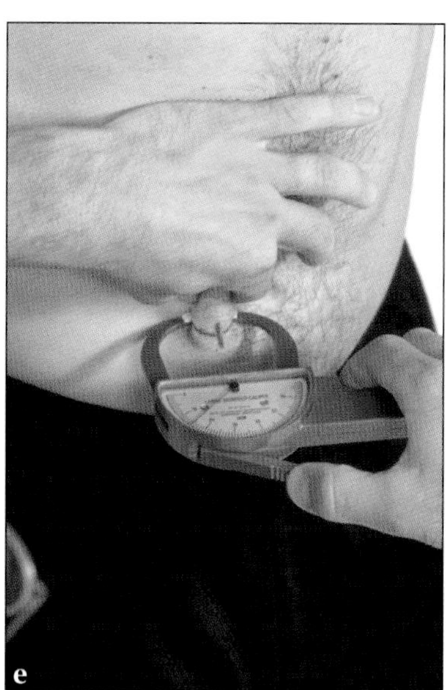

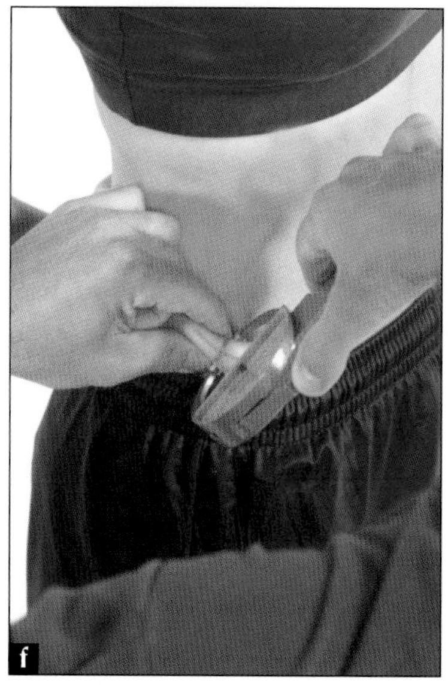

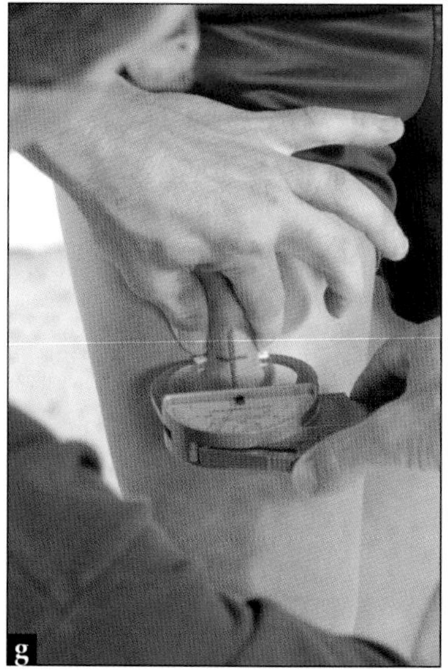

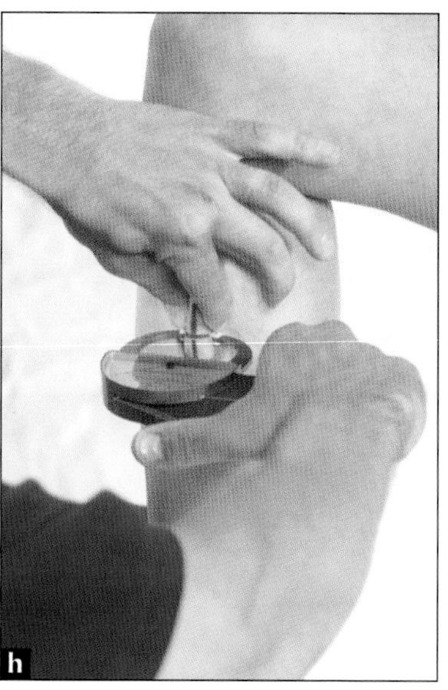

Figure 11.2 Skinfold measurements: *(a)* chest skinfold, *(b)* midaxilla skinfold, *(c)* triceps skinfold, *(d)* subscapula skinfold, *(e)* abdomen skinfold, *(f)* suprailium skinfold, *(g)* thigh skinfold, and *(h)* medial calf skinfold.

body at various anatomical sites, such as the biceps, triceps, subscapula, suprailium, and thigh [7]. Equipment for NIR consists of a fiber-optic probe or "light wand" that emits low-level electromagnetic radiation light waves [7]. Most authors [7, 17] agree, however, that NIR body composition measurements (a) are not as accurate as skinfolds, (b) are not sensitive to changes in body composition, and (c) can produce large measurement errors.

Waist-to-Hip Girth Ratio

Although not truly a measure of body composition per se, the measurement of the waist-to-hip ratio is a valuable tool for assessing relative fat distribution and risk of disease. People with more fat in the trunk, particularly abdominal fat, are at increased risk for a variety of cardiovascular and metabolic diseases [2].

Equipment

- Nonelastic (i.e., plastic or metal) tape measure

Procedure

1. Place tape measure around girth of waist (smallest girth around the abdomen) and hip (largest girth measured around the buttocks). See figures 11.3 and 11.4.
2. Hold zero end of tape in one hand, positioned below the other part of the tape, which is held in the other hand.
3. Apply tension to the tape so that it fits snugly around the body part but does not indent the skin or compress the subcutaneous tissue.
4. Align the tape in a horizontal plane, parallel to the floor.
5. To determine the waist-to-hip ratio, divide the waist circumference by the hip circumference.
6. Use table 11.15 (page 247) to assess risk.

From Heyward 1998 [10].

Cardiovascular Endurance

The personal trainer can use submaximal cardiovascular endurance tests to attain a reasonably accurate estimation of a client's $\dot{V}O_2$max [2]. Submaximal exercise tests are used most often because of high equipment expenses, the personnel needed, and the increased risks associated with maximal tests. Table 10.3 on page 209 provides a list of indicators a personal trainer should look for that would require an exercise test to be terminated immediately.

The concept behind a submaximal test is to monitor HR, BP, and/or rating of perceived exertion (RPE) during exercise until a predetermined percentage of the client's predicted maximal HR

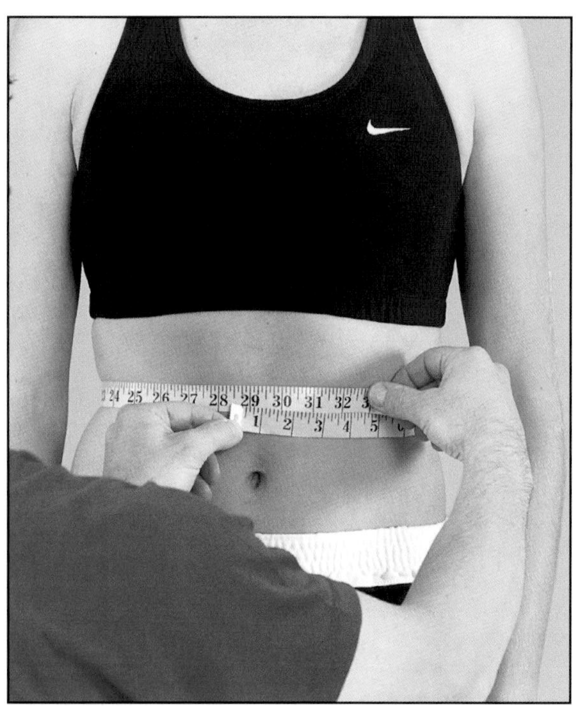

Figure 11.3 Waist circumference measurement.

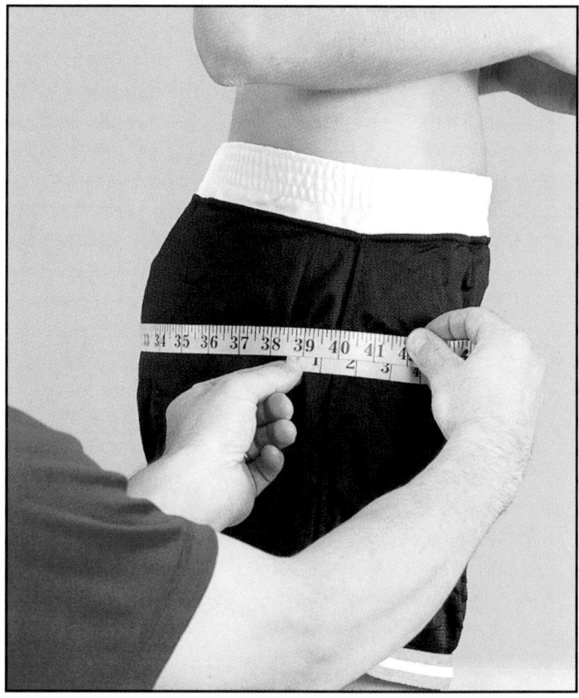

Figure 11.4 Hip circumference measurement.

Assumptions and Solutions for Submaximal Exercise Tests

Assumption 1: Heart rate measurements must be **steady state.**

Solution: Heart rate can fluctuate dramatically with sudden changes in work rate. To ensure that HR has achieved steady state, personal trainers should record HR values at the end of a constant work rate stage or after two to three minutes of exercise at a constant work rate [2]. Steady-state HR is defined as two consecutive HR measurements that are within 6 beats/min of each other [2].

Assumption 2: True maximal HR for a given age must be the same for all clients.

Solution: For any given age, maximal HR can vary as much as ±10 beats/min across individuals [2]; therefore, the typical equation to calculate age-predicted maximal HR can introduce an unknown error into the model for submaximal estimation of $\dot{V}O_2$max.

$$\text{age-predicted maximal HR (beats/min)} = 220 - \text{age (years)} \quad \textbf{(11.3)}$$

Assumption 3: The relationship between HR and work rate must be strong, positive, and linear.

Solution: The positive relationship between HR and workload is most linear between 50% and 90% of maximal HR [1]. One should consider this when extrapolating HR versus work rate data points. In example 11.4, only the HR values at work rates 2, 3, and 4 should be used to estimate $\dot{V}O_2$max since those HR values are between 50% and 90% of the age-predicted maximal HR.

Assumption 4: Mechanical efficiency ($\dot{V}O_2$ at a given work rate) is the same for all clients.

Solution: Personal trainers should choose a test that is specific to the client's existing cardiovascular exercise mode(s), daily activities, or both. For example, if a client typically goes for long walks three or four times per week, the Rockport walking test or a submaximal treadmill walking test might be the best indicator of that client's $\dot{V}O_2$max.

is achieved, at which point the test is terminated. To get a true measure of a client's cardiovascular endurance, one would need to conduct a maximal test, taking the client to their extreme limits of HR and oxygen consumption rate ($\dot{V}O_2$max). Maximal tests, however, are not safe or necessary for many clients and sometimes cannot be conducted without physician supervision; thus submaximal tests are used instead. By their very nature, submaximal tests provide *estimations* of a client's $\dot{V}O_2$max. However, most submaximal exercise testing protocols, such as those presented in this chapter, provide a valid, reliable, specific, and sensitive estimation of $\dot{V}O_2$max. And, like many estimation techniques, there are certain assumptions that must be considered. Therefore, refer to the above outline to understand the basic assumptions underlying a submaximal exercise test as well as some potential solutions that the personal trainer should consider.

General Procedures for Cycle Ergometer Testing

1. Ensure that the cycle ergometer has been recently and correctly calibrated.
2. Adjust the seat height so that there is a slight flexion at the knee joint (about 5 degrees) at maximal leg extension (lowest pedal position) with the ball of the foot on the pedal [11].
3. The client should be seated on the cycle ergometer in an upright position with the hands properly positioned on the handlebars [11]. Ask the client to maintain the same grip and posture throughout the duration of the test.
4. Establish the pedaling cadence before setting the resistance [11]. If a metronome is necessary to set the pedaling cadence, set it at twice the desired cadence so that one full pedal revolution occurs for every two metronome beats (e.g., set the metronome at 100 for a test requiring a pedaling cadence of 50 revolutions per minute [rpm]) [11].
5. Set the workload. The workload on a cycle ergometer usually refers to the work rate. Work rate is defined as a power output and is measured in units of kilogram-meters per minute ($kg \cdot m \cdot min^{-1}$) or watts (W) that can be calculated with the following equations:

$$\text{work rate (kg} \cdot \text{m} \cdot \text{min}^{-1}) = \text{res. (kg)} \times \text{dis. (m)} \times \text{cad. (rpm)} \quad \textbf{(11.4)}$$

where resistance (res.) = the amount of friction placed on the flywheel (usually in kilograms or kiloponds)

distance (dis.) = the distance the flywheel travels as a result of one pedal revolution (meters)

cadence (cad.) = the pedaling cadence (rpm)

$$\text{work rate (W)} = \text{work rate (kg} \cdot \text{m} \cdot \text{min}^{-1}) \div 6.12 \quad \textbf{(11.5)}$$

- Setting the work rate on an electronically braked cycle ergometer is usually simple, because these expensive ergometers often have computer- or digitally interfaced work rate settings that automatically adjust the resistance based on the pedaling cadence to maintain a predetermined work rate.
- On a mechanically braked ergometer, maintaining a work rate is more difficult. Mechanically braked cycle ergometers have a flywheel "braked" by a belt that adds resistance by friction as it is tightened. Since the work rate is controlled by the resistance and the pedaling cadence, both must remain constant to maintain the work rate.

6. Check the resistance setting frequently during the test to avoid the unexpected increases or decreases that are common with use of mechanically braked cycle ergometers [11].
7. Continuously monitor the appearance and symptoms of the client (see table 10.3 on page 209 for general indications for stopping an exercise test in low-risk adults [2]).
8. During multistage tests (i.e., the YMCA cycle ergometer test):
   - Assess HR during the end of each stage or until steady-state HR is achieved. For example, if the client is working through a three-minute stage, measure their HR during the final 15-30 seconds of the second and third minutes. If the consecutive HR measurements are not within six beats/min of each other, continue the stage for one more minute and measure HR again (see HR testing protocol [2]).
   - Assess BP near the end of each stage and repeatedly in the case of a hypo- or hypertensive response (see BP testing protocol [2]).
   - Assess RPE near the end of each stage using either the 6-20 or the 0-10 scale [2] (see figure 16.3 on page 407).
9. Terminate the test if the client (a) reaches 85% of his or her predicted maximal HR or (b) meets only one of the criteria on table 10.3 [2].
10. Once you have terminated the test, initiate an appropriate cool-down. The cool-down can be an active recovery period consisting of light pedaling at a resistance equal to or less than the starting resistance. Or, if the client is uncomfortable or is experiencing signs and symptoms (table 10.3), a passive recovery may be necessary [2].
11. During the cool-down, monitor HR, BP, and signs and symptoms regularly for at least four minutes. If unusual or abnormal responses occur, further monitoring of the recovery period will be necessary [2].

YMCA Cycle Ergometer Test

The YMCA cycle ergometer test is a submaximal, multistage exercise test for cardiovascular endurance. This is a traditionally popular test that was designed to progress the client to reach 85% of his or her predicted maximal HR using three-minute stages of increasing work rate.

Equipment

- Mechanically or electrically braked cycle ergometer
- Metronome (if the cycle ergometer does not have an rpm gauge)
- Stopwatch
- Heart rate and BP measurement equipment (see "Heart Rate" and "Blood Pressure" sections earlier in this chapter)
- Rating of perceived exertion scale

Procedure

Table 11.16 (page 248) contains the protocol for the YMCA cycle ergometer test for submaximal estimations of $\dot{V}O_2$max.

Estimating $\dot{V}O_2$max From the YMCA Cycle Ergometer Test

When the test is complete, the personal trainer should have the following data:

- Body weight (kg)
- Age-predicted maximal HR
- At least two HR measurements at each work rate up to 85% of the age-predicted maximal HR
- A BP measurement at each work rate
- An RPE assessment at each work rate

To attain an estimation of the client's $\dot{V}O_2max$:

1. Plot the HR (Y-axis in beats/min) versus work rate (X-axis in kg · m · min^{-1} or W) on a graph (example 11.4).
2. Construct a horizontal line at the age-predicted maximal HR value (A in figure 11.5).
3. Extrapolate the data by drawing a line of best fit for the HR values between 50% and 90% of the age-predicted maximal HR (B in figure 11.5).
4. Continue the line of best fit (B) beyond the final data point until it crosses the horizontal line (A) representing the age-predicted maximal HR.
   - Construct a vertical line from the intersection (C in figure 11.5) of the line of best fit and the horizontal age-predicted maximal HR line. Extend the vertical line to the X-axis and record the corresponding work rate value (D in figure 11.5). This X value is the predicted maximal work rate that will be used to calculate the estimated $\dot{V}O_2max$ (E in figure 11.5).
5. If the predicted maximal work rate is in kg · m · min^{-1}, it will need to be converted to watts (W). Use equation 11.5 to convert the kg · m · min^{-1} value to W.
6. Use the following equation (from [2]) to calculate the predicted $\dot{V}O_2max$ value in milliliters per kilogram per minute (ml · kg^{-1} · min^{-1}):

   $$\dot{V}O_2max\ (ml \cdot kg^{-1} \cdot min^{-1}) = [(10.8 \times W) \div BW] + 7 \quad \textbf{(11.6)}$$

   where W = the predicted maximal work rate (in watts) and BW = body weight (kg).
7. Once a client's $\dot{V}O_2max$ has been estimated (ml · kg^{-1} · min^{-1}), use table 11.17 (page 249) to rank the client's $\dot{V}O_2max$ based on his or her age. For example, if the $\dot{V}O_2max$ has just been estimated to be 36.0 ml · kg^{-1} · min^{-1} for a 46-year-old male client, that client would rank among the 35th percentile when compared to others his age. In other words, one can say that 35% of men his age have a lower $\dot{V}O_2max$, while 65% have a higher $\dot{V}O_2max$.

Example 11.4

Client A, a 23-year-old male client who weighs 181 pounds (82 kilograms), has just completed a YMCA cycle ergometer test with the following data:

Resting HR = 62 beats/min

Resting BP = 124/78 mmHg

Age-predicted maximal HR = 197 beats/min

$$220 - 23 = 197 \text{ beats/min} \quad \textbf{(11.3)}$$

85% age-predicted maximal HR = 167 beats/min

$$0.85 \times 197 \text{ beats/min} = 167 \text{ beats/min}$$

50% age-predicted maximal HR = 99 beats/min

$$0.50 \times 197 \text{ beats/min} = 99 \text{ beats/min}$$

90% age-predicted maximal HR = 177 beats/min

$$0.90 \times 197 \text{ beats/min} = 177 \text{ beats/min}$$

Stage	Work rate	Elapsed time	HR	Average HR*	BP	RPE
1	150 kg · m · min^{-1}	2:00	88 beats/min			
1	150 kg · m · min^{-1}	3:00	88 beats/min	88 beats/min*	134/82 mmHg	9
2	600 kg · m · min^{-1}	5:00	132 beats/min			

(continued)

Example 11.4 *(continued)*

Stage	Work rate	Elapsed time	HR	Average HR*	BP	RPE
2	600 kg · m · min^{-1}	6:00	136 beats/min	134 beats/min*	148/76 mmHg	13
3	750 kg · m · min^{-1}	8:00	154 beats/min			
3	750 kg · m · min^{-1}	9:00	158 beats/min	156 beats/min*	152/80 mmHg	15
4	900 kg · m · min^{-1}	11:00	164 beats/min			
4	900 kg · m · min^{-1}	12:00	168 beats/min	166 beats/min*	160/82 mmHg	17

*Average HR was calculated by averaging the two consecutive HR values at each work rate.

Step 1: Plot all of the average HR measurements (Y-axis) versus the corresponding work rates (X-axis) on a graph.
Step 2: Construct a horizontal line (A in figure 11.5) at 197 beats/min (the age-predicted maximum heart rate).
Step 3: Construct a line of best fit (B in figure 11.5) for the plotted data points (from step 1) and extend the line beyond the horizontal line at 197 beats/min (A in figure 11.5).
Step 4: Construct a vertical line (D in figure 11.5) from the intersection (C in figure 11.5) of lines A and B that extends to the X-axis.
Step 5: Identify the X-axis value that corresponds with the vertical line D. This value is the predicted maximal work rate that will be used to calculate the estimated $\dot{V}O_2max$ (E in figure 11.5). In this example, it is 1,172 kg · m · min^{-1}.

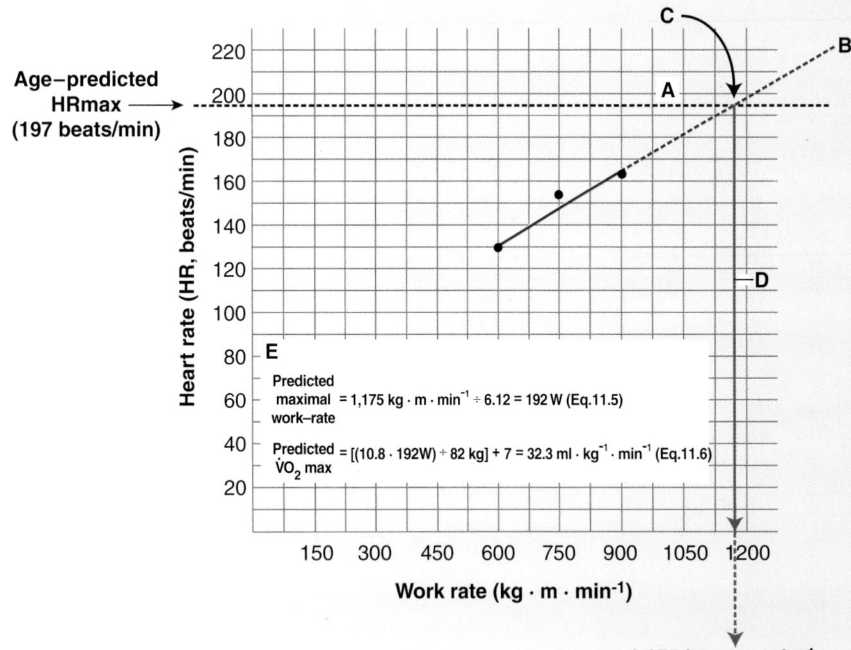

Figure 11.5 Using data from example 11.4, this figure illustrates how to graph a client's submaximal YMCA test data and how to construct the horizontal line for predicted maximal HR (A), extrapolate the line of best fit (B), identify the intersection (C), construct a vertical line for predicted maximal work rate (D), and use equations 11.5 and 11.6 to determine the predicted $\dot{V}O_2max$ (E).

Step 6: Use equation 11.5 to convert the kg · m · min^{-1} value to watts.

Work rate (W) = work rate (kg · m · min^{-1}) ÷ 6.12 **(11.5)**

from step 5, predicted maximal work rate (kg · m · min^{-1}) = 1,175 kg · m · min^{-1}

predicted maximal work rate (W) = 1,175 kg · m · min^{-1} ÷ 6.12

predicted maximal work rate (W) = 192 W

Step 7: Use equation 11.2 to convert the client's body weight in pounds to kilograms.

pounds (lb) ÷ 2.2046 = kilograms (kg) **(11.2)**

body weight (lb) = 181 lb

181 lb ÷ 2.2046 = kilograms (kg)

body weight (kg) = 82 kg

Step 8: Use equation 11.6 (from [2]) to determine the predicted $\dot{V}O_2$max score in $ml \cdot kg^{-1} \cdot min^{-1}$.

$\dot{V}O_2max\ (ml \cdot kg^{-1} \cdot min^{-1}) = [(10.8 \times W) \div BW] + 7$ **(11.6)**

from step 6, predicted maximal work rate (W) = 192 W

body weight (kg) = 82 kg

$\dot{V}O_2max\ (ml \cdot kg^{-1} \cdot min^{-1}) = [(10.8 \times 192) \div 82] + 7$

$\dot{V}O_2max\ (ml \cdot kg^{-1} \cdot min^{-1}) = 32.3\ ml \cdot kg^{-1} \cdot min^{-1}$

Step 9: Use table 11.17 [2] to compare this client's predicted $\dot{V}O_2$max of 32.3 $ml \cdot kg^{-1} \cdot min^{-1}$ to normative values. 32.3 $ml \cdot kg^{-1} \cdot min^{-1}$ for a 23-year-old male ranks at less than the 10th percentile. Therefore, more than 90% of the population [2] have higher $\dot{V}O_2$max scores, while less than 10% have a lower $\dot{V}O_2$max.

Åstrand-Ryhming Cycle Ergometer Test

The Åstrand-Ryhming cycle ergometer test is a single-stage test [3]. Total duration of the test is six minutes.

Equipment

- Mechanically or electrically braked cycle ergometer
- Metronome (if the cycle ergometer does not have an rpm gauge)
- Stopwatch

Procedure

1. Set the pedaling cadence at 50 rpm.
2. Set the work rate. Work rates used for the Åstrand-Ryhming test are chosen based on gender and fitness level [1]. Note that when estimating a client's fitness level (unconditioned vs. conditioned) prior to the Åstrand-Ryhming test to determine the starting work rate, the recommendation is to always choose the more conservative work rate (unconditioned) if there is any question about the client's current status.

Males, unconditioned	300 or 600 $kg \cdot m \cdot min^{-1}$
Males, conditioned	600 or 900 $kg \cdot m \cdot min^{-1}$
Females, unconditioned	300 or 450 $kg \cdot m \cdot min^{-1}$
Females, conditioned	450 or 600 $kg \cdot m \cdot min^{-1}$

3. Instruct the client to begin pedaling. Once the proper cadence is achieved, start the stopwatch. After two minutes, take a HR measurement.
   - If the HR is ≥120 beats/min, have the client continue the selected work rate throughout the six-minute test duration.
   - If the HR after two minutes is <120, increase the resistance to the next highest increment or until the HR measurement is ≥120 beats/min after two minutes of riding at a constant work rate.
4. Take HR measurements at the end of the fifth and sixth minutes of the test, average them, and use this average value to estimate $\dot{V}O_2$max in liters per minute ($L \cdot min^{-1}$) from table 11.18 (page 250) for males and table 11.19 (page 251) for females.
5. Once the $\dot{V}O_2$max is estimated, it must be corrected for the age of the client. To obtain the age-corrected $\dot{V}O_2$max estimation, multiply the unaltered $\dot{V}O_2$max value ($L \cdot min^{-1}$) from table 11.18 or table 11.19 by the appropriate age correction factor in table 11.20 (page 252).
6. After age correction of the $\dot{V}O_2$max estimation ($L \cdot min^{-1}$), it can then be converted to $ml \cdot kg^{-1} \cdot min^{-1}$ by the following equation:

$$\dot{V}O_2max\ (ml \cdot kg^{-1} \cdot min^{-1}) = \dot{V}O_2max \text{ in } L \cdot min^{-1} \times 1{,}000 \div BW \quad \textbf{(11.7)}$$

where BW = body weight in kilograms (kg).

7. Compare the age-corrected $\dot{V}O_2$max estimations ($ml \cdot kg^{-1} \cdot min^{-1}$) from the Åstrand-Ryhming test to the normative values listed in table 11.21 (page 252) [1].

Example 11.5

A 57-year-old female client who weighs 145 pounds (66 kilograms) has just completed the Åstrand-Ryhming cycle ergometer test. The following data were recorded:

Work rate = 450 kg · m · min^{-1}

Heart rate after 2nd min = 122 beats/min

Heart rate after 5th min = 129 beats/min

Heart rate after 6th min = 135 beats/min

Step 1. (129 beats/min + 135 beats/min) ÷ 2 = 132 beats/min average.

Step 2. Estimated $\dot{V}O_2max$ value from table 11.19 for an average HR of 132 beats/min and a work rate of 450 kg · m · min^{-1} = 2.7 L · min^{-1}.

Step 3. Age correction factor from table 11.20 for a 57-year-old client = 0.70.

Step 4. 2.7 L · min^{-1} × 0.70 age correction factor = 1.89 L · min^{-1}.

Step 5. (1.89 L · min^{-1} × 1,000) ÷ 66 kilograms = 28.64 ml · kg^{-1} · min^{-1}.

Step 6. Aerobic fitness category from table 11.21 for 28.64 ml · kg^{-1} · min^{-1} for a 57-year-old female = Good.

Step 7. Percentile rank from table 11.17 for 28.64 ml · kg^{-1} · min^{-1} for a 57-year-old female: ~ 55%.

YMCA Step Test

The YMCA step test is a basic, inexpensive cardiovascular endurance test that can be easily administered individually or to large groups. This test classifies fitness levels based on the postexercise HR response but does not provide an estimation of $\dot{V}O_2max$. The objective of the YMCA step test is to have the client step up and down to a set cadence for three minutes and to measure the HR recovery response immediately after the test.

Equipment

- 12-inch (30-centimeter) step bench or box
- Metronome set at 96 beats/min
- Stopwatch

Procedure

1. For familiarization, the client should listen to the cadence prior to stepping.
2. Instruct the client to step "up, up, down, down" to a cadence of 96 beats/min, which allows 24 steps per minute.
3. Have the client continue stepping for three minutes.
4. Immediately after the final step, help the client sit down and, within five seconds, measure the HR for one minute.
5. Compare the one-minute recovery HR value to the normative values in table 11.22 (page 253).

Distance Run and Walk Test Considerations

Distance run tests are based on the assumption that a more "fit" client will be able to run a given distance in less time or run a greater distance in a given period of time. These tests are practical, inexpensive, less time-consuming than other tests, and easy to administer to large groups. They also can be used to classify the cardiovascular endurance level of healthy men under 40 years of age and healthy women under 50 years of age. The personal trainer cannot, however, use field tests to detect or control for cardiac episodes because HR and BP are typically not monitored during the performance of these tests.

It is important to note that these field tests are effort-based assessments and are suited for clients who can run (or walk briskly) for either 12 minutes, 1.5 miles (2.4 kilometers), or 1 mile (1.6 kilometers). Examples of clients for whom these tests are appropriate are those who have been training for several weeks and those who regularly use running or fast walking as a mode of cardiovascular exercise. Other tests for $\dot{V}O_2max$ such as the Åstrand-Ryhming cycle ergometer test or the YMCA step test are recommended for clients who do not meet these criteria.

12-Minute Run/Walk

The 12-minute run/walk test is a field test designed to measure the distance traveled over 12 minutes of running/walking. After distance is recorded as the test score, it is used in a regression equation (equation 11.8) to estimate $\dot{V}O_2max$.

Equipment

- 400-meter (437-yard) track or flat course with measured distances so that the number of laps completed can be easily counted and multiplied by the course distance

- Visible place markers—may be necessary to divide the course into predetermined section lengths (e.g., every one-fourth or one-half of a lap) so that the exact distance covered in 12 minutes can be determined quickly
- Stopwatch

Procedure

1. Instruct the client to run as far as possible during the 12-minute duration. Walking is allowed; however, the objective of this test is to cover as much distance as possible in 12 minutes.
2. Record the total distance completed in meters. For example, a client has just completed five full laps and one-fourth of the last lap (5.25 laps). Since there are 400 meters per lap, the client completed 2,100 meters (5.25 laps × 400 meters = 2,100 meters).
3. Use the following equation (from [11]) to estimate the client's $\dot{V}O_2max$ ($ml \cdot kg^{-1} \cdot min^{-1}$):

$$\dot{V}O_2max\ (ml \cdot kg^{-1} \cdot min^{-1}) = [0.0268 \times (D)] - 11.3 \quad \textbf{(11.8)}$$

where D = distance completed in meters.

4. You can then compare estimated $\dot{V}O_2max$ scores to the normative values listed in table 11.17 [2].

Example 11.6

A 31-year-old female client who weighs 128 pounds (58 kilograms) has just completed the 12-minute run. The following data were recorded:

12-min run distance = 1.16 miles (6,109 ft; 1,862 m)

1. [0.0268 × (1,862 meters)] – 11.3 = 38.60 ml · $kg^{-1} \cdot min^{-1}$.
2. Percentile rank from table 11.17 for 38.60 ml · $kg^{-1} \cdot min^{-1}$ for a 31-year-old female = 80th percentile.

1.5-Mile Run

The 1.5-mile run is a field test designed to measure the time it takes for a client to run 1.5 miles. Once the time is recorded as the test score, it is used in a regression equation (equation 11.9) to estimate $\dot{V}O_2max$.

Equipment

- 400-meter (437-yard) track or flat course with the 1.5-mile (2.4-kilometer) distance measured (to measure the course, use an odometer or measuring wheel [11])
- Stopwatch

Procedure

1. Instruct clients to cover the 1.5-mile (2.4-kilometer) distance in the fastest possible time. Walking is allowed, but the objective is to complete the distance in as short a time as possible.
2. Call out or record the elapsed time (in minutes and seconds, 00:00) as the client crosses the finish line.
3. Convert the seconds to minutes by dividing the seconds by 60. For example, if a client's time for the test is 12:30, the run time is converted to 12.5 minutes (30 ÷ 60 seconds = 0.5 minutes).
4. Use the following equation (from [11]) to estimate the client's $\dot{V}O_2max$ ($ml \cdot kg^{-1} \cdot min^{-1}$):

$$\dot{V}O_2max\ (ml \cdot kg^{-1} \cdot min^{-1}) = 88.02 - (0.1656 \times BW) - (2.76 \times (time) + (3.716 \times gender^{*}) \quad \textbf{(11.9)}$$

where BW = body weight in kilograms (kg), and time = 1.5-mile run time to completion (to the nearest hundredth of a minute, 0.00 min).

*For gender, substitute 1 for males and 0 for females.

5. Estimated $\dot{V}O_2max$ scores can be compared to the normative values listed in table 11.17 [2].

Example 11.7

A 28-year-old male client who weighs 171 pounds (77.6 kilograms) has just completed the 1.5-mile (2.4-kilometer) run. The following data were recorded:

1.5-mile run time = 8:52 min:sec

1. 52 seconds ÷ 60 seconds = 0.87 minutes, so 8:52 min:sec = 8.87 minutes.
2. 88.02 – [0.1656 × (77.6)] – [2.76× (8.87)] + [3.716 × (1 *for males*)] = 54.40 ml · kg^{-1} · min^{-1}.
3. Percentile rank from table 11.17 for 54.40 ml · $kg^{-1} \cdot min^{-1}$ for a 28-year-old male = over 90th percentile.

Rockport Walking Test

The Rockport walking test has been developed to estimate $\dot{V}O_2max$ for men and women ages 18 to 69 years [12]. Because this test requires only walking at a fast pace, it is useful for testing older or sedentary clients.

Equipment

- Stopwatch
- Measured 1.0-mile (1.6-kilometer) walking course that is flat and uninterrupted (preferably an outdoor track)

Procedure

1. Instruct the client to walk 1.0 mile (1.6 kilometers) as briskly as possible.
2. Immediately after the test, calculate the client's HR (in beats per minute) using a 15-second HR count duration (see "Heart Rate" section earlier in this chapter).
3. Convert the seconds to minutes by dividing the seconds by 60 (see step 3 for the 1.5-mile run procedure).
4. Estimate the client's $\dot{V}O_2max$ ($ml \cdot kg^{-1} \cdot min^{-1}$) using the following equation (from [18]):

$$\dot{V}O_2max\ (ml \cdot kg^{-1} \cdot min^{-1}) = 132.853 - (0.0769 \times BW) - (0.3877 \times age) + (6.315 \times gender^*) - (3.2649 \times time) - (0.1565 \times HR) \quad \textbf{(11.10)}$$

where BW = body weight in pounds,
age = age in years,
time = 1.0-mile walk time to completion (to the nearest hundredth of a minute, 0.00 minutes), and
HR = heart rate in beats per minute.

*For gender, substitute 1 for males and 0 for females.

5. Estimated $\dot{V}O_2max$ scores can be compared to the normative values listed in table 11.17 [2].
6. 1.0-mile walk times can also be compared to the normative values listed in table 11.23 (page 253) [18].

1-Mile Run

The 1-mile run has been developed to estimate cardiovascular endurance for children ages 6 to 17 years [22].

Equipment

- Stopwatch
- A flat and uninterrupted 1.0-mile (1.6-kilometer) course (e.g., an outdoor track)

Example 11.8

A 52-year-old male client who weighs 228 pounds (103.4 kilograms) has just completed the Rockport walking test. The following data were recorded:

Posttest HR = 159 beats/min

1.0-mile walk time = 10:35 min:sec

1. 35 seconds ÷ 60 seconds = 0.58 minutes; 10:35 min:sec = 10.58 minutes.
2. 132.853 – [0.0769 × (228 pounds)] – [0.3877× (52)] + [6.315 × (1 *for males*)] – [3.2649 × (10.58 minutes)] – [0.1565 × (159)] = 42.05 $ml \cdot kg^{-1} \cdot min^{-1}$.
3. Percentile rank from table 11.17 for 42.05 $ml \cdot kg^{-1} \cdot min^{-1}$ for a 52-year-old male = 80th to 90th percentile.
4. Rating from table 11.23 for 10:35 min:sec = Good.
5. Percentile rank from table 11.23 for 10:35 min:sec = over 90th percentile.

Procedure

1. Instruct clients to cover the one-mile (1.6-kilometer) distance in the fastest possible time. Walking may be interspersed with running, but the client should try to complete the distance in the fastest time possible.
2. Record the elapsed time (in minutes and seconds, 00:00) as the client crosses the finish line.
3. Convert the seconds to minutes by dividing the seconds by 60 (see step 3 for the 1.5-mile run procedure).
4. Compare the recorded time to the normative values listed in table 11.24 (page 254) [22].

Muscular Strength

Muscular strength is an important component of physical fitness. A minimal level of muscular strength is needed to perform daily activities, especially as one ages, and to participate in recreational or occupational activities without undue risk of injury. Strength may be expressed either as absolute strength or as relative strength. Absolute strength is simply the raw strength score a person achieves. Relative strength is usually expressed relative to body weight.

1-Repetition Maximum Bench Press

A 1-repetition maximum (1RM) bench press test may be used to measure upper body strength. Because free weights are used, this test requires skill on the part of the client being tested.

Equipment

- Adjustable barbell and weight plates that allow resistance increments of 5 to 90 pounds (approximately 2.5-40 kilograms).

Procedure

1. Provide a spotter and closely observe technique. See page 314 for proper bench press technique.
2. Follow these steps for determining a 1-repetition maximum (1RM):
   a. Instruct the client to warm up with a light resistance that easily allows 5 to 10 reps.
   b. Provide a one-minute rest period.
   c. Estimate a warm-up load that will allow the client to complete three to five reps by adding:

Body area	Absolute increase or percent increase
Upper body exercise	10-20 lb (4-9 kg) or 5-10%
Lower body exercise	30-40 lb (14-18 kg) or 10-20%

   d. Provide a two-minute rest period.
   e. Estimate a conservative, near-maximum load that will allow the client to complete two to three reps by adding:

Body area	Absolute increase or percent increase
Upper body exercise	10-20 lb (4-9 kg) or 5-10%
Lower body exercise	30-40 lb (14-18 kg) or 10-20%

   f. Provide a two- to four-minute rest period.
   g. Make a load increase:

Body area	Absolute increase or percent increase
Upper body exercise	10-20 lb (4-9 kg) or 5-10%
Lower body exercise	30-40 lb (14-18 kg) or 10-20%

   h. Instruct the client to attempt a 1RM.
   i. If the client was successful, provide a two- to four-minute rest period and go to back to step 2g. If the client failed, provide a two- to four-minute rest period, and decrease the load by subtracting:

Body area	Absolute decrease or percent decrease
Upper body exercise	5-10 lb (2-4 kg) or 2.5-5%
Lower body exercise	15-20 lb (7-9 kg) or 5-10%

   And then go back to step 2h.
   Continue increasing or decreasing the load until the client can complete one repetition with proper exercise technique. Ideally, the client's 1RM will be measured within three testing sets.
   j. Record the 1RM value as the maximum weight lifted (i.e., the client's absolute strength) for the last successful attempt.
3. Divide the 1RM value by the client's body weight to determine relative strength.
4. Compare the relative strength value to values in table 11.25 (page 255).

From Baechle, Earle, and Wathen 2000 [4] and Kraemer and Fry 1995 [15].

1-Repetition Maximum Leg Press

The 1RM leg press may be used to measure lower body strength. Chapter 13 provides a detailed account of client and spotter responsibilities during most lower body exercises. Personal trainers should be familiar with the guidelines in chapter 13 before attempting 1RM trials.

Equipment

- Universal® leg press machine. This resistance training device is less common than many others and therefore may be difficult to find. The personal trainer can instead opt to use a different exercise such as an angled hip sled or horizontal leg press to assess a client's lower body muscular strength. Note, however, that even if one follows the testing protocol described here, the normative data shown in table 11.26 (page 256) do not apply.

Procedure

1. Have the client sit in the seat of the leg press machine and place the feet on the upper pair of foot plates.
2. Adjust the seat to standardize the knee angle at approximately 120 degrees.
3. Follow the steps for determining a 1RM described in the "1-Repetition Maximum Bench Press" section to assess the client's leg press 1RM [4].

4. Divide the 1RM value by the client's body weight to determine relative strength.
5. Compare the relative strength value to values in table 11.26.

From Baumgartner and Jackson 1999 [5].

Estimating a 1-Repetition Maximum

For safety, technique reasons, or both, many personal trainers prefer not to have their clients perform 1RM testing. Fortunately, it is possible to estimate a client's 1RM from a submaximal resistance. This involves having the client perform as many repetitions as possible with a submaximal resistance. More detailed instructions can be found elsewhere [4], and the process to estimate starting loads for a resistance training program is described in chapter 15.

Muscular Endurance

Muscular endurance is the ability of a muscle or muscle group to exert submaximal force for extended periods. Along with muscular strength, muscular endurance is important for performing the activities of daily living, as well as in recreational and occupational pursuits. Muscular endurance may be assessed during static and dynamic muscle contractions.

YMCA Bench Press Test

The YMCA bench press test is used to measure upper body muscular endurance. This is a test of absolute muscular endurance, that is, the resistance is the same for all members of a given gender.

Equipment

- Adjustable barbell and weight plates
- Metronome

Procedure

1. Spot the client and closely observe the technique.
2. Set the resistance at 80 pounds (36.3 kilograms) for male clients, 35 pounds (15.9 kilograms) for female clients.
3. See page 314 for proper bench press technique.
4. Set the metronome cadence at 60 beats/min to establish a rate of 30 repetitions per minute.
5. Have the client, beginning with the arms extended and a shoulder-width grip, lower the weight to the chest. Then, without pausing, the client should raise the bar to full arm's length. The movement should be smooth and controlled, with the bar reaching its highest and lowest positions with each beat of the metronome.
6. Terminate the test when the client can no longer lift the barbell in cadence with the metronome.
7. Compare the client's score to values in table 11.27 (page 257).

Partial Curl-Up Test

The partial curl-up test measures the muscular endurance of the abdominal muscles. It is often favored over the sit-up test because it eliminates the use of the hip flexor muscles.

Equipment

- Metronome
- Ruler
- Masking tape
- Mat

Procedures

1. Direct the client to assume a supine position on a mat with the knees at 90 degrees (figure 11.6a). The arms are at the side (on the floor), with the fingers touching a four-inch (10-centimeter) piece of masking tape (that is placed on the floor perpendicular to the fingers). A second piece of masking tape is placed 8 centimeters (three inches; for those who are ≥45 years) or 12 centimeters (five inches; for those who are <45 years) beyond (but parallel to) the first.
2. Set a metronome to 40 beats/min and have the individual do slow, controlled curl-ups to lift the shoulder blades off the mat (trunk makes a 30 degrees angle with the mat; figure 11.6b) in time with the metronome (20 curl-ups per minute). The low back should be flattened before curling up.
3. Direct the client to perform as many curl-ups as possible without pausing, up to a maximum of 75.
4. Compare the client's score to table 11.28 (page 257).

Adapted from American College of Sports Medicine 2000 [2].

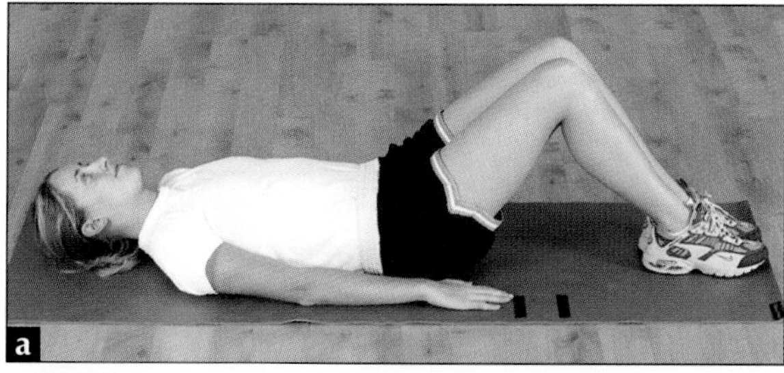

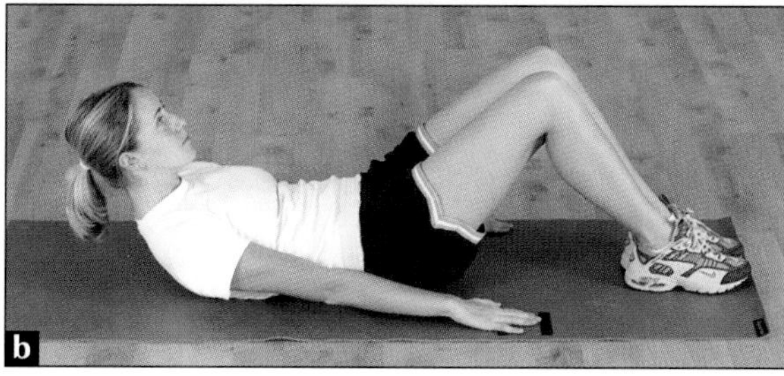

Figure 11.6 Curl-up: *(a)* beginning position and *(b)* end position.

One-Minute Sit-Up Test

The one-minute sit-up test measures the muscular endurance of the abdominal and hip flexor muscle groups.

Equipment

- Stopwatch
- Mat

Procedure

1. Direct the client to assume a supine position on a mat with arms crossed on chest, hands touching the shoulders. The hips and knees should be flexed, with the heels approximately 12 to 18 inches (30-45 centimeters) from the buttocks.
2. On a signal (i.e., "Go"), the client raises the torso until it is perpendicular to the floor. The chin should be tucked in to the chest, and the hands should stay in contact with the shoulders. The client then lowers the torso until the shoulders are once again in contact with the floor. Rest periods are allowed.
3. This is repeated for the maximum number of repetitions possible in 60 seconds.
4. Compare the client's score to values in table 11.29 (page 258).

Push-Up Test

Some muscular endurance tests may involve resistances heavy enough to permit only a limited number of repetitions to be performed by untrained clients. For example, clients with weak or smaller upper body muscles (e.g., younger and older clients, women, sedentary clients) may not be able to complete very many repetitions (e.g., ≤6) in the push-up test because their body weight—even using the modified body position—is simply too heavy. For these clients, the push-up test becomes one that can be used to assess muscular *strength.*

Equipment

- Foam roller (for a female client)

Procedure

1. Have the client assume the standard push-up starting position. For men, the hands are shoulder-width apart, the back is straight, and the head is up. For women, modify this position by having the client in a kneeling position, with the knees flexed at 90 degrees and the ankles crossed. See the photos on page 287 for proper positioning.
2. For a male client, place a fist on the floor beneath his chest, counting the repetitions only when the chest touches the fist. There are no criteria for establishing when the female client has lowered far enough [11]. One suggestion is to use a foam roller and instruct the female client to lower her torso until she lightly touches it. The body should then be raised to full arm's length.
3. Record the maximum number of repetitions performed without resting.
4. Compare the client's score to the values in table 11.30 (page 259).

Flexibility

Flexibility refers to the range of motion (ROM) around a joint (shoulder) or a series of joints (vertebral column). It is believed to be related to the development of a number of musculoskeletal disorders, for example low back pain. There is no single test that can measure whole-body flexibility. Separate tests need to be administered for each area of interest. Traditionally, personal trainers have focused on tests that measure the flexibility of joints believed to be associated with risk of developing low back pain.

Sit and Reach

Many believe that the sit and reach test is a measure of hip and low back flexibility. However, it may not be an adequate measure of low back function because it determines only the distance reached [2]. Nonetheless, a lack of hip and low back flexibility, along with poor muscular strength and endurance of the abdominal muscles, is believed to be predictive of low back pain.

Equipment

- Yardstick or sit and reach box
- Adhesive tape
- Measuring tape

Procedures

1. Have the client warm up and perform some moderate stretching prior to the test. All testing should be done without shoes. The test should be performed with slow, controlled stretches.
2. For the YMCA sit and reach test, place a yardstick on the floor and place tape across the yardstick at a right angle to the 15-inch (38-centimeter) mark (see figure 11.7a). The client then sits with the yardstick between the legs, extending the legs at right angles to the taped line on the floor. The heels should touch the edge of the taped line and should be about 10 to 12 inches (25-30 centimeters) apart. With use of a sit and reach box, the heels should be placed against the edge of the box (see figure 11.8a).
3. Have the client reach forward slowly with both hands, moving as far as possible and holding the terminal position. The fingers should overlap and should be in contact with the yardstick (figure 11.7b) or sit and reach box (figure 11.8b).
4. The score is the most distant point reached. Use the best of three trials as the score. The knees must stay extended throughout the test, but the tester should not press the client's legs down.
5. Compare the test results using either table 11.31 (YMCA sit and reach test) or 11.32 (sit and reach box) on page 260. Note that the norms for the YMCA sit and reach test use a "zero" point (the "zero" point is the point at which the client reaches the toes) of 15 inches (38 centimeters), while the sit and reach box typically uses a "zero point" set at 26 centimeters. When using a different zero point, be sure to adjust the client's score before using the norm tables. For example, if the box has a zero point of 23 centimeters, add 3 centimeters to the client's score before consulting table 11.32 (or subtract 3 centimeters from the norms in the table before comparing the client's score to table 11.32).

From ACSM 2000 [2].

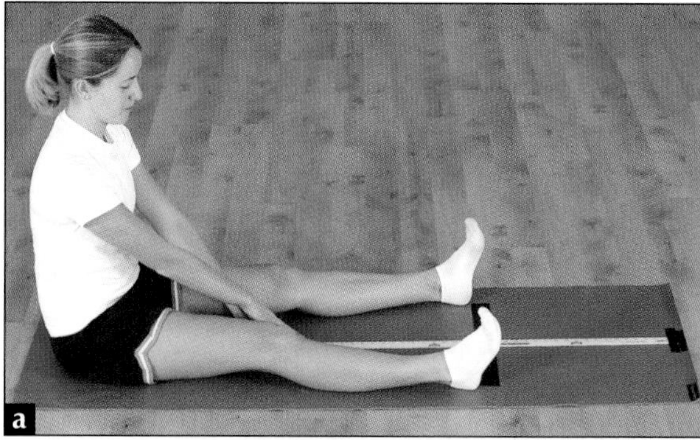

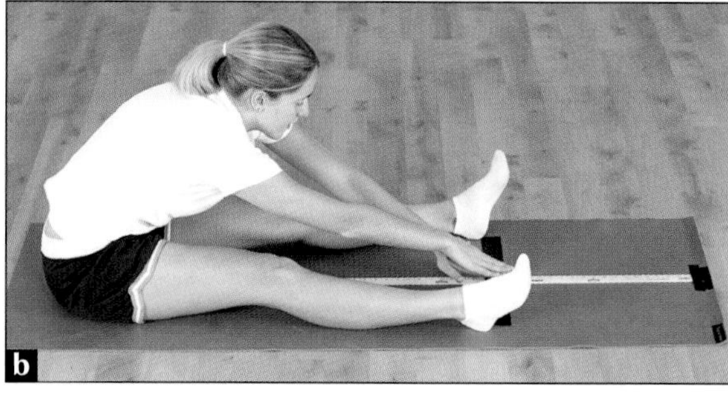

Figure 11.7 Sit and reach positioning with a yardstick: *(a)* beginning position and *(b)* end position.

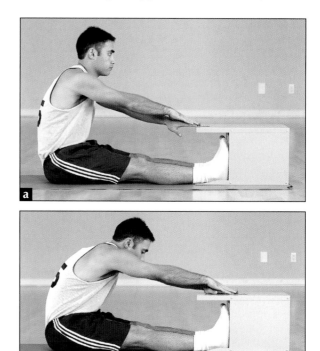

Figure 11.8 Sit and reach positioning with a sit and reach box: *(a)* beginning position and *(b)* end position.

CONCLUSION

Typically the personal trainer has the challenge of working with clients who have a broad spectrum of fitness or exercise capabilities. To gather baseline assessments, the personal trainer may test for a variety of fitness parameters such as HR, BP, body composition, cardiovascular endurance, muscular strength, muscular endurance, and flexibility and then make comparisons to established sets of descriptive or normative data. The resulting conclusions can then form the basis for the client's exercise prescription.

TABLE 11.1

Resting Heart Rate Classification

Resting Heart Rate Classification
<60 beats/min = bradycardia (slow heart rate)
60 to 100 beats/min = normal heart rate
>100 beats/min = tachycardia (fast heart rate)

Reprinted from Heyward 2002.

TABLE 11.2

Norms for Resting Heart Rate in Men and Women, Ages 18+ Years

Heart rate category	Heart rates (beats/min)	
	Men	Women
Low	35-56	39-58
Moderately low	57-61	59-63
<Average	62-65	64-67
Average	66-71	68-72
>Average	72-75	73-77
Moderately high	76-81	78-83
High	82-103	84-104

Data from Golding, Myers, and Sinning 1989.

Reprinted from Adams 2002.

TABLE 11.3

Conversion Equations for Heart Rate Count Durations

Heart rate count duration	×	Correct multiplier	=	HR (beats/min)
6 sec	×	10	=	60 sec (beats/min)
10 sec	×	6	=	60 sec (beats/min)
15 sec	×	4	=	60 sec (beats/min)
30 sec	×	2	=	60 sec (beats/min)

TABLE 11.4

Classification of Blood Pressure for Adults Age 18 and Older

Category	Systolic (mmHg)		Diastolic (mmHg)
Optimal*	<120	and	<80
Normal	<130	and	<85
High-normal	130-139	or	85-89
	*Hypertension***		
Stage 1	140-159	or	90-99
Stage 2	160-179	or	100-109
Stage 3	≥180	or	≥110

Note: Values are for adults not taking antihypertensive drugs and not acutely ill. When systolic and diastolic blood pressures fall into different categories, the higher category should be selected to classify the client's blood pressure status. For example, 160/92 mmHg should be classified as stage 2 hypertension, and 174/120 mmHg should be classified as stage 3 hypertension. Isolated systolic hypertension is defined as SBP of 140 mmHg or greater and DBP below 90 mmHg and staged appropriately (e.g., 170/82 mmHg is defined as stage 2 isolated systolic hypertension). In addition to classifying stages of hypertension on the basis of average blood pressure levels, the client's physician should verify presence or absence of target organ disease and additional risk factors. This specificity is important for risk classification and treatment.

*Optimal blood pressure with respect to cardiovascular risk is below 120/80 mmHg. However, unusually low readings should be evaluated for clinical significance.

**Based on the average of two or more readings taken at each of two or more visits after an initial screening.

Reprinted from National Institutes of Health; National Heart, Lung, and Blood Institute; National High Blood Pressure Education Program 1997.

TABLE 11.5

Guidelines for Type of Blood Pressure Cuff According to Limb Circumference

Limb size (cm)	Type of cuff*	Bladder size (cm)	
		Length	Width
	Upper arm circumference		
32-42	Large adult	33 or 42	15
24-32	Adult (standard)	24	12.5
18-24	Child	21.5	10
	Thigh circumference		
42-50	Thigh	37	18.5

*Other types of cuffs are newborn and infant.

Reprinted from Adams 2002.

TABLE 11.6

Percentile Norms for Blood Pressure in Active Men and Women

	Men				Women			
	Ages (years)				Ages (years)			
	20-29	30-39	20-29	30-39	20-29	30-39	20-29	30-39
Percentile	Systolic		Diastolic		Systolic		Diastolic	
90	110	108	70	70	99	100	63	65
80	112	110	72	74	101	104	68	70
70	118	116	78	78	106	110	70	70
60	120	120	80	80	110	110	72	74
50	121	120	80	80	112	114	75	76
40	128	124	80	81	118	118	78	80
30	130	130	84	85	120	120	80	80
20	136	132	88	90	122	122	80	82
10	140	140	90	92	130	130	82	90

Data from Pollock, Wilmore, and Fox 1978.

Reprinted from Adams 2002.

TABLE 11.7

Classification of Overweight and Obese by Body Mass Index (BMI), Waist Circumference, and Associated Disease Risks

			Disease* risk relative to normal weight and waist circumference	
	BMI (kg/m[2])	Obesity class	Men ≤102 cm (≤40 in.) Women ≤88 cm (≤35 in.)	Men >102 cm (>40 in.) Women >88 cm (>35 in.)
Underweight	<18.5		–	–
Normal	18.5-24.9		–	–
Overweight	25.0-29.9		Increased	High
Obesity	30.0-34.9	I	High	Very high
	35.0-39.9	II	Very high	Very high
Extreme obesity	≥40.0	III	Extremely high	Extremely high

*Disease risk for type 2 diabetes, hypertension, and coronary heart disease.

Reprinted from National Institutes of Health; National Heart, Lung, and Blood Institute 1998.

TABLE 11.8

Average Stature and Percentiles for American Men

Age (years)	Centi-meters	Percentiles								
		5	10	15	25	50	75	85	90	95
18-24.9	176.6	165.4	167.8	169.5	171.9	176.6	181.2	183.7	185.5	188.6
25-29.9	176.7	165.1	167.8	169.4	172.0	176.6	181.5	184.0	185.7	188.0
30-34.9	176.2	164.8	167.4	169.0	171.5	176.2	180.9	183.3	184.8	187.2
35-39.9	176.1	164.0	166.8	168.8	171.9	176.1	181.0	183.5	185.0	187.7
40-44.9	175.9	165.0	167.2	168.9	171.4	176.0	180.3	182.7	184.2	186.9
45-49.9	175.2	163.8	166.5	168.0	170.6	174.8	180.2	182.9	184.5	186.6
50-54.9	174.6	164.2	166.4	167.8	170.2	174.6	178.8	181.4	183.2	185.3
55-59.9	173.9	163.2	165.0	166.8	169.3	173.8	178.7	181.0	182.3	184.6
60-64.9	173.0	161.9	165.0	166.4	168.7	173.0	177.4	179.8	181.3	183.7
65-69.9	171.5	159.7	162.9	164.5	166.7	171.6	176.3	178.6	180.1	182.5
70-74.9	170.6	159.5	162.0	163.6	165.8	170.7	175.0	177.4	179.4	182.0

Inches (in.) × 2.54 = centimeters (cm).
Inches (in.) × 0.0254 = meters (m).
Reprinted from Frisancho 1990.

TABLE 11.9

Average Stature and Percentiles for American Women

Age (years)	Centi-meters	Percentiles								
		5	10	15	25	50	75	85	90	95
18-24.9	163.0	152.3	154.8	156.4	158.8	163.1	167.1	169.6	171.0	173.6
25-29.9	162.9	152.6	155.2	153.6	156.6	162.8	167.1	169.5	170.9	173.3
30-34.9	162.6	152.9	155.2	156.4	158.4	162.4	166.8	169.2	171.2	173.1
35-39.9	162.8	152.0	155.0	156.4	158.6	162.7	167.0	169.4	171.0	173.5
40-44.9	162.6	151.6	154.3	156.2	158.1	162.7	166.7	168.8	170.5	173.2
45-49.9	161.2	151.7	154.0	155.4	157.9	162.0	166.3	168.4	169.9	172.2
50-54.9	161.2	151.3	153.8	155.3	156.9	161.1	165.1	167.3	169.2	171.0
55-59.9	160.3	149.8	152.7	154.1	156.7	160.3	164.4	166.6	167.8	170.1
60-64.9	159.6	149.2	151.4	153.0	155.6	160.0	163.7	166.1	167.3	169.8
65-69.9	158.6	148.5	150.7	152.4	154.8	158.8	162.6	164.8	166.2	168.1
70-74.9	157.6	147.2	150.0	151.7	153.7	157.4	161.5	163.8	165.5	167.5

Inches (in.)× 2.54 = centimeters (cm).
Inches (in.) × 0.0254 = meters (m).
Reprinted from Frisancho 1990.

TABLE 11.10

Average Weight for American Men

Height		Age group (years)											
		18-24		25-34		35-44		45-54		55-64		65-74	
in.	cm	lb	kg	lb	kg	lb	kg	lb	kg	lb	kg	lb	kg
62	157.5	130	59.1	141	64.1	143	65.0	147	66.8	143	65.0	143	65.0
63	160.0	135	61.4	145	65.9	148	67.3	152	69.1	147	66.8	147	66.8
64	162.6	140	63.6	150	68.2	153	69.5	156	70.9	153	69.5	151	68.6
65	165.1	145	65.9	156	70.9	158	71.8	160	72.7	158	71.8	156	70.9
66	167.6	150	68.2	160	72.7	163	74.1	164	74.5	163	74.1	160	72.7
67	170.2	154	70.0	165	75.0	169	76.8	169	76.8	168	76.4	164	74.5
68	172.8	159	72.3	170	77.3	174	79.1	173	78.6	173	78.6	169	76.8
69	175.3	164	74.5	174	79.1	179	81.4	177	80.5	178	80.9	173	78.6
70	177.8	168	76.4	179	81.4	184	83.6	182	82.7	183	83.2	177	80.5
71	180.3	173	78.6	184	83.6	190	86.4	187	85.0	189	85.9	182	82.7
72	182.9	178	80.9	189	85.9	194	88.2	191	86.8	193	87.7	186	84.5
73	185.4	183	83.2	194	88.2	200	90.9	196	89.1	197	89.5	190	86.4
74	188.0	188	85.5	199	90.5	205	93.2	200	90.9	203	92.3	194	88.2

Note: Weights include clothing weight between 0.1 and 0.3 kg; pound-to-kilogram conversion uses 2.2.

Reprinted from Abraham, Johnson, and Najjar 1979.

TABLE 11.11

Average Weight for American Women

Height		Age group (years)											
		18-24		25-34		35-44		45-54		55-64		65-74	
in.	cm	lb	kg	lb	kg	lb	kg	lb	kg	lb	kg	lb	kg
57	144.8	114	51.8	118	53.6	125	56.8	129	58.6	132	60.0	130	59.1
58	147.3	117	53.2	121	55.0	129	58.6	133	60.5	136	61.8	134	60.9
59	149.9	120	54.5	125	56.8	133	60.5	136	61.8	140	63.6	137	62.3
60	152.4	123	55.9	128	58.2	137	62.3	140	63.6	143	65.0	140	63.6
61	154.9	126	57.3	132	60.0	141	64.1	143	65.0	147	66.8	144	65.5
62	157.5	129	58.6	136	61.8	144	65.5	147	66.8	150	68.2	147	66.8
63	160.0	132	60.0	139	63.2	148	67.3	150	68.2	153	69.5	151	68.6

(continued)

TABLE 11.11 *(continued)*

Height		Age group (years)											
		18-24		25-34		35-44		45-54		55-64		65-74	
in.	cm	lb	kg	lb	kg	lb	kg	lb	kg	lb	kg	lb	kg
64	162.6	135	61.4	142	64.5	152	69.1	154	70.0	157	71.4	154	70.0
65	165.1	138	62.7	146	66.4	156	70.9	158	71.8	160	72.7	158	71.8
66	167.6	141	64.1	150	68.2	159	72.3	161	73.2	164	74.5	161	73.2
67	170.2	144	65.5	153	69.5	163	74.1	165	75.0	167	75.9	165	75.0
68	172.8	147	66.8	157	71.4	167	75.9	168	76.4	171	77.7	169	76.8

Note: Weights include clothing weight between 0.1 and 0.3 kg; pound-to-kilogram conversion uses 2.2.

Reprinted from Abraham, Johnson, and Najjar 1979.

TABLE 11.12

Equations for Calculating the Estimated Body Density From Skinfold Measurements Among Various Populations

SKF sites*	Sex	Age	Equation
Σ7SKF (chest + abdomen + thigh + triceps + subscapula + suprailium + midaxilla	Women	18-55 years	$Db\ (g \cdot cc^{-1})^{**} = 1.0970 - 0.00046971(\Sigma 7SKF) + 0.00000056(\Sigma 7SKF)^2 - 0.00012828(age)$
	Men	18-61 years	$Db\ (g \cdot cc^{-1})^{**} = 1.1120 - 0.00043499(\Sigma 7SKF) + 0.00000055(\Sigma 7SKF)^2 - 0.00028826(age)$
Σ4SKF (triceps + suprailium + abdomen + thigh)	Women	18-29 years	$Db\ (g \cdot cc^{-1})^{**} = 1.096095 - 0.0006952(\Sigma 4SKF) - 0.0000011(\Sigma 4SKF)^2 - 0.0000714(age)$
Σ3SKF (triceps + suprailium + thigh)	Women	18-55 years	$Db\ (g \cdot cc^{-1})^{**} = 1.0994921 - 0.0009929(\Sigma 3SKF) + 0.0000023(\Sigma 3SKF)^2 - 0.0001392(age)$
(chest + abdomen + thigh)	Men	18-61 years	$Db\ (g \cdot cc^{-1})^{**} = 1.109380 - 0.0008267(\Sigma 3SKF) + 0.0000016(\Sigma 3SKF)^2 - 0.0002574(age)$
Σ2SKF (triceps + medial calf)	Boys	6-17 years	$\%\ BF = 0.735(\Sigma 2SKF) + 1.0$
	Girls	6-17 years	$\%\ BF = 0.610(\Sigma 2SKF) + 5.1$

*ΣSKF = sum of skinfolds (mm).

**Use population-specific conversion formulas (see table 11.13) to calculate % BF (percent body fat) from Db (body density).

Adapted from Heyward 2002.

TABLE 11.13

Population-Specific Equations for Calculating the Estimated Percent Body Fat From Body Density (Db)

Population	Age	Sex	% BF*
Race			
American Indian	18-60	Female	(4.81 ÷ Db) – 4.34
Black	18-32	Male	(4.37 ÷ Db) – 3.93
	24-79	Female	(4.85 ÷ Db) – 4.39
Hispanic	20-40	Female	(4.87 ÷ Db) – 4.41
Japanese native	18-48	Male	(4.97 ÷ Db) – 4.52
		Female	(4.76 ÷ Db) – 4.28
	61-78	Male	(4.87 ÷ Db) – 4.41
		Female	(4.95 ÷ Db) – 4.50
White	7-12	Male	(5.30 ÷ Db) – 4.89
		Female	(5.35 ÷ Db) – 4.95
	13-16	Male	(5.07 ÷ Db) – 4.64
		Female	(5.10 ÷ Db) – 4.66
	17-19	Male	(4.99 ÷ Db) – 4.55
		Female	(5.05 ÷ Db) – 4.62
	20-80	Male	(4.95 ÷ Db) – 4.50
		Female	(5.01 ÷ Db) – 4.57
Levels of body fatness			
Anorexic	15-30	Female	(5.26 ÷ Db) – 4.83
Obese	17-62	Female	(5.00 ÷ Db) – 4.56
Athletes	High school and college age	Male and female	(4.57 ÷ Db) – 4.142

*Multiply the value from this column's calculations by 100 to yield the percentage value.

Adapted from Heyward and Stolarczyk 1996.

TABLE 11.14

Criterion Scores and Normative Values for Percent Body Fat for Males and Females

Male rating (criterion scores)	Age (years)						
	6-17**	18-25	26-35	36-45	46-55	56-65	66+
Very lean	<5 (not recommended)	4-7	8-12	10-14	12-16	15-18	15-18
Lean (low)	5-10	8-10	13-15	16-18	18-20	19-21	19-21
Leaner than average	–	11-13	16-18	19-21	21-23	22-24	22-23
Average (mid)	11-25	14-16	19-21	22-24	24-25	24-26	24-25
Fatter than average	–	18-20	22-24	25-26	26-28	26-28	25-27
Fat (upper)	26-31	22-26	25-28	27-29	29-31	29-31	28-30
Overfat (obesity)	>31	28-37	30-37	30-38	32-38	32-38	31-38

Male percentiles (normative references)***	20-29	30-39	40-49	50-59	60+
90	7.1	11.3	13.6	15.3	15.3
80	9.4	13.9	16.3	17.9	18.4
70	11.8	15.9	18.1	19.8	20.3
60	14.1	17.5	19.6	21.3	22.0
50	15.9	19.0	21.1	22.7	23.5
40	17.4	20.5	22.5	24.1	25.0
30	19.5	22.3	24.1	25.7	26.7
20	22.4	24.2	26.1	27.5	28.5
10	25.9	27.3	28.9	30.3	31.2

Female rating (criterion scores)*	6-17**	18-25	26-35	36-45	46-55	56-65	66+
Very lean	<12 (not recommended)	13-17	13-18	15-19	18-22	18-23	16-18
Lean (low)	12-15	18-20	19-21	20-23	23-25	24-26	22-25
Leaner than average	–	21-23	22-23	24-26	26-28	28-30	27-29
Average (mid)	16-30	24-25	24-26	27-29	29-31	31-33	30-32
Fatter than average	–	26-28	27-30	30-32	32-34	34-36	33-35
Fat (upper)	31-36	29-31	31-35	33-36	36-38	36-38	36-38
Overfat (obesity)	>36	33-43	36-48	39-48	40-49	39-46	39-40

Female percentiles (normative references)***	20-29	30-39	40-49	50-59	60+
90	14.5	15.5	18.5	21.6	21.1
80	17.1	18.0	21.3	25.0	25.1
70	19.0	20.0	23.5	26.6	27.5
60	20.6	21.6	24.9	28.5	29.3
50	22.1	23.1	26.4	30.1	30.9
40	23.7	24.9	28.1	31.6	32.5
30	25.4	27.0	30.1	33.5	34.3
20	27.7	29.3	32.1	35.6	36.6
10	32.1	32.8	35.0	37.9	39.3

When personal trainers assess a client's body composition, they must account for a standard error of the estimate (SEE) and report a range of percentages that the client falls into. Note that the minimum SEE for population-specific skinfold equations is ±3-5%. Therefore, if a 25-year-old male client's body fat is measured at 24%, there is a minimum of a 6% range (21%-27%) that suggests a criterion-reference score of "fat." Note that reporting a client's body fat percentage with an SEE range can also cover any gaps and overlaps in the criterion-referenced norms shown. For example, what is the criterion score for a 30-year-old male with 29% body fat? The minimum SEE of ±3% places this client between 26% and 32% and therefore would suggest a criterion-reference score of "fat-overfat" or "borderline overfat."

*Data for male and female rating (criterion scores), ages 18-66+, are adapted from Morrow, Jackson, Disch, and Mood 2000.

**Data for male and female rating (criterion scores), ages 6-17, are from Lohman, Houtkooper, and Going 1997.

***Data for male and female percentiles (normative references) are reprinted from ACSM 2000.

Adapted from Golding, Myers, and Sinning 1989.

TABLE 11.15

Waist-to-Hip Circumference Ratio Norms for Men and Women

Age	Risk			
	Low	Moderate	High	Very high
		Men		
20-29	<0.83	0.83-0.88	0.89-0.94	>0.94
30-39	<0.84	0.84-0.91	0.92-0.96	>0.96
40-49	<0.88	0.88-0.95	0.96-1.00	>1.00
50-59	<0.90	0.90-0.96	0.97-1.02	>1.02
60-69	<0.91	0.91-0.98	0.99-1.03	>1.03
		Women		
20-29	<0.71	0.71-0.77	0.78-0.82	>0.82
30-39	<0.72	0.72-0.78	0.79-0.84	>0.84
40-49	<0.73	0.73-0.79	0.80-0.87	>0.87
50-59	<0.74	0.74-0.81	0.82-0.88	>0.88
60-69	<0.76	0.76-0.83	0.84-0.90	>0.90

Adapted from Bray and Gray 1988.

TABLE 11.16

YMCA Cycle Ergometry Protocol

	HR <80 beats/min	HR 80-89 beats/min	HR 90-100 beats/min	HR >100 beats/min
1st stage	150 kg · m · min^{-1} (0.5 kg)			
2nd stage	750 kg · m · min^{-1} (2.5 kg)*	600 kg · m · min^{-1} (2.0 kg)	450 kg · m · min^{-1} (1.5 kg)	300 kg · m · min^{-1} (1.0 kg)
3rd stage	900 kg · m · min^{-1} (3.0 kg)	750 kg · m · min^{-1} (2.5 kg)	600 kg · m · min^{-1} (2.0 kg)	450 kg · m · min^{-1} (1.5 kg)
4th stage	1,050 kg · m · min^{-1} (3.5 kg)	900 kg · m · min^{-1} (3.0 kg)	750 kg · m · min^{-1} (2.5 kg)	600 kg · m · min^{-1} (2.0 kg)

Directions:

1. Instruct the client to begin pedaling at 50 rpm and maintain this cadence throughout the duration of the test.
2. Set the work rate for the 1st three-minute stage at 150 kg · m · min^{-1} (0.5 kg at 50 rpm).
3. Measure the client's HR during the final 15-30 seconds of the second and third minute of the 1st stage; if they are not within six beats/min of each other, continue the stage for one more minute.
4. If the client's HR at the end of the 1st stage is:

   <80 beats/min, set the work rate for the 2nd stage at 750 kg · m · min^{-1} (2.5 kg at 50 rpm)

   80-89 beats/min, set the work rate for the 2nd stage at 600 kg · m · min^{-1} (2.0 kg at 50 rpm)

   90-100 beats/min, set the work rate for the 2nd stage at 450 kg · m · min^{-1} (1.5 kg at 50 rpm)

   >100 beats/min, set the work rate for the 2nd stage at 300 kg · m · min^{-1} (1.0 kg at 50 rpm)
5. Measure the client's HR during the final 15-30 seconds of the second and third minute of the 2nd stage; if they are not within six beats/min of each other, continue the stage for one more minute.
6. Set the 3rd and 4th three-minute stages (if required) according to the table above (work rates for the 3rd and 4th stages are located in the rows below the 2nd stage). Be sure to measure the client's HR in the final 15-30 seconds of the second and third minute of each stage; if they are not within six beats/min of each other, continue each stage for one more minute.
7. Terminate the test when the client reaches 85% of his or her age-predicted maximal HR or if the client meets one of the criteria listed in table 10.3.

*Resistance settings shown here are appropriate for an ergometer with a flywheel that is geared to travel 6 meters per pedal revolution.

Reprinted from ACSM 2000.

TABLE 11.17

Percentile Values for Maximal Aerobic Power (ml · kg^{-1} · min^{-1})

Percentile*	Age (years)				
	20-29	30-39	40-49	50-59	60+
			Men		
90	51.4	50.4	48.2	45.3	42.5
80	48.2	46.8	44.1	41.0	38.1
70	46.8	44.6	41.8	38.5	35.3
60	44.2	42.4	39.9	36.7	33.6
50	42.5	41.0	38.1	35.2	31.8
40	41.0	38.9	36.7	33.8	30.2
30	39.5	37.4	35.1	32.3	28.7
20	37.1	35.4	33.0	30.2	26.5
10	34.5	32.5	30.9	28.0	23.1
			Women		
90	44.2	41.0	39.5	35.2	35.2
80	41.0	38.6	36.3	32.3	31.2
70	38.1	36.7	33.8	30.9	29.4
60	36.7	34.6	32.3	29.4	27.2
50	35.2	33.8	30.9	28.2	25.8
40	33.8	32.3	29.5	26.9	24.5
30	32.3	30.5	28.3	25.5	23.8
20	30.6	28.7	26.5	24.3	22.8
10	28.4	26.5	25.1	22.3	20.8

Note: Data provided by Institute for Aerobics Research, Dallas, TX, 1994.

Study population for the data set was predominately white and college educated. A modified Balke treadmill test was used with $\dot{V}O_2max$ estimated from the last grade/speed achieved.

*Descriptors for percentile rankings: 90 = well above average; 70 = above average; 50 = average; 30 = below average; 10 = well below average.

Adapted from ACSM 2000.

TABLE 11.18

Prediction of Maximal Oxygen Consumption From Heart Rate and Cycling Power in Men

Maximal oxygen consumption ($L \cdot min^{-1}$)						Maximal oxygen consumption ($L \cdot min^{-1}$)				
	Power ($kg \cdot m \cdot min^{-1}$; Watts)						Power ($kg \cdot m \cdot min^{-1}$; Watts)			
HR (beats/min)	300; 50	600; 100	900; 150	1,200; 200	1,500; 250	HR (beats/min)	600; 100	900; 150	1,200; 200	1,500; 250
120	2.2	3.5	4.8			146	2.4	3.3	4.4	5.5
121	2.2	3.4	4.7			147	2.4	3.3	4.4	5.5
122	2.2	3.4	4.6			148	2.4	3.2	4.3	5.4
123	2.1	3.4	4.6			149	2.3	3.2	4.3	5.4
124	2.1	3.3	4.5	6.0		150	2.3	3.2	4.2	5.3
125	2.0	3.2	4.4	5.9		151	2.3	3.1	4.2	5.2
126	2.0	3.2	4.4	5.8		152	2.3	3.1	4.1	5.2
127	2.0	3.1	4.3	5.7		153	2.2	3.0	4.1	5.1
128	2.0	3.1	4.2	5.6		154	2.2	3.0	4.0	5.1
129	1.9	3.0	4.2	5.6		155	2.2	3.0	4.0	5.0
130	1.9	3.0	4.1	5.5		156	2.2	2.9	4.0	5.0
131	1.9	2.9	4.0	5.4		157	2.1	2.9	3.9	4.9
132	1.8	2.9	4.0	5.3		158	2.1	2.9	3.9	4.9
133	1.8	2.8	3.9	5.3		159	2.1	2.8	3.8	4.8
134	1.8	2.8	3.9	5.2		160	2.1	2.8	3.8	4.8
135	1.7	2.8	3.8	5.1		161	2.0	2.8	3.7	4.7
136	1.7	2.7	3.8	5.0		162	2.0	2.8	3.7	4.6
137	1.7	2.7	3.7	5.0		163	2.0	2.8	3.7	4.6
138	1.6	2.7	3.7	4.9		164	2.0	2.7	3.6	4.5
139	1.6	2.6	3.6	4.8		165	2.0	2.7	3.6	4.5
140	1.6	2.6	3.6	4.8	6.0	166	1.9	2.7	3.6	4.4
141		2.6	3.5	4.7	5.9	167	1.9	2.6	3.5	4.4
142		2.5	5.5	4.6	5.8	168	1.9	2.6	3.5	4.3
143		2.5	3.4	4.6	5.7	169	1.9	2.6	3.5	4.3
144		2.5	3.4	4.5	5.7	170	1.8	2.6	3.4	4.3
145		2.4	3.4	4.5	5.6					

Modified from nomogram in I. Åstrand 1960.

Reprinted from Adams 2002.

TABLE 11.19

Prediction of Maximal Oxygen Consumption From Heart Rate and Cycling Power in Women

Maximal oxygen consumption ($L \cdot min^{-1}$)						Maximal oxygen consumption ($L \cdot min^{-1}$)					
	Power ($kg \cdot m \cdot min^{-1}$; Watts)						Power ($kg \cdot m \cdot min^{-1}$; Watts)				
HR (beats/min)	300; 50	450; 75	600; 100	750; 125	900; 150	HR (beats/min)	300; 50	450; 75	600; 100	750; 125	900; 150
120	2.6	3.4	4.1	4.8		146	1.6	2.2	2.6	3.2	3.7
121	2.5	3.3	4.0	4.8		147	1.6	2.1	2.6	3.1	3.6
122	2.5	3.2	3.9	4.7		148	1.6	2.1	2.6	3.1	3.6
123	2.4	3.1	3.9	4.6		149		2.1	2.6	3.0	3.5
124	2.4	3.1	3.8	4.5		150		2.0	2.5	3.0	3.5
125	2.3	3.0	3.7	4.4		151		2.0	2.5	3.0	3.4
126	2.3	3.0	3.7	4.4		152		2.0	2.5	2.9	3.4
127	2.2	2.9	3.5	4.2		153		2.0	2.4	2.9	3.3
128	2.2	2.8	3.5	4.2		154		2.0	2.4	2.8	3.3
129	2.2	2.8	3.4	4.1		155		1.9	2.4	2.8	3.2
130	2.1	2.7	3.4	4.0	4.7	156		1.9	2.3	2.8	3.2
131	2.1	2.7	3.4	4.0	4.6	157		1.9	2.3	2.7	3.2
132	2.0	2.7	3.3	4.0	4.5	158		1.8	2.3	2.7	3.1
133	2.0	2.6	3.2	3.8	4.4	159		1.8	2.2	2.7	3.1
134	2.0	2.6	3.2	3.8	4.4	160		1.8	2.2	2.6	3.0
135	2.0	2.6	3.1	3.7	4.3	161		1.8	2.2	2.6	3.0
136	1.9	2.5	3.1	3.6	4.2	162		1.8	2.2	2.6	3.0
137	1.9	2.5	3.0	3.6	4.2	163		1.7	2.2	2.6	2.9
138	1.8	2.4	2.9	3.5	4.1	164		1.7	2.1	2.5	2.9
139	1.8	2.4	2.8	3.5	4.0	165		1.7	2.1	2.5	2.9
140	1.8	2.4	2.8	3.4	4.0	166		1.7	2.1	2.5	2.8
141	1.8	2.3	2.8	3.4	3.9	167		1.6	2.1	2.4	2.8
142	1.7	2.3	2.8	3.3	3.9	168		1.6	2.0	2.4	2.8
143	1.7	2.2	2.7	3.3	3.8	169		1.6	2.0	2.4	2.8
144	1.7	2.2	2.7	3.2	3.8	170		1.6	2.0	2.4	2.7
145	1.6	2.2	2.7	3.2	3.7						

Modified from nomogram in I. Åstrand 1960.

Reprinted from Adams 2002.

TABLE 11.20

Age Correction Factors (CF) for Age-Adjusted Maximal Oxygen Consumption

Age	CF	Age	CF	Age	CF	Age	CF	Age	CF
15	1.10	25	1.00	35	0.87	45	0.78	55	0.71
16	1.10	26	0.99	36	0.86	46	0.77	56	0.70
17	1.09	27	0.98	37	0.85	47	0.77	57	0.70
18	1.07	28	0.96	38	0.85	48	0.76	58	0.69
19	1.06	29	0.95	39	0.84	49	0.76	59	0.69
20	1.05	30	0.93	40	0.83	50	0.75	60	0.68
21	1.04	31	0.93	41	0.82	51	0.74	61	0.67
22	1.03	32	0.91	42	0.81	52	0.73	62	0.67
23	1.02	33	0.90	43	0.80	53	0.73	63	0.66
24	1.01	34	0.88	44	0.79	54	0.72	64	0.66

Adapted from Åstrand 1960.

TABLE 11.21

Norms for Evaluating Åstrand-Ryhming Cycle Test Performance

Age	Aerobic fitness categories					
	Very high	High	Good	Average	Fair	Low
	Maximal oxygen consumption ($ml \cdot kg^{-1} \cdot min^{-1}$)					
			Men			
20-29	>61	53-61	43-52	34-42	25-33	<25
30-39	>57	49-57	39-48	31-38	23-30	<23
40-49	>53	45-53	36-44	27-35	20-26	<20
50-59	>49	43-49	34-42	25-33	18-24	<18
60-69	>45	41-45	31-40	23-30	16-22	<16
			Women			
20-29	>57	49-57	38-48	31-37	24-30	<24
30-39	>53	45-53	34-44	28-33	20-27	<20
40-49	>50	42-50	31-41	24-30	17-23	<17
50-59	>42	38-42	28-37	21-27	15-20	<15
60-69	>39	35-39	24-34	18-23	13-17	<13

Reprinted from Adams 2002.

TABLE 11.22

Male and Female Norms for Recovery Heart Rate Following the 3-Minute Step Test (beats/min)

Rating	Heart rate					
	Age (years)					
	18-25	26-35	36-45	46-55	56-65	66+
Male rating						
Excellent	70-78	73-79	72-81	78-84	72-82	72-86
Good	82-88	83-88	86-94	89-96	89-97	89-95
Above average	91-97	91-97	98-102	99-103	98-101	97-102
Average	101-104	101-106	105-111	109-115	105-111	104-113
Below average	107-114	109-116	113-118	118-121	113-118	114-119
Poor	118-126	119-126	120-128	124-130	122-128	122-128
Very poor	131-164	130-164	132-168	135-158	131-150	133-152
Female rating						
Excellent	72-83	72-86	74-87	76-93	74-92	73-86
Good	88-97	91-97	93-101	96-102	97-103	93-100
Above average	100-106	103-110	104-109	106-113	106-111	104-114
Average	110-116	112-118	111-117	117-120	113-117	117-121
Below average	118-124	121-127	120-127	121-126	119-127	123-127
Poor	128-137	129-135	130-138	127-133	129-136	129-134
Very poor	142-155	141-154	143-152	138-152	142-151	135-151

Reprinted from Morrow, Jackson, Disch, and Mood 2000.

TABLE 11.23

Norms for the Rockport Walk Test

Clients aged 30-69 years (min:sec)		
Rating	Males	Females
Excellent	<10:12	<11:40
Good	10:13-11:42	11:41-13:08
High average	11:43-13:13	13:09-14:36
Low average	13:14-14:44	14:37-16:04
Fair	14:45-16:23	16:05-17:31
Poor	>16:24	>17:32

(continued)

TABLE 11.23 *(continued)*

Clients aged 18-30 years (min:sec)		
Percentile	**Males**	**Females**
90	11:08	11:45
75	11:42	12:49
50	12:38	13:15
25	13:38	14:12
10	14:37	15:03

Reprinted from Morrow, Jackson, Disch, and Mood 2000.

TABLE 11.24

Norms for 1-Mile Run (min:sec)

	Percentile			
	Boys		**Girls**	
Age	**85**	**50**	**85**	**50**
6	10:15	12:36	11:20	13:12
7	9:22	11:40	10:36	12:56
8	8:48	11:05	10:02	12:30
9	8:31	10:30	9:30	11:52
10	7:57	9:48	9:19	11:22
11	7:32	9:20	9:02	11:17
12	7:11	8:40	8:23	11:05
13	6:50	8:06	8:13	10:23
14	6:26	7:44	7:59	10:06
15	6:20	7:30	8:08	9:58
16	6:08	7:10	8:23	10:31
17	6:06	7:04	8:15	10:22

Reprinted from the U.S. Department of Health and Human Services and the President's Council on Physical Fitness and Sports 2002.

TABLE 11.25

Relative Strength Norms for 1RM Bench Press

Men						
	Age (years)					
Percentile*	20-29	30-39	40-49	50-59	60+	
90	1.48	1.24	1.10	0.97	0.89	
80	1.32	1.12	1.00	0.90	0.82	
70	1.22	1.04	0.93	0.84	0.77	
60	1.14	0.98	0.88	0.79	0.72	
50	1.06	0.93	0.84	0.75	0.68	
40	0.99	0.88	0.80	0.71	0.66	
30	0.93	0.83	0.76	0.68	0.63	
20	0.88	0.78	0.72	0.63	0.57	
10	0.80	0.71	0.65	0.57	0.53	
Women						
	Age (years)					
Percentile*	20-29	30-39	40-49	50-59	60-69	70+
90	0.54	0.49	0.46	0.40	0.41	0.44
80	0.49	0.45	0.40	0.37	0.38	0.39
70	0.42	0.42	0.38	0.35	0.36	0.33
60	0.41	0.41	0.37	0.33	0.32	0.31
50	0.40	0.38	0.34	0.31	0.30	0.27
40	0.37	0.37	0.32	0.28	0.29	0.25
30	0.35	0.34	0.30	0.26	0.28	0.24
20	0.33	0.32	0.27	0.23	0.26	0.21
10	0.30	0.27	0.23	0.19	0.25	0.02

*Descriptors for percentile rankings: 90 = well above average; 70 = above average; 50 = average; 30 = below average; 10 = well below average.

Data for men provided by The Cooper Institute for Aerobics Research, Dallas, TX, 1994. Data for women provided by the Women's Exercise Research Center, The George Washington Medical Center, Washington, DC, 1998. Published in *The Physical Fitness Specialist Certification Manual,* The Cooper Institute for Aerobics Research, Dallas, TX, revised 1997.

Reprinted from Heyward 2002.

TABLE 11.26

Relative Strength Norms for 1RM Leg Press

Men						
	Age					
Percentile*	20-29	30-39	40-49	50-59	60+	
90	2.27	2.07	1.92	1.80	1.73	
80	2.13	1.93	1.82	1.71	1.62	
70	2.05	1.85	1.74	1.64	1.56	
60	1.97	1.77	1.68	1.58	1.49	
50	1.91	1.71	1.62	1.52	1.43	
40	1.83	1.65	1.57	1.46	1.38	
30	1.74	1.59	1.51	1.39	1.30	
20	1.63	1.52	1.44	1.32	1.25	
10	1.51	1.43	1.35	1.22	1.16	
Women						
	Age					
Percentile*	20-29	30-39	40-49	50-59	60-69	70+
90	2.05	1.73	1.63	1.51	1.40	1.27
80	1.66	1.50	1.46	1.30	1.25	1.12
70	1.42	1.47	1.35	1.24	1.18	1.10
60	1.36	1.32	1.26	1.18	1.15	0.95
50	1.32	1.26	1.19	1.09	1.08	0.89
40	1.25	1.21	1.12	1.03	1.04	0.83
30	1.23	1.16	1.06	0.95	0.98	0.82
20	1.13	1.09	0.94	0.86	0.94	0.79
10	1.02	0.94	0.76	0.75	0.84	0.75

*Descriptors for percentile rankings: 90 = well above average; 70 = above average; 50 = average; 30 = below average; 10 = well below average.

Data for men provided by The Cooper Institute for Aerobics Research, Dallas, TX, 1994. Data for women provided by the Women's Exercise Research Center, The George Washington Medical Center, Washington, DC, 1998. Published in *The Physical Fitness Specialist Certification Manual,* The Cooper Institute for Aerobics Research, Dallas, TX, revised 1997.

Reprinted from Heyward 2002.

TABLE 11.27

YMCA Bench Press Norms

Percentile	Age 18-25		26-35		36-45		46-55		56-65		>65	
Sex	M	F	M	F	M	F	M	F	M	F	M	F
90	44	42	41	40	36	33	28	29	24	24	20	18
80	37	34	33	32	29	28	22	22	20	20	14	14
70	33	28	29	28	25	24	20	18	14	14	10	10
60	29	25	26	24	22	21	16	14	12	12	10	8
50	26	21	22	21	20	17	13	12	10	9	8	6
40	22	18	20	17	17	14	11	9	8	6	6	4
30	20	16	17	14	14	12	9	7	5	5	4	3
20	16	12	13	12	10	8	6	5	3	3	2	1
10	10	6	9	6	6	4	2	1	1	1	1	0

Note: Score is number of repetitions completed in 1 minute using 80-lb barbell for men and 35-lb barbell for women.

Adapted from Golding, Meyers, and Sinning 2000.

TABLE 11.28

Percentiles by Age Groups and Gender for Partial Curl-Up

Percentile*	Age 20-29		30-39		40-49		50-59		60-69	
Sex	M	F	M	F	M	F	M	F	M	F
90	75	70	75	55	75	50	74	48	53	50
80	56	45	69	43	75	42	60	30	33	30
70	41	37	46	34	67	33	45	23	26	24
60	31	32	36	28	51	28	35	16	19	19
50	27	27	31	21	39	25	27	9	16	13
40	23	21	26	15	31	20	23	2	9	9
30	20	17	19	12	26	14	19	0	6	3
20	13	12	13	0	21	5	13	0	0	0
10	4	5	0	0	13	0	0	0	0	0

*Descriptors for percentile rankings: 90 = well above average; 70 = above average; 50 = average; 30 = below average; 10 = well below average.

Based on data from *Canadian Standardized Test of Fitness Operations Manual,* 3rd ed. Ottawa: Canadian Society for Exercise Physiology in cooperation with Fitness Canada, Government of Canada, 1986.

Reprinted from ACSM 2000.

TABLE 11.29

YMCA Norms for the Sit-Up Test (number of repetitions)

Percentile	Age											
	18-25		26-35		36-45		46-55		56-65		>65	
Sex	M	F	M	F	M	F	M	F	M	F	M	F
90	77	68	62	54	60	54	61	48	56	44	50	34
80	66	61	56	46	52	44	53	40	49	38	40	32
70	57	57	52	41	45	38	51	36	46	32	35	29
60	52	51	44	37	43	35	44	33	41	27	31	26
50	46	44	38	34	36	31	39	31	36	24	27	22
40	41	38	36	32	32	28	33	28	32	22	24	20
30	37	34	33	28	29	23	29	25	28	18	22	16
20	33	32	30	24	25	20	24	21	24	12	19	11
10	27	25	21	20	21	16	16	13	20	8	12	9

Adapted from Golding, Myers, and Sinning 2000.

Percentile	85	50	85	60
Age (years)	Boys		Girls	
6	33	22	35	30
7	36	28	35	30
8	40	31	36	31
9	41	32	36	31
10	45	35	36	31
11	47	37	37	32
12	50	40	39	33
13	53	42	41	34
14	56	45	43	36
15	57	45	46	39
16	56	45	45	37
17	55	44	45	38

U.S. Department of Health and Human Services 2002.

TABLE 11.30

Age-Gender Norms for Push-Up Test (number of repetitions)

Men					
Percentile*	Age (years)				
	20-29	30-39	40-49	50-59	60-69
90	41	32	25	24	24
80	34	27	21	17	16
70	30	24	19	14	11
60	27	21	16	11	10
50	24	19	13	10	9
40	21	16	12	9	7
30	18	14	10	7	6
20	16	11	8	5	4
10	11	8	5	4	2

Women						
Percentile*	Age (years)					
	20-29	30-39	40-49	50-59	60-69	70+
90	31	27	25	19	18	24
80	27	22	21	17	15	17
70	21	20	17	13	13	11
60	19	17	16	12	11	9
50	18	16	14	11	9	7
40	14	13	11	9	6	2
30	13	10	10	6	4	0
20	10	7	8	3	0	0
10	6	1	4	0	0	0

*Descriptors for percentile rankings: 90 = well above average; 70 = above average; 50 = average; 30 = below average; 10 = well below average.

Data for men from the Canada Fitness Survey 1981. Data for modified push-up test for women provided by the Women's Exercise Research Center 1998.

Reprinted from Health Canada 1986 and Heyward 2002.

TABLE 11.31

Percentiles by Age Groups and Gender for YMCA Sit and Reach Test (inches)

Percentile	Age											
	18-25		26-35		36-45		46-55		56-65		>65	
Sex	M	F	M	F	M	F	M	F	M	F	M	F
90	22	24	21	23	21	22	19	21	17	20	17	20
80	20	22	19	21	19	21	17	20	15	19	15	18
70	19	21	17	20	17	19	15	18	13	17	13	17
60	18	20	17	20	16	18	14	17	13	16	12	17
50	17	19	15	19	15	17	13	16	11	15	10	15
40	15	18	14	17	13	16	11	14	9	14	9	14
30	14	17	13	16	13	15	10	14	9	13	8	13
20	13	16	11	15	11	14	9	12	7	11	7	11
10	11	14	9	13	7	12	6	10	5	9	4	9

These norms are based on a yardstick placed so that the "zero" point is set at 15 in. (38 cm).

Adapted from Golding, Myers, and Sinning 2000.

TABLE 11.32

Percentiles by Age Groups for Trunk Forward Flexion Using a Sit and Reach Box (cm)

Percentile*	Age									
	20-29		30-39		40-49		50-59		60-69	
Sex**	M	F	M	F	M	F	M	F	M	F
90	42	43	40	42	37	40	38	40	35	37
80	38	40	37	39	34	37	32	37	30	34
70	36	38	34	37	30	35	29	35	26	31
60	33	36	32	35	28	33	27	32	24	30
50	31	34	29	33	25	31	25	30	22	28
40	29	32	27	31	23	29	22	29	18	26
30	26	29	24	28	20	26	18	26	16	24
20	23	26	21	25	16	24	15	23	14	23
10	18	22	17	21	12	19	12	19	11	18

These norms are based on a sit and reach box in which the "zero" point is set at 26 cm. When using a box in which the "zero" point is set at 23 cm, subtract 3 cm from each value in this table.

*Descriptors for percentile rankings: 90 = well above average; 70 = above average; 50 = average; 30 = below average; 10 = well below average.

**Data for men from the Canada Fitness Survey 1981.

Reprinted from Health Canada 1986.

Percentile	85	50	85	50
Age (years)	Boys		Girls	
6	34	29	35	30
7	33	28	35	30
8	34	28	36	31
9	34	28	36	31
10	33	28	36	31
11	34	28	37	32
12	34	29	39	33
13	36	29	41	34
14	39	31	43	36
15	40	33	46	39
16	41	33	45	37
17	44	37	45	38

Adapted from U.S. Department of Health and Human Services 2002.

STUDY QUESTIONS

1. A 52-year-old male client's resting blood pressure was 130/82 during the initial assessment. When measuring his blood pressure one month later, to what level of mercury (Hg) should the bladder be inflated?

   A. 130 mm
   B. 150 mm
   C. 170 mm
   D. 200 mm

2. Which of the following skinfold sites should a personal trainer select when applying a three-site SKF equation to a 45-year-old female client?

   I. triceps
   II. subscapula
   III. suprailium
   IV. thigh

   A. I, II, and III only
   B. I, III, and IV only
   C. II, III, and IV only
   D. I, II, and IV only

3. A 39-year-old female client performed a submaximal bicycle ergometer test and had her $\dot{V}O_2$ max estimated as 30.2 ml · kg^{-1}· min^{-1}. She weighs 136 pounds (62 kilograms) and is 66 inches (168 centimeters) tall. Her body fat is 24% and resting blood pressure is 124/84 mmHg. Which of the following should be her primary exercise goal?

   A. lowering body fat
   B. increasing aerobic endurance

C. increasing lean body mass
D. lowering BMI

4. A 21-year-old male client had the following results during his initial assessment:

   Height: 72 inches (183 centimeters)

   Body weight: 210 pounds (95 kilograms)

   1RM bench press: 200 pounds (91 kilograms)

   1RM leg press: 400 pounds (192 kilograms)

   Sit-ups (1 minute): 50

   Sit and reach: 15 inches (38 centimeters) (using a sit and reach box)

Which of the following should be his primary exercise goal?

A. upper body strength
B. lower body strength
C. muscular endurance
D. hip/low back flexibility

APPLIED KNOWLEDGE QUESTION

A personal trainer assessed the aerobic endurance of a male client using the YMCA Cycle Ergometer test with these results:

Body weight: 167 pounds (76 kilograms)

Age: 36

Resting BP: 122/76

Test data:

Stage	Work rate ($kg \cdot m \cdot min^{-1}$)	Elapsed time	HR (beats/min)	Average HR* (beats/min)	BP (mmHg)	RPE
1	150	2:00	80			
1	150	3:00	84	82	134/78	8
2	600	5:00	128			
2	600	6:00	132	130	148/78	13
3	750	8:00	156			
3	750	9:00	160	158	152/74	16

*Average HR was calculated by averaging the two consecutive HR values at each work rate.

What is this client's estimated $\dot{V}O_2$max and how does it compare (i.e., what is his percentile rank)?

REFERENCES

1. Adams, G.M. 2002. *Exercise Physiology Laboratory Manual,* 4th ed. New York: McGraw-Hill.
2. American College of Sports Medicine. 2000. *ACSM's Guidelines for Exercise Testing and Prescription,* 6th ed., B.A. Franklin, M.H. Whaley, E.T. Howley, and G.J. Balady, eds. Philadelphia: Lippincott Williams & Wilkins.
3. Åstrand, P.-O., and I. Ryhming. 1954. A nomogram for calculation of aerobic capacity (physical fitness) from pulse rate during submaximal work. *Journal of Applied Physiology* 7: 218-221.
4. Baechle, T.R., R.W. Earle, and D. Wathen. 2000. Resistance training. In: *Essentials of Strength Training and Conditioning,* 2nd ed., T.R. Baechle and R.W. Earle, eds. Champaign, IL: Human Kinetics, pp. 395-425.
5. Baumgartner, T.A., and A.S. Jackson. 1999. *Measurement for Evaluation in Physical Education and Exercise Science.* Boston: McGraw-Hill.
6. Brooks, G.A., T.D. Fahey, T. P. White, and K.M. Baldwin. 2000. *Exercise Physiology: Human Bioenergetics and Its Applications,* 3rd ed. Mountain View, CA: Mayfield.

7. Devries, H.A., and T.J. Housh. 1994. *Physiology of Exercise for Physical Education, Athletics, and Exercise Science,* 5th ed. Madison, WI: Brown and Benchmark.
8. Eckerson, J.M., J.R. Stout, T.K. Evetovich, T.J. Housh, G.O. Johnson, and N. Worrell. Validity of self-assessment techniques for estimating percent fat in men and women. *Journal of Strength and Conditioning Research* 12: 243-247.
9. Harrison, G.G., E.R. Buskirk, J.E. Carter Lindsay, F.E. Johnston, T.G. Lohman, M.L. Pollock, A.F. Roche, and J.H. Wilmore. 1988. Skinfold thicknesses and measurement technique. In: *Anthropometric Standardization Reference Manual,* T.G. Lohman, A.F. Roche, and R. Martorell, eds. Champaign, IL: Human Kinetics, pp. 55-70.
10. Heyward, V.H. 1998. *Advanced Fitness Assessment and Exercise Prescription.* Champaign, IL: Human Kinetics.
11. Heyward, V.H. 2002. *Advanced Fitness Assessment and Exercise Prescription,* 4th ed. Champaign, IL: Human Kinetics.
12. Kline, G.M., J.P. Porcari, R. Hintermeister, P.S. Freedson, A. Ward, R.F. McCarron, J. Ross, and J.M. Rippe. 1987. Estimation of VO_2max from a one-mile track walk, gender, age, and body weight. *Medicine and Science in Sports and Exercise* 19: 253-259.
13. Kofler, M., A. Kreczy, and A. Gschwendtner. 2002. "Occupational backache"—surface electromyography demonstrates the advantage of an ergonomic versus a standard microscope workstation. *European Journal of Applied Physiology* 86: 492-497.
14. Kordich, J.A. 2002. *Evaluating Your Client: Fitness Assessment and Protocol Norms.* Lincoln, NE: NSCA Certification Commission.
15. Kraemer, W.J., and A.C. Fry. 1995. Strength testing: Development and evaluation of methodology. In: *Physiological Assessment of Human Fitness,* P.J. Maud and C. Foster, eds. Champaign, IL: Human Kinetics, pp. 115-138.
16. Leger, L., and M. Thivierge. 1988. Heart rate monitors: Validity, stability, and functionality. *Physician and Sportsmedicine* 16: 143-151.
17. McArdle, W.D., F.I. Katch, and V.L. Katch. 2001. *Exercise Physiology: Energy, Nutrition, and Human Performance,* 5th ed. Philadelphia: Lippincott Williams & Wilkins.
18. Morrow, J.R. Jr., A.W. Jackson, J.G. Disch, and D.P. Mood. 2000. *Measurement and Evaluation in Human Performance,* 2nd ed. Champaign, IL: Human Kinetics.
19. National Institutes of Health and National Heart, Lung, and Blood Institute. 1997. The sixth report of the Joint National Committee on Prevention, Detection, Evaluation, and Treatment of High Blood Pressure; and National High Blood Pressure Education Program. *Archives of Internal Medicine* 157: 2413-2446. Retrieved December 31, 2002, from www.nhlbi.nih.gov/guidelines/hypertension/index.htm. NIH Pub. No. 98-4080.
20. Prisant, L.M., B.S. Alpert, C.B. Robbins, A.S. Berson, M. Hayes, M.L. Cohen, and S.G. Sheps. 1995. American National Standard for nonautomated sphygmomanometers. Summary report. *American Journal of Hypertension* 8: 210-213.
21. Schmidt, P.K., and J.E. Carter. 1990. Static and dynamic differences among five types of skinfold calipers. *Human Biology* 62: 369-388.
22. U.S. Department of Health and Human Services. 2002. *The President's Challenge.* The President's Council on Physical Fitness and Sports.

PART III

Exercise Technique

CHAPTER 12

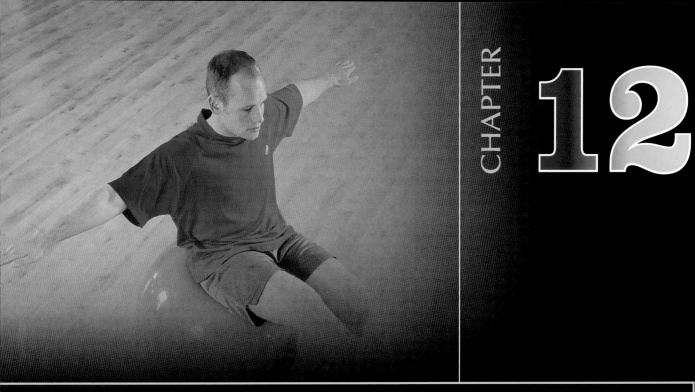

Flexibility, Body-Weight, and Stability Ball Exercises

Allen Hedrick

After completing this chapter, you will be able to

- describe the benefits of participating in a flexibility training program;
- understand the factors that affect flexibility;
- explain the value of warming up before participating in flexibility training;
- list and explain the various types of flexibility training;
- supervise a flexibility training program emphasizing a combination of dynamic and static stretching; and
- supervise exercises using body weight only and stability balls.

Personal trainers recognize that improving flexibility is an important aspect of the overall exercise program. The personal trainer needs to be able to communicate to clients why time devoted to improving flexibility will enhance other aspects of their program. This chapter deals first with flexibility training, including its benefits, the factors that influence flexibility, and the tissue adaptations that flexibility training targets. It then addresses the importance of warm-up, the types of flexibility training, and program design considerations. A final section of the chapter covers body-weight and stability ball exercises. At times personal trainers may need to be able to provide resistance training to clients in nontraditional settings where little or no equipment is available. The information in this section provides relevant information and practical training suggestions for this type of training. Exercise instructions and illustrations of common flexibility, body-weight, and stability ball exercises are provided at the end of the chapter.

Flexibility Training

Those involved in supervising conditioning or rehabilitation programs typically use some form of stretching. Nevertheless, there is still much confusion about flexibility training in terms of its scientific basis [5, 6]. Much of the confusion is the result of the notion that people must achieve extreme levels of flexibility in order to reduce the opportunity for injury and improve movement capabilities [9]. This is not an accurate representation of the role that flexibility plays. Flexibility is an important piece of the training puzzle. But, like other aspects of training, it must be based on the needs of the client.

A logical starting point in alleviating some of the confusion is to provide a definition of flexibility. Most commonly, **flexibility** is defined as the range of motion of a joint or a series of joints [1, 3, 4]. Perhaps a more relevant definition for personal trainers, in terms of improving movement performance or reducing the opportunity for injury, is the ability of a joint to move freely through the full normal range of motion (ROM) [22].

Although every training session should begin with a warm-up, designed to elevate core temperature, not every activity needs to be preceded by flexibility training. After the warm-up session is completed, the client may or may not need to participate immediately in a flexibility training program, depending on the nature of the activity to follow. For example, if the client is going to participate in a dynamic activity (e.g., basketball, racquetball) after the warm-up, then participating in flexibility training before the activity is necessary. In contrast, if the client will be participating in a less dynamic activity (e.g., stationary bike), then flexibility training can take place after the training session. In either case, flexibility training is part of the total exercise program and part of each workout.

Benefits of Flexibility Training

Flexibility is an important aspect of any training program. Achieving optimum flexibility helps eliminate awkward and inefficient movement by allowing joints to move freely through a full normal ROM, and may also provide increased resistance to muscle injury [2, 16, 17, 18, 25]. Improving flexibility is a fundamental element of any training program, because good flexibility may enhance the ability to perform various movement skills, especially those that require a high level of flexibility (e.g., serving a tennis ball, picking up a bag of groceries off the floor) [1, 4, 5, 15, 22, 26, 29, 32]. However, it is important to note that although there have been great athletes who have been able to exhibit amazing flexibility, this is not usually why they are great athletes. The ability to move effectively depends on strength with coordination, and being flexible can enhance this ability in certain situations [9]. The goal of flexibility training is not to achieve a point at which the client has no joint stability, but rather to achieve strength intertwined with flexibility that can allow the client to better control his or her movements [9].

Flexibility training is also important in injury prevention [1, 4, 5, 6, 19, 22, 26, 29, 32]. The more common problems in clients with poor flexibility include lower back pain potentially resulting from tight quadriceps, iliopsoas, and back muscles (and possibly a corresponding weakness in the abdominal muscles and hamstrings). A lack of flexibility may also increase the incidence of muscle tears resulting from tight muscles on one or both sides of a joint [5]. The accepted rule regarding the role of flexibility in injury prevention is that a normal ROM in each joint will reduce the opportunity for injury [6]. If a client is involved in a sport or activity that requires a greater-than-normal ROM, greater

Some portions of this chapter are adapted from A. Hedrick, 2002, "Flexibility training for range of motion," *NSCA's Performance Training Journal* 1 (2): 13-20.

emphasis will need to be placed on increasing flexibility to help protect against injury.

Because of these important benefits, it is recommended that personal trainers supervise stretching sessions as they would any other part of the training session. Doing so communicates the importance of the warm-up/stretching period and may encourage clients to keep their attention focused on the task at hand [19].

Flexibility training is important to those interested in fitness because of the role that optimum flexibility plays in improving movement performance and reducing the opportunity for injury.

Factors Affecting Flexibility

A number of factors influence flexibility. Some of these factors cannot be affected by training, such as joint structure, age, and sex. However, other factors can be influenced by training, including muscle and connective tissue, core temperature, activity level, participation in a well-designed resistance training program, and of course participation in a flexibility training program [1, 14].

Joint Structure

One of the primary limiting factors in static ROM is the structure of the joint itself [6]. Because of joint structure there is a limit to how much movement is available. Joint structures vary between clients, and the personal trainer must consider this variation when evaluating flexibility.

Joint structure also varies between joints. Some joints offer a reduced range of movement compared to others by virtue of their construction. The hinge-type joints of the knee and elbow allow only backward and forward movements (flexion and extension), so knee and elbow ROM is significantly less than that of the shoulder or hip [1]. In contrast, the ball and socket joints of the hip and shoulder allow movements in all anatomical planes and have the greatest ROM of all joints [1, 5, 14, 22].

Flexibility is joint specific. That is, it is common to have above-average flexibility in one joint and below-average ROM in another [3, 7]. As a result, flexibility needs to be thought of not as a general characteristic but instead as a characteristic that is specific to a particular joint and joint action [22]. Being flexible in one joint does not guarantee a high degree of flexibility in another joint [22]. Because of this, performing a single flexibility test as a measure of overall flexibility is based on a fallacy [7, 19].

Muscle and Connective Tissue

Connective tissue (muscles, ligaments, and tendons) is the area of emphasis during ROM exercise. Muscle is not thought of as a connective tissue structure. However, evidence indicates that during ROM exercise, when a relaxed muscle is stretched, the majority of the resistance to the stretch comes from the extensive connective tissue framework and sheathing within and around the muscle [18].

Under normal circumstances, connective tissue is the major structure limiting joint ROM. Range of motion is primarily limited by one or more connective issue structures, including ligamentous joint capsules, tendons, and muscles [18, 19]. Thus improvements in ROM as a result of stretching are primarily due to the connective tissue adaptations [1].

Most of the difference between individuals in static ROM is attributable to the elastic properties of the muscle and tendons attached across the joints [6]. "Stiff" muscles and tendons reduce the ROM while "compliant" muscles and tendons increase ROM.

It is these elastic properties that are altered as a result of stretching exercises. When a muscle is held for a period of time under tension in a static stretch, the passive tension in the muscle declines; that is, the muscle "gives" a little. This is called a "viscoelastic stretch relaxation response" [6]. Passive tension is defined as the amount of external force required to lengthen the relaxed muscle. Obviously, the less external force required, the more pliable the muscle. This increased pliability is maintained for up to 90 minutes after the stretch.

The muscles crossing over or adjacent to a joint also affect flexibility [3]. In any movement, the active contraction of a muscle (agonistic) occurs simultaneously with the relaxation or stretching of the antagonistic muscle. The more easily the antagonistic muscles yield, the less energy is spent in overcoming their resistance. The capacity of a muscle fiber to lengthen improves as a result of flexibility training. However, flexibility is often limited, regardless of the amount of training, if the antagonistic muscles are not relaxed or if there is a lack of coordination between contraction (agonists) and relaxation (antagonists).

Hyperlaxity

Although not commonly, some people are born with a tissue structure that predisposes them to

hyperlaxity. Hyperlaxity allows the joints of the body to achieve a ROM that exceeds the normal ROM [26]. With someone in whom joint hyperlaxity has been determined, the personal trainer needs to use caution when implementing the stretching program. It is important to not overstretch the client and create even greater levels of laxity in the surrounding supportive tissues. Problems can arise when clients with hyperlaxity are placed in a stretching program without being properly assessed by a health care professional. Poor selection of stretching exercises can cause even more problems for the client.

Age

Age also plays a role in flexibility. Investigators have found that elementary school children become less flexible with age, reaching a low point between the ages of 10 and 12 [1, 4, 7, 19, 22]. Flexibility normally improves after this point, but never again reaches the level seen during early childhood [18]. This decrease in flexibility is due to a gradual loss of elasticity in the muscle [3].

From the anatomical point of view, childhood is the ideal time to start a flexibility program [3, 4]. During this stage, training programs should be aimed at developing flexibility in all joints.

Sex

Sex also plays a role in flexibility; typically females are more flexible than males [1, 5, 7, 16, 19]. Research shows that elementary school girls are superior to boys in flexibility, and it is likely that this difference exists throughout adult life [18]. This higher degree of flexibility in females is generally attributable to anatomical variations in joint structures [16]. The biggest differences in flexibility are seen in the trunk (flexion and extension), hips, and ankles [3]. The decrease in flexibility in boys at puberty is thought to be related to increases in muscle size, stature, and muscle strength.

Temperature

Core temperature is also a factor in flexibility, as ROM is positively affected by an increase in either core temperature [1, 5, 7, 22] or external temperature [22]. The positive effect that increasing core temperature has on ROM points to the importance of warming up before participation in flexibility training. Warm-up is discussed later in the chapter.

Activity Level

As one would expect, evidence indicates that people who are physically active tend to be more flexible than inactive individuals. The decrease in flexibility in inactive individuals occurs because connective tissues tend to become less pliable when exposed only to limited ROMs [1, 18, 22]. A decrease in activity level results in an increase in percent body fat and a decrease in the pliability of connective tissue. Further, an increase in fat deposits around the joints creates obstructions to ROM [18].

Resistance Training

A well-designed and properly executed resistance training program can have the effect of increasing flexibility. However, a resistance training program emphasizing high loads performed through less than full ROM can decrease flexibility [1]. Therefore resistance training programs should be designed to develop both agonist and antagonist muscles, and all exercises must be performed through the full available ROM of the involved joints [1]. It is important to point out that while improper resistance training can impair flexibility, this generally does not occur because a person has become too muscular or muscle bound. Instead, the decrease in flexibility occurs because of the improper development of a muscle or a group of muscles around a joint, resulting in a restriction of motion at that joint [5, 9]. For example, a person with large biceps and deltoids may experience difficulty in stretching the triceps, racking a power clean, or holding the bar while performing the front squat [1].

Flexibility is influenced by a variety of factors. Some of the factors (joint structure, age, and sex) cannot be affected by training. However, the client's core temperature during flexibility training, overall activity level, participation in a well-designed resistance training program, and stretching on a regular basis can all affect flexibility and can all be positively influenced by the personal trainer.

Elasticity and Plasticity

Flexibility training targets two different tissue adaptations, elastic and plastic. **Elasticity** refers to the ability to return to original resting length after a passive stretch [1]. As a result, elasticity provides a temporary change in length. In contrast, **plasticity** refers to the tendency to assume a new and greater length after a passive stretch, even after the load is removed [1, 18].

Muscle has elastic properties only. However, ligaments and tendons have both plastic and elastic properties. When connective tissue is stretched, some of the elongation occurs in the elastic tissue elements and some occurs in the plastic elements. When the stretch is removed, the elastic deformation recovers, but the plastic deformation remains [18].

Obviously stretching techniques should be designed primarily to produce a plastic deformation, because a permanent increase in ROM is the goal. During stretching, the proportion of elastic and plastic deformation can vary, depending on how and under what conditions the flexibility training occurs. Emphasizing stretching to the point of mild discomfort, holding the stretched position for a period of time, and stretching only when the core temperature has been elevated will assist in maximizing plastic stretch [18].

Warm-Up

It is commonly accepted that clients should engage in some form of preparatory exercises before undertaking vigorous activities. These types of preparatory exercises or movements are generally referred to as **warm-up.**

It needs to be made clear that warm-up and stretching are not the same thing. Warm-up is an activity that raises the total body temperature, as well as temperature of the muscles, to prepare the body for vigorous exercise [1]. Warming up is part of the foundation of a successful exercise session. Getting fully warmed up, mentally and physically, is a key aspect of attaining the training intensity required to achieve optimal results. A warm-up period is also important before physical activity because it may help protect against injury by improving flexibility of the muscles [10, 18, 28, 32, 38]. This increase in flexibility as a result of warming up is due to the fact that muscle elasticity is dependent on blood flow to the target muscle [35]. Accordingly, cold muscles with low blood flow are more susceptible to injury or damage than muscles at higher temperature and an associated blood saturation [35].

To date the psychological aspects of warm-up have not been adequately investigated. However, most individuals who perform a warm-up prior to their main activity tend to be more mentally tuned or prepared [35].

Unfortunately, many clients attempt to take shortcuts in the warm-up procedure, which translates into a poor workout or competition [27]. In fact, every workout, regardless of the time constraints of the client, needs to be preceded by a warm-up session. If the client does not have time to warm up, then he or she does not have time to work out.

Clients should, as a matter of routine, perform warm-up activities to prepare themselves more suitably for strenuous exercise. Most research clearly indicates that the major benefits of warm-up are very much related to temperature-dependent physiological processes.

Effects of Increased Body Temperature After Warm-Up

An increase in body temperature after a warm-up helps to produce the following effects [28]:

- An increase in muscle blood flow
- An increase in the sensitivity of nerve receptors
- An increase in the disassociation of oxygen from hemoglobin and myoglobin
- An increase in the speed of nerve impulse transmissions
- A reduction in muscle viscosity
- A lowering of the energy rates of metabolic chemical reactions

The increase in tissue temperature that occurs during warm-up is the result of three physiological processes [14]. The first is the friction of the sliding filaments during muscular contraction. In addition, the metabolism of fuels and the dilation of intramuscular blood vessels contribute to increased tissue temperature [14].

Theoretically, the following physiological changes take place during warm-up and should enhance performance [19]:

1. The temperature increases within the muscles that are being recruited during the warm-up session. A warmed muscle contracts more forcefully and relaxes more quickly. As a result, both speed and strength should be enhanced during exercise.

2. The temperature of the blood as it travels through the working muscle increases. As blood temperature rises, more oxygen is unloaded to the working muscles.
3. The ROM around joints is increased as a result of the warm-up.

Range of motion is increased after a warm-up period. The reason is that elevated core temperatures lower muscle, tendon, and ligament viscosity, leading to increased ROM [35]. This will enable achievement of best possible results and reduce the potential risk of stretching-induced injuries. It has been reported that excessive stretching, when the tissue temperatures are relatively low, increases the risk of connective tissue damage [35].

For this reason many authors believe that stretching should occur only after warm-up [4, 8, 22, 35] or post-workout [14]. Post-workout flexibility training also has a regenerative effect, restoring the muscles to their resting length, stimulating blood flow, and reducing muscle spasm [14]. The physiological responses that occur due to warming up warrant its continuation as a method to prepare the body for flexibility training [12]. Body temperature should be elevated to a point that the client has started sweating before beginning flexibility exercises[19].

Unfortunately, often the pre-exercise warm-up program consists primarily of static stretching. There are three distinct disadvantages to using static stretching to increase core temperature [11]:

1. Because static stretching is a passive activity, minimal friction of the muscle's sliding filaments occurs.
2. There is little, if any, increase in the rate of fuels being metabolized.
3. There is no need for the intramuscular blood vessels to dilate in response to static stretching.

For these reasons, clients using static stretching to warm up begin an exercise session with only a minimal increase in core body temperature [23]. This means they are missing out on the benefits of increased core temperature, decreased viscosity of the muscle, and reduced muscle and joint stiffness. The decrease in viscosity leads to increases in ROM, which protects the body against sudden, unexpected movements [14]. Getting fully warmed up, mentally and physically, is a key aspect of achieving a training intensity required to achieve optimal results.

Flexibility training should never be used as a method to warm up. Instead, flexibility training should occur only after core temperature has been elevated to a point where the client is beginning to perspire.

Types of Warm-Up

Most agree that there are three types of warm-up methods, namely passive, general, and specific [23, 35], although some authors use only two categories, active and passive. Regardless of the warm-up method chosen, the general purpose of warming up before physical activity is to increase muscle temperature [17].

Passive Warm-Up

Passive warm-up involves such methods as hot showers, heating pads, or massage. Much of the research [13, 31, 33], but not all [19], has shown that passive warm-up methods can have a positive effect. One obvious advantage of a passive warm-up is that it does not prefatigue a client before an exercise session; once elevated temperatures are achieved, this increase in temperature can be preserved prior to physical activity with minimal energy expenditure [35]. Unfortunately, the procedures of a passive warm-up (e.g., using a moist heat pack) may not be practical in many settings.

General Warm-Up

General warm-up involves basic activities that require movement of the major muscle groups, such as jogging, cycling, or jumping rope [35]. General warm-up increases heart rate, blood flow, deep muscle temperature, respiration rate, viscosity of joint fluids, and perspiration [1]. The increase in muscle temperature allows a greater amount of flexibility [1], which prepares the body for movements [1]. Thus, general warm-up seems more appropriate than passive when the goal is preparing the body for demanding physical activity.

Specific Warm-Up

Unlike general warm-up, **specific warm-up** includes movements that are an actual part of the activity, such as slow jogging before going out on a run or performing light repetitions of bench presses before progressing to the workout weight [1, 19, 35]. Specific warm-up appears to be the method that is most desirable because it increases the temperature of the specific muscles that will be used in subsequent, more strenuous activity, as well as serving as a mental rehearsal of the upcoming activity [23]. See chapter 17 for examples of specific warm-up drills for plyometric and speed training.

Warm-Up Guidelines

The amount, intensity, and duration of warm-up must ideally be adjusted to every individual depending on the client's current level of fitness. The length of the warm-up period depends on climate and physical conditioning level. In general the warm-up activity should last approximately 5 to 15 minutes, long enough for the client to break out in a sweat [32].

Also, as a client's training status improves, the intensity and duration of the warm-up should increase. Compared to an untrained client, a well-conditioned client probably requires a longer or more intense warm-up, or one that is both longer and more intense, to achieve an optimal level of body temperature [35].

Types of Flexibility Training

A number of stretching techniques are used to maintain or increase flexibility. The most common of these methods are ballistic, static, and various proprioceptive neuromuscular facilitation (PNF) techniques [4, 18, 19, 22]. Dynamic flexibility, while not as common as the three methods just mentioned, is gaining acceptance and is discussed in greater detail further into the chapter.

Flexibility training can be further categorized into active and passive stretching exercises. **Active stretching** occurs when the person who is stretching supplies the force of the stretch. For example, during the sitting toe touch, the client supplies the force for the forward lean that stretches the hamstrings and low back [1]. In contrast, **passive stretching** occurs when a partner or stretching device provides the force for the stretch [1].

The most important aspect of designing an effective flexibility training program is to ensure correct performance of the exercises, regardless of which flexibility training method is used [6]. For example, one technique commonly used to stretch the hamstrings is the toe touch stretch. However, this position requires lower back flexion, which posteriorly rotates the pelvis, decreasing the effectiveness of the stretch for the hamstrings. A better method to stretch the hamstrings is to place one foot slightly in front of the other, leaning forward from the hips and keeping the back arched. Supporting upper-body weight with the hands on the rear leg, the client should feel the stretch in the front leg. This position ensures that the back does not flex and that the pelvis remains tilted forward, keeping the hamstrings optimally lengthened [6]. The point is that it is necessary to perform the stretch with good technique to bring about optimal increases in flexibility.

Ballistic Stretching

Ballistic stretching (bouncing) is a rapid, jerky, uncontrolled movement. During ballistic stretching the body part is put into motion and momentum takes it through the ROM until the muscles are stretched to the limits [1, 3, 4, 18, 22, 32].

A negative aspect of ballistic stretching is that the increased flexibility is achieved through a series of jerks or pulls on the resistant tissue. Because these movements are performed at high speeds, the rate and degree of stretch, as well as the force applied to induce the stretch, are difficult to control [18]. Another negative aspect of ballistic stretching is that this type of stretching may injure muscles or connective tissues, especially when there has been a previous injury [1, 22]. This increased opportunity for injury occurs because there is a danger of exceeding the extensibility limits of the tissue being stretched [32].

Ballistic stretching, though widely used in the past, is no longer considered an acceptable method for increasing ROM in any joint. When one is comparing static and ballistic stretching techniques, there are four distinct disadvantages of ballistic stretching to consider [2]:

1. Increased danger of exceeding the extensibility limits of tissues involved
2. Higher energy requirements
3. Greater likelihood of causing muscular soreness than with static stretching
4. Activation of the stretch reflex

Two of the sensory organs within skeletal muscles that function as protective mechanisms against injury during passive and active stretching are the muscle spindles and the Golgi tendon organs. Muscle spindles are located within the center of a muscle [22]. When the muscle spindles are not stimulated, the muscle relaxes, allowing a greater stretch. However, as the client bounces, the muscles respond by contracting to protect themselves from overstretching. Thus, internal tension develops in the muscle and prevents it from being fully stretched [18]. A familiar example of this stretch reflex is the knee jerk response. When the patellar tendon is struck, the tendon, and consequently the quadriceps muscle, experience a slight but rapid stretch. The induced stretch results in activation of muscle spindle receptors within the quadriceps [18], and the knee extends. Stimulation of the muscle spindle and the subsequent activation of the stretch reflex should be avoided during stretching, as motion will be limited by the reflexive muscle action.

The other sensory organ, the Golgi tendon organ, is located at the musculotendinous junction. When excessive force is generated in the muscle, the Golgi tendon organ causes a reflex opposite that of the muscle spindle by inhibiting muscle contraction and causing the muscle to relax. The Golgi tendon organ helps to prevent injury by preventing the muscle from developing too much force or tension during active stretching [22].

Static Stretching

The most commonly used method of increasing flexibility is **static stretching**. A slow constant speed is used during static stretching, with the stretched position generally held for 30 seconds [1]. Static stretching involves relaxing and simultaneous lengthening of the stretched muscle. Because of the slow speed at which the stretches are performed, static stretching does not activate the stretch reflex of the stretched muscle. Thus the opportunity for injury is lower than during ballistic stretching [1]. Although injury to muscles or connective tissue may result if the static stretch is too intense, there are no real disadvantages to static stretching in terms of injury potential as long as proper technique is used. However, recent research suggests that performing static flexibility before taking part in a dynamic activity (running, jumping, throwing) may have a negative effect on performance [10, 24].

It is important to note that increasing the length of time that the stretched position is held beyond 30 seconds is not necessarily advantageous. For example, it has been found that increasing the time from 30 seconds to 60 seconds does not result in improved flexibility [22]. Those just starting a flexibility training program may find it difficult to hold a stretch for 30 seconds. In these cases the personal trainer may wish to start the client out with 15 or 20 seconds of holding and gradually progress to 30 seconds as the client gains experience and focus.

Moving into the final static stretch position should occur slowly and only to a point of minor discomfort. As the stretched position is held, the feeling of tension should diminish. If the feeling of tension does not diminish, the stretched position should be slightly reduced. Use of this procedure should assist in eliminating activation of the stretch reflex [18]. Instructions for static stretches can be found on pages 278 to 281.

To avoid activation of the stretch reflex, the client should move into the final static stretch position slowly and only to a point of minor discomfort. As the stretched position is held, the feeling of tension should diminish. If the feeling of tension does not diminish, the stretched position should be slightly reduced.

Proprioceptive Neuromuscular Facilitation

Proprioceptive neuromuscular facilitation (PNF) stretching was originally developed as a technique to relax muscles with increased tone or activity. It has since expanded to the conditioning of both athletes and the general population as a method of increasing ROM [1].

Proprioneuromuscular facilitation is widely accepted as an effective method of increasing ROM [9, 13, 21, 30, 36]. These techniques, normally performed with a partner, make use of both passive movement and active (concentric and isometric) muscle actions [6, 19, 22]. Although there are a variety of PNF techniques, perhaps the most common method involves taking the muscle or joint into a static stretch position while keeping the muscle relaxed. After this static stretch position is held for about 10 seconds, the muscle is contracted for 6 seconds with a strong isometric contraction against an external fixed object (i.e., a partner) acting in the direction of the stretch. The partner should not allow the client to have any movement in the joint. Following a very brief (1-2 second) rest, another 30-second passive stretch is performed, potentially resulting in a greater stretch. The isometric contraction will result in the stimulation of the respective Golgi tendon organs; this may help to maintain low muscle tension during the second stretching maneuver, allowing connective tissue length to further increase and resulting in increased ROM [18].

PNF stretching may be superior to other stretching methods because it assists muscular relaxation, potentially assisting in increased ROM [9, 20, 21, 26, 30, 36]. A study evaluating increases in ROM resulting from static and PNF stretching procedures showed that while both procedures resulted in increased flexibility, subjects using the PNF method gained the most ROM. Despite this, not everyone agrees that PNF is the best method. Although some studies suggest that PNF produces better results than other forms of stretching, PNF techniques can be impractical to use. One limitation is that a partner is usually required. The partner has to take great care not to overstretch the muscle. In addition, PNF can be dangerous unless each person is familiar with the appropriate techniques, because too much emphasis can be placed on flexibility and not enough on correct technique [8]. The injury potential from PNF may be a concern especially with children or with groups of youngsters because of the need for close supervision. For this reason, and because the research advocating PNF as an effective technique has been disputed in some studies, caution is necessary when one is implementing a PNF program with this age group [5].

Because of the limitations just mentioned, PNF methods have limited application in personal training settings. A significant level of training is needed to safely implement PNF methods. Because a partner is needed, use of PNF can be more time-consuming than other methods. Further, because static and dynamic flexibility methods are effective at increasing flexibility, and because most clients do not need to achieve superior flexibility levels, PNF methods are generally not required in this setting. If the personal trainer has been trained in PNF methods, and if the client has a drastic lack of ROM in one or more joints, PNF methods might be used in these limited applications.

Dynamic Stretching

Dynamic flexibility is not new, but it is not as common as the other flexibility training methods that have been discussed. **Dynamic stretching** and ballistic stretching are similar in that both allow faster movements to occur during training. However, dynamic stretching avoids bouncing and includes movements specific to a sport or movement pattern [1]. An example of a dynamic stretch is a lunge walk, in which the client exaggerates the length of the stride and bends the back leg so that he or she ends up in a position in which the front knee is over the toe (but not in front of it) and the back knee is just off the floor with the torso held in an upright position.

As the client becomes better able to perform each drill, he or she can perform the exercises in combinations. For example, a knee tuck can be combined with a lunge walk, alternating legs after each movement has been performed. The possible combinations of exercises are nearly limitless. Combining movements has two primary advantages. First, it provides greater variety so that the flexibility training program does not become monotonous to the client. Second, it becomes a more time-efficient way to train because a larger number of muscle groups are stretched during a combination of stretches. This is important because many clients have a limited amount of time to devote to their training programs.

The use of dynamic flexibility is still somewhat controversial. However, applying the specificity of training principle to flexibility training may help reduce the controversy [6]. For example, no personal trainer would use only isometric training to develop a client's muscular strength. Rather, a goal of resistance training is to build a client's *usable, functional* strength. This makes one wonder why so many people use only static stretches to develop flexibility [6].

Similarly, dynamic flexibility may be more appropriate because it more closely simulates movements that occur in daily activities. For example, consider the everyday movement of reaching for an item on the top shelf in the grocery store, home, or workplace. Dynamic arm circles, which are done with fluidity of movement, may more closely resemble reaching overhead in everyday life than would a position in which the arms are held statically over the head.

There is still much about stretching methods to be investigated before all the definitive answers can be given. In particular, static stretching as part of a warm-up is very common; and yet the research, and logic, suggest that static stretches will do little to help prevent injuries or improve muscle function before an activity. Instead, active mobility exercises, those that take the muscles dynamically through the full ROM, starting slowly and building up to movement-specific speeds, are appropriate when preparing to exercise and when developing active ROM for daily activities [6].

Dynamic stretching puts an emphasis on functionally based movements. As training progresses, advancing from a standing position to a walk or a skip (e.g., repeated over a distance of 20 to 25 yards, or 18 to 23 meters) can enhance the effectiveness of the dynamic stretching exercises. Adjusting from static stretching exercises to dynamic exercises is not difficult. Often the stretching exercise is the same, but it is preceded and followed by some form of movement.

Personal trainers who wish to implement dynamic flexibility training in a client's program should begin with low-volume, low-intensity exercises. Dynamic flexibility exercises require balance and coordination, so the client may experience muscle soreness for a short period of time during the introduction of dynamic flexibility training.

Four primary types of flexibility training methods are used: ballistic, static, PNF, and dynamic.

Body-Weight and Stability Ball Exercises

The personal trainer may work with a client who does not have access to traditional resistance training equipment or who simply prefers not to train in a health club setting. This does not mean that the client does not have the opportunity to perform resistance training activities; it does mean that the client's personal trainer will have to be creative in his or her approach.

One possible solution is to have the client perform a series of either body-weight exercises, stability ball exercises, or both. The type of exercise is not the most important criterion; for example, the pectoralis and triceps muscle groups can be trained by performing the free weight bench press exercise, the chest bench press exercise on a variety of selectorized machines, or push-ups on the floor or off of a stability ball. As long as the intensity is at the necessary threshold and applied to the correct muscles, adaptation will occur, regardless of the type of exercise.

Although body-weight, calisthenic types of exercises have been used for years, one might think of stability ball training as a relative innovation. In reality, stability ball training has been used since the 1960s [8], though originally it was used as a method of orthopedic and neuro-development treatment. More recently the stability ball has been used in general fitness programs and in the conditioning programs of athletes [34].

As with any training method, it is important to adhere to training guidelines (see "Guidelines for Stability Ball Exercises," below) to assure that clients are maximizing the time and effort they spend training with the stability ball.

Guidelines for Stability Ball Exercises

- Make sure the stability ball is fully inflated, so that it is firm.
- To determine the correct-size ball, have the client sit on the ball with feet flat on the floor. The thighs should be parallel to the ground. If the client has low back pain, the thighs should be slightly above parallel, with the knees lower than the hips.
- Clients should warm up for 5 to 15 minutes before doing a complete stability ball workout. Activities such as brisk walking or jogging, walking up stairs, or calisthenic-type activities (i.e., jumping jacks, mountain climbers) can be used during this warm-up period. Warm-up activities performed on the stability ball can also be used, as they have the advantage of training the stabilizing muscle groups, improving balance and coordination [37].
- Beginning clients should start with low volume and low intensity and progress gradually as strength and stamina allow.
- Do not allow the client to use poor form as a result of fatigue. Even well-trained clients may fatigue quickly when beginning stability ball exercises. Instead, help clients to progress gradually so as to maintain correct form on each repetition.
- Ensure correct technique. Because of the "unstable" nature of the ball, even the slightest deviation from correct technique or position can have a negative effect on performance of the exercise.

The number of sets and repetitions depends on the fitness level of the client. Depending on their fitness goals, clients can either do the exercises in circuit training-type fashion or do the full number of sets on each exercise before advancing to the next exercise. As with beginning any exercise routine, the client should start with a low-volume, low-intensity training plan (e.g., 1 set × 8 repetitions) and gradually adjust the training variables as the fitness level improves (e.g., 3 × 15). Descriptions of body-weight exercises appear on pages 286 to 287, and stability ball exercise instructions can be found on pages 288 to 292. Also, several of the resistance training exercises shown in chapter 13 can be performed with the client's body weight only (e.g., lunge, squat, and calf raise).

CONCLUSION

Personal trainers typically incorporate some form of stretching into their clients' programs, and it is important that personal trainers and their clients have a clear understanding of what flexibility is and how it relates to conditioning in general. Defined as the range of motion of a joint or a series of joints, flexibility helps a joint to move freely through a full normal ROM and helps to improve performance and prevent injury. Many factors affect a client's flexibility, including joint structure, muscle and connective tissue, sex, temperature, and resistance training. Warm-up—which is not to be confused with stretching—is part of the foundation of an effective workout, increasing the client's body temperature and range of motion.

Ballistic, static, and various PNF techniques are the stretching techniques most commonly used to maintain or increase flexibility, although dynamic stretching, while still somewhat controversial, is also gaining acceptance. In designing flexibility programs the personal trainer is well advised to incorporate a combination of dynamic and static flexibility training. For some clients, it is appropriate to use a series of body-weight or stability ball exercises or to use a combination of these two forms of exercise.

Flexibility, Body-Weight, and Stability Ball Exercises

Static Flexibility Exercises

Dynamic Flexibility Exercises

Body-Weight Exercises

Stability Ball Exercises

Static Flexibility Exercises

Hands Behind Back

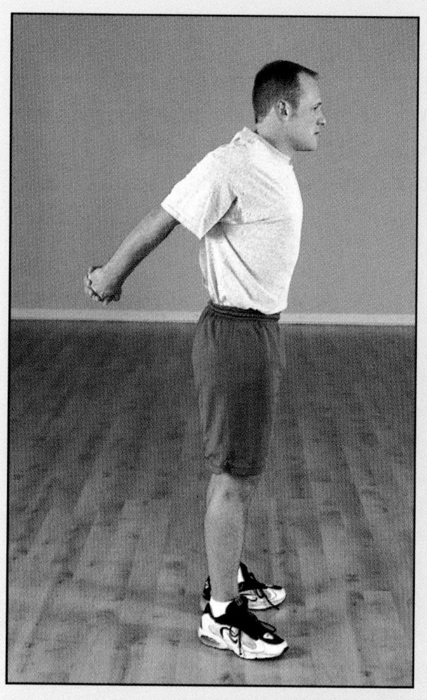

1. Stand erect and reach behind the back with both arms.
2. Clasp the hands together and fully extend the elbows.
3. Slightly flex the knees and look straight ahead.
4. Raise the arms until a stretch is felt.

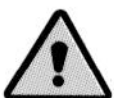 **Common Errors**

- Allowing the elbows to flex
- Flexing the torso forward or looking down at the floor

Primary Muscles Stretched:
Anterior deltoids, pectoralis major

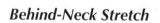

Behind-Neck Stretch

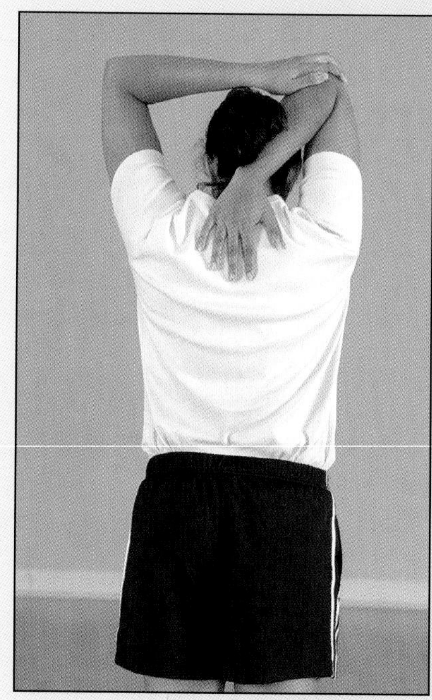

1. Stand erect and raise the right arm to position it next to the right side of the head.
2. Flex the right elbow to allow the right hand to touch the back of the neck or upper back.
3. Raise the left arm to grasp the right elbow with the left hand.
4. Pull the right elbow toward (and behind) the head with the left hand (i.e., increase shoulder abduction) until a stretch is felt.
5. Repeat the stretch with the right hand grasping and pulling the left elbow.

 **Common Error**

- Flexing the torso forward or rounding the shoulders

Primary Muscles Stretched:
Triceps brachii, latissimus dorsi

Pretzel

1. Sit on the floor with the legs next to each other and extended away from the body.
2. With the torso upright, flex the right knee, cross it over the left leg, and place the right foot on the floor to the outside of the left knee.
3. Twist the torso to the right to position the back of the left elbow against the outside of the right knee.
4. Place the right palm on the floor 12 to 16 inches (30-40 centimeters) behind the hips.
5. Keeping the buttocks on the floor, use the right knee to hold the left elbow stationary while twisting the head and shoulders to the right until a stretch is felt.
6. Repeat the stretch with the left foot placed to the outside of the right knee and the right elbow against the outside of the left knee.

Primary Muscles Stretched:
Internal oblique, external oblique, piriformis, erector spinae

 **Common Errors**

- Placing the elbow on the front of the thigh (rather than to the outside of the knee)
- Allowing the buttocks to rise off of the floor

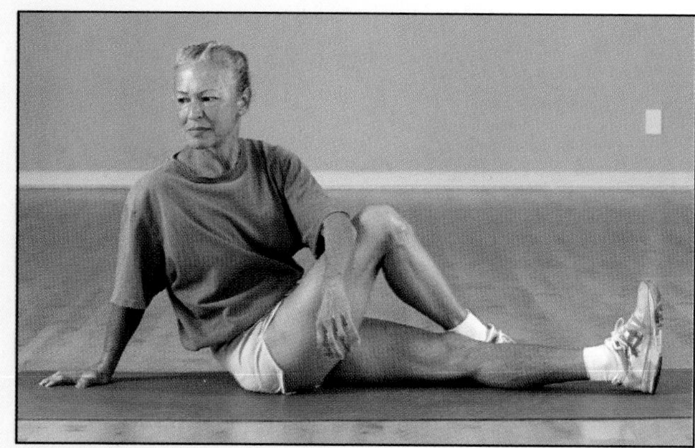

Forward Lunge

1. From a standing position, take an exaggerated step forward with the right leg.
2. Flex the right knee until it is positioned over the right foot.
3. Keep the right foot on the floor with both feet pointed straight ahead.
4. Keep the left leg almost fully extended; the heel can be off the floor, if needed.
5. Place the hands on the top of the right thigh or on the hips and look straight ahead.
6. With the torso fully upright, move the hips forward and slightly downward until a stretch is felt.
7. Repeat the stretch with the left leg positioned ahead of the body (i.e., lunge with the left leg).

 **Common Errors**

- Allowing the lead knee to flex beyond the toes of the lead foot
- Allowing the heel of the lead foot to lift off of the floor
- Flexing the torso forward or looking down at the floor

Primary Muscles Stretched:
Iliopsoas, rectus femoris, gluteus maximus, hamstrings

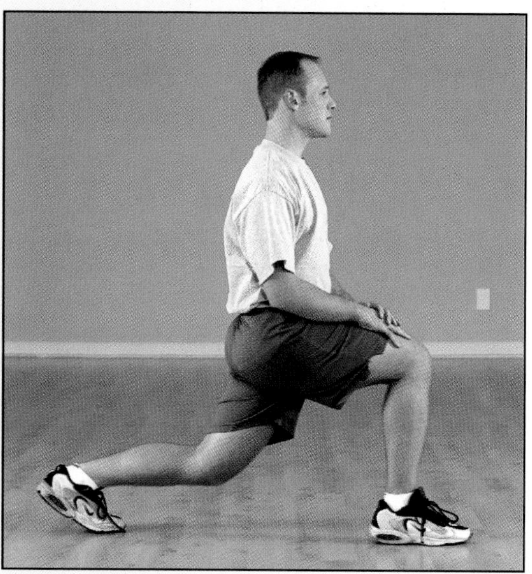

Lying Knee to Chest

1. Lie supine with the legs next to each other and extended away from the body.
2. Flex the right knee and hip to elevate the right thigh toward the chest.
3. Grasp the back of the right thigh (underneath the right knee).
4. Keep the left leg in the same starting position.
5. Use the arms to pull the right thigh further toward the chest until a stretch is felt.
6. Repeat the stretch with the left knee pulled to the chest and the right leg extended away from the body.

Common Errors

- Grasping the front of the flexed knee (rather than the back of the thigh)
- Flexing the neck or arching the back
- Lifting the opposite leg off of the floor

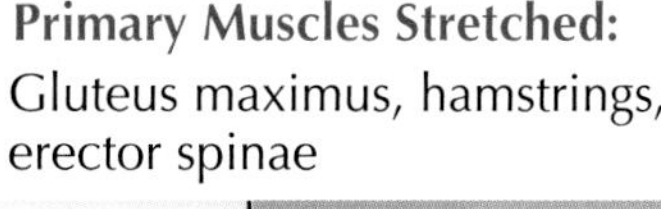

Primary Muscles Stretched:
Gluteus maximus, hamstrings, erector spinae

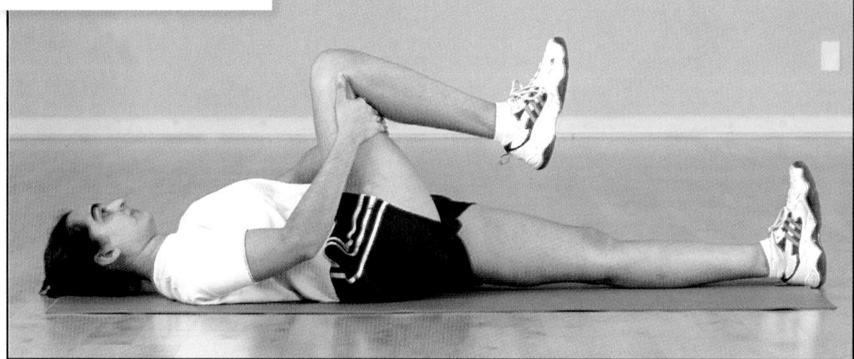

Semistraddle (Modified Hurdler's Stretch)

1. Sit on the floor with the left leg extended away from the body and the sole of the right foot pressed against (or near to) the inside of the left knee.
2. The outside of the right leg will be touching or nearly touching the floor.
3. Keeping the back flat, lean forward at the hips and grasp the toes of the left foot with the left hand.
4. Pull the toes of the left foot toward the upper body as the torso is flexed toward the left leg until a stretch is felt.
5. Repeat the stretch with the right leg extended away from the body and the sole of the left foot pressed against (or near to) the inside of the right knee.

Common Errors

- Allowing the extended thigh to externally rotate
- Rounding the shoulders or curling the torso toward the extended leg (rather than flexing the torso at the hips)
- Allowing the knee of the extended leg to flex

Primary Muscles Stretched:
Hamstrings, erector spinae, gastrocnemius

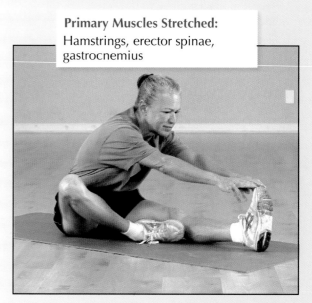

Butterfly

1. Sit on the floor with the torso upright.
2. Flex the hips and knees and externally rotate the thighs to bring the soles of the feet together.
3. Lean forward at the hips and grasp the feet and move them toward the body.
4. Place the elbows on the inside of the legs.
5. Keeping the back flat, slightly push the elbows down, pull the feet toward the upper body, and flex the torso forward until a stretch is felt.

 **Common Error**

- Rounding the shoulders or curling the torso toward the feet (rather than flexing the torso at the hips)

Primary Muscles Stretched:
Hip adductors, gracilis

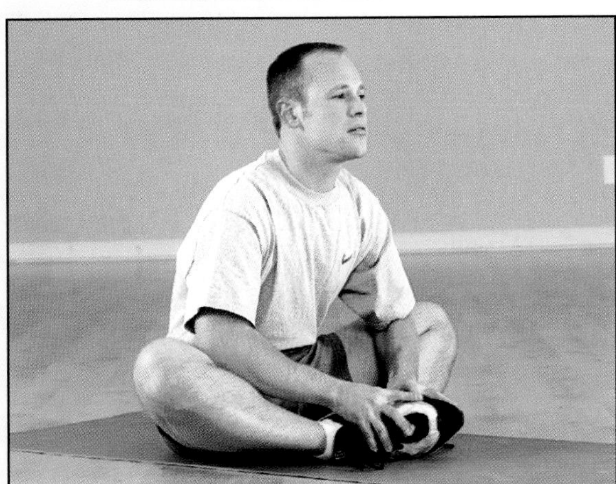

Wall Stretch

1. Stand facing a wall with the feet shoulder-width apart and the toes about 12 inches (30 centimeters) from the wall.
2. Lean forward and place the hands on the wall.
3. Step back about two feet (61 centimeters) with the left leg and slightly flex the right knee.
4. Fully extend the left knee and keep the left heel on the floor.
5. Allow the elbows to flex to move the hips and torso closer to the wall until a stretch is felt.
6. Repeat the stretch with the right leg positioned behind the body (i.e., step back with the right leg).

 **Common Errors**

- Moving the torso closer to the wall without also moving the hips forward
- Allowing the heel of the stepped-back foot to lift off of the floor

Primary Muscles Stretched:
Gastrocnemius, soleus (and Achilles tendon)

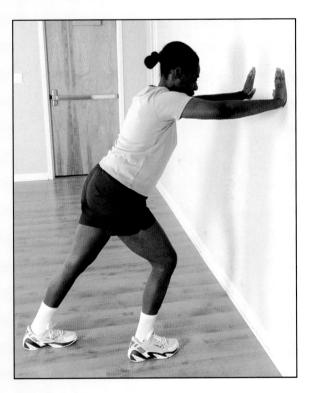

Dynamic Flexibility Exercises

Arm Circle

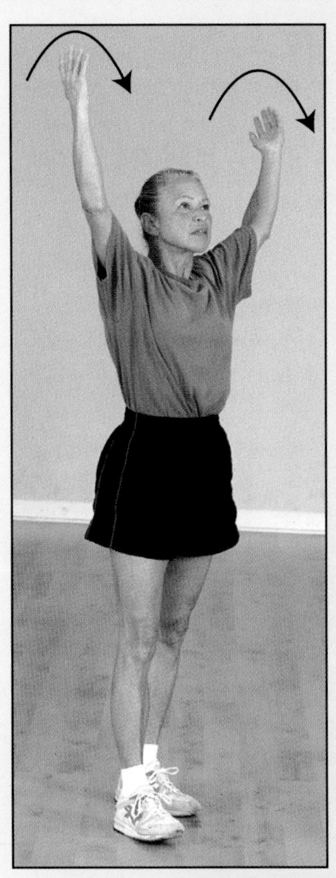

1. While slowly walking over the prescribed distance, move the arms in wide circles progressing from a position in which the arms are directly at the sides to a position in which the arms are directly overhead.
2. Allow movement to occur only at the shoulder joints (i.e., keep the elbows fully extended).
3. Perform the arm circles both forward and backward through a full comfortable range of motion.

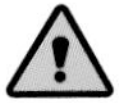 **Common Error**

- Allowing the torso to flex and extend as the arms move in circles

Primary Muscles Stretched:
Deltoids, latissimus dorsi, pectoralis major

Arm Swing

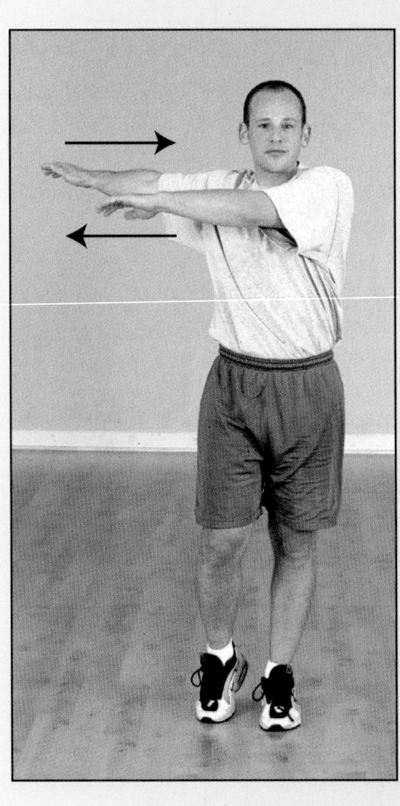

1. Flex the arms at the shoulders to position the arms parallel to the floor in front of the body.
2. While slowly walking over the prescribed distance, swing the arms in unison to the right so the left arm is in front of the chest, the fingers of the left hand are pointing directly lateral to the right shoulder, and the right arm is behind the body.
3. Immediately reverse the movement direction to swing the arms in unison to the left.
4. Allow movement to occur only at the shoulder joints (i.e., keep the torso and head facing forward).
5. Alternate the arm swings to the right and left through a full comfortable range of motion.

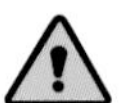 **Common Error**

- Allowing the torso or neck to rotate in the direction of the arm swing

Primary Muscles Stretched:
Latissimus dorsi, teres major, anterior and posterior deltoids, pectoralis major

Lunge Walk

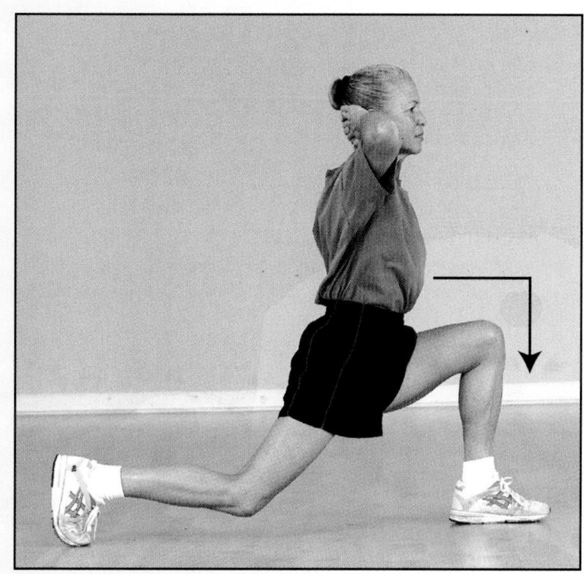

1. Clasp the hands behind the head.
2. From a standing position, take an exaggerated step forward with the left leg.
3. Flex the left knee until it is positioned over the left foot.
4. Slightly flex the right knee to be just off the floor; both feet should be pointed straight ahead.
5. Keep the torso erect (or leaning back slightly) and look straight ahead.
6. Pause for a count in the bottom lunged position, stand up, and then repeat with the right leg, progressing forward with each step.

 **Common Errors**

- Allowing the lead knee to flex beyond the toes of the lead foot
- Touching the knee of the trailing leg to the floor
- Flexing the torso forward or looking down at the floor

Primary Muscles Stretched:
Iliopsoas, rectus femoris, gluteus maximus, hamstrings

Variation: Reverse Lunge Walk

1. Clasp the hands behind the head.
2. From a standing position, take an exaggerated step backward with the right leg.
3. Flex the left knee until it is positioned over the left foot.
4. Slightly flex the right knee to be just off the floor; both feet should be pointed straight ahead.
5. Keep the torso erect (or leaning back slightly) and look straight ahead.
6. Pause for a count in the bottom lunged position, stand up, and then repeat with the left leg, progressing backward with each step.

 **Common Errors**

- Allowing the lead knee to flex beyond the toes of the lead foot
- Touching the knee of the trailing leg to the floor
- Flexing the torso forward or looking down at the floor

Primary Muscles Stretched:
Iliopsoas, rectus femoris, gluteus maximus, hamstrings

Hockey Lunge Walk

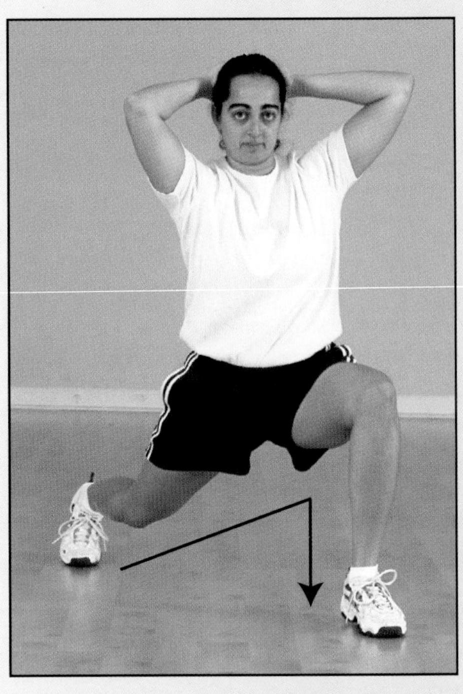

1. Clasp the hands behind the head.
2. From a standing position, take an exaggerated step forward and diagonally to the right with the right leg.
3. Place the right foot on the floor 10 to 12 inches (25-30 centimeters) wider than the placement of the lead foot during the Lunge Walk exercise (page 283).
4. Keep the toes of both feet pointing straight ahead.
5. Flex the right knee until it is positioned over the right foot.
6. Slightly flex the left knee to be just off the floor.
7. Keep the torso erect (or leaning back slightly) and look straight ahead.
8. Pause for a count in the bottom lunged position, stand up, and then repeat with the left leg, progressing forward with each step.

 **Common Errors**

- Allowing the lead knee to flex beyond the toes of the lead foot
- Touching the knee of the trailing leg to the floor
- Flexing the torso forward or looking down at the floor
- Stepping too laterally or pointing the feet medially or laterally

Primary Muscles Stretched:
Iliopsoas, rectus femoris, gluteus maximus, hamstrings, hip adductors

Variation: Walking Side Lunge

1. Clasp the hands behind the head.
2. Turn sideways, with the right shoulder pointing in the desired movement direction.
3. From a standing position, take an exaggerated lateral step to the right with the right foot.
4. Keeping the left knee straight, flex the right knee until it is positioned over the right foot and allow the hips to sink back and to the right.
5. Keep the torso erect and look straight ahead.
6. Pause for a count in the bottom lunged position then stand back up, pivot on the right foot, and repeat with the left leg.

 **Common Errors**

- Allowing the lead knee to flex beyond the toes of the lead foot
- Flexing the knee of the trailing leg
- Flexing the torso forward or looking down at the floor

Primary Muscles Stretched:
Iliopsoas, rectus femoris, gluteus maximus, hamstrings, hip adductors

Walking Knee Tuck

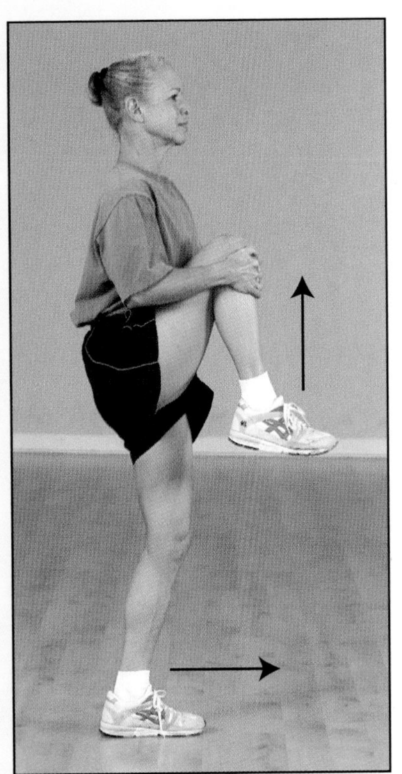

1. From a standing position, step forward with the left leg and flex the right hip and knee to move the right thigh toward the chest.
2. Grasp the front of the right knee/upper shin.
3. Use the arms to pull the right knee further up and squeeze the right thigh against the chest.
4. Pause for a count in the knee tuck position then step back down with the right leg, shift the bodyweight to the right leg, and repeat with the left leg, progressing forward with each step.
5. Try to pull the knee slightly higher with each repetition.

 **Common Error**

- Flexing the torso forward or looking down at the floor

Primary Muscles Stretched:
Gluteus maximus, hamstrings

Walking Knee Over Hurdle

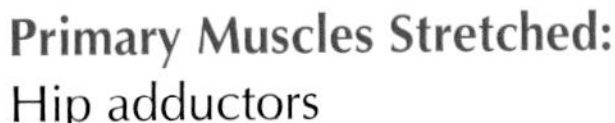

Primary Muscles Stretched:
Hip adductors

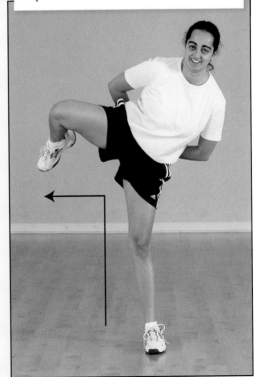

1. Imagine a line of hurdles approximately 3 feet (91 centimeters) tall placed on alternating sides of the body (i.e., a hurdle on the right, followed by a short space, and then a hurdle on the left, followed by a short space, and so on).
2. From a standing position, flex the right hip and knee then abduct the right thigh to be parallel with the floor.
3. Lead the right knee over the first imaginary hurdle that is on the right.
4. Pause for a count in the highest thigh position then step back down with the right leg, shift the bodyweight to the right leg, and repeat with the left leg, progressing forward with each step.
5. Try to lift the thigh slightly higher over the hurdle with each repetition.

 **Common Errors**

- Leaning the torso too far away from the hurdle (rather than emphasizing hip abduction)
- Leading the torso or the head over the hurdle (rather than the lead knee)

Body-Weight Exercises

Abdominal Crunch

Primary Muscle Trained:
Rectus abdominis

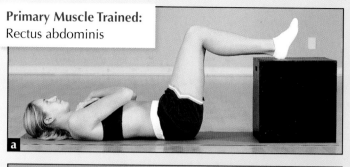

1. Assume a supine position on the floor.
2. Flex the hips and knees and place the heels on a box.
3. Place the hands behind or at the sides of the head (to hold its weight only) or fold the arms across the chest or abdomen.
4. Curl the torso until the upper back is off of the floor.
5. Keep the feet, buttocks, and lower back stationary at all times.
6. After completing the crunch, allow the torso to uncurl back down to the starting position.

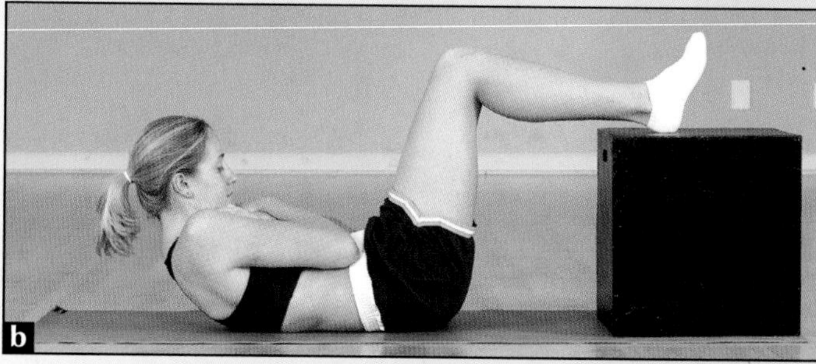

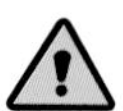 **Common Errors**

- Raising the hips or feet
- Pulling the head with the hands
- Flexing the torso to a fully seated position

Variation: Twisting Crunch

1. Assume a supine position on the floor.
2. Flex the hips and knees and place the heels on a box or bench.
3. Place the hands behind or at the sides of the head (to hold its weight only) or fold the arms across the chest or abdomen.
4. Twist (rotate) the torso to move the right shoulder toward the left thigh.
5. Continue flexing and twisting the torso until the upper back is off of the floor.
6. Keep the feet, buttocks, and lower back stationary at all times.
7. After completing the crunch, allow the torso to uncurl and untwist back down to the starting position.
8. Alternate the direction of the twist with each repetition.

 **Common Errors**

- Raising the hips or feet
- Pulling the head with the hands

Primary Muscles Trained:
Rectus abdominis, internal and external oblique

Back Extension

1. Assume a prone position on the floor with the knees fully extended and the toes pointed down to the floor.
2. Clasp the hands behind the head.
3. Keeping the toes in contact with the floor, extend the torso (i.e., arch the back) to lift the chest off the floor.
4. After completing the extension, allow the chest to lower and return to the starting position.

 **Common Errors**

- Flexing the knees or lifting the toes off the floor
- Rapidly rocking up and down on the hips (rather than performing the movement under control)

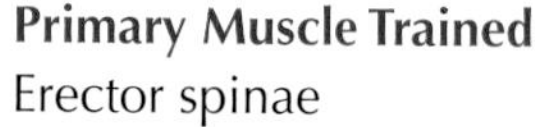

Primary Muscle Trained:
Erector spinae

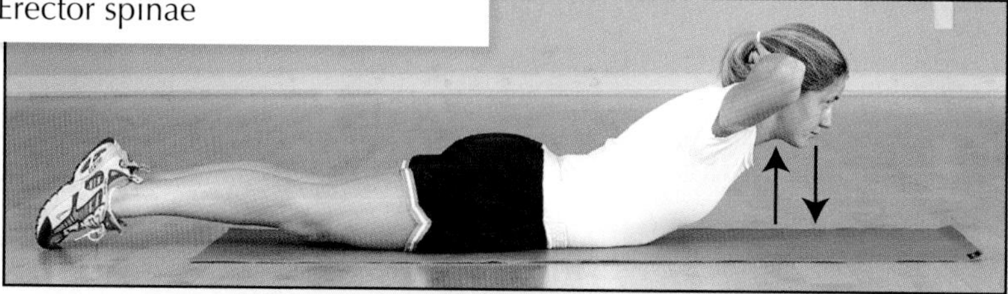

Variation: Twisting Back Extension

1. Assume a prone position on the floor with the knees fully extended and the toes pointed down to the floor.
2. Clasp the hands behind the head.
3. Keep the toes in contact with the floor.
4. Extend and twist (rotate) the torso to move the right shoulder up and to the left.
5. Continue extending and twisting the torso until the chest is off of the floor.
6. Keep the feet, buttocks, and lower back on the floor at all times.
7. After completing the extension, allow the chest to lower and untwist back down to the starting position.
8. Alternate the direction of the twist with each repetition.

Common Errors

- Flexing the knees or lifting the toes off the floor
- Rapidly rocking back and forth on the hips (rather than performing the movement under control)

Primary Muscle Trained:
Erector spinae

Push-Up

1. Assume a prone position on the floor with the knees fully extended and the toes pointed down to the floor.
2. Place the hands on the floor, palms down, about two to three inches (5-8 centimeters) wider than shoulder-width apart with the elbows pointed outward.
3. Keeping the body in a straight line and the toes in contact with the floor, push against the floor with the hands to fully extend the elbows.
4. After completing the push-up, lower the body by allowing the elbows to flex to a 90 degree angle. Alternatively, the personal trainer can place a soft object about the size of rolled-up socks or a foam half-roller on the floor beneath the client's chest and count the repetitions only when the client's chest touches the socks or roller.

 **Common Errors**

- Allowing the hips to sag or rise up (rather than keeping the body in a straight line)
- Performing the exercise through a reduced range of motion

Primary Muscles Trained:
Pectoralis major, anterior deltoid, triceps brachii

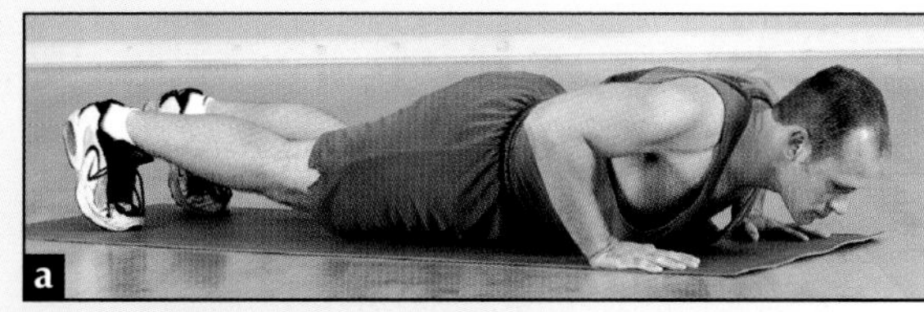
a

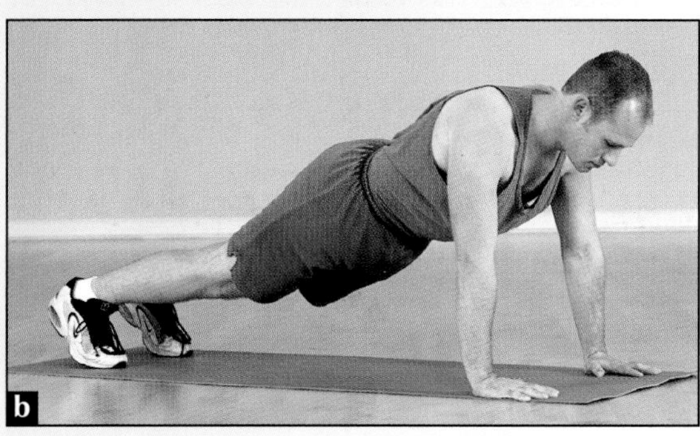
b

Variation: Modified Push-Up

1. Modify the standard push-up technique by having the client in a kneeling position, with the knees flexed to 90 degrees and the ankles crossed.

Primary Muscles Trained:
Pectoralis major, anterior deltoid, triceps brachii

 **Common Errors**

- Allowing the hips to sag or rise up (rather than keeping the body in a straight line)
- Performing the exercise through a reduced range of motion

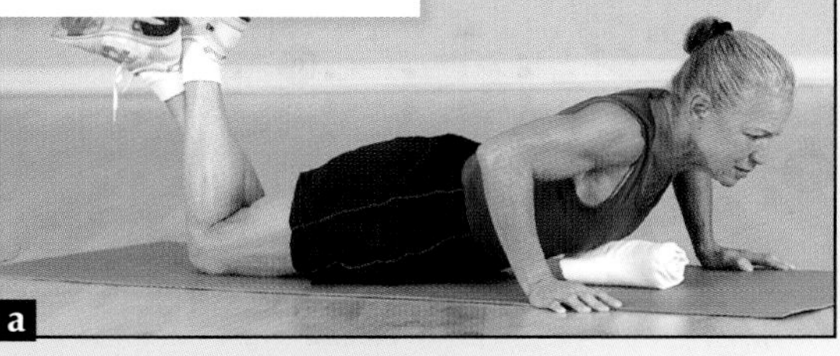
a

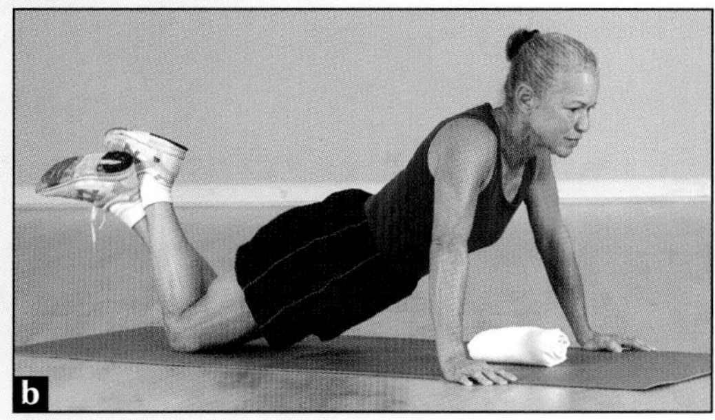
b

Stability Ball Exercises

Extended Abdominal Crunch

1. Lie supine on the stability ball with the lower-to-middle section of the back on the apex of the ball.
2. Place the feet flat on the floor about hip-width apart with the thighs, hips, and lower abdomen approximately parallel to the floor.
3. Place the hands behind or at the sides of the head (to hold its weight only) or fold the arms across the chest or abdomen.
4. Curl the torso to raise it 30 degrees to 40 degrees from the starting position.
5. Keep the feet on the floor and the thighs and hips stationary.
6. After completing the crunch, allow the torso to uncurl back down to the starting position.

 **Common Errors**

- Raising the feet off the floor
- Allowing the hips to drop down off the side of the ball
- Pulling the head with the hands

Primary Muscle Trained:
Rectus abdominis

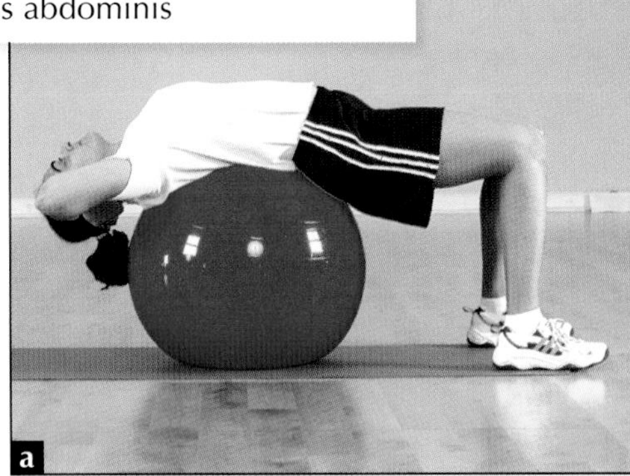
a

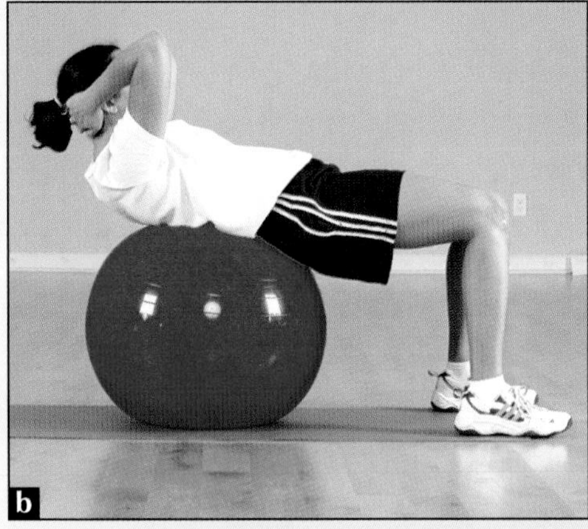
b

Supine Leg Curl

1. Lie supine on the floor with the legs next to each other and extended away from the body.
2. Abduct the arms 90 degrees away from the torso with the palms facing the floor.
3. Lift the hips off the floor to position the lower calves and back of the heels on the apex of the stability ball.
4. Begin the exercise with the feet, knees, hips, and shoulders in a straight line.
5. Keeping the upper body in the same position, flex the knees (which will cause the ball to roll backward) to bring the heels toward the buttocks.
6. Continue flexing the knees to a 90 degree angle; the soles of the feet will finish near the apex of the ball.
7. Keep the knees, hips, and shoulders in a straight line.
8. After completing the leg curl, allow the knees to extend and the ball to roll forward to the starting position.

 **Common Error**

- Allowing the hips to flex or sag (rather than keeping them in line with the knees and shoulders)

Primary Muscles Trained:
Hamstrings, gluteus maximus, erector spinae

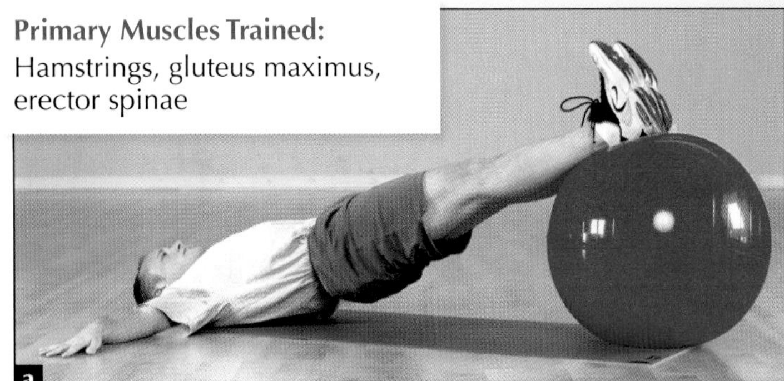
a

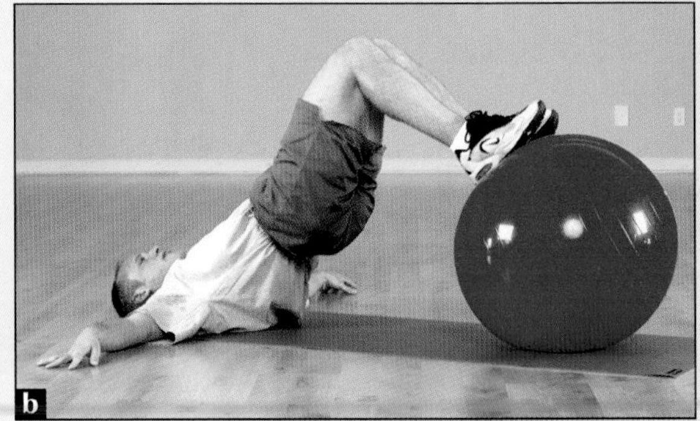
b

Supine Hip Lift

1. Lie supine on the floor with the legs next to each other and extended away from the body.
2. Abduct the arms 90 degrees away from the torso with the palms facing the floor.
3. Keeping the hips on the floor, position the back of the heels on the apex of the stability ball.
4. Begin the exercise with the feet, knees, and hips in a straight line.
5. Keeping the upper body in the same position, lift (extend) the hips until the feet, knees, hips, and shoulders are in a straight line.
6. After completing the hip lift, allow the hips to lower and return to the starting position.

 **Common Error**

- Allowing the knees to flex (rather than keeping them in line with the feet and hips)

Primary Muscles Trained:
Erector spinae, gluteus maximus, hamstrings

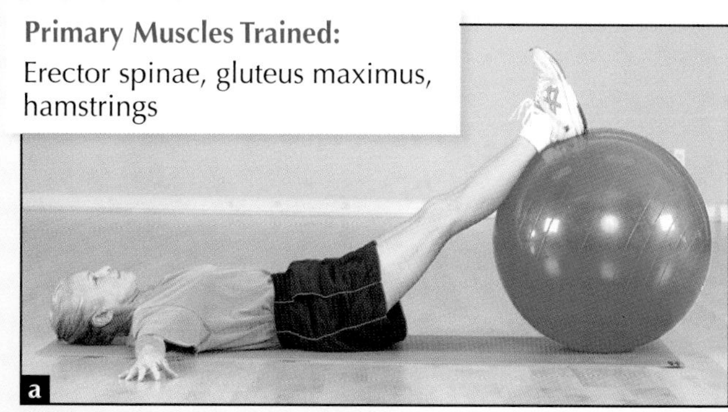

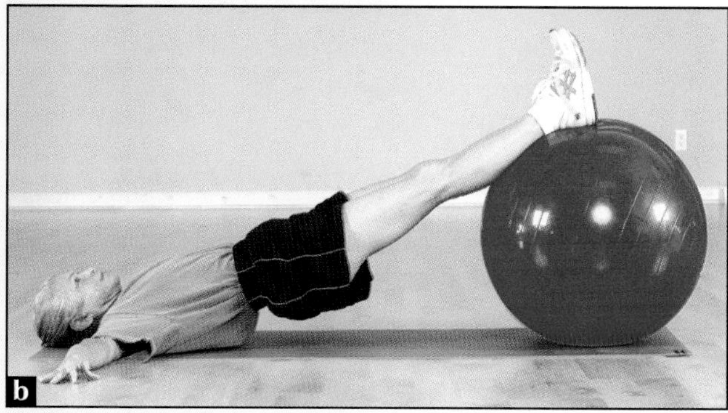

Back Hyperextension

1. Lie prone on the stability ball with the navel positioned on the apex of the ball.
2. Place the feet (toes) on the floor at least 12 inches (30 centimeters) apart with the knees fully extended.
3. Clasp the hands behind the head.
4. Keeping the toes in contact with the floor, elevate torso until it is fully extended (arched) and the chest is off the ball.
5. After completing the extension, allow the torso to lower and return to the starting position.

Common Errors

- Flexing the knees or lifting the toes off the floor
- Allowing the navel to move off the apex of the ball as the torso extends

Primary Muscle Trained:
Erector spinae

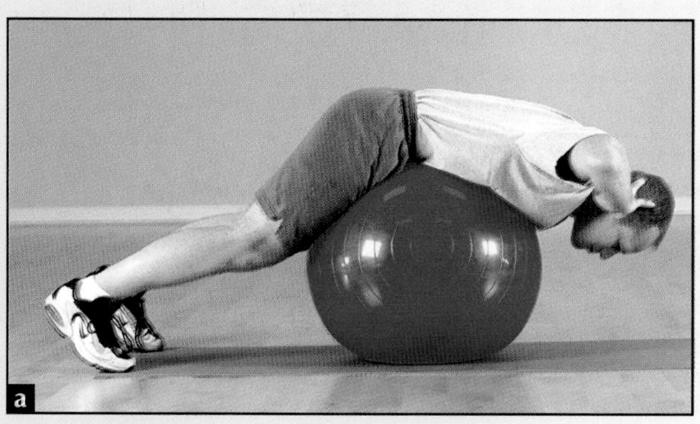

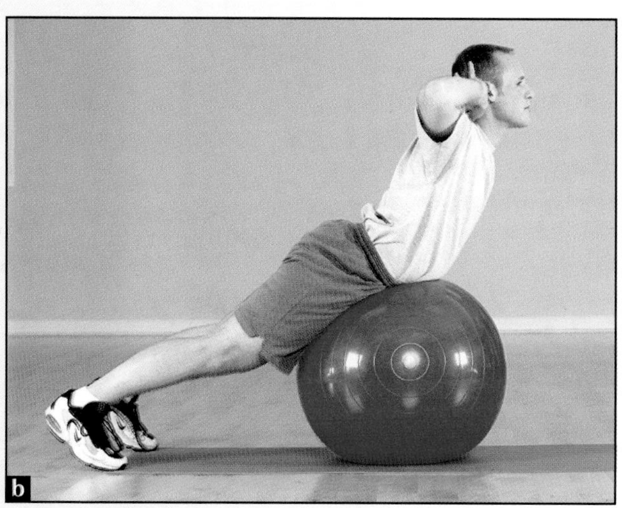

Reverse Back Hyperextension

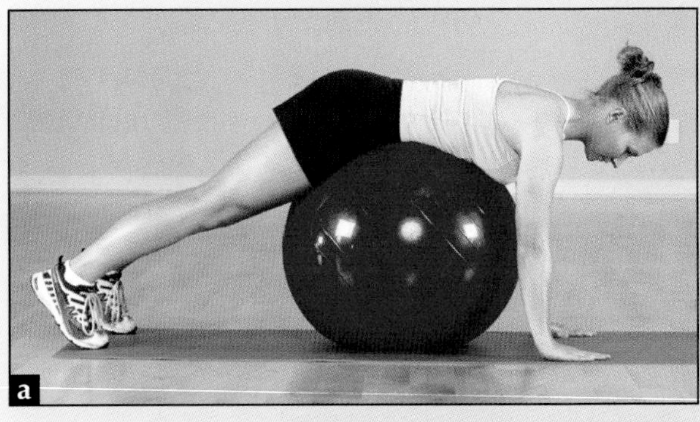

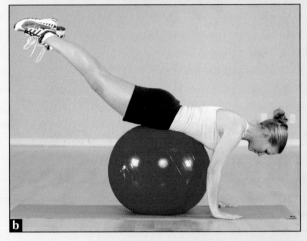

1. Lie prone on the stability ball with the navel positioned on the apex of the ball.
2. Place the hands (palms) on the floor at least 12 inches (30 centimeters) apart with the elbows fully extended.
3. Begin the exercise with the knees extended and the toes in contact with the floor.
4. Keeping the hands in contact with the floor, elevate legs with the knees held in extension until the hips are fully extended.
5. After completing the reverse extension, allow the legs to lower and return to the starting position.

 **Common Errors**

- Flexing the knees or lifting the hands off the floor
- Allowing the navel to move off the apex of the ball as the legs are raised

Primary Muscles Trained:
Gluteus maximus, erector spinae, hamstrings

Elbow Bridge

1. Kneel next to the stability ball and place the elbows and the back of the upper forearms on the ball.
2. While keeping the elbows/forearms on the ball, roll the ball forward or reposition the kneeling location to create about a 90 degree angle at the elbows, shoulders, and knees.
3. Keeping the knees and toes on the floor and the elbows on the ball, begin the exercise by extending the knees to roll the ball forward until the elbows, shoulders, hips, and knees are nearly in a straight line and the back of the upper arms are on the ball.
4. After completing the elbow bridge, flex the knees to roll the ball backward to return to the starting position.

 **Common Errors**

- Arching the back as the knees extend
- Raising the feet off the floor

Primary Muscles Trained:
Rectus abdominis, internal and external obliques, quadratus lumborum, latissimus dorsi, teres major, erector spinae

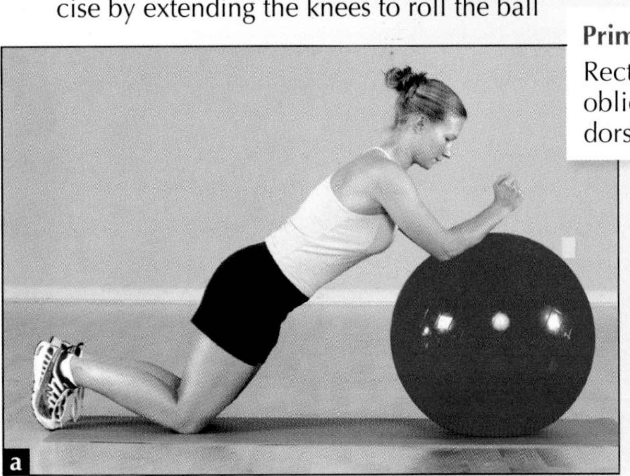

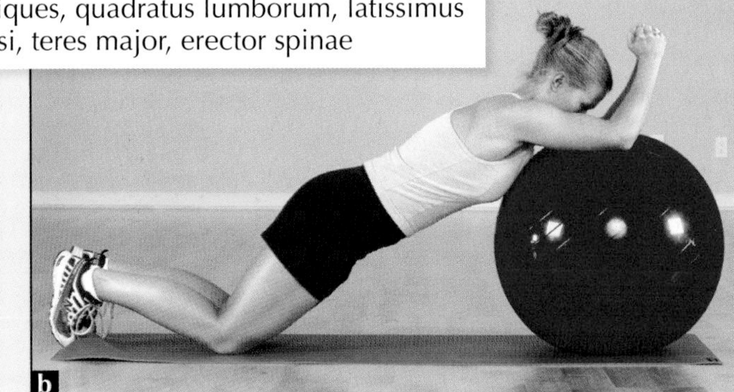

Variation: Straight Arm Roll-Out

1. Kneeling next to the stability ball, fully extend the elbows and place the hands on the stability ball.
2. While keeping the hands on the ball, roll the ball forward or reposition the kneeling location to create about a 90 degree angle at the shoulders and knees.
3. Keeping the knees and toes on the floor, begin the exercise by extending the knees to roll the ball forward until the hands, elbows, shoulders, hips, and knees are nearly in a straight line and the arms are across the ball.
4. After completing the roll-out, flex the knees to roll the ball backward to return to the starting position.

 **Common Errors**

- Arching the back as the knees extend
- Raising the feet off the floor

Primary Muscles Trained:
Rectus abdominis, internal and external obliques, quadratus lumborum, latissimus dorsi, teres major, erector spinae

---

Stability Ball Push-Up

1. Assume a push-up position (see page 287) with the shins and the instep of the feet on the stability ball and the elbows fully extended.
2. Position the feet, knees, hips, and shoulders in a straight line.
3. Allow the elbows to flex to lower the face to a position one to two inches (2.5-5 centimeters) from the floor while keeping the body in a straight line.
4. After reaching the lowest position, push with the arms to extend the elbows back to the starting position.

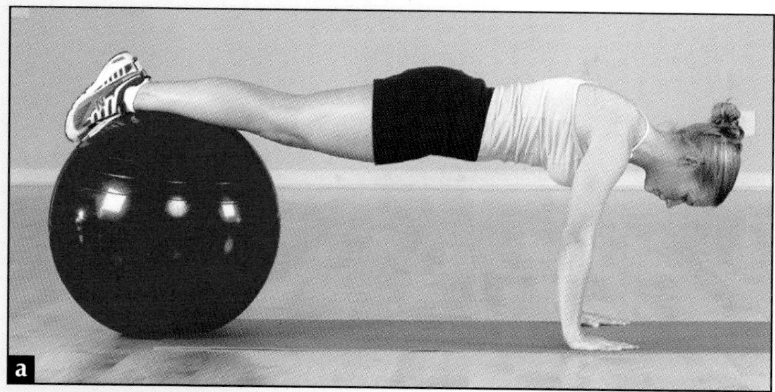
a

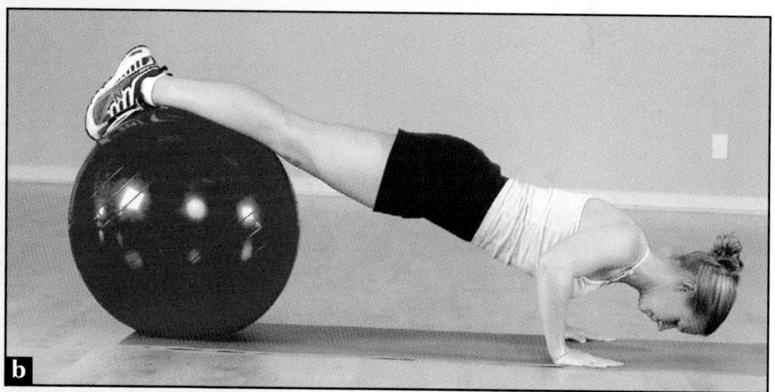
b

 **Common Errors**

- Allowing the hips to sag or rise up (rather than keeping the body in a straight line)
- Pushing slightly backward with the arms to move the body backward or roll the knees onto the ball

Primary Muscles Trained:
Pectoralis major, anterior deltoid, triceps brachii

Pike Roll Out and In

1. Assume a push-up position (see page 287) with the instep of the feet on the stability ball and the elbows fully extended.
2. Position the feet, knees, hips, and shoulders in a straight line.
3. Keeping the knees and elbows fully extended, begin the exercise by flexing the hips to roll the ball forward until the toes are on top of the ball and the hips are directly over the shoulders.
4. After reaching the pike position, allow the hips to extend back to the starting position.

Common Errors

- Arching the back in the push-up position
- Hyperextending the neck in the pike position

Primary Muscles Trained:
Rectus abdominis, internal and external obliques, quadratus lumborum, hip flexors

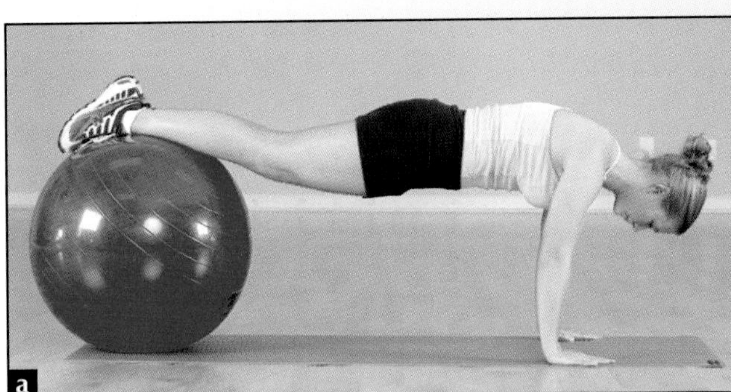
a

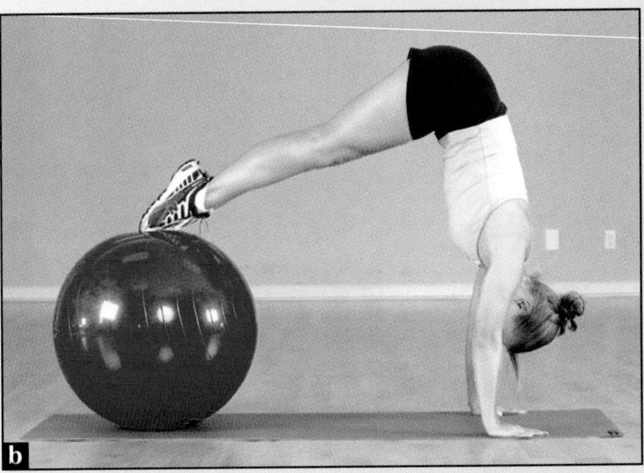
b

Variation: Knee to Chest (Jackknife)

1. Assume a push-up position (see page 287) with the instep of the feet on the stability ball and the elbows fully extended.
2. Position the feet, knees, hips, and shoulders in a straight line.
3. Keeping the elbows fully extended, begin the exercise by raising the hips slightly and flexing the hips and knees to roll the ball forward until the hips and knees are fully flexed and the knees are near the torso.
4. After reaching the knee-to-chest position, allow the hips and knees to extend back to the starting position.

Common Errors

- Arching the back in the push-up position
- Allowing the elbows to flex in the knee-to-chest position

Primary Muscles Trained:
Rectus abdominis, internal and external obliques, quadratus lumborum, hip flexors

STUDY QUESTIONS

1. After completing a warm-up, a client should immediately perform flexibility exercises before which of the following activities?
   A. singles tennis
   B. rowing machine
   C. stationary bike
   D. stair climber
2. Which of the following is a benefit of performing warm-up activities?
   A. muscle blood flow increases
   B. muscle viscosity increases

C. nerve impulse velocity decreases
D. nerve receptor sensitivity decreases

3. Compared to static stretching, which of the following is a disadvantage of ballistic stretching?
   A. decreased danger of overstretching the target tissues
   B. increased amount of energy is needed to perform the exercises
   C. decreased likelihood of becoming sore after stretching
   D. increased passivity of the stretch reflex
4. A 6-foot, 9-inch (206 centimeter), 230-pound (105-kilogram) male client has been preparing for the upcoming basketball season and has been performing traditional resistance training for the past six months. His personal trainer decides to introduce stability ball exercises into the client's program. Which of the following guidelines apply to this client?
   A. Due to the client's weight, the personal trainer should slightly under inflate the ball.
   B. When determining correct ball size, the client's thighs should be parallel to the ground when sitting on the ball with the feet flat on the floor.
   C. Because the ball is unstable and the client is so tall, slight deviations from correct technique are acceptable.
   D. Since the client had been performing resistance training exercises for so long, the personal trainer should direct the client to stop resistance training and perform only stability ball exercises.

APPLIED KNOWLEDGE QUESTION

The personal trainer determines that a client needs to emphasize the flexibility and muscular fitness of the hip extensors so the client can become better conditioned to play tennis.

a. What static flexibility exercises focus on the hip extensors?
b. What dynamic flexibility exercises involve the hip extensors?
c. What body-weight exercises strengthen the hip extensors?
d. What stability ball exercises actively (concentrically, not isometrically) train the hip extensors?

REFERENCES

1. Baechle, T.R., and R.W. Earle, eds. 2000. *Essentials of Strength Training and Conditioning,* 2nd ed. Champaign, IL: Human Kinetics.
2. Bandy, W.D., J.M. Irion, and M. Briggler. 1998. The effect of static and dynamic range of motion training on the flexibility of the hamstring muscles. *Journal of Orthopaedic and Sports Physical Therapy* 27 (4): 295-300.
3. Bompa, T.O. 1995. *From Childhood to Champion Athlete.* Toronto: Veritas.
4. Bompa, T.O. 2000. *Total Training for Young Champions.* Champaign, IL: Human Kinetics.
5. Bourne, G. 1995. The basic facts about flexibility in a nutshell. *Modern Athlete and Coach* 33 (2): 3-4, 35.
6. Brandon, R. 1998. What science has to say about the performance benefits of flexibility training. *Peak Performance* (September): 6-9.
7. Chek, P. 1998. Swiss ball exercise. *Sports Coach* 21 (3): 27-29.
8. Collins, P. 2001. How to make use of Swiss ball training. *Modern Athlete and Coach* 39 (4): 34-36.
9. Cornelius, W.J., and M.M. Hinson. 1980. The relationship between isometric contractions of hip extensions and subsequent flexibility in males. *Sports Medicine and Physical Fitness* 20: 75-80.
10. Cornwell, A., A.G. Nelson, and B. Sideaway. 2002. Acute effects of stretching on the neuromuscular properties of the triceps surae muscle complex. *European Journal of Applied Physiology* 86 (5): 428-434.
11. DiNubile, N., ed. 1991. Scientific, medical, and practical aspects of stretching. In: *Clinics in Sports Medicine.* Philadelphia: Saunders, pp. 63-86.
12. Franklin, A.J., C.F. Finch, and C.A. Sherman. 2001. Warm-up practices of golfers: Are they adequate? *British Journal of Sports Medicine* 35 (2): 125-127.
13. Funk, D., A.M. Swank, K.J. Adams, and D. Treolo. 2001. Efficacy of moist heat pack application over static stretching on hamstring flexibility. *Journal of Strength and Conditioning Research* 15 (1): 123-126.
14. Gambetta, V. 1997. Stretching the truth; The fallacies of flexibility. *Sports Coach* 20 (3): 7-9.
15. Gesztesi, B. 1999. Stretching during exercise. *Strength and Conditioning Journal* 21 (6): 44.
16. Hardy, L., and D. Jones. 1986. Dynamic flexibility and proprioceptive neuromuscular facilitation. *Research Quarterly for Exercise and Sport* 57 (2): 150-153.
17. Hedrick, A. 1992. Physiological responses to warm-up. *NSCA Journal* 14 (5): 25-27.
18. Hedrick, A. 1993. Flexibility and the conditioning program. *NSCA Journal* 15 (4): 62-66.
19. Hedrick, A. 2000. Dynamic flexibility training. *Strength and Conditioning Journal* 22 (5): 33-38.
20. Hedrick, A. 2000. Volleyball coaches guide to warm-up and flexibility training. *Performance Conditioning Volleyball* 8 (3): 1-4.
21. Holt, L.E., T.M. Travis, and T. Okia. 1970. Comparative study of three stretching techniques. *Perceptual & Motor Skills* 31: 611-616.

22. Karp, J.R. 2000. Flexibility for fitness. *Fitness Management* (April): 52-54.
23. Kato, Y., T. Ikata, H. Takia, S. Takata, K. Sairyo, and K. Iwanaga. 2000. Effects of specific warm-ups at various intensities on energy metabolism during subsequent exercise. *Journal of Sports Medicine and Physical Fitness* 40 (2): 126-130.
24. Kokkonen, J., A.G. Nelson, and A. Cornwell. 1998. Acute muscle stretching inhibits maximal strength performance. *Research Quarterly for Exercise and Sport* 69 (4): 411-415.
25. McBride, J. 1995. Dynamic warm-up and flexibility: A key to basketball success. *Coaching Women's Basketball* (Summer): 15-17.
26. Ninos, J. 1999. When could stretching be harmful? *Strength and Conditioning Journal* 21 (5): 57-58.
27. O'Brien, B., W. Payne, P. Gastin, and C. Burge. 1997. A comparison of active and passive warm-ups in energy system contribution and performance in moderate heat. *Australian Journal of Science and Medicine in Sport* 29 (4): 106-109.
28. Poe, C.M. 1995. Principles of off-ice strength, power, and flexibility training for figure skaters. *Skating* 72 (9): 43-50.
29. Ross, M. 1999. Stretching the hip flexors. *Strength and Conditioning Journal* 21 (3): 71-72.
30. Sady, S.P., M. Wortman, and D. Blanke. 1982. Flexibility training: Ballistic, static, or proprioceptive neuromuscular facilitation? *Archives of Physical Medicine and Rehabilitation* 63: 261-263.
31. Shellock, F.G., and W.E. Prentice. 1985. Warming-up and stretching for improved physical performance and prevention of sports-related injuries. *Sports Medicine* 2 (4): 267-278.
32. Sobel, T., T.S. Ellenbecker, and E.P. Roetert. 1995. Flexibility training for tennis. *Strength and Conditioning* 17 (6): 43-51.
33. Stricker, T., T. Malone, and W.E. Garrett. 1990. The effects of passive warming on muscle injury. *American Journal of Sports Medicine* 18 (2): 141-145.
34. Takkinen, A., and J. Fleming. 1998. Swiss ball training. *Sports Coach* 21 (2): 6-7.
35. Tancred, T., and B. Tancred. 1995. An examination of the benefits of warm-up: A review. *New Studies in Athletics* 10 (4): 35-41.
36. Tanigawa, M.C. 1972. Comparison of the hold relax procedure and passive mobilization on increasing muscle length. *Physical Therapy* 52: 725-735.
37. Thomas, M. 2000. The functional warm-up. *Strength and Conditioning Journal* 22 (2): 51-53.
38. Wirth, V.J., B.L. Van Luten, D. Mistry, E. Saliba, and F.C. McCue. 1998. Temperature changes in deep muscles during upper and lower extremity exercise. *Journal of Athletic Training* 33 (3): 211-215.

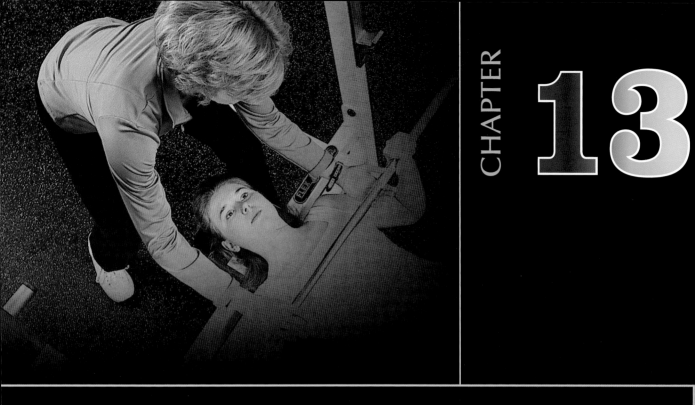

CHAPTER 13

Resistance Training Exercise Techniques

Thomas R. Baechle | Roger W. Earle

After completing this chapter, you will be able to

- understand the basic techniques for properly performing and teaching common resistance training exercises;
- provide proper breathing guidelines;
- determine when it is appropriate to wear a weight belt;
- describe the conditions and techniques for spotting free weight exercises; and

One of a personal trainer's primary responsibilities is to teach and supervise a client's resistance training exercise technique to create the safest possible training environment. The first part of this chapter provides guidelines and strategies for teaching, critiquing, and spotting safe and effective resistance training exercises, and provides recommendations for using a weight belt and breathing during an exercise. The last section presents checklists and shows photographs of proper resistance training exercise and spotting techniques, and also lists common technique errors and the primary muscles involved in the exercises.

Basic Exercise Technique Guidelines

Several basic guidelines apply to performing nearly all resistance (weight) training exercises. The client has to grasp some type of bar, dumbbell, or handle; place his or her body in an optimal position; and follow a recommended movement and breathing pattern to promote safe and effective exercise technique. Additionally, some exercises may require the use of a weight belt.

Handgrip Types and Widths

The two most common handgrips used in nearly all resistance training exercises are the **pronated grip,** with the palms down and the knuckles up (also called the **overhand grip**), and the **supinated grip,** with the palms up and the knuckles down (also called the **underhand grip**) (figure 13.1, a and b). Examples of exercises that use these handgrips are the bench press, which uses a pronated grip, and the biceps curl, which uses a supinated grip. Some exercises such as the dumbbell hammer curl and a version of the machine seated shoulder press use a **neutral grip.** With this grip, the palms face in and the knuckles point out to the side, as in a handshake.

A grip that is often recommended for spotting the bar (e.g., for the free weight bench press exercise) is the **alternated grip,** in which one hand is pronated and the other is supinated (figure 13.1c). In the pronated, supinated, and alternated grips, the thumb is wrapped around the bar so that the bar is fully held by the hand. This thumb position creates a **closed grip.** When the thumb does not wrap around the bar but instead is placed next to the index finger, the position is called an **open** or **false grip** (figure 13.1d).

When a client is preparing to perform a free weight resistance training exercise using a bar, it is also important for the personal trainer to instruct the client to place the hands a certain distance from each other. This placement is called the **grip width.** The four standard grip widths, shown in figure 13.2, are close, hip-width, shoulder-width, and wide. For most exercises, the hands are placed shoulder-width apart on the bar. A client's body dimensions influence the decisions regarding actual hand placement, however. For all of the grip widths, the hand position should result in an evenly balanced bar.

Starting Position

For all resistance training exercises, it is critical that the personal trainer instruct the client to "assume" or get into a correct initial body position. Every

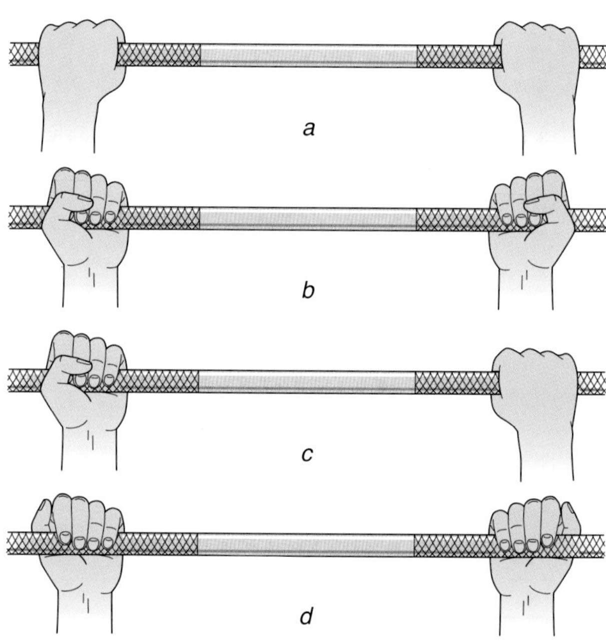

Figure 13.1 Recommended grips: *(a)* pronated, closed; *(b)* supinated, closed; *(c)* alternated, closed; *(d)* supinated, open.

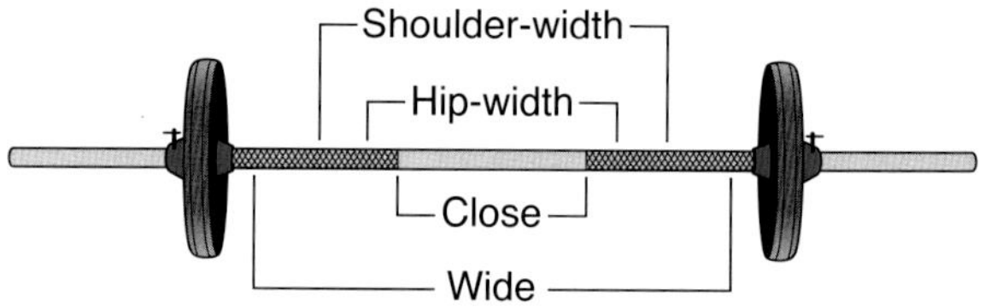

Figure 13.2 Choices for grip widths: close, hip-width, shoulder-width, wide.

demonstration of a new exercise given to a client should begin with how to establish a stable starting position. From this position, the client is able to maintain proper body alignment throughout the exercise, thereby placing the stress only on the targeted muscles.

Standing exercises (e.g., biceps curl, squat, dumbbell lateral raise, shoulder press) typically require the client's feet to be at or between hip-width or shoulder-width apart with the feet flat on the floor. Establishing a stable position in or on a machine typically requires the personal trainer to change the seat height, the position of all adjustable body and limb pads, or both the seat height and pad positions, to align the joint(s) involved in the exercise with the axis of the machine. For example, preparing a client to perform the leg (knee) extension exercise requires the personal trainer to adjust the position of the back pad forward or backward and the ankle pad up or down to place the client's knee joints in line with the machine axis.

Every demonstration of a new exercise given to a client should begin with establishing a stable starting position.

Five-Point Body Contact Position

Some free weight and machine exercises are performed while the client is seated (e.g., vertical chest press, leg press, shoulder press) or lying down on the back facing up (**supine;** e.g., bench press, lying triceps extension, dumbbell fly). The exercises performed on a chairlike seat or a torso-length bench require the personal trainer to instruct the client to position his or her body in a **five-point body contact position** so that these body parts or segments contact the seat or bench and the floor or foot platform:

- Back of the head
- Upper back and shoulders
- Lower back and buttocks
- Right foot
- Left foot

For **prone** exercises, that is, exercises the client does while lying facedown (e.g., leg [knee] curl, back hyperextension), most of the front surface of the client's body is in contact with the floor or machine pads and handles. For example, the proper position for the leg (knee) curl exercise involves these five contact points:

- Chin (or one cheek if the head is turned to the side)
- Chest/Stomach
- Hips/Front of the thighs
- Right hand
- Left hand

Breathing Considerations

The best general recommendation personal trainers can give to their clients about when and how to breathe during a resistance exercise is to exhale through the **sticking point** (the most difficult part of the exercise) during the concentric or exertion phase and inhale during the easier part of the exercise (the eccentric phase). Typically, the sticking point occurs soon after the transition from the eccentric to the concentric phase. For example, since the sticking point of the shoulder press exercise is reached when the bar or machine handles are about halfway up, the client should exhale through this portion of the movement. As the bar or handles are lowered back down to the starting position, the client should inhale. This breathing strategy applies to nearly all resistance training exercises.

The best general breathing recommendation is to exhale through the sticking point during the concentric phase and inhale during the eccentric phase. A personal trainer can tell a client to "breathe out during the hardest part of the exercise and to breathe in during the easier part of the exercise."

Valsalva Maneuver

There are situations in which variations to the breathing method just explained may be helpful for the personal trainer to explain to certain clients. For example, clients who are resistance trained and will perform **structural exercises** (those that load the vertebral column; e.g., back squat, push press) or exercises that stress the lower back (e.g., bent-over row, deadlift, shoulder press) may benefit from temporarily holding their breath during the exercise. This course of action creates what is referred to as the **Valsalva maneuver.** In this breathing technique, the glottis (the narrowest part of the larynx) is closed to keep air from escaping the lungs while the muscles of the abdomen and rib cage contract. In other words, a person is trying to exhale against a closed "throat." The result is that the diaphragm and the deep muscles of the torso contract and generate intra-abdominal pressure against the **fluid ball,** which aids in supporting the vertebral column internally, from the inside out and significantly reduces the compressive forces on the vertebral column and the effort required by other muscles (e.g., the low back muscles during the back squat exercise) to perform the exercise [1.7]. Thus, the client is better able to maintain correct posture and body alignment.

The following are two breathing options, with sample verbal directions, that a personal trainer can give to advanced clients who are performing exercises that involve the Valsalva maneuver.

- Option 1: Inhale during the eccentric phase until just before starting the concentric phase; hold the breath through the sticking point; then exhale. Verbal directions: "Take a breath in during the easiest part of the exercise; hold your breath until the hardest part of the exercise is completed, and then exhale."
- Option 2: Inhale prior to beginning a repetition; hold the breath through the sticking point of the concentric phase; then exhale. Verbal directions: "Take a breath in before starting a repetition; hold your breath until the hardest part of the exercise is completed, and then exhale."

For an example of option 1, advanced clients attempting to lift heavy loads for the back squat exercise can take a breath in as they descend to the bottom or low position, perform the Valsalva maneuver and continue to hold the breath until right after the sticking point of the upward movement, and then exhale through the rest of the concentric phase back up to the starting or standing body position.

Advanced clients may benefit from breath-holding during structural exercises and those that place stress on the lower back.

Despite its advantages, the Valsalva maneuver causes an increase in the pressure in the chest that can have the undesirable side effect of exerting compressive forces on the heart, making venous return more difficult. Also, the Valsalva maneuver can momentarily raise blood pressure to high levels that may cause dizziness, rapid-onset fatigue, blood vessel rupture, disorientation, and blackouts. Therefore, a personal trainer should not permit clients with any known or suspected cardiovascular, metabolic, respiratory, or orthopedic conditions to hold their breath during resistance exercise.

Personal trainers who conduct maximum or near-maximum muscular strength tests need to be aware of the advantages and disadvantages of encouraging or allowing their clients to use the Valsalva maneuver. While it is important that the vertebral column be internally supported during these testing situations for safety and technique reasons, it is recommended that a client not overextend the time that the breath is held. Even resistance-trained and technique-experienced clients should be advised to hold their breath only momentarily (e.g., one to two seconds).

A personal trainer should not permit clients with any known or suspected cardiovascular, metabolic, respiratory, or orthopedic conditions to breath-hold during resistance exercise.

Weightlifting Belt Recommendations

Weight belts have been shown to increase intra-abdominal pressure during performance of a resistance training exercise [4, 5, 6]. Therefore, the use of a weight belt can contribute to injury-free training by decreasing the compressive forces on the vertebral column. Despite this benefit, if a client uses a weight belt for all resistance training exercises, the muscles of the lower back and abdomen may become unaccustomed to supporting the torso [4]. Then, if the client performs an exercise without a weight belt, the weaker torso muscles may not be capable of generating enough intra-abdominal pressure to decrease the chance of injury.

When determining whether or not a client should wear a weight belt during a resistance training exercise, the personal trainer should base the decision on the following guidelines:

- A weight belt is recommended for ground-based, structural exercises that load the trunk and place stress on the lower back (e.g., back and front squat, standing shoulder press, deadlift) *and* involve lifting maximal or near-maximal loads. (Both conditions should exist; it is not necessary, for example, for the client to wear a weight belt when lifting lighter loads even when performing a structural exercise.)
- A weight belt is not needed for an exercise that does not directly load the trunk even if it places stress on the lower back (e.g., lat pulldown, bench press, biceps curl, leg extension).

A weight belt is recommended for ground-based, structural exercises that involve lifting maximal or near-maximal loads.

Spotting Resistance Training Exercises

When a client is performing a resistance training exercise, the personal trainer's primary responsibility is the client's safety. In addition to teaching and reinforcing proper exercise technique, the personal trainer may also serve as a spotter by physically assisting the client in completing the exercise to help protect the client from injury. This need for a spotter is typically associated with free weight exercises. Bars, dumbbells, and weight plates that are not restricted to a fixed movement path increase the possibility that a client will lose control and become injured. A spot can be given for a machine exercise, but it is not as necessary because clients are not exposed to the possibility that a bar, dumbbell, or weight plate could fall on them. This advantage does not imply that machine exercises do not require supervision or assistance, however (e.g., a client may need help with maintaining proper speed and range of motion).

A personal trainer may assist a client with **forced repetitions** (repetitions that are successfully performed with help from another person), but this type of assistance should not be confused with or substituted for spotting for safety.

Four free weight exercise conditions require a spotter. These include exercises that are performed

- overhead (e.g., standing shoulder press),
- over the face (e.g., bench press, lying triceps extension),
- with a bar on the upper back and shoulders (e.g., back squat), or
- with a bar positioned on the front of the shoulders or clavicles (e.g., front squat).

Spotting Overhead or Over-the-Face Exercises

Many overhead and over-the-face resistance training exercises place the client in a sitting or standing position (e.g., shoulder press, overhead dumbbell triceps extension) or a supine position (e.g., bench press, dumbbell chest fly, lying triceps extension, dumbbell pullover). Because of the location of the barbell or dumbbell above the client's head or face, the potential for serious injury is greater during the performance of these exercises compared to most others. Also, to be effective at providing enough assistance to spot an overhead exercise, the personal trainer must be at least the same height as the client. If this is not the case, then the personal trainer should modify the exercise so that the client is in a seated position. Some types of bench press and shoulder press benches have a small platform that places the spotter in a better position for spotting overhead or over-the-face exercises.

Barbell Exercises

When spotting over-the-face barbell exercises, the personal trainer should grasp the bar between the client's hands using an alternated grip. This helps to keep the bar from rolling out of the personal trainer's hands and onto the client's head, face, or neck. Also the personal trainer should take a position as close to the client as possible—without creating a distraction—in order to be able to grab the bar quickly if necessary. Finally, to create a stable base of support, the personal trainer, if possible, should be in a flat-back rather than rounded-back position, with the feet flat on the floor in a staggered stance. With some bench frames there may not be enough room for the staggered stance, however.

Dumbbell Exercises

It is common to see people receiving spotting assistance at their upper arms or elbows while performing an overhead or over-the-face dumbbell exercise. This spotting technique may lead to injury if the individual's elbows quickly collapse while the spotter is lifting the upper arms or elbows. If that happens, the spotter probably will not be able to prevent the dumbbells from landing on the client's head, face, neck, or chest. The personal trainer should instead spot the client's wrists (figure 13.3) very near to the dumbbell. For exercises that require the client to use two hands to hold one dumbbell (e.g., dumbbell pullover) or only one hand at a time to perform an exercise (e.g., overhead dumbbell triceps extension), the personal trainer should spot the lowest half of the dumbbell itself, that is, the end closest to the floor.

When a client is performing an overhead or over-the-face dumbbell exercise, the personal trainer should spot the client's wrists close to the dumbbell, not the upper arms or elbows.

Spotting Exercises With the Bar on the Back or Front Shoulders

Exercises that involve placing the bar across the shoulders at the base of the neck or the upper back (e.g., back squat, lunge, step-up) or on the front of the shoulders and across the clavicles (e.g., front squat)

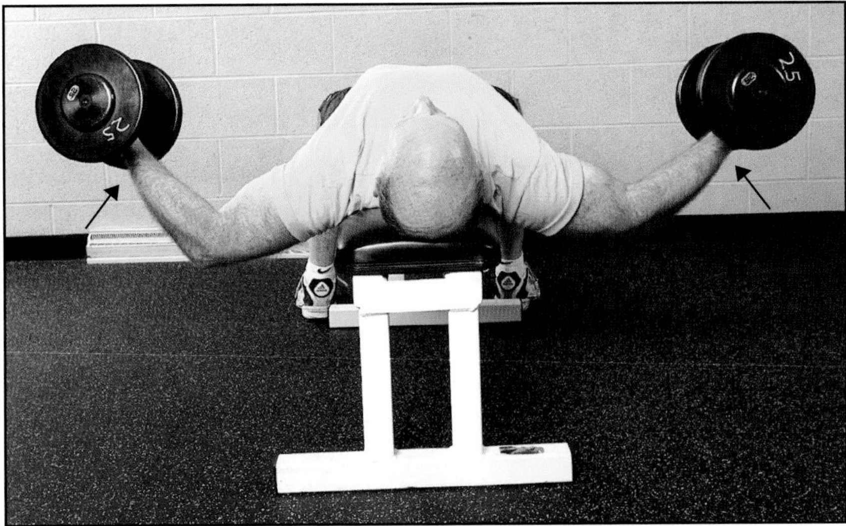

Figure 13.3 The arrows point to where the personal trainer should grasp the client's wrists when spotting a dumbbell exercise.

should also be spotted. As with the overhead or over-the-face exercises, in order to be an effective spotter the personal trainer needs to be strong enough to handle the load lifted and needs to be at least as tall as the client. To further guard against injury or accident, these types of exercises should be performed, if possible, inside a squat rack with the crossbars placed just below the lowest position the bar will reach during the downward movement phase.

Spotting Power Exercises

As a rule, "explosive" or simply "power" exercises (e.g., power clean, hang clean, push jerk, high pull, snatch) should not be spotted. Fast-moving bars are difficult for a personal trainer to spot and catch; trying to do so may result in injury to one or both parties. Because of this dynamic situation, power exercises should be performed in a segregated area or on a lifting platform in case the client "misses" (fails to complete a repetition) or loses control of the bar. Instead of physically spotting the bar during a missed lift, the personal trainer should teach the client to push the bar away or simply drop it. Clients should be instructed that if the bar begins to fall behind their head, they should simultaneously let go of the bar and step or jump forward. It is also important to remove any equipment from the area in and around the space where power exercises are performed.

Power exercises should be performed in a segregated area or on a lifting platform without the use of a spotter.

Number of Spotters

Once a personal trainer decides that a client requires a spot for an exercise, the next step is to determine how many spotters are necessary. If the load is beyond the personal trainer's ability to handle it effectively, an additional spotter must be used. For example, it is common to use one spotter at each end of the bar during the front or back squat exercise. This technique requires spotters who are experienced, because the spotters have to perfectly synchronize when and how much they assist the client to keep the bar even and balanced. When excessively heavy loads are involved, three spotters may be appropriate.

Communication

Communication is the responsibility of both the client and the personal trainer. A client should be instructed to tell the personal trainer when he or she is ready to move the bar, dumbbells, or machine handles into the starting position (called a **liftoff**). If the client needs help during the set, he or she should quickly ask or signal the personal trainer; and after the last repetition the personal trainer should help the client move the bar back onto the supports (called **racking the bar**). Poor communication may cause the personal trainer to spot the client too soon, too late, or improperly. Therefore, the personal trainer should discuss all of these issues with the client before the beginning of a set.

Additional Resistance Training Safety Guidelines

The personal trainer and the client should do the following:

- Check to see if there is sufficient floor-to-ceiling space before performing a standing exercise that finishes with the bar positioned over the head.
- Use a bar with revolving sleeves for power exercises.
- When performing exercises in which the client will step out and return to a rack (e.g., back squat, lunge), clients should be instructed to always step back (i.e., away from the bar's supports) to get into starting position at the beginning of the set, and step forward at the end of the set; do not walk backward to return the bar to the rack when performing an exercise in a squat or power rack.
- Always use collars and locks to secure free weight plates on the bar.
- Fully insert the selectorized pin or key (usually L- or T-shaped) into the weight stack for machine exercises.

CONCLUSION

Personal trainers are responsible for teaching clients proper resistance training exercise technique to maximize the training effect of the exercises and create the safest training environment. This includes not only instructions on how to perform an exercise, but also proper breathing guidelines and weight belt recommendations. The personal trainer must also know when and how to spot a client during a resistance training exercise and how to recognize and correct mistakes in a client's exercise technique.

A personal trainer should be familiar with all of the exercises described in this chapter and should realize that there has been no attempt to explain or provide photos of all possible technique and spotting variations. The checklists on the following pages offer the most commonly accepted guidelines for resistance training exercise technique [2, 3, 8].

Resistance Training Exercises

Abdominals

Back

Arms (Biceps)

Arms (Triceps)

Calves

Chest

Hip and Thigh

Shoulders

Whole Body

Abdominals

Bent Knee Sit-Up

Starting Position

Assume a supine position on a floor mat.

Flex the knees to bring the heels near the buttocks.

Fold the arms across the chest or abdomen.

Upward Movement Phase

Flex the neck to move the chin to the chest.

Keeping the feet, buttocks, and lower back flat and stationary on the mat, curl the torso toward the thighs until the upper back is off the mat.

Keep the arms folded across the chest or abdomen.

Downward Movement Phase

Allow the torso, then the neck, to uncurl and extend back to the starting position.

Keep the feet, buttocks, lower back, and arms in the same position.

Common Errors

- Raising the feet off the mat during the upward movement phase
- Raising the hips off the mat during the downward movement phase

Primary Muscle Trained:
Rectus abdominis

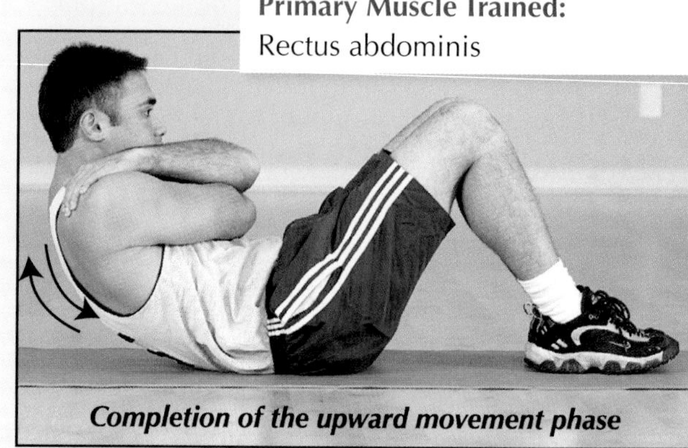

Completion of the upward movement phase

Machine Abdominal Crunch

Primary Muscle Trained:
Rectus abdominis

Starting Position

Sit in the machine with the upper chest pressed against the chest pad; if there are handles instead, grasp them with a closed, pronated or neutral grip.

Forward Movement Phase

Flex the neck to move the chin to the chest.

Keeping the feet, legs, and buttocks stationary, curl the torso toward the thighs.

Keep the upper chest pressed against the pad (or keep a grip on the handles).

Backward Movement Phase

Allow the torso, then the neck, to uncurl and extend back to the starting position.

Keep the feet, legs, buttocks, and arms in the same position.

Keep the upper chest pressed against the pad (or keep a grip on the handles).

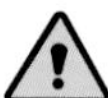

Common Errors

- Raising the hips off the seat during the forward movement phase
- Pulling with the legs or hands to help curl the torso forward

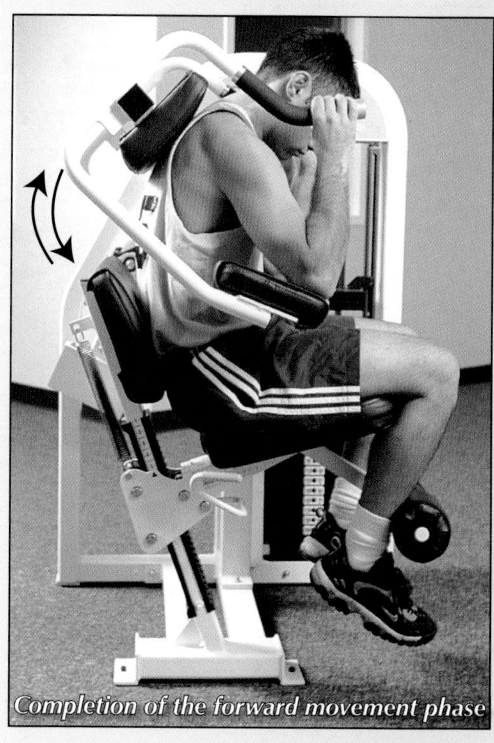

Completion of the forward movement phase

Back

Bent-Over Row

Starting Position

Grasp the bar with a closed, pronated grip wider than shoulder-width.

Lift the bar from the floor to a position at the front of the thighs using the first pull phase of the power clean exercise.

Adjust the feet to assume a shoulder-width stance with the knees slightly to moderately flexed.

Flex the torso forward so that it is slightly above parallel to the floor.

Assume a flat-back torso position with the shoulders back and the chest out.

Focus the eyes a short distance ahead of the feet.

Allow the bar to hang with the elbows fully extended.

Adjust the position of the knees, hips, and torso to suspend the weight plates off the floor.

Upward Movement Phase

Pull the bar up toward the lower chest or upper abdomen.

Keep the elbows pointed away from the sides of the body with the wrists straight.

Keep the torso rigid, back flat, and knees in the same flexed position.

Touch the bar to the sternum or upper abdomen.

At the highest bar position, the elbows should be higher than the torso.

Downward Movement Phase

Allow the elbows to slowly extend back to the starting position.

Keep the torso rigid, back flat, and knees in the same flexed position.

After the set is completed, squat down to return the bar to the floor.

Common Errors

- Jerking the upper body, shrugging the shoulders, extending the torso, extending the knees, curling the bar in the hands, or rising up on the toes to help raise the bar
- Allowing the upper back to round (losing the flat-back position) during the movement

Primary Muscles Trained:
Latissimus dorsi, teres major, rhomboid, posterior deltoid

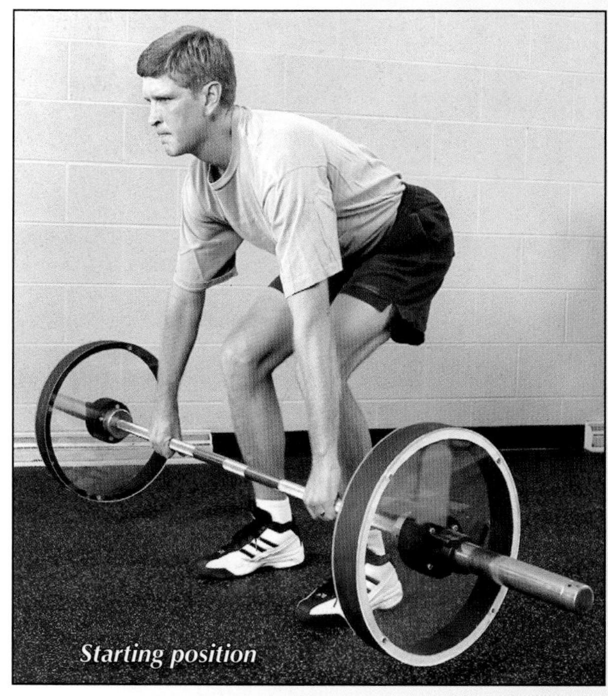
Starting position

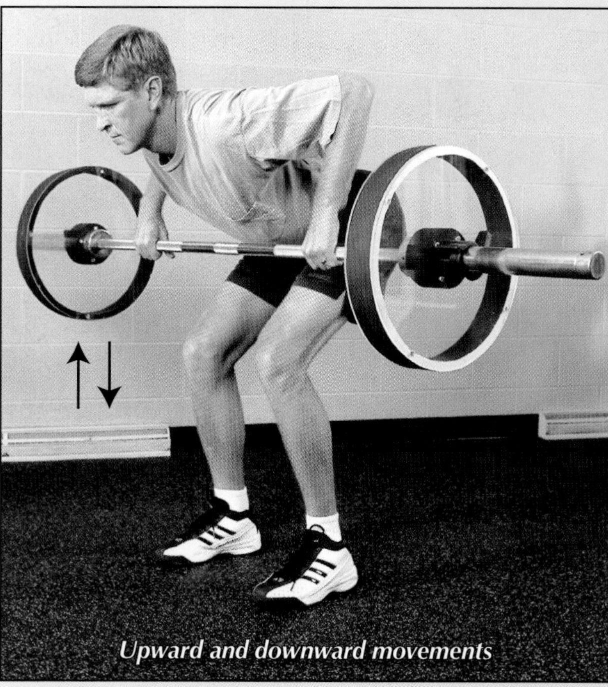
Upward and downward movements

Lat Pulldown

Starting Position

Grasp the bar with a closed, pronated grip wider than shoulder-width.

Sit facing the machine stack with the legs under the thigh pads and the feet flat on the floor.

Slightly lean the torso backward to create a path for the bar to pass by the face.

Allow the elbows to fully extend.

In this position, the weight to be lifted will be suspended above the rest of the stack.

Downward Movement Phase

Pull the bar down and toward the upper chest; the elbows should move down and back and the chest up and out as the bar is lowered.

Keep the feet, legs, and torso in the same position.

Touch the bar to the clavicles or upper chest.

Upward Movement Phase

Allow the elbows to slowly extend back to the starting position.

Keep the feet, legs, and torso in the same position.

After the set is completed, stand up and return the weight to its resting position.

Common Errors

- Using an open grip on the bar
- Contracting the abdominal muscles and flexing the torso to assist in the downward movement phase
- Not fully extending the elbows during the upward movement phase

Primary Muscles Trained:
Latissimus dorsi, teres major, rhomboid, posterior deltoid

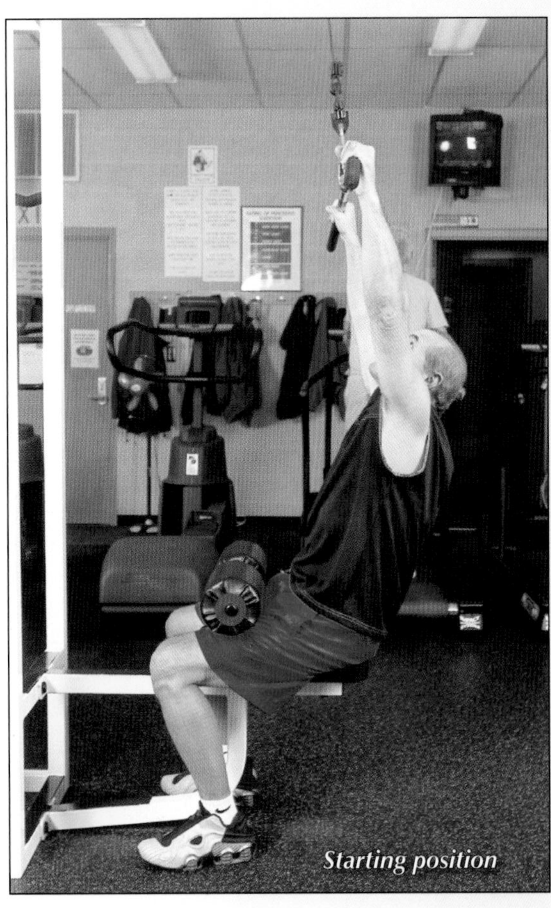

Starting position

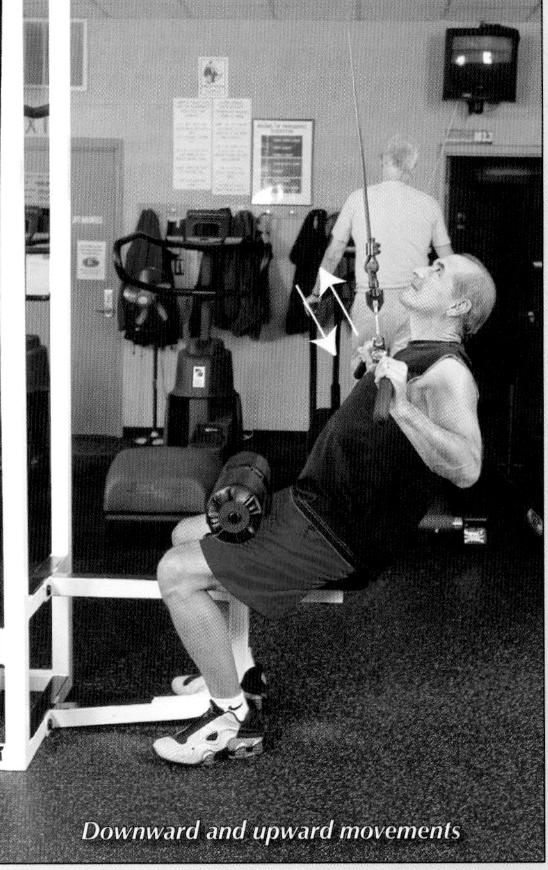

Downward and upward movements

Low Pulley Seated Row

Starting Position

Facing the machine, sit on the floor (or on the long seat pad, if available).

Place the feet on the machine frame or foot supports.

Flex the knees and hips to reach forward and grasp the handle with a closed, neutral grip.

Pull the handle back and assume an erect seated position with the torso perpendicular to the floor, knees slightly flexed, and the feet and legs parallel to each other.

Allow the elbows to fully extend with the arms about parallel to the floor.

In this position, the weight to be lifted will be suspended above the rest of the stack.

Backward Movement Phase

Pull the handle toward the chest or upper abdomen.

Maintain an erect torso position with the knees in the same slightly flexed position.

Touch the handle to the sternum or abdomen.

Forward Movement Phase

Allow the elbows to slowly extend back to the starting position.

Maintain an erect torso position with the knees in the same slightly flexed position.

After the set is completed, flex the knees and hips to reach forward and return the weight to its resting position.

Common Errors

- Jerking the upper body or leaning back during the backward movement phase
- Curling the handle toward the torso during the backward movement phase
- Flexing the torso forward during the forward movement phase

Primary Muscles Trained:
Latissimus dorsi, teres major, rhomboid, posterior deltoid

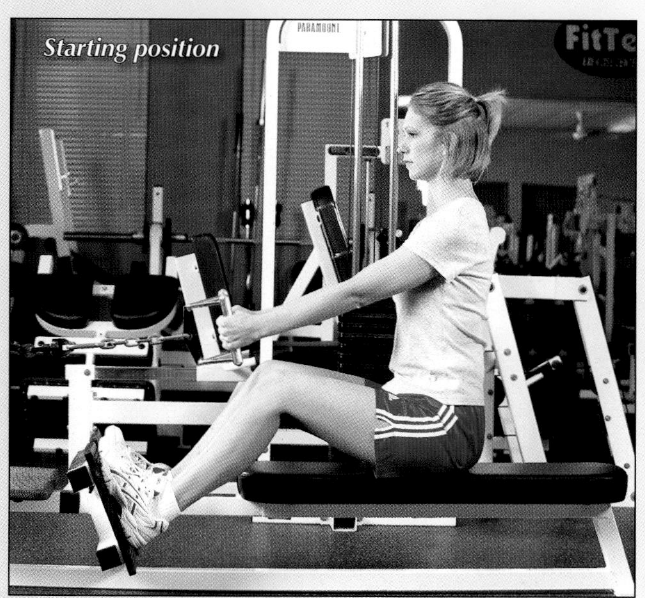

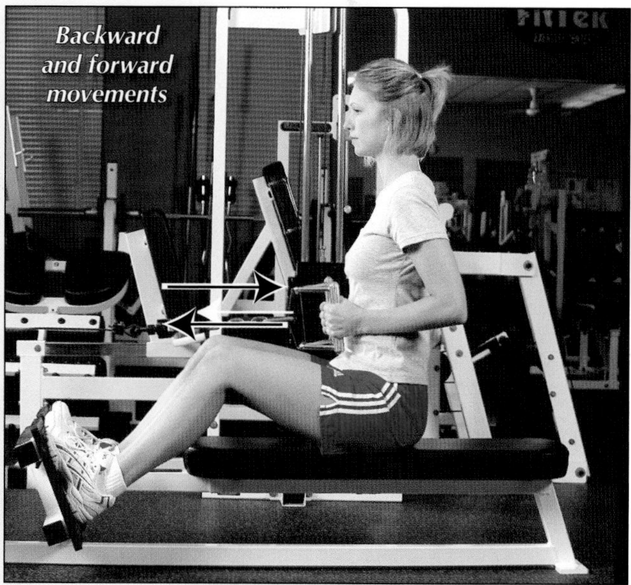

Seated Row (Resistance Band)

Starting Position

Grasp the handles of the resistance band with a closed, neutral grip.

Sit on the floor or mat with the knees slightly flexed, and evenly wrap the resistance band around the insteps of the feet.

Assume an erect position with the torso perpendicular to the floor.

Hold on to the handles with the elbows fully extended, the arms about parallel to the floor, and the palms facing each other.

In this position, the resistance band should be nearly taut (not stretched); if it is not, take up the slack by wrapping the resistance band further around the feet.

Backward Movement Phase

Pull the handles toward the chest or upper abdomen.

Maintain an erect torso position with the knees in the same slightly flexed position.

Touch the hands to the sides of the torso.

Forward Movement Phase

Allow the elbows to slowly extend back to the starting position.

Maintain an erect torso position with the knees in the same slightly flexed position.

Common Errors

- Jerking the upper body or leaning back during the backward movement phase
- Curling the handles toward the torso during the backward movement phase
- Flexing the torso forward during the forward movement phase

Primary Muscles Trained:
Latissimus dorsi, teres major, rhomboid, posterior deltoid

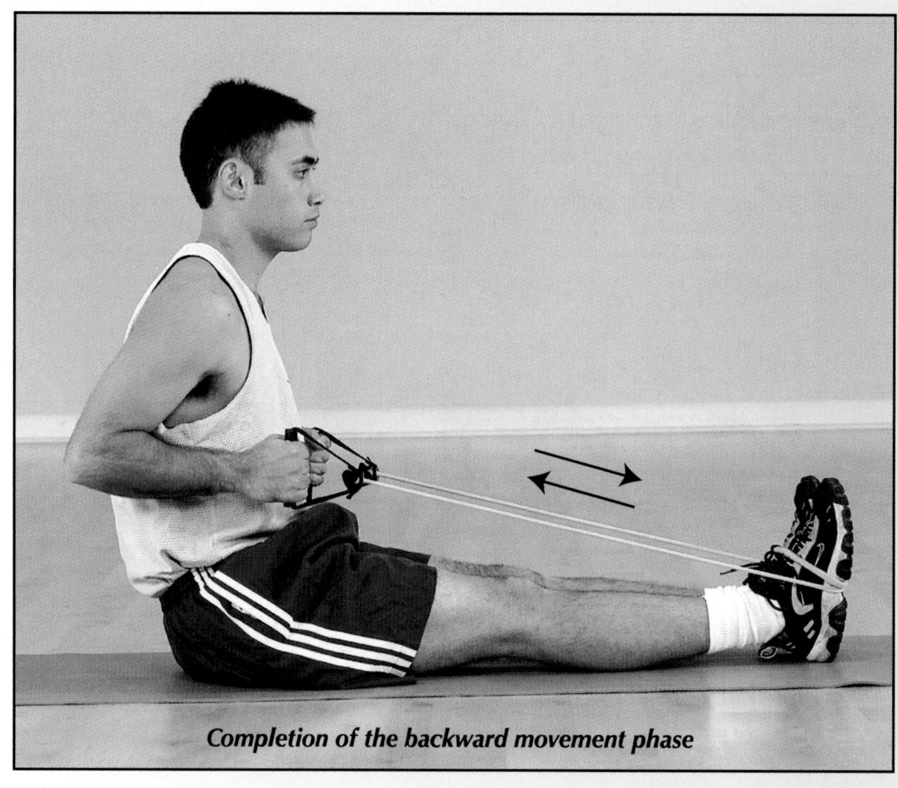
Completion of the backward movement phase

Machine Back Extension

Starting Position

Sit in the machine with the upper back pressed against the back pad.

Flex the torso forward and move the body back to align the hips with the axis of the machine.

Place the feet on the machine frame or foot supports.

Grasp the handles or the sides of the seat.

Backward Movement Phase

Keeping the thighs and feet stationary, extend the torso (lean backward).

Keep the upper back firmly pressed against the back pad.

Maintain a tight grip on the handles or the sides of the seat.

Forward Movement Phase

Allow the torso to flex (lean forward) back to the starting position.

Keep the upper back firmly pressed against the back pad and the thighs and feet stationary.

Maintain a tight grip on the handles or the sides of the seat.

Common Errors

- Pushing with the legs or rising off the seat during the backward movement phase
- Arching the back at the end of the backward movement phase

Primary Muscle Trained:
Erector spinae

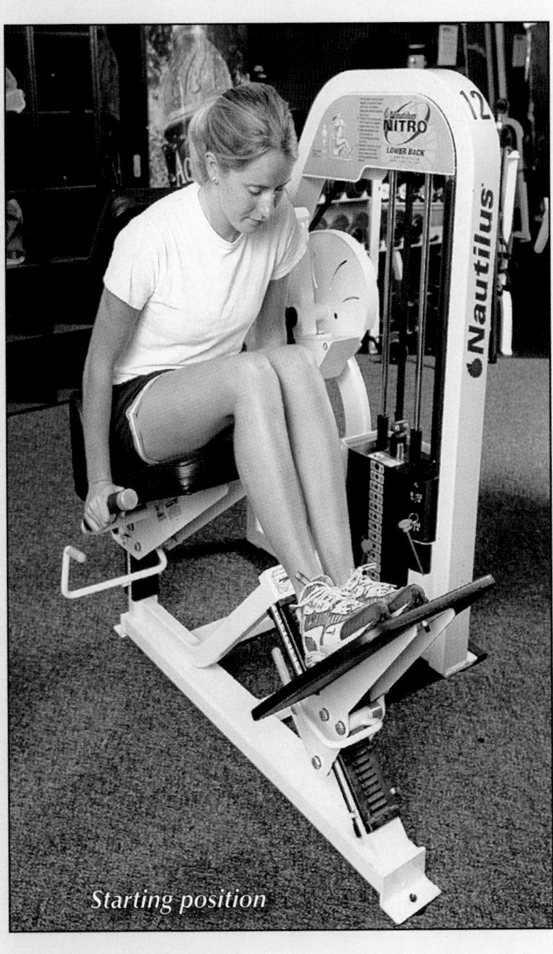

Starting position

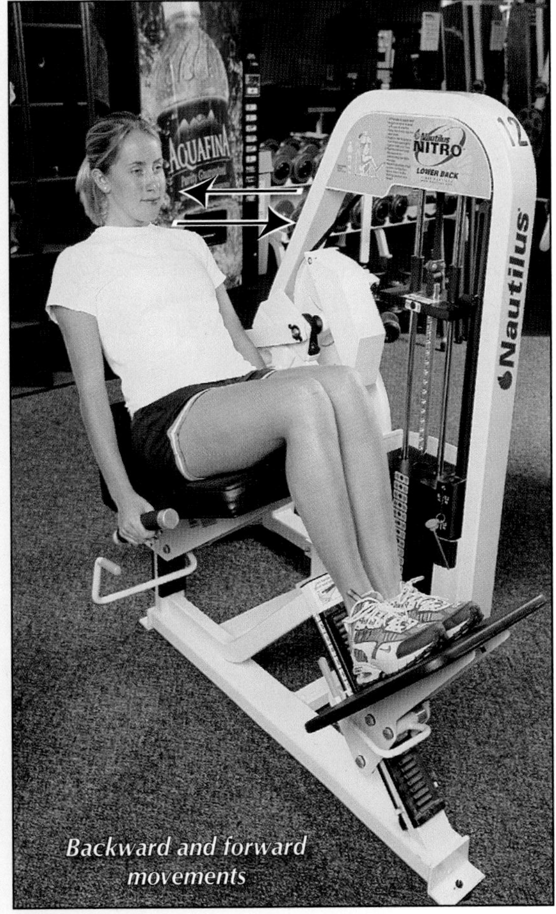

Backward and forward movements

Arms (Biceps)

Biceps Curl (Bar)

Starting Position

Grasp the bar with a closed, supinated grip at or slightly wider than shoulder-width.

Stand erect with the feet shoulder-width apart and knees slightly flexed.

Position the bar in front of the thighs with the elbows fully extended.

Position the upper arms against the sides of the torso and perpendicular to the floor.

Upward Movement Phase

Flex the elbows to move the bar in an upward arc toward the shoulders.

Keep the torso erect, the upper arms stationary, and the knees in the same slightly flexed position.

Flex the elbows until the bar is within four to six inches (10-15 centimeters) of the shoulders.

Downward Movement Phase

Allow the elbows to slowly extend back to the starting position.

Keep the torso, upper arms, and knees in the same position.

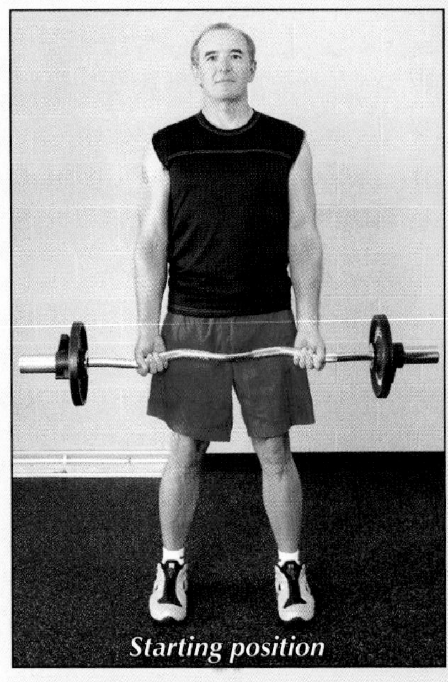
Starting position

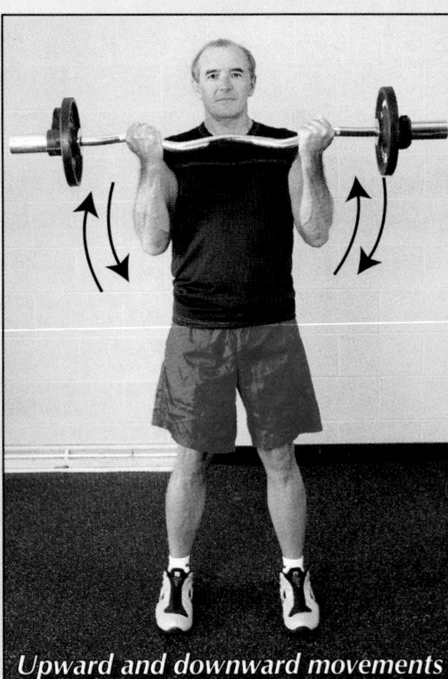
Upward and downward movements

Primary Muscles Trained:
Brachialis, biceps brachii (especially), brachioradialis

 **Common Errors**

- Jerking the upper body, shrugging the shoulders, extending the torso, extending the knees, swinging the bar, or rising up on the toes to help raise the bar
- Moving the elbows away from the sides of the torso (backward during the downward movement phase or forward during the upward movement phase)
- Keeping the elbows partially flexed at the end of the downward movement phase (a shortened range of motion)
- Bouncing the bar off the thighs to add momentum to help with the next repetition.

Biceps Curl (Resistance Band)

Starting Position

Grasp the handles of the resistance band with a closed, supinated grip.

Position the feet shoulder-width apart with the arches of both feet on top of a middle section of the resistance band.

Stand erect with the knees slightly flexed.

Position the handles outside of the thighs with the arms at the sides and the palms facing forward.

In this position, the resistance band should be nearly taut (not stretched); if not, take up the slack by widening the stance or selecting a shorter band.

Upward Movement Phase

Flex the elbows to move the handles in an upward arc toward the shoulders.

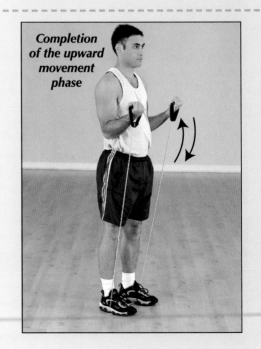
Completion of the upward movement phase

Keep the torso erect, the upper arms stationary, and the knees in the same slightly flexed position.

Flex the elbows until the hands are within four to six inches (10-15 centimeters) of the shoulders.

Downward Movement Phase

Allow the elbows to slowly extend back to the starting position.

Keep the torso, upper arms, and knees in the same position.

 **Common Errors**

- Shrugging the shoulders to help raise the handles upward
- Moving the elbows away from the sides of the torso (backward during the downward movement phase or forward during the upward movement phase)
- Keeping the elbows partially flexed at the end of the downward movement phase (a shortened range of motion)

Primary Muscles Trained:
Brachialis, biceps brachii (especially), brachioradialis

Machine (Preacher) Biceps Curl

Starting Position

Assume a seated position facing the chest pad of the machine.

Grasp the handles with a closed, supinated grip with the elbows fully extended.

Position the upper arms on the angled upper arm pad(s), and align the elbows with the axis of the machine.

Place the feet on the machine frame, foot supports, or floor.

Sit erect and press the torso against the chest pad. If necessary, adjust the pad to position the torso perpendicular to the floor.

Upward Movement Phase

Keeping the torso, thighs, and feet stationary, flex the elbows to move the handles toward the face and shoulders.

Keep the torso and upper arms firmly pressed against their pads.

Flex the elbows until the handles are within four to six inches (10-15 centimeters) of the face and shoulders.

Downward Movement Phase

Allow the elbows to slowly extend back to the starting position.

Keep the torso and upper arms firmly pressed against their pads.

 **Common Errors**

- Lifting the upper arms off the angled upper arm pad(s) during the upward movement phase
- Jerking the upper body or leaning back during the upward movement phase
- Rising off the seat during the downward movement phase
- Keeping the elbows partially flexed at the end of the downward movement phase (a shortened range of motion)

Primary Muscles Trained:
Brachialis, biceps brachii (especially), brachioradialis

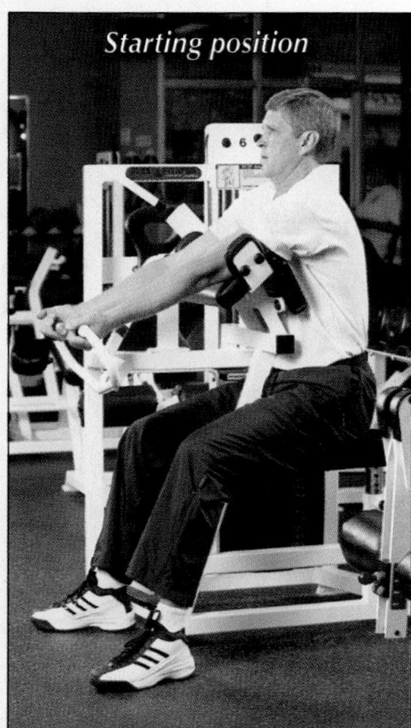
Starting position

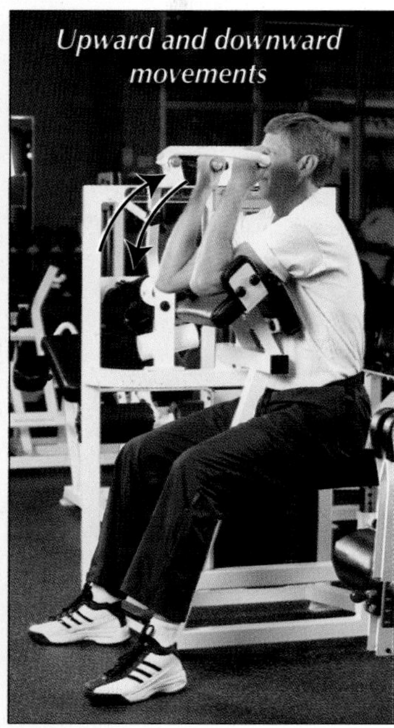
Upward and downward movements

Arms (Triceps)

Lying Triceps Extension

A spotter is required for this exercise, but in order to show proper exercise technique the head-on photo does not include the spotter.

Client: Starting Position

Assume a supine position on a bench in the five-point body contact position.

On a signal, take the bar from the personal trainer.

Grasp the bar with a closed, pronated grip about 12 inches (30 centimeters) apart.

Position the bar over the chest with the elbows fully extended and the arms parallel.

Point the elbows away from the face.

Personal Trainer: Starting Position

At the client's signal, grasp the bar with a closed, alternated grip (not where the client will grasp the bar, however) and lift it from the floor.

Stand erect and very close to the head of the bench (but not so close as to distract the client).

Place the feet shoulder-width apart with the knees slightly flexed.

At the client's signal, place the bar in the client's hands.

Guide the bar to a position over the client's chest.

Release the bar smoothly.

Client: Downward Movement Phase

Allow the elbows to slowly flex to lower the bar toward the nose, eyes, forehead, or the top of the head depending upon the length of the arms.

Keep the wrists rigid and the elbows pointing away from the face.

Keep the upper arms parallel to each other and perpendicular to the floor.

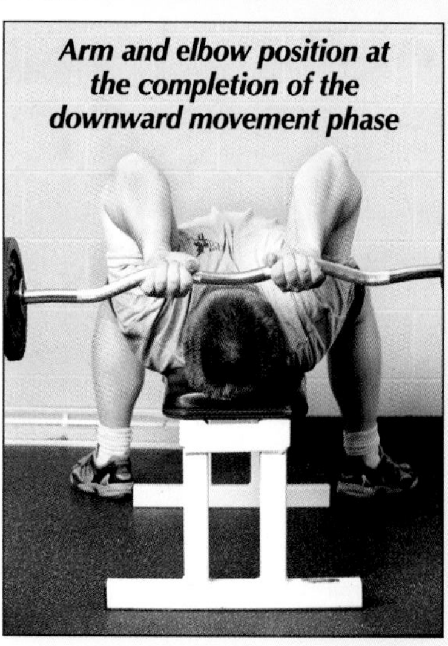

Arm and elbow position at the completion of the downward movement phase

Lower the bar to touch the top of the head or forehead.

Maintain the five-point body contact position.

Personal Trainer: Downward Movement Phase

Keep the hands in the alternated grip position close to—but not touching—the bar as it descends.

Slightly flex the knees, hips, and torso and keep the back flat when following the bar.

Client: Upward Movement Phase

Push the bar upward until the elbows are fully extended.

Keep the wrists rigid and the elbows pointing away from the face.

Keep the upper arms parallel to each other and perpendicular to the floor.

Maintain the five-point body contact position.

At the completion of the set, signal the personal trainer to take the bar.

Primary Muscle Trained:
Triceps brachii

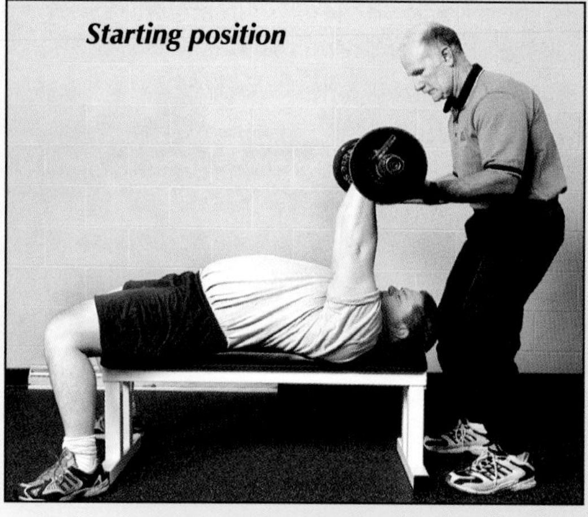

Starting position

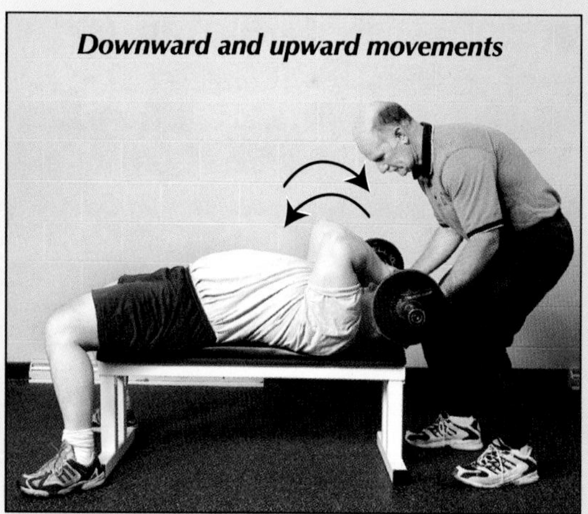

Downward and upward movements

Personal Trainer: Upward Movement Phase

Keep the hands in the alternated grip position close to—but not touching—the bar as it ascends.

Slightly extend the knees, hips, and torso and keep the back flat when following the bar.

At the client's signal, grasp the bar with an alternated grip, take it from the client, and return it to the floor.

Common Errors

- Allowing the elbows to flare out to the sides during the movement
- Moving the upper arms away from their perpendicular position in relation to the floor
- Arching the back or raising the hips off the bench during the upward movement phase

Triceps Pushdown

Starting Position

Grasp the bar with a closed, pronated grip 6 to 12 inches (15-30 centimeters) apart. A minimum recommended grip width is close enough for the tips of the thumbs to touch each other when they are extended along the bar. A maximum grip width is one in which the forearms are parallel to each other.

Stand erect with feet shoulder-width apart and knees slightly flexed.

Pull the bar down and position the upper arms against the sides of the torso with the arms flexed.

Adjust the degree of elbow flexion to position the forearms approximately parallel to the floor.

Stand close enough to the machine to allow the cable to hang straight down when it is held in the starting position.

Keep the head in a neutral position with the cable directly in front of the nose.

Keep the torso in position by holding the

- shoulders back,
- upper arms and elbows against the sides of the body, and
- abdominal muscles contracted throughout the exercise.

In this position, the weight to be lifted will be suspended above the rest of the stack.

Downward Movement Phase

Push the bar down until the elbows are fully extended.

Keep the torso and the upper arms stationary.

Upward Movement Phase

Allow the elbows to slowly flex back to the starting position.

Keep the torso, upper arms, and knees in the same position.

After the set is completed, guide the bar upward to move the weight back to its resting position.

Common Errors

- Moving the elbows away from the sides of the torso (backward during the downward movement phase or forward during the upward movement phase)
- Flexing the torso during the downward movement phase
- Forcefully locking out the elbows during the downward movement phase
- Turning the head to the side during the movement

Primary Muscles Trained:
Triceps brachii

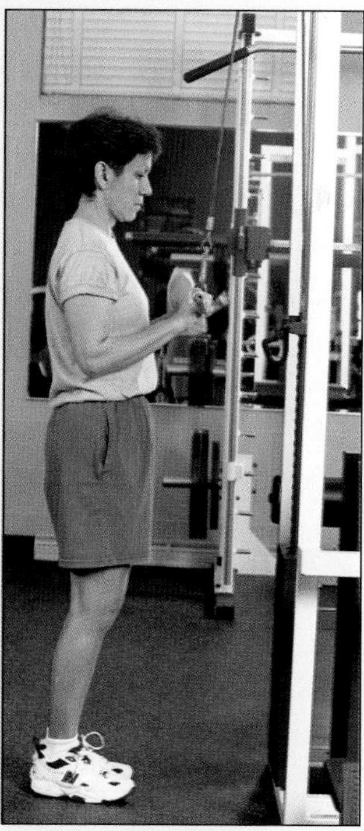

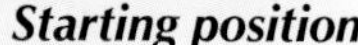

Starting position

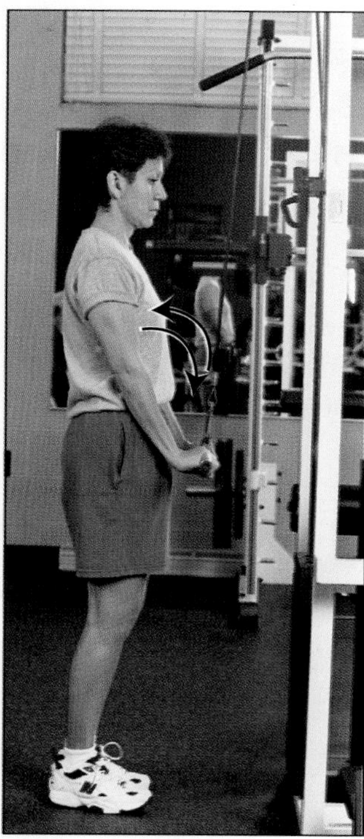

Downward and upward movements

Triceps Extension (Resistance Band)

Starting Position

Grasp the handles of the resistance band with a closed, pronated grip.

Sit on the floor or mat with the buttocks on top of a middle section of the resistance band.

Assume an erect position with the torso perpendicular to the floor and the legs crossed in front the body.

Position the arms and handles behind the head and upper back with the elbows flexed and the palms facing up.

In this position, the resistance band should be nearly taut (not stretched); if not, select a shorter band.

Upward Movement Phase

Keeping the wrist rigid, push one handle upward until the elbow is fully extended.

Maintain an erect torso position with the legs in the same position.

Downward Movement Phase

Allow the elbow to flex to slowly move the handle down to the starting position.

Maintain an erect torso position with the legs in the same position.

At the completion of the set, repeat the movement with the other arm.

 **Common Errors**

- Excessively arching the back during the upward movement phase
- Flexing the torso or head forward during the downward movement phase

Primary Muscles Trained:
Triceps brachii

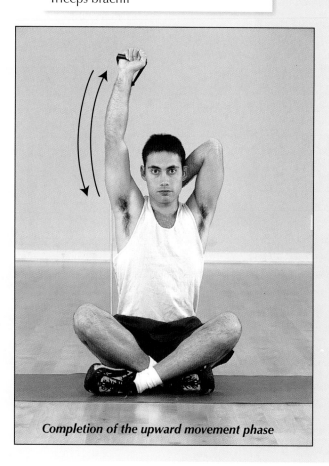

Completion of the upward movement phase

Calves

Machine Standing Calf (Heel) Raise

Starting Position

Facing the machine, place the balls of the feet on the nearest edge of the step with the toes pointing straight ahead.

Move under the shoulder pads and stand erect with the hips under the shoulders.

Position the feet and legs parallel to each other.

Slightly plantar flex the feet and ankles to lift the thigh pads to remove the supports. If there are none, then the position of the shoulder pads needs to be low enough that the exercise can be performed through a full range of motion.

Extend the knees fully, but not forcefully.

Allow the heels to drop down lower than the step in a comfortable, stretched position.

Upward Movement Phase

Fully plantar flex the feet and ankles.

Keep the torso erect, legs and feet parallel, and knees extended.

Downward Movement Phase

Allow the heels to slowly lower back to the starting position.

Maintain the same body position.

After the set is completed, slightly flex the knees, replace the supports, and move out from under the shoulder pads.

Common Errors

- Allowing the ankles to invert or evert (i.e., rising up on the big or little toes, respectively) during the upward movement phase
- Allowing the knees to flex during the downward movement phase or extend during the upward movement phase
- Bouncing the weight to add momentum to help with the next repetition

Primary Muscles Trained:
Soleus, gastrocnemius (especially)

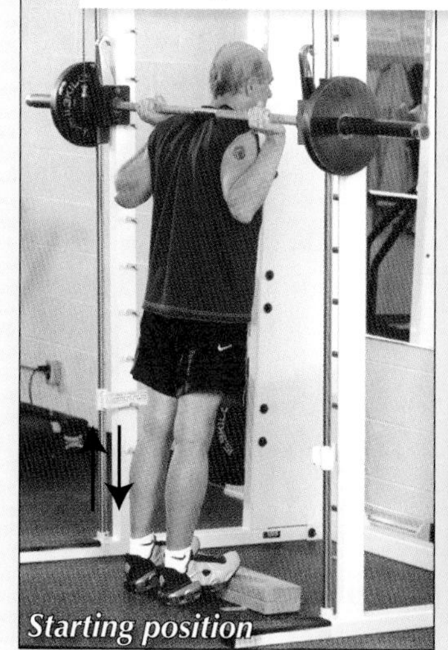
Starting position

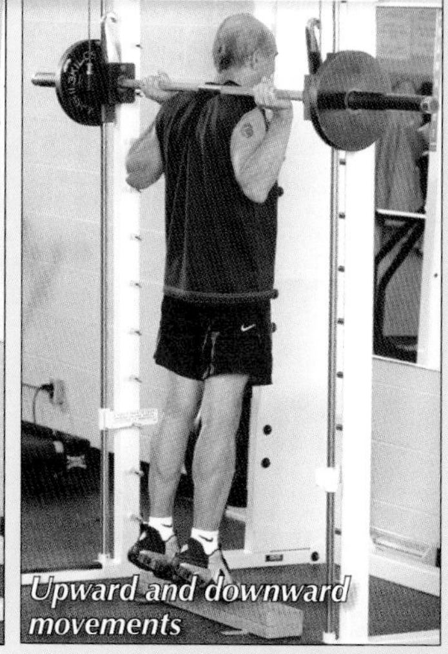
Upward and downward movements

Machine Seated Calf (Heel) Raise

Starting Position

Sit erect on the seat and place the knees and lower thighs under the pads with the thighs parallel to the floor.

Place the balls of the feet on the nearest edge of the step with the toes pointing straight ahead.

Position the feet and legs parallel to each other.

Slightly plantar flex the feet/ankles to lift the thigh pads to remove the supports.

Allow the heels to drop down lower than the step in a comfortable, stretched position.

Upward Movement Phase

Keeping the torso erect and the legs and feet parallel, fully plantar flex the feet/ankles.

Downward Movement Phase

Allow the heels to slowly lower back to the starting position.

Maintain the same body position.

After the set is completed, replace the supports and remove the feet.

Common Errors

- Allowing the ankles to invert or evert (i.e., rising up on the big or little toes, respectively) during the upward movement phase
- Pulling with the hands or jerking the torso to help raise the weight
- Bouncing the weight to add momentum to help with the next repetition

Primary Muscles Trained:
Soleus (especially), gastrocnemius

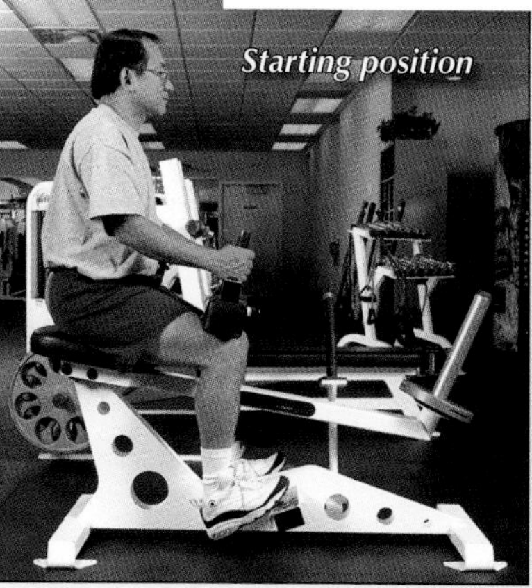
Starting position

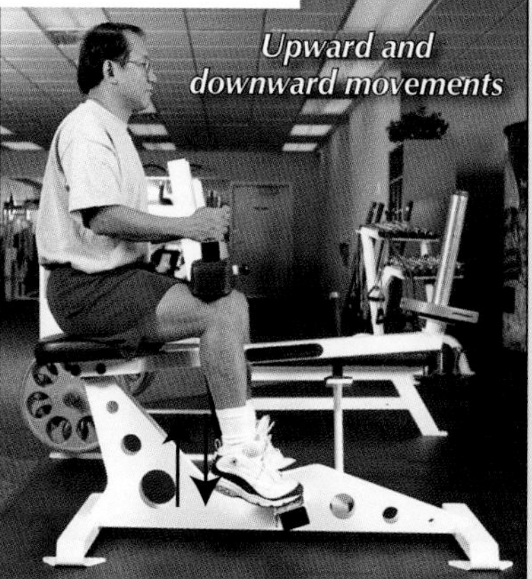
Upward and downward movements

Chest

Flat Barbell Bench Press

Client: Starting Position

Assume a supine position on a bench in the five-point body contact position.

Place the body on the bench so that the eyes are below the bar.

Grasp the bar with a closed, pronated grip slightly wider than shoulder-width.

Signal the personal trainer for a liftoff.

Guide the bar to a position over the chest with the elbows fully extended.

Personal Trainer: Starting Position

Stand erect and very close to the head of the bench (but not so close as to distract the client).

Place the feet shoulder-width apart with the knees slightly flexed.

Grasp the bar with a closed, alternated grip inside the client's hands.

At the client's signal, assist with moving the bar off the supports and to a height that allows the client's elbows to be fully extended.

Guide the bar to a position over the client's chest.

Release the bar smoothly.

Client: Downward Movement Phase

Allow the bar to lower to touch the chest at approximately nipple level.

Allow the elbows to move down past the torso and slightly away from the body.

Keep the wrists rigid and directly above the elbows.

Keep the forearms approximately perpendicular to the floor and parallel to each other.

Maintain the five-point body contact position.

Personal Trainer: Downward Movement Phase

Keep the hands in the alternated grip position close to—but not touching—the bar as it descends.

Slightly flex the knees, hips, and torso and keep the back flat when following the bar.

Client: Upward Movement Phase

Push the bar upward and very slightly backward until the elbows are fully extended.

Keep the wrists rigid and directly above the elbows.

Maintain the five-point body contact position.

After the set is completed, signal the personal trainer for assistance in racking the bar.

Keep a grip on the bar until it is racked.

Personal Trainer: Upward Movement Phase

Keep the hands in the alternated grip position close to—but not touching—the bar as it ascends.

Slightly extend the knees, hips, and torso and keep the back flat when following the bar.

At the client's signal after the set is completed, grasp the bar with an alternated grip inside the client's hands and help to rack the bar.

Common Errors

- Bouncing the bar on the chest during the upward movement phase to help raise the bar past the sticking point
- Lifting the buttocks off the bench
- Raising the head off the bench during the movement

Primary Muscles Trained:
Pectoralis major, anterior deltoid, serratus anterior, pectoralis minor, triceps brachii

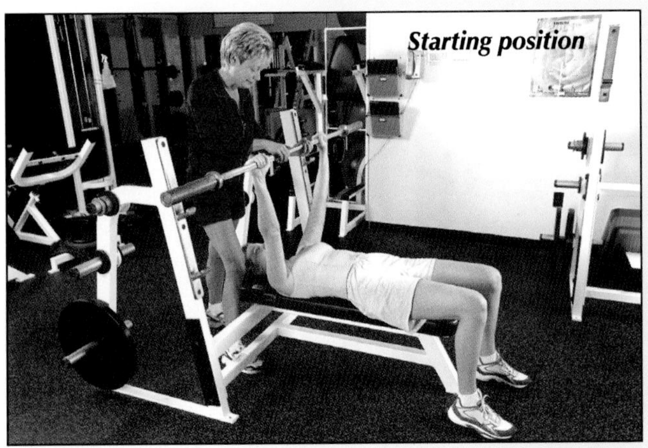
Starting position

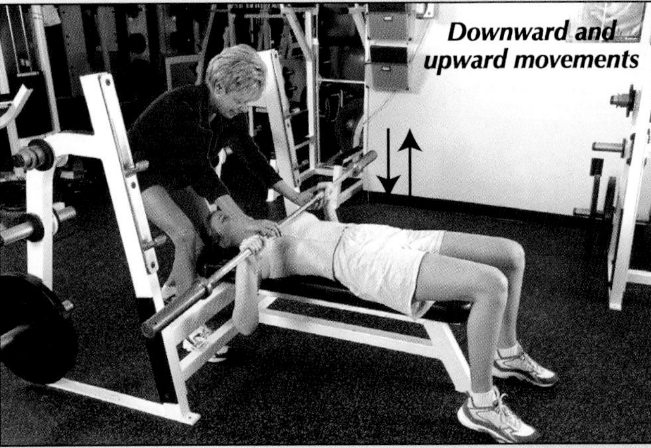
Downward and upward movements

Flat Dumbbell Fly

A spotter is required for this exercise, but in order to show proper exercise technique the photos do not include the spotter.

Client: Starting Position

Assume a supine position on a bench in the five-point body contact position.

On a signal, take the dumbbells from the personal trainer (one at a time) and position them near to or on the chest.

Rotate the dumbbells to a neutral grip position.

Signal the personal trainer for assistance to move the dumbbells into an extended elbow position over the chest with the arms parallel to each other.

Slightly flex the elbows and point them out to the sides.

Personal Trainer: Starting Position

At the client's signal, lift the dumbbells from the floor into the client's hands (one at a time).

While the client adjusts the dumbbells, position one knee on the floor with the foot of the other leg forward and flat on the floor (or kneel on both knees) very close to the head of the bench (but not so close as to distract the client).

Grasp the client's wrists.

At the client's signal, assist with moving dumbbells to a position over the client's chest.

Release the client's wrists smoothly.

Client: Downward Movement Phase

Allow the dumbbells to lower at the same rate in a wide arc until they are level with the shoulders or chest.

Keep the dumbbell handles parallel to each other as the elbows move downward.

Keep the wrists rigid and the elbows held in a slightly flexed position.

Keep the dumbbells in line with the elbows and shoulders.

Maintain the five-point body contact position.

Personal Trainer: Downward Movement Phase

Keep the hands near—but not touching—the client's wrists as the dumbbells descend.

Client: Upward Movement Phase

Pull the dumbbells up toward each other in a wide arc back to the starting position; imagine the arc formed by the arms when hugging a very large tree trunk.

Keep the wrists rigid and the elbows held in a slightly flexed position.

Keep the dumbbells in line with the elbows and shoulders.

Maintain the five-point body contact position.

At the completion of the set, first slowly lower the dumbbells to the chest and armpit area then signal the personal trainer to return them to the floor.

Personal Trainer: Upward Movement Phase

Keep the hands near—but not touching—the client's wrists as the dumbbells ascend.

At the client's signal, take the dumbbells from the client and return them to the floor.

Common Errors

- Allowing the elbows to flex and extend during the movement
- Lifting the buttocks off the bench
- Raising the head off the bench during the movement
- Lowering the dumbbells below chest level.

Primary Muscles Trained:
Pectoralis major, anterior deltoid

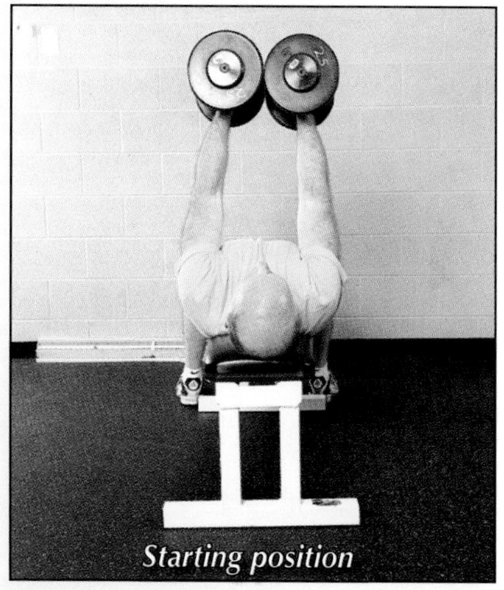

Starting position

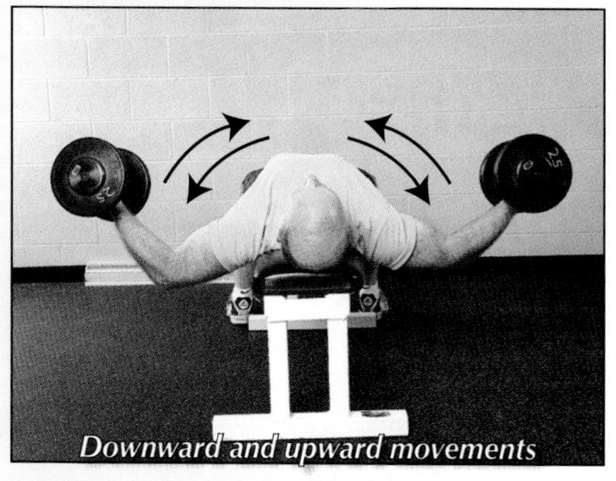

Downward and upward movements

Pec Deck (Butterfly)

Starting Position

Sit in the machine with the head, back, hips, and buttocks pressed against their pads.

If the seat is adjustable, move it up or down to

- position the thighs parallel to the floor with the feet flat in the starting seated position,
- position the shoulders slightly above the bottom of the forearm pads (or in line with the elbow pads, depending upon the type of machine), and
- position the upper arms parallel to the floor (or slightly above parallel) when the elbows are flexed to 90 degrees with the hands holding on to the handles.

Grasp the handles with

- a closed, neutral grip;
- the elbows flexed at right angles (90 degrees); and
- the forearms pressed against the small vertical pads near the handgrips. (If the machine has elbow pads, press the inside of the elbows against them.)

If the handles are too far back to be grasped from the seated position, push down on the foot pedal (if available), or request the assistance of a spotter.

Begin the exercise with the handles together in front of the face.

Backward Movement Phase

Begin the exercise by allowing both handles to swing out and back slowly and under control.

Keep the wrists erect, the forearms and elbows next to the arm pads, and the upper arms approximately parallel to the floor.

Allow the handles to move back so they are level with the chest.

Primary Muscle Trained:
Pectoralis major

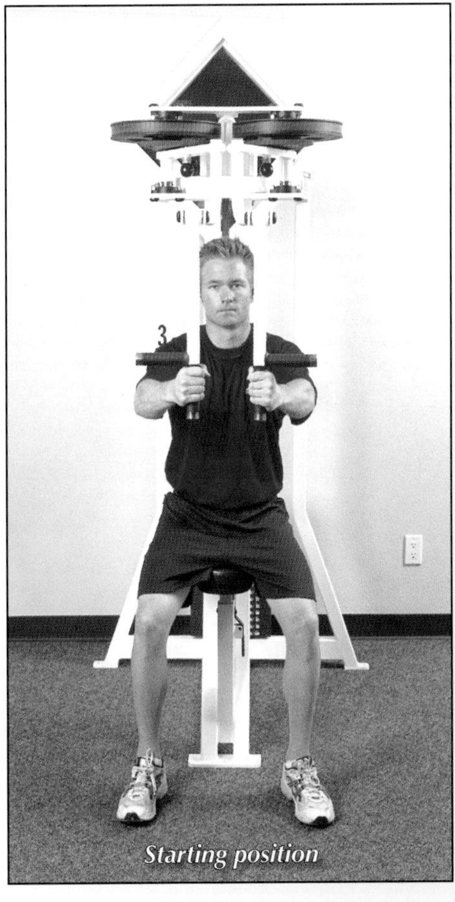

Starting position

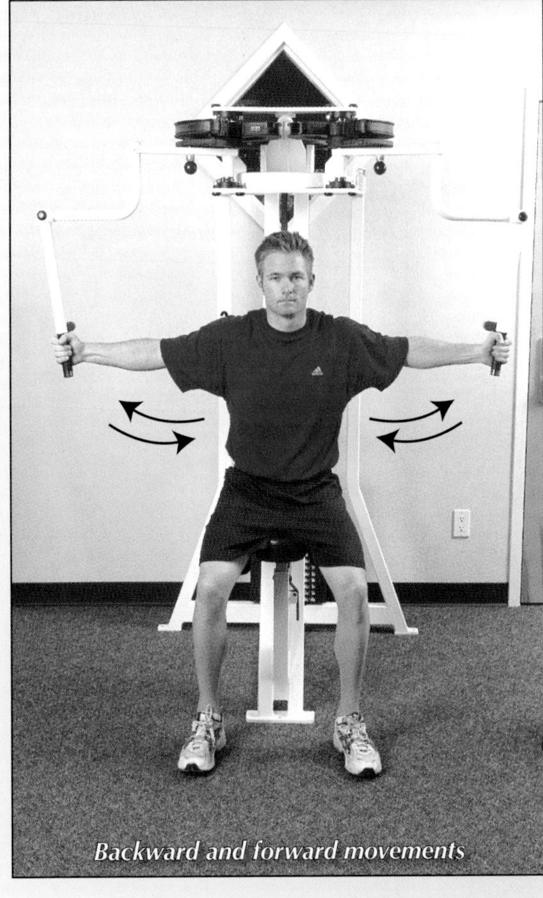
Backward and forward movements

Forward Movement Phase

Move the handles out and then toward each other, under control, by squeezing the forearms and elbows together.

Use the entire arm to exert pressure against the pads to squeeze the handles together.

At the completion of the set, guide the handles backward to their resting position.

 **Common Errors**

- Positioning the seat too low or too high
- Pushing the handles together with the hands or the palms of the hands
- Swinging the handles back to add momentum to help with the next repetition
- Flexing the torso forward to help move the handles together

Chest Press (Resistance Band)

Primary Muscles Trained:
Pectoralis major, anterior deltoid, triceps brachii

Starting Position

Grasp the handles of the resistance band with a closed, pronated grip, and evenly wrap the band around the upper back at nipple height.

Stand erect with the feet shoulder-width apart and the knees slightly flexed.

Position the handles to the outside of the chest at nipple height with the palms facing down.

In this position, the resistance band should be nearly taut (not stretched); if not, select a shorter band.

Forward Movement Phase

Push the handles away from the chest until the elbows are fully extended.

Keep the arms parallel to the floor.

Maintain the erect standing position with the heels on the floor and the knees slightly flexed.

Backward Movement Phase

Allow the handles to slowly move backward to the starting position.

Keep the arms parallel to the floor.

Maintain the erect standing position with the heels on the floor and the knees slightly flexed.

 **Common Errors**

- Forcefully locking out the elbows at the end of the forward movement phase
- Shortening the range of motion during the backward movement phase

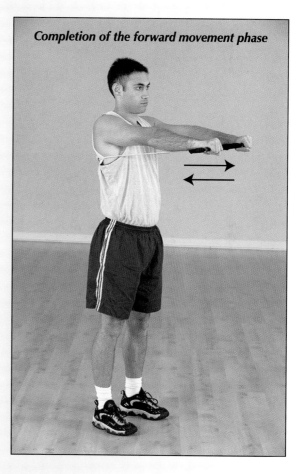

Completion of the forward movement phase

Vertical Chest Press

Starting Position

Sit in the machine with the head, back, hips, and buttocks pressed against their pads.

If the seat is adjustable, move it up or down to

- position the thighs parallel to the floor with the feet flat in the starting seated position,
- put the body in line with the handgrips (an imaginary line connecting both handgrips should cross the front of the chest at nipple height), and
- position the arms parallel to the floor with the elbows extended and holding on to the handgrips.

Grasp the handles with a closed, pronated grip. If the handles are too far back to be grasped from the seated position, push down on the foot pedal (if available) or request the assistance of a spotter to move the handles slightly forward.

Primary Muscles Trained:
Pectoralis major, anterior deltoid, triceps brachii

Forward Movement Phase

Push the handles away from the chest until the elbows are fully extended.

Maintain the five-point body contact position.

Backward Movement Phase

Allow the handles to slowly move backward so that they are level with the chest.

Maintain the five-point body contact position.

At the completion of the set, guide the handles backward to their resting position.

Common Errors

- Positioning the seat too low or too high
- Arching the back or pushing with the legs during the forward movement phase
- Flexing the torso forward to help move the handles forward
- Forcefully locking out the elbows at the end of the forward movement phase
- Shortening the range of motion during the backward movement phase

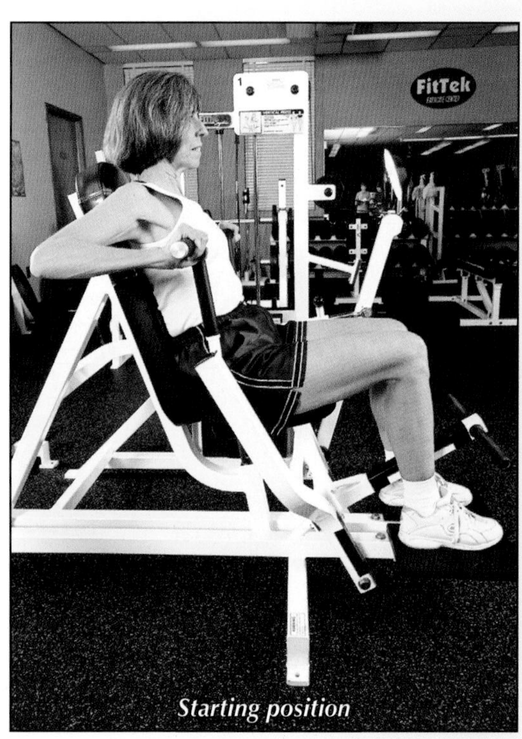

Starting position

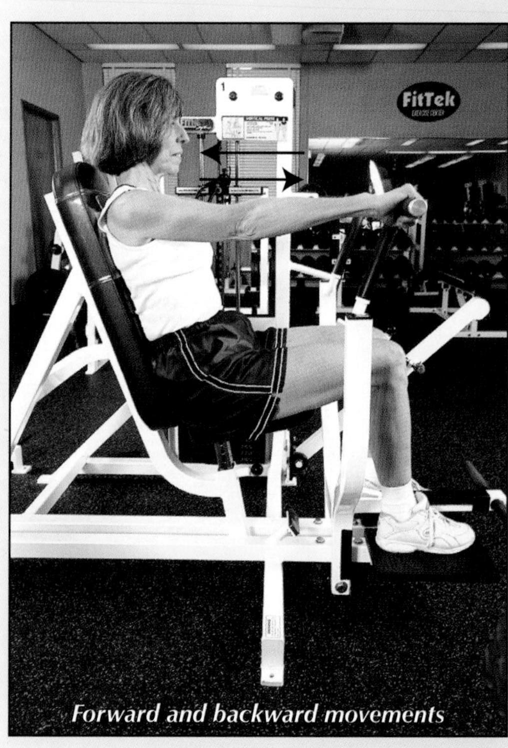

Forward and backward movements

Hip and Thigh

Leg Press

Starting Position

Sit in the machine with the back, hips, and buttocks pressed against their pads. (If the horizontal position of the foot platform or the seat is adjustable, move it forward or backward to allow the thighs to be parallel to the foot platform when seated in the starting position.)

Place the feet flat in the middle of the platform in a hip-width position with the toes slightly pointed out.

Position the thighs and lower legs parallel to each other.

Grasp the handles or the sides of the seat.

Forward Movement Phase

Extend the hips and knees to push the foot platform forward (note that in some machines, the foot platform is fixed and the seat will move *backward* during this phase).

Push to a fully extended position while maintaining the same upper body position and the heels in contact with the platform.

Backward Movement Phase

Allow the hips and knees to slowly flex to lower the weight.

Keep the hips and buttocks on the seat and the back flat against the back pad.

Keep the legs parallel to each other.

Continue flexing the hips and knees until the thighs are parallel to the foot platform.

Common Errors

- Allowing the heels to lift off the platform, the buttocks to lose contact with the seat, or the hands to let go during the movement
- Allowing the knees to move in (via hip adduction) or out (hip abduction) during the movement
- Locking the knees out at the end of the forward movement phase

Primary Muscles Trained:
Gluteus maximus, hamstrings, quadriceps

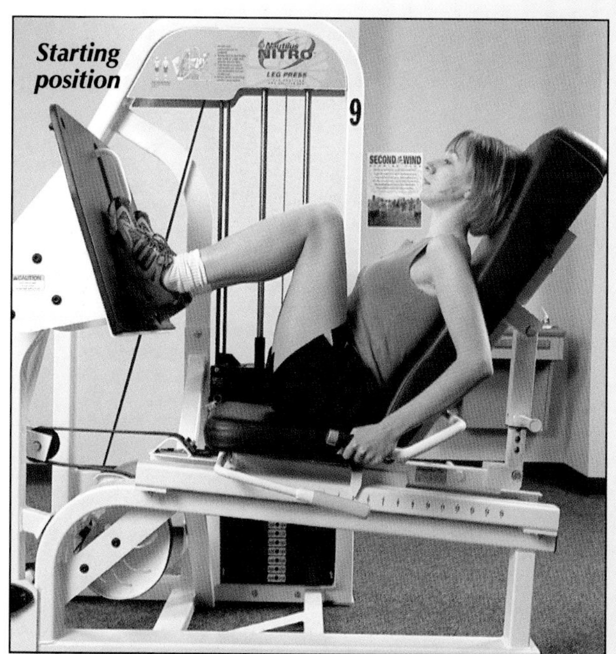

Starting position

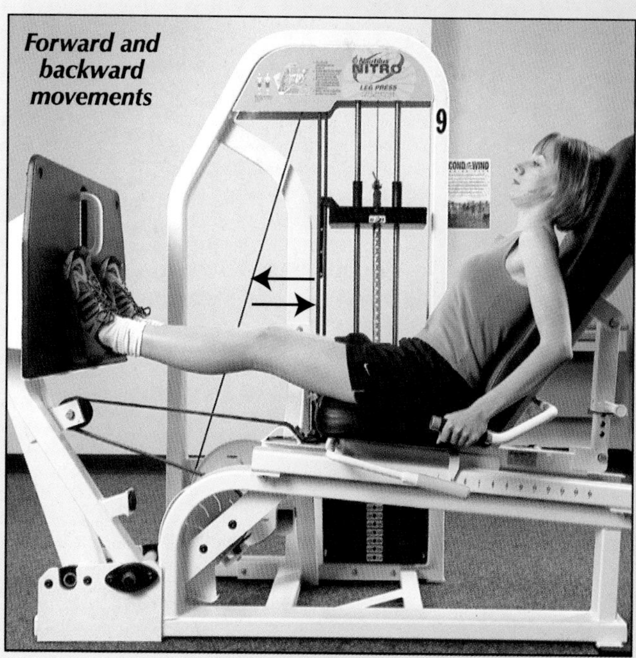

Forward and backward movements

Back Squat

Client: Starting Position

Step under the bar and position the feet parallel to each other.

Place the hands on the bar using the "high bar position" technique:

- Grasp the bar with a closed, pronated grip slightly wider than shoulder-width.
- Dip the head under the bar and move the body to place the bar evenly above the posterior deltoids at the base of the neck.

Lift the elbows up to create a shelf for the bar to rest on.

Hold the chest up and out.

Pull the scapulae toward each other.

Tilt the head slightly up.

Once in position, signal the spotters for a liftoff.

Extend the hips and knees to lift the bar off the racks, and take one or two steps backward.

Position the feet shoulder-width or wider apart and even with each other, with the toes slightly pointed outward.

Keep the elbows lifted up and backward to keep the bar on the shoulders.

Two Spotters: Starting Position

Stand erect at opposite ends of the bar with the feet shoulder-width apart and the knees slightly flexed.

Grasp the end of the bar by cupping the hands together with the palms facing upward.

At the client's signal, assist with lifting and balancing the bar as it is moved out of the rack.

Release the bar smoothly in unison with the other spotter.

Hold the hands two to three inches (five to eight centimeters) below the ends of the bar.

Move sideways in unison with the client as the client moves backward.

Once the client is in position, assume a hip-width stance with the knees slightly flexed and the torso erect.

Client: Downward Movement Phase

Allow the hips and knees to slowly flex while keeping the torso-to-floor angle constant.

Maintain a position with the back flat, elbows high, and the chest up and out.

Keep the heels on the floor and the knees aligned over the feet.

Continue allowing the hips and knees to flex until *one* of these three events first occurs (this determines client's maximum range of motion; the lowest or "bottom" position):

- The thighs are parallel to the floor.
- The trunk begins to round or flex forward.
- The heels rise off the floor.

Two Spotters: Downward Movement Phase

Keep the cupped hands close to—but not touching—the bar as it descends.

Slightly flex the knees, hips, and torso and keep the back flat when following the bar.

Client: Upward Movement Phase

Extend the hips and knees at the same rate to keep the torso-to-floor angle constant.

Maintain a position with the back flat, elbows high, and the chest up and out.

Primary Muscles Trained:
Gluteus maximus, hamstrings, quadriceps

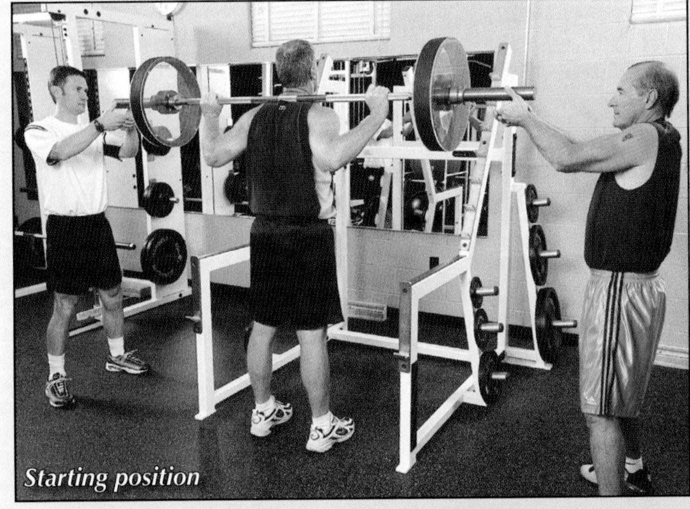

Starting position

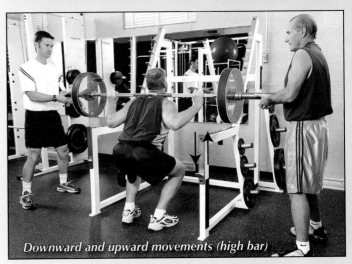

Downward and upward movements (high bar)

Keep the heels on the floor and the knees aligned over the feet.

Continue extending the hips and knees to reach the starting position.

After the set is completed, step forward and rack the bar.

Two Spotters: Upward Movement Phase

Keep the cupped hands close to—but not touching—the bar as it ascends.

Slightly extend the knees, hips, and torso and keep the back flat when following the bar.

After the set is completed, help the client rack the bar.

 **Common Errors**

- Allowing the heels to lift off the floor, the torso to flex further forward, or the upper back to round during the upward movement phase
- Allowing the knees to move in (via hip adduction) or out (hip abduction) during the movement
- Allowing the arms to relax or the elbows to drop down and forward

Squat (Resistance Band)

Starting Position

Grasp the handles of the resistance band with a closed, pronated grip.

Position the feet shoulder-width apart with the toes slightly pointed outward and the arches of both feet on top of a middle section of the resistance band.

Position the handles to the outside and level with the top of the shoulders, palms facing forward.

Create a flat-back position with the chest held up and out and the shoulders back.

Flex the hips and knees to assume the lowest desired squat position.

In this position, the resistance band should be nearly taut (not stretched); if not, select a shorter band.

Upward Movement Phase

Extend the hips and knees at the same rate to keep the torso-to-floor angle constant.

Maintain the flat-back position with the chest held up and out.

Keep the heels on the floor and the knees aligned over the feet.

Continue extending the hips and knees to a fully standing position.

Downward Movement Phase

Allow the hips and knees to slowly flex while keeping the torso-to-floor angle relatively constant.

Maintain the flat-back position with the chest held up and out.

Keep the heels on the floor and the knees aligned over the feet.

Continue allowing the hips and knees to flex until reaching the lowest desired squat position.

Common Errors

- Allowing the heels to lift off the floor, the torso to flex further forward, or the upper back to round during the upward movement phase
- Allowing the knees to move in (via hip adduction) or out (hip abduction) during the movement

Primary Muscles Trained:
Gluteus maximus, hamstrings, quadriceps

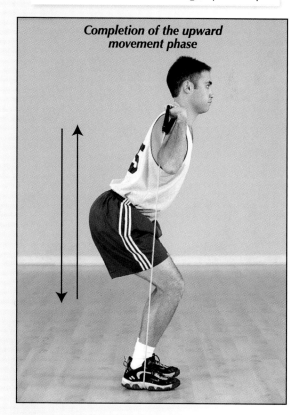

Front Squat

Client: Starting Position

Walk up to the bar and position the feet parallel to each other.

Place the hands on the bar using the "parallel arm position" technique:

- Grasp the bar with a closed, pronated grip slightly wider than shoulder-width.
- Move the body to place the bar evenly on top of the anterior deltoids and clavicles.
- Fully flex the elbows and hyperextend the wrists to position the upper arms parallel to the floor. The back of the hands should be either on top of or just to the outside of the shoulders, right next to where the bar is resting on the deltoids.

Hold the chest up and out.

Pull the scapulae toward each other.

Tilt the head slightly up.

Once in position, signal the spotters for a liftoff.

Extend the hips and knees to lift the bar off the racks, and take one or two steps backward.

Position the feet shoulder-width or wider apart, and even with each other, with the toes slightly pointed outward.

Keep the elbows lifted up and forward to keep the bar on the shoulders.

Two Spotters: Starting Position

Stand erect at opposite ends of the bar with the feet shoulder-width apart and the knees slightly flexed.

Grasp the end of the bar by cupping the hands together with the palms facing upward.

At the client's signal, assist with lifting and balancing the bar as it is moved out of the rack.

Release the bar smoothly in unison with the other spotter.

Hold the hands two to three inches (five to eight centimeters) below the ends of the bar.

Move sideways in unison with the client as the client moves backward.

Once the client is in position, assume a hip-width stance with the knees slightly flexed and the torso erect.

Client: Downward Movement Phase

Allow the hips and knees to slowly flex while keeping the torso-to-floor angle relatively constant.

Maintain a position with the back flat, elbows high, and the chest up and out.

Keep the heels on the floor and the knees aligned over the feet.

Continue allowing the hips and knees to flex until *one* of these three events first occurs (this determines client's maximum range of motion; the lowest or "bottom" position):

- The thighs are parallel to the floor.
- The trunk begins to round or flex forward.
- The heels rise off the floor.

Two Spotters: Downward Movement Phase

Keep the cupped hands close to—but not touching—the bar as it descends.

Slightly flex the knees, hips, and torso and keep the back flat when following the bar.

Client: Upward Movement Phase

Extend the hips and knees at the same rate to keep the torso-to-floor angle constant.

Primary Muscles Trained:
Gluteus maximus, quadriceps, hamstrings

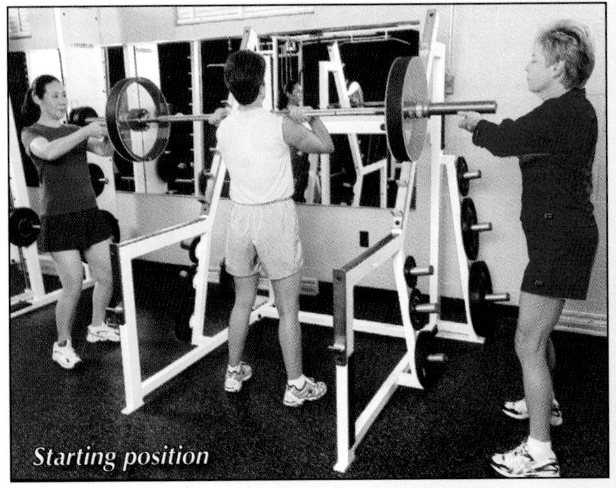

Starting position

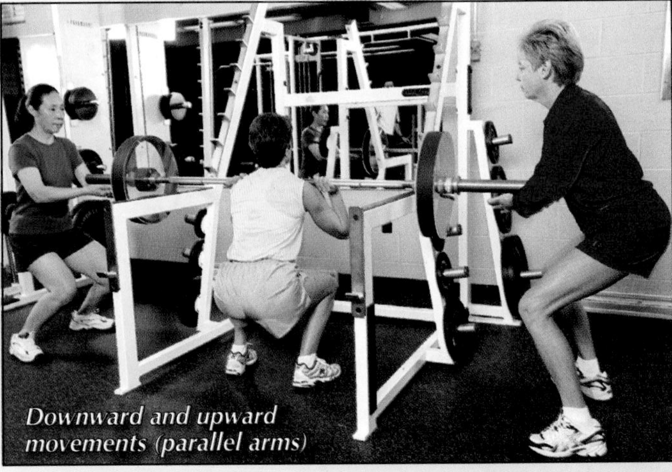

Downward and upward movements (parallel arms)

Maintain a position with the back flat, elbows high (higher than the photos show), and the chest up and out.

Keep the heels on the floor and the knees aligned over the feet.

Continue extending the hips and knees to reach the starting position.

After the set is completed, step forward and rack the bar.

Two Spotters: Upward Movement Phase

Keep the cupped hands close to—but not touching—the bar as it ascends.

Slightly extend the knees, hips, and torso and keep the back flat when following the bar.

After the set is completed, help the client rack the bar.

Common Errors

- Allowing the heels to lift off the floor, the torso to flex forward, or the upper back to round during the upward movement phase
- Allowing the knees to move in (via hip adduction) or out (hip abduction) during the movement
- Allowing the arms to relax or the elbows to drop down and backward

Leg (Knee) Extension

Starting Position

Sit in the machine with the thighs and back in the center of their pads (not to the left or right side) and the knees aligned with the axis of the machine. If the back pad is adjustable, move it forward or backward to

- align the knees with the axis of the machine and
- position the buttocks and thighs so that the backs of the knees are touching the front end of the seat.

Hook the feet under the ankle pad or pads; if the pad is adjustable, position it so it is in contact with the instep of the foot.

Position the thighs, lower legs, and feet parallel to each other.

Grasp the handles or the sides of the seat.

Upward Movement Phase

Keeping the thighs, lower legs, and feet parallel to each other, extend the knees until they are straight.

Keep the torso erect and the back firmly pressed against the back pad.

Maintain a tight grip on the handles or the sides of the seat.

Downward Movement Phase

Allow the knees to slowly flex back to the starting position.

Keep the thighs, lower legs, and feet parallel to each other.

Keep the torso erect and the back firmly pressed against the back pad.

Maintain a tight grip on the handles or the sides of the seat.

Common Errors

- Allowing the hips or buttocks to lift off the seat during the upward movement phase
- Swinging the legs or jerking the torso backward to help raise the weight
- Forcefully locking out the knees at the end of the upward movement phase

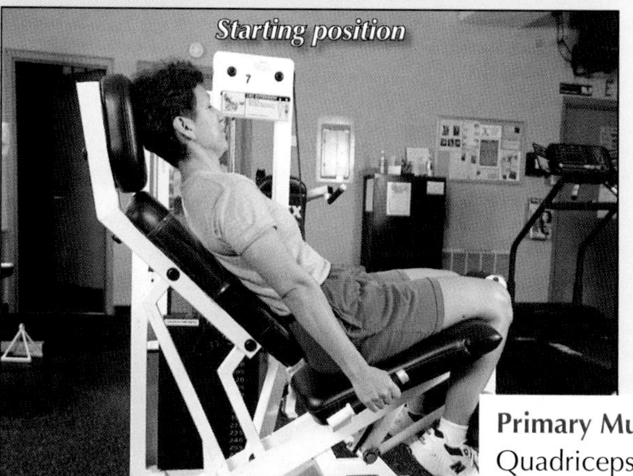

Starting position

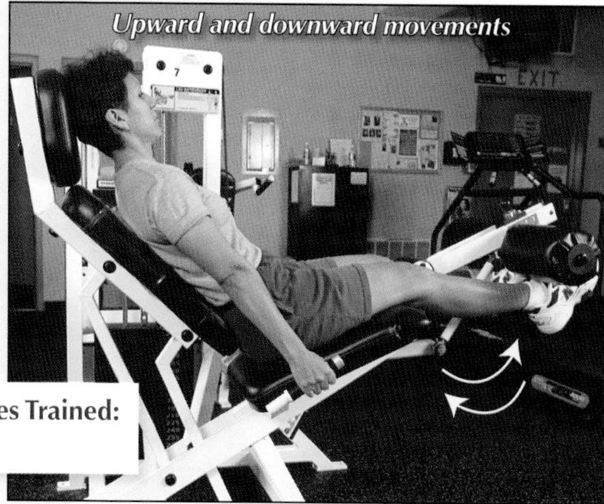

Upward and downward movements

Primary Muscles Trained:
Quadriceps

Forward Lunge

Client: Starting Position

Grasp the bar with a closed, pronated grip slightly wider than shoulder-width.

Step under the bar and position the feet parallel to each other.

Place the bar evenly on the upper back and shoulders above the posterior deltoids at the base of the neck.

Lift the elbows up to create a shelf for the bar to rest on.

Hold the chest up and out.

Pull the scapulae toward each other.

Tilt the head slightly up.

Once in position, signal the personal trainer for a liftoff.

Extend the hips and knees to lift the bar off the racks, and take two or three steps backward.

Place the feet hip-width apart with the toes pointed ahead.

Personal Trainer: Starting Position

Stand erect and very close to the client (but not close enough to be a distraction).

Place the feet shoulder-width apart with the knees slightly flexed.

At the client's signal, assist with lifting and balancing the bar as it is moved out of the rack.

Move in unison with the client as the client moves backward to the starting position.

Once the client is in position, assume a hip-width stance with the knees slightly flexed and the torso erect.

Position the hands near the client's hips, waist, or torso.

Client: Forward Movement Phase

Take one exaggerated step directly forward with one leg (the lead leg).

Keep the torso erect as the lead foot moves forward and contacts the floor.

Keep the trailing foot in the starting position, but allow the trailing knee to slightly flex.

Plant the lead foot flat on the floor pointing straight ahead or slightly inward. To help maintain balance, place this foot directly ahead from its initial position with the lead ankle, knee, and hip in one vertical plane.

Allow the lead hip and knee to slowly flex. Once balance has shifted to be even on both feet, flex the lead knee to lower the trailing knee toward the floor. The trailing knee will flex somewhat further, but not to the same degree as the lead knee.

Keep the lead knee directly over the lead foot (which remains flat on the floor).

Lower the trailing knee—still slightly flexed—until it is one to two inches (three to five centimeters) above the floor. At this point, the lead knee will be flexed to about 90 degrees with the lower leg perpendicular to the floor.

Balance the weight evenly between the ball of the trailing foot and the entire lead foot.

Keep the torso perpendicular to the floor by "sitting back" on the trailing leg. Actual lunge depth, however, depends primarily upon individual hip joint flexibility.

Personal Trainer: Forward Movement Phase

Step forward with the same foot as the client.

Plant the lead foot 12 to 18 inches (30-45 centimeters) behind the client's foot.

Flex the lead knee as the client's lead knee flexes.

Keep the torso erect.

Keep the hands near, but not touching, the bar.

Assist only when necessary to keep the client balanced.

Client: Backward Movement Phase

Shift the balance forward to the lead foot, and forcefully push off the floor by extending the lead hip and knee. As the lead foot moves back toward the trailing foot, balance will shift back to the trailing foot. This will cause the heel of the trailing foot to regain contact with the floor.

Maintain the same torso position.

Bring the lead foot back to a position next to the trailing foot.

Stand erect in the starting position, pause, and then alternate lead legs.

After the set is completed, step forward and rack the bar.

Personal Trainer: Backward Movement Phase

Push backward with the lead leg in unison with the client.

Bring the lead foot back to a position next to the trailing foot.

Keep hands near, but not touching, the bar.

Stand erect in the starting position, pause to wait for the client, and alternate lead legs.

Assist only when necessary to keep the client balanced.

After the set is completed, help the client rack the bar.

Common Errors

- Stepping out too shallowly, causing the lead knee to extend past the lead foot
- Allowing the torso to flex forward during the forward movement phase
- Quickly jerking the torso backward during the backward movement phase
- Stutter-stepping backward during the backward movement phase

Primary Muscles Trained:
Gluteus maximus, hamstrings, quadriceps, iliopsoas (of the trailing leg), soleus and gastrocnemius (of the lead leg)

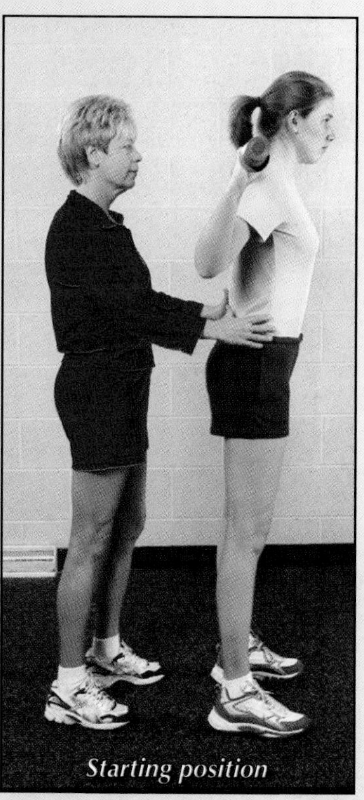
Starting position

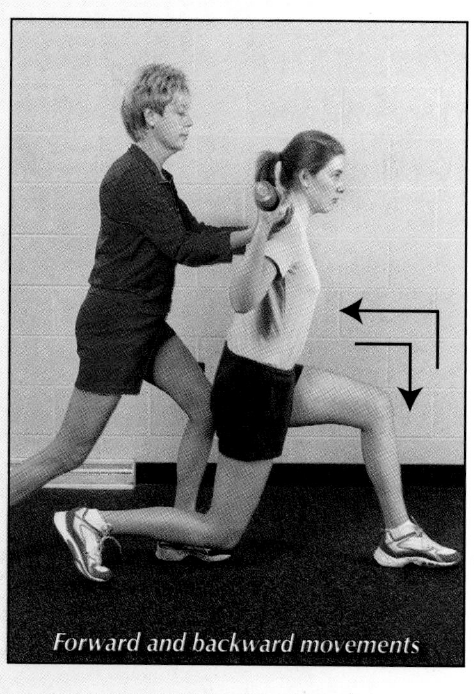
Forward and backward movements

Leg (Knee) Curl

Starting Position

Assume a prone position on the machine with the hips and torso in the center of their pads (not to the left or right side) and the knees aligned with the axis of the machine.

Hook the feet under the ankle pad or pads; if the pad is adjustable, position it so it is in contact with the back of the heel just above the top of the shoe.

Once in proper position, the knees should be hanging slightly off the bottom edge of the thigh pad.

Position the thighs, lower legs, and feet parallel to each other.

Grasp the handles or the sides of the chest pad.

Upward Movement Phase

Keeping the thighs, lower legs, and feet parallel to each other, flex the knees until the ankle pad nearly touches the buttocks.

Keep the torso stationary.

Maintain a tight grip on the handles or the sides of the chest pad.

Downward Movement Phase

Allow the knees to slowly extend back to the starting position.

Keep the thighs, lower legs, and feet parallel to each other.

Keep the torso stationary.

Maintain a tight grip on the handles or the sides of the chest pad.

Common Errors

- Allowing the hips to rise (using hip flexion) during the upward movement phase
- Swinging the legs backward to help raise the weight
- Locking out the knees at the end of the downward movement phase

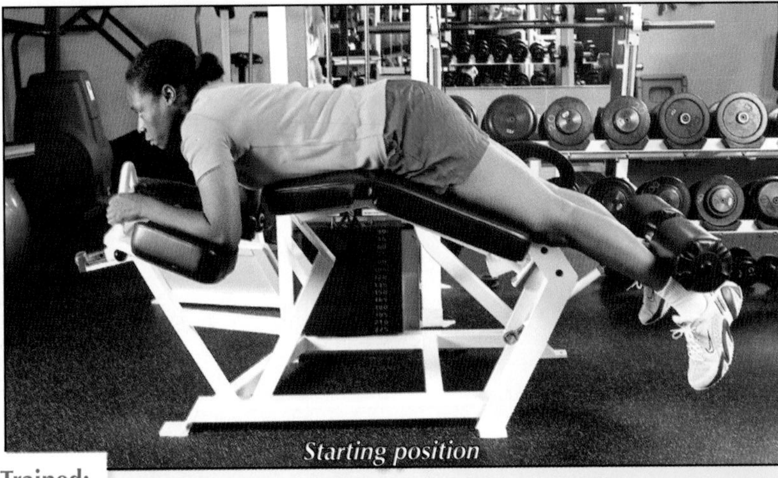

Starting position

Primary Muscles Trained:
Hamstrings

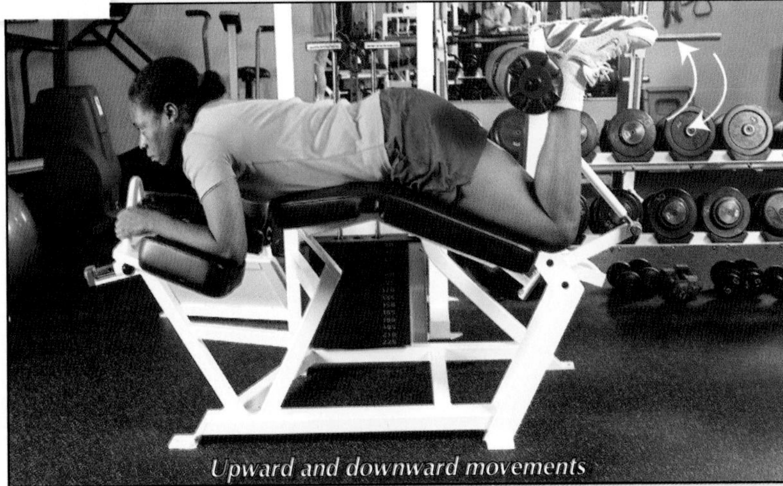

Upward and downward movements

Shoulders

Shoulder Press (Bar)

Note: It is recommended that this exercise be performed with a shoulder press bench with upright supports to hold the bar. One was not available when the photograph was taken however.

Client: Starting Position

Sit on a shoulder press bench and lean back to assume the five-point body contact position. If the seat can be adjusted, modify its height to

- position the thighs parallel to the floor (with the feet flat) and
- allow the bar to move in and out of the rack without hitting the top of the head (the seat is too high) or having to half-stand up to reach the racks (the seat is too low).

Grasp the bar with a closed, pronated grip slightly wider than shoulder-width.

Signal the personal trainer for a liftoff.

Press the bar over the head until the elbows are fully extended.

Personal Trainer: Starting Position

Stand erect on the step at the back of the bench or on the spotter's platform (if present) with the feet shoulder-width apart, if there is enough room, and the knees slightly flexed.

Grasp the bar with a closed, alternated grip inside the client's hands (or spot the client's wrists as shown in the photo).

At the client's signal, assist with moving bar off the racks.

Guide the bar to a position over the client's head.

Release the bar (or wrists) smoothly.

Client: Downward Movement Phase

Allow the elbows to slowly flex to lower the bar toward the head.

Keep the wrists rigid and directly above the elbows. The width of the grip will determine how parallel the forearms are to each other.

Extend the neck slightly to allow the bar to pass by the face as the bar is lowered to touch the clavicles and anterior deltoids.

Maintain the five-point body contact position.

Personal Trainer: Downward Movement Phase

Keep the hands in the alternated grip position close to—but not touching—the bar as it descends.

Slightly flex the knees, hips, and torso and keep the back flat when following the bar.

Client: Upward Movement Phase

Push the bar upward until the elbows are fully extended.

Extend the neck slightly to allow the bar to pass by the face as it is raised.

Keep the wrists rigid and directly above the elbows.

Maintain the five-point body contact position.

After the set is completed, signal the personal trainer for assistance in racking the bar.

Keep a grip on the bar until it is racked.

Upward Movement Phase: Personal Trainer

Keep the hands in the alternated grip position close to—but not touching—the bar as it ascends.

Slightly extend the knees, hips, and torso and keep the back flat when following the bar.

After the set is completed, help the client rack the bar.

Common Errors

- Pushing with the legs or rising off the seat to help raise the bar upward
- Excessively arching the back during the upward movement phase

Primary Muscles Trained:
Anterior and medial deltoids, trapezius, triceps brachii

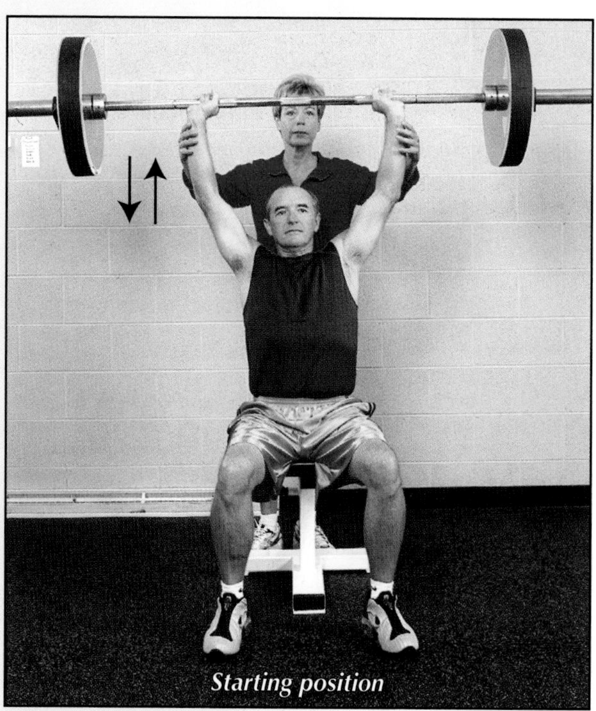

Starting position

Shoulder Press (Resistance Band)

Starting Position

Grasp the handles of the resistance band with a closed, pronated grip.

Sit on the floor or mat with the buttocks on top of a middle section of the resistance band.

Assume an erect position with the torso perpendicular to the floor and the legs together and extended away from the body.

Slightly flex the hips and knees for balance.

Position the handles to the outside and level with the top of the shoulders with the palms facing forward.

In this position, the resistance band should be nearly taut (not stretched); if not, select a shorter band.

Upward Movement Phase

Push the handles upward until the elbows are fully extended.

Keep the wrists rigid and directly above the elbows.

Maintain an erect torso position with the legs in the same position.

Downward Movement Phase

Allow the handles to slowly move backward to the starting position.

Maintain an erect torso position with the legs in the same position.

 **Common Errors**

- Excessively arching the back during the upward movement phase
- Flexing the torso forward during the downward movement phase

Primary Muscles Trained:
Anterior and medial deltoids, trapezius, triceps brachii

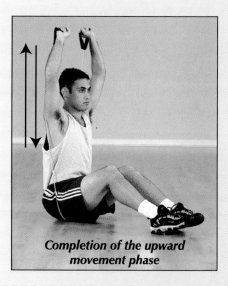

Completion of the upward movement phase

Dumbbell Lateral Raise

Starting Position

Grasp two dumbbells with a closed, neutral grip.

Position the feet shoulder- or hip-width apart, knees slightly flexed, torso erect, shoulders back, and eyes focused ahead.

Move the dumbbells to the front of the thighs, positioning them with the palms facing each other.

Slightly flex the elbows and hold this flexed position throughout the exercise.

Upward Movement Phase

Raise the dumbbells up and out to the sides; the elbows and upper arms should rise together and ahead of (and slightly higher than) the forearms and hands/dumbbells. This movement is similar to pouring liquid out of a plastic jug.

Maintain an erect upper body position with the knees slightly flexed and feet flat.

Continue raising the dumbbells until the arms are approximately parallel to the floor or nearly level with the shoulders. At the highest position, the elbows and upper arms will be slightly higher than the forearms and hands/dumbbells.

Downward Movement Phase

Allow the dumbbells to lower slowly back to the starting position.

Keep the knees slightly flexed, feet flat on the floor, and eyes focused ahead.

 **Common Errors**

- Extending or flexing the elbows during the movement
- Shrugging the shoulders, flexing the torso backward, extending the knees, or rising up on the toes to help raise the dumbbells upward
- Flexing the torso forward or allowing the body's weight to shift toward the toes during the downward movement phase

Primary Muscles Trained:
Deltoids, trapezius

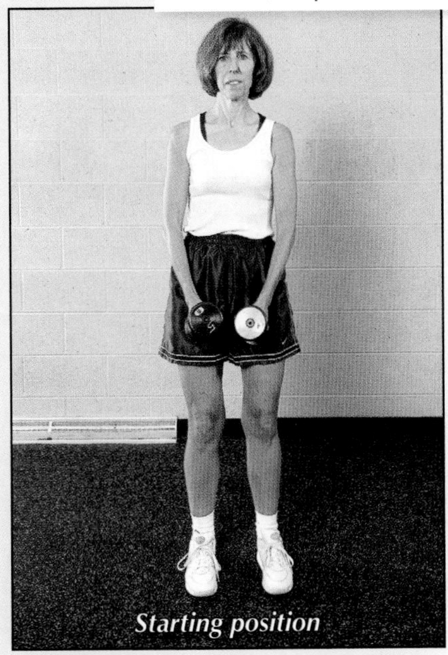
Starting position

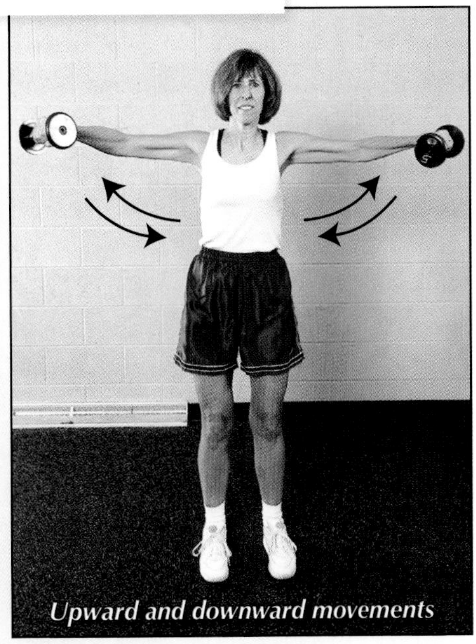
Upward and downward movements

Lateral Raise (Resistance Band)

Starting Position

Grasp the handles of the resistance band with a closed, neutral grip.

Position the feet shoulder-width apart with the arches of both feet on top of a middle section of the resistance band.

Stand erect with the knees slightly flexed.

Position the handles outside of the thighs with the arms at the sides and the palms facing inward.

In this position, the resistance band should be nearly taut (not stretched); if not, take up the slack by widening the stance or selecting a shorter band.

Upward Movement Phase

Pull the handles up and out to the sides; the hands, forearms, elbows, and upper arms should rise together.

Maintain an erect body position with the knees slightly flexed and feet flat.

Continue raising the handles until the arms are approximately parallel to the floor or nearly level with the shoulders.

Downward Movement Phase

Allow the handles to slowly move back to the starting position.

Maintain an erect body position with the knees slightly flexed and feet flat.

Common Errors

- Extending or flexing the elbows during the movement
- Shrugging the shoulders to help raise the handles upward

Primary Muscles Trained:
Deltoids, trapezius

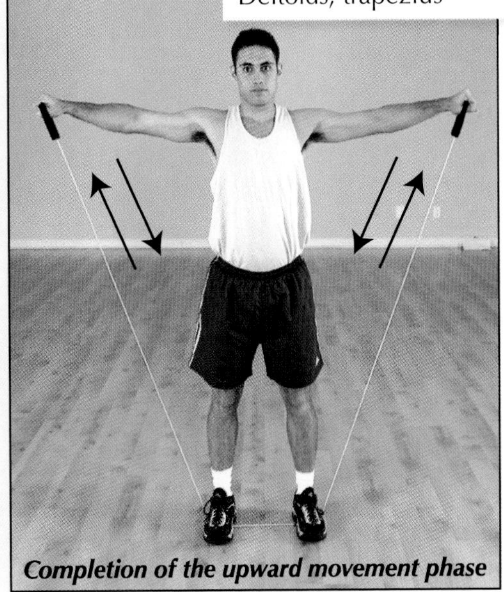
Completion of the upward movement phase

Whole Body

Power Clean

This exercise consists of four phases (first pull, scoop, second pull, and catch), but there is no pause between them; the bar is lifted (pulled up) from the floor to the front of the shoulders in one continuous movement.

Starting Position

Stand with the feet placed between hip- and shoulder-width apart with the toes pointed slightly outward.

Squat down with the hips lower than the shoulders and grasp the bar with a closed, pronated grip.

Place the hands on the bar slightly wider than shoulder-width apart, outside of the knees, with the elbows fully extended.

Place the feet flat on the floor and position the bar approximately one inch (three centimeters) in front of the shins and over the balls of the feet.

Position the body with the

- back flat or slightly arched,
- trapezius relaxed and slightly stretched,
- chest held up and out,
- scapulae retracted,
- head in line with the spine or slightly hyperextended,
- shoulders over or slightly in front of the bar, and
- eyes focused straight ahead or slightly upward.

Upward Movement Phase: First Pull

Lift the bar off the floor by forcefully extending the hips and knees.

Keep the torso-to-floor angle constant.

Do not let the hips rise before the shoulders.

Maintain a flat-back position.

Keep the elbows fully extended, the head neutral in relation to the spine, and the shoulders over or slightly ahead of the bar.

As the bar is raised, keep it as close to the shins as possible.

Upward Movement Phase: Scoop (Transition)

As the bar rises just above the knees, thrust the hips forward and slightly re-flex the knees to move the thighs against and the knees under the bar.

Keep the back flat or slightly arched, the elbows fully extended and pointing out to the sides, and the head in line with the spine.

Upward Movement Phase: Second Pull

Forcefully and quickly extend the hips and knees and plantar flex the ankles.

Keep the bar near to or in contact with the front of the thighs.

Keep the bar as close to the body as possible.

Keep the back flat, the elbows pointing out to the sides, and the head in line with the spine.

Keep the shoulders over the bar and the elbows extended as long as possible.

When the lower body joints reach full extension, rapidly shrug the shoulders upward, but do not allow the elbows to flex yet.

As the shoulders reach their highest elevation, flex the elbows to begin pulling the body under the bar.

Because of the explosive nature of this phase, the torso will be erect or slightly hyperextended, the head will be tilted slightly back, and the feet may lose contact with the floor.

Upward Movement Phase: Catch

After the lower body has fully extended and the bar reaches near-maximal height, pull the body under the bar and rotate the arms around and under the bar.

Simultaneously, the hips and knees flex into a quarter-squat position.

Once the arms are under the bar, lift the elbows to position the upper arms parallel to the floor.

Rack the bar across the front of clavicles and anterior deltoids.

The bar should be caught at the anterior deltoids and clavicles with the

- head facing forward,
- neck neutral or slightly hyperextended,
- wrists hyperextended,
- elbows fully flexed,
- upper arms parallel to the floor,
- back flat or slightly arched,
- knees and hips slightly flexed to absorb the impact of the weight,
- feet flat on the floor, and
- the body's weight over the middle of the feet.

Stand up by extending the hips and knees to a fully erect position.

Downward Movement Phase

Lower the bar to the thighs by gradually reducing the muscular tension of the arms to allow a controlled descent.

Simultaneously flex the hips and knees to cushion the impact of the bar on the thighs.

Squat down with the elbows fully extended until the bar touches the floor.

Common Errors

- Allowing the hips to rise before the shoulders during the first pull
- Allowing the upper back to round (i.e., losing the flat-back position), especially during the first pull
- Extending the knees faster than the hips, before the hips, or both
- Allowing the bar to travel upward too far away from the body
- Using a "reverse curl" movement to move the bar into the catch position

Primary Muscles Trained:
Gluteus maximus, hamstrings, quadriceps, soleus, gastrocnemius, deltoids, trapezius

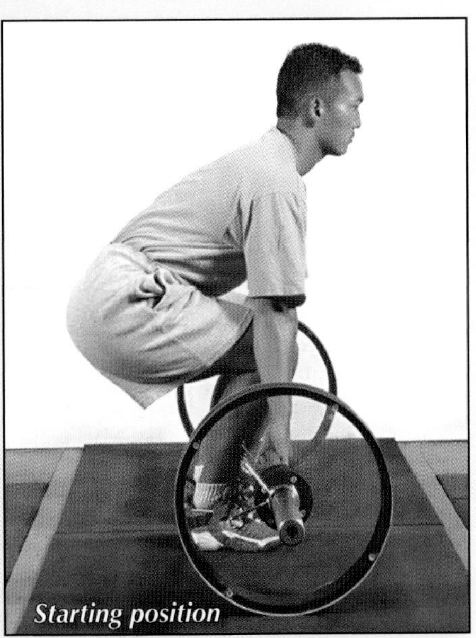
Starting position

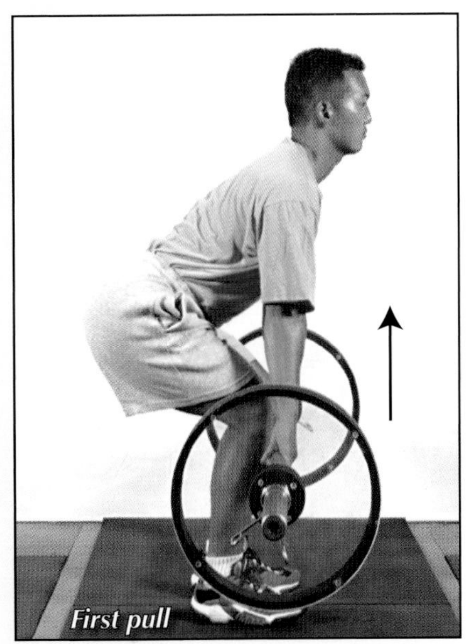
First pull

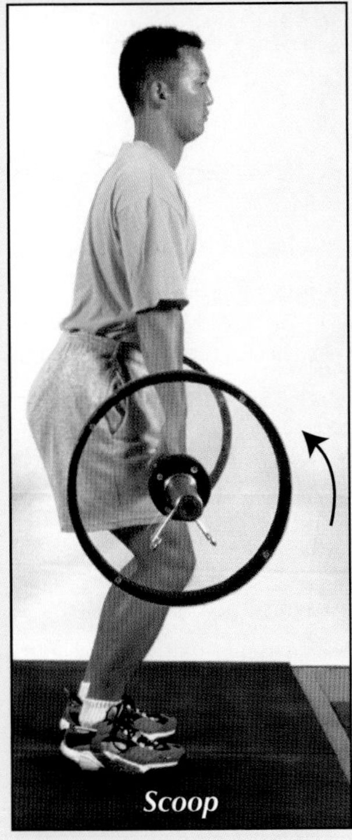
Scoop

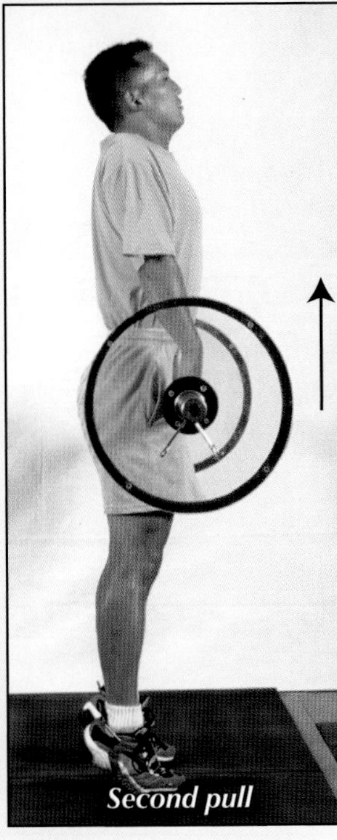
Second pull

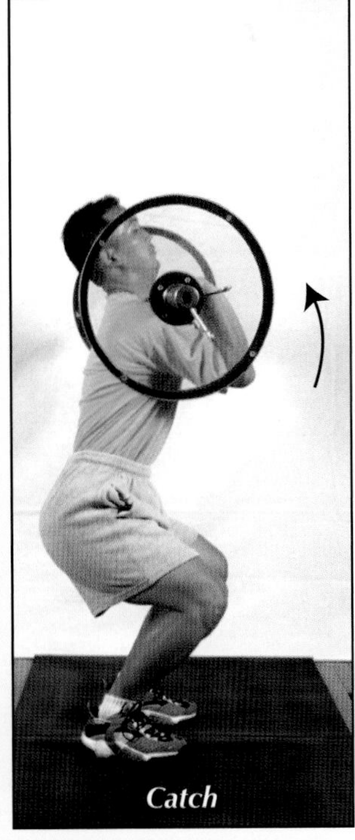
Catch

STUDY QUESTIONS

1. Which of the following phases of the power clean involves hip and knee extension and plantar flexion?
   A. first pull
   B. transition
   C. second pull
   D. catch

2. Which of the following are conditions (or examples of conditions) that must be met before a personal trainer should recommend a client to use the Valsalva maneuver during a resistance training exercise?
   I. the client will perform the bench press exercise
   II. the client has exercise technique experience
   III. the client does not have hypertension
   IV. the client is resistance-trained

   A. I, II, and III only
   B. I, III, and IV only
   C. II, III, and IV only
   D. I, II, and IV only

3. Which of the following are conditions (or examples of conditions) that must be met before a personal trainer should recommend a client to use a weight belt during a resistance training exercise?
   I. the client will be performing 3 repetitions with a 3RM load
   II. the client will be performing an exercise that places stress on the lower back
   III. the client will be performing an exercise that directly loads the trunk
   IV. the client will be performing 5 repetitions with a 15RM load

   A. I, II, and III only
   B. II, III, and IV only
   C. I, III, and IV only
   D. I, II, and IV only

4. Which of the following exercises should be spotted?
   I. power clean
   II. lateral raise
   III. seated shoulder press
   IV. forward lunge

   A. I and II only
   B. III and IV only
   C. I and IV only
   D. II and III only

APPLIED KNOWLEDGE QUESTION

Describe two more common technique mistakes inexperienced clients make when they perform these exercises: (1) bench press, (2) back squat, (3) front squat, (4) shoulder press, and (5) power clean.

REFERENCES

1. Bartelink, D.L. 1957. The role of abdominal pressure in relieving the pressure on the lumbar intervertebral discs. *Journal of Bone and Joint Surgery* 39B (4): 718-725.
2. Earle, R.W., and T.R. Baechle. 2000. Resistance training and spotting techniques. In: *Essentials of Strength Training and Conditioning*, 2nd ed., T.R. Baechle and R.W. Earle, eds. Champaign, IL: Human Kinetics.
3. Faigenbaum, A., and W. Westcott. 2000. *Strength and Power for Young Athletes.* Champaign, IL: Human Kinetics.
4. Harman, E.A., R.M. Rosenstein, P.N. Frykman, and G.A. Nigro. 1989. Effects of a belt on intra-abdominal pressure during weight lifting. *Medicine and Science in Sports and Exercise* 21 (2): 186-190.
5. Lander, J.E., J.R. Hundley, and R.L. Simonton. 1990. The effectiveness of weight-belts during multiple repetitions of the squat exercise. *Medicine and Science in Sports and Exercise* 24 (5): 603-609.
6. Lander, J.E., R.L. Simonton, and J.K.F. Giacobbe. 1990. The effectiveness of weight-belts during the squat exercise. *Medicine and Science in Sports and Exercise* 22 (1): 117-126.
7. Morris, J.M., D.B. Lucas, and B. Bresler. 1961. Role of the trunk in stability of the spine. *Journal of Bone and Joint Surgery* 43A: 327-351.
8. NSCA Certification Commission. 2001. *Exercise Technique Checklist Manual.* Lincoln, NE: NSCA Certification Commission.

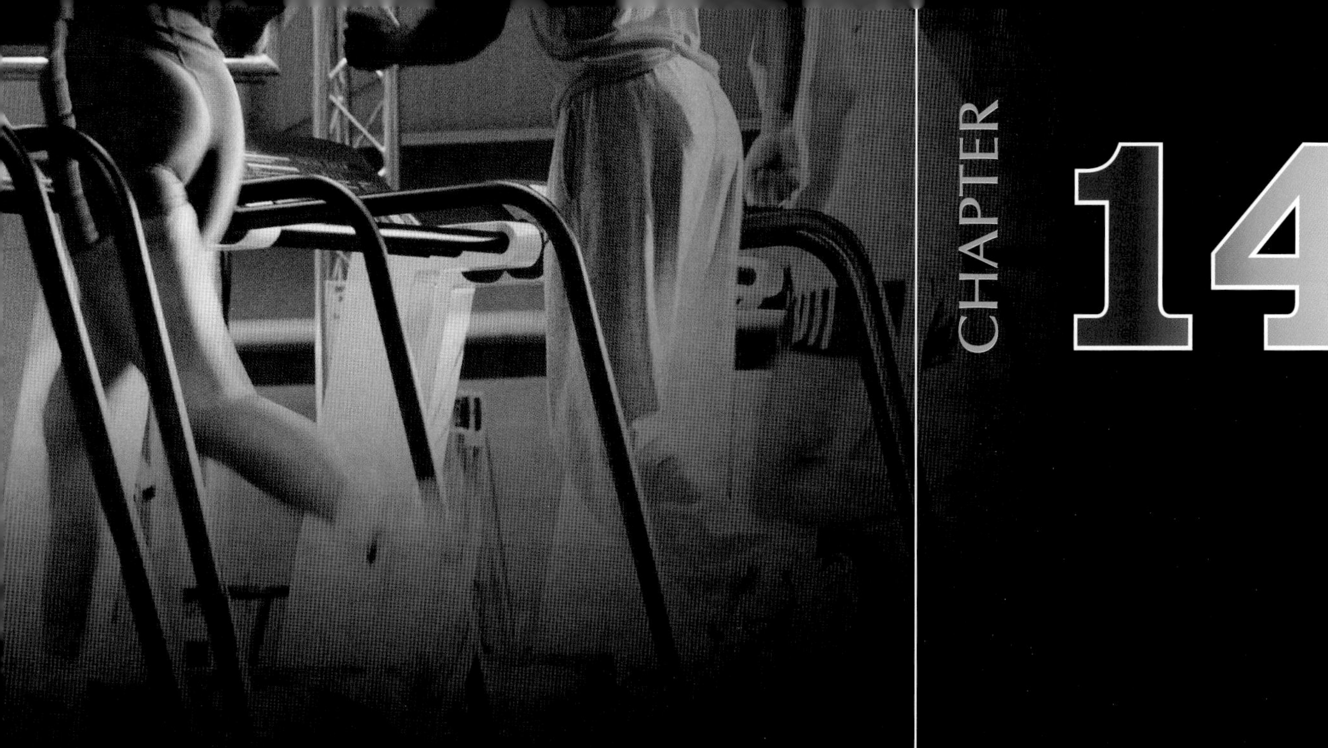

CHAPTER 14

Cardiovascular Activity Techniques

J. Henry "Hank" Drought

After completing this chapter, you will be able to

- recognize general guidelines for safe participation in cardiovascular activities, including proper hydration, clothing, and footwear; warm-up and cool-down; and exercise frequency, intensity, and duration;
- teach proper technique for a number of cardiovascular machines (treadmill, stair climber, stationary bicycle, elliptical trainer, and rowing machine);
- teach proper technique for a number of cardiovascular non-machine activities (walking, running, and swimming);
- guide clients on safe participation in group exercise classes and aquatic exercise; and
- help direct individuals to cardiovascular activities that match their preferences and physical capabilities.

Including aerobic exercise as a component of a client's training program requires proper cardiovascular exercise technique. As with resistance training exercises, correct aerobic exercise technique is important for safety and helps clients achieve maximum benefits. Poor technique can lead to injuries and may hinder progress and goal attainment.

Typically, personal trainers work with clients having a wide range of physical fitness capabilities and interests. Personal trainers should help clients choose exercise activities that are appropriate for their physical fitness capabilities, exercise preferences, and time available for exercise. Some clients have physical limitations or orthopedic problems suggesting that a given type of exercise may be preferable for safety reasons. Personal trainers should involve clients in choosing the exercise modality, however, since personal preference may encourage greater adherence to the program [66]. New exercise activities can be introduced when appropriate. Variety in programming allows muscles to be worked differently, reduces repetitive orthopedic stresses, and may contribute to exercise adherence [1].

Cardiovascular activities can be divided into machine and non-machine exercises. Cardiovascular machine exercises discussed in this chapter include those using the treadmill, stair climber, elliptical trainer, stationary bicycle, and rowing machine. The cardiovascular non-machine exercises include walking, running, group fitness classes, swimming, and aqua exercise. Other popular cardiovascular activities that merit mentioning, but are beyond the scope of this chapter, include cross-country skiing, hiking, basketball, racquetball, squash, tennis, mountaineering, rope skipping, and in-line skating. Covering the entire scope of exercise technique for all of these activities might require a whole book. The purpose of this chapter is to give an overview of important technique considerations in some of the more popular activities.

General Guidelines for Safe Participation in Cardiovascular Activities

Several general guidelines for safe participation apply to all cardiovascular activities. These include intake of plenty of fluids for optimal hydration; appropriate clothing and footwear; proper warm-up and cool-down; appropriate exercise frequency, intensity, and duration; proper breathing; and proper program progression. Clients should warm up prior to any cardiovascular activity and should cool down afterward, and they should be advised of appropriate breathing during the workout. The personal trainer will have developed an exercise prescription for each client, with appropriate frequency, intensity, and duration to meet the client's goals. As the client improves in technique or conditioning, the personal trainer may enhance progression by carefully adding new techniques or activities.

Hydration

Clients should drink plenty of fluids. Water is the body's most important nutrient and is an important regulator of body temperature. Water carries other nutrients and actively participates in many chemical reactions throughout the body. Water also serves as a solvent for vitamins, amino acids, glucose, and minerals and acts as a lubricant and cushion around joints [60]. During heavy exercise, such as high-intensity group cycling classes and running, clients can lose as much as 2 to 4 quarts (1.9-3.8 liters) of fluid every hour, but the digestive system can only absorb approximately 1 quart (0.95 liters) per hour [60]. Therefore, it is important for clients to hydrate before, during, and after exercise. It is also important to drink fluids *before* the onset of thirst, since exercise may blunt the thirst mechanism [60]. The amount of fluid replacement is determined by the amount of fluid lost during exercise activity. Heavy exercise in hot weather demands greater fluid replacement than low to moderate exercise in cooler weather. Core temperature, heart rate, and perceived exertion all remain lower when fluid replacement closely matches fluid loss [23, 40].

Plain, cool water is perhaps the best fluid replacement because it leaves the digestive tract and enters the tissues the fastest. Generally, water is a fine fluid replacement for exercise durations of less than one hour. Sport drinks may also provide rapid fluid replacement with the addition of sodium and glucose for electrolyte replacement and may be recommended for exercise durations of longer than one hour [23, 60]. See chapter 7 for additional hydration guidelines.

Clothing

Exercisers should wear appropriate clothing for the activity, temperature, and weather conditions. Comfortable, loose-fitting clothing allows greater movement than tighter clothing. Light clothing is preferable in the heat, while layered clothing provides warmth in the cold. Much of the body's heat is lost through the head and extremities in cold weather; therefore, covering the head, neck, hands, and feet with warm clothing is especially important.

People may use a face mask or scarf to cover the mouth and nose during very cold weather if desired. Usually, cold air is sufficiently warmed and humidified by the nasal passages, but clients who have asthma may experience some bronchoconstriction in cold dry air, especially with prolonged mouth breathing [47].

Footwear

Proper footwear is essential for weight-bearing exercises like walking, running, and aerobic dance (table 14.1). Proper footwear promotes better performance and safety. In general, shoes should provide comfort, cushioning, stability, flexibility, and durability. Walking shoes should have an adequate combination of all these characteristics. Running shoes should have greater cushioning because of the greater impact forces—between two and four times body weight at each foot strike [51]. Aerobic dance shoes should have better lateral stability because of the lateral movement required.

One cannot judge the wear on a pair of shoes by outward appearance alone. Even if a shoe does not look worn, compression capabilities may still be severely compromised. Running shoes generally lose some of their midsole conditioning as early as 150 miles (240 kilometers) and may lose up to 50% of their compression capability by 300 to 500 miles (480-800 kilometers) [28]. Therefore, most running shoes should be replaced after 300 to 500 miles, or every six months, whichever comes sooner. Heavy runners or over- or underpronators may need to replace shoes more often [28].

Generally, normal (neutral) foot strike mechanics during running involve a gentle inward rolling action (pronation) from the heel to the ball of the foot. Overpronation occurs when the foot collapses too far inward on the arch with each foot strike. Conversely, the underpronator (supinator) tends to run too much on the outsides of the feet with little inward roll (table 14.2). Neither of these abnormal foot strike characteristics (see figure 14.1) is desirable, and each may lead to injuries to the foot, knee, hip, and back. Athletic shoes with the correct motion-control features, last construction, and in some cases orthotics, may help encourage a more neutral foot strike and may reduce the likelihood of injury [26, 28].

TABLE 14.1

Shoe Selection Based on Activity

	General shoe characteristics	
Activity	**Cushion**	**Lateral stability**
Walking	Moderate	Moderate
Running	High	Low
Aerobics	Moderate-high	Moderate-high
Racket sports	Moderate	High
Cross-training	Moderate-high	Moderate-high

TABLE 14.2

Shoe Selection Based on Foot Strike

Type of foot strike	Specific shoe characteristics
Neutral	Semicurved last; moderate motion control
Overpronators	Straight last; high motion control
Underpronators (supinators)	Curved last; high motion flexibility

Running shoes are generally made with three different types of lasts, or forms: curved, semicurved, or straight (figure 14.2). Overpronators may benefit from a motion-control shoe with a straight last. Underpronators may favor a shoe with a curved last that allows greater foot range of motion flexibility. Neutral foot strikers may benefit from shoes with a semicurved last and moderate direction- and foot-control features [26]. A consultation with a podiatrist to analyze running biomechanics may be helpful for proper shoe selection.

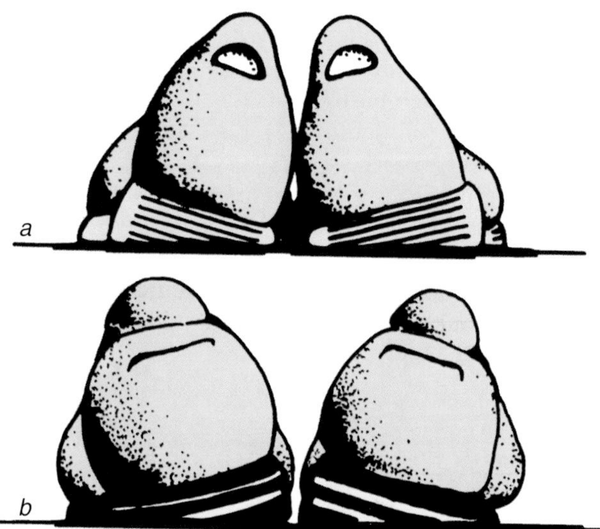

Figure 14.1 *(a)* Overpronation and *(b)* underpronation (supination).
Adapted from Town and Kearney 1994.

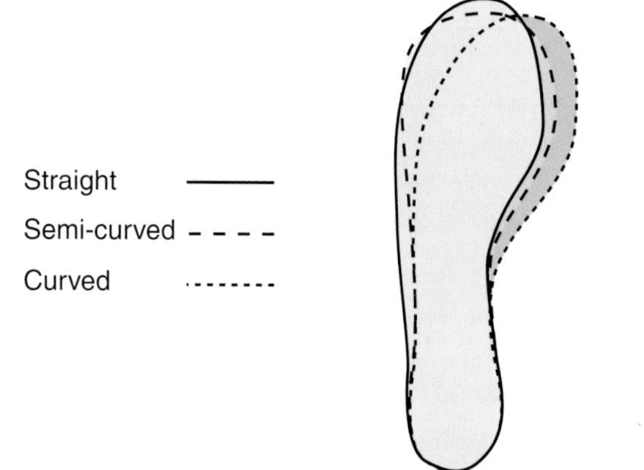

Figure 14.2 The shapes of straight, semicurved, and curved lasts. Overpronators may benefit from straight lasts, neutral foot strikers from semicurved lasts, and underpronators (supinators) from curved lasts.
Adapted from Kreighbaum and Smith 1996.

Warm-Up and Cool-Down

All exercises should begin with a warm-up and end with a cool-down. A proper warm-up begins with low-intensity activity, and the workload is increased incrementally for a minimum of 5 to 10 minutes until the desired intensity is reached. A warm-up gives the cardiovascular and musculoskeletal systems the opportunity to acclimate to the increased demands of the exercise. If target heart rate exercise is the goal, the intensity should be maintained for the prescribed duration. A cool-down of 5 to 10 minutes or more is recommended to allow the heart rate and blood pressure to recover toward resting levels before exercise stops completely. Stretching may also be added to the warm-up and cool-down phases [1]. See chapter 12 for more information on warm-up and stretching.

Exercise Frequency, Intensity, and Duration

General frequency, intensity, and duration guidelines for cardiovascular exercise are as follows:

Frequency: Two to five sessions per week
Intensity: 50% to 85% of heart rate reserve (HRR)
Duration: 20 to 60 minutes

Moderate-to-vigorous exercise is recommended for most clients. However, deconditioned clients may benefit from lower-intensity activity for shorter durations. Intermittent bouts of at least 10 minutes of exercise throughout the day (totaling 20-60 minutes) may also be effective for improving cardiovascular health [1]. For more information, please refer to chapter 16.

Breathing

In general, breathing during all cardiovascular activities should be relaxed and regular. Personal trainers should emphasize (especially to novice clients) that it is not necessary to train in a state of breathlessness to achieve cardiovascular benefits. Well-trained clients interested in maximizing performance may use advanced training techniques that require higher heart and breathing rates for sustained or intermittent periods. These advanced training techniques differ from steady-state target heart rate training and may include sprint, interval, and fartlek training (refer to chapter 16). Higher-intensity training methods require more vigorous breathing than steady-state target heart rate training.

Breathing during cardiovascular activities should be relaxed and regular. Except for well-trained clients who are following a vigorous training program, it is not necessary to train in a state of breathlessness to achieve cardiovascular benefits. Clients should be able to carry on a casual conversation while exercising.

Clients training at low to moderate levels may be able to breathe solely through the nose. As the intensity and duration of exercise increase, however, breathing through both the nose and mouth is preferable since this will allow a greater volume of air to pass into the lungs [49].

Adding or Substituting New Exercises

Personal trainers should pay special attention to proper progression when adding or substituting new activities into the client's program. New exercises stress the body and muscles in new ways. Although there is some crossover effect for general fitness improvement, a client's ability to perform one exercise modality does not completely transfer to another [1].

For example, a middle-aged client who has been riding a stationary bike for 30 minutes three times a week may not be able to immediately switch to treadmill running for 30 minutes three times a week. "General" cardiovascular benefits to the lungs and heart will transfer to other cardiovascular activities, and some training adaptations in the lower extremities from cycling may help in running. However, each exercise modality presents a unique stress to the body and produces "specific" training adaptations in the working muscles, connective tissues, and skeletal system. In this case, the client's stationary bicycling program has produced a training stimulus specific to cycling; but the client's muscles, connective tissues, and skeletal system may not be accustomed to the specific stresses and impact forces of running. Therefore, the client may need time to acclimate to the new running program. When adding or substituting new exercises into the program, it may be necessary to initially decrease the frequency, intensity, and/or duration of the new activity in order to reduce the risk of injury and promote adherence.

In keeping with the principle of specificity, a client's ability to perform one exercise modality does not completely transfer to another. Personal trainers should pay special attention to proper progression when adding or substituting new activities into the client's program.

Cardiovascular Machine Exercise Technique

Cardiovascular machines offer the convenience of indoor exercise; handrail support; and adjustable speed, elevation, and resistance for precise manipulations of workout training intensity. Cardiovascular machine training as discussed in this chapter includes use of the treadmill, stair climber, elliptical trainer, stationary bicycle, and rowing machine.

Treadmill

Primary muscles used: quadriceps, hamstrings, gluteals, iliopsoas, tibialis anterior, gastrocnemius, and soleus

Treadmill exercises include walking and running. In addition to the conveniences of indoor exercise, handrail support, and controlled speed and elevation, treadmill exercise offers a soft landing surface on a flexible deck to reduce foot strike impact forces. Older clients and cardiac rehabilitation patients may benefit from treadmill exercise because it is easy to supervise and the handrail allows for support and balance.

Stepping on the Belt

Personal trainers often work with a clientele that spans a wide range of ages and fitness capabilities, and many clients will have no problem walking or running on a treadmill. However, some clients who have never used a treadmill may initially be intimidated by the revolving belt and may need more detailed instructions on getting started. For these clients, the following progression for beginning treadmill exercise may be helpful [39]:

1. Before starting the machine, instruct the client to hold on to the handrails while straddling the belt. When the belt begins moving, have the client step on with one foot, then the other, and begin walking. If necessary, encourage the client to "paw" the treadmill belt with the dominant leg several times before stepping on to help build confidence.
2. Have the client continue to hold the handrail if balance is an issue. The handrail should be held with a firm enough grip to maintain balance, but not too tightly. If handrail holding is unnecessary, encourage the client to release the handrail and to swing the arms in a natural walking manner.

3. Instruct the client to walk/run toward the front part of the treadmill deck and to stay in the center. Warn the client to avoid "drifting" back, or from side to side, since this increases the risk of falling.

Handrail Holding

Novice treadmill users, cardiac rehabilitation patients, and severely deconditioned clients with balance problems may benefit from holding the handrails for greater safety and better stability. However, many clients support too much of their body weight on the handrails, which decreases the intensity of the workout, especially when the platform is inclined [21]. Handrail holding should be light, with as little pressure as necessary. Clients who are able to balance by themselves should be encouraged to release the handrail and swing the arms naturally at their sides in a normal walking or running manner. See "Weaning Clients From Handrail Usage" for a progression from handrail holding to not using the handrails.

Treadmill Running

The energy cost of running indoors on a treadmill is slightly lower than that for running outdoors at the same velocity, for two reasons: (1) there is no air resistance on an indoor treadmill, and (2) the body must only keep up with the belt rather than propel itself forward. Therefore, runners often notice that they can run at a slightly faster pace on a treadmill than they can outdoors. Runners who wish to offset this difference may use a slight inclination—1% grade—when running on a treadmill to increase the energy cost of treadmill running to a level more closely resembling that attained during outdoor running [38].

For detailed instruction on walking and running technique, refer to the "Walking" and "Running" sections under "Cardiovascular Non-Machine Exercise Technique."

Stair Climber

Primary muscles used: quadriceps, hamstrings, gluteals, erector spinae, gastrocnemius, and soleus

Biomechanical analysis of traditional non-machine stair climbing shows that reaction forces at the knee can reach approximately three to four times body weight [52]. However, stair climber machines can help reduce these knee stresses [61, 63]. Stair climber machines that use a revolving "escalator" mechanism slightly decrease knee stress because the downward stroke of the leg is assisted by the moving step (similar to the moving belt on a treadmill). However, escalator-style stair climbers do not allow variation in step height, and there is some impact because the foot leaves and recontacts the revolving surface. Stair climbers using pedals do a better job of reducing impact and knee stress because the foot rarely leaves the pedal surface [61]. Stair climbers with pedals allow the client to control the stepping depth. In general, muscle activation (especially of the gluteals) increases with a larger stepping depth. However, a stepping depth that is too large may lead to premature fatigue and technique errors. Individual control of stepping depth allows taller and shorter clients to work at a comfortable range of motion.

Stair climbing is challenging because it requires vertical force production from the legs and hips. The drawback is that severely deconditioned clients may not be able to perform at even the lowest levels [3]. Like treadmills, stair climbers have handrails for balance. For clients who need extra support and help with balance, this is an advantage. However, many clients tend to lean heavily on the

Weaning Clients From Handrail Usage

A gradual progression may be used to "wean" clients from handrail assistance. Personal trainers should instruct clients to hold the handrails with

1. two hands lightly;
2. the fingers of two hands;
3. one hand, while swinging the other arm naturally at the side;
4. the fingers of one hand; and then
5. only one finger of one hand.

The final instruction is to release the handrails completely and swing both arms naturally at the sides in a normal walking or running manner.

handrails and therefore may support too much of their body weight. This reduces the intended workload and may compromise proper upright **postural alignment.** In addition, excessive forward lean can stress the lower back and cause injury. Clients who use the handrails on stair climbers should hold the handrails lightly, and just enough for balance. Clients who can safely balance by themselves should release the handrails completely and pump the arms, with elbows held at about 90 degrees from relaxed shoulders.

Body Position

Good postural alignment and body position are essential during exercise on stair climbers. Personal trainers should instruct clients to hold the handrails while stepping *forward* onto the pedals and to follow proper body position recommendations. Reversing body position and "facing out" on the stair climber is not recommended. Empirical evidence suggests that a "facing-out" position (in which the heels and back, instead of the toes and chest, face the console of the machine) results in poor postural body alignment characterized by an exaggerated forward lean. This excessive forward lean happens because the body has to counterbalance the reverse angle of the pedal moment arms. The client usually is forced to support too much body weight on the handrails for stability. Because extreme forward lean in the "facing-out" position may place more stress on the low back and may result in injury, the facing-out position is not recommended.

Proper exercise techniques on stair climbers include the following (figure 14.3):

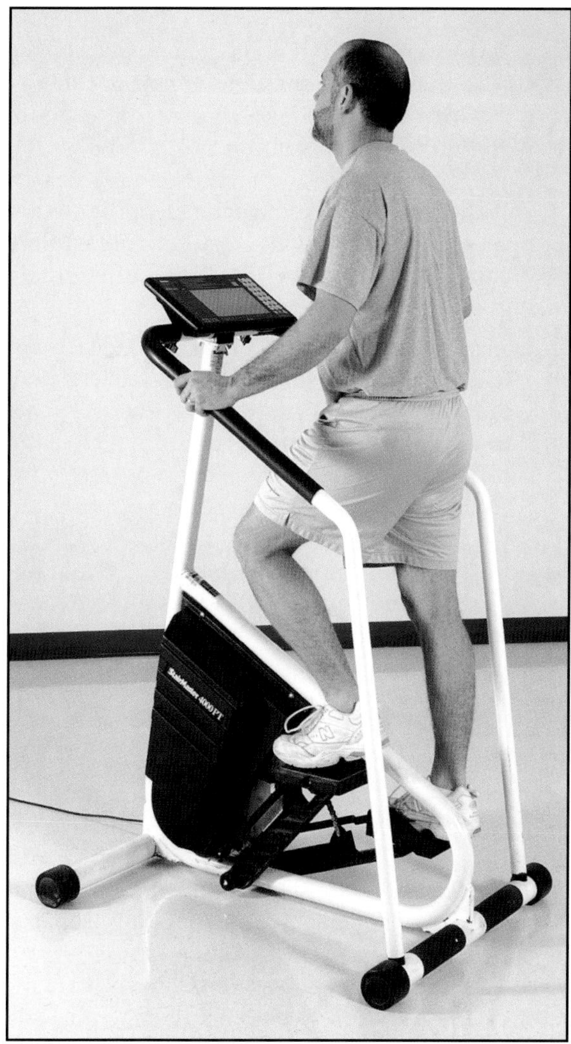

Figure 14.3 Proper stair climbing exercise technique: head up, torso over hips, no excessive forward lean, flexed knee no further forward from toe, extended knee slightly bent, no hyperextension.

Feet: With the toes facing forward, the client should place the whole foot on each pedal.

Arms/Hands: The hands should hold on to the handrails lightly, just enough for balance. Excessive leaning on the handrails and supporting of the body weight can reduce workout caloric consumption by up to 20% [63]. If handrail holding is unnecessary, instruct the client to release the handrail completely. Have the client hold the elbows at about 90 degrees and swing the arms naturally from relaxed shoulders.

Upper body: Instruct the client to hold the head upright, looking straight ahead. The shoulders should be square and relaxed. The posture is upright, with the torso positioned over the hips. An upright body position enables the vertebrae and erector spinae muscles to share body weight equally. Many clients lean too far forward, flexing the torso at the waist. Forward lean can create stress on the lower back and should be discouraged. Often, excessive forward lean and handrail holding occur because a novice client is working at an intensity that is too high [61]. Recommending a slower stepping speed with greater control may alleviate the problem.

Hips: The hips should be positioned directly under the torso to encourage good postural alignment and reduce low back arching. Some hip movement during stair-climbing activity is beneficial. However, uncontrolled and exaggerated hip movement should be discouraged. Extreme side-to-side rocking at the hips indicates excessive stepping depth and usually results in compromised postural alignment due to too much forward flexion at the spine [63]. Reduce the stepping depth, speed, or both until the client can comfortably balance the torso over the hips and maintain good postural alignment.

Knees: The knees should be aligned with the feet, toes pointed forward. With knee flexion, the knees should not move forward of the toes. With knee extension, there is no locking or hyperextension. The extending (straightening) leg should never be locked out, and the knee should remain slightly flexed in the fully extended position. Exaggerated and improper knee flexion and extension can cause increased stress at the knee and may cause injury [63].

Range of Movement

Stair-stepping depth is influenced by the client's height and fitness level. An appropriate range of movement allows proper intensity without compromising upright posture. Stepping depth usually ranges between four and eight inches (10 and 20 centimeters) [39]. Side-to-side rocking from the hips, indicating excessive stepping depth, should be discouraged. The pedals should not contact the floor or the upper limit stop of the machine, but should allow maximum range of movement without producing excessive fatigue or forward body lean. A stepping depth that is too shallow is also undesirable. A very short range of motion will not properly engage the quadriceps, hamstring, and gluteal muscles.

Stepping Speed

Stepping speed also depends on the fitness level of the client. Appropriate **cadence** allows the individual to sustain exercise for the prescribed duration without undue fatigue or deviations in postural alignment.

Generally, stair-stepping speed can range anywhere from 43 to 95 steps per minute [61]. Beginners should start with a slower cadence. Speed may be increased when the client is comfortable with balance and the pedal movement. A stepping speed that is too fast usually results in two mistakes: (1) excessive side-to-side hip movement in order to keep up with stepping depth or (2) short, fast, choppy steps that result in a stepping depth that is too shallow. Both of these extremes should be discouraged.

Manual settings on stair climber machines make it easy to adjust stepping speed. When performing preprogrammed exercises or interval training programs, the client must be able to tolerate the range of changing stepping speeds. The personal trainer needs to instruct the client that stepping speed may be reduced at any time.

Elliptical Trainer

Primary muscles used: quadriceps, hamstrings, gluteals, iliopsoas, tibialis anterior, gastrocnemius, and soleus

Elliptical trainers have become popular because this nonimpact exercise blends the motions of stair climbing with walking or running. Some elliptical trainers have fixed pedals and a restricted range of motion. Newer models have movable foot pedals and allow the range of motion to be determined by the client. Generally, the elliptical movement of the pedals can remain flatter to resemble walking or running or can be inclined to resemble stair climbing. Forward and backward foot and leg motions are also allowed on elliptical trainers. Elliptical trainers can be an effective low-impact substitute for running, walking, and stair climbing.

Foot Placement

The whole foot should be placed on the pedal surface, and full contact should be maintained at all times unless the design of the machine causes the heel of the rear foot to lift (e.g., figure 14.4).

Handrail Holding

Similar to the situation with the treadmill and stair climber, handrail holding on elliptical trainers should be just light enough to maintain balance. Excessive leaning on the handrails reduces work output and may compromise proper body alignment. Clients who need to hold on to the handrail for balance should do so. However, if handrail holding is unnecessary, the individual should be encouraged to release the hold completely and pump the arms in a walking or running manner.

Body Position

The body position on elliptical trainers is upright, with the torso properly balanced directly over the hips. The head is held high, and the shoulders are relaxed but not rounded (figure 14.4).

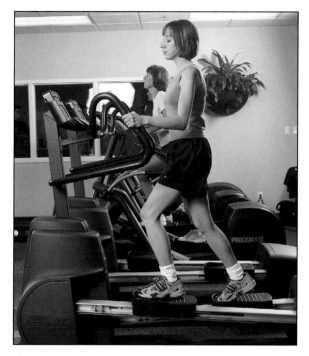

Figure 14.4 Proper elliptical trainer exercise technique: head up, looking straight ahead, torso balanced over hips with no excessive forward lean.

Knees

The knees should not come forward of the toes in the flexed position. This places strain at the knee joint and may cause injury.

Cadence, Elevation, and Resistance

The pedaling motion is elliptical and nonimpact. At a slower cadence, with little or no inclination, the motion resembles walking. When the cadence is faster, the exercise resembles running. Midlevel inclines at slow and faster cadences result in motions similar to walking and running up hills. Very high inclines increase vertical force production, and the motion approximates stair climbing. Resistance at all inclines and speeds can be adjusted to increase workload.

Direction of Movement

Elliptical trainers allow both forward and backward pedaling motions. Performing both directions of movement gives the muscles a chance to work in a slightly varying manner. In general, empirical evidence suggests that the backward motion (simulating backward walking, running, or stair climbing) may slightly increase the involvement of the gluteals and hamstrings. Changing between forward and backward pedaling directions may reduce the potential for repetitive stress injuries and can help prevent boredom.

While some individuals may require handrail holding for balance and safety during treadmill, stair climbing, and elliptical trainer exercise, excessive forward lean and support of body weight compromise proper upright body position and decrease energy expenditure.

Stationary Bicycles

Primary muscles used: quadriceps, hamstrings, gluteals, tibialis anterior, gastrocnemius, and soleus

The stationary bicycle is popular because the cycling motion is familiar to most people. In addition, stationary cycling is a non-weight-bearing and nonimpact exercise. Overweight clients may benefit from stationary cycling because their body weight is supported on the bicycle seat. Stationary cycling may also benefit clients who cannot participate in walking programs because of foot problems or injuries. The drawback of stationary cycling is that local leg muscle fatigue may prevent severely deconditioned clients from being able to sustain exercise or achieve or maintain target heart rate [3].

Seat Height

The seat height on a stationary bicycle should be adjusted to allow a slight bend in the knee at the bottom of the pedal stroke. This produces maximum extension of the leg without locking the knee joint. Technically, this slight bend in the knee should measure approximately 25 to 35 degrees with a goniometer. This angle is formed from the bony point on the hip (the greater trochanter), to the side of the knee, to the lateral malleolus (anklebone) [62].

To set the seat height (figure 14.5, a-c), the personal trainer instructs the client to place a heel on the downward pedal at 6 o'clock while the client is sitting on the seat. With the heel on the pedal, the leg should be straight. Then, when the ball of the foot is positioned on the pedal, there should be a slight bend in the knee. With the ball of the foot on the upward pedal at 12 o'clock (at maximum knee flexion), the knee should be about even with the height of the hips, with the upper leg approximately parallel to the floor.

If the seat is too low, the knee may be higher than the hips with the pedal at 12 o'clock. This puts too much strain on the knee during the powerful downstroke and can result in injury. Also, if the seat is too low, the other leg on the downward pedal at 6 o'clock cannot extend properly. This creates a "cramped" feeling because the whole pedaling action is too high toward the upper body, with too

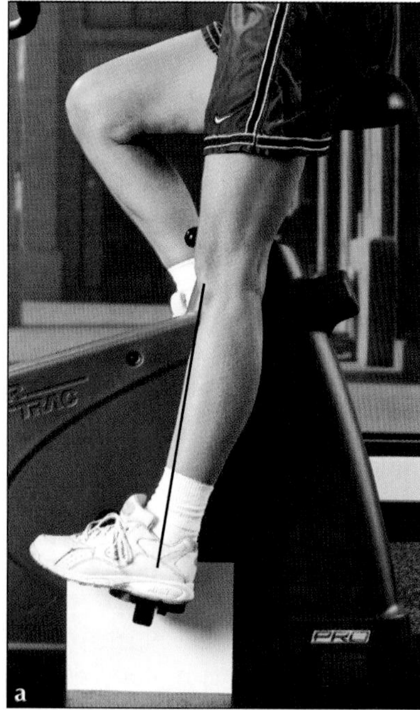
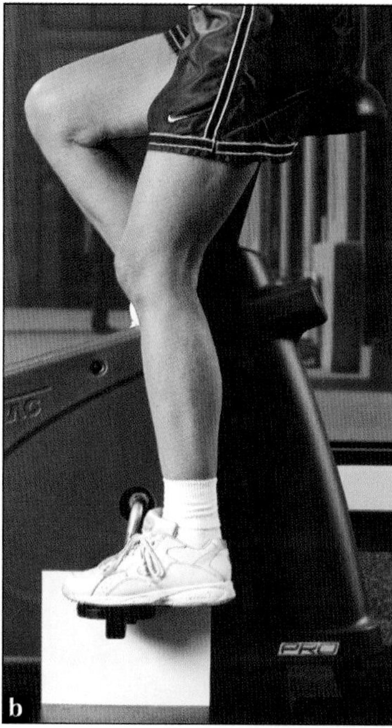
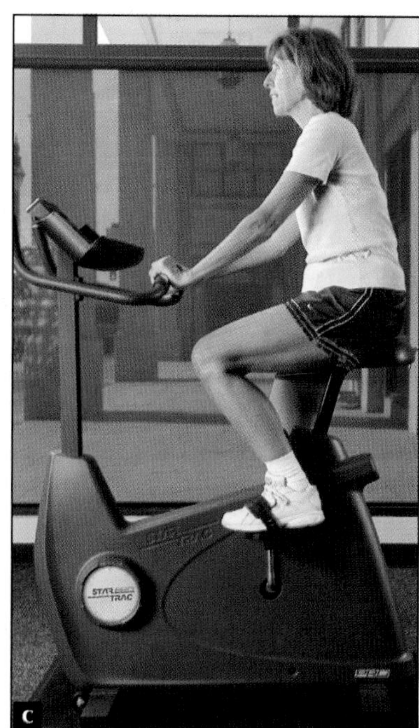

Figure 14.5 Proper seat height adjustment: *(a)* leg straight with knee locked and heel on pedal; *(b)* knee slightly bent with ball of foot on pedal; and *(c)* with the pedal at 12 o'clock, the knee will be about even with the hips and approximately parallel with the floor.

much knee flexion and not enough knee extension. Conversely, a feeling of "reaching" for the pedals or a swaying of the hips indicates that the seat is too high. The hips should not rock back and forth as the cyclist attempts to reach the pedals, and the extending leg should never lock out. This can cause seat irritation as well as knee and low back pain [62]. Finally, it is important to ask the client if the seat position is comfortable, since personal preference should also be taken into consideration.

Handlebars and Body Position

In general, the handlebar position for a stationary bicycle should allow the back to be tilted forward from the hips, but the back should not be rounded. Ideally, the upper arm and torso will form an angle of approximately 90 degrees (or slightly less) [18, 62]. Many stationary bicycles feature "bullhorn" handlebars that enable the rider to hold on with a variety of hand positions. Bullhorn handlebars have a front bar that curves 90 degrees on either side and extends forward, ending with a slight upward tilt. These handlebars allow a variety of hand positions, including the following:

1. A pronated palms-facing-down grip on the front of the handlebar, allowing a more upright posture
2. A neutral palms-facing-in grip on the sides of the handlebar, encouraging more forward lean
3. A "racing" position with maximum forward lean, in which the forearms rest on the sides of the handlebar and support much of the upper body weight

During longer rides, changes in hand positions are highly recommended to alter the pressure on the wrists and hands [18, 62]. Most novices generally prefer a more upright sitting posture, but there will still be a slight forward body lean. Unfortunately, many electronic and generator-driven stationary bicycles do not allow handlebar height or fore-and-aft adjustments.

Cadence

Pedaling cadence on a stationary bike is measured by the number of pedal revolutions per minute (rpm). Generally, the most economical pedaling cadence ranges from 60 to 100 rpm. Novice and intermediate cyclists tend to pedal between 60 and 80, while elite cyclists are often closer to 90 to 100 rpm. Pedaling at too low a cadence overloads the working muscles and results in premature lactate production and leg fatigue. Pedaling at too high a cadence results in wasted energy, too, due to added muscular work needed to stabilize the trunk [29, 41, 42, 50, 64].

Pedaling Action

The pedaling action in cycling is a fluid *circular* 360-degree motion. However, the majority of force is applied forward and downward during the downstroke. If the downstroke begins at 0 degrees (12 o'clock) and finishes at 180 degrees (6 o'clock), then the most powerful force in the pedaling action is applied from approximately 45 degrees (between 1 and 2 o'clock) to 135 degrees (between 4 and 5 o'clock) [18, 19, 26] (see figure 14.6). During the downstroke, the hip extends, and the powerful quadriceps and gluteal muscles assist the hamstrings, gastrocnemius, and soleus. The forward and downward force contributes more than 96% of the total force output, while the upstroke contributes less than 4% [26]. The personal trainer should instruct the client to think of the thighs as pistonlike levers, rhythmically driving up and down, and doing most of the work, and the calves as connecting rods, traveling in a nice relaxed circle [35].

Foot position angle changes slightly with the circular pedaling action. The toe points slightly up on the downstroke, and slightly down on the upstroke. The involved calf muscles help provide some force, and the foot should be allowed some movement at the ankle; but it is unnecessary to overly emphasize calf involvement [26].

Semi-Recumbent Bikes

Semi-recumbent stationary bikes provide back support and a wider seat for greater comfort (figure 14.7). These advantages may be particularly beneficial for special populations including deconditioned and overweight clients, persons with low back pain, cardiac rehabilitation patients, and pregnant women. In general, heart rate, blood pressure, oxygen consumption ($\dot{V}O_2$), rate-pressure product, and rating of perceived exertion are lower on semi-recumbent bikes than they are on upright bikes [15]. The reasons for this are twofold: (1) back support on semi-recumbent bikes alleviates the workload on postural muscles, and (2) the reclining position reduces the need for the heart to pump blood vertically against gravity [15].

Group Indoor Cycling

On the opposite end of the spectrum from the generally lower-intensity workout with semi-recumbent biking is a higher-intensity cycling workout commonly known as *group indoor cycling*. Group indoor cycling offers a challenging workout, usually set to music, on flywheel bikes in a class atmosphere. Instructors lead the participants on a simulated outdoor training ride or road race with periods of level touring, hills, valleys, and finish lines. Classes often last 40 to 45 minutes, but some beginner sessions may be 30 minutes [17].

As with standard stationary bicycles, seat height positions for group indoor cycling bikes should be set to allow a slight bend in the knee at the bottom of the pedal stroke (about 25-35 degrees with a goniometer). With the pedal at 12 o'clock, the knee should be about level with the hips, with the upper leg approximately parallel to the floor. The methods for setting the seat height are the same as for standard stationary bicycles (refer to the "Seat Height" section under "Stationary Bicycle").

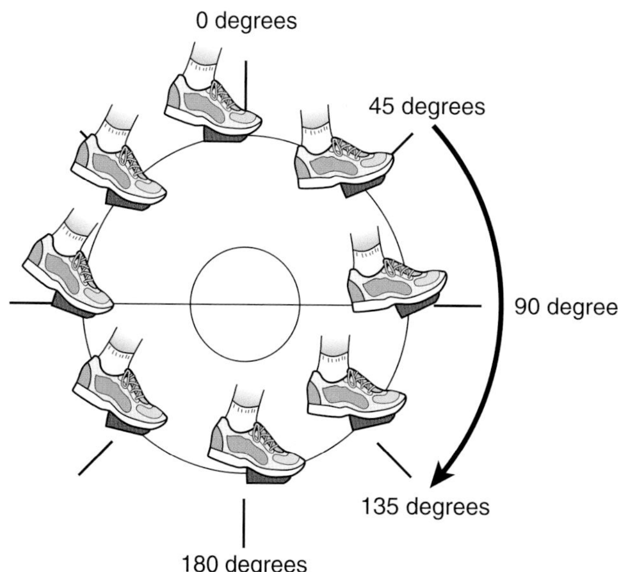

Figure 14.6 The most powerful pedaling force occurs during the downstroke from approximately 45 degrees to 135 degrees.
Adapted from Evans 1997.

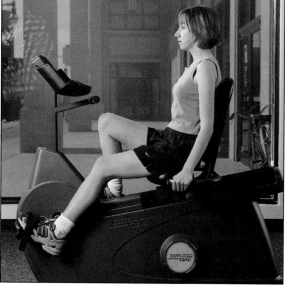

Figure 14.7 The upper body is supported in a reclining position on a semi-recumbent bike; the seat is adjusted to allow a slight bend at the knee (similar to standard stationary bicycle).

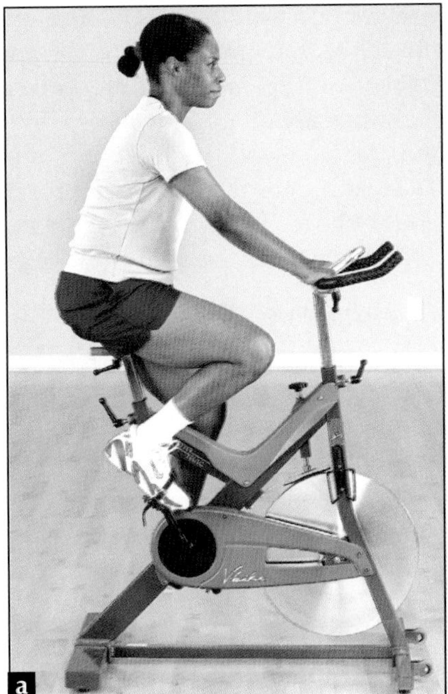

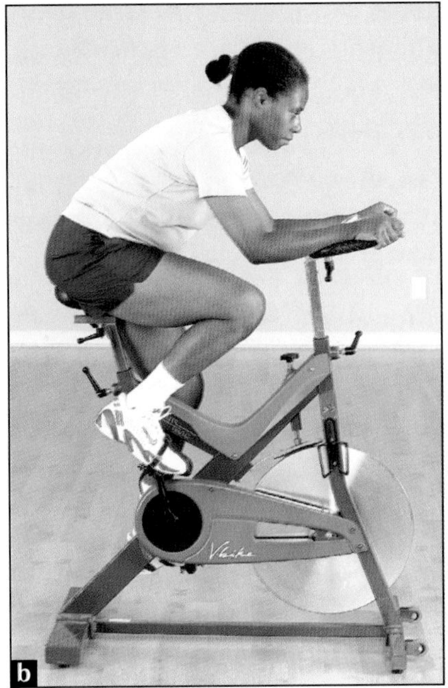

Figure 14.8 Proper body position on group cycling bike *(a)* when not racing and *(b)* when racing.

Group indoor cycling bikes typically additionally allow fore (forward) and aft (backward) seat adjustments. When set properly, fore and aft seat adjustments encourage optimal force production on the downstroke and better safety for the knee. To adjust the fore and aft seat position, the client should set the pedals parallel to the floor at 3 and 9 o'clock, then adjust the seat forward or backward so that at 3 o'clock the knee does not come forward in front of the toe. A plumb line dropped from the tibial tuberosity (small bump just below the kneecap) should contact the ball of the foot at the center of the pedal [62]. The knee should not come forward in front of the toe, since this reduces optimal force output and may lead to knee injuries [43, 62].

Group indoor cycling bikes also allow handlebar height adjustments. Handlebar height is largely a function of individual preference, but normally the handlebar should be set level with the tip of the saddle. Novices and clients with poor back flexibility may prefer the handlebar higher to allow a more upright sitting posture (figure 14.8a). Either way, the arms should be a comfortable distance from the handlebar with the elbows slightly bent at a minimum of 15 degrees [62]. The angle between the torso and the upper arm typically measures approximately 90 degrees (or slightly less) [18, 43, 62]. Some bikes also include handlebar fore and aft positioning, which further allows proper adjustment to maximize comfort. In general, a more forward-leaning upper body "racing" posture (figure 14.8b) is used more often during group indoor cycling than it is for standard stationary bicycling on electronic and generator-driven bikes.

Although group indoor cycling participants are instructed to set their own intensity levels by adjusting the bike's resistance, many individuals may want to first build a foundation of cycling fitness by training on a standard stationary bicycle [62]. After getting into "cycling shape" on a standard stationary bicycle, the novice should start with a group indoor cycling beginner class. Many novices need time to get accustomed to the more forward-leaning racing positions, as well as "out of the saddle" standing pedal positions that are used for simulated hill climbing and sprinting. In beginner classes, the instructor spends more time demonstrating proper seat and handlebar adjustments and typical riding techniques and positions. Beginner classes also enable the client to acclimate to the higher-intensity training techniques that are regularly used in group indoor cycling [17, 43].

When clients are performing stair climbing, elliptical trainer, or stationary bicycling exercise, the knee should not come forward in front of the toe when the knee is in the flexed position. This produces added strain on the knee and can cause injury.

Rowing Machine

Primary muscles used: quadriceps, hamstrings, gluteals, tibialis anterior, gastrocnemius, soleus, biceps brachii, brachioradialis, brachialis, rectus abdominis, posterior and medial deltoids, trapezius, latissimus dorsi, teres major, erector spinae, and flexor and extensor carpi ulnaris

Indoor rowing provides an excellent upper and lower body non-weight-bearing and nonimpact aerobic workout. Like biking, indoor rowing requires the client to be in a seated position; and therefore the risk of body-weight impact injuries to the hips, knees, ankles, and feet is greatly reduced. Indoor rowing, like swimming, is a full-body aerobic workout. The exercise uses the large hip, gluteal, and leg muscles of the lower body, as well as the muscles of the upper and lower back and arms. The proper rowing stroke is a coordinated, rhythmic pulling action that maximizes efficiency.

The drawback of rowing is that most clients are not familiar with the rowing motion. Novice rowers often pull too much with the upper body. Proper rowing technique dictates that approximately 70% to 75% of the pulling actions come from the stronger leg and hip muscles [30]. It is also important to pay attention to clients with lower back problems who choose to perform rowing exercise. Although rowing can improve lower back strength and muscular endurance, it can also aggravate problems if proper technique is not followed. Forward and backward lean comes primarily from the hips, and the back should maintain lumbar lordosis (not be rounded). Proper body position is shown in figure 14.9, a-d.

The Starting Position

In the starting (or "catch") position, the client should be instructed to hold the head upright, looking straight ahead. The back should be upright but not rounded, with a slight forward lean from the hips. The arms are straightened in front of the body, and the hips and knees are flexed at the knees with the shins vertical [22, 45].

The Drive

During the drive, the client should extend the hips and knees forcefully, using the muscles of the hips, gluteals, and quadriceps. At the same time, the torso leans back slightly. After the hips and knees are extended, the arms pull the handle to the abdomen below the rib cage [22, 45].

Note: The arms must not be flexed during the leg drive. This positioning pits the strength of the legs against the strength of the arms. If the arms are pulling while the legs are pressing, the weaker and smaller arm muscles will fatigue quickly.

The Finish

In the finish, the client's legs are fully extended, with the torso leaning slightly backward. The arms are bent at the elbows, and the handle comes to the abdomen just under the rib cage [22, 45].

The Recovery

During the recovery, the client's arms extend forward, followed by a forward lean of the torso from the hips. When the handle passes over the client's knees, the knees flex and allow the body to slide forward until the shins are vertical [22, 45].

Note: Rowing exercise is a smooth well-coordinated movement of the upper and lower body. Many novice rowers make the mistake of "humping" the handle over the knees during the recovery. This happens because they flex the knees too soon after the finish. For proper recovery, the knees should flex only after the handle crosses the knees with the arms coming forward and the back gradually leaning forward.

The Catch

At the end of the recovery, the rower is back to the starting position. The client's body leans slightly forward from the hips, with the arms straight and the shins vertical. The next stroke is then ready to begin [22, 45].

Resistance

Rowing resistance is controlled by the amount of air admitted to the flywheel. The more open the air vent, the greater the resistance. If the air vent is closed (less air admitted), the resistance is decreased. Resistance is determined by personal preference, but should generally allow the client to row rhythmically, without strain or undue effort [30]. Novices may want to set the flywheel at lower resistances. Even elite rowers often train at moderate resistances. Heavy resistances may be used for periodic high-intensity efforts for short durations.

Cadence

The cadence, in rowing, is the number of strokes per minute. Recreational rowers, using a moderate pace, row at a cadence of approximately 20 to 25 strokes per minute [30]. Elite rowers may use higher cadences, generally from 25 to 35 strokes per minute. A faster cadence, however, does not necessarily mean faster times. A slow, smooth, efficient stroke is often better (faster) than a fast cadence done with poor technique. A trained rower maximizes the force production of each pull, and maintains stroke efficiency at higher cadences.

Note: Although rowing may strengthen the low back area, rowing exercise may be contraindicated for some clients with low back problems. Clients who are overweight, are severely deconditioned, or have minor low back discomfort may be advised to build a foundation of fitness before beginning rowing exercise. Strengthening the low back and

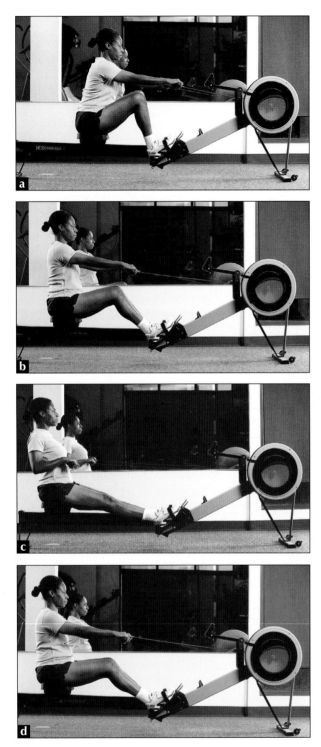

Figure 14.9 Proper body position on the rowing machine: *(a)* starting position (and the catch); *(b)* the drive; *(c)* the finish; and *(d)* the recovery.

abdominal area and improving low back flexibility may be particularly important. The personal trainer may also want to instruct some clients to row with an upright back instead of with slight forward and backward lean from the hips. Rowing with an upright back lowers the intensity of the exercise and reduces the workload on the lower back extensor muscles. While power output may be compromised without the forward and backward torso lean from the hips, indoor rowing remains an effective exercise for the major muscle groups of the lower and upper body and may still produce cardiovascular benefits.

Cardiovascular Non-Machine Exercise Technique

Many clients may wish to include non-machine training and outdoor exercise in their programs. Non-machine exercises like outdoor walking and running may be less expensive than other options because no equipment is necessary other than a good pair of shoes; clients who enjoy water activities may enjoy swimming or aqua exercise; and group fitness classes offer a variety of popular exercise choices. Non-machine cardiovascular activities discussed in this chapter include walking, running, swimming, group exercise classes, and aqua exercise.

Walking

Primary muscles used: quadriceps, hamstrings, gluteals, iliopsoas, tibialis anterior, gastrocnemius, and soleus

Beginner walkers may simply put one foot in front of the other without any special attention to *how* they are doing it. However, as with all forms of exercise, walking with proper biomechanics improves performance, increases benefits, and decreases the risk of injury. Good walking technique allows for greater efficiency in work output over longer distances. Walking is a convenient, safe, and low-cost exercise. The only equipment necessary is a good pair of comfortable shoes.

Body Position

Good postural alignment is essential during walking. Good posture aids performance and decreases strain on the spine and lower back muscles. The head should be held upright, eyes looking straight ahead. The shoulders should be relaxed, but not rounded. The upper body should be positioned directly over the hips. It is helpful to encourage clients to "walk tall" and imagine a string pulling up from the top of the head that elongates the spine upward. From a side view, imagine a plumb line dropping from the ear, aligning the client's ear, shoulder, and hip. Body position during walking should be upright, with the torso positioned directly over the hips. This allows the vertebrae and erector spinae muscles to share the weight and impact equally.

Foot Strike

Proper **foot strike** during walking occurs when the heel strikes the ground (or treadmill belt) and the weight is then immediately spread over the foot by a gentle "rolling" *heel-to-ball* action. Primarily, this heel-to-ball roll starts near the outer side of the heel and continues forward and slightly inward toward the middle of the ball of the foot at push-off [48]. Abnormal foot strike patterns include overpronation and underpronation or supination. (See pages 333-334 for more details). Neither of these exaggerated foot strike patterns is desirable, and each may lead to injury.

Hip Action

Walking speed is controlled by a combination of **stride length** and **stride frequency.** Stride length is the distance covered with each step. Stride frequency is the number of steps per minute. A given distance can be covered in a shorter period of time (faster pace) through increasing stride length, stride frequency, or both. To increase stride frequency, one simply takes faster steps. To increase stride length, the person allows greater hip action in the movement with each step. It is not necessary to adopt the highly noticeable pelvic roll of a racewalker (unless racewalking is the goal), but freer movement at the hips allows a more elongated walking gait [37]. (For specific information on racewalking, refer to the "Racewalking" section further on.)

Arm Action

Basically, the arm swing and leg stride during walking are coordinated movements, with the left arm swinging forward when the right foot strides forward, and the right arm swinging forward when the left foot strides forward. The arms swing naturally from relaxed shoulders. This pendulum swinging of the arms becomes more pronounced at faster speeds.

Because arm and leg action must be coordinated, arm-swing length and speed will increase proportionally with leg stride length and speed. At faster walking speeds, it becomes more efficient to hold the arms bent at the elbow at 90 degrees. This bent arm swinging action allows the arms to swing faster through a shorter arc. The elbows pass fairly close to the sides of the body, and the arms and hands swing primarily in a forward and backward motion to help propel the body forward. The hands and arms also move slightly inward, but the hands should not cross the midline of the body. On the forward swing with the arms bent at the elbow to 90°, the hands come to the level of the chest at the nipple line. On the backward swing, the hands reach the hipbone at the side of the body. The hands are "cupped" loosely, with the thumb gently touching the side of the forefinger and the thumbnail pointing upward [37].

Racewalking

Although a complete explanation of racewalking is beyond the scope of this chapter, a couple of notable differences between racewalking and walking are worth mentioning. Two race-walking rules prevent fast walking from turning into running. First, in competitive racewalking, one foot must always be in contact with the ground; that is, from one step to another there can be no airborne movement (as in running). In addition, the knee must remain straight from the time the foot lands until the body passes over the supporting leg. (A bent leg will also produce running.)

To optimize proper racewalking performance, it is necessary to maximize stride length. To achieve this, racewalkers increase hip rotation with each stride. This hip rotation produces the distinctive "pelvic roll" that enables racewalkers to cover more ground with each step (figure 14.10). In racewalking, correct hip rotation moves the hip through three phases:

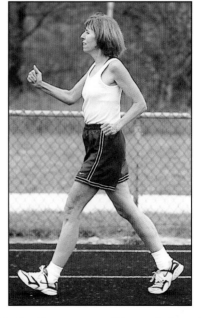

Figure 14.10 Proper racewalking technique dictates that one foot must always be in contact with the ground, and the support leg must remain straight. Racewalkers increase stride length with increased hip rotation.

1. The hip inwardly rotates and flexes to allow the striding leg to reach out as far as possible.
2. The hip relaxes to a neutral position, in midstance, with the body coming directly over the support leg.
3. The hip opens and extends during propulsion, when the ball of the foot pushes off.

The extra few inches gained from rotating the hips in order to increase stride length are crucial to the success of competitive racewalkers [37].

Walking Technique

Good postural alignment: The client should be instructed to "walk tall" by holding the head upright and looking straight ahead; shoulders are relaxed, but not rounded; upper body is positioned directly over the hips. The client should imagine a plumb line aligning the ear, shoulder, and hip.

Stride: Encourage the client to take long, relaxing strides; lift the knees; and engage the hips and gluteals in the movement.

Arm swing: Have the client swing the arms from relaxed shoulders; the amplitude of the arm swing is increased with higher walking speeds and longer strides; at faster speeds, instruct the client to pump the arms bent at the elbow at 90 degrees.

Foot strike: Teach the client to allow the heel to strike the ground gently, and then roll to the middle of the ball of the foot for push-off.

Running

Primary muscles used: quadriceps, hamstrings, gluteals, iliopsoas, tibialis anterior, gastrocnemius, and soleus.

Running produces outstanding cardiovascular benefits and, like walking, is a low-cost exercise. Running is time efficient for conditioned clients and is sport specific for recreational athletes whose sport involves running.

The net energy cost of running is generally greater than for walking and therefore requires greater cardiovascular fitness. The reason is the vertical component in running when the body propels itself forward [2, 54]. When a client can walk about four miles (6.4 kilometers) without fatigue, a walk/run program may be substituted, if desired [55]. In a walk/run program, clients alternate periods of running and walking (e.g., a one- to two-minute run followed by three to five minutes of walking). The sequence is then repeated for the prescribed duration. Clients gradually increase running time (i.e., three minutes, four minutes, etc.) every few weeks until they can sustain continuous running for 15 to 20 minutes. Other walk/run periods may be tailored to fit the client's fitness capability and preference.

The disadvantage of running is that it is high impact. With each foot strike, the impact can range between two and four times body weight [51]. This increased wear and tear on the structural anatomy of the body may result in injury. Overweight clients or clients with orthopedic problems in the low back, hips, knees, ankles, and feet may be better off choosing lower-impact activities such as walking, biking, swimming, or aqua exercise.

Body Position

Like walking, running demands proper attention to posture (figure 14.11). The best posture for a distance runner is an upright one. Good upright postural alignment increases running efficiency and puts less strain on the vertebrae and erector spinae muscles. The head is held upright, eyes looking straight ahead. The shoulders are relaxed, but not rounded. The lower back should *not* be arched during running. Instead, the torso should be balanced directly over the hips. One should instruct the client to "run tall" by imagining a string pulling from the top of the head, elongating the spine upward. From the side, imagine a plumb line dropped from the ear, aligning the ear with the shoulder and hip.

Foot Strike

Most long-distance runners use the **heel-to-ball** foot strike. With this method, the heel touches the ground first, and the weight is immediately spread over the foot by a gentle "rolling" action. This heel-to-ball roll starts primarily near the outer side of the heel and continues forward and inward toward the middle of the ball of the foot at push-off. The heel should not be "jammed" into the ground, nor should the forefoot be "slapped" down hard. The client should be encouraged to "run lightly" and "glide" along in order to create a gentler foot strike,

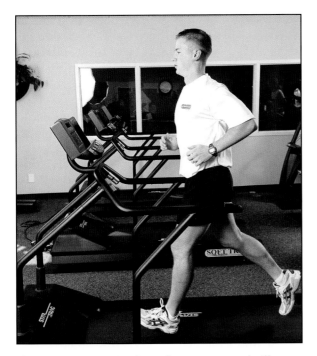

Figure 14.11 During long distance or treadmill running, proper foot strike involves contact with the heel and then a gentle "rolling" action toward the ball of the foot for push-off.

conserve energy, and reduce the risk of impact injury. Bouncing with each step should be avoided because it wastes energy by vertical displacement and increases shock. The heel-ball method is the safest foot strike for running long distances because the impact is well absorbed by the entire foot.

Foot strike abnormalities, like overpronation and underpronation (refer to the section on footwear in "General Guidelines for Safe Participation in Cardiovascular Activities"), have greater consequences during running than during walking because of the foot strike impact.

Arm Action

During long-distance running, the arms hang from relaxed shoulders and are bent at the elbows. Some arm action occurs from the shoulders, but too much shoulder movement wastes energy. Much of the arm movement comes from the lower arm (forearm, wrist, and hand) by means of hinging at the elbow. In this way, the elbow is unlocked, and the angle at the elbow opens during the arm downswing and closes during the upswing.

The forearms are carried between the waist and chest. If the arms are carried too high, the shoulders and upper back become fatigued. If the arms are carried too low, excessive forward lean may occur. The hands are gently cupped, and the thumb softly touches the index finger. The hands should not be clenched into fists. On the forward swing, the hands reach chest height. On the backward swing, the hands reach the hips at the side of the body. The arms and hands also move slightly inward, but the hands do not cross the midline of the body. The wrists should be relaxed but not held too loosely [28].

Stride Length

Running speed, like walking speed, is determined by stride length and stride frequency. To improve running performance, it is necessary to increase stride length, stride frequency, or both. A client's exact stride length depends on leg length, flexibility, strength, coordination, and level of fatigue.

With each running step, the body should land approximately under the hips. If the foot hits too far in front of the body's center of gravity, greater shock and a slight *braking* effect will result. This is **overstriding.** Braking, as well as too much time spent in the air, makes overstriding inefficient. Many runners overreach with the front leg and foot in an effort to improve stride length. This is counterproductive and will likely cause braking. Conversely, **understriding** (taking too short a stride) also wastes energy, since it prevents the body from advancing far enough with each stride.

The best way to improve stride length is to increase rear leg drive by improving strength and to increase range of motion by improving flexibility. Plyometric exercises may also increase rear leg drive and may be added to the program when appropriate [28]. See chapter 17 for plyometric exercise techniques.

Stride Frequency

To increase stride frequency, the client should be instructed to simply take quicker, softer, relaxed steps and keep the feet low to the ground. Plyometric exercises, when appropriate, may also be used to increase stride frequency.

People who are running for health benefits may not see the importance of improving stride frequency and stride length, since speed and racing are not the goal. One safety reason is worth mentioning, though. A slow overstride usually results in a raised center of gravity and more time spent in the air. This results in a harder landing and greater impact. Therefore, a slow overstride may cause not only loss of speed, but also an increased risk of injury. Finding one's optimal stride frequency and stride length can produce better performance and also leads to greater safety [28].

Swimming

Primary muscles used: can be nearly a full-body activity depending on the swimming strokes performed

Swimming is an excellent, full-body, non-weight-bearing aerobic activity that is a good alternative to land-based aerobic activities. As with any exercise activity, the benefits of swimming are equal to the time and effort invested and the efficacy of one's performance.

Personal trainers with swimming experience may be able to prescribe general swimming program design and may be able to help with basic swimming stroke technique improvement. However, it is recommended that American Red Cross-certified Water Safety Instruction (WSI) instructors teach clients who do not know how to swim at all [7].

The four competitive swimming strokes are freestyle (front crawl), backstroke, breaststroke, and butterfly. Sidestroke and elementary backstroke are also strokes that may be taught to recreational swimmers. The topic of instruction in all strokes is beyond the scope of this chapter. Therefore this section is limited to a brief discussion of instruction on freestyle (front crawl).

Freestyle, or the Front Crawl

Freestyle (the **front crawl**) is the most popular and fastest swimming stroke. Freestyle uses both the upper and lower body and, like all strokes, depends on the efficiency of motion and the coordinated efforts of stroke components including correct body position, leg and arm action, and good breathing rhythm [6].

Body Position In freestyle swimming the body is prone and straight. Any extraneous lateral or up-and-down movement causes turbulence and resistance. The head should be held in a natural position with the eyes looking at the bottom of the pool or slightly forward. Depending on the swimmer's buoyancy, the water level should come somewhere between the middle of the forehead to the hairline or crown of the head [6, 25, 32, 36].

Although the body is straight and streamlined, there is a good amount of body roll (a transverse plane rotating around the body's midline) that occurs with every stroke. This body roll involves the whole body. Body roll is initiated by the hips and includes the shoulder turn, hips, legs, and feet. The head remains still and rotates only to take a breath. When taking a breath the turning of the head should be a natural extension of body roll. Body roll results because (1) the hips rotate, (2) the recovery arm is lifted, (3) the pulling arm is providing propulsion at a slight angle, and (4) the leg kick produces some sideways force as the legs roll with the rest of the body. Body roll also helps these movements occur, so it is difficult to know exactly which comes first. Most likely the movements happen together, synergistically [6, 25, 31, 32, 33, 36]. Body roll is important because it aids in relaxed recovery, allows easier breathing, improves arm propulsion in the power phase, decreases the effect of drag forces, and reduces the stresses on the shoulder and therefore helps prevent injury [6].

Arm Stroke The arm stroke action of freestyle swimming is extremely important because it accounts for the majority (as much as 80%-90%) of the propulsion force needed to move the body through the water [36]. The arm stroke includes three major phases: the entry/catch phase, the power phase, and the recovery phase [6].

The **entry/catch phase** begins the underwater portion of the arm stroke when the forward-reaching hand and arm enter the water and the hand and forearm "catches" the water.

The **entry** of the hand is made in front of the shoulder (or somewhere between the shoulder and head) [6, 25, 31, 32, 33]. The reaching hand should not cross the midline of the body or come in front of the head. The hand enters the water at about three-fourths the length of the fully outstretched arm because the elbow is held high and slightly bent and because the hand needs to break the surface of the water smoothly, at an angle of about 40 degrees [6, 25]. A high elbow during the entry phase is important because it allows the arm to enter the water cleanly, without resistance, and ensures an effective pulling position [32]. The hand is in a slightly pronated position so that the index finger and thumb enter the water first. The fingertips, hand, forearm, elbow, and shoulder should all enter the water in the same location, following one another in a streamlined manner. After entry, the arm extends forward into the water without producing turbulence (i.e., the hand and arm should *not* be slapped on top of the water [6, 25, 36].

The **catch** occurs just after entry, when the elbow of the reaching arm flexes, allowing the hand and forearm to "catch" the water in front of the shoulder. The catch phase is not propulsive, but it properly positions the hand and arm so they can pull effectively during the remainder of the stroke. This "feeling" for the water—in which the hand seems to have grabbed a semi-solid mass of water—can be likened to the way a mountain climber grabs a piece of rock with an outstretched arm to pull the body upward. If the arm has made a good entry into the water, the elbow will be higher than the hand at the catch and should remain higher throughout the arm stroke [6, 25, 36].

The **power phase** is the propulsive phase of the arm stroke. After the forward-reaching hand and forearm "catches" the water, the power phase occurs when the swimmer pulls the body forward through the water by accelerating the hand and arm by means of a forceful backward pull. The pulling movement of both the hand and forearm are important for generating propulsion. In general, the propulsive phase of the arm stroke traces a subtle curvilinear "S"-shaped pattern (reverse"S" for the right hand). This "S"-shaped pattern (see figure 14.12) begins when the hand sweeps downward and slightly outward (the top of the "S"shape). Then the hand and arm sweep slightly inward and backward toward the chest and middle of the body as the elbow bends to about 90 degrees (the diagonal part of the "S"shape). Finally, the hand rotates to a neutral position with the palm facing backward, and the arm extends and sweeps forcefully outward, upward, and backward past the thigh (the bottom of the "S"-shape). This final backward thrust past the thigh is the most forceful portion of the power phase, when the arm reaches its maximum (controlled) pulling capacity. The finish of the stroke should be coupled with body roll to maximize propulsion [6, 25, 36].

It is important to keep in mind that these "S"-shaped movements are subtle and should not be exaggerated. The lateral portion of the "S"-movement occurs only from slightly outside of the shoulder (the catch, top of the "S"), toward the chest at middle of the body (the insweep, diagonal portion of the "S"), and then outward and backward past the thigh (the outsweep, the bottom of the "S"). This out-in-out movement spans a width of only about four to eight inches (10-20 centimeters), so the movement makes a very skinny "S." These "sculling" movements of the hand and forearm produce hydrodynamic "lift" forces that may add to the forward propulsion [58, 69]. Lift forces are generated by the hand "slicing" through the water and are similar to the forces that lift a plane off the ground. A more in-depth discussion of lift versus paddle hydrodynamics is beyond the scope of this chapter.

Recent research has shown that a wide "S"-shape pull may not be the most effective means of generating propulsion since most propulsion is generated by pushing water straight towards the feet [12]. The best arm pull should include a small "S"-pattern to it, but for the most part should be directed towards the feet. One can observe the effectiveness of this technique in many of today's elite swimmers. Proponents of a more linear pulling motion feel that the "S"-shape sweeping movements are less efficient and that a more linear backward power phase arm movement leads to a more powerful stroke. These coaches and elite swimmers believe that the more linear pulling arm stroke, which maximizes paddle forces, is superior to the sculling movements of the "S"-shaped sweeping movements [32].

It is not necessary to hold the fingers tightly together during the arm stroke. A slight amount of space between the fingers increases the pulling surface area. Because of the speed with which the hands move through the water, there is a "web effect," and water does not pass between fingers that are slightly apart [6, 36]. The hands should be comfortable and relaxed.

The recovery phase of the arm stroke prepares the arm for another pull; it is not propulsive. The first movement in the recovery is to lift the elbow high out of the water. The forearm and hand

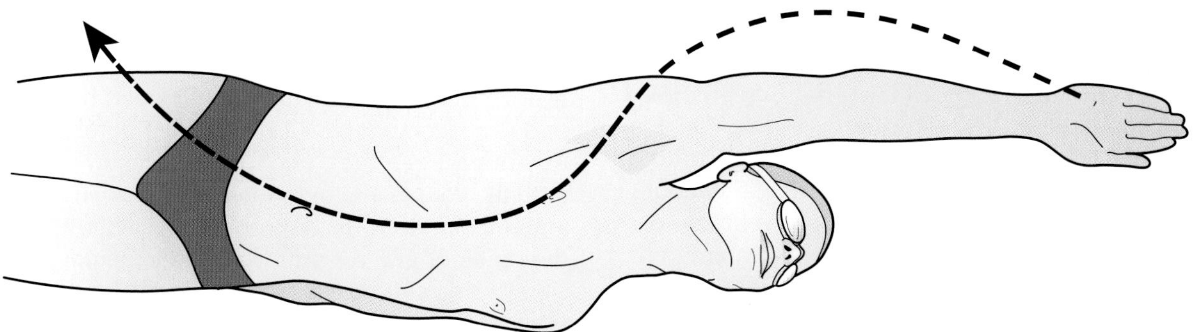

Figure 14.12 The subtle "S"-shaped hand pattern during the power phase of the freestyle (front crawl) arm stroke in swimming.
Adapated from American Red Cross 1992.

follow the elbow out of the water, and the hand is turned toward the legs so that the little finger exits first. This relaxed high elbow position allows the forearm to "hang" downward. After the hand clears the water, it moves forward to a position for another entry and the next pulling power phase [6, 25, 31, 32, 33, 36].

Leg Kick In most swimmers, the leg kick does not contribute substantially to the swimmer's propulsion (perhaps only about 10%-20%), but it is still important [24, 36]. The main functions of the leg kick are to balance the body and help maintain a horizontal position.

The leg movement in freestyle swimming is described as a flutter kick. The amplitude of this up-and-down kicking movement is not great and ranges from about 12 to 15 inches (30-38 centimeters) [6].

The power part of the flutter kick is the downbeat. The kick originates from the hips and continues with slight knee flexion and extension. In general, the ankles remain plantar flexed to allow the feet to provide an effective kicking surface. In the recovery part of the kick (the upbeat), the leg rises with little or no flexion at the knee until the heel just breaks the surface of the water [6].

Many recreational swimmers swim with a two-beat kick. This means that the feet kick two times with each arm cycle (from the time one arm starts to pull on one stroke until it starts to pull on the next stroke). For long-distance swimming, the idea is to kick only fast enough to keep afloat since this ratio conserves energy. However, elite swimmers may place a greater emphasis on kicking propulsion. Elite long distance swimmers may use a two-four-, or six-beat kick. Elite sprinters primarily use a six-beat kick because they are not concerned with conserving energy and attempt to utilize every bit of propulsion available [6, 31, 32, 33, 36].

Breathing When breathing, the head turns to the side as a natural extension of the body rotation. The head remains fairly level, with the forehead just higher than the chin. The swimmer breathes in the trough created by the head as it turns to breathe [31]. Too often, swimmers lift the head, causing the hips to sink. The swimmer's eyes should focus on the water surface just a few inches ahead of the mouth [31, 32]. After the inhalation, the body rolls and the head turns back into the water. The out-breath underwater should be through the mouth and nose [6, 25, 36]. At low intensities it may be possible to exhale through the nose only; but at higher intensities it is necessary to forcefully exhale through the mouth and nose in order to make sure that all the air is expelled.

Group Exercise Classes

Primary muscles used: can be nearly a full-body activity depending on the exercises involved

Group exercise classes provide a variety of cardiovascular activities in a group setting, usually choreographed with music. Traditional "aerobics classes" have expanded to include a variety of group exercise classes such as step classes, kickboxing, group resistance training, fitness yoga, aqua exercise, and tai chi [5, 16]. This section cannot cover the various types of classes in depth. Rather it presents a brief description of traditional aerobics, step classes, kickboxing, and aqua exercise because these classes can feature a prominent cardiovascular conditioning component.

Safety priorities for all group exercise classes include good posture and proper body position. The head should be held upright, with the eyes looking straight ahead. The shoulders should be relaxed, but not rounded. The ear, shoulder, and hip should be aligned. Abdominal and gluteal muscles should be slightly contracted to prevent excessive back arching. With knee flexion the knee should not come in front of the toe [5, 16]. Participants should always begin new exercise activities by learning proper exercise technique at a comfortable pace.

Clients in group exercise classes should maintain good posture, aligning the ear, shoulder, and hip; slightly contract abdominal and gluteal muscles to prevent excessive back arching; and ensure that when they flex the knee, the knee does not come in front of the toe.

Traditional Aerobics

Typically, traditional aerobics classes last for 60 minutes, but some classes may range from 45 to 75 minutes. Most classes include a warm-up, preperformance stretching, an aerobic activity, cooldown, muscular conditioning, and flexibility. The time spent on each section depends on the emphasis of the class [16].

Traditional aerobics is further broken into classes featuring low-impact, moderate-impact, high-impact, and combination hi/lo-impact aerobics. In **low-impact aerobics,** one foot remains in contact with the floor at all times. Intensity is varied by the amount of muscle mass used, raising and lowering the center of gravity, range of motion, tempo, and side-to-side and forward and backward traveling. Lower-intensity low-impact classes are especially good for beginning, deconditioned, or obese clients; senior clients; and pregnant women. The vertical impact forces of low-impact aerobics range from 1 to 1 1/4 times body weight [16].

In **moderate-impact aerobics,** one foot remains in contact with the floor at all times, but the center of gravity is raised and lowered on the balls of the feet. This technique gives the feeling of "bounce" without the extreme impact of high-impact aerobics. Vertical impact forces of moderate-impact aerobics range from 2 to 2 1/2 times body weight [16].

In **high-impact aerobics,** both feet leave the floor as the body is lifted into the air. Examples of training moves include running, jumping, hopping, and leaping. High-impact aerobics provides a vigorous workout for injury-free, well-conditioned clients but is not suited for clients who are deconditioned or obese, senior clients, or pregnant women. Vertical impact forces of high-impact aerobics are greater than three times body weight [16].

Combination hi/lo-impact aerobic classes alternate high- and low-impact movements and are popular with a wide range of clients because of the diversity of movements.

Step Training

Step training is a relatively low-impact group exercise class that utilizes a step platform ranging from 4 to 12 inches (10 to 30 centimeters) in height. Participants step up and down to music while performing a variety of movements and sequences using large muscle groups. Step training conditions the cardiovascular and muscular systems, and the range of stepping height allows beginners to gradually acclimate to greater intensity demands. Step training may not be suitable for individuals with chronic knee problems, however, since step training requires repeated bouts of knee flexion and extension [14].

Basic (nonpropulsive) stepping up and down on a moderately high bench of 6 to 8 inches (15 to 20 centimeters) involves impact forces of about 1.4 to 1.5 times body weight (when all four foot strikes are averaged). This resembles the approximate impact forces of brisk walking [14, 27]. However, when stepping speeds are increased and vigorous propulsive moves are added, the impact forces may increase to 2.5 times body weight, or the level of running or high-impact aerobic classes [14, 46, 59]. Therefore, propulsive, or power moves should be included only in classes for intermediate and advanced exercisers. Additionally, repetitive propulsive moves should always be directed up onto the platform, which absorbs impact, and never down onto the floor [14].

Proper platform stepping heights are important to reduce knee compression forces. Step training studies have shown that when the knee is flexed 60 degrees from a fully extended position, patellar compression forces are only slightly more than body weight. However, compression forces increase quickly as deeper full flexion occurs, especially beyond 90 degrees [14, 56]. Therefore, it is recommended that a beginner's step platform height allows a maximum of 60 degrees knee flexion for maximal comfort and safety. Stepping heights for advanced exercisers may be higher but should be restricted to knee flexion of no more than 90 degrees [14].

In every session, start with simple movements to get clients familiar with the step. Encourage clients to "eye" the step occasionally to make sure balance and foot postion are maintained. When landing on the step, the entire foot should land on the step and close to the center, not hanging off an edge.

Kickboxing

Kickboxing is a cardiovascular workout that simulates martial arts training by using choreographed kicks and punching moves for health and fitness benefits [53] (figure 14.13). Typically, these classes are performed like group "shadow boxing" sessions and do not involve actual contact sparring against an opponent. In addition to cardiovascular fitness, kickboxing training can increase dynamic strength and flexibility, improve coordination, and sharpen reflexes [5, 53]. Kickboxing classes are normally 60 minutes in duration but may vary from 45 to 90 minutes. All classes should devote adequate time to warm-up, conditioning, cool-down, flexibility, and strengthening phases [53].

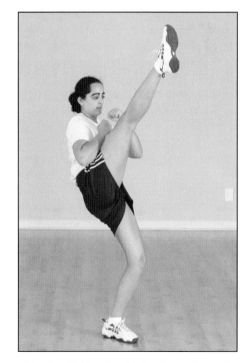

Figure 14.13 Kickboxing kicks above the waist provide a challenging workout for experienced exercisers.

As with any group exercise, kickboxing beginners should be encouraged to learn the moves correctly at their own comfortable pace. Most injuries occur when beginners try to do too much too soon. A combination of fatigue, poor technique, and excessive force will increase the likelihood of injury [53]. Beginners should also be encouraged to have at least one day of rest between kickboxing classes in order to adapt to the new movement stresses and allow recovery of their musculoskeletal systems [53].

For more experienced kickboxing class participants, speed combinations, speed kicking, and kicks above the waist provide a challenging workout. These moves should be performed only after a proper warm-up when participants are working in their target heart rate zones [53].

Some kickboxing programs may progress to equipment-based classes that teach skills using heavy bags, speed bags, punching mitts, and kicking pads. These classes should be taught only by experienced kickboxing or boxing instructors who are familiar with safe and proper use of the equipment. The popularity of health club–based kickboxing classes may encourage some individuals to enroll in traditional kickboxing, boxing, and martial arts specialty schools in order to learn these martial arts skills at more advanced levels.

Aquatic Exercise

Aquatic exercise is one of the safest exercise training modalities because the buoyancy of the water reduces the impact of land-based exercise and is easier on the joints [13]. Aquatic exercise improves cardiorespiratory conditioning, muscular strength, muscular endurance [57], and flexibility [11]. Many populations can benefit from aquatic exercise including older adults, obese individuals, individuals with arthritis and back pain [10], pregnant women [34], and elite athletes training long hours or rehabilitating injuries [65].

Aquatic exercise uses the benefits of working in the water while eliminating the need for swimming expertise. Additionally, exercise in water may be less intimidating because it offers a greater degree of privacy. With much of the body submerged in the water, some clients may feel more comfortable while exercising [13].

Proper hydration is as important with aquatic exercise as it is when exercising on land. Sweat loss occurs while performing exercise in the water, and participants should be encouraged to drink fluids before, during, and after water workouts [13].

Heart rate responses are slightly blunted while exercising in the water (similar to swimming). Aquatic exercise heart rates can be up to 13% or 17 beats per minute lower than during similar land-based exercise [13, 44]. Therefore, rate of perceived exertion and talk test methods should be used to gauge intensity levels rather than relying solely on pulse rates. Lower heart rate responses will generally occur in deeper water because more of the body weight is supported by buoyancy. Water temperature can also affect heart rate response. In general, exercising in cooler water produces lower heart rates than exercising in warmer water [13, 68].

Like other exercise activities, good technique helps maximize the benefits of aquatic exercise while reducing the risk of injury. Participants should be able to perform the exercise movements safely while maintaining proper upright spinal alignment and correct body position. Locking of the knees and joint hyperextension should be avoided. Additionally, participants should avoid spending too much time in excessive plantar flexion, where the body is supported on the toes with the calves in constant contraction [13].

Common Aquatic Exercise Movements Aquatic exercises are performed in shallow or deep water, typically in an upright body position. The effects of gravity are dependent on how far the body is immersed in the water. In general (without taking into effect body composition) a body submerged to the waist bears 50% of its weight; submersion to the chest bears 25-35%; and submersion to the neck bears only 10% of body weight [8, 9, 13]).

Basic aquatic exercise movements include walking, jogging, kicking, jumping, and scissors [13].

Walking involves striding in waist-to-chest deep water with good upright posture and proper spinal alignment. Walking with high knees, backwards, sideways, and on toes provide several variations. Additional variety can be accomplished by including arm movements, with the arms either in or out of the water [13].

Jogging can be done in place or with traveling movement. Erect posture is important for safety. Greater speed of movement increases intensity. Like walking, additional arm movements with the arms in and out of the water can add variety and increase intensity [13].

Kicking movements with one leg can include forward, sideways, and backward kicks, knee lifts, and hamstring curls. When kicking, participants should maintain good postural alignment and avoid hyperextending the knees. Swimming flutter kicks may also be performed from a seated position while at the side of the pool or in a prone position while holding on to the side of the pool [13].

Jumping can be performed on one or both feet. Rebounding from the pool bottom increases intensity. All participants should learn proper landing technique before performing jumping movements. A proper landing involves a toe-ball-heel landing with "soft" knees (extended but not locked) directly over the ankles to absorb body-weight impact and reduce the risk of injury. Jumping variations include jumping jacks, traveling jumps, jumping with a twist, frog jumps, and leaps [13].

Scissors movements involve simultaneous arm and leg actions that resemble cross-country skiing. Larger movements, rebounding off the pool bottom, and traveling may be used to increase workout intensity [13].

Other Moves in Aquatic Exercise Other basic moves for the upper and lower body may include squats, lunges, knee flexion/extension, elbow flexion/extension, shoulder flexion/extension, horizontal shoulder abduction/adduction, and deltoid lateral raises [13]. Increasing the range of motion, increasing the tempo or speed of movement, adding traveling (e.g., walking while doing bicep curls), or adding the use of aquatic resistance equipment will increase workout intensity and resistance of each exercise [13].

Aquatic exercise includes callisthenic-type exercises, simulated weight training movements, and dance and leg movements in shallow or deep water. The water provides resistance against working muscles. Equipment devices can be worn on the arms or legs to further increase resistance. Shallow water programming is performed in waist-to-chest deep water [8, 9]. The feet remain in contact with the pool bottom for most of the workout, providing low impact training.

Aquatic Exercise and Elite Athletes Elite running athletes and other runners may use deep-water running as a supplement to dry-land training in order to reduce impact forces on the feet, knees, hips, and low back. Deeper water programs are performed in chest-to-neck high water [8, 9]. Deep-water programs may include exercise moves with feet touching or not touching the pool bottom. Elite runners and other runners may also use deep-water running as a temporary alternative to dry-land running during periods of injury and rehabilitation. Deep-water running allows athletes to retain cardiovascular conditioning while maintaining some level of running specificity. The running motion is mimicked while suspended in the water with the aid of flotation vests or belts to keep the body buoyant and vertical [13]. Studies have shown that elite runners can maintain dry-land running performance for 4-6 weeks with deep-water running [20, 67]. Slow long distance, interval, fartlek, and sprint training can all be employed in a well-designed deep-water running program.

CONCLUSION

As with any form of exercise, cardiovascular activities should be performed with proper technique. Good form is important for safety and helps achieve maximum benefits. Poor technique can lead to injuries and may hinder progress and goal attainment.

Personal trainers should help clients choose activities that are appropriate for their physical capabilities, exercise preference, and time available for exercise. Clients should perform activities they enjoy, and new exercises should be added when appropriate, since exercise preference and variety in programming contribute to exercise adherence. Having a variety of cardiovascular activities to choose from can eliminate psychological and physiological boredom. Changing activities can also help prevent overuse injuries. Therefore, both the personal trainer who has the diverse knowledge to teach a variety of cardiovascular activities, and the client who is motivated to learn them, will benefit in the long run. Participation in a wide range of activities combined with a long-term exercise program is the best way to achieve physical fitness while reducing the risks of injury.

STUDY QUESTIONS

1. While watching a client's running gait, the personal trainer notices that the client's feet and ankles roll in excessively as they strike the ground. Which of the following combinations of foot strike classifications and shoe lasts apply to this client?

	Foot strike classification	Shoe last
A.	supinator	straight
B.	pronator	straight
C.	supinator	curved
D.	pronator	curved

2. Which of the following is the first action to perform when using a treadmill?
   A. set the treadmill incline to 0 degrees
   B. hold on to the handrails while straddling the belt
   C. walk/run toward the front part of the treadmill deck
   D. turn on the machine to a speed of no more than 1 mph (0.6 kph)
3. Which of the following instructions should be given to a client for using a stair climber?
   A. "Place your entire foot on the pedal to start but allow the heels to lift off as each pedal rises."
   B. "Lean forward slightly, especially as the workout becomes harder."
   C. "Lock out the knees at the bottom of each step."
   D. "Hold the handrails for balance, if necessary."
4. Which of the following describes correct body position on a stationary bicycle?
   A. with the ball of the foot on the upward pedal, the knee is above the height of the hips
   B. with the heel of the foot on the downward pedal, the leg is straight
   C. with the heel of the foot on the upward pedal, the knee is even with height of the hips
   D. with the ball of the foot on the downward pedal, the leg is straight

APPLIED KNOWLEDGE QUESTION

Explain the similarities and differences in the exercise technique guidelines (e.g., body position, foot strike, arm action) that a personal trainer gives a client for *walking* and *running*.

REFERENCES

1. American College of Sports Medicine. 2000. *ACSM's Guidelines for Exercise Testing and Prescription,* 6th ed. Philadelphia: Lippincott Williams & Wilkins, pp. 144-151.
2. American College of Sports Medicine. 2000. *ACSM's Guidelines for Exercise Testing and Prescription,* 6th ed. Philadelphia: Lippincott Williams & Wilkins, p. 303.
3. American College of Sports Medicine. 2001. *ACSM's Resource Manual for Guidelines for Exercise Testing and Prescription,* 4th ed. Philadelphia: Lippincott Williams & Wilkins, p. 642.
4. American Council on Exercise. 1999. Cardio kickboxing packs a punch. *ACE FitnessMatters.* San Diego: American Council on Exercise, pp. 4-5.
5. American Council on Exercise. 2000. *Group Fitness Instructor Manual.* San Diego: American Council on Exercise, pp. 141-204.
6. American Red Cross. 1992. *Swimming and Diving.* Boston: American Red Cross, pp. 112-119, 236.
7. American Red Cross. 1995. *Water Safety Instructor's Manual,* rev. ed. Boston: American Red Cross.
8. Aquatic Exercise Association. 2000. *Aquatic Fitness Professional Manual,* 2nd ed. Nokomis, Fla: Aquatic Exercise Association.
9. Aquatic Exercise Association. 2001. *The Water Well Newsletter* 6.
10. Ariyoshi, M., K. Sonoda, K. Nagata, T. Mashima, M. Zenmyo, C. Paku, Y. Takamiya, H. Yoshimatsu, Y. Hirai, H. Yasunaga, H. Akashi, H. Imayama, T. Shimokobe, A. Inoue, and Y. Mutoh. 1999. Efficacy of aquatic exercises for patients with low-back pain. *Kurume Medical Journal* 46 (2): 91-96.
11. Baretta, R., and R. Robergs. 1995. Physiological training adaptations to a 14-week deep water exercise program. *Aquatic Physical Therapy Report* 3.
12. Bixler B., and S. Riewald. 2002. Analysis of a swimmer's hand and arm in steady flow conditions using computational fluid dynamics. *Journal of Biomechanics* 35 (5): 713-717.
13. Bonelli, S. 2001. *Aquatic Exercise.* American Council on Exercise Group Fitness Specialty Series. San Diego: American Council on Exercise.
14. Bonelli, S. 2000. *Step Training.* American Council on Exercise Group Fitness Specialty Series. San Diego: American Council on Exercise.
15. Bonzheim, S.C., B.A. Franklin, C. Dewitt, C. Marks, B. Goslin, R. Jarski, and S. Dann. 1992. Physiologic responses to recumbent versus upright cycle ergometry, and implications

for exercise prescription in patients with coronary artery disease. *American Journal of Cardiology* 69 (1): 40-44.

16. Bricker, K. 2000. *Traditional Aerobics*. American Council on Exercise Group Fitness Specialty Series. San Diego: American Council on Exercise.
17. Bryant, C.X., J. Wenson, and J.A. Peterson. 2000. Safe and enjoyable group cycling for your members. StairMaster Health & Fitness Products Web site. Retrieved November 13, 2002, from www.stairmaster.com/consumer/lifestyles/index.html.
18. Burke, E.R., ed. 1988. *The Science of Cycling*. Champaign, IL: Human Kinetics.
19. Burke, E.R. 1998. *Cycling Health and Physiology: Using Sports Science to Improve Your Riding and Racing*, 2nd ed. Montpelier, VT: Vitesse Press.
20. Bushman, B.A., M.G. Flynn, F.F. Andres, C.P. Lambert, M.S. Taylor, and W.A. Braun. 1997. Effect of four weeks of deep water run training on running performance. *Medicine and Science in Sports and Exercise* 29 (5): 694-699.
21. Christman, S.K., A.F. Fish, L. Bernhard, D.J. Frid, B.A. Smith, and L. Mitchell. 2000. Continuous handrail support, oxygen uptake, and heart rate in women during sub-maximal step treadmill exercise. *Research in Nursing and Health* 23 (1): 35-42.
22. Concept2. 2001. *Rowing Instruction Information*. Morrisville, VT: Concept2.
23. Convertino, V.A., L.E. Armstrong, E.F. Coyle, G.W. Mack, M.N. Sawka, L.C. Senay Jr., and W.M. Sherman. 1996. American College of Sports Medicine position stand. Exercise and fluid replacement. *Medicine and Science in Sports and Exercise* 28 (1): i-vii.
24. Deschodt, V.J., L.M. Arsac, and A.H. Rouard. 1999. Relative contribution of arms and legs in humans to propulsion in 25-m sprint front-crawl swimming. *European Journal of Applied Physiology and Occupational Physiology* 80 (3): 192-199.
25. Evans, M. 1997. *Endurance Athlete's Edge*. Champaign, IL: Human Kinetics, pp. 40-49.
26. Evans, M. 1997. *Endurance Athlete's Edge*. Champaign, IL: Human Kinetics, pp. 75-77, 93.
27. Francis, P., J. Poliner, M. Buono, and L. Francis. 1992. Effects of choreography, step height, fatigue and gender on metabolic cost of step training (abstract). *Medicine and Science in Sports and Exercise* 23 (S839).
28. Glover, B., and S.L. Florence Glover. 1999. *The Competitive Runner's Handbook*, rev. ed. New York: Penguin Books, pp. 336-337.
29. Hagberg, J.M., J.P. Mullin, M.D. Giese, and E. Spitznagel. 1981. Effect of pedaling rate on submaximal exercise responses of competitive cyclists. *Journal of Applied Physiology* 51 (2): 447-451.
30. Hagerman, F.C. 1994. *The Benefits of Indoor Rowing*. Morrisville, VT: Concept2.
31. Hannula, D. 1995. *Coaching Swimming Successfully*. Champaign, IL: Human Kinetics.
32. Hannula, D. 2003. *Coaching Swimming Successfully*, 2nd ed. Champaign, IL: Human Kinetics.
33. Hannula, D. and N. Thornton, eds. 2001. *The Swim Coaching Bible*. Champaign, IL: Human Kinetics.
34. Hartmann, S., and P. Bung. 1999. Physical exercise during pregnancy: Physiological considerations and recommendations. *Journal of Perinatal Medicine* 27 (3): 204-215.
35. Hobson, W., C. Cambell, and M. Vickers. 2001. *Swim, Bike, Run*. Champaign, IL: Human Kinetics, pp. 111-112.
36. Hobson, W., C. Cambell, and M. Vickers. 2001. *Swim, Bike, Run*. Champaign, IL: Human Kinetics, pp. 45-54.
37. Iknoian, T. 1998. *Walking Fast*. Champaign, IL: Human Kinetics, p. 40.
38. Jones, A.M., and J.H. Doust. 1996. A 1% treadmill grade most accurately reflects the energetic cost of outdoor running. *Journal of Sports Science* 14 (4): 321-327.
39. Kordich, J.A. 1994. *Stair Machine. Treadmill. Teaching Technique Series*. Colorado Springs, CO: National Strength and Conditioning Association.
40. Latzka, W.A., and S.J. Montain. 1999. Water and electrolyte requirements for exercise. *Clinical Sports Medicine* 18 (3): 513-524.
41. Lepers, R., G.Y. Millet, N.A. Maffiuletti, C. Hausswirth, and J. Brisswalter. 2001. Effect of pedaling rates on physiological response during endurance cycling. *European Journal of Applied Physiology* 85 (3-4): 392-395.
42. Lucia, A., J. Hoyos, and J.L. Chicharro. 2001. Preferred pedaling cadence in professional cycling. *Medicine and Science in Sports and Exercise* 33 (8): 1361-1366.
43. Mad Dogg Athletics. 2001. (Spinning) Safety guidelines. Spinning Web site. Retrieved November 13, 2002 from www.spinning.com.
44. Maybeck, J. 2000. Aqua beat—heart rate monitors make a splash! *The AKWA Letter* 6 (9): 13.
45. Mazzone, T. 1988. Kinesiology of the rowing stroke. *NSCA Journal* 10 (2): 4-13.
46. Michaud, T., J. Rodriguez-Zavas, C. Armstrong, et al. 1993. Ground recation forces in high impact and low impact aerobic dance. *The Journal of Sports Medicine and Physical Fitness* 33: 359-366.
47. Millqvist, E., B. Blake, U. Bengtsson, and O. Lowhagen. 1995. Prevention of asthma induced by cold air by cellulose-fabric face mask. *Allergy* 50 (3): 221-224.
48. Miyazaki, K. 1998. Impact loading on the foot and ankle and its attenuation during level walking. *Kurume Medical Journal* 45 (1): 75-80.
49. Morton, A.R., K. King, S. Papalia, C. Goodman, K.R. Turley, and J.H. Wilmore. 1995. Comparison of maximal oxygen consumption with oral and nasal breathing. *Australian Journal of Science and Medicine in Sport* 27 (3): 51-55.
50. Neptune, R.R., and W. Herzog. 1999. The association between negative muscle work and pedaling rate. *Journal of Biomechanics* 32 (10): 1021-1026.
51. Nilsson, J., and A. Thorstensson. 1989. Ground reaction forces at different speeds of human walking and running. *Acta Physiologica Scandinavica* 136 (2): 217-227.
52. Nordin, M., and V.H. Frankel. 1989. *Basic Biomechanics of the Musculoskeletal System*. Philadelphia: Lea & Febiger.
53. Ordas, T., and T. Rochford. 2000. *Kickboxing Fitness*. American Council on Exercise Group Fitness Specialty Series. San Diego: American Council on Exercise.
54. Powers, S.K., and E.T. Howley. 1990. *Exercise Physiology*. Dubuque, IA: Brown, p. 336.
55. Powers, S.K., and E.T. Howley. 1990. *Exercise Physiology*. Dubuque, IA: Brown, p. 332.
56. Reilly, D., and M. Martens. 1972. Experimental analysis of quadriceps muscle force and patellofemoral joint reaction force for various activities. *Acta Orthopedic Scandanavia* 43: 16-37.
57. Sanders, M.E., and N.E. Rippee. 1993. *Aquatic Fitness Instructor's Training Manual*. London: Speedo International, Limited.

58. Sanders, R. H., and A.M. Stewart. 1992. The biomechanics of swimming (part 1). *Swimming Technique (magazine)* May-June.

59. Scharff-Olson, M., and H. Williford. 1998. Step aerobics fulfills its promise. *ACSM's Health & Fitness Journal* 2: 32-37.

60. Sizer, F., and E. Whitney. 1994. *Nutrition: Concepts and Controversies,* 6th ed. St. Paul, MN: West, pp. 264-265.

61. Shih, J., Y.T. Wang, and M.H. Moeinzadeh. Effects of speed and experience on kinetic and kinematic factors during exercise on a stair-climbing machine. Unpublished. Department of Kinesiology, University of Illinois, Urbana, and Department of Research & Development/Sports Medicine, StairMaster Sports/Medical Products, Inc., Kirkland, WA.

62. Stairmaster Health & Fitness Products. 2000. *Lemond RevMaster Spin Bike Instructor's Manual.* Kirkland, WA: Stairmaster Health & Fitness Products.

63. Stairmaster Health & Fitness Products. 2001. *Stair Climbing: From Head to Toe.* Kirkland, WA: Stairmaster Health & Fitness Products.

64. Takaishi, T., Y. Yasuda, T. Ono, and T. Moritani. 1996. Optimal pedaling rate estimated from neuromuscular fatigue for cyclists. *Medicine and Science in Sports and Exercise* 28 (12): 1492-1497.

65. Thein, J.M., and L.T. Brody. 1998. Aquatic-based rehabilitation and training for the elite athlete. *Journal of Orthopaedic and Sports Physical Therapy* 27 (1): 32-41.

66. Thompson, C.E., and L.M. Wankel. 1980. The effects of perceived choice upon frequency of exercise behavior. *Journal of Applied Social Psychology* 10: 436-443.

67. Wilber, R.K., R.J. Moffatt, B.E. Scott, D.T. Lee, and N.A. Cucuzzo. 1996. Influence of water run training on the maintenance of aerobic performance. *Medicine and Science in Sports and Exercise* 28 (8): 1056-1062.

68. YMCA of the USA. 2000. *YMCA Water Fitness for Health.* Champaign, IL: Human Kinetics.

69. Zatsiorsky, V. M., ed. 2000. *Biomechanics in Sport: Performance Enhancement and Injury Prevention.* London: Blackwell Science.

PART IV

Program Design

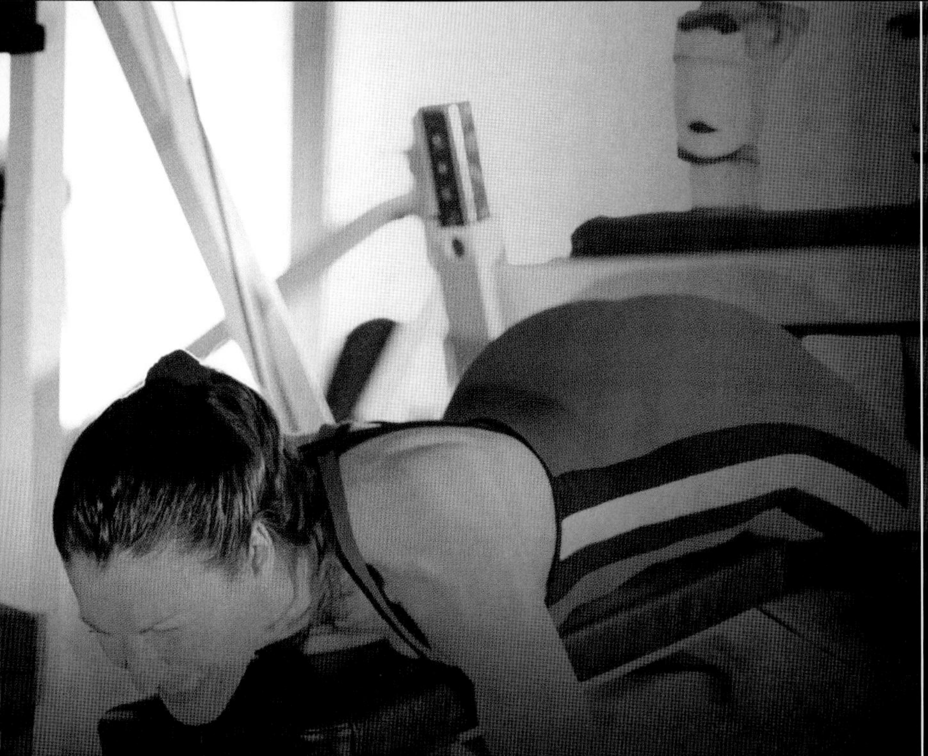

CHAPTER 15

Resistance Training Program Design

Roger W. Earle | Thomas R. Baechle

After completing this chapter, you will be able to

- understand the application of specificity, overload, and progression;
- select exercises, determine training frequency, and arrange exercises in a specific sequence;
- gather load-related information by performing 1-repetition maximum, percent of body weight, or repetition maximum testing;
- assign training loads, volume (as repetitions and sets), and rest period lengths;
- add variation to a client's resistance training program; and
- know when and how much to increase a training load.

Designing a safe and effective resistance training program involves the consideration and manipulation of certain variables that make resistance training programs more complex than aerobic exercise programs. The process begins with an initial consultation and fitness assessment to determine a client's resistance training status, exercise technique experience, and primary resistance training goal. The personal trainer then needs to consider what exercises to include in the program; how often the client will resistance train; the sequence of the selected exercises; the load, repetition, and set assignments; and the length of the rest periods. To promote the client's ongoing improvements and minimize overtraining, the personal trainer can apply the principles of variation and progression to the resistance training program.

General Training Principles

All effective exercise programs are based on three general training principles: specificity, overload, and progression. A program that attends to only one or two of the three principles can result in unmet client goals, poor adherence, and possible litigation due to injury.

Specificity

An important training principle was first identified 50 years ago [17] and is the foundation of every effective exercise program today. **Specificity** refers to training a client in a specific way to produce a specific change or result. For example, if a client wants to strengthen the muscles of the hips and thighs, he or she must perform an exercise such as the back squat that recruits the muscles of the hips and thighs, not the lat pulldown exercise, which trains the upper back.

Specificity also applies when a personal trainer needs to design a program for a client's activity or sport. The movement patterns of selected exercises should be very similar to the movements of the activity or sport. For example, if a client is a basketball player, the personal trainer should recognize that basketball involves repeated jumping movements. To mimic the lower body movements of jumping, the client could perform the power clean or the front (or back) squat exercise.

Overload

Even the most muscle- or activity-specific resistance training program will produce only limited results unless the client experiences **overload** (a training stress or intensity greater than what a client is used to). The most common application of overload is the amount of weight lifted in an exercise, but a personal trainer can also increase training stress by scheduling more workouts in a week, by having a client perform more sets of exercises, or by shortening the rest periods between sets.

Progression

Since a client's training status will improve over time, the personal trainer needs to apply the principle of **progression** so the training stress or intensity continues to be greater than what the client is accustomed to. The personal trainer, however, needs to be careful to overload and advance a client's program gradually and at a level that is proportionate to the client's training status.

All effective exercise programs are based on three general training principles: specificity, overload, and progression. A program that attends to only one or two of the three principles can result in unmet client goals, poor adherence, and possible litigation due to injury.

Components of a Resistance Training Program

Designing a resistance training program requires a personal trainer to manipulate or make decisions about the **program design variables**—certain components that create a safe, effective, and goal-specific exercise program. The rest of this chapter describes the components (listed in the box on page 363) that a personal trainer needs to consider when designing a resistance training program.

Initial Consultation and Fitness Evaluation

Before developing any exercise program, the personal trainer must conduct an initial client consultation to assess compatibility, establish a client-trainer agreement, and discuss exercise goals (see chapter 9). Following this, the personal trainer needs to evaluate the client's exercise history and current level of fitness to determine a baseline for improvement comparisons, identify current strengths and weaknesses, identify areas of potential injury or contraindications, and refine exercise goals (see chapter 10).

Components of a Resistance Training Program

- Initial consultation and fitness evaluation
- Choice (exercise selection)
- Frequency
- Order (exercise arrangement)
- Load (weight)
- Volume: repetitions (reps) and sets
- Rest periods
- Variation
- Progression

As the initial evaluation applies to designing a resistance training program, the personal trainer specifically needs to assess a client's initial resistance training status and exercise technique experience, conduct a fitness evaluation and analyze the results, and determine the client's primary goal for resistance training.

Initial Resistance Training Status and Experience

Two important factors that affect the design of the resistance training program are a client's current training status and exercise technique experience. Information about both is often revealed during the initial meeting between the personal trainer and the client (or soon thereafter) when the client's exercise history is discussed.

To determine a client's resistance training status, the client should answer the general exercise history questions listed on the Health/Medical Questionnaire (page 184). Then, to obtain more specific information, the personal trainer should ask the client these five questions:

- Are you currently following a resistance training program?
- How long have you been following a regular resistance training program?
- How many times per week do you resistance train?
- How difficult or intense are your resistance training workouts?
- What types and how many of resistance training exercises can you perform with proper technique?

It can be difficult to pigeonhole a specific client into a generalized training status classification; the professional knowledge and experience of the personal trainer are needed to interpret and objectify the client's responses. Table 15.1 provides one approach to classify a client's training status as beginner, intermediate, or advanced. The personal trainer asks the client the five assessment questions, and when the client's answers match the answers shown in at least three out of the five columns in one row, the estimated or predicted resistance training status is provided in the right-hand column.

Note that if a client is not currently resistance training but was following a regular resistance training program within the past four to six weeks, the personal trainer could consider the answer to question 1 a "yes" and the client could answer questions 2 through 5 based on that recent program. The decision to equate participation in a recent program with participation in a current resistance training program is based entirely on the personal trainer's professional judgment regarding that particular client.

The personal trainer should realize that one method of classifying resistance training status will not apply to *every* client; the unique characteristics of *each* client need to be considered.

Fitness Evaluation

In the fitness evaluation, the personal trainer typically measures a client's heart rate, blood pressure, body composition, height, weight, girth, muscular strength and endurance, cardiovascular endurance, and flexibility. In the context of this chapter, the fitness evaluation focuses on assessing or estimating a client's muscular strength. Personal trainers should refer to the "Load and Repetitions" discussion on page 370 and chapters 10 and 11 for a complete explanation.

After testing is complete, the personal trainer should compare the results with the normative or descriptive data presented in chapter 11 to assess a client's current level of fitness, set a baseline for future comparison as training status improves, and identify current strengths and weaknesses for goal setting.

TABLE 15.1

A Method to Classify Resistance Training Status

Question 1 Are you currently following a resistance training program?*	Question 2 How long have you been following a regular (1 or more times per week) resistance training program?	Question 3 How many times per week do you resistance train?	Question 4 How difficult or intense are your resistance training workouts?	Question 5 What types and how many of resistance training exercises can you perform with proper technique?**	Estimated resistance training status***
No	N/a	N/a	N/a	None	Beginner
Yes	≤2 months	1-2	Low	3-5 machine exercises	
Yes	4-6 months	2-3	Low to medium	6-10 machine core and assistance exercises; 3-5 free weight assistance exercises	
Yes	8-10 months	3	Medium	11-15 machine core and assistance exercises; 6-10 free weight assistance exercises; 3-5 free weight core exercises	Intermediate
Yes	1 year	4	Medium to high	>15 free weight and machine core and assistance exercises	
Yes	1-1 1/2 years	4	High	>15 free weight and machine core and assistance exercises; 3-5 power/explosive exercises	Advanced
Yes	2+ years	5+	Very high	>15 free weight and machine core and assistance exercises; most power/explosive exercises	

*If a client is not currently resistance training but was following a regular resistance training program within the past four to six weeks, the personal trainer could consider the answer to question 1 as a "yes" and the client could answer questions 2 through 5 based on that recent program. The decision to equate participation in a recent program with participation in a current resistance training program is based entirely on the personal trainer's professional judgment regarding that particular client.

**As determined or evaluated by a qualified personal trainer; refer to the section "Types of Resistance Training Exercises" on page 365 for a description of the various types of resistance exercises.

***Classification of resistance training status is determined when the client's answers match the answers shown in at least three out of the five columns in one row pertaining to resistance training exercise history and technique experience.

Note: The personal trainer should realize that this method of classifying resistance training status will not apply to *every* client; the unique characteristics of *each* client need to be considered.

Adapted from Baechle and Earle 2000.

Primary Resistance Training Goal

The critical piece of information personal trainers need to have before designing the resistance training program is a client's primary training goal or outcome. The specificity principle dictates that training a client in a specific way will produce a specific result, but also that to reach a specific goal a client has to follow a specific type of program. The three primary resistance training goals are muscular endurance, hypertrophy (muscle size or tone), and muscular strength.

Personal trainers may have to educate their clients about the specific results of the three primary goals of resistance training; it is uncommon for a client to say, for example, "I want to follow a resistance training program for hypertrophy." Often, the client's training goal is not clearly identified until after the initial client consultation and fitness evaluation.

Muscular Endurance

A client may allude to muscular endurance as the desired resistance training goal by saying, for example, "I want to have better endurance" or "I want to have more stamina." The outcome of training for greater muscular endurance is an enhanced ability of the targeted muscles to perform at a submaximal level for many repetitions or for an extended duration. A common example is what the muscles do during an aerobic workout: the lower body muscles contract and relax thousands of times during a 20-minute run.

Hypertrophy

Statements like "I want my arms to be bigger," "I want more size," "I want to be more sculpted," or "I want to change my appearance" may signal that a client wants to follow a resistance training program that will result in increased muscular hypertrophy.

Muscular Strength

Often clients who wish to gain muscular strength will state directly, "I want to get stronger." Commonly these individuals are athletes who are interested in following a resistance training program to encourage improvements in athletic performance. Compared to training for muscular endurance and hypertrophy, training loads used for developing strength are heavier. Therefore, unless the client is already well resistance trained, he or she should become accustomed to "strength" training by following a hypertrophy or muscular endurance training program first.

The three primary resistance training goals are muscular endurance, hypertrophy (muscle size or tone), and muscular strength.

Choice

Exercise choice (also called **exercise selection**) involves picking exercises that a client will perform during a resistance training workout. Exercise selection is influenced by the specificity principle, how much time the client has to exercise, what equipment is available, and the client's experience with correctly performing resistance exercises. After consideration of these issues, the personal trainer selects resistance exercises based on their characteristics or type.

Influential Factors

First, the personal trainer should choose exercises based on the specificity principle; to train certain muscle groups, the personal trainer should select only those exercises that will actually encourage improvements in those muscle groups.

The personal trainer should also choose exercises based on how much time a client has available for each session. This factor affects not only the number of exercises that can be performed, but also the complexity of the exercises. Some exercises simply take longer to do. For example, a set of the alternating dumbbell curl exercise takes longer than a set of the (two-armed) barbell biceps curl exercise.

The personal trainer must also consider equipment availability when choosing resistance exercises. Despite any outstanding or goal-specific benefit of an exercise, the personal trainer cannot include a given exercise in a client's program if the equipment is not available. An inventory list of the equipment at a client's facility can be a helpful resource for a personal trainer to refer to when selecting exercises.

The most important factor is that the client can perform the exercises correctly. If a client is inexperienced in or not familiar with the proper technique of a certain exercise, or if the extent of a client's experience is unknown, the personal trainer must provide a thorough demonstration and complete instruction. This precaution is an effective strategy to reduce litigation, promote adherence, and improve success. Inexperienced clients are often taught machine exercises or free weight assistance exercises first because these require less skill than free weight core exercises [24, 27, 77, 89].

Exercise selection is influenced by the specificity principle, how much time a client has to exercise, what equipment is available, and the client's experience at correctly performing resistance exercises.

Types of Resistance Training Exercises

A personal trainer can select from among many resistance exercises, but all can be classified as either *core* or *assistance* based on the extent of joint involvement, size of the recruited muscle areas, and degree of contribution toward the client's exercise goals.

Core Exercises

A personal trainer should preferentially choose **core exercises** for a client's program because they are typically more effective at helping clients reach their exercise goals. A core exercise must meet these two criteria:

- It should involve movement at two or more primary joints (a **multijoint exercise**).
- It should recruit one or more large muscle groups or areas (i.e., chest, shoulders, upper back, hips/thighs) with the synergistic help of one or more smaller muscle groups or areas (i.e., biceps, triceps, abdominals, calves, neck, forearms, lower back, or shins). One core exercise can affect as many muscles or muscle groups as four to eight assistance exercises [75].

For example, the bench press exercise is a core exercise because it involves movement principally at the shoulder and elbow joints and recruits the large chest muscles with the synergistic help of the anterior deltoids and the triceps brachii muscles.

A core exercise that places an axial stress (or load) on the spine (e.g., power clean, shoulder press, back squat) is also called a **structural exercise.** More exactly, a structural exercise requires the torso muscles to maintain an erect or near-erect posture when performing the exercise (e.g., keeping the upper body in the correct vertical position during the upward and downward movement phases of the shoulder press exercise). A structural exercise that is performed very quickly is further classified as a **power** or **explosive exercise** (e.g., push press, power clean, snatch, high pull).

Assistance Exercises

Not all exercises need to be precisely applicable to reaching a client's exercise goals. Often, clients perform **assistance exercises** to maintain muscular balance across joints, help prevent injury or rehabilitate a previous injury, or isolate a specific muscle or muscle group. An assistance exercise must meet these two criteria:

- It must involve movement at only one primary joint (a **single-joint exercise**).
- It must recruit a smaller muscle group or only one large muscle group or area.

For example, the barbell biceps curl exercise involves movement only at the elbow joints and recruits a small muscle group (i.e., the biceps brachii). The pec deck and dumbbell fly are also assistance exercises because they involve movement only at the shoulders and primarily focus on the muscles of the chest, despite the fact that the chest is a large muscle area.

Guidelines to Follow When Choosing Exercises

There are two main strategies that a personal trainer can use when selecting exercises for a client's resistance training program. These guidelines can be used together or independently depending on the unique needs of the client.

One Exercise per Muscle Group

This guideline can be used with a beginner (i.e., untrained). It is a basic approach that involves choosing one exercise for each muscle group or area commonly trained in a resistance workout: chest, shoulders, upper back, hips/thighs, biceps, triceps, abdominals, and calves [4, 65]. An intermediate program may include two exercises per muscle group, different exercises for each muscle group throughout the week, or both [65].

Client-Specific Exercises

For a client with a specialized condition like severe deconditioning, low back pain, or recent injury, or for a client on the opposite end of the wellness continuum (i.e., a well-trained athlete), the resistance training program can be "specialized" to concentrate directly (or only) on the client's particular needs. Thus, the personal trainer selects exercises—under the guidance of a medical professional, if necessary—that include movements addressing the client's specialized condition and exclude movements that are contraindicated or not recommended.

For example, if a client was recently released from the care of a physical therapist for a shoulder impingement, the dumbbell lateral raise could be an effective exercise to select, but the overhead shoulder press exercise would not be recommended. For an athlete, the more closely the resistance exercises mimic the movement patterns of the sport, the greater their enhancive carryover to that sport [11, 20, 24, 27, 42, 59, 62, 77, 84]. Therefore, a personal trainer would include the power clean exercise in a program for a basketball or volleyball player to imitate the jumping movements of those sports. (Refer to chapter 23 for guidelines on selecting exercises for a sport.)

Frequency

Training **frequency** commonly refers to the number of workouts a client performs in one week. Actual frequency is influenced by a client's training status, the impact of other activities or exercise, and the client's personal schedule.

Influential Factors

The personal trainer should determine training frequency based primarily on a client's resistance training status. Less-trained clients require more rest between workouts, which lowers the training frequency. Conversely, the more highly trained the client is, the fewer rest days he or she needs between training sessions and the more sessions the personal trainer can schedule in a week. Note, however, that the frequency of resistance training workouts may need to be reduced if the client's overall amount of physical stress is high [16] as a consequence of other demands (e.g., job responsibilities, other forms of exercise, or both). For example, if the client is a construction worker or is already running for 30 minutes three days a week, he or she may not want (or feel up to) resistance training three additional days a week.

Training frequency is influenced by a client's training status, the impact of other activities or exercise, and the client's personal schedule.

Guidelines to Follow When Determining Training Frequency

To allow sufficient recovery, the personal trainer should schedule the training sessions so there is at least one day (but not more than three) between workouts that stress the same muscle group or groups [3, 10, 40, 65]. More specific guidelines depend on a client's resistance training status. A beginner client (as classified during the initial consultation) can usually resistance train two or three times per week, an intermediate client three or four times per week, and an advanced client four or more times per week (table 15.2) [3, 28, 45, 65].

Beginner Resistance Training Status

A beginner program involves two or three sessions per week that are evenly spaced out (e.g., Monday and Thursday; Monday, Wednesday, and Friday). This spacing is important because, for example, a Monday and Wednesday training schedule allows too much rest from the Wednesday workout to the following Monday (i.e., more than three days) [28, 40].

TABLE 15.2

Guidelines for Resistance Training Frequency

Resistance training status	Recommended number of sessions per week
Beginner	2-3
Intermediate	3-4
Advanced	4+

Adapted from Atha 1981; Graves, Pollock, Leggett, Braith, Carpenter, and Bishop 1988; Kraemer, Noble, Clark, and Culver 1987; and Pearson, Faigenbaum, Conley, and Kraemer 2000.

Intermediate or Advanced Status: Split Routine

Better-trained clients can tolerate more than three sessions per week, but the odd number of days in a week means that clients in this category have to train multiple days in a row to increase frequency. A **split routine** schedules four or more workouts evenly spread out in one week but with each workout including exercises that train only a part of the body (e.g., upper body or lower body) or certain muscle areas (e.g., chest, back, or legs). The result is an increased training frequency with sufficient recovery between workouts that involve the same exercises [65].

A common example of a four times per week split routine for intermediate or advanced clients is upper body exercises on Monday and Thursday and lower body exercises on Tuesday and Friday. Although the client resistance trains two days in a row (e.g., Monday and Tuesday), the workouts stress different muscle groups (e.g., upper body on Monday and lower body on Tuesday), and there are two days of rest before the client has to repeat the same workout (e.g., after Monday, the next upper body day is not until Thursday). The rest days (or at least the non-resistance training days) in this example are consistently Sundays, Wednesdays, and Saturdays. (A second option is to perform the chest and shoulder exercises twice a week and the lower body and back exercises twice a week [65].)

The next progression in training frequency for an advanced client is a "three days on, one day off" split routine that yields five to six workouts per week. The personal trainer creates three distinct workouts that train different muscle groups, and the client completes one workout on three consecutive days and rests on the fourth day. A common strategy is to divide the resistance training program into upper body "push" exercises (i.e., chest, shoulders, and triceps), lower body exercises, and upper body "pull" exercises (i.e., upper back, trapezius, and biceps). In contrast to the previous examples, the workouts are on unspecified days; that is, the rest days are not the same each week.

Order

Exercise order or **arrangement** refers to placing the exercises in a specific sequence within a resistance training workout. Exercise arrangement is influenced by the specificity principle but is primarily dictated by the type and characteristics of the selected exercises.

Influential Factors

Exercises can be arranged in order of descending priority or application to a client's training goal, activity, or sport. Thus, the client performs the more goal-specific exercises earlier in the workout and the less goal-specific exercises toward the end of the workout. (Refer to the discussion of training specificity at the beginning of the chapter for examples.)

To maximize a client's ability to complete all the exercises in one workout, the personal trainer should arrange the selected exercises in an order such that fatigue caused by one exercise has the least possible impact on the quality of effort or the technique of the next exercise [6]. The way to reach this goal is to arrange exercises based on their type (core or assistance) and other characteristics such as the targeted muscle area and the nature of the exercise movement.

> Exercise arrangement is influenced by the specificity principle but is dictated primarily by the type and characteristics of the selected exercises.

Guidelines to Follow When Arranging Exercises

There are many ways to arrange exercises within a resistance training session [24], but most can be categorized within several primary methods (see "Examples of Ordering Resistance Training Exercises" on page 369 for examples) and two secondary methods.

Power, Other Core, Then Assistance Exercises

One guideline directs the personal trainer to arrange all of the power exercises at the beginning of the resistance training session, the remaining core exercises (note that power exercises are also classified as core exercises) next, and the assistance exercises last [24, 71, 79]. This is an effective exercise sequence because power exercises require more effort, skill, and focus than non-power core or assistance exercises [24] and thus should be performed first. Most clients, unless they are athletes, probably will not have power exercises assigned to them, so the exercise arrangement becomes *core exercises and then assistance exercises.*

It is important to mention that many references also include *multijoint exercises first and then single-joint exercises,* or *exercises that train large muscle groups first and then exercises that train small muscle groups,* as ways to arrange exercises [7, 19, 24, 62, 65, 71, 77, 81]. Both of these additional methods are effective, but their applications are nearly parallel to those of the *power, other core, and then assistance exercises* method because power and core exercises are multijoint and train large muscle areas. Further, assistance exercises are single-joint movements stressing smaller muscle groups.

Alternate "Push" and "Pull" Exercises

Another method that provides necessary rest between exercises to maintain effort and technique is to alternate "pushing" exercises (e.g., vertical chest press and triceps pushdown) with "pulling" exercises (e.g., seated row and dumbbell biceps curl) [7]. This push-pull sequencing guarantees that the same muscle group will not be used for two exercises in a row, thus diminishing fatigue in the involved muscles [6]. This arrangement is a good option for untrained individuals or clients resuming resistance training after an injury or a vacation [7, 24].

Alternate Upper and Lower Body Exercises

If an untrained client is not able to tolerate performing several upper or lower body exercises in a row [24, 62], or if a trained client with less available training time wants to cut back on the length of the rest intervals to shorten the workout, he or she can alternate upper body exercises with lower body exercises. If a client is somewhat conditioned, a lower body exercise can immediately follow an upper body exercise without needing to rest very long.

Examples of Ordering Resistance Training Exercises

Power, other core, then assistance exercises

1. Power clean
2. Push press
3. Front squat
4. Bench press
5. Seated row
6. Triceps pushdown
7. Wrist curl
8. Seated heel raise

Multijoint exercises first and then single-joint exercises

1. Back squat
2. Leg press
3. Bench press
4. Lat pulldown
5. Biceps curl
6. Lying triceps extension
7. Lateral raise
8. Wrist extension

Exercises that train large muscle groups first and then exercises that train small muscle groups

1. Front squat
2. Back squat
3. Bench press
4. Shoulder press
5. Seated row
6. Abdominal crunch
7. Biceps curl
8. Triceps pushdown

Alternate "push" and "pull" exercises

1. Back squat
2. Leg curl
3. Standing heel raise
4. Upright row
5. Incline bench press
6. Dumbbell biceps curl
7. Shoulder press
8. Lat pulldown

Alternate upper body exercises and lower body exercises

1. Hip sled
2. Bench press
3. Lunge
4. Shoulder shrug
5. Leg (knee) extension
6. Dumbbell shoulder press
7. Leg (knee) curl
8. Triceps extension

Core exercises and then assistance exercises combined with alternated "push" and "pull" exercises

1. Back squat
2. Leg (knee) curl
3. Standing heel raise
4. Incline bench press
5. Lat pulldown
6. Shoulder press
7. Hammer curl
8. Overhead triceps extension

These lists are *not* representative of a *complete* resistance training workout.

Combination of Arrangement Methods

One of the most common methods of arranging exercises is to combine two of the previously mentioned methods: *core exercises and then assistance exercises* and *alternate "push" and "pull" exercises.* Often the lower body exercises are performed first and then the upper body exercises within the context of the combined arrangement methods. This sequencing offers one of the best strategies for minimizing the effect of fatigue for clients of all resistance training levels.

Compound Sets and Supersets

Two secondary methods of ordering exercises that involves completing a set of two different exercises in succession without an intervening rest period. If the two exercises train the same primary muscle group (e.g., bench press and dumbbell fly), the set is called a **compound set** [7]. If the two exercises stress opposing or antagonistic muscle groups (e.g., bench press and seated row), the set is called a **superset** [7, 77]. These methods of ordering and completing both exercises are time efficient and purposely more demanding, and consequently may not be appropriate for untrained clients [6].

Load and Repetitions

Determining the **load** or proper amount of weight for a client to lift is the most difficult but arguably the most important program design variable that the personal trainer considers when developing a resistance training program [24, 27, 55, 63, 77]. Then, lifting a given load, a client will be able to perform an exercise only a certain number of times (**repetitions** or **reps**). The assigned load lifted and the number of repetitions that can be performed are influenced by a client's primary resistance training goal and by each other (i.e., the percent of 1RM-repetition relationship).

Determining a client's load and repetition scheme is a two-step process. First, the personal trainer needs to perform some type of testing to gather information about a client's capability or ability to handle loads for the selected exercises. The personal trainer then assigns the actual training loads.

Influential Factors

As dictated by the specificity principle, load and repetitions are intimately associated with a client's primary resistance training goal. For example, lifting heavy loads for a low number of repetitions increases muscular strength, whereas lifting light loads for a high number of repetitions increases muscular endurance. Alternatively, focusing on the client's primary training goal automatically implies or requires a certain load and a certain number of repetitions: Increasing muscular strength requires lifting heavy loads for few repetitions, and increasing muscular endurance requires lifting light loads for many repetitions.

Load and repetitions should be based on the client's primary resistance training goal.

Percent of 1RM-Repetition Relationship

There is an inverse relationship between the load assigned and the number of repetitions a client can perform with that load; that is, the lighter the load assigned for any exercise, the greater the number of repetitions that can be performed. Conversely, the heavier the load, the lower the number of repetitions that can be performed. This association is referred to as the **percent of 1RM-repetition relationship.** As a load becomes heavier, the number of repetitions a client can lift it decreases; eventually the load becomes so heavy that the client can perform only one repetition with proper technique. This maximum load is the client's **one-repetition maximum (1RM)** for that exercise.

Resistance training loads are assigned either as a percentage of the 1RM (%1RM) or as a specified **repetition maximum (RM)** that is the heaviest load lifted for a certain number of repetitions [17]. For example, if a client provides a maximal effort to complete 15 repetitions—not more or less than 15—with 100 pounds (45 kilograms) in the leg press exercise, the client's 15RM (in that exercise only) is 100 pounds.

Table 15.3 presents the relationship between a given %1RM and the number of repetitions that can be performed with that load. At 100% of the 1RM, only one repetition can be performed. As the loads become lighter (i.e., the %1RM decreases), more repetitions can be performed, but there are slight variations in the specific numbers according to the reference [4, 6, 13, 14, 21, 47, 53, 57, 86]. The intent in table 15.3 is to report the most common values.

Limitations in the %1RM-Repetition Relationships

A %1RM-repetition relationship table (e.g., table 15.3) is a valuable tool for determining training loads, but a personal trainer must be aware of a

TABLE 15.3

Percent of 1RM-Repetition Relationship

%1RM*	Estimated number of repetitions that can be performed
100	1
95	2
93	3
90	4
87	5
85	6
83	7
80	8
77	9
75	10
70	11
67	12
65	15

*The percentages vary slightly (±0.5-2%) based upon the reference. Refer to the section "Limitations in the %1RM-Repetition Relationships" that begins on page 370 for discussion about the limitations of this table.

Adapted from Baechle and Earle 1995; Baechle and Earle 2000; Brzycki 1993; Chapman, Whitehead, and Binkert 1998; Epley 1985; Lander 1984; Mayhew, Ball, Arnold, and Bowen 1992; Morales and Sobonya 1996; and Wathen 1994.

number of limitations that influence the accuracy of this relationship:

- The %1RM-repetition tables imply a direct association between the loads lifted and the number of repetitions that can be performed, but several studies do not support this [49, 53, 54].
- Well-trained clients often can perform more repetitions at a given %1RM [38, 39].
- The number of repetitions that can be performed at a certain %1RM applies only to one set, not multiple sets (i.e., fatigue typically leads to fewer repetitions in sequential sets) [86].
- The associations between the loads lifted and the number of repetitions that can be performed largely stem from research involving only three resistance exercises (bench press, back squat, power clean) [24, 81]; the same %1RM-repetition relationship does not apply to all exercises [38, 39].
- It has been reported [38, 39] that more repetitions at any %1RM can be completed with a machine version (e.g., vertical chest press) of a free weight exercise (e.g., barbell bench press).
- Often, a client cannot perform as many repetitions for an assistance exercise at any %1RM as he or she can for a core exercise [66, 81].

A personal trainer will likely have the most success with table 15.3 for loads ≥75% of the 1RM for ≤10 repetitions [2, 13, 14, 73, 85], because it appears that the %1RM-repetition relationship loses its level of accuracy as the loads decrease and the repetitions increase [6]. Therefore, the personal trainer should use table 15.3 as a guideline rather than a rule.

Guidelines to Follow When Assessing Load Capabilities

Before assigning a training load, the personal trainer needs to perform an assessment to determine a client's capability to handle loads for the selected exercises using one or more of these primary methods:

- Directly testing or estimating the 1RM
- Using a percentage of a client's body weight for testing
- Performing RM testing

The personal trainer chooses one method or a combination of all these methods based on a client's training status, exercise technique experience, and the characteristics and type of exercises selected [6].

1-Repetition Maximum Determination

To be able to use table 15.3, the personal trainer must first determine a client's 1RM. Some clients are able to tolerate the progressively increasing loads of 1RM testing; but for others, either because their training status is too low or because they lack sufficient exercise technique experience, such an assessment is not warranted. Although it is more accurate to assign loads based on a percentage of a test-established 1RM than on a 1RM estimated from a submaximal load [37, 39, 59, 72], both of the following methods can be used at the personal trainer's discretion.

Directly Testing the 1-Repetition Maximum Clients who are untrained, have little or no experience, are currently or were recently injured, or are under medical supervision are not recommended to perform maximal strength testing. This type of evaluation is more often recommended and more effective for intermediate or advanced clients who also have experience with properly performing the exercise used for testing. Further, only core exercises qualify for safe and effective 1RM testing; maximal strength testing for assistance exercises is typically not recommended [7, 19] due to the high physiological stress that would be applied to smaller muscle groups across a single joint. The larger and multiple muscle groups involved in a core exercise can tolerate heavy loads, but the personal trainer should still examine each exercise for suitability for 1RM testing. Above all, an exercise should be selected for 1RM testing only if it can safely, accurately, and consistently assess maximal strength [6].

For example, although the bent-over row exercise involves the large upper back muscles that function across several joints, the weaker lower back muscles may not be able to maintain proper body position after several testing sets, and the 1RM would be compromised. Furthermore, even though multijoint exercises like the lunge or the step-up use large and multiple muscle groups, they should not be selected for 1RM testing because they apply uneven loads to the lower body that can result in accident or injury. If, after the consideration of these limitations, an exercise still qualifies for 1RM testing, the personal trainer can refer to chapter 11 for a suggested protocol.

1RM testing is not recommended for clients who are untrained, have little or no experience, are currently or were recently injured, or are under medical supervision.

Estimating the 1-Repetition Maximum An indirect method to determine a client's 1RM is to first perform 10RM testing (i.e., the heaviest load that can be lifted 10 times with proper technique) and then estimate the 1RM from the 10RM. This method is acceptable for nearly all exercises and for most clients, as long as they know how to properly perform the exercise; only those who may become quickly fatigued from the multiple repetitions and testing sets should be excluded (their results would likely be inaccurate). For any client or exercise, the personal trainer should determine the 10RM within three testing sets.

The personal trainer follows the same approach for 10RM testing as for 1RM testing, except that the client is directed to perform 10 repetitions in each testing set instead of one. Also, because more repetitions are performed, the load changes across testing sets should be smaller (about 50% of the amounts suggested in the 1RM testing protocol described in chapter 11).

After determining a client's 10RM, the personal trainer can use table 15.4 to estimate the 1RM. In the "Max reps (RM) 10, %1RM 75" column, read down to locate the number closest to (but not greater than) the client's 10RM; then read left across the row to the "Max reps (RM) 1, %1RM 100" column to see the client's estimated 1RM. For example, if a client's 10RM for the leg press exercise is 105 pounds, the estimated 1RM is 140 pounds. (See the section "Based on the 1-Repetition Maximum" for a further application of this example for assigning an actual training load.)

Percent of Body-Weight Testing

A second method for gathering information needed to assign a training load is to perform testing using a certain percentage of a client's body weight (%BWT) [5, 7]. This type of assessment is acceptable for core or assistance exercises and for clients who are untrained or inexperienced (the personal trainer can explain and demonstrate proper technique) because the calculated testing loads are often relatively light. Well-trained clients should not use this method because of their greater ratio of strength to body weight and because the training loads will end up being too light.

The protocol for this assessment method is shown in "Protocol for Testing with a Percentage of a Client's Body Weight" on page 376. In short, the personal trainer uses an exercise-specific numerical factor from table 15.5 to determine a **trial load** for a client to try out during testing that is a certain percent of the client's body weight. To account for differences in body composition, the personal trainer should use a maximum body weight of 175 pounds (79 kilograms) for male clients and 140 pounds (64 kilograms) for female clients. Following instruction and warm-up, the client performs as many consecutive repetitions as possible with proper exercise technique.

TABLE 15.4

Estimating a 1-Repetition Maximum From a Training Load

Max reps (RM)	1	2	3	4	5	6	7	8	9	10	12	15
%1RM*	**100**	**95**	**93**	**90**	**87**	**85**	**83**	**80**	**77**	**75**	**67**	**65**
Load** (lb or kg)	5	5	5	5	4	4	4	4	4	4	3	3
	10	10	9	9	9	9	8	8	8	8	7	7
	15	14	14	14	13	13	12	12	12	11	10	10
	20	19	19	18	17	17	17	16	15	15	13	13
	25	24	23	23	22	21	21	20	19	19	17	16
	30	29	28	27	26	26	25	24	23	23	20	20
	35	33	33	32	30	30	29	28	27	26	23	23
	40	38	37	36	35	34	33	32	31	30	27	26
	45	43	42	41	39	38	37	36	35	34	30	29
	50	48	47	45	44	43	42	40	39	38	34	33
	55	52	51	50	48	47	46	44	42	41	37	36
	60	57	56	54	52	51	50	48	46	45	40	39
	65	62	60	59	57	55	54	52	50	49	44	42
	70	67	65	63	61	60	58	56	54	53	47	46
	75	71	70	68	65	64	62	60	58	56	50	49
	80	76	74	72	70	68	66	64	62	60	54	52
	85	81	79	77	74	72	71	68	65	64	57	55
	90	86	84	81	78	77	75	72	69	68	60	59
	95	90	88	86	83	81	79	76	73	71	64	62
	100	95	93	90	87	85	83	80	77	75	67	65
	105	100	98	95	91	89	87	84	81	79	70	68
	110	105	102	99	96	94	91	88	85	83	74	72
	115	109	107	104	100	98	95	92	89	86	77	75
	120	114	112	108	104	102	100	96	92	90	80	78
	125	119	116	113	109	106	104	100	96	94	84	81
	130	124	121	117	113	111	108	104	100	98	87	85
	135	128	126	122	117	115	112	108	104	101	90	88
	140	133	130	126	122	119	116	112	108	105	94	91

(continued)

TABLE 15.4 *(continued)*

Max reps (RM)	1	2	3	4	5	6	7	8	9	10	12	15
%1RM*	**100**	**95**	**93**	**90**	**87**	**85**	**83**	**80**	**77**	**75**	**67**	**65**
Load** (lb or kg)	145	138	135	131	126	123	120	116	112	109	97	94
	150	143	140	135	131	128	125	120	116	113	101	98
	155	147	144	140	135	132	129	124	119	116	104	101
	160	152	149	144	139	136	133	128	123	120	107	104
	165	157	153	149	144	140	137	132	127	124	111	107
	170	162	158	153	148	145	141	136	131	128	114	111
	175	166	163	158	152	149	145	140	135	131	117	114
	180	171	167	162	157	153	149	144	139	135	121	117
	185	176	172	167	161	157	154	148	142	139	124	120
	190	181	177	171	165	162	158	152	146	143	127	124
	195	185	181	176	170	166	162	156	150	146	131	127
	200	190	186	180	174	170	166	160	154	150	134	130
	210	200	195	189	183	179	174	168	162	158	141	137
	220	209	205	198	191	187	183	176	169	165	147	143
	230	219	214	207	200	196	191	184	177	173	154	150
	240	228	223	216	209	204	199	192	185	180	161	156
	250	238	233	225	218	213	208	200	193	188	168	163
	260	247	242	234	226	221	206	208	200	195	174	169
	270	257	251	243	235	230	224	216	208	203	181	176
	280	266	260	252	244	238	232	224	216	210	188	182
	290	276	270	261	252	247	241	232	223	218	194	189
	300	285	279	270	261	255	249	240	231	225	201	195
	310	295	288	279	270	264	257	248	239	233	208	202
	320	304	298	288	278	272	266	256	246	240	214	208
	330	314	307	297	287	281	274	264	254	248	221	215
	340	323	316	306	296	289	282	272	262	255	228	221
	350	333	326	315	305	298	291	280	270	263	235	228
	360	342	335	324	313	306	299	288	277	270	241	234
	370	352	344	333	322	315	307	296	285	278	248	241
	380	361	353	342	331	323	315	304	293	285	255	247

Max reps (RM)	1	2	3	4	5	6	7	8	9	10	12	15
%1RM*	**100**	**95**	**93**	**90**	**87**	**85**	**83**	**80**	**77**	**75**	**67**	**65**
Load** (lb or kg)	390	371	363	351	339	332	324	312	300	293	261	254
	400	380	372	360	348	340	332	320	308	300	268	260
	410	390	381	369	357	349	340	328	316	308	274	267
	420	399	391	378	365	357	349	336	323	315	281	273
	430	409	400	387	374	366	357	344	331	323	288	280
	440	418	409	396	383	374	365	352	339	330	295	286
	450	428	419	405	392	383	374	360	347	338	302	293
	460	437	428	414	400	391	382	368	354	345	308	299
	470	447	437	423	409	400	390	376	362	353	315	306
	480	456	446	432	418	408	398	384	370	360	322	312
	490	466	456	441	426	417	407	392	377	368	328	319
	500	475	465	450	435	425	415	400	385	375	335	325
	510	485	474	459	444	434	423	408	393	383	342	332
	520	494	484	468	452	442	432	416	400	390	348	338
	530	504	493	477	461	451	440	424	408	398	355	345
	540	513	502	486	470	459	448	432	416	405	362	351
	550	523	512	495	479	468	457	440	424	413	369	358
	560	532	521	504	487	476	465	448	431	420	375	364
	570	542	530	513	496	485	473	456	439	428	382	371
	580	551	539	522	505	493	481	464	447	435	389	377
	590	561	549	531	513	502	490	472	454	443	395	384
	600	570	558	540	522	510	498	480	462	450	402	390

*The percentages vary slightly (±0.5-2%) based on the reference. Refer to the section "Estimating the 1-Repetition Maximum" on page 372 for an explanation of how to estimate a client's 1RM from a 10RM load.

**When possible, the personal trainer should round the load *down* to the nearest 5-pound (or 5-kilogram) increment.

Adapted from Baechle and Earle 1989; Baechle and Earle 2000; Brzycki 1993; Chapman, Whitehead, and Binkert 1998; Epley 1985; Lombardi 1989; Mayhew, Ball, Arnold, and Bowen 1992; Morales and Sobonya 1996; and Wathen 1994.

The goal or intended outcome of %BWT testing is that a client can perform between 12 and 15 repetitions with the trial load. Despite this, resistance training equipment variety and client individuality make perfect calculated testing loads impossible. The results of the %BWT testing protocol can, however, serve as a valuable starting point for determining training loads.

For example, suppose that a 165-pound male client will be %BWT tested in the free weight standing shoulder press exercise. According to table 15.5, his trial load is 60 pounds (i.e., 165 × 0.38 = 62.7;

Protocol for Testing With a Percentage of a Client's Body Weight

1. Locate the exercise to be tested in the middle column of table 15.5. There are two types of machine exercises, so the personal trainer should examine the actual piece of equipment to differentiate a cam machine (CM) from a pivot machine (PM).
2. Fill in the client's body weight (BWT); note that there are separate sections for men and women. The personal trainer should use a maximum body weight of 175 pounds (79 kilograms) for male clients and 140 pounds (64 kilograms) for female clients. Clients weighing less than these amounts should use their actual body weight.
3. Multiply the body weight by the "factor" (i.e., the percentage expressed as a decimal), round down to the nearest 5-pound increment or the closest weight stack plate, and fill in this number in the "Trial load" column.
4. Explain and demonstrate proper technique; then ask the client to perform several repetitions with little or no weight. If the client can perform the exercise correctly, have him or her warm up by performing about 10 repetitions with approximately one-half of the trial load.
5. Allow a one- to three-minute rest period; then change the weight to the calculated trial load and direct the client to perform as many consecutive repetitions as possible with proper exercise technique.
6. Record the number of repetitions the client was able to perform in the "Reps completed" column.

Adapted from Baechle and Groves 1998 and Baechle and Earle 1995.

TABLE 15.5

Determining Loads for Percent of Body-Weight Testing

BWT	Factor	Trial load	Reps completed	Adjustment	Training load	Exercise	BWT	Factor	Trial load	Reps completed	Adjustment	Training load
	Women					**Chest**			**Men**			
____	× 0.35 =	____	____	____	____	Bench press (FW)	____	× 0.60 =	____	____	____	____
____	× 0.27 =	____	____	____	____	Bent-arm fly (CM)	____	× 0.55 =	____	____	____	____
____	× 0.27 =	____	____	____	____	Chest press (PM)	____	× 0.55 =	____	____	____	____
						Back						
____	× 0.35 =	____	____	____	____	Bent-over row (FW)	____	× 0.45 =	____	____	____	____
____	× 0.20 =	____	____	____	____	Seated row (CM)	____	× 0.40 =	____	____	____	____
____	× 0.20 =	____	____	____	____	Pull-over exercise (CM)	____	× 0.40 =	____	____	____	____
____	× 0.25 =	____	____	____	____	Seated row (PM)	____	× 0.45 =	____	____	____	____
						Shoulders						
____	× 0.22 =	____	____	____	____	Standing press (FW)	____	× 0.38 =	____	____	____	____
____	× 0.15 =	____	____	____	____	Seated press (PM)	____	× 0.35 =	____	____	____	____
____	× 0.25 =	____	____	____	____	Shoulder press (CM)	____	× 0.40 =	____	____	____	____
						Biceps						
____	× 0.23 =	____	____	____	____	Biceps curl (FW)	____	× 0.30 =	____	____	____	____
____	× 0.12 =	____	____	____	____	Preacher curl (CM)	____	× 0.20 =	____	____	____	____

BWT	Factor	Trial load	Reps completed	Adjust-ment	Training load	Exercise	BWT	Factor	Trial load	Reps completed	Adjust-ment	Training load
	Women					**Biceps**		Men				
___	× 0.15 =	___	___	___	___	Low pulley curl (PM)	___	× 0.25 =	___	___	___	___
						Triceps						
___	× 0.12 =	___	___	___	___	Triceps extension (FW)	___	× 0.21 =	___	___	___	___
___	× 0.13 =	___	___	___	___	Triceps extension (CM)	___	× 0.35 =	___	___	___	___
___	× 0.19 =	___	___	___	___	Triceps pushdown (PM)	___	× 0.32 =	___	___	___	___
						Legs						
___	× 1.0 =	___	___	___	___	Dual leg press (CM)	___	× 1.3 =	___	___	___	___
___	× 1.0 =	___	___	___	___	Leg press (PM)	___	× 1.3 =	___	___	___	___
						Abdominals						
___	× 0.20 =	___	___	___	___	Trunk curl (CM)	___	× 0.20 =	___	___	___	___

The calculated trial load is designed to allow 12-15 repetitions. FW: free weight exercise; CM: cam-based machine exercise; PM: pivot-based machine exercise; BWT: body weight (to account for differences in body composition when calculating testing loads, the personal trainer should use a maximum body weight of 175 pounds [79 kilograms] for male clients and 140 pounds [64 kilograms] for female clients).

Adapted from Baechle and Groves 1998 and Baechle and Earle 1995.

rounded down to 60 pounds). After a warm-up set of 30 pounds and a two-minute rest period, the client completes 12 repetitions with the trial load of 60 pounds. (Refer to the section "Based on Percent of Body Weight Testing" for an example of how the personal trainer can adjust the trial load to match the client's primary training goal.)

Repetition Maximum Testing

A third method to assess a client's capability to handle loads requires that the personal trainer decides—in advance—the number of **goal repetitions** for the exercise being tested, that is, how many repetitions of that exercise the client will perform in the actual program. For example, if an advanced resistance-trained client will perform four repetitions in the back squat exercise for the actual resistance training workout, the personal trainer 4RM tests the client. (See the section "Based on Repetition Maximum Testing" to continue this example for assigning an actual training load.)

This method of assessment is appropriate for all core exercises, although higher RMs (i.e., eight or more) can cause considerable fatigue if a client has to perform multiple trial sets [77]. Assistance exercises can also be RM tested but using only 8RMs or higher (i.e., an 8RM load or lighter) [7], for the same reasons they should not be 1RM tested. Comparable guidelines apply to the appropriateness of testing clients. That is, RM testing is effective for nearly all intermediate or advanced resistance-trained clients; but untrained or inexperienced clients should be limited to the lower loads of higher RM testing (≥8RM), although, again, the personal trainer must use caution to ensure that the client does not become overfatigued. For any client, the personal trainer should determine the RM within three testing sets.

Repetition maximum testing is similar to 1RM testing (see chapter 11), but a client performs the number of goal repetitions for each trial set with smaller load changes (about 50-75%) than recommended for 1RM testing.

Guidelines to Follow When Assigning Loads

As previously explained, the specificity principle dictates that a personal trainer needs to know a client's primary training goal (muscular endurance, hypertrophy, or muscular strength) before he or she can assign loads. To reach the desired training outcome, the client must train within a certain load and repetition scheme (table 15.6).

Based on results from the three methods of assessing load capabilities, the three primary methods to assign training loads are derived from the 1RM, %BWT testing, or RM testing.

Based on the 1-Repetition Maximum

After identifying the training goal and directly testing or estimating a client's 1RMs, the personal trainer needs to decide the goal repetitions for each exercise within the range shown in table 15.6. Then, to calculate a certain load for an exercise, the personal trainer can use table 15.3 ("Percent of 1RM-Repetition Relationship") to discover what specific 1RM percentage will allow the goal number of repetitions. To make the calculation, simply multiply the 1RM load (directly tested or estimated) by the percent of the 1RM that is associated with the goal repetitions to yield the training load.

For example, table 15.6 shows that the load and repetition scheme of 67% to 85%1RM for 6 to 12 repetitions will improve a client's muscular size. If the results of the fitness evaluation include an estimated 1RM of 140 pounds for the leg press exercise, and if the personal trainer has decided that the client will perform eight repetitions per set in the actual program, the load as seen in table 15.3 should be 80%1RM or 112 pounds (i.e., 140 × 0.80 = 112). Since it is unlikely that the machine can be set to this exact load, a rounded-down load of 110 pounds becomes the assigned load. Note that this training load may have to be adjusted (decreased) in subsequent sets if the client will complete multiple sets.

Based on Percent of Body-Weight Testing

Once the training goal and the number of goal repetitions within the range shown in table 15.6 are decided for each exercise, the personal trainer needs to compare the number of repetitions a client completed during %BWT testing with the goal number of repetitions. Although the factors listed in table 15.5 are designed to produce 12 to 15 repetitions, it is not uncommon for clients to perform less than 12 or more than 15 repetitions. Also, it is possible that the completed repetitions will not match the goal repetitions in the same exercise of the client's actual program. As a result of these discrepancies, the trial load from %BWT testing has to be adjusted to produce a corrected load that will allow the right number of goal repetitions. Table 15.7 provides one approach to increasing the trial load if the client performed too many repetitions, or decreasing the trial load if it was too heavy and resulted in an insufficient number of repetitions. These load adjustments are not completely without error (e.g., multijoint exercises training large muscles may require greater load changes), but the process can still serve as a method of honing in on an appropriate training load.

For example, if a client wants to improve muscular endurance, table 15.6 advises a load and repetition scheme of ≤67%1RM for ≥12 repetitions. If a 165-pound male client completed 12 repetitions in the free weight standing shoulder press exercise with a trial load of 60 pounds during %BWT testing, and if the personal trainer has decided that the client will perform 15 repetitions per set in the actual program, table 15.7 can be used to adjust (decrease) the load.

TABLE 15.6

Assigning Loads and Repetitions Based on the Training Goal

Training goal	Load (%1RM)	Goal repetitions
Muscular endurance	≤67	≥12
Hypertrophy	67-85	6-12
Muscular strength*	≥85	≤6

*The %1RM loads for muscular strength training apply only to core exercises; assistance exercises should be limited to 8RMs or higher (i.e., an 8RM load or lighter).

Adapted from Berger 1972; Fleck and Kraemer 1987; Fleck and Kraemer 1997; Garhammer 1986; Hedrick 1995; Herrick and Stone 1996; Kraemer and Koziris 1992; Lombardi 1989; O'Shea 1976; Stone and O'Bryant 1987; Tesch 1993; Tesch and Larson 1982; and Verhoshansky 1976.

TABLE 15.7

Adjusting the Trial Load to Allow the Goal Number of Repetitions

Goal repetitions	Repetitions completed with the trial load									
	>18	16-17	14-15	12-13	10-11	8-9	6-7	4-5	2-3	<2
14-15	+10	+5		−5	−10	−15	−15	−20	−25	−30
12-13	+15	+10	+5		−5	−10	−15	−15	−20	−25
10-11	+15	+15	+10	+5		−5	−10	−15	−15	−20
8-9	+20	+15	+15	+10	+5		−5	−10	−15	−15
6-7	+25	+20	+15	+15	+10	+5		−5	−10	−15
4-5	+30	+25	+20	+15	+15	+10	+5		−5	−10
2-3	+35	+30	+25	+20	+15	+15	+10	+5		−5

Load increase (+) or decrease (−)

Adapted from Baechle and Earle 1995.

Since the client performed 12 repetitions with the trial load, find the "12-13" column under "Repetitions completed with the trial load." Because the client will perform 15 repetitions in the resistance training program, locate the "14-15" row for the "Goal repetitions." Then read down the column and across the row to where they intersect at the −5 box; this is the number of pounds that need to be subtracted from the trial load to allow the client to perform the desired number of repetitions. Thus, the assigned training load is 55 pounds (i.e., 60 − 5 = 55). The personal trainer can use the "Adjustment" and "Training load" columns in table 15.5 ("Determining Loads for Percent of Body-Weight Testing") to record these load corrections. If the client has difficulty performing two or more sets with the 55-pound load, table 15.7 can be used again to adjust the training load, even during a workout session.

Based on Repetition Maximum Testing

The advantage of RM testing is that the personal trainer arrives at the assigned training load without performing any calculations. Since the RM testing protocol uses the same number of repetitions per trial set as the number a client will perform in that exercise for the actual program, the RM load *is* the assigned training load.

For example, table 15.6 shows that muscular strength is specifically improved by loads ≥85%1RM of ≤6 repetitions. If the personal trainer performed 4RM testing in the back squat exercise with a result of 225 pounds, that means a client will perform four repetitions with 225 pounds in this exercise as part of a muscular strength training program (although fatigue due to multiple sets may necessitate a slightly lighter load to still allow four repetitions per set).

Volume: Repetitions and Sets

There are two different definitions of **volume** as it relates to resistance training: the total amount of weight lifted in a training session (i.e., the total number of repetitions times the weight lifted per repetition) [24, 58, 75, 86] or the total number of repetitions completed in a training session (i.e., the number of repetitions performed in each set times the number of sets) [8, 24, 61, 77]. A **set** is a group of repetitions that are performed consecutively [24]. Although the previous section provided guidelines for assigning repetitions for a client's program, training volume also encompasses repetition assignments. Volume is influenced by a client's resistance training status and primary training goal.

Influential Factors

Because the number of assigned or goal repetitions is directly linked to the primary training goal, the personal trainer cannot assign goal repetitions outside of the ranges shown in table 15.6 without affecting the training outcome. So, for a given goal, the personal trainer modifies training volume largely by altering the number of assigned sets to match the training status of a client (i.e., the more well trained a client, the more sets he or she can and can perform).

Set assignments are not as directly influenced by a client's primary resistance training goal as, for example, the number of assigned repetitions. Although research has shown that performing only one set per exercise can promote increases in hypertrophy [12, 41, 90] and muscular strength [1, 28, 51, 52], intermediate and advanced resistance-trained clients will need to perform additional sets to continue to make improvements [43, 46, 56, 80, 91].

Volume is influenced by a client's resistance training status and primary training goal.

Guidelines to Follow When Assigning Volume

A client's training volume will be partially determined when the personal trainer makes the load and repetition assignments based on the %1RM-repetition relationship. A range for the number of assigned sets is also linked to the training goal, but it may be reduced based on the training status of a client.

Resistance Training Status

An untrained client often cannot complete multiple sets of the same exercise with an RM load; fortunately, a single set may be appropriate up through the first several months of training [24, 28]. As training status improves, clients can perform additional sets until they meet the guidelines shown in table 15.8.

Resistance Training Goal

As previously explained, the specificity principle requires a client to perform the correct number of repetitions (within a range), and the overload principle requires the client to complete enough sets to create a sufficient training stimulus. A program that attends to both of these principles—along with progression—will allow the client to reach his or her resistance training goal. The repetition and set assignments designed to improve muscular endurance, hypertrophy, and muscular strength, shown in table 15.8, are as follows:

- Muscular endurance: a greater number of repetitions (i.e., ≥12 repetitions per set) [10, 23, 24, 27, 44, 50, 59, 78, 82, 83, 84] but with fewer sets (typically two or three per exercise) [44]
- Hypertrophy: a higher training volume [34, 55] due to a moderate to higher number of repetitions per set and three to six sets per exercise [23, 35, 36, 60, 82]
- Muscular strength: for core exercises, sets of ≤6 repetitions [9, 10, 23, 24, 27, 35, 36, 44, 50, 59, 77, 78, 82, 83, 84] and three to six sets per exercise [24, 81]; for assistance exercises, ≥8 repetitions [7] and one to three sets [7, 44]

Rest Periods

The time interval between multiple sets of the same exercise is the **rest period** [6]. If a client performs more than one exercise for the same muscle group or body area, the rest period also refers to the time between exercises. Rest period lengths, like load assignments, are predominantly influenced by a client's primary resistance training goal and secondarily by the client's resistance training status.

Influential Factors

There is a direct relationship between an assigned load and the needed rest between sets with that load; that is, the heavier a load is for a client, the

TABLE 15.8

Assigning Volume Based on the Training Goal

Training goal	Goal repetitions	Sets*
Muscular endurance	≥12	2-3
Hypertrophy	6-12	3-6
Muscular strength	≤6	2-6

*These assignments do not include warm-up sets and typically apply to core exercises only [4, 44].

Adapted from Berger 1972; Fleck and Kraemer 1997; Garhammer 1986; Hedrick 1995; Lombardi 1989; O'Shea 1976; Stone and O'Bryant 1987; Tesch 1993; Tesch and Larson 1982; and Verhoshansky 1976.

longer the client will need to rest before lifting it again (and the lighter the load is, the less rest is needed) [24, 27, 50, 64, 77, 89]. Therefore, the rest period length is directly related to the number of goal repetitions and, ultimately, the primary resistance training goal [65]. A factor that also has a strong influence is the client's resistance training status; untrained or deconditioned clients initially will require longer rest periods than those shown in table 15.9.

Rest period lengths, like load assignments, are predominantly influenced by a client's primary resistance training goal and secondarily by the client's resistance training status.

Guidelines to Follow When Assigning Rest Periods

Because a client's resistance training goal determines the load and repetition assignments, it also dictates the amount of rest that is needed between sets and exercises.

Resistance Training Status

An intermediate or advanced trained client will tolerate the rest period lengths shown in table 15.9, but empirical evidence suggests that untrained clients may need at least twice as much rest as trained individuals. As a client becomes better trained, he or she will be able to perform multiple sets and longer sequences of exercises with less rest between sets.

Resistance Training Goal

To create the correct goal-specific resistance training stimulus, the personal trainer must allow sufficient rest between sets and exercises so that a client can lift the assigned training load for the targeted number of repetitions. The recommended rest period lengths for muscular endurance, hypertrophy, and muscular strength training programs, shown in table 15.9, are assigned as follows:

- Muscular endurance: a very short rest period, often 30 seconds or less [68, 69, 70]
- Hypertrophy: a short to moderate rest period [24, 27, 44, 45, 64, 77] within a range of 30 to 90 seconds [35, 65, 82]
- Muscular strength: a long rest period, especially for lower body or whole-body exercises [87], that spans two to five minutes [45, 48, 65] or three to five minutes [24, 50, 74, 77, 88, 89]

Variation

To develop a complete resistance training workout, the personal trainer needs to consider each of the program design variables discussed so far: choice, frequency, order, load, volume, and rest periods. But even the most effective and individualized program cannot increase muscular endurance, hypertrophy, or muscular strength for an indefinite period. In time, a client's progress will level off or possibly decrease if he or she becomes bored or overtrained (see chapter 5). Even intermediate or advanced

TABLE 15.9

Assigning Rest Periods Based on the Training Goal

Training goal*	Rest period length
Muscular endurance	≤30 seconds
Hypertrophy	30-90 seconds
Muscular strength	2-5 minutes

*To create the correct goal-specific resistance training stress, the personal trainer must allow sufficient rest between sets and exercises so that a client can lift the training load for the targeted number of repetitions. Note that the actual %1RM or RM load for each exercise is the basis for the rest period lengths, more so than the overall training goal. For example, assistance exercises that are performed within a muscular strength training program are not assigned loads heavier than an 8RM load [4], so the rest periods will be shorter than the guidelines for muscular strength (i.e., 30-90 seconds because an 8RM load is associated with a hypertrophy training program).

Adapted from Fleck and Kraemer 1997; Kraemer, Noble, Clark, and Culver 1987; Larson and Potteiger 1997; Lombardi 1989; Spassov 1989; Stone and O'Bryant 1987; Weiss 1991; and Wescott 1982.

resistance-trained clients who are exposed to, for example, several months of heavy resistance training (e.g., ≤6RMs) can experience decreases in muscular strength and neuromuscular activation [29, 30, 31, 32, 33] and increases in the frequency of overtraining symptoms [25, 29, 33, 76].

To help a client experience ongoing improvements, lower the risk of overtraining, relieve boredom, and maintain training intensity, the personal trainer needs to add variation to the program [15, 26]. **Variation** is the purposeful change of the program design variable assignments to expose a client to new or different training stressors [43, 46, 75]. The personal trainer can vary a resistance training program by periodically altering a client's frequency, load, volume, or rest period [15, 22, 65, 67, 75]. This manipulation can result in variation within a training session or between the workouts in one training week. A variety of methods can be used to provide this variation; two of them are highlighted here. (See chapter 23 for a detailed discussion on **periodization,** a training variation commonly used for athletes.)

Pyramid Training

A personal trainer can add variation within a workout by directing a client to perform **pyramid training.** In one common type of pyramid training, the load is progressively increased while the number of repetitions in sequential sets of an exercise is progressively decreased [18, 24, 61, 63, 81]. For example, the client may perform three sets of the back squat exercise with the first set consisting of a 75%1RM load for 10 repetitions, the second set consisting of 80%1RM for 8 repetitions, and the third set consisting of 85%1RM for 6 repetitions. The personal trainer can use table 15.3 ("Percent of 1RM-Repetition Relationship") or table 15.4 ("Estimating a 1-Repetition Maximum From a Training Load") to calculate or find the load and repetition assignments.

Within-the-Week Variation

The personal trainer can also vary a client's program across the sessions of a training week. For example, a personal trainer may want to design a four-days-a-week split routine (e.g., lower body on Mondays and Thursdays; upper body on Tuesdays and Fridays) that focuses on muscular strength, but most clients typically cannot tolerate the same workout with the assigned heavy loads with only one or two rest days between sessions [18, 46, 63].

One approach to alleviate this concern and reduce the risk of overtraining is to vary the loads for some or all of the core exercises so that only the first training session for each muscle group or body area (e.g., Mondays for lower body and Tuesdays for upper body) is assigned the loads from table 15.3 or those obtained through testing. These "heavy day" loads are designed to be 100% of the calculated RMs (i.e., the result of the decisions and calculations from the section "Guidelines to Follow When Assigning Loads"). The loads for the other two training days (e.g., Thursdays for lower body and Fridays for upper body) are intentionally reduced to allow a client to recover after the "heavy" day. These "light day" loads for the core exercises are 80% of the loads lifted on the "heavy days," but the client will still complete the same number of goal repetitions [4, 7,

Example of Within-the-Week Training Variation

If a client's 1RM in the bench press exercise is 230 pounds and the repetition goal for a muscular strength training program is five per set, the assigned loads for a "heavy" and "light" training day are as follows:

"Heavy" Training Day

- A repetition goal of five is associated with 87%1RM (table 15.3).
- If the 1RM is 230 pounds, then the calculated load for a "heavy" day is:

$$230 \times 0.87 = 200 \text{ pounds (or use table 15.4)}$$

- Therefore, the assigned load (i.e., 100% of the calculated load) is 200 pounds for sets of five repetitions.

"Light" Training Day

- If the calculated load from the "heavy" day is 200 pounds, then the calculated load for a "light" day is:

$$200 \times 0.80 = 160 \text{ pounds}$$

- Therefore, the assigned load (i.e., 80% of the calculated load) is 160 pounds for sets of five repetitions. The client should not perform more repetitions just because the load is lighter!

77, 86]. (See "Example of Within-the-Week Training Variation" on the previous page.)

This strategy can be used for other training frequencies. For example, if the client is training three times per week, the personal trainer can design a "heavy, light, medium" program in which the loads for the "medium day" are 90% of the assigned "heavy day" training loads [4, 7, 18, 63].

To help a client experience ongoing improvements, lower the risk of overtraining, relieve boredom, and maintain training intensity, the personal trainer needs to add variation to the program.

Progression

Although progression was discussed earlier as one of the three general training principles, it is also considered a program design variable. Just as variation is essential to improvement, even the most effective and individualized program will not allow a client to meet his or her training goal unless the resistance training workouts provide a progressive stimulus. Progression can be applied to a client's training frequency, number or difficulty of exercises, number of sets, or any combination of these or other changes; but the most frequently used method is to regularly and appropriately increase the weight lifted for each exercise.

When to Increase Training Loads

It can be difficult for a personal trainer to know when a client is ready for an increase in the training load for one or more sets of an exercise. One approach that is helpful yet conservative for many clients is the **2-for-2 rule** [7], which is based on the number of goal repetitions assigned for an exercise. If a client can complete *two more* repetitions than the repetition goal in the *final set* of an exercise for *two consecutive* training sessions, then the personal trainer should increase the load in all of the sets of that exercise for the next training session (see "Using the 2-for-2 Rule to Increase the Training Load (an Example)" on the next page).

Even the most effective and individualized program will not allow a client to meet his or her training goal unless the resistance training workouts provide a progressive stimulus.

How Much to Increase Training Loads

Because of the large assortment of resistance training exercises and the varied resistance training status of clients performing those exercises, it is often difficult to assign an appropriate and effective load increase. Table 15.10 provides guidelines based on training status, targeted body area, and exercise

TABLE 15.10

Examples of Load Increases

Resistance training status	Body area	Type of exercise	Approximate load increase*: Absolute increase (add weight)	Approximate load increase*: Relative increase (add a percent of the previous load)
Beginner	Upper body	Core	2.5-5 pounds (1-2 kilograms)	2.5%
	Upper body	Assistance	1.25-2.5 pounds (0.6-1 kilograms)	1-2%
	Lower body	Core	10-15 pounds (4-7 kilograms)	5%
	Lower body	Assistance	5-10 pounds (2-4 kilograms)	2.5-5%
Intermediate or advanced	Upper body	Core	5-10+ pounds (2-4+ kilograms)	2.5-5+%
	Upper body	Assistance	5-10 pounds (2-4 kilograms)	2.5-5%
	Lower body	Core	15-20+ pounds (7-9+ kilograms)	5-10+%
	Lower body	Assistance	10-15 pounds (4-7 kilograms)	5-10%

*Although these load increases are appropriate for training programs with volumes of approximately three sets of 5 to 10 repetitions, they should be regarded only as guidelines.

Adapted from Baechle and Earle 2000 and Earle 1999.

Using the 2-for-2 Rule to Increase the Training Load (an Example)

If a beginner client's repetition goal in the back squat exercise is 10:

Training session 1

Set 1	Set 2	Set 3
135 pounds	135 pounds	135 pounds
10 reps	10 reps	11 reps ←Exceeded the repetition goal by only one rep

Training session 2

Set 1	Set 2	Set 3
135 pounds	135 pounds	135 pounds
12 reps	11 reps	10 reps ←Did not exceed the repetition goal

Training session 3

Set 1	Set 2	Set 3
135 pounds	135 pounds	135 pounds
12 reps	12 reps	12 reps ←Successfully exceeded the repetition goal by two reps

Training session 4

Set 1	Set 2	Set 3
135 pounds	135 pounds	135 pounds
12 reps	12 reps	12 reps ←Successfully exceeded the repetition goal by two reps in a consecutive training session

Next training session

Set 1	Set 2	Set 3
145 pounds	145 pounds	145 pounds ←10 pounds is added to all three sets for next training session

type. The load changes can be made in terms of an actual (absolute) pound or kilogram increase or as a certain (relative) percentage increase.

For instance, the example above shows a client following the 2-for-2 rule to increase the load in the back squat exercise from 135 pounds to 145 pounds. According to table 15.10, this 10-pound load increase is appropriate for a lower body core exercise performed by a client with a beginner training status.

CONCLUSION

Designing a resistance training program requires a personal trainer to understand how specificity, overload, and progression influence the effectiveness of a number of program design variables: choice, frequency, order, load, volume, and rest periods. Once a program is developed, the personal trainer needs to vary and advance the assigned load or the other variables to provide a continual and dynamic training stimulus. An example of a resistance training program for each primary training goal (using only those exercises included in chapter 13) is shown on pages 385-394.

Sample Muscular Endurance Program: Alternate Upper Body Exercises and Lower Body Exercises

Tuesdays and Fridays

Bench press (FW)	2 sets × 15 repetitions @ 45 pounds
Leg press (PM)	2 × 15 @ 145 pounds
Seated row (CM)	2 × 15 @ 30 pounds
Leg (knee) curl (CM)	2 × 15 @ a 15RM load
Shoulder press (CM)	2 × 15 @ 15 pounds
Leg (knee) extension (CM)	2 × 15 @ a 15RM load
Biceps curl (FW)	2 × 15 @ 25 pounds
Seated heel raise (PM)	2 × 15 @ a 15RM load
Triceps pushdown (PM)	2 × 15 @ 20 pounds
Abdominal crunch	2 × 15

Rest period length: 30 seconds

Explanation

Initial consultation and fitness evaluation

Initial resistance training status and experience: beginner (table 15.1)

Fitness evaluation: %BWT and 15RM testing (see "Load")

Primary resistance training goal: muscular endurance

Choice

Mixture of free weight (FW), cam machine (CM), and pivot machine (PM) exercises

Core exercises: bench press, leg press, seated row, shoulder press

Assistance exercises: leg (knee) curl, leg (knee) extension, biceps curl, seated heel raise, triceps pushdown, abdominal crunch

One exercise per muscle group (the selected exercises were limited to those included in chapter 13)

Frequency

Frequency range to match training status: 2-3 times per week (table 15.2)

Assigned frequency: 2 times per week, spaced evenly throughout the week (Tuesdays and Fridays)

Order

Alternate upper body exercises and lower body exercises

Complete one set of each exercise, then repeat

Load

Assessing load capabilities (testing methods and results)

Percent of body-weight testing (protocol—"Protocol for Testing With a Percentage of a Client's Body Weight" on page 376, %BWT factors—table 15.5)

- Body weight (for a female client): 135 pounds
- Factors, calculations, trial loads, and number of completed repetitions for these exercises:

(continued)

Exercise	Calculation	Trial load	Number of completed repetitions
Bench press (FW)	135 × 0.35	47.25 pounds (round down to 45)	15
Leg press (PM)	135 × 1.00	135 pounds	20
Seated row (CM)	135 × 0.20	27 pounds (round down to 25)	16
Shoulder press (CM)	135 × 0.25	33.75 pounds (round down to 30)	8
Biceps curl (FW)	135 × 0.23	31.05 pounds (round down to 30)	12
Triceps pushdown (PM)	135 × 0.19	25.65 pounds (round down to 25)	13

15RM testing for these exercises (conservative testing to avoid client fatigue; limited to 3 testing sets): leg (knee) curl, leg (knee) extension, seated heel raise

Assigning loads

Based on %BWT testing: goal repetitions (see "Repetitions") = 15

Adjust the loads from %BWT testing to assign loads (to adjust—table 15.7; to record—table 15.5):

Exercise	Load adjustment	Equation	Assigned training load
Bench press (FW)	None needed	N/a	45 pounds
Leg press (PM)	+ 10 pounds	135 + 10 = 145	145 pounds
Seated row (CM)	+ 5 pounds	25 + 5 = 30	30 pounds
Shoulder press (CM)	– 15 pounds	30 – 15 = 15	15 pounds
Biceps curl (FW)	– 5 pounds	30 – 5 = 25	25 pounds
Triceps pushdown (PM)	– 5 pounds	25 – 5 = 20	20 pounds

Based on RM testing (note that the RM loads may have to be decreased due to the multiple assigned sets): assign loads from 15RM testing for leg (knee) curl, leg (knee) extension, and seated heel raise

Repetitions

Repetition range to match training goal: ≥12 per set (table 15.6 or table 15.8)

Goal repetitions: 15

Sets

Set range to match training goal: 2-3 per exercise (table 15.8)

Assigned sets: 2 (note that warm-up sets are not included in the set assignments)

Rest periods

Rest period range to match training goal: ≤30 seconds (table 15.9)

Assigned rest: 30 seconds between exercises

Sample Hypertrophy Program: Four Times Per Week Split Routine

Upper Body Workout (Mondays and Thursdays)

Incline bench press (FW)[a]	3 sets × 8 repetitions @ 175 pounds
Dumbbell fly[b]	3 × 12 @ a 12RM load
Lat pulldown[b]	3 × 12 @ 120 pounds
Seated row[b]	3 × 12 @ 90 pounds
Shoulder press (FW)[a]	3 × 8 @ 95 pounds
Superset	
Biceps curl + Lying triceps extension[b]	3 × 12 @ a 12RM load (for each exercise)
Bent-knee sit-up[c]	2 × 15

Rest period lengths: [a]90 seconds; [b]60 seconds; [c]30 seconds

Lower Body Workout (Tuesdays and Fridays)

Back squat[a]	3 × 8 @ 240 pounds
Lunge[b]	3 × 12 @ 65 pounds
Leg press[a]	3 × 8 @ 400 pounds
Leg (knee) curl[b]	3 × 12 @ a 12RM load
Leg (knee) extension[b]	3 × 12 @ a 12RM load
Compound set	
Standing heel raise + seated heel raise[c]	2 × 15 @ a 15RM load (for each exercise)
Abdominal crunch[c]	2 × 15

Rest period lengths: [a]90 seconds; [b]60 seconds; [c]30 seconds

Explanation

Initial consultation and fitness evaluation

Initial resistance training status and experience: intermediate (table 15.1)

Fitness evaluation: 10RM testing (to estimate a 1RM), 12RM testing, and 15RM testing (see "Load")

Primary resistance training goal: hypertrophy

Choice

Primarily free weight (FW) exercises, but some machine exercises (especially for the assistance exercises)

Core exercises: incline bench press, lat pulldown, seated row, shoulder press, back squat, lunge, leg press

Assistance exercises: dumbbell fly, biceps curl, lying triceps extension, bent-knee sit-up, leg (knee) curl, leg (knee) extension, standing heel raise, seated heel raise, abdominal crunch

1-2 exercises per muscle group (the selected exercises were limited to those included in chapter 13)

Frequency

Frequency range to match training status: 3-4 times per week (table 15.2)

Assigned frequency: a split routine of 4 times per week; 2 times per week for upper body exercises (Mondays and Thursdays) and 2 times per week for lower body exercises (Tuesdays and Fridays)

Order

Primary methods

Core exercises and then assistance exercises

Exercises that train large muscle groups first and then exercises that train small muscle groups

Multijoint exercises first and then single-joint exercises

(An exception: the dumbbell fly is a single-joint exercise)

Secondary methods

Exercises performed in a superset: biceps curl, lying triceps extension

Exercises performed in a compound set: standing heel raise, seated heel raise

(continued)

Load

Assessing load capabilities (testing methods and results)

10RM testing to estimate a 1RM (protocol—chapter 11, but modified; estimation chart—table 15.4)

10RM loads and their estimated 1RMs for these exercises:

Exercise	10RM	Estimated 1RM
Incline bench press	165 pounds	220 pounds
Lat pulldown	135 pounds	180 pounds
Seated row	105 pounds	140 pounds
Shoulder press	90 pounds	120 pounds
Back squat	225 pounds	300 pounds
Lunge	75 pounds	100 pounds
Leg press	375 pounds	500 pounds

12RM testing for these exercises (limited to 3 testing sets): dumbbell fly, biceps curl, lying triceps extension, leg (knee) curl, leg (knee) extension

15RM testing for these exercises (limited to 3 testing sets): standing heel raise, seated heel raise

Assigning loads based on the 1RM

Primary resistance training goal: hypertrophy (but exercises at a 15RM load will improve muscular endurance)

Repetition range to match training goal: 6-12 per set (table 15.6 or table 15.8)

- Goal repetitions: 8—for these exercises: incline bench press, shoulder press, back squat, leg press
- Goal repetitions: 12—for these exercises: lat pulldown, seated row, lunge

Loading (%1RM; see table 15.3) range to match the training goal: 67-85%1RM (table 15.6)

- Percentage of the 1RM associated with 8 goal repetitions (i.e., an 8RM load): 80%
- Percentage of the 1RM associated with 12 goal repetitions (i.e., a 12RM load): 67%

Calculate training loads from the estimated 1RM:

Exercise	Goal repetitions	Calculation	Assigned training load
Incline bench press	8	220 × 0.80	176 (round down to 175 pounds)
Lat pulldown	12	180 × 0.67	120.6 (round down to 120 pounds)
Seated row	12	140 × 0.67	93.8 (round down to 90 pounds)
Shoulder press	8	120 × 0.80	96 (round down to 95 pounds)
Back squat	8	300 × 0.80	240 pounds
Lunge	12	100 × 0.67	67 (round down to 65 pounds)
Leg press	8	500 × 0.80	400 pounds

Assigning loads based on RM testing (note that the RM loads may have to be decreased due to the multiple assigned sets)

Assign loads from 12RM testing for dumbbell fly, biceps curl, lying triceps extension, leg (knee) curl, leg (knee) extension

Assign loads from 15RM testing for standing heel raise, seated heel raise

Repetitions

Repetition range to match training goal: 6-12 per set for hypertrophy training (but exercises assigned ≥12 repetitions are associated with muscular endurance training) (table 15.6 or table 15.8)

Goal repetitions: 8, 12, or 15 (depending on the exercise; see "Load")

Sets

Set range to match training goal: 3-6 per exercise for hypertrophy training (but exercises assigned 2-3 sets are associated with muscular endurance training) (table 15.8)

Assigned sets: 3 per exercise at an 8RM or 12RM load, 2 per exercise at a 15RM load, and 2 sets for abdominal exercises (note that warm-up sets are not included in the set assignments)

Rest periods

Rest period range to match training goal: 30-90 seconds for hypertrophy training (but exercises assigned ≤30 seconds rest are associated with muscular endurance training) (table 15.9)

Assigned rest between sets and exercises: 90 seconds for 8RM loads, 60 seconds for 12RM loads, and 30 seconds for 15RM loads and abdominal exercises

Sample Muscular Strength Program: Pyramid Training and Within-the-Week Variation

Lower Body Workout (Mondays)

"Heavy" day
100% of calculated loads in the core exercises

Back squat	1 set × 6 repetitions @ 340 pounds[c]
	2 × 4 @ 360 pounds[b]
	2 × 2 @ 380 pounds[a]
Leg press	1 × 6 @ 510 pounds[c]
	2 × 4 @ 540 pounds[b]
	2 × 2 @ 570 pounds[a]
Leg (knee) curl	1 × 12 @ 105 pounds[e]
	1 × 10 @ 120 pounds[d]
	1 × 8 @ 125 pounds[d]
Leg (knee) extension	1 × 12 @ 130 pounds[e]
	1 × 10 @ 150 pounds[d]
	1 × 8 @ 160 pounds[d]
Abdominal crunch[f]	3 × 25

Rest period lengths: [a]5 minutes; [b]4 minutes; [c]3 minutes; [d]90 seconds; [e]60 seconds; [f]30 seconds

Lower Body Workout (Thursdays)

"Light" day
80% of calculated loads in the core exercises

Back squat	1 × 6 @ 270 pounds[c]
	2 × 4 @ 285 pounds[b]
	2 × 2 @ 300 pounds[a]
Leg press	1 × 6 @ 405 pounds[c]
	2 × 4 @ 430 pounds[b]
	2 × 2 @ 455 pounds[a]
Leg (knee) curl	1 × 12 @ 105 pounds[e]
	1 × 10 @ 120 pounds[d]
	1 × 8 @ 125 pounds[d]
Leg (knee) extension	1 × 12 @ 130 pounds[e]
	1 × 10 @ 150 pounds[d]
	1 × 8 @ 160 pounds[d]
Abdominal crunch[f]	3 × 25

Rest period lengths: [a]5 minutes; [b]4 minutes; [c]3 minutes; [d]90 seconds; [e]60 seconds; [f]30 seconds

Upper Body Workout (Tuesdays)

"Heavy" day
100% of calculated loads in selected core exercises

Bench press	1 × 6 @ 265 pounds[c]
	2 × 4 @ 280 pounds[b]
	2 × 2 @ 295 pounds[a]
Bent-over row[d]	3 × 8 @ 175 pounds
Shoulder press	1 × 6 @ 165 pounds[c]
	2 × 4 @ 175 pounds[b]
	2 × 2 @ 185 pounds[a]
Lat pulldown[d]	3 × 8 @ 180 pounds
Lying triceps extension	1 × 12 @ 90 pounds[e]
	1 × 10 @ 105 pounds[d]
	1 × 8 @ 110 pounds[d]
Biceps curl	1 × 12 @ 90 pounds[e]
	1 × 10 @ 105 pounds[d]
	1 × 8 @ 110 pounds[d]
Bent-knee sit-up[f]	3 × 25

Rest period lengths: [a]5 minutes; [b]4 minutes; [c]3 minutes; [d]90 seconds; [e]60 seconds; [f]30 seconds

Upper Body Workout (Fridays)

"Light" day
80% of calculated loads in selected core exercises

Bench press	
1 × 6 @ 210 pounds[c]	2 × 4 @ 220 pounds[b]
	2 × 2 @ 235 pounds[a]
	Bent-over row[d]
3 × 8 @ 175	pounds
Shoulder press	1 × 6 @ 130 pounds[c]
	2 × 4 @ 140 pounds[b]
	2 × 2 @ 145 pounds[a]
Lat pulldown[d]	3 × 8 @ 180 pounds
Lying triceps extension	1 × 12 @ 90 pounds[e]
	1 × 10 @ 105 pounds[d]
	1 × 8 @ 110 pounds[d]
Biceps curl	1 × 12 @ 90 pounds[e]
	1 × 10 @ 105 pounds[d]
	1 × 8 @ 110 pounds[d]
Bent-knee sit-up[f]	3 × 25

Rest period lengths: [a]5 minutes; [b]4 minutes; [c]3 minutes; [d]90 seconds; [e]60 seconds; [f]30 seconds

Explanation

Initial consultation and fitness evaluation

Initial resistance training status and experience: advanced (table 15.1)

Fitness evaluation: 1RM testing and 10RM testing (see "Load")

Primary resistance training goal: muscular strength

Choice

Mostly structural free weight exercises, some machine assistance exercises

Core exercises: back squat, leg press, bench press, bent-over row, shoulder press, lat pulldown

Assistance exercises: leg (knee) curl, leg (knee) extension, abdominal crunch, lying triceps extension, biceps curl, bent-knee sit-up

1-2 exercises per muscle group (the selected exercises were limited to those included in chapter 13)

Frequency

Frequency range to match training status: 4+ times per week (table 15.2)

Assigned frequency: a split routine of 4 times per week; 2 times per week for lower body exercises (Mondays and Thursdays) and 2 times per week for upper body exercises (Tuesdays and Fridays)

Order

Core exercises and then assistance exercises

Exercises that train large muscle groups first and then exercises that train small muscle groups

Multijoint exercises first and then single-joint exercises

Alternate "push" and "pull" exercises (on upper body days)

Load

Assessing load capabilities (testing methods and results)

1RM testing (protocol—chapter 11) for these selected core exercises:

- Back squat: 1RM = 400 pounds
- Leg press: 1RM = 600 pounds
- Bench press: 1RM = 315 pounds
- Shoulder press: 1RM = 195 pounds

10RM testing to estimate a 1RM (protocol—chapter 11, but modified; estimation chart—table 15.4)

10RM loads and their estimated 1RMs for these exercises:

Exercise	10RM	Estimated 1RM
Leg (knee) curl	120 pounds	160 pounds
Leg (knee) extension	150 pounds	200 pounds
Bent-over row	165 pounds	220 pounds
Lat pulldown	175 pounds	230 pounds
Lying triceps extension	105 pounds	140 pounds
Biceps curl	105 pounds	140 pounds

Assigning loads based on the 1RM

Primary resistance training goal: muscular strength (but exercises at an 8RM, 10RM, or 12RM load are associated with hypertrophy training; abdominal exercises are designed to improve muscular endurance)

Repetition range to match training goal: ≤6 per set (table 15.6 or table 15.8)

(continued)

- Goal repetitions: 6, 4, 2 (pyramid)—for these exercises: back squat, leg press, bench press, shoulder press
- Goal repetitions: 8—for these exercises: bent-over row, lat pulldown (because they should not be loaded heavier than an 8RM)
- Goal repetitions: 12, 10, 8 (pyramid)—for these assistance exercises: leg (knee) curl, leg (knee) extension, lying triceps extension, biceps curl (because they should not be loaded heavier than an 8RM)

Loading (%1RM; see table 15.3) range to match the training goal: ≥85%1RM (table 15.6)

Repetition and load goal	Associated percentage of the 1RM
2 repetitions (2RM load)	95%
4 repetitions (4RM load)	90%
6 repetitions (6RM load)	85%
8 repetitions (8RM load)	80%
10 repetitions (10RM load)	75%
12 repetitions (12RM load)	67%

Calculate training loads from the directly tested or the estimated 1RM (for the "heavy" day):

Exercise	Goal repetitions	Calculation	Assigned training load
Back squat	6	400 × 0.85	340 pounds
	4	400 × 0.90	360 pounds
	2	400 × 0.95	380 pounds
Leg press	6	600 × 0.85	510 pounds
	4	600 × 0.90	540 pounds
	2	600 × 0.95	570 pounds
Leg (knee) curl	12	160 × 0.67	107.2 pounds (round down to 105)
	10	160 × 0.75	120 pounds
	8	160 × 0.80	128 pounds (round down to 125)
Leg (knee) extension	12	200 × 0.67	134 pounds (round down 130)
	10	200 × 0.75	150 pounds
	8	200 × 0.80	160 pounds
Bench press	6	315 × 0.85	267.75 pounds (round down 265)
	4	315 × 0.90	283.5 pounds (round down to 280)
	2	315 × 0.95	299.25 pounds (round down to 295)
Bent-over row	8	220 × 0.80	176 pounds (round down to 175)

Exercise	Goal repetitions	Calculation	Assigned training load
Shoulder press	6	195 × 0.85	165.75 pounds (round down to 165)
	4	195 × 0.90	175.5 pounds (round down to 175)
	2	195 × 0.95	185.25 pounds (round down to 185)
Lat pulldown	8	230 × 0.80	184 pounds (round down to 180)
Lying triceps extension	12	140 × 0.67	93.8 pounds (round down to 90)
	10	140 × 0.75	105 pounds
	8	140 × 0.80	112 (round down to 110)
Biceps curl	12	140 × 0.67	93.8 pounds (round down to 90)
	10	140 × 0.75	105 pounds
	8	140 × 0.80	112 pounds (round down to 110)

Calculate training loads for the "light" training days (80% of the "heavy" day loads) for selected core exercises:

Exercise	Number of repetitions	Calculation	Assigned training load
Back squat	6	340 × 0.80	272 pounds (round down to 270)
	4	360 × 0.80	288 pounds (round down to 285)
	2	380 × 0.80	304 pounds (round down to 300)
Leg press	6	510 × 0.80	408 pounds (round down to 405)
	4	540 × 0.80	432 pounds (round down to 430)
	2	570 × 0.80	456 pounds (round down to 455)
Bench press	6	265 × 0.80	212 pounds (round down to 210)
	4	280 × 0.80	224 pounds (round down to 220)
	2	295 × 0.80	236 pounds (round down to 235)
Shoulder press	6	165 × 0.80	132 pounds (round down to 130)
	4	175 × 0.80	140 pounds
	2	185 × 0.80	148 pounds (round down to 145)

(continued)

Repetitions

Repetition range to match training goal: ≤6 per set for muscular strength training (but exercises assigned 6-12 repetitions are associated with hypertrophy training and exercises assigned ≥12 repetitions are associated with muscular endurance training) (table 15.6 or table 15.8)

Goal repetitions: 2, 4, 6, 8, 10, 12, or 25 (depending on the exercise—some have pyramid sets; see "Load")

Sets

Set range to match training goal: 2-6 for muscular strength training (but exercises assigned 3-6 sets are associated with hypertrophy training and exercises assigned 2-3 sets are associated with muscular endurance training) (table 15.8)

Assigned sets: 5 per exercise at 2-6RM loads (pyramids) for selected core exercises, 3 per exercise at an 8RM load, 3 per exercise at 8-12RM loads (pyramids), and 3 sets for abdominal exercises (note that warm-up sets are not included in the set assignments)

Rest periods

Rest period range to match training goal: 2-5 minutes for muscular strength training (but exercises assigned 30-90 seconds rest are associated with hypertrophy training and exercises assigned ≤30 seconds rest are associated with muscular endurance training) (table15.9)

Assigned rest between sets and exercises: 5 minutes for 2RM loads, 4 minutes for 4RM loads, 3 minutes for 6RM loads, 90 seconds for 8RM and 12RM loads, 60 seconds for 12RM loads, and 30 seconds for abdominal exercises

Variation

In each training session

Pyramid sets: 6, 4, 2 repetitions or 12, 10, 8 repetitions with progressively heavier loads

Within-the-week

Once per week: upper body "heavy" day (100% of calculated loads in selected core exercises)

Once per week: upper body "light" day (80% of calculated loads in selected core exercises)

Once per week: lower body "heavy" day (100% of calculated loads in selected core exercises)

Once per week: lower body "light" day (80% of calculated loads in selected core exercises)

STUDY QUESTIONS

1. When a client progresses to follow a split routine, all of the following describe the changes in the program EXCEPT:
   - A. increased weekly training frequency
   - B. decreased overall training volume
   - C. decreased training frequency of each muscle group's workout
   - D. increased number of rest days between each muscle group's workout
2. Which describes the arrangement of exercises performed in this order: bench press, bent-over row, lying triceps extension, biceps curl, shoulder press?
   - A. multijoint exercises first and then single-joint exercises
   - B. exercises that train large muscle groups first and then exercises that train small muscle groups
   - C. core exercises then assistance exercises
   - D. alternate "push" and "pull" exercises
3. A personal trainer wants to include the lateral shoulder raise exercise in a client's program. Which of the following is an appropriate testing method that will produce a test result that allows the most accurate assigned training load for a repetition goal of 10 per set?
   - A. directly testing the 1RM
   - B. estimating the 1RM from a 15RM

C. percent of body-weight testing
D. 10RM testing

4. What is the load for the bench press exercise on a "light" day of a strength training program if the client's 1RM is 200 pounds (91 kilograms) and the number of goal repetitions is 6 per set?
   A. 170 pounds (77 kg)
   B. 160 pounds (73 kg)
   C. 135 pounds (61 kg)
   D. 130 pounds (59 kg)

APPLIED KNOWLEDGE QUESTION

Based on the following initial consultation and fitness testing information, fill in the empty spaces to determine the client's training loads for selected exercises.

Initial resistance training status and exercise technique experience: intermediate

Fitness evaluation: 10RM testing to estimate a 1RM

Primary resistance training goal: hypertrophy

Assessing load capabilities

10RM loads and their estimated 1RMs for these selected exercises:

Exercise (all are cam machines)	10RM (pounds)	Estimated 1RM (pounds)
Vertical chest press	60	
Seated row	50	
Shoulder press	45	
Biceps curl	35	
Triceps extension	30	
Leg (knee) extension	70	
Leg (knee) curl	60	

Assigning loads

Repetition range to match training goal: ______to______per set

Goal repetitions: 8

Loading (%1RM) range to match the training goal: ______ % to ______%1RM

%1RM associated with 8 goal repetitions: ______%1RM

Calculate training loads from the estimated 1RM

Exercise (all are cam machines)	Estimated 1RM (pounds)	×	%1RM associated with 8 goal repetitions (in decimal form)	=	Calculated trial load	Assigned training load (rounded down, if needed)
Vertical chest press		×		=		
Seated row		×		=		
Shoulder press		×		=		
Biceps curl		×		=		

(continued)

(continued)

Exercise (all are cam machines)	Estimated 1RM (pounds)	×	%1RM associated with 8 goal repetitions (in decimal form)	=	Calculated trial load	Assigned training load (rounded down, if needed)
Triceps extension		×		=		
Leg (knee) extension		×		=		
Leg (knee) curl		×		=		

REFERENCES

1. Alén, M., A. Pakarinen, K. Häkkinen, and P.V. Komi. 1988. Responses of serum androgenic-anabolic and catabolic hormones to prolonged strength training. *International Journal of Sports Medicine* 9: 229-233.
2. Arnold, M.D., J.L. Mayhew, D. LeSuer, and J. McCormick. 1995. Accuracy of predicting bench press and squat performance from repetitions at low and high intensity. *Journal of Strength and Conditioning Research* 9: 205-206. (abstract)
3. Atha, J. 1981. Strengthening muscle. *Exercise and Sport Science Review* 9: 1-73.
4. Baechle, T.R., and R.W. Earle. 1989. *Weight Training: A Text Written for the College Student.* Omaha, NE: Creighton University Press.
5. Baechle, T.R., and R.W. Earle. 1995. *Fitness Weight Training.* Champaign, IL: Human Kinetics.
6. Baechle, T.R., and R.W. Earle, eds. 2000. *Essentials of Strength Training and Conditioning,* 2nd ed. Champaign, IL: Human Kinetics.
7. Baechle, T.R., and B.R. Groves. 1998. *Weight Training: Steps to Success,* 2nd ed. Champaign, IL: Human Kinetics.
8. Baker, D., G. Wilson, and R. Carlyon. 1994. Periodization: The effect on strength of manipulating volume and intensity. *Journal of Strength and Conditioning Research* 8: 235-242.
9. Berger, R.A. 1962. Effect of varied weight training programs on strength. *Research Quarterly* 33: 168-181.
10. Berger, R.A. 1972. Strength improvement. *Strength and Health,* August.
11. Bompa, T.A. 1983. *Theory and Methodology of Training.* Kendall/Hunt: Dubuque, IA.
12. Brzycki, M. 1988. Accent on intensity. *Scholastic Coach.* 97: 82-83.
13. Brzycki, M. 1993. Strength testing: Predicting a one-rep max from reps-to-fatigue. *JOHPERD* 64: 88-90.
14. Chapman, P.P., J.R. Whitehead, and R.H. Binkert. 1998. The 225-lb reps-to-fatigue test as a submaximal estimate of 1RM bench press performance in college football players. *Journal of Strength and Conditioning Research* 12 (4): 258-261.
15. Craig, B.W. 2000. Variation: An important component of training. *Strength and Conditioning Journal* 22 (15): 22-23.
16. Craig, B.W., J. Lucas, R. Pohlman, and H. Schilling. 1991. The effect of running, weightlifting and a combination of both on growth hormone release. *Journal of Applied Sport Science Research* 5 (4): 198-203.
17. DeLorme, T.L. 1945. Restoration of muscle power by heavy-resistance exercises. *Journal of Bone and Joint Surgery* 27: 645.
18. Duval, J. 1998. Traditional and unique approaches to strength training programs. *Strength and Conditioning* 20 (5): 28-29.
19. Earle, R.W. 1999. Weight training exercise prescription. In: *Essentials of Personal Training Symposium Workbook.* Lincoln, NE: NSCA Certification Commission.
20. Edgerton, V.R. 1976. Neuromuscular adaptation to power and endurance work. *Canadian Journal of Applied Sports Sciences* 1: 49-58.
21. Epley, B. 1985. Poundage chart. *Boyd Epley Workout.* Lincoln, NE: University of Nebraska.
22. Fleck, S.J. 1999. Periodized strength training: A critical review. *Journal of Strength and Conditioning Research* 13 (1): 82-89.
23. Fleck, S.J., and W.J. Kraemer. 1987. *Designing Resistance Training Programs.* Champaign, IL: Human Kinetics.
24. Fleck, S.J., and W.J. Kraemer. 1997. *Designing Resistance Training Programs,* 2nd ed. Champaign, IL: Human Kinetics.
25. Fry, A.C., W.J. Kraemer, B. Femke, J.M. Lynch, J.L. Marsit, E.P. Roy, N.T. Triplett, and H.G. Knuttgen. 1994. Performance decrements with high-intensity resistance exercise overtraining. *Medicine and Science in Sports and Exercise* 26: 1165-1173.
26. Garhammer, J. 1979. Periodization of strength training for athletes. *Track Techniques* 73: 2398-2399.
27. Garhammer, J. 1986. *Sports Illustrated Strength Training.* New York: Harper & Row.
28. Graves, J.E., M.L. Pollock, S.H. Leggett, R.W. Braith, D.M. Carpenter, and L.E. Bishop. 1988. Effect of reduced training frequency on muscular strength. *International Journal of Sports Medicine* 9: 316-319.
29. Häkkinen, K. 1994. Neuromuscular adaptation during strength training, aging, detraining and immobilization. *Critical Reviews in Physical and Rehabilitation Medicine* 6: 161-198.
30. Häkkinen, K., M. Alen, and P. Komi. 1985. Changes in isometric force- and relaxation-time. Electromyographic and muscle fibre characteristics of human skeletal muscle during strength training and detraining. *Acta Physiologica Scandinavica* 125: 573-586.
31. Häkkinen, K., M. Alen, and P. Komi. 1985. Effect of explosive type strength training on isometric force and relaxation time, electromyographic and muscle fiber characteristics of leg extensor muscle. *Acta Physiologica Scandinavica* 125: 587-592.
32. Häkkinen, K., and P.V. Komi. 1983. Electromyographic changes during strength training and detraining. *Medicine and Science in Sports and Exercise* 15: 455-501.

33. Harris, G.R, M.H. Stone, M.H. O'Bryant, H.S. Proulx, C.M. Johnson, and L. Robert. 2000. Short-term performance effects of high power, high force, or combined weight-training methods. *Journal of Strength and Conditioning Research* 14 (1): 14-20.

34. Hather, B.M., P.A. Teach, P. Buchanan, and G.A. Dudley. 1992. Influence of eccentric actions on skeletal muscle adaptations to resistance training. *Acta Physiologica Scandinavica* 143: 177-185.

35. Hedrick, A. 1995. Training for hypertrophy. *Strength and Conditioning* 17 (3): 22-29.

36. Herrick, A.R., and M.H. Stone. 1996. The effects of periodization versus progressive resistance exercise on upper and lower body strength in women. *Journal of Strength and Conditioning Research* 10 (2): 72-76.

37. Hickson, R., M.A. Rosenkoetter, and M.M. Brown. 1980. Strength training effects on aerobic power and short-term endurance. *Medicine and Science in Sports and Exercise* 12: 336-339.

38. Hoeger, W., S.L. Barette, D.F. Hale, and D.R. Hopkins. 1987. Relationship between repetitions and selected percentages of one repetition maximum. *Journal of Applied Sport Science Research* 1 (1): 11-13.

39. Hoeger, W., D.R. Hopkins, S.L. Barette, and D.F. Hale. 1990. Relationship between repetitions and selected percentages of one repetition maximum: A comparison between untrained and trained males and females. *Journal of Applied Sport Science Research* 4: 47-54.

40. Hoffman, J.R., C.M. Maresh, L.E. Armstrong, and W.J. Kraemer. 1991. Effects of off-season and in-season resistance training programs on a collegiate male basketball team. *Journal of Human Muscle Performance* 1: 48-55.

41. Jones, A. 1971. *Nautilus Training Principles.* Bulletin No. 2. Deland, FL: Nautilus.

42. Kraemer, W.J. 1992. Endocrine responses and adaptations to strength training. In: *Strength and Power in Sports,* P. Komi, ed. Oxford, England: Blackwell Scientific.

43. Kraemer, W.J. 1997. A series of studies: The physiological basis for strength training in American football: Fact over philosophy. *Journal of Strength and Conditioning Research* 11 (3): 131-142.

44. Kraemer, W.J., and L.P Koziris. 1992. Muscle strength training: Techniques and considerations. *Physical Therapy Practice* 2: 54-68.

45. Kraemer, W.J., B.J. Noble, M.J. Clark, and B.W. Culver. 1987. Physiologic responses to heavy resistance exercise with very short rest periods. *International Journal of Sports Medicine* 8: 247-252.

46. Kramer, J.B., M.H. Stone, H.S. O'Bryant, M.S. Conley, R.L. Johnson, D.C. Nieman, D.R. Honeycutt, and T.P. Hoke. 1997. Effects of single vs. multiple sets of weight training: Impact of volume, intensity, and variation. *Journal of Strength and Conditioning Research* 11 (3): 143-147.

47. Lander, J. 1984. Maximum based on reps. *NSCA Journal* 6 (6): 60-61.

48. Larson, G.D., Jr., and J.A. Potteiger. 1997. A comparison of three different rest intervals between multiple squat bouts. *Journal of Strength and Conditioning Research* 11 (2): 115-118.

49. LeSuer, D.A., J.H. McCormick, J.L. Mayhew, R.L. Wasserstein, and M.D. Arnold. 1997. The accuracy of predicting equations for estimating 1RM performance in the bench press, squat, and deadlift. *Journal of Strength and Conditioning Research* 11 (4): 211-213.

50. Lombardi, V.P. 1989. *Beginning Weight Training.* Dubuque, IA: Brown.

51. Luthi, J.M., H. Howald, H. Claassen, K. Rosler, P. Vock, and H. Hoppler. 1986. Structural changes in skeletal muscle tissue with heavy-resistance exercise. *International Journal of Sports Medicine* 7: 123-127.

52. Marcinik, E.J., J. Potts, G. Schlabach, S. Will, P. Dawson, and B.F. Hurley. 1991. Effects of strength training on lactate threshold and endurance performance. *Medicine and Science in Sports and Exercise* 23: 739-743.

53. Mayhew, J.L., T.E. Ball, M.E. Arnold, and J.C. Bowen. 1992. Relative muscular endurance performance as a predictor of bench press strength in college men and women. *Journal of Applied Sport Science Research* 6 (4): 200-206.

54. Mayhew, J.L., J.R. Ware, and J.L. Prinster. 1993. Using lift repetitions to predict muscular strength in adolescent males. *NSCA Journal* 15 (6): 35-38.

55. McDonagh, M.J.N., and C.T.M. Davies. 1984. Adaptive response of mammalian skeletal muscle to exercise with high loads. *European Journal of Applied Physiology* 52: 139-155.

56. McGee, D., T.C. Jessee, M.H. Stone, and D. Blessing. 1992. Leg and hip endurance adaptations to three weight-training programs. *Journal of Applied Sport Science Research* 6: 92-95.

57. Morales, J., and S. Sobonya. 1996. Use of submaximal repetition tests for predicting 1-RM strength in class athletes. *Journal of Strength and Conditioning Research* 10 (3): 186-189.

58. O'Bryant, H.S., R. Byrd, and M.H. Stone. 1988. Cycle ergometer performance and maximum leg and hip strength adaptations to two different methods of weight training. *Journal of Applied Sport Science Research* 2: 27-30.

59. O'Shea, J.P. 1976. *Scientific Principles and Methods of Strength Fitness.* Reading, MA: Addison-Wesley.

60. Ostrowski, K.J., G.J. Wilson, R. Weatherby, P.W. Murphy, and A.D. Lyttle. 1997. The effect of weight training volume on hormonal output and muscular size and function. *Journal of Strength and Conditioning Research* 11 (3): 148-154.

61. Pauletto, B. 1985. Sets and repetitions. *NSCA Journal* 7 (6): 67-69.

62. Pauletto, B. 1986. Choice and order of exercise. *NSCA Journal* 8 (2): 71-73.

63. Pauletto, B. 1986. Intensity. *NSCA Journal* 8 (1): 33-37.

64. Pauletto, B. 1986. Rest and recuperation. *NSCA Journal* 8 (3): 52-53.

65. Pearson, D., A. Faigenbaum, M. Conley, and W.J. Kraemer. 2000. The National Strength and Conditioning Association's basic guidelines for the resistance training of athletes. *Strength and Conditioning Journal* 22 (4): 14-27.

66. Poliquin, C. 1988. Five steps to increasing the effectiveness of your strength training program. *NSCA Journal* 10 (3): 34-39.

67. Rhea, M.R., W.T. Phillips, L.N. Burkett, W.J. Stone, S.D. Ball, B.A. Alvar, and A.B. Thomas. 2003. A comparison of linear and daily undulating periodized programs with equated volume and intensity for local muscular endurance. *Journal of Strength and Conditioning Research* 17 (1): 82-87.

68. Richardson, T. 1993. Program design: Circuit training with exercise machines. *NSCA Journal* 15 (5): 18-19.

69. Roundtable: Circuit training. 1990. *NSCA Journal* 12 (2): 16-27.

70. Roundtable: Circuit training—Part II. 1990. *NSCA Journal* 12 (3): 10-21.

71. Sforzo, G.A., and P.R. Touey. 1996. Manipulating exercise order affects muscular performance during a resistance exercise training session. *Journal of Strength and Conditioning Research* 10 (1): 20-24.

72. Simmons, L. 1988. Training by percents. *Powerlifting U.S.A.* 12 (2): 21.
73. Sobonya, S., and J. Morales. 1993. The use of maximal repetition test for prediction of 1 repetition maximum loads. *Sports Medicine Training and Rehabilitation* 4: 154. (abstract)
74. Spassov, A. June 1989. Bulgarian training methods. Paper presented at the symposium of the National Strength and Conditioning Association, Denver.
75. Stone, M.H., D. Collins, S. Plisk, G. Haff, and M.E. Stone. 2000. Training principles: Evaluation of modes and methods of resistance training. *Strength and Conditioning Journal* 22 (3): 65-76.
76. Stone, M.H., R. Keith, J.T. Kearney, G.D. Wilson, and S.J. Fleck. 1991. Overtraining: A review of the signs and symptoms of overtraining. *Journal of Applied Sport Science Research* 5: 35-50.
77. Stone, M.H., and H.S. O'Bryant. 1987. *Weight Training: A Scientific Approach.* Minneapolis: Burgess.
78. Stone, M.H., H.S. O'Bryant, J. Garhammer, J. McMillan, and R. Rozenek. 1982. A theoretical model of strength training. *National Strength and Conditioning Association Journal* 4 (4): 36-40.
79. Stone, M.H., and D. Wilson. 1985. Resistive training and selected effects. *Medical Clinics of North America* 69: 109-122.
80. Stowers, T., J. McMillan, D. Scala, V. Davis, D. Wilson, and M.H. Stone. 1983. The short-term effects of three different strength-power training methods. *NSCA Journal* 5 (3): 24-27.
81. Tan, B. 1999. Manipulating resistance training program variables to optimize maximum strength in men. *Journal of Strength and Conditioning Research* 13 (3): 289-304.
82. Tesch, P.A. 1993. Training for bodybuilding. In: *Strength and Power in Sports,* P.V. Komi, ed. London, England: Blackwell Scientific.
83. Tesch, P., and L. Larson. 1982. Muscle hypertrophy in body builders. *European Journal of Applied Physiology* 49: 301-306.
84. Verhoshansky, Y. 1976. *Fundamentals of Special Strength Training in Sport.* Livonia, MI: Sportivny Press.
85. Ware, J.S., C.T. Clemens, J.L. Mayhew, and T.J. Johnston. 1995. Muscular endurance repetitions to predict bench press and squat strength in college football players. *Journal of Strength and Conditioning Research* 9 (2): 99-103.
86. Wathen, D. 1994. Load assignment. In: *Essentials of Strength Training and Conditioning,* T.R. Baechle, ed. Champaign, IL: Human Kinetics.
87. Weir, J.P., L.L. Wagner, and T.J. Housh. 1994. The effect of rest interval length on repeated maximal bench presses. *Journal of Strength and Conditioning Research* 8 (1): 58-60.
88. Weiss, L. 1991. The obtuse nature of muscular strength: The contribution of rest to its development and expression. *Journal of Applied Sport Science Research* 5 (4): 219-227.
89. Wescott, W. 1982. *Strength Fitness.* Boston: Allyn & Bacon.
90. Wescott, W.L. 1986. Four key factors in building a strength program. *Scholastic Coach.* 55: 104-105.
91. Willoughby, D.S. 1993. The effects of mesocycle-length weight training programs involving periodization and partially equated volumes on upper and lower body strength. *Journal of Strength and Conditioning Research* 7: 2-8.

CHAPTER 16

Aerobic Endurance Training Program Design

Patrick S. Hagerman

After completing this chapter, you will be able to

- design aerobic endurance training programs based on the principle of specificity and individual client goals;
- select the appropriate mode of aerobic exercise;
- determine aerobic endurance training frequency, duration, and intensity and understand their interactions and effects on the training outcome;
- determine training intensity using calculated target heart rate zones, ratings of perceived exertion, or metabolic equivalents;
- design programs with proper warm-up, cool-down, and exercise progression; and
- apply long slow distance, pace/tempo, interval training, cross-training, arm exercise, and combination training in accord with client goals.

Aerobic endurance training is an essential component of any general exercise program. Health clubs and gyms dedicate large sections of their facilities to **aerobic endurance training** equipment, and the majority of athletic competitions for the general public are designed around aerobic endurance exercise (10K [6.2-mile] runs, marathons, cycling tours). To underscore the importance of aerobic endurance activities, the 1996 Surgeon General's report on physical activity and health emphasized the recommendation that everyone engage in some form of aerobic exercise on most days of the week [107]. Additionally, in its *Healthy People 2010,* the U.S. Department of Health and Human Services listed lack of physical activity and obesity as the top two major health issues facing the nation [108]. As a result, the goals for Healthy People 2010 include increasing (1) "the proportion of adults who engage regularly, preferably daily, in moderate physical activity for *at least* 30 minutes per day" and (2) "the proportion of adolescents who engage in vigorous physical activity that promotes cardiorespiratory fitness 3 or more days per week for 20 or more minutes per occasion" [108]. There can be no doubt as to the importance of proper aerobic endurance training.

Aerobic endurance training is often referred to as **aerobic exercise, cardiovascular exercise,** or **cardiorespiratory exercise.** These terms are used throughout this chapter and should be considered synonymous because they all refer to exercise that involves the cardiovascular and respiratory systems, including the heart, blood vessels, and lungs.

Designing an aerobic endurance training program necessitates looking at the client's present level of fitness, exercise history, and fitness goals. One of the more common health-related goals among the general population is fat loss, and a well-designed aerobic endurance training program should be a part of workouts for clients with this goal. Likewise, clients who wish to compete in the local 10K (6.2-mile) race or to be able to complete a marathon will need specific training guidelines in order to meet their goals.

Previous chapters have already dealt with determining fitness level and appropriateness of exercise levels. This chapter is devoted to putting together proper aerobic exercise programs for a variety of clients.

Specificity of Aerobic Endurance Training

The same principle of **specificity** that applies to resistance training also applies to aerobic endurance training. The principle of specificity states that the results of a training program will be directly related to the type of training performed [27, 112]. The results of a resistance training program will be specific to resistance training, and the results of aerobic training will be specific to aerobic training. In other words, resistance training does not significantly improve maximal aerobic power ($\dot{V}O_2max$) [51, 56, 73]. In addition, training that involves one mode of aerobic exercise will not guarantee equal improvement with a different aerobic exercise mode [12, 119]. For instance, a person who has achieved a high level of aerobic conditioning through cycling will not necessarily be able to produce the same aerobic performance, as measured by peak $\dot{V}O_2$ capability, during a running workout [90, 103, 118]. The muscle activation patterns and oxygen requirements among exercise modes are not equal, so the responses and adaptations are not equal [16, 84, 88, 104, 120]. Even though improvements in $\dot{V}O_2$ elicited from one exercise mode will help in other exercise modes, they will not do so to the same extent [13, 19, 78, 92, 110].

Components of an Aerobic Endurance Training Program

An aerobic endurance training program consists of several components that can be manipulated in a variety of ways to produce a number of particular outcomes. These components include the mode of exercise, frequency of exercise sessions, duration of each exercise session, and intensity of training during each session. The personal trainer needs to consider each component in relation to the client's personal goals, as well as in terms of how each component interacts with the other components.

Two hypothetical clients will serve throughout the remainder of this chapter to highlight some practical examples of integrating the components into an overall aerobic endurance training program. The first client, Becky, has a goal of completing a local 10K (6.2-mile) race in less than 50 minutes. The second client is Floyd, who wants to lose about 30 pounds (14 kilograms) of body fat. Neither client has any musculoskeletal dysfunction, and each has received physician clearance for exercise. See the next page for the initial status and goals of these two hypothetical clients.

Initial Client Status and Goals

Client: Becky

Age: 30

Height: 5 feet 5 inches (165 centimeters)

Weight: 120 pounds (55 kilograms)

Goal: Complete 10K (6.2-mile) race in less than 50 minutes

Training status: Intermediate. Has run three to five miles (4.8-8.1 kilometers) an average of two times a week for the past three years. Her 10K (6.2-mile) personal best is 56 minutes.

Other activities: Works as a receptionist, mostly sitting from 8 a.m. to 5 p.m. No other structured exercise or activities.

Client: Floyd

Age: 52

Height: 6 feet 0 inches (183 centimeters)

Weight: 230 pounds (105 kilograms)

Goal: Lose about 30 pounds (14 kilograms) of body fat

Training status: Beginner (untrained), former college baseball player. Has not been involved in a regular exercise program since college.

Other activities: Works long hours as bank officer. Walks throughout the office during the day, but no more than 40 feet (12 meters) at a time, and is usually sitting in his office. Teaches at the community college at night. No structured exercise or activity.

Exercise Mode

The first step in designing aerobic endurance training programs is to decide on the mode of exercise. Exercise **mode** refers simply to what exercise or activity will be performed. As discussed in chapter 14, cardiovascular exercise modes include machine and non-machine exercises. Athletes should choose the exercise mode that most closely mimics their specific sport or the movement that they perform during competition. The decision about which exercise mode to use depends on several factors, including equipment availability, personal preference, the client's ability to perform the exercise, and the client's goals.

The machine exercise modes use cardiovascular equipment and depend on what is available at the facility where the training will take place (figure 16.1). Most health clubs have a variety of cardiovascular equipment that typically includes treadmills, stair climbers, and stationary bikes. Advances in cardiovascular equipment have expanded the choices to include cross-country ski simulators, elliptical trainers, rowing ergometers, upper body ergometers, semi-recumbent bikes, rotating climbing walls, and others.

If cardiovascular equipment is not available, non-machine exercises can provide a variety of

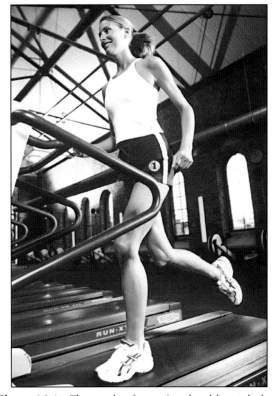

Figure 16.1 The mode of exercise should match the client's goals, physical abilities, and preferences.

options as well. Non-machine exercises comprise anything that allows the person to move freely and independently of equipment. This includes walking, jogging, running, swimming, water-resisted walking or running, skating, cardio kickboxing, and aerobic dance or step classes.

Choosing a mode of exercise, whether it is machine or non-machine, is more than simply using whatever is available. The client's personal preference has a great influence on how well he or she will adhere to the program [5, 93]. Selecting activities or exercises that clients enjoy will help them complete the training program as it was designed, and not cut corners to shorten the exercise session or decrease the intensity.

The mode of exercise must also be matched to the client's physical abilities. A client with lower body orthopedic concerns may be limited in his or her ability to perform certain exercises because of impact strain on the foot or shear forces across the knee. These clients would be better served by a non-impact form of exercise. Clients who have limitations in joint range of motion need an exercise that works within their capacity. For instance, a client with diagnosed shoulder impingement may not be able to use a VersaClimber®.

The initial exercise mode must also be within the client's current $\dot{V}O_2$ capacity. In many cases the client has not had a graded exercise test to determine his or her $\dot{V}O_2$max. Without actual data to help determine what a client is capable of, it is always prudent to begin with an enjoyable exercise mode. A client who used to walk or ride a bike might begin a new exercise program by resuming those activities. This method will prevent situations in which clients are instructed to perform an activity that is inappropriate for them. For instance, if one assigns a running program to a client who does not have the fitness capacity to even walk briskly, the client will not be able to adhere to or participate in an exercise session of sufficient duration to elicit any improvement. A different, less demanding exercise mode is needed instead.

Finally, exercise mode should match the client's ultimate goals for specificity of training. For instance, Becky, who wishes to complete a 10K (6.2-mile) race, will spend a good deal of time running either on a treadmill or on an outdoor track. In a different approach, Floyd, who is interested in losing body fat, will need to purposely expend calories, which does not necessitate any particular piece of equipment or mode of exercise. Several different modes of exercise could be added to promote variety in his workouts.

The decision which exercise mode to use depends on several factors, including equipment availability, personal preference, the client's ability to perform the exercise, and the client's goals.

Exercise Intensity

The **intensity** of exercise sessions is the main determinant of both exercise duration and training frequency. Before the personal trainer establishes duration and frequency of exercise sessions, he or she must determine the intensity level required to reach the client's goals.

Regulating and monitoring exercise intensity are key to prescribing the correct aerobic endurance training program and preventing over- or undertraining. A certain threshold of $\dot{V}O_2$ or **heart rate reserve (HRR)**, which is the difference between a client's maximal heart rate and his or her resting heart rate, must be attained during an aerobic exercise session before improvements in the cardiorespiratory system are seen [8, 48, 60, 65, 98, 116]. A person's **oxygen uptake reserve** (**$\dot{V}O_2$R** = difference between $\dot{V}O_2$max and resting $\dot{V}O_2$) has been shown to equate fairly evenly to the HRR. Since it is not common to have laboratory-assessed $\dot{V}O_2$max or $\dot{V}O_2$R data for a personal training client, the use of HRR for determining exercise intensity is acceptable [4, 83, 102].

Ultimately, the necessary aerobic exercise threshold depends on a client's initial fitness level, but for the apparently healthy adult the threshold is generally considered to be approximately 50% to 85% of HRR [3, 29, 67, 101, 102]. Depending on a client's fitness level, some may find 50% of HRR to be strenuous, while more advanced clients may find 85% of HRR insufficient to elicit cardiorespiratory system improvements. If the exercise intensity is too high, overtraining and injury may result. If the intensity is too low, the physiological stimulus to improve will be insufficient, and it will take longer to reach the goals that have been set. The key to knowing where to begin lies in examining the client's exercise and medical history and in the results of any recent exercise testing. It is always smart to begin conservatively and have to increase the intensity rather than beginning too high and risk overtraining and poor adherence.

Target Heart Rate

Heart rate and oxygen consumption ($\dot{V}O_2$) are closely related. During exercise, heart rate increases linearly with increases in workload, and an increase in workload necessitates an increase in oxygen consumption [32, 40]. Therefore, as heart rate increases to the client's **maximal heart rate (MHR)**, a greater percentage of $\dot{V}O_2max$ is being utilized. Table 16.1 shows a range of age-predicted maximal heart rates (APMHR) and their related percentages of $\dot{V}O_2max$. This relationship has been shown to be consistent across age, sex, coronary artery disease status, fitness level, training status, muscle groups exercised, and testing mode [32, 40, 67, 99, 117]. Because of this relationship, heart rate is often used as a quick and easy way to measure exercise intensity.

The only way to determine a person's true MHR is to perform a graded exercise test that takes the client to the point where the heart rate does not increase with an increase in workload. At this point the heart has reached its maximal beat per minute (beat/min) capacity. For safety's sake, it may be recommended that a physician be present during a **maximal graded exercise test** on a client [83]. Refer to chapter 10 for discussion on the conditions warranting the presence of a physician during exercise testing. Instead of performing a maximal graded exercise test, the personal trainer can use an estimate of a client's MHR in most cases. The most commonly used **age-predicted maximal heart rate (APMHR)** equation is as follows:

$$\text{APMHR} = 220 - \text{age} \qquad \textbf{(16.1)}$$

This is only an estimate, with an error range of ±10 to 15 beats/min [54, 79, 113]. The APMHR will therefore actually be maximal for some, unattainable for others, and submaximal for the rest [68]. However, it will be rare for a client ever to experience an MHR during the course of submaximal aerobic training, so the age-predicted estimate provides a close approximation that is acceptable for designing aerobic exercise programs [113]. An exception to using APMHR exists for clients who are taking medications such as beta-blockers that blunt the heart rate response to exercise. Before using APMHR to prescribe exercise intensity, the personal trainer must determine that the client is not using any such heart rate-altering medications; and if the client is doing so, use of alternative intensity prescriptions not based on heart rate is necessary. (Refer to chapter 20 for discussion about heart rate-altering medications.) Furthermore, with clients whose body fat is greater than 30%, a variation of equation 16.1 is more accurate than the traditional APMHR equation [79]:

$$\text{modified APMHR} = 200 - (0.5 \times \text{age}) \qquad \textbf{(16.2)}$$

If the use of APMHR is appropriate and this value has been calculated, an appropriate exercise intensity **"training zone"** or **target heart rate range (THRR)** can be determined through one of two dif-

TABLE 16.1

Relationship Between Percentages of $\dot{V}O_2max$ and Age-Predicted Maximal Heart Rate (APMHR)

%$\dot{V}O_2max$	%APMHR*
50	66
55	70
60	74
65	77
70	81
75	85
80	88
85	92
90	96
100	100

*The percentages vary slightly (±0.5-2%) according to the reference.

Adapted from Londeree and Ames 1976; Pollock and Wilmore 1990.

ferent calculations. (Refer to chapter 11 for a further discussion that includes converting the THRR in beats/min to beats-per-10 [or 15] second intervals that are more appropriate to use when exercising.)

Percent of APMHR Once the APMHR is known, a range of exercise intensities based on known relationships between percentages of the APMHR and $\dot{V}O_2$max can be used. For the apparently healthy adult, 55% to 75% of $\dot{V}O_2$max approximates to 70% to 85% of the APMHR, which provides the appropriate stimulus to improve aerobic function (figure 16.2). Other ranges may be calculated depending on the client's medical history, any complications present, and physician recommendations. This is especially appropriate for clients who are very deconditioned, because initial fitness level greatly affects the minimal threshold for cardiovascular improvement [62, 74, 94]. In these cases, a lower range of 55% to 65% of APMHR may be more appropriate [2].

To determine the intensity training zone using a percent of APMHR for an apparently healthy adult, multiply the client's APMHR by 70% and 85% (called the **percent of APMHR method**). The results will be the lower and upper limits of exercise heart rate needed for improving cardiovascular function (table 16.2).

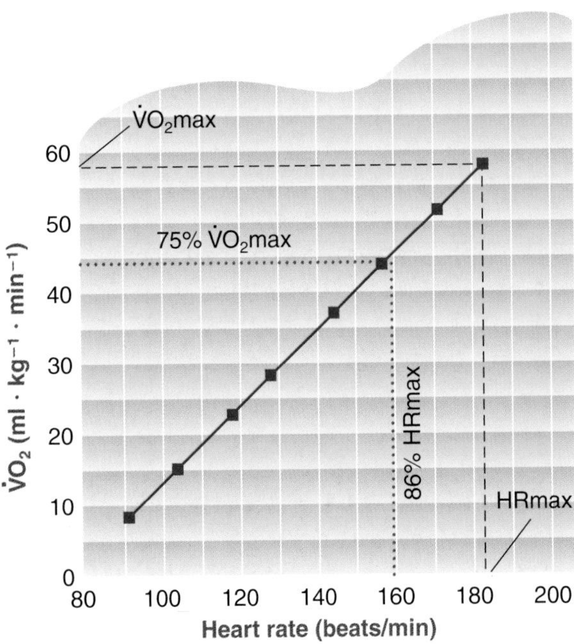

Figure 16.2 An example of the relationship between $\dot{V}O_2$max and age-predicted maximal heart rate.
Reprinted from Wilmore and Costill 1999.

$$\text{THR} = \text{APMHR} \times \text{exercise intensity} \quad \textbf{(16.3)}$$

Percent of Heart Rate Reserve: The Karvonen Formula The **Karvonen formula** is related to the percent of APMHR formula, except that the Karvonen formula allows for differences in **resting heart rate (RHR)** [60, 61]. To use this formula, first measure the client's RHR and then subtract the RHR from the APMHR to obtain the HRR:

$$\text{HRR} = \text{APMHR} - \text{RHR} \quad \textbf{(16.4)}$$

The HRR is the available increase in heart rate over the RHR, up to the APMHR. In other words, the HRR is the number of beats per minute that the heart rate can increase from resting up to maximal. For instance, a 40-year-old client with an RHR of 70 has an APMHR of 180 and an HRR of 110 beats/min (an APMHR of 180 minus an RHR of 70). As mentioned earlier, 50% to 85% of HRR is needed to improve cardiovascular function. To determine the target training zone, multiply the HRR by 50% and 85%, and then add the RHR back to each answer to obtain the lower and upper heart rate limits. Failure to add the RHR back to the answer will result in a underestimated training zone that will not provide the desired improvements.

$$\text{THR} = (\text{HRR} \times \text{exercise intensity}) + \text{RHR} \quad \textbf{(16.5)}$$

The benefit to using HRR is that it is specific to the client because it is based on his or her baseline RHR. As a person becomes more fit and the RHR decreases, the HRR will increase; this represents a greater "reserve" to draw from.

In most situations, using the Karvonen formula provides slightly larger training ranges than the percent of APMHR formula does (table 16.2) [39, 83]. To calculate exercise heart rate range, use 70% to 85% of APMHR or 50% to 85% of HRR. Both will provide a heart rate range that produces an appropriate exercise stimulus to improve cardiovascular fitness [3, 60, 65, 67]. Note that untrained or beginning clients probably should begin with a THRR based on the lower half of the APMHR intensity range (e.g., 70% to 80%) and more trained clients typically can tolerate intensities in the upper half of the HRR range (e.g., 70% to 85%). See "Exercise Intensity Calculations Using Heart Rate" on page 406 for exercise intensity formulas and sample calculations for both methods.

To calculate exercise heart rate range, assign an exercise intensity of 70% to 85% of APMHR or 50% to 85% of HRR.

TABLE 16.2

Aerobic Endurance Training Exercise Heart Rates

Age	APMHR* (beats/min)	Percent of APMHR method		Karvonen formula method**	
		70%	85%	50%	85%
80	140	98	119	105	130
75	145	102	123	108	134
70	150	105	128	110	138
65	155	109	132	113	142
60	160	112	136	115	147
55	165	116	140	118	151
50	170	119	145	120	155
45	175	123	149	123	160
40	180	126	153	125	164
35	185	130	157	128	168
30	190	133	162	130	172
25	195	137	166	133	176
20	200	140	170	135	181
15	205	144	174	138	185

*APMHR = Age-predicted maximal heart rate.

**Assumes a resting heart rate of 70 beats/min.

Percent of Functional Capacity

If a client's **functional capacity** (measured as $\dot{V}O_2max$) has been determined through a physician-supervised graded exercise test, the true MHR will be known. In this situation, it is best to use the measured MHR rather than an estimate. Either the Karvonen formula or the percent of APMHR formula (using the actual MHR in place of the APMHR) can be used to determine the aerobic exercise training zone.

Ratings of Perceived Exertion

An additional method, to be used along with heart rate calculation methods, is known as the rating of perceived exertion scale, or more commonly as the Borg **Rating of Perceived Exertion (RPE)** scale [15]. The RPE scales are designed to help clients monitor their exercise intensities through a rating system that accounts for all of the body's responses to a particular exercise intensity. A client must be taught to quantify the stress of the exercise session in terms of both physiological and psychological factors, based on the mode of exercise; environment (temperature, humidity, etc.); intensity of the effort; and extent of strain, discomfort, or fatigue [38, 72, 91]. Basically, an RPE is not just a measure of how fast the heart is beating, but is meant to include exertion, respiration, and emotional responses to exercise.

Often during graded exercise testing, clients are asked to give an RPE during each successive workload. These RPEs are paired to the $\dot{V}O_2$ of that workload so that when the test is completed, any given workload and $\dot{V}O_2$ has a known RPE. Because the personal trainer now knows what exertion rating corresponds to a given workload, the RPE can be used to determine approximate $\dot{V}O_2$ during exercise without the need to directly measure $\dot{V}O_2$. For example, if the personal trainer knows that a

Exercise Intensity Calculations Using Heart Rate

Percent of APMHR Method

Formula: age-predicted maximal heart rate (APMHR) = 220 – age

target heart rate (THR) = (APMHR × exercise intensity)

Do this calculation twice for the lower and upper limits to determine the target heart rate range (THRR).

Example: 30-year-old client; 70% to 85% of APMHR

APMHR = 220 – 30 = 190 beats/min

THR (70%) = 190 × 0.70 = 133 beats/min

THR (85%) = 190 × 0.85 = 162 beats/min

THRR = 133 to 162 beats/min

Karvonen Method

Formula: age-predicted maximal heart rate (APMHR) = 220 – age

heart rate reserve (HRR) = APMHR – resting heart rate (RHR)

target heart rate (THR) = (HRR × exercise intensity) + RHR

Do this calculation twice for the lower and upper limits to determine the target heart rate range (THRR).

Example: 30-year-old client; 50% to 85% of HRR; RHR = 70 beats/min

APMHR = 220 – 30 = 190 beats/min

HRR = 190 – 70 = 120 beats/min

THR (50%) = (120 × 0.50) + 70 = 130 beats/min

THR (85%) = (120 × 0.85) + 70 = 172 beats/min

THRR = 130 to 172 beats/min

particular $\dot{V}O_2$ elicited an RPE of 13 (on the 6-20 scale) during the YMCA cycle ergometer test (see chapter 11), during the next exercise session he or she should attempt to approximate that same $\dot{V}O_2$ intensity with a different exercise mode. The personal trainer must simply adjust the intensity of the machine to the point where the client rates the exercise at an RPE of 13.

In exercise settings in which the client's $\dot{V}O_2max$ is not known, the RPE scale can be used as an approximation of heart rate to monitor a client's exercise heart rate. Each number on the original 6-20 RPE scale corresponds to an approximate heart rate, found by simply multiplying the RPE by 10 [25, 34, 66]. An RPE of 6 approximates a heart rate of 60 beats/min, whereas an RPE of 20 approximates a heart rate of 200 beats/min. Obviously, the "RPE × 10 = exercise heart rate" formula is just an estimate; it is influenced by many factors (e.g., the client's age and fitness level).

Figure 16.3 shows the original RPE scale of 6-20 with the new scale of 0-10 [15]. There are several notable differences between the two scales. As mentioned before, the 6-20 scale is associated with approximate heart rates; the 0-10 scale is not. The 6-20 scale was designed primarily for graded exercise, as each increase in rating is proportional to an increase in heart rate caused by an increased workload [91]. A problem with using the 6-20 scale arises with older clients whose MHR lies somewhere below 200 beats/min. If a client has an APMHR of 160 beats/min, then an RPE of 20, which is associated with maximal exertion, should occur at a heart rate of 160 beats/min, not 200 beats/min (RPE of 20 ×

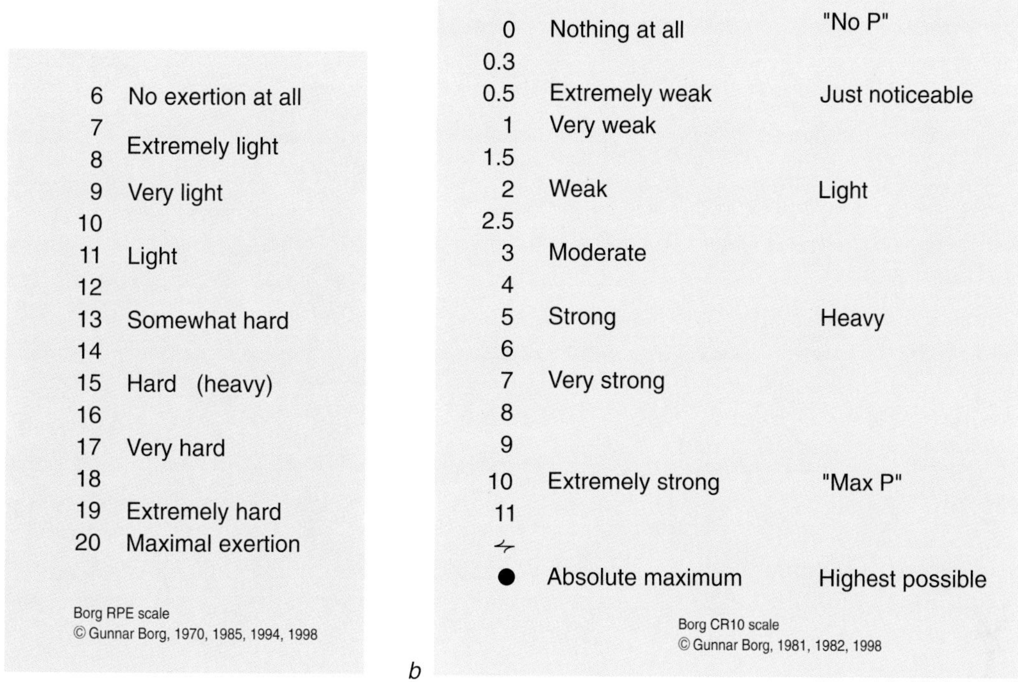

6 No exertion at all
7
8 Extremely light
9 Very light
10
11 Light
12
13 Somewhat hard
14
15 Hard (heavy)
16
17 Very hard
18
19 Extremely hard
20 Maximal exertion
Borg RPE scale
© Gunnar Borg, 1970, 1985, 1994, 1998
a
0 Nothing at all "No P"
0.3
0.5 Extremely weak Just noticeable
1 Very weak
1.5
2 Weak Light
2.5
3 Moderate
4
5 Strong Heavy
6
7 Very strong
8
9
10 Extremely strong "Max P"
11
● Absolute maximum Highest possible
Borg CR10 scale
© Gunnar Borg, 1981, 1982, 1998
b

Figure 16.3 *(a)* Rating of perceived exertion scale and *(b)* category-ratio scale. On the category-ratio scale, "P" represents perceived intensity.

For correct usage of the Borg scales, it is necessary to follow the administration and instructions given in G. Borg, 1998, *Borg's Perceived Exertion and Pain Scales*. Champaign, IL: Human Kinetics.

10 = 200 beats/min). In these situations, the 0-10 scale is more appropriate. The 0-10 scale ratings are not associated with a particular heart rate; rather they indicate how stressful the perceived exertion is above a resting level, or how much harder the exercise is than a minimal level of exertion.

Regardless of which scale is used, the numerical ratings on each are associated with adjectives that describe the level of exertion. These ratings range from "No exertion at all" to "Maximal exertion" [15] (for the 6-20 scale) or "Nothing at all" to "Absolute maximum" (for the 0-10 scale). Teaching a client to differentiate between exertion levels may take some time. To untrained, deconditioned clients, an exercise level that produces a heart rate of 60% HRR may seem maximal because they are unaccustomed to exercise and do not really know what a maximal effort is. Only through training and changes in exercise intensities will such clients learn the true meaning of the rating adjectives and how to accurately report their RPE.

In settings where the client's $\dot{V}O_2max$ is not known, the 6-20 RPE scale can be used as an approximation of heart rate to monitor a client's exercise heart rate.

To make this learning easier, RPE scales should be used along with heart rate measurements, so that over time, a pattern of exercise intensity for a given client can be established. A downside to using RPEs is that they vary between clients and between exercise modes for any given heart rate [80]. Therefore, the personal trainer should avoid general exercise prescriptions based on an RPE, as they do not take individual differences into account.

The strength of RPE scales is that they allow for more than just a measurement of heart rate. These scales can be used when traditional heart rate intensity prescriptions are inaccurate due to the influence of medications or illness. When combined with heart rate, RPE allows assessments of whether the exercise intensity is providing enough of a stimulus for a particular client [14]. For instance, if an advanced client is exercising at 80% of HRR and indicates an RPE of 4 on the 0-10 scale, an increase in exercise intensity is appropriate. In contrast, if a new client indicates a rating of 18 on the 6-20 scale but has an actual exercise heart rate equal to 70% of HRR, the personal trainer should reduce exercise intensity until the client becomes better trained.

Finally, an RPE of "somewhat hard" (13-14 on the 6-20 scale) or "strong" (4-5 on the 0-10 scale) has been found to equate with the lactate threshold in both trained and untrained men and women [91]. Training at or just below the lactate threshold is considered the most efficient exercise intensity for increasing cardiovascular fitness and losing body fat [52, 53, 75].

Metabolic Equivalents

Exercise intensity can also be prescribed in terms of **metabolic equivalents (METs)**. One MET is equal to 3.5 $ml \cdot kg^{-1} \cdot min^{-1}$ of oxygen consumption and is considered the amount of oxygen required by the body to function when at rest [76]. Therefore, any given MET level is an indication of how much harder than rest a particular activity is. For example, an activity that has a 4-MET rating is four times harder than rest, meaning that it requires the body to work four times harder than at rest. In order to accurately prescribe an exercise intensity based on METs, the personal trainer or physician must perform a maximal graded exercise test on a client to obtain the maximal MET level possible for that client (i.e., $\dot{V}O_2max$ divided by 3.5). Without this information, assigning a percentage of maximal METs is not possible.

The data displays on cardiovascular equipment often show the METs for given exercise levels and thus allow comparison of exercise intensities between different pieces of equipment. For instance, a personal trainer may set up a client on a treadmill whose display indicates that the intensity is 4 METs. When the client then moves to a semi-recumbent bike, the intensity may also be set at 4 METs. There are also published MET approximations as shown in "Estimated Metabolic Equivalents for Various Activities," below. These approximations can be used to prescribe a variety of activities for the client's total exercise program. The "Client Update" on page 410 shows sample intensity prescriptions based on various methods for the hypothetical clients.

Estimated Metabolic Equivalents for Various Activities

METs	Activity
1.0	Lying or sitting quietly, doing nothing, lying in bed awake, listening to music, watching a movie
2.0	Walking, <2 mph (<3.2 km/hr), level surface
2.5	Stretching, hatha yoga
2.5	Walking, 2 mph (3.2 km/hr), level surface
3.0	Resistance training (free weight, Nautilus® or Universal® type), light or moderate effort
3.0	Stationary cycling, 50 watts, very light effort
3.0	Walking, 2.5 mph (4 km/hr)
3.3	Walking, 3 mph (4.8 km/hr), level surface
3.5	Calisthenics, home exercise, light or moderate effort
3.5	Golf, using a power cart
3.5	Rowing machine, 50 watts, light effort
3.5	Stair stepping (with a 4-inch [10-centimeter] step height), 20 steps per minute
3.8	Walking, 3.5 mph (5.6 km/hr), level surface
4.0	Water aerobics, water calisthenics
4.5	Badminton, social singles and doubles
4.5	Golf, walking and carrying clubs
4.8	Stair stepping (with a 4-inch [10-centimeter] step height), 30 steps per minute
4.9	Stair stepping (with a 8-inch [20-centimeter] step height), 20 steps per minute
5.0	Aerobic dance, low impact
5.0	Tennis, doubles
5.0	Walking, 4 mph (6.4 km/hr), level surface
5.5	Stationary cycling, 100 watts, light effort
6.0	Basketball, non-game
6.0	Outdoor cycling, 10 to 11.9 mph (16.1-19.2 km/hr)
6.0	Resistance training (free weight, Nautilus® or Universal® type), power lifting or body building, vigorous effort

METs	Activity
6.3	Stair stepping (with a 12-inch [30-centimeter] step height), 20 steps per minute
6.3	Walking, 4.5 mph (7.2 km/hr), level surface
6.9	Stair stepping (with a 8-inch [20-centimeter] step height), 30 steps per minute
7.0	Aerobic dance, high impact
7.0	Badminton, competitive
7.0	Cross-country skiing, 2.5 mph (4 km/hr), slow or light effort, ski walking
7.0	Rowing machine, 100 watts, moderate effort
7.0	Stationary cycling, 150 watts, moderate effort
7.0	Swimming laps, freestyle, slow, moderate or light effort
8.0	Basketball, game
8.0	Calisthenics (e.g., pushups, sit-ups, pull-ups, jumping jacks), vigorous effort
8.0	Circuit training, including some aerobic stations, with minimal rest
8.0	Cross-country skiing, 4.0 to 4.9 mph (6.4-7.9 km/hr), moderate speed and effort
8.0	Outdoor cycling, 12 to 13.9 mph (19.3-22.4 km/hr)
8.0	Tennis, singles
8.0	Walking, 5 mph (3.2 km/hr)
8.5	Rowing machine, 150 watts, vigorous effort
8.5	Step aerobics (with a 6- to 8-inch [15- to 20-centimeter] step)
9.0	Cross-country skiing, 5 to 7.9 mph (8.1-12.7 km/hr), brisk speed, vigorous effort
9.0	Running, 5.2 mph (3.2 km/hr) (11.5-minute mile)
9.0	Stair stepping (with a 12-inch [30-centimeter] step height), 30 steps per minute
10.0	Outdoor cycling, 14 to 15.9 mph (22.5-25.6 km/hr)
10.0	Running, 6 mph (9.7 km/hr) (10-minute mile)
10.0	Step aerobics (with a 10- to 12-inch [25- to 30-centimeter] step)
10.0	Swimming laps, freestyle, fast, vigorous effort
10.5	Stationary cycling, 200 watts, vigorous effort
11.0	Running, 6.7 mph (10.8 km/hr) (9-minute mile)
11.5	Running, 7 mph (11.3 km/hr) (8.5-minute mile)
12.0	Outdoor cycling, 16 to 19 mph (25.7-30.6 km/hr)
12.0	Roller-blading (in-line skating), not coasting
12.0	Rowing machine, 200 watts, very vigorous effort
12.5	Running, 7.5 mph (12.1 km/hr) (8-minute mile)
12.5	Stationary cycling, 250 watts, very vigorous effort
13.5	Running, 8 mph (12.9 km/hr) (7.5-minute mile)
14.0	Cross-country skiing, >8 mph (>12.9 km/hr), racing
14.0	Running, 8.5 mph (13.7 km/hr) (7-minute mile)
15.0	Running, 9 mph (14.5 km/hr) (6-min, 40-sec mile)
16.0	Outdoor cycling, >20 mph (>32.2 km/hr)
16.0	Running, 10 mph (16.1 km/hr) (6-minute mile)
18.0	Running, 10.9 mph (17.5 km/hr) (5.5-minute mile)

MET = metabolic equivalent.

Adapted from Ainsworth et al. 2000 (consult this reference for a comprehensive list of the MET level for 605 specific activities) and ACSM 2000 (consult this reference for more MET levels for stair stepping).

Training Frequency

Training **frequency** refers to how often the workouts are performed (e.g., the number of training sessions per week). The frequency of training sessions depends on the client's goals, current fitness level, duration, intensity, and recovery time required for the exercise.

As noted earlier, the U.S. Surgeon General has recommended that all people over the age of 2 years

Client Update: Exercise Intensity

A variety of intensities are provided for each client. The personal trainer should choose one based on the mode of exercise and the intensity monitoring tools that are available (e.g., heart rate monitor, MET readout on a machine, RPE chart). (Refer to chapters 2 and 11 for illustrations and directions of how to measure a client's heart rate manually.)

Becky

Age: 30

RHR: 65

APMHR: 190 beats/min

70% to 85% HRR = 153 to 171 beats/min

RPE = 4-5 (0-10 scale)

METs = 12.5 (8-minute-mile pace)

Because Becky is somewhat trained, her THRR can be based on the upper half (e.g., 70% to 85%) of her HRR. Her current 10K (6.2-mile) personal best time is 56 minutes which is about nine minutes per mile. Although Becky's workouts may vary from day-to-day, to reach her goal time of under 50 minutes, she needs to increase her average training pace to eight minutes per mile. Her personal trainer can monitor Becky's ability to tolerate this increase in exercise intensity by either an RPE or heart rate.

Floyd

Age: 52

RHR: 74

APMHR: 168 beats/min

70% to 80% APMHR = 118 to 134 beats/min

RPE = 11-13 (6-20 scale)

METs = 3 to 3.8 (walking at 2.5-3.5 miles [4-5.6 kilometers] per hour); 5.5 (stationary cycling at 100 watts; refer to chapter 11 to convert watts to an exercise work rate)

Because Floyd is untrained, his THRR can be based on the lower half (70% to 80%) of his APMHR. The MET intensities chosen for Floyd will allow him to exercise at a pace he can sustain as a beginner for weight-bearing exercises, and a little harder (5.5 METs) for non-weight-bearing exercises. Until Floyd becomes accustomed to exercise and can give accurate RPEs, his personal trainer should monitor Floyd's exercise intensity by regularly measuring his heart rate during the exercise session.

should accumulate at least 30 minutes of aerobic endurance-type of physical activity, of at least moderate intensity, on most—preferably all—days of the week [107]. In a 1998 position stand, the American College of Sports Medicine stated that aerobic exercise should be done three to five days per week; that training for less than two days per week is generally not a sufficient stimulus for developing and maintaining fitness [2]. So a minimum of two days per week, up to five days per week, is suggested for general fitness goals. Some advanced clients may be able to tolerate more than five days per week if the rest between sessions is sufficient to prevent overuse injury.

Beginning clients (e.g., no participation in a regular aerobic exercise program for the past six months) should start with the minimum number of sessions per week, spaced out evenly. As fitness levels improve, the frequency of training can increase (see the "Sample Exercise Frequency Options" below). As the number of exercise sessions per week increases, the frequency should not exceed the frequency that a client is willing to adopt and maintain [4]. For example, despite the common examples shown, some clients may only have the weekdays (or just the weekends) to exercise so the personal trainer will need to design an exercise schedule around when the client is available. Most desirably, however, the client's rest days should be placed in between exercise days to space them evenly throughout the week.

In the case of Becky, because she is already running twice a week, her exercise prescription can begin at three to four days per week. Floyd, on the other hand, as a nonexerciser, will begin with two days per week, although he reports that he has the flexibility and desire to exercise in the morning before work and during his lunch hour (not on the weekends, though).

Ultimately, the frequency of exercise must be balanced with the duration and intensity of exercise. In general, exercise sessions of longer duration or higher intensity require more recovery time and are therefore performed less frequently, whereas exercise sessions of shorter duration or less intensity do not require as much recovery time and can be performed more often [87].

In general, exercise sessions of longer duration or higher intensity necessitate more recovery time between sessions and are therefore performed less frequently; whereas exercise sessions of shorter duration or less intensity do not require as much recovery time and can be performed more often.

Exercise Duration

Exercise **duration** is a measure of how long an exercise session lasts. Along with training frequency, exercise duration depends on the client's goals, current fitness levels, and the intensity of the exercise. The greater the intensity of an aerobic exercise session, the greater the $\dot{V}O_2$ requirement and the less time a client will be able to spend exercising at that level [96].

Sample Exercise Frequency Options

Sunday	Monday	Tuesday	Wednesday	Thursday	Friday	Saturday
Beginner: two days exercise, five days rest						
Rest	Exercise	Rest	Rest	Exercise	Rest	Rest
Beginner: three days exercise, four days rest						
Rest	Exercise	Rest	Exercise	Rest	Exercise	Rest
Intermediate: four days exercise, three days rest						
Rest	Exercise	Exercise	Rest	Exercise	Exercise	Rest
Intermediate: five days exercise, two days rest						
Rest	Exercise	Exercise	Rest	Exercise	Exercise	Exercise
Advanced: six days exercise, one day rest						
Exercise	Exercise	Exercise	Rest	Exercise	Exercise	Exercise

The National Institutes of Health Consensus Development Panel on Physical Activity and Cardiovascular Health agrees with the Surgeon General's report in stating that duration of aerobic endurance training should be at least 30 minutes [82]. The American Heart Association recommends between 30 to 60 minutes for the purposes of health promotion and cardiovascular disease prevention [28]. Finally, the American College of Sports Medicine recommends 20 to 60 minutes of continuous or intermittent bouts accumulated throughout the day [3].

If time constraints prevent a client from dedicating a block of time large enough to meet exercise duration needs, or if the client is very deconditioned, shorter **intermittent exercise** bouts can be substituted. If the intensity is moderate to high, intermittent exercise bouts of at least 10 minutes each can improve the aerobic fitness of all but the most advanced clients [24, 43, 81]. Intermittent bouts have also been shown to improve adherence to exercise in those people who are unaccustomed to exercise [57]. For clients who are severely deconditioned and unable to complete even a 10-minute exercise bout, several shorter bouts of exercise with rest periods in between will allow them to build up to a continuous bout.

Beyond the recommended minimum of 30 minutes, the human body is capable of withstanding hours of aerobic endurance exercise, as is evident in athletes who complete full triathlons, 24-hour ultramarathons, or bike races of 100 miles (160 kilometers) or more. The total duration of a given client's program is ultimately determined by that client's personal goals, the intensity level of a given workout, and the client's ability to fit the training session into his or her schedule. In the case of Becky, she has been running three to five miles (4.8-8.1 kilometers) at about a nine-minute-mile pace for an exercise duration of 27 to 45 minutes. Since her goal of completing a 10K (6.2 miles) in less than 50 minutes requires a continuous exercise bout, intermittent training throughout the day will not offer her sufficient training specificity; therefore, she must adjust her schedule (e.g., exercise before or after work) to allow for longer exercise sessions. In contrast, Floyd's goal of weight loss does not require sustained bouts of exercise; and although he will be able to eventually sustain a longer exercise bout, he has decided that he would like to begin with two 10- to 15-minute sessions each exercise day.

Exercise duration is inversely related to exercise intensity.

Progression

One of the keys to designing a proper aerobic endurance training program is exercise **progression.** For purposes of training the general population, aerobic endurance training programs can be divided into two distinct types: *improvement* and *maintenance.* The type of program the personal trainer designs for a client depends on the client's initial fitness level and training background. The untrained beginner will start with an improvement program because "you can't maintain what you don't have;" a client who has been exercising but wants to improve will use an improvement program; and a client who just wishes to maintain his or her current level of aerobic endurance will use a maintenance program.

Improvement in aerobic endurance training can be measured as an increase in $\dot{V}O_2$ capacity or increased tolerance for longer durations or higher intensities. The time spent in an improvement program depends on the client's goals and initial fitness level. In some cases, a client may follow only an improvement program. If the goal is to continually increase aerobic capacity, by definition a maintenance program is not required. Following an improvement program requires making periodic, progressive increases in exercise frequency, duration, or intensity. As a general rule, increases in frequency, intensity, or duration should be limited to 10% per week. Constraints on a client's available training time, along with the fact that there are only seven days in a week, often mean that exercise frequency and duration reach their upper limits before exercise intensity after which improvements in aerobic capacity will have to result from increases in intensity. In other words, the client will have only so much time available to exercise, but he or she can continually (albeit gradually) increase exercise intensity.

The maintenance program is reserved for clients who want to maintain their current level of fitness or who have progressed through the improvement program and have reached the upper limits of how intensely they wish to train. Maintenance of aerobic capacity requires significantly less effort than trying to improve (raise) it. Over the long term, clients can maintain improvements from an aerobic endurance training program if they reduce the frequency of training to no less than two sessions per week but maintain the duration and (especially) the intensity during the exercise sessions that they do perform [17, 48, 49, 50]. Additionally, to keep a client motivated during a maintenance program and to facilitate continued adherence, the personal trainer can design the program to use a

Client Update: Six-Week Progression

Becky

Becky indicated that she can work out only three days a week. Since she has been running three to five miles (4.8-8.1 kilometers) at about a nine-minute-mile pace (27-45 minutes) twice a week, her six-week program will concentrate on gradually increasing the distance she runs while maintaining the faster training pace (8 minutes per mile) needed to prepare her for running a 10K (6.2 miles) in her goal time.

Week 1: three days (Mon, Wed, Fri): running 3 to 4 miles (4.8-6.4 kilometers) in 24 to 32 minutes

Week 2: three days (Sun, Tue, Thur): running 3 to 4 miles (4.8-6.4 kilometers) in 24 to 32 minutes

Week 3: three days (Mon, Wed, Fri): running 4 to 5 miles (6.4-8.1 kilometers) in 32 to 40 minutes

Week 4: three days (Sun, Tue, Thur): running 4 to 5 miles (6.4-8.1 kilometers) in 32 to 40 minutes

Week 5: three days (Mon, Wed, Fri): running 5 to 6 miles (6.4-9.7 kilometers) in 40 to 48 minutes

Week 6: three days (Sun, Tue, Thur): running 5 to 6 miles (6.4-9.7 kilometers) in 40 to 48 minutes

Floyd

Floyd indicated that he can begin with working out two days a week (although he has each weekday available), in two 15-minute sessions each exercise day. His six-week program will concentrate on increasing the number of days and the duration of exercise while keeping him within his APMHR training zone of 118 to 134 beats/min.

Week 1: two days (Mon, Thur), two times each day (in the morning before work and during the lunch hour): walking on a treadmill at 2.5-3.5 miles [4-5.6 kilometers] per hour for 10 to 15 minutes

Week 2: three days (Tue, Thur, Sat), two times each day: in the morning before work: riding the stationary bike at 100 watts for 10 to 15 minutes; during the lunch hour: walking on a treadmill at 2.5-3.5 miles [4-5.6 kilometers] per hour for 10 to 15 minutes

Week 3: four days (Mon, Tue, Thu, Fri), once each day (Floyd can decide when): riding the stationary bike at 100 watts for 20 to 25 minutes

Week 4: four days (Mon, Tue, Thu, Fri), once each day (Floyd can decide when): walking on a treadmill at 2.5-3.5 miles [4-5.6 kilometers] per hour for 15 to 20 minutes

Week 5: five days (Mon, Tue, Wed, Thu, Fri), once each day (Floyd can decide when): three times a week (Mon, Wed, Fri), walking on a treadmill at 2.5-3.5 miles [4-5.6 kilometers] per hour for 20 to 25 minutes; two times a week (Tue, Thurs), riding the stationary bike at 100 watts for 25 to 30 minutes

Week 6: five days (Mon, Tue, Wed, Thu, Fri), once each day (Floyd can decide when): walking on a treadmill at 2.5-3.5 miles [4-5.6 kilometers] per hour for 25 to 30 minutes

variety of exercise modes [5, 42]. Another use of a maintenance program is for a client who wishes to take some time off from training (or needs to because of a business trip or vacation); this person can decrease the total volume of aerobic exercise for a few weeks by as much as 70% without negatively affecting $\dot{V}O_2$max [77].

As a general rule, increases in frequency, intensity, or duration should be limited to 10% per week.

Warm-Up and Cool-Down

Regardless of which program a client is using, appropriate **warm-up** and **cool-down** procedures should be integrated into the exercise sessions. The purpose of a warm-up is to increase blood flow to the muscles that will be used during the workout, slowly increase heart rate so that oxygen debt is minimized, prepare the nervous system for action, and increase muscle core temperature to cause more complete unloading of oxygen from the blood to the muscles [41, 95, 97, 109]. Proper warm-up involves a slow progression from small, simple movements to the larger, more complicated movements that mimic those used during the exercise session [33]. For instance, if a client will be running, a proper warm-up will include progression from normal walking with the arms at the sides, to slow jogging with a swinging of slightly bent arms, to running with full pumping of the arms at a 90° bend in the elbows. The client should allow enough time in each activity for the heart rate to increase to meet metabolic demands before progressing further.

The cool-down uses the same progression in reverse. The client progresses from running, to jogging, to walking, again allowing the heart rate to decrease and reach a lower steady state before slowing down. Clients can do additional flexibility exercises after the cool-down. See chapter 12 for more information on warm-up, cool-down, and flexibility exercises.

Types of Aerobic Training Programs

There are many ways to design aerobic endurance training programs, but all will contain the components previously discussed. As mentioned earlier, the first step is deciding which mode or modes of exercise to use. Sometimes choosing more than one mode is appropriate. For instance, outdoor running, cycling, and swimming are all dependent on the weather. Combining machine and non-machine exercises that mimic each other can provide a continued training stimulus when the environment is not conducive to outdoor workouts. Running outside or on a treadmill, cycling or riding a stationary bike, and swimming in a lake or in a pool can all provide the stimulus needed for improvement if adjustments for duration and intensity are made. The exercise mode must be one that the client will enjoy and can perform without any problems or pain, and one that provides enough of a challenge to stimulate improvement.

After exercise modes have been selected, the frequency, duration, and intensity can be combined in a number of ways, each of which will produce a different effect. The final program may take the form of long slow distance training, pace/tempo training, interval training, circuit training, or cross-training. The most important determinant of how to combine these components is the goal of the client.

Long Slow Distance

In **long slow distance (LSD)** training, once intensity is achieved, the exercise can continue as long as the client is able to maintain his or her heart rate within the prescribed zone and energy is available. When heart rate increases beyond the training zone, the anaerobic systems begin to provide energy at the expense of carbohydrate and glycogen stores, and volitional fatigue will eventually follow. Once the client's heart rate begins to increase without an increase in workload, the exercise session is complete. For the beginning exerciser, this may occur after only a brief period of time (10 to 15 minutes). With subsequent exercise sessions, the client can increase the duration of exercise as cardiorespiratory system improvements allow for greater perfusion of oxygenated blood, delivery of energy substrates, and removal of waste products.

Long slow distance training sessions should be performed at an intensity less than that normally used so that the duration of the workout can be longer. For example, during LSD training, a client capable of running at a six-minute-mile pace would exercise at an eight-minute-mile pace for a longer distance. A client who normally rides a stationary bike for 30 minutes at 150 watts would ride for one hour at 100 watts. The basic idea is to exercise for a longer duration than normal but at a lower intensity than normal. A good indicator of proper intensity other than percent of HRR is whether the client can carry on a conversation during the exercise session. The idea is not to speak at length, but to be able to talk without becoming short of breath. The goals of LSD training include improvements in the anaerobic threshold, development of endurance in supporting musculature, and fat utilization with corresponding glycogen sparing. Typical training sessions last between 30 minutes and two hours and, to prevent overtraining, should not take place more than twice a week [22, 111].

One should note that not all clients will initially be able to achieve the 50% to 85% HRR training zone or be able to continue the exercise for more than a short time period. Seriously deconditioned clients will require a lower starting point and a slower increase in both intensity and duration.

Pace/Tempo Training

For clients who wish to improve their cardiorespiratory endurance, and who are capable of working at the highest percentages of their heart rate range, **pace/tempo training** can help improve $\dot{V}O_2max$. Pace/tempo training sessions typically last between 20 and 30 minutes and require clients to exercise at their lactate threshold [20, 22]. As mentioned earlier, an RPE of 13-14 on the 6-20 scale, or 4-5 on the 0-10 scale, is considered an approximation of the lactate threshold. The workout can be performed either intermittently or steadily. Intermittent pace/tempo training involves work bouts of three to five minutes with rest periods of 30 to 90 seconds, repeated until the desired pace cannot be maintained. Steady pace/tempo training involves one bout of exercise lasting 20 to 30 minutes, sustained at the desired pace. Because pace/tempo training requires that a higher intensity be achieved during a workout session, the duration of the workout is reduced. Pace/tempo training should be performed only one to two times a week. Below is an example of an intermittent pace/tempo workout.

Interval Training

Interval training programs get their name from the alternating periods of high- and low-intensity exercise they include. Interval training can involve short periods of exercise at intensities at or above the lactate threshold and $\dot{V}O_2max$, alternated with long periods of lesser intensities (a combination of pace/tempo and LSD training). Interval training can also involve high-intensity exercise (90-100% HRR) with periods of rest in between. The benefit of interval training is that with the correct spacing of work and rest, clients can accomplish a great amount of work that normally is not possible with a continuous program. Normally, exercising at such a high intensity (90-100% HRR) would cause a client to tap into the anaerobic energy systems and fatigue quickly. With interval training, fatigue is a result; but the length of time spent exercising is kept relatively short, and the rest periods are lengthened to allow for more complete recovery between exercise intervals. Thus complete fatigue is delayed. For instance, clients who want to increase their running or cycling speed would use intervals of faster running or cycling that push their HRR limits, alternated with rest periods in which they continue moving at a pace that is equal to the lower end of their HRR. A client who wishes to burn a maximum number of calories in a set amount of time could employ interval training also. In this case, alternating high and low intensities, instead of using one set intensity, allows the client to burn a greater number of calories during a workout [6, 7, 18].

Properly adjusting the **work-to-rest ratio** is essential to allow the client to complete the prescribed exercise session. High-intensity intervals should last between three and five minutes, with a rest period of 1:1 to 1:3 depending on the ability of the client to perform successive high-intensity intervals. As the client fatigues, the rest interval

Sample Intermittent Pace/Tempo Workout for Becky

Intervals: 3 to 5 minutes
Intensity: 80 to 85% HRR or 8 METs
Rest between intervals: 60 seconds
Mode: Elliptical machine

Elliptical Machine

Warm-up
Three minutes at MET level 8, 60 seconds rest
Four minutes at MET level 8, 60 seconds rest
Five minutes at MET level 8, 60 seconds rest
Five minutes at MET level 8, 60 seconds rest
Five minutes at MET level 8, 60 seconds rest
Four minutes at MET level 8, 60 seconds rest
Three minutes at MET level 8
Cool-down

can be lengthened to allow for greater recovery between work bouts. Extending the rest interval beyond 1:3 reduces the amount of time that can be spent in high-intensity work bouts during a fixed-length exercise session, and thus reduces the total amount of work done and improvement made. The 1:1 to 1:3 work-to-rest ratios cause improvements in cardiorespiratory endurance mainly through raising the lactate threshold and enhancing the body's ability to clear lactate from the bloodstream [111, 115].

Clients should use interval training only after they have established a firm aerobic base and are able to maintain exercise intensity within the HRR training zone for a period of time roughly equal to the total time that will be spent on interval training [64]. As an example, a client who is able to maintain a steady-state HRR training zone for 60 minutes could perform interval training for up to 60 minutes.

Almost any cardiovascular exercise can be selected for an interval training workout. If the intensity can be adjusted quickly and easily, cardiovascular machines can be used in the same way that outdoor exercises are used for interval training. For variety, the high-intensity bouts can be done on one machine and the rest bouts performed with another exercise. For example, an interval training program could involve using the VersaClimber for the work period and the treadmill for the rest period.

Long slow distance, interval, and pace/tempo programs are advanced aerobic exercise programs that should be used only after an initial aerobic training program has been completed.

Circuit Training

Circuit training combines resistance training with cardiovascular training; the client performs short

Client Update: Sample Training Programs With Long Slow Distance, Interval, and Pace/Tempo

Because LSD, interval, and pace/tempo programs require a firm aerobic base, these sample programs should be viewed as a progression to be used after some tolerance for exercise has been established through consistent and regular aerobic training.

Becky (Rest Days: Tuesday, Thursday, Friday, Sunday)

Monday	Wednesday	Saturday
Long slow distance	Interval	Pace/tempo
Outdoor running	Treadmill	Outdoor running
15K to 20K (9.3-12.4 miles)	60 minutes	30 minutes steady
9- to 10-minute-mile pace	5-minute work period at a 6-minute-mile pace (10 mph [16.1 km/hr]) alternated with a 5-minute rest period at a 12-minute-mile pace (5 mph [8.1 km/hr])	8-minute-mile pace

Floyd (Rest Days: Sunday, Saturday)

Monday/Thursday	Tuesday/Friday	Wednesday
Interval	Long slow distance	Pace/tempo
Stationary cycle	Treadmill	Stationary cycle
30 minutes	60 minutes	20 minutes intermittent
5-minute work period at 150 watts alternated with a 5-minute rest period at 75 watts	3 miles [4.8 kilometers] per hour	5-minute work period at 80% to 85% HRR alternated with a 1-minute rest period

intervals of cardiovascular training between the resistance training sets. The goal is to increase heart rate to the training zone and keep it there for the duration of the exercise session, thus inducing improvement in cardiorespiratory endurance and muscular endurance at the same time [37, 56]. Unfortunately, most investigations on variations of circuit training have shown that although strength increased, $\dot{V}O_2max$ did not significantly improve compared that for participants in an aerobic exercise-only program [36, 106]. Those research studies that did show small improvements in $\dot{V}O_2max$ due to circuit training required the subjects to train at heart rates close to 90% HRR [21]. However, although circuit training has not been shown to significantly increase $\dot{V}O_2$ in many cases, there is no evidence that $\dot{V}O_2$ decreases during a circuit training program. Therefore, it may be a useful tool in a maintenance program. Circuit training can also be used with beginning clients as a means of introducing them to both resistance and aerobic training when their available time for training is short.

Cross-Training

Cross-training is a method of combining several exercise modes for aerobic endurance training. In order for cross-training to be effective in maintaining or improving $\dot{V}O_2max$, the intensity and duration of each exercise must be of sufficient quantity with respect to the client's fitness level [35, 70, 114]. For clients who wish to do cross-training, the personal trainer must prescribe the intensity and duration of each mode of exercise individually while keeping the combined volume of exercise within the client's capabilities. The benefit of cross-training is that it distributes the physical stress of training to different muscle groups during the different activities and increases the adaptations of the cardiorespiratory and musculoskeletal systems [63, 85, 121].

The result of cross-training is that it overcomes the limitations of specificity of training. That is, when a client has a goal that cannot be met with use of one particular exercise, increased running and swimming speed for instance, cross-training is a way of obtaining both of those goals.

Aerobic endurance cross-training can be accomplished by two different means: (1) utilizing different modes of exercise each training period, rotating through two or more modes within a week; or (2) utilizing several different exercise modes within the same workout. With the first option, a client may train on the treadmill one day, cycle outdoors the next, and then finish the week on a rowing machine. The second option entails setting up a series of exercise modes that can be completed back to back. For example, instead of doing 30 minutes on the treadmill, the client might do 10 minutes each on the treadmill, elliptical trainer, and arm ergometer.

Client Update: Sample Cross-Training Workouts

Cross-training workouts should be designed around the total volume or duration of exercise that the client is capable of. The following examples are progressions to be used after some tolerance for exercise duration has been established through consistent and regular aerobic training.

Becky

Monday: 60 minutes on the treadmill

Wednesday: 60 minutes on the stationary bike

Friday: 30 minutes on the stair climber

Floyd

Monday: 10 minutes on the treadmill, 10 minutes on the stationary bike, 10 minutes on the stair climber

Tuesday: 10 minutes on the rowing ergometer, 10 minutes on the elliptical trainer, 10 minutes on the treadmill

Thursday: 30 minutes on the stationary bike

Saturday: 20 minutes walking outdoors, 15 minutes on the rowing machine

The key to making cross-training effective is ensuring that with each exercise mode the client works within his or her prescribed training zone. Different exercises may elicit different heart rates for a given workload or speed, so individualization of the program for each mode is necessary.

Arm Exercise

Many aerobic endurance activities primarily involve the major muscles of the lower body. Arm exercises are becoming more popular, are often part of cardiac rehabilitation programs, and are a contributing source of power for swimming. When prescribing a THRR based on a percent of APMHR, it is necessary to make a downward adjustment of 10 to 13 beats/min in calculating the APMHR because during **arm exercise,** heart rate is higher than during leg exercise for any given workload [26, 30, 31, 58, 71, 105]. Additionally, the $\dot{V}O_2$max for arm exercise is significantly lower than that for leg exercise [26, 58]. The result is that the lactate threshold is reached at lower intensities than during leg exercise [89]. It is possible to use ratings of perceived exertion with arm exercise, but the guidelines given earlier will not apply [26, 58, 59]. Ratings of perceived exertion may used as an accurate indicator of exercise stress if they are established specifically for arm exercise.

Upper body ergometers (arm bikes) are the most common type of arm-specific equipment found in fitness centers. Stationary bicycles with an attachment to the pedals that allow the arms to work with the legs, such as the Schwinn® Airdyne®, can be used in an arms-only mode for upper body cardiovascular exercise. Likewise, the arm portion of a rowing ergometer can be used if the feet are placed on the floor so that the body does not slide back and forth.

Arm exercise is probably the most underutilized type of cardiovascular exercise. To increase variety, arm work can be added to current programs that mainly use lower body exercises. Arm exercise is especially helpful in providing some cardiovascular exercise to clients who have orthopedic problems with their lower body, such as an injury to the foot, knee, or hip.

Combined Aerobic and Resistance Training

Quite often, clients undertake aerobic endurance and resistance training programs simultaneously. While the benefits of both are clear, and there is no doubt that both should be part of a complete training program, there is a downside to combining these two different types of training. Research has shown that when properly designed resistance training and aerobic training programs are combined, the increase in strength gains will be blunted, while $\dot{V}O_2$ increases normally. Clients will see increases in aerobic endurance similar to those they would have seen if they had done only aerobic endurance training, but the increases in strength from the resistance training portion of their program will be smaller than if they had done only resistance training [11, 23, 44, 45, 55]. Along with reduced maximum strength gains, combined programs result in reductions in the amount of muscle girth gains and in specific speed- and power-related performances [21, 23, 45]. On the other hand, the addition of anaerobic resistance training to an aerobic endurance training program seems to improve low-intensity aerobic endurance [46, 51, 100].

A relatively sedentary client who is just beginning to exercise will show improvements from both aerobic and resistance training when using both programs within a total workout. However, for more advanced clients who are reaching plateaus in improvement, it is doubtful that they can get the full benefits of both programs at the same time because there will be little to no recovery time (days off to rest).

To remedy this problem, the personal trainer can design a program to allow the client to complete the aerobic endurance training program before beginning the resistance training program. For instance, a client could perform eight weeks of aerobic endurance training only, followed by eight weeks of resistance training with only the minimal amount of aerobic endurance training needed for maintenance. This would allow the client to increase $\dot{V}O_2$max and establish an aerobic base first, then work on increasing his or her muscular fitness (e.g., strength) while maintaining the improved $\dot{V}O_2$ [9, 10, 46]. After the initial 16 weeks, the client could begin alternating periods of aerobic endurance training (with minimal resistance training for maintenance of strength) with periods of resistance training (with minimal aerobic endurance training for maintenance) [47]. This style of program provides continued increases in both aerobic endurance and muscular strength, although at a reduced rate in comparison to training only for one or the other, but also allows for changes in program variables such as mode and intensity to enhance variety. See the "Sample Combined Aerobic and Resistance Training Programs" on the next page for sample combined training programs based on differing training goals.

Sample Combined Aerobic and Resistance Training Programs

Goal: Increased Muscular Strength, Maintenance of Aerobic Endurance

1. Perform initial aerobic training for 8 to 10 weeks: three to four days a week, 50% to 85% HRR, 30 to 60 minutes.
2. Reduce aerobic training to two days per week, 50% to 85% HRR, 30 minutes, and begin resistance training.

Goal: Increased Aerobic Endurance, Maintenance of Muscular Strength

1. Perform 8 to 10 weeks of initial resistance training.
2. Reduce resistance training to two days per week and begin aerobic training three to four days per week, 50% to 85% HRR, 30 to 60 minutes.

CONCLUSION

Designing aerobic endurance training programs that meet clients' goals and improve the working capacity of the cardiovascular and cardiorespiratory systems requires careful thought and accurate calculations. Because of the individual differences clients exhibit in regard to exercise preference, long-term goals, and current training status, the personal trainer must take care when manipulating the components of intensity, duration, and frequency. When program components are properly aligned, improvements in $\dot{V}O_2$max for an individual are limited only by genetics. Incorporation of different training methods such as long slow distances, pace/tempo training, interval training, circuit training, cross-training, arm exercises, and the combination of aerobic and resistance training will allow clients to continue making improvements as the body has to continually adapt to ever changing program components.

STUDY QUESTIONS

1. A client is preparing for her first marathon, and she wants to complete the 26.2-mile (42-kilometer) distance in four hours. Which of the following sample workouts will be the most effective to reach her goal?
   A. cycling 26.2 miles (42 kilometers)
   B. stair climbing for four hours
   C. running 20 miles (32 kilometers)
   D. freestyle swimming for four hours
2. The personal trainer is designing an aerobic exercise program for a 50-year-old client who has a resting heart rate of 70 beats/min. What is the THRR if the personal trainer assigns an intensity of 60% to 70% of the client's HRR?
   A. 102 to 119 beats/min
   B. 110 to 120 beats/min
   C. 130 to 140 beats/min
   D. 132 to 154 beats/min

3. The personal trainer is designing an aerobic exercise program for a 30-year-old client who has a resting heart rate of 50 beats/min. What is the THRR if the personal trainer assigns an intensity of 75% to 85% of the client's APMHR?
   A. 155 to 169 beats/min
   B. 143 to 162 beats/min
   C. 135 to 149 beats/min
   D. 105 to 119 beats/min
4. A sedentary 35-year-old client is morbidly obese and would like to lose weight. The personal trainer selected treadmill walking as the exercise mode. Which of the following is an appropriate exercise duration for the first exercise session?
   A. 10 minutes
   B. 20 minutes
   C. 25 minutes
   D. 30 minutes

APPLIED KNOWLEDGE QUESTION

Fill in the chart to describe the types of aerobic training programs.

Type	Intensity	Duration	Frequency	Goals
LSD				
Pace/tempo: intermittent				
Pace/tempo: steady				
Interval				

REFERENCES

1. Ainsworth, B.E., W.L. Haskell, M.C. Whitt, M.L. Irwin, A.M. Swartz, S.J. Strath, W.L. O'Brien, D.R. Bassett, K.H. Schmitz, P.O. Emplaincourt, D.R. Jacobs, and A.S. Leon. 2000. Compendium of physical activities: An update of activity codes and MET intensities. *Medicine and Science in Sports and Exercise* 32 (9 Suppl): S498-S516.
2. American College of Sports Medicine. 1998. The recommended quantity and quality of exercise for developing and maintaining cardiorespiratory and muscular fitness, and flexibility in healthy adults. *Medicine and Science in Sports and Exercise* 30 (6): 975-991.
3. American College of Sports Medicine. 2000. *Guidelines for Exercise Testing and Prescription*, 6th ed. Philadelphia: Lippincott Williams & Wilkins.
4. American College of Sports Medicine. 2001. Appropriate intervention strategies for weight loss and prevention of weight regain for adults. *Medicine and Science in Sports and Exercise* 33 (12): 2145-2156.
5. Annesi, J.J., and J. Mazas. 1997. Effects of virtual reality-enhanced exercise equipment on adherence and exercise-induced feeling states. *Perceptual and Motor Skills* 85: 835-844.
6. Åstrand, I., P.O. Åstrand, E.H. Christensen, and R. Hedman. 1960. Intermittent muscular work. *Acta Physiologica Scandinavica* 48: 443.
7. Åstrand, P.O., and K. Rodahl. 1986. *Textbook of Work Physiology*. New York: McGraw-Hill.
8. Atomi, Y., K. Ito, H. Iwasaski, and M. Miyashita. 1978. Effects of intensity and frequency of training on aerobic work capacity of young females. *Journal of Sports Medicine* 18: 3-9.
9. Bell, G.J., S.R. Petersen, and H.A. Quinner. 1988. Sequencing of endurance and high-velocity strength training. *Canadian Journal of Sport Science* 13: 214-219.
10. Bell, G.J., S.R. Petersen, J. Wessel, K. Bagnall, and H.A. Quinner. 1991. Adaptations to endurance and low velocity resistance training performed in a sequence. *Canadian Journal of Sport Science* 16 (3): 186-192.
11. Bell, G.J., S.R. Petersen, J. Wessel, K. Bagnall, and H.A. Quinner. 1991. Physiological adaptations to concurrent endurance training and low velocity resistance training. *International Journal of Sports Medicine* 12: 384-390.
12. Ben-Ezra, V., C. Lacy, and D. Marshall. 1992. Perceived exertion during graded exercise: Treadmill vs step ergometry. *Medicine and Science in Sports and Exercise* 24 (5 Suppl): S136.
13. Ben-Ezra, V., and R. Verstraete. 1991. Step ergometry: Is it task-specific training? *European Journal of Applied Physiology* 63: 261-264.

14. Borg, G. 1985. *An Introduction to Borg's RPE-Scale.* Ithaca, NY: Mouvement.

15. Borg. G. 1998. *Borg's Perceived Exertion and Pain Scales.* Champaign, IL: Human Kinetics.

16. Bressel, E., G.D. Heise, and G. Bachman. 1998. A neuromuscular and metabolic comparison of forward and reverse pedaling. *Journal of Applied Biomechanics* 14 (4): 401-411.

17. Brynteson, P., and W.E. Sinning. 1973. The effects of training frequencies on the retention of cardiovascular fitness. *Medicine and Science in Sports* 4: 29-33.

18. Christensen, E.H., R. Hedman, and B. Saltin. 1960. Intermittent and continuous running. *Acta Physiologica Scandinavica* 50: 269.

19. Clausen, J.P., D. Klausen, B. Rasmussen, and J. Trap-Jensen. 1973. Central and peripheral circulatory changes after training of the arms or legs. *American Journal of Physiology* 225: 675-682.

20. Costill, D.L. 1986. *Inside Running: Basics of Sports Physiology.* Indianapolis: Benchmark Press.

21. Craig, B.W., J. Lucas, R. Pohlman, and H. Stelling. 1991. The effects of running, weightlifting and a combination of both on growth hormone release. *Journal of Applied Sport Science Research* 5 (4): 198-203.

22. Daniels, J. 1989. Training distance runners—a primer. *Gatorade Sports Science Exchange* 1: 1-5.

23. Dudley, G.A., and R. Djamil. 1985. Incompatibility of endurance and strength training modes of exercise. *Journal of Applied Physiology* 59: 1446-1451.

24. Ebisu, T. 1985. Splitting the distance of endurance running: On cardiovascular endurance and blood lipids. *Japanese Journal of Physical Education* 30: 37-43.

25. Edwards, R.H., A. Melcher, C.M. Hesser, O. Wegebtz, and L.G. Ekelund. 1972. Physiological correlates of perceived exertion in continuous and intermittent exercise with the same average power output. *European Journal of Clinical Investigation* 2: 108-114.

26. Eston, R.G., and D.A. Brodie. 1986. Responses to arm and leg ergometry. *British Journal of Sports Medicine* 20 (1): 4-6.

27. Fleck, S.J., and W.J. Kraemer. 1987. *Designing Resistance Training Programs.* Champaign, IL: Human Kinetics.

28. Fletcher, G.F., G. Balady, S.N. Blair, J. Blumenthal, C. Caspersen, B. Chaitman, S. Epstein, E.S. Sivarajen Froelicher, V.F. Froelicher, I.L. Pina, and M.L. Pollock. 1996. Benefits and recommendations for physical activity programs for all Americans. A statement for health professionals by the Committee on Exercise and Cardiac Rehabilitation of the Council on Clinical Cardiology, American Heart Association. *Circulation* 94: 857-862.

29. Fox, S.M., J.P. Naughton, and P.A. Gorman. 1972. Physical activity and cardiovascular health III. The exercise prescription: Frequency and type of activity. *Modern Concepts of Cardiovascular Disease* 41 (6): 25-30.

30. Franklin, B.A. 1983. Aerobic requirements of arm ergometry: Implications for testing and training. *Physician and Sportsmedicine* 11: 81.

31. Franklin, B.A. 1989. Aerobic exercise training programs for the upper body. *Medicine and Science in Sports and Exercise* 21: S141.

32. Franklin, B.A., J. Hodgson, and E.R. Buskirk. 1980. Relationship between percent maximal O2 uptake and percent maximal heart rate in women. *Research Quarterly* 51: 616-624.

33. Franks, B.D. 1983. Physical warm-up. In: *Ergogenic Aids in Sport,* M.H. Williams, ed. Champaign, IL: Human Kinetics, pp. 340-375.

34. Gamberale, F. 1972. Perception of exertion, heart rate, oxygen uptake and blood lactate in different work operations. *Ergonomics* 15: 545-554.

35. Gergley, T.J., W.D. McArdle, P. DeJesus, M.M. Toner, S. Jacobowitz, and R.J. Spina. 1984. Specificity of arm training on aerobic power during swimming and running. *Medicine and Science in Sports and Exercise* 16: 349-354.

36. Gettman, L.R., J.J. Ayres, and M.L. Pollock. 1979. Physiologic effects on adult men of circuit strength training and jogging. *Archives of Physical Medicine and Rehabilitation* 60: 115-120.

37. Gettman, L.R., J.J. Ayres, M.L. Pollock, and A. Jackson. 1978. The effect of circuit weight training on strength, cardiorespiratory function, and body composition of adult men. *Medicine and Science in Sports and Exercise* 10: 171-176.

38. Glass, S.C., R.G. Knowlton, and M.D. Becque. 1994. Perception of effort during high-intensity exercise at low, moderate, and high wet bulb globe temperatures. *European Journal of Applied Physiology* 68: 519-524.

39. Goldberg, L., D.L. Elliot, and K.S. Kuehl. 1988. Assessment of exercise intensity formulas by use of ventilatory threshold. *Chest* 94 (1): 95-98.

40. Green, J.H., N.T. Cable, and N. Elms. 1990. Heart rate and oxygen consumption during walking on land and in deep water. *Journal of Sports Medicine and Physical Fitness* 30: 49-52.

41. Gutin, B., K. Stewart, S. Lewis, and J. Kruper. 1976. Oxygen consumption in the first stages of strenuous work as a function of prior exercise. *Journal of Sports Medicine and Physical Fitness* 16 (1): 60-65.

42. Hanson, J.M. 1994. *The Relationship Between Personal Incentives for Exercise and the Selection of Activity Among Patrons of Fitness Centers and Recreation Centers.* Microform Publications. Eugene, OR: University of Oregon, International Institute for Sport and Human Performance.

43. Hardman, A.E. 2001. Issues of fractionization of exercise (short vs long bouts). *Medicine and Science in Sports and Exercise* 33 (6 Suppl): S421-S427.

44. Hennessy, L.C., and A.W.S. Watson. 1994. The interference effects of training for strength and endurance simultaneously. *Journal of Strength Conditioning Research* 8 (1): 12-19.

45. Hickson, R.C. 1980. Interference of strength development by simultaneous training for strength and endurance. *European Journal of Applied Physiology* 45: 255-263.

46. Hickson, R.C., B.A. Dvorak, E.M. Gorostiaga, T.T. Kurowski, and C. Foster. 1988. Potential for strength and endurance training to amplify endurance performance. *Journal of Applied Physiology* 65 (5): 2285-2290.

47. Hickson, R.C., B.A. Dvorak, E.M. Gorostiaga, T.T. Kurowski, and C. Foster. 1988. Strength training and performance in endurance-trained subjects. *Medicine and Science in Sports and Exercise* 20: S86.

48. Hickson, R.C., C. Foster, M.L. Pollock, T.M. Galassi, and S. Rich. 1985. Reduced training intensities and loss of aerobic power, endurance, and cardiac growth. *Journal of Applied Physiology* 58 (2): 492-499.

49. Hickson, R.C., C. Kanakis Jr., J.R. Davis, A.M. Moore, and S. Rich. 1982. Reduced training duration effects on aerobic power, endurance, and cardiac growth. *Journal of Applied Physiology* 53: 225-229.

50. Hickson, R.C., and M.A. Rosenkoetter. 1981. Reduced training frequencies and maintenance of increased aerobic power. *Medicine and Science in Sports and Exercise* 13: 13-16.

51. Hickson, R.C., M.A. Rosenkoetter, and M.M. Brown. 1980. Strength training effects on aerobic power and short-term

endurance. *Medicine and Science in Sports and Exercise* 12 (5): 336-339.

52. Holloszy, J.O., and F.W. Booth. 1976. Biochemical adaptations to endurance exercise in muscle. *Annual Review in Physiology* 38: 273-291.
53. Holloszy, J.O., and E.F. Coyle. 1984. Adaptations of skeletal muscle to endurance exercise and their metabolic consequences. *Journal of Applied Physiology* 56: 831-838.
54. Howley, E.T. 2000. You asked for it: Question authority. The equation "220-age" is used to estimate maximal heart rate, but there is potential error in the estimate. Where did that equation come from, and are better equations available? *ACSM's Health and Fitness Journal* 4 (4): 6-18.
55. Hunter, G., R. Dement, and D. Miller. 1987. Development of strength and maximum oxygen uptake during simultaneous training for strength and endurance. *Journal of Sports Medicine and Physical Fitness* 27: 269-275.
56. Hurley, B.F., D.R. Seals, A.A. Ehsani, L.-J. Cartier, G.P. Dalsky, J.M. Hagberg, and J.O. Holloszy. 1984. Effects of high-intensity strength training on cardiovascular function. *Medicine and Science in Sports and Exercise* 16 (5): 483-488.
57. Jakicic, J.M., R.R. Wing, B.A. Butler, and R.J. Robertson. 1995. Prescribing exercise in multiple short bouts versus one continuous bout: Effects on adherence, cardiorespiratory fitness, and weight loss in overweight women. *International Journal of Obesity* 19: 893-901.
58. Kang, J., E.C. Chaloupka, M.A. Mastrangelo, and J. Angelucci. 1999. Physiological responses to upper body exercise on an arm and a modified leg ergometer. *Medicine and Science in Sports and Exercise* 31 (10): 1453-1459.
59. Kang, J., E.C. Chaloupka, M.A. Mastrangelo, M.S. Donnelly, W.P. Martz, and R.J. Robertson. 1998. Regulating exercise intensity using ratings of perceived exertion during arm and leg ergometry. *European Journal of Applied Physiology and Occupational Physiology* 78 (3): 241-246.
60. Karvonen, M., K. Kentala, and O. Mustala. 1957. The effects of training on heart rate: A longitudinal study. *Annales Medicinae Experimentalis et Biologial Fennial* 35: 307-315.
61. Karvonen, J., and T. Vuorimaa. 1988. Heart rate and exercise intensity during sports activities. Practical application. *Sports Medicine* 5 (5): 303-311.
62. Kearney, J.T., A.G. Stull, and J.L. Ewing. 1976. Cardiorespiratory responses of sedentary college women as a function of training intensity. *Journal of Applied Physiology* 41: 822-825.
63. Kohrt, W.M., D.W. Morgan, B. Bates, and J.S. Skinner. 1987. Physiological responses of triathletes to maximal swimming, cycling, and running. *Medicine and Science in Sports and Exercise* 19: 51-55.
64. Lamb, D.R. 1995. Basic principles for improving sport performance. *Sports Science Exchange* 8: 1-5.
65. Liang, M.T.C., J.F. Alexander, H.L. Taylor, R.C. Serfass, and A.S. Leon. 1982. Aerobic training threshold: Intensity, duration and frequency of exercise. *Scandinavian Journal of Sports Sciences* 4 (1): 5-8.
66. Lollgen, H., H.V. Ulmer, and G. von Nieding. 1977. Heart rate and perceptual responses to exercise with different pedaling speed in normal subjects and patients. *European Journal of Applied Physiology* 37: 297-304.
67. Londeree, B.R., and S.A. Ames. 1976. Trend analysis of the $\%VO_2$max-HR regression. *Medicine and Science in Sports* 8: 122-125.
68. Londeree, B.R., and M.L. Moeschberger. 1982. Effect of age and other factors on maximal heart rate. *Research Quarterly in Exercise and Sport* 53 (4): 297-304.
69. Loy, S.F., G. Holland, D. Mutton, J. Snow, W. Vincent, J. Hoffmann, and S. Shaw. 1993. Effects of stair-climbing vs. run training on treadmill and track running performance. *Medicine and Science in Sports and Exercise* 25: 1275-1278.
70. Magel, J.R., G.F. Foglia, W.D. McArdle, B. Gutin, and G.S. Pechar. 1975. Specificity of swim training on maximal oxygen uptake. *Journal of Applied Physiology* 38: 151-155.
71. Magel, J.R., W.D. McArdle, M. Toner, and D.J. Delio. 1978. Metabolic and cardiovascular adjustment to arm training. *Journal of Applied Physiology* 45: 75.
72. Mahon, A.D., K.O. Stolen, and J.A. Gay. 2001. Differentiated perceived exertion during submaximal exercise in children and adults. *Journal of Pediatric Exercise Science* 13: 145-153.
73. Marcinik, E.J., J. Potts, G. Schlabach, S. Will, P. Dawson, and B.F. Hurley. 1991. Effects of strength training on lactate threshold and endurance performance. *Medicine and Science in Sports and Exercise* 23 (6): 739-743.
74. Marigold, E.A. 1974. The effect of training at predetermined heart rate levels for sedentary college women. *Medicine and Science in Sports* 6: 14-19.
75. Matoba, H., and P.D. Gollnick. 1984. Response of skeletal muscle to training. *Sports Medicine* 1: 240-251.
76. McArdle, W.D., F.I. Katch, and V.L. Katch. 1991. In: *Exercise Physiology: Energy, Nutrition, and Human Performance,* 3rd ed. Philadelphia: Lea & Febiger.
77. McConell, G.K., D.L. Costill, J.J. Widrick, M.S. Hickey, H. Tanaka, and P.B. Gastin. 1993. Reduced training volume and intensity maintain aerobic capacity but not performance in distance runners. *International Journal of Sports Medicine* 14 (1): 33-37.
78. McKenzie, D.C., E.L. Fox, and K. Cohen. 1978. Specificity of metabolic and circulatory responses to arm or leg interval training. *European Journal of Applied Physiology* 39: 241-248.
79. Miller, W.C., J.P. Wallace, and K.E. Eggert. 1993. Predicting max HR and the HR-VO_2 relationship for exercise prescription in obesity. *Medicine and Science in Sports and Exercise* 25 (9): 1077-1081.
80. Moyna, N.M., R.J. Robertson, C.L. Meckes, J.A. Peoples, N.B. Millich, and P.D. Thompson. 2001. Intermodal comparison of energy expenditure at exercise intensities corresponding to perceptual preference range. *Medicine and Science in Sports and Exercise* 33: 1404-1410.
81. Murphy, M.H., and A.E. Hardman. 1998. Training effects of short and long bouts of brisk walking in sedentary women. *Medicine and Science in Sports and Exercise* 30: 152-157.
82. National Institutes of Health: Consensus Development Panel on Physical Activity and Cardiovascular Health. 1996. Physical activity and cardiovascular health. *Journal of the American Medical Association* 276: 214-246.
83. Nieman, D.C. 2003. *Exercise Testing and Prescription,* 5th ed. Boston: McGraw-Hill.
84. Nilsson, J., A. Thorstensson, and J. Halbertsma. 1985. Changes in leg movements and muscle activity with speed of locomotion and mode of progression in humans. *Acta Physiologica Scandinavica* 123: 457-475.
85. O'Toole, M.L., P.S. Douglas, and W.D.B. Hiller. 1989. Applied physiology of a triathlon. *Sports Medicine* 8: 201-225.

86. Pollock, M.L., and J.H. Wilmore. 1990. *Exercise in Health and Disease: Evaluation and Prescription for Prevention and Rehabilitation,* 2nd ed. Philadelphia: Saunders.

87. Potteiger, J.A. 2000. Aerobic endurance exercise training. In: *Essentials of Strength Training and Conditioning,* 2nd ed., T.R. Baechle and R.W. Earle, eds. Champaign, IL: Human Kinetics, pp. 495-509.

88. Raasch, C.C., and F.E. Zajac. 1999. Locomotor strategy for pedaling: Muscle groups and biomechanical functions. *Journal of Neurophysiology* 82 (5): 515-525.

89. Reybrouck, T., G.F. Heigenhauser, and J.A. Faulkner. 1975. Limitations to maximum oxygen uptake in arms, leg, and combined arm-leg ergometry. *Journal of Applied Physiology* 38 (5): 774-779.

90. Riddle, S., and C. Orringer. 1990. Measurement of oxygen consumption and cardiovascular response during exercise on the Stairmaster 4000PT versus the treadmill. *Medicine and Science in Sports and Exercise* 22 (2 Suppl): S65.

91. Robertson, R.J., and B.J. Noble. 1997. Perception of physical exertion: Methods, mediators, and applications. *Exercise and Sport Science Reviews* 25: 407-452.

92. Rosentswieg, J., D. Verstraete, and G. Bassett. 1986. Stair-climbing as a training modality for women (abstract). *Medicine and Science in Sports and Exercise* 18: S28.

93. Ryan, R.M., C.M. Frederick, D. Lepes, N. Rubio, and K.M. Sheldon. 1997. Intrinsic motivation and exercise adherence. *International Journal of Sport Psychology* 28 (4): 335-354.

94. Saltin, B., L. Hartley, A. Kilbom, and I. Åstrand. 1969. Physical training in sedentary middle-aged and older men. *Scandinavian Journal of Clinical and Laboratory Investigation* 24: 323-334.

95. Semenick, D. 1986. Warmup and flexibility. *Sports Medicine Guide* 5 (1): 4.

96. Sharkey, B.J. 1970. Intensity and duration of training and the development of cardiorespiratory fitness. *Medicine and Science in Sports* 2: 197-202.

97. Shellock, F.G., and W.E. Prentice. 1985. Warming-up and stretching for improved physical performance and prevention of sports-related injuries. *Sports Medicine* 2: 267.

98. Shepard, R.J. 1969. Intensity, duration, and frequency of exercise as determinants of the response to a training regime. *Internationale Zeitschrift fur Angewandte Physiologie* 26: 272-278.

99. Springer, C., T.J. Barstow, K. Wasserman, and D.M. Cooper. 1991. Oxygen uptake and heart rate responses during hypoxic exercise in children and adults. *Medicine and Science in Sports and Exercise* 23: 71-79.

100. Stone, M.H., S.J. Fleck, W.J. Kraemer, and N.T. Triplett. 1991. Health and performance related adaptations to resistive training. *Sports Medicine* 11 (4): 210-231.

101. Swain, D.P., K.S. Abernathy, C.S. Smith, S.J. Lee, and S.A. Bunn. 1994. Target heart rates for the development of cardiorespiratory fitness. *Medicine and Science in Sports and Exercise* 26: 112-116.

102. Swain, D.P., and B.C. Leutholtz. 1997. Heart rate reserve is equivalent to VO2 reserve, not % VO2 max. *Medicine and Science in Sports and Exercise* 29: 837-843.

103. Thomas, T., G. Ziogas, T. Smith, Q. Zhang, and B. Londeree. 1995. Physiological and perceived exertion responses to six modes of submaximal exercise. *Research Quarterly in Exercise and Sport* 66 (3): 239-246.

104. Thorstensson, A. 1986. How is the normal locomotor program modified to produce backward walking? *Experimental Brain Research* 61: 664-668.

105. Tulppo, M.P., T.H. Makikallio, R.T. Laukkanen, and H.V. Huikuri. 1999. Differences in autonomic modulation of heart rate during arm and leg exercise. *Clinical Physiology* 19 (4): 294-299.

106. Turcotte, L., W. Byrnes, P. Frykman, P. Freedson, and F. Katch. 1984. The effects of hydraulic resistive training on maximal oxygen uptake and anaerobic threshold. *Medicine and Science in Sports and Exercise* 16: S183.

107. U.S. Department of Health and Human Services. 1996. *Physical Activity and Health: A Report of the Surgeon General.* Atlanta: U.S. Department of Health and Human Services, Centers for Disease Control and Prevention, National Center for Chronic Disease Prevention and Health Promotion.

108. U.S. Department of Health and Human Services. 2000. *Healthy People 2010: Understanding and Improving Health,* 2nd ed. Washington, DC: U.S. Government Printing Office.

109. Van de Graff, K.M., and S.J. Fox. 1989. *Concepts of Human Anatomy and Physiology,* 2nd ed. Dubuque, IA: Brown.

110. Velasquez, K.S., and J.H. Wilmore. 1993. Changes in cardiorespiratory fitness and body composition after a 12-week bench step training program. *Medicine and Science in Sports and Exercise* 24 (Suppl): S78.

111. Wells, C.L., and R.R. Pate. 1995. Training for performance of prolonged exercise. In: *Perspectives in Exercise Science and Sports Medicine,* D.R. Lamb and R. Murray, eds. Indianapolis: Benchmark Press, pp. 357-388.

112. Westcott, W. 1983. *Strength Fitness.* Boston: Allyn & Bacon.

113. Whaley, M.H., L.A. Kaminsky, G.B. Dwyer, L.H. Getchell, and L.A. Norton. 1992. Predictors of over- and under-achievement of age-predicted maximal heart rate. *Medicine and Science in Sports and Exercise* 24 (10): 1173-1179.

114. Wilber, R.L., R.J. Moffatt, B.E. Scott, D.T. Lee, and N.A. Cucuzzo. 1996. Influence of water run training on maintenance of aerobic performance. *Medicine and Science in Sports and Exercise* 28: 1056-1062.

115. Wilmore, J.H., and D.L. Costill. 1988. *Training for Sport and Activity,* 3rd ed. Champaign, IL: Human Kinetics.

116. Wilmore, J.H., and D.L Costill. 1999. *Physiology of Sport and Exercise,* 2nd ed. Champaign, IL: Human Kinetics.

117. Yamaji, K., M. Greenley, D.R. Northey, and R.L. Houghson. 1990. Oxygen uptake and heart rate responses to treadmill and water running. *Canadian Journal of Sport Science* 15: 96-98.

118. Zeni, A., M. Hoffman, and P. Clifford. 1996. Energy expenditure with indoor exercise machines. *Journal of the American Medical Association* 275: 1424-1427.

119. Zeni, A., M. Hoffman, and P. Clifford. 1996. Relationships among heart rate, lactate concentration, and perceived effort for different types of rhythmic exercise in women. *Archives of Physical Medicine and Rehabilitation* 77: 237-241.

120. Zimmerman, C.L., T.M. Cook, M.S. Bravard, M.M. Hansen, R.T. Honomichl, S.T. Karns, M.A. Lammers, S.A. Steele, L.K. Yunker, and R.M. Zebrowski. 1994. Effects of stair-stepping exercise direction and cadence on EMG activity of selected lower extremity muscle groups. *Journal of Occupations and Sports Physical Therapy* 19 (3): 173-180.

121. Zupan, M.F., and P.S. Petosa. 1995. Aerobic and resistance cross-training for peak triathlon performance. *Strength and Conditioning* 17: 7-12.

CHAPTER 17

Plyometric and Speed Training

David H. Potach

After completing this chapter, you will be able to

- explain the mechanics and physiology of plyometric and speed-enhancing exercises;
- identify the phases of the stretch-shortening cycle;
- understand the different roles of plyometric and speed training;
- recommend proper equipment for use during plyometric exercise performance;
- design safe and effective plyometric and speed training programs; and
- provide instruction in correct plyometric and speed training technique and recognize common errors.

In an effort to improve sport performance, athletes at all levels want an advantage that allows them to outplay their opponent. Obtaining this edge through the use of plyometric and speed training has commonly been available to only high-level athletes, with the training provided by a team of strength and conditioning professionals [3]. Although not typically emphasized in the design of programs for personal training clients, plyometric and speed training are fast becoming important components of a well-balanced plan to improve not only sport performance, but function during job and activities of daily living. Exercises designed to train clients to jump higher and run faster are becoming popular, and arguably essential, program components. Further, because so many injuries occur as the result of an inability to control decelerative forces, the use of both plyometric and speed training, with their emphasis on the efficient production and use of ground reaction forces, should be considered an integral part of any program whose goal is injury prevention.

A practical definition of plyometric exercise is a quick, powerful movement preceded by a prestretch, or countermovement, and involving the **stretch-shortening cycle (SSC)** [84], while speed is simply the ability to achieve high velocity. Though its definition may be simpler, speed training also relies heavily on the SSC to elicit its desired outcome, that is, the achievement of higher velocity. The purpose of plyometric exercise is to use the stretch reflex and natural elastic components of both muscle and tendon to increase the power of subsequent movements; speed training exercises are designed to use these same mechanical and neurophysiological components, in concert with technique and muscular strength, to produce larger ground forces, thereby allowing clients to run faster. This chapter describes how to use plyometric and speed training exercise effectively as part of an overall training program.

Plyometric Mechanics and Physiology

To be successful, goal-directed movements—athletic, job-related, and functional—depend on all active musculotendinous structures working in concert at appropriate velocities. The term used to define this force-speed relationship is **power** (see chapter 4 for a definition of power). When used correctly, plyometric training has consistently demonstrated the ability to improve the production of muscle force and power [6, 44, 69, 78]. This increased production of muscular power is best explained by two proposed models as discussed in this section—mechanical and neurophysiological [84]. Each model's function is then summarized by a description of the SSC.

Mechanical Model of Plyometric Exercise

In the *mechanical model*, elastic energy is stored following a rapid stretch and then released during a subsequent concentric muscle action, thereby increasing the total force production [2, 16, 45]. A common model presents the function of the musculotendinous unit as a relationship between three mechanical components, the series and parallel elastic components and the contractile component (CC) (figure 17.1, second row). While the **series elastic component (SEC)**—a primary contributor to force production during plyometric exercise—includes some muscular components, it is composed mainly of tendons. When the musculotendinous unit is stretched, as during an eccentric muscle action, the SEC acts as a spring and is lengthened, storing elastic energy. If the muscle then *immediately* begins a concentric muscle action, the stored energy is released, contributing to the total force production by naturally returning the muscles and tendons to their resting configuration. If a concentric muscle action does not occur immediately following the eccentric action, or if the eccentric phase is too long or requires too great a motion about the given joint, the stored energy dissipates and is lost as heat.

Neurophysiological Model of Plyometric Exercise

The *neurophysiological element* involves a change in the force-velocity characteristics of the muscle's contractile components caused by stretch [30]; concentric muscle force is increased with the use of the stretch reflex (figure 17.1, third row) [9, 10, 11, 12]. The **stretch reflex** is the body's involuntary response to an external stimulus [40, 60]. This reflexive component of plyometric exercise is composed primarily of muscle spindle activity. **Muscle spindles** are intramuscular organs that are sensitive to the rate and magnitude of a stretch; when a quick stretch is detected, muscular activity reflexively increases [40, 60]. This reflexive response **potentiates,** or increases, the activity in the agonist muscle, thereby increasing the force the muscle produces [9, 10, 11, 12, 49]. As with the mechanical model, if a concentric muscle action does not immediately follow a

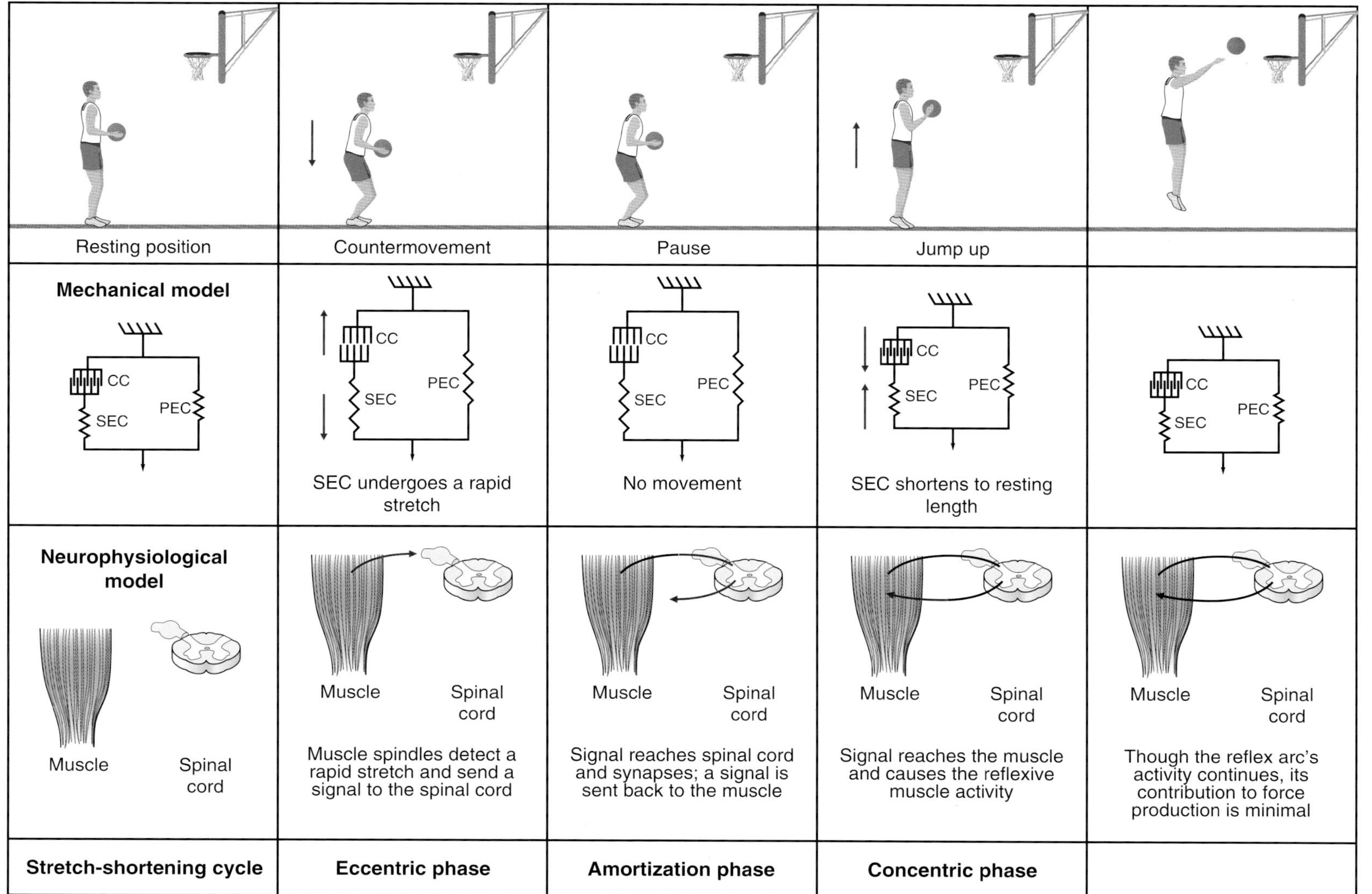

Figure 17.1 Illustration of the stretch-shortening cycle (SSC) with the events of the mechanical model (row two) and neurophysiological model (row three) that occur during each of its three phases (row four). For example, during the eccentric phase of the SSC (column two)—ie., the client's countermovement shown above—the series elastic component (SEC) undergoes a rapid stretch that the muscle spindles detect and send a signal to the spinal cord.

Mechanical model (middle row of figure) adapted from Albert 1995.

stretch (e.g., due to an excessive delay between the stretch and concentric action or with a movement occurring over too large a range), the potentiating ability of the stretch reflex is negated.

Stretch-Shortening Cycle

The SSC is a model explaining the energy-storing capabilities of the SEC and stimulation of the stretch reflex that facilitate a maximal increase in muscle recruitment over a minimal amount of time. The SSC involves three distinct phases (table 17.1). While these phases outline the SSC's individual mechanical and neurophysiological events, it is important to remember that all of the events listed do not necessarily occur within the given phase, as some events may last longer or require less time than the given phase allows. The **eccentric phase—**the first phase—involves preloading the agonist muscle group(s). During this phase, the SEC stores elastic energy and the muscle spindles are stimulated [7, 41]. To visualize the eccentric phase, think about a basketball jump shot. The person quickly performs a half-squat and immediately jumps up to shoot the ball. The time from the beginning of the squat—or countermovement—to the bottom of the movement is the eccentric phase (figure 17.1, second column).

The **amortization**, or transition, **phase** is the time between the eccentric and concentric phases—the time from the end of the eccentric phase to the initiation of the concentric muscle action. There is a delay between the eccentric and concentric muscle actions during which the spinal cord begins to transmit signals to the agonist—stretched—muscle group. This phase must be kept short in duration. If the amortization phase lasts too long, the energy stored during the eccentric phase will be dissipated as heat, and the stretch reflex will not increase muscle activity during the concentric phase [14]. Consider again the basketball jump shot. Once the person's downward half-squat has stopped, the amortization phase has begun. As soon as upward movement begins, the amortization phase has ended (figure 17.1, third column).

The **concentric phase** is the body's response to the events occurring during the eccentric and amortization phases. During this final phase of the SSC, the energy stored in the SEC during the eccentric phase is either used to increase the force of the subsequent movement or is dissipated as heat. Use of the stored elastic energy increases the force produced during the concentric phase movement to a level above that of an isolated concentric muscle action [15, 78, 82]. In addition, the agonist muscle group performs a reflexive concentric muscle action as a result of the stretch reflex. Again visualize the jump shot. Following the half-squat movement, as soon as movement begins in an upward direction, the concentric phase of the SSC has begun and the amortization phase has ended (figure 17.1, fourth column). In this example, one of the agonist muscles is the quadriceps femoris. During the countermovement, quadriceps femoris undergoes a rapid stretch (eccentric phase); there is a delay in movement (amortization phase); then the muscle acts concentrically to extend the knee, allowing the person to push off the ground (concentric phase) (figure 17.1 second, third, and fourth columns, respectively).

The stretch-shortening cycle describes the stretch reflex and stored elastic energy-induced increases in concentric force production that follow a rapid eccentric muscle action.

TABLE 17.1

Stretch-Shortening Cycle

Phase	Action	Physiological event
I—Eccentric	Stretch of the agonist muscle	• Elastic energy is stored. • Muscle spindles are stimulated. • Signal is sent to spinal cord.
II—Amortization	Pause between phases I and III	• Nerves synapse (meet) in spinal cord. • Signal is sent to stretched muscle.
III—Concentric	Shortening of agonist muscle fibers	• Elastic energy is released from the SEC. • The stretched muscle is stimulated by nerve.

When to Use Plyometric Exercise

It should seem obvious that plyometric training offers significant benefits to athletic clients in that most sporting movements rely on quick, powerful movements to be successful [3]. What other populations may benefit from use of these types of movements is less clear. This bias has allowed plyometric exercise to become an ignored training modality for the general population. Many nonathletic clients, however, may benefit from the increases in muscular power production that plyometric training provides. The ability of the personal trainer to identify nonathletic clients who may benefit from plyometrics, as well as those for whom plyometrics are not needed or are contraindicated, is an essential skill for designing individualized exercise programs.

Plyometric Training and Sport Performance

Increased production of muscular power is an established outcome of participation in a plyometric training program [2, 16, 43, 44, 45, 59, 64, 78, 85]. The ability to produce more muscular power has been associated with improved sport performance [4, 5, 54, 77]. Plyometric training, then, is an ideal exercise mode when the goal is to improve muscular power production. In addition to bringing about this increase in muscular power, plyometric training prepares athletes for the deceleration-acceleration and change-of-direction requirements in most sports by improving their ability to perform these types of tasks.

Plyometric Training and Work Performance

In addition to sport performance, participation in a plyometric training program has the potential to improve performance at work [52]. Though this has not been sufficiently examined in the literature, an analysis of some job requirements indicates that the production of muscular power is a key to movement efficiency and may improve job output. For example, police officers must be able to run quickly, change directions effectively, and jump onto or over objects (e.g., fences) in preparation for their occupational demands.

Plyometric Exercise and Injury Prevention

Decreasing the incidence of injury, especially in populations who are at a greater risk of injury than others, is an important consideration when one is designing an exercise training program. Specifically, there is great interest in the utility of plyometric training in decreasing risk of injury. Studies have shown that athletic injury rates decrease following participation in a plyometric training program [8, 43, 44]. It is difficult, however, to extrapolate the results of these studies to different populations. Further, researchers have yet to examine the effect of plyometric training on nonathletic populations. A component of plyometric training is eccentric control of movement, which research has shown may decrease the risk of injury [74]. Eccentric training may therefore be a compromise for clients who wish to engage in injury prevention activities but for whom plyometric training is not appropriate. For example, although plyometric training may not be appropriate for a 75-year-old female client, this client would benefit from eccentric training to lessen her chance of falling.

Contraindicated Populations

There has been no research to delineate populations for whom plyometric training is contraindicated, though analysis of a client's age, experience, and current training level may help identify those clients who are and are not ready for plyometric training.

Age

Plyometric training alters bone structure; spine height has been shown to decrease by up to two millimeters following a depth jumping program [36, 37]. Plyometric training also reportedly increased bone mineral content by up to 7%, though the changes were similar in the non-plyometrically trained control group [88]. Given these limited findings, research has yet to determine the age at which one is physically able to participate in a plyometric training program without experiencing deleterious effects on growing (or aging) muscles, bones, and joints. However, the body's development provides insight into the issue. Clients at both extremes of age should avoid plyometric training for primarily the same reason. Because the epiphyseal plates of the bones of prepubescent children have yet to close [48, 56], and because bones weaken with osteoporosis, depth jumps and other high-intensity lower body plyometric drills are contraindicated for these clients [1, 46, 53]. The personal trainer needs to take care regarding the level of plyometric training appropriate for these client types. For clients younger than 14 years and those older than 60 years, the personal trainer should use caution when prescribing plyometric exercise as a training modality.

Experience and Current Training Level

Clients who have never participated in a resistance training program should be precluded from taking part in a plyometric training program. Plyometric training requires significant strength and muscle control, especially during the eccentric phase. For this reason, clients should be encouraged to take part in a resistance training program that includes core exercises (e.g., squat, bench press, deadlift) before beginning a plyometric training program.

Plyometric Program Design

Plyometric exercise prescription is similar to resistance and aerobic exercise prescriptions [34]. After an evaluation of the client's needs, the mode, intensity, frequency, duration, recovery, progression, and a warm-up period must all be included in the design of a sound plyometric training program. Unfortunately, there is little research demarcating optimal program variables for the design of plyometric exercise programs. Therefore, in addition to the available research, personal trainers must rely on the methodology used during the design of resistance and aerobic training programs and on practical experience when prescribing plyometric exercise. The guidelines that follow are based in part on Chu's work [18, 19, 20, 21, 23, 24] and the National Strength and Conditioning Association's position statement [63].

Needs Analysis

As with other training modalities, when incorporating plyometric exercise into a training program the personal trainer must perform a needs analysis to evaluate a client's current abilities. Specifically, the personal trainer determines the client's needs and the requirements of the client's activities and lifestyle. A combination of the following factors helps in the analysis of a client's needs:

- **Age**—Does the client's age predispose the client to injury and therefore preclude plyometric training?
- **Training experience and current training level**—Has the client been resistance training? If so, what types of exercises has the client been performing? Has he or she participated in a plyometric training program? If so, when?
- **Injury history**—Is the client currently injured? Has the client experienced an injury that might affect his or her ability to participate in a plyometric training program?
- **Physical testing results**—What are the client's current abilities as they relate to muscular power production (e.g., vertical and standing long jump results)?
- **Training goals**—What does the client want to improve? A specific movement (e.g., throwing)? A particular skill (e.g., volleyball hitting)? An on-the-job activity (e.g., loading a truck)?
- **Incidence of injury in a client's job or chosen activity**—What is the risk of injury in the client's chosen activity? Is the activity relatively sedentary (e.g., student or office worker)? Does the activity require constant change of direction (e.g., racquetball player or construction worker)? If the activity is dynamic, is the client prepared for it physically?

"Client Examples—Needs Analysis" on the facing page illustrates one form of the plyometric needs analysis. At the end of this discussion of program design are sample programs for each of these six clients, illustrating the "how" of program design.

Mode

The *mode* of plyometric training is determined by the general part(s) of the body that are performing the given exercise. For example, a **depth jump** is a *lower body* plyometric exercise, whereas a medicine ball chest pass is an *upper body* exercise.

Lower Body Plyometrics

Lower body plyometrics are appropriate for clients involved in virtually any sport—including soccer, volleyball, basketball, and baseball—as well as in nonathletic activities or occupations that require muscular power production or quick changes of direction. These types of activities require participants to produce a maximal amount of force in a minimal amount of time. Soccer and basketball require quick, powerful movements and changes of direction from competitors. A client who plays basketball is an example of one who would benefit greatly from a plyometric training program, as basketball players must jump repeatedly for rebounds.

Client Examples—
Needs Analysis for Plyometric Exercise

Sport Client A. A healthy, 30-year-old male has been fairly active all of his life and joins a YMCA basketball league. He is currently in a resistance training program and performed plyometrics two years ago. He is six feet (182 centimeters) tall, weighs 200 pounds (91 kilograms), and has a 16-inch (40-centimeter) vertical jump and 180-pound (82-kilogram) 1-repetition maximum (1RM) squat. He wants to

1. increase his vertical jump to improve his ability to rebound the basketball and
2. run up and down the court faster as well as change directions quickly.

Sport Client B. A healthy, 28-year-old female fast pitch softball player has played first base for the past five years but is transitioning to an outfield position. She trains with weights one to two times a week, with a circuit weight training program for both the upper and lower body. She is five feet, three inches (160 centimeters) tall and weighs 125 pounds (57 kilograms). Her testing session reveals a 60-pound (27-kilogram) 1RM bench press and an 11-inch (28-centimeter) vertical jump. She requests help in improving her

1. ability to cover right field and
2. arm strength to help throw the ball to the infield.

Work Client A. A 35-year-old firefighter participates in a resistance training program five days a week with both upper and lower body exercises. He was in a plyometric training program six months ago. He is six feet, two inches (187 centimeters) and weighs 225 pounds (102 kilograms). He has a 5.3-second 40-yard (37-meter) dash time, 225-pound (102-kilogram) squat, and 20-inch (51-centimeter) vertical jump. In addition to the necessary cardiovascular training, he has requested help in improving his

1. lifting ability and
2. speed while carrying the hose.

Work Client B. A 40-year-old female warehouse worker has had difficulty the past two months lifting boxes up and onto shelves at or above shoulder level. She has no complaints of pain and has been cleared by the company physician of any musculoskeletal dysfunction. She is five feet, 10 inches (177 centimeters) and weighs 150 pounds (68 kilograms). Her estimated 1RM bench press is 70 pounds (32 kilograms); estimated 1RM squat is 135 pounds (61 kilograms); and vertical jump is 13 inches (33 centimeters). She has never participated in a resistance training program. She has come to a personal trainer to assist her in improving her

1. arm strength, especially when pushing the boxes onto a shelf and
2. leg strength to assist her in lifting the heavier boxes.

Injury Prevention Client A. A healthy 14-year-old female soccer player is preparing to try out for her high school soccer team. She is five feet, seven inches (170 centimeters) and weighs 110 pounds (50 kilograms). She has not performed 1RM testing, but her vertical jump is 12 inches (30 centimeters). Her parents are concerned that she will get hurt playing with girls who are so much older than she. She has been involved in a general resistance training program for the past six months but has never participated in a plyometric training program. The parents have requested help for their daughter to

1. reduce her risk of injury and
2. "get in shape."

Injury Prevention Client B. A 55-year-old female Master's level tennis player is returning to play following a year-long layoff and is concerned about "losing a step" and injuring herself. She has not had any serious injuries. She is five feet, six inches (168 centimeters) and weighs 150 pounds (68 kilograms). Physical testing reveals an estimated 1RM squat of 140 pounds (64 kilograms), vertical jump of 10 inches (25 centimeters), and 40-yard (37-meter) dash of 7.0 seconds. She has been resistance training for the past four months. She would like to

1. improve her speed when coming to the net and
2. reduce her risk of injury.

Lower body plyometric training allows the client's muscles to produce more force in a shorter amount of time, thereby allowing the person to jump higher. There are a wide variety of lower body plyometric drills with various intensity levels and directional movements. Descriptions of different types of lower body plyometric drills are provided in table 17.2 and in general are listed from lower to higher intensities.

Upper Body Plyometrics

Rapid, powerful upper body movements are requisites of several sports and activities, including golf, baseball, softball, and tennis. As an example, a baseball pitcher routinely throws a baseball at 80 to 100 miles per hour (129-161 kilometers per hour). To reach velocities of this magnitude, the pitcher's shoulder joint must move at over 6,000 degrees per second [27, 32, 35, 68]. Plyometric training of the shoulder joint would not only increase pitching velocity it may also prevent injury to the shoulder and elbow joints, although further research is needed to substantiate the role of plyometrics in injury prevention.

Plyometric drills for the upper body are not used as often as those for the lower body and have been studied less vigorously. Nonetheless, they are essential to athletes requiring upper body power [65] and may help clients who need greater levels of upper body strength. Plyometrics for the upper body include medicine ball **throws,** catches, and push-up variations.

Intensity

Plyometric *intensity* refers to the amount of stress placed on muscles, connective tissues, and joints,

TABLE 17.2

Lower Body Plyometric Drills

Type of jump	Definition	Examples
Jumps-in-place	Jumping and landing in the same spot, performed repeatedly, without rest between jumps	Squat jump, tuck jump
Standing jumps	Maximal effort jumps involving either vertical or horizontal components Recovery between repetitions is required	Vertical jump, jump over barrier
Multiple hops and jumps	Drills involving repeated movements Commonly viewed as a combination of jumps-in-place and standing jumps	Double-leg hop, front barrier hop
Bounds	Drills that involve exaggerated movements with greater horizontal speed than other drills Volume for bounding is typically measured by distance and is normally greater than 30 meters (98 feet)	Skip and alternate-leg bound
Box drills	Multiple hops and jumps using a box to jump on or off The height of the box depends on the size of the client, the landing surface, and goals of the program	Jump to box, jump from box
Depth jumps	Drills in which the client assumes a position on a box, steps off, lands, and immediately jumps vertically, horizontally, or to another box	Depth jump, depth jump to second box

TABLE 17.3

Factors Affecting the Intensity of Lower Body Plyometric Drills

Factor	Methods to increase plyometric drill intensity
Points of contact	Progress from double- to single-leg support.
Speed	Increase the drill's speed of movement.
Height of the drill	Raise the body's center of gravity by increasing the height of a drill (e.g., depth jump).
Participant's weight	Add weight (in the form of weight vests, ankle weights, and wrist weights).

and is controlled both by the type of drill performed and by the distance covered (e.g., height of a jump) (table 17.3). The intensity of plyometric drills ranges from low-level skipping to depth jumps that apply significant stress to the agonist muscles and joints.

Intensity should be kept at a low level for those just beginning a plyometric program. Double-leg **jumps-in-place,** double-leg **standing jumps,** and simple skips are appropriate for such clients. Rather than concentrating on advancing intensity, efforts should focus on ensuring proper technique to prevent injury when the client is ready for more advanced drills.

Frequency

Frequency is the number of plyometric training sessions per week and depends on the client's goals. As with other program variables, research is limited on the optimal frequency for plyometric training sessions, again necessitating reliance on practical experience when one is determining the appropriate plyometric training frequency. Rather than concentrating on the *frequency,* many authors and personal trainers rely more on the *recovery time* between plyometric training sessions [19, 20, 21, 23]. Forty-eight to 72 hours between plyometric sessions (i.e., recovery time) is a typical guideline when one is prescribing plyometrics [19, 20, 21, 23]; using these typical recovery times, most clients should perform one to three plyometric sessions per week.

Recovery

Because plyometric drills involve maximal efforts to improve anaerobic power, a complete, adequate *recovery* (the time between repetitions, sets, and workouts) is required [63, 83]. Recovery for depth jumps may consist of 5 to 10 seconds of rest between repetitions and two to three minutes between sets. The time between sets is determined by a proper work-to-rest ratio (i.e., a range of 1:5 to 1:10) and is specific to the volume and type of drill being performed. That is, the higher the intensity of a drill, the more rest a client requires. For example, rest between sets of a plyometric skip will be shorter than the rest between sets of a depth jump.

Volume

Plyometric *volume* is typically expressed as the number of repetitions and sets performed during a given training session. Lower body plyometric volume is normally expressed as the number of foot contacts (each time a foot, or feet together, contact the surface) per workout [1, 19, 20, 21, 23], but may also be expressed as distance, as with plyometric bounding. For example, a client beginning a plyometric training program may start with a double-arm **bound** for 30 meters (33 yards) per repetition but advance to 100 meters (109 yards) per repetition for the same drill. Lower body plyometric volumes vary for clients of different needs (i.e., client age and goals; resistance training and plyometric experience); suggested volumes are provided in table 17.4. Upper body plyometric volume is typically expressed as the number of throws or catches per workout.

The guidelines of mode, intensity, frequency, and volume can now be applied to the sample clients, first introduced on page 431. See the chart on page 435 for sample plyometric programs designed for these clients.

Progression

Plyometric exercise is a form of resistance training and thus must follow the principles of progressive overload—a systematic increase in training frequency, volume, and intensity through the use of various combinations. Typically, as intensity

TABLE 17.4

General Plyometric Volume Guidelines Based on Age and Experience

Age	No resistance training experience	More than 3 months general resistance training experience	More than 3 months resistance training experience, including power exercises	More than 1 year general resistance training experience	More than 1 year resistance training experience, including power exercises	Resistance training but no plyometric training experience	Resistance training and plyometric training more than 1 year ago	Resistance training and plyometric training within past year
≤13	Nr*	Nr	Nr	Nr	Nr	Nr	Nr	Nr
14-17	Nr	40-60	40-60	60-80	80-100	40-60	60-80	80-100
18-30	Nr	60-80	60-80	80-100	100-120	80-100	100-120	120-140
31-40	Nr	40-60	60-80	60-80	80-100	60-80	80-100	100-120
41-60	Nr	40-60	40-60	60-80	60-80	40-60	60-80	80-100

Note: Volume is expressed as number of foot contacts (lower body plyometrics) or throws and catches (upper body plyometrics). Beginning plyometric training volume may be based on a variety of factors. The volumes included in this table may be modified according to individual client goals and abilities.

*Nr = not recommended (i.e., no plyometric training for a client in this situation).

increases, volume decreases, progressing from low to moderate volume of low-intensity plyometrics to low to moderate volumes of moderate to high intensity.

Warm-Up

As with any training program, the plyometric exercise session must begin with general and specific warm-ups (refer to chapter 12 for discussion of warm-up). The general warm-up may consist of light jogging or using a stationary bicycle at low intensity, while a specific warm-up for plyometric training should consist of low-intensity, dynamic movements similar in style to those performed during plyometric exercises. Refer to table 17.5 for a description of dynamic warm-up drills that are generally appropriate for most clients.

Plyometric programs must include the many elements essential to effective training program design. Following a needs analysis, the variables to be included in the program design are mode, intensity, frequency, recovery, volume, program length, progression, and warm-up.

Safety Considerations

Plyometric exercise is not inherently dangerous; however, as with all modes of exercise, injury risk is present. Injuries may occur following an accident, but they more typically occur when training procedures are violated and may result from an improper program design, inadequate instruction and supervision, or inappropriate training environment. Personal trainers must understand and address these and other risk factors to improve the safety of the client performing plyometric exercise.

Pretraining Evaluation

To reduce the risk of injury and to improve the performance of plyometric exercises, the client must understand proper plyometric technique and possess a sufficient base of strength, speed, and balance. In addition, the client must be sufficiently mature both physically and psychologically to participate in a plyometric training program. The following evaluative items will help determine whether these conditions have been met.

Sample Plyometric Programs for Client Examples

	Mode	Intensity*	Frequency (sessions per week)*	Volume*	Activity-specific drills**
Sport Client A	LB***	Medium	2	100 contacts	Double-leg tuck jump Standing long jump Double-leg vertical jump Double-leg hop Jump to box Jump from box
Sports Client B	LB and UB	Low	1	60 contacts 20 throws for UB	Standing long jump Double-leg hop Skip Jump to box Chest pass Two-hand overhead throw
Work Client A	LB and UB	Medium-high	2	100 contacts for LB 20 throws for UB	Split squat jump Standing long jump Double-leg vertical jump Single-leg push-off Jump to box Chest pass Depth push-up
Work Client B	Though this client would benefit from plyometrics eventually, because she has not previously participated in a resistance training program she must begin there and can progress to plyometric training after three months.				
Injury Prevention Client A	LB	Low	1	40 contacts	Split squat jump Double-leg vertical jump Skip Jump from box
Injury Prevention Client B	LB and UB	Low	1	40 contacts	Split squat jump Standing long jump Single-leg push-off Lateral push-off

*The values for these variables represent beginning levels; each will be advanced according to client tolerance and performance. (See page 431 for a description of these clients.)

**The drills provided for each client are examples of exercises that are appropriate, based on the client's background, goals, and experience. The client is not expected to include all of the listed drills in his or her program.

***LB = lower body; UB = upper body.

Landing Position

Before the personal trainer adds any drill to a client's plyometric program, it is necessary to demonstrate proper technique in order to maximize the drill's effectiveness and minimize the risk of injury. For lower body plyometrics, proper landing technique is essential and is of particular importance for depth jumps. If the center of gravity is offset from the base of support, performance will be hindered and injury may occur. During the landing the shoulders should be over the knees, and the knees should be over the toes, with the ankles, knees, and hips flexed (figure 17.2).

Strength

One must consider the client's level of strength before the client performs plyometrics. If the

TABLE 17.5

Plyometric Warm-Up Drills

Dynamic warm-up drill	Description
Lunging	Performed to improve the client's readiness to move into a variety of positions May be performed in a variety of directions (e.g., forward, diagonal, backward)
Toe jogging	Jogging while not allowing the heels to touch the ground
Straight-leg jogging	Jogging while maintaining an extended (or nearly extended) knee
"Butt-kicker"	Jogging and allowing the heel to touch the buttocks through leg flexion
Skipping	Exaggerated mode of reciprocal upper and lower body movements
Footwork	A variety of drills that require changes in direction (e.g., shuffling, sliding, carioca, backward running)

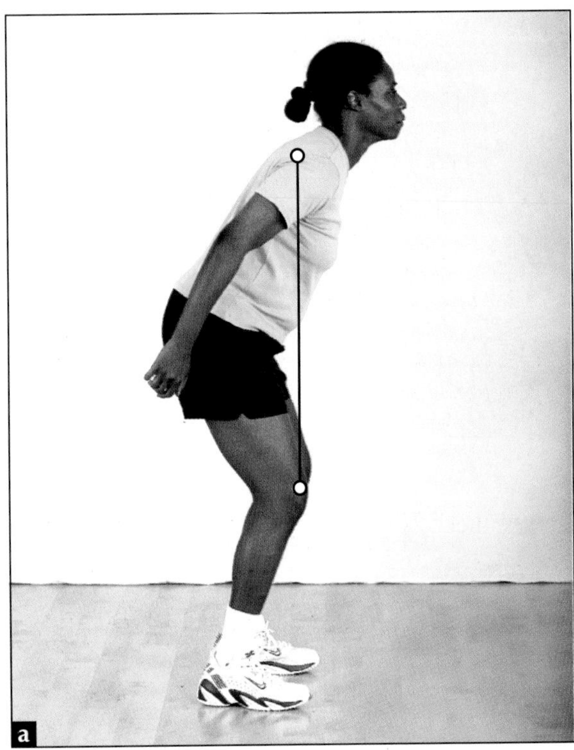

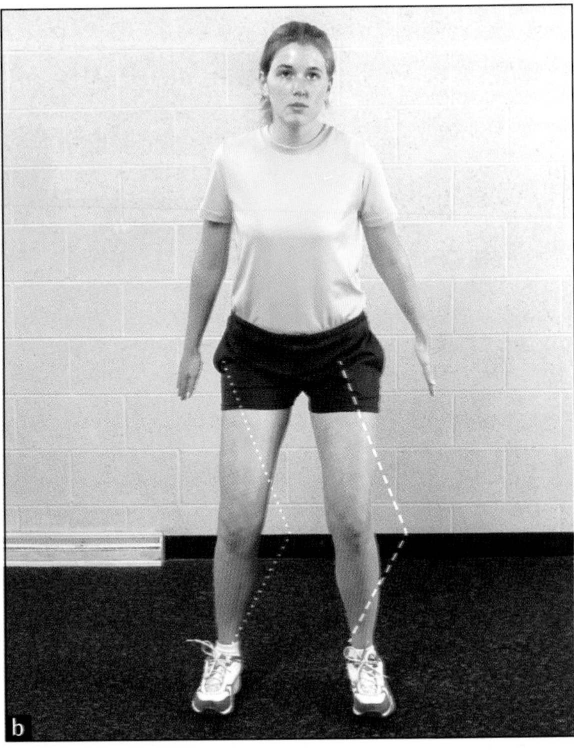

Figure 17.2 Proper plyometric landing position. *(a)* The shoulders are in line with the knees, which helps place the center of gravity over the body's base of support. *(b)* The knees are in line with the feet. There is no valgus (·········) or varus (------) deviation.

client does not possess sufficient muscular strength, plyometrics should be delayed until certain standards—originally intended for athletes—are met. Because research has yet to define a prerequisite level of strength, the following guidelines offer the only published recommendations available for personal trainers to use when determining a client's readiness to participate in a plyometric training program.

For lower body plyometrics, the client's 1RM squat should be at least 1.5 times his or her body weight [17, 29, 46, 63, 83]. For upper body plyometrics, clients weighing more than 220 pounds (100 kilograms) should have a bench press 1RM of at least

1.0 times their body weight, while those under 220 pounds should have a bench press 1RM of at least 1.5 times their body weight [46, 63, 83]. An alternative measure of prerequisite upper body strength is the ability to perform five clap push-ups in a row [63, 83]. These guidelines assure that the client has sufficient strength to engage in plyometric exercises; but if this is not the case, the client may begin a plyometric training program using a low volume of low-intensity exercises provided that he or she has been consistently involved in a resistance training program. Table 17.4 provides suggested volumes according to different training experiences.

Speed

Perhaps a more specific need for plyometric training participants is speed of exercise movement. Because plyometric exercise relies on quick movements, the ability to move rapidly is essential before a client begins a plyometric program. Again, in the absence of research specifying the level of speed necessary to perform plyometric exercise, the following requirements provide an acceptable speed base. For lower body plyometrics, the client should be able to perform five repetitions of the squat with 60% body weight in five seconds or less [63, 83]. To satisfy the speed requirement for upper body plyometrics, the client should be able to perform five repetitions of the bench press with 60% body weight in five seconds or less. Like the strength guidelines mentioned previously, the speed requirements provided here were originally intended for athletic populations. As with the strength requirement, should a client lack the speed of movement described here, he or she may begin a plyometric training program provided that the program starts with lower-intensity drills that do not rely as heavily on speed of movement (e.g., two-foot ankle hop, standing long jump, double-leg vertical jump).

Balance

A less obvious lower body plyometric requirement is **balance**—the ability to maintain a position for a given period of time without moving. Many lower body plyometric drills require the client to move in nontraditional movement patterns (e.g., double-leg zigzag hop and backward skip) or on a single leg (e.g., single-leg tuck jump and single-leg hop). These types of drills necessitate a solid, stable base of support upon which the client can safely and correctly perform the plyometric exercises. Even lower-intensity drills performed by clients just beginning a plyometric program require sufficient balance to prevent injury.

Three balance tests are provided in table 17.6 and are divided into level of difficulty; each test position must be held for 30 seconds [81]. For example, a client beginning plyometric training with double-leg drills for the first time is required to stand on one leg for 30 seconds without falling. An experienced client beginning an advanced plyometric training program involving single-leg drills must maintain a single-leg half-squat for 30 seconds without falling. The surface on which the balance testing is performed must be the same as that for the plyometric drills.

TABLE 17.6

Balance Tests

Level*	Position**	Drill variation***
Beginning	Standing	Double leg Single leg
Intermediate	Quarter-squat	Double leg Single leg
Advanced	Half-squat	Double leg Single leg

*Each of these levels corresponds with a drill's intensity level (e.g., beginning-level balance corresponds with low-intensity plyometric drills).

**The client is required to maintain each position with each variation for 30 seconds before attempting plyometric exercises of the same intensity and the more difficult balance test.

***The type of balance test (i.e., how many legs are used) needs to match the intended type of plyometric drill (e.g., the beginning client has to pass the standing single-leg balance test to qualify to perform single-leg plyometric drills).

Maturity

Though one guideline is to exercise caution with use of plyometric training for clients under 14 years and older than 60 years of age, physical maturity should not be the sole determinant of plyometric preparedness; psychological and mental maturity are necessary before someone begins plyometric training. The client must respond positively to the personal trainer's instructions to proceed with plyometric training. If he or she does not, plyometric training should be postponed. Injury, overtraining, or undertraining may result if the client is inattentive to instructions.

Physical Characteristics

As with other forms of exercise, joint structure, posture, body type, and previous injuries must be examined and reviewed prior to beginning a plyometric training program. Previous injuries or abnormalities of the spine, lower extremities, or upper extremities may increase a client's risk of injury during performance of plyometric exercise. Specifically, clients with a history of muscle strains, pathological joint laxity, or spinal dysfunction, including vertebral disc dysfunction or compression injuries [36, 37], should exercise caution when beginning plyometric training [46, 72].

A specific characteristic requiring a personal trainer's caution is client size. Clients weighing more than 220 pounds (100 kilograms) may be at an increased risk for injury when performing plyometric exercises [63, 83]. Because greater weight increases joint compressive forces, these clients are at increased risk of injuring their lower extremity joints. Therefore, clients weighing over 220 pounds (100 kilograms) should avoid high-volume, high-intensity plyometric exercises. For the same reason, clients weighing over 220 pounds should not perform depth jumps from heights greater than 18 inches (46 centimeters) [63, 83].

Equipment and Facilities

In addition to proper participant fitness and health, the area where the client performs plyometric drills and the equipment used may significantly affect his or her safety.

Landing Surface

To prevent injuries, the landing surface used for lower body plyometrics must possess adequate shock-absorbing properties but must not be so absorbent as to significantly increase the transition between eccentric and concentric phases. A grass field, a suspended floor, and rubber mats are good surface choices [46]. Surfaces such as concrete, tile, and hardwood are not recommended because they lack effective shock-absorbing properties [46]. Excessively thick (greater than or equal to six inches [15 centimeters]) exercise mats and mini-trampolines may extend the amortization phase, thus not allowing efficient use of the stretch reflex.

Minimum Requirements for Participation in a Plyometric Training Program

- Proper technique for each drill
- More than three months of resistance training experience
- Sufficient strength, speed, and balance for the level of drill used
- Over 13 years of age
- No current injuries to involved body segments

Training Area

The amount of space needed depends on the drill. Most bounding and running drills require at least 30 meters (33 yards) of straightaway, though some drills may require a straightaway of 100 meters (109 yards). For most standing, box, and depth jumps, only a minimal surface area is needed; but adequate height—three to four meters (9.8 to 13.2 feet)—is required.

Equipment

Boxes used for box jumps and depth jumps must be sturdy and should have a nonslip top. Box heights should range from 6 to 42 inches (15-107 centimeters) [3, 24, 38, 50, 57] with landing surfaces of at least 18 by 24 inches (46 by 61 centimeters) [20]. The box should be constructed of sturdy wood (e.g., 3/4-inch [1.9-centimeter] plywood) or heavy gauge metal. To further reduce injury risk, ways to make the landing surface nonslip are to (1) add nonslip treads, (2) mix sand into the paint used on the box, or (3) affix rubberized flooring to the top of the box [20].

Proper Footwear

Plyometrics require footwear with good ankle and arch support, good lateral stability, and a wide, nonslip sole [63, 83]. Shoes with a narrow sole and poor upper support (e.g., running shoes) may invite ankle problems, especially with excessive lateral movements.

Supervision

In addition to the safety considerations already mentioned, clients must be closely monitored to ensure proper technique. Plyometric exercise is not intrinsically dangerous when performed correctly; but as with other forms of training, poor technique may unnecessarily predispose a client to injury. It is especially important for personal trainers to monitor client jumping and landing technique for lower extremity drills. In particular, personal trainers must instruct clients to avoid extremes of lateral knee motion (i.e., valgus and varus movements (see figure 17.2)) and to minimize time spent on the ground. While not passing them in the front (anteriorly), knees should line up with the second and third toes, with the amortization phase kept as short as possible. Should the client deviate from these norms, drill intensity should be lowered to allow successful completion of each drill. Common technique errors are provided for each drill at the end of this chapter.

Speed Training Mechanics and Physiology

All sports depend on the speed of execution; that is, whether a client is a sprinter, cross country runner, or swimmer, success depends on the ability to perform a given task in the shortest time possible. Speed training has been classically considered a modality used to improve sport function. Indeed, many of the concepts discussed in the paragraphs that follow are difficult to incorporate into personal training programs for those uninvolved in sport. For example, training to improve speed in soccer and baserunning in baseball should seem obvious. Training to improve speed in a work setting is more challenging to envision and difficult to defend as an appropriate exercise mode for the personal trainer to choose. The paragraphs that follow, then, use primarily athletic settings and situations as examples. Some nonsporting applications, however, are provided as appropriate.

Speed Training Definitions

The basis of speed training is the application of maximal force in a minimal amount of time. Accomplished in a variety of ways, this simply means that if a client is to move more quickly, he or she must *explode* when his or her feet are on the ground. **Speed-strength** is this application of maximum force at high velocities [79, 80]. People improve speed-strength in essentially the same way they improve muscular power production, by performing rapid movements both with and without resistance. Examples include weightlifting-type movements (e.g., power clean, hang clean, snatch) and plyometric exercise; each of these exercise modes is performed quickly to potentiate muscle force through the release of stored elastic energy and the stretch reflex. Therefore, to improve speed-strength, the exercise prescription should rely on powerful exercises and avoid those requiring slow movement [76].

Speed-endurance is the ability to maintain running speed over an *extended duration* (typically longer than six seconds) [28]. The development of speed-endurance helps prevent a client from slowing down during a maximal-speed effort. Consider a soccer player caught from behind on a breakaway or a police officer on foot who is unable to keep up with a fleeing suspect. Each of these illustrates poor speed-endurance; that is, each person either slowed down or was unable to accelerate due to fatigue.

Sprinting Technique

Technique evaluation is an important tool to use when assessing movement efficiency and, ultimately, when training to improve speed. The basic techniques of running are presented in chapter 14; running for speed, or sprinting, though similar, is a considerably different form of training. Like running, sprinting is a somewhat natural activity, though it may be performed in a variety of ways. Because of this relative normalcy, technique training should initially focus on optimizing form and correcting faults [22]; developing completely new movement patterns is typically unnecessary. The form and faults that characteristically need correction center on posture and action of the legs and arms. Maximizing sprinting speed, therefore, depends on a combination of optimal body posture, leg action, and arm action (figure 17.3, a-b) [26, 39, 47, 58, 70, 75].

Posture

While maintaining a relaxed, upright position, the head, torso, and legs should be aligned at all times. Although commonly viewed as a controlled fall [13], sprinting may be more accurately described as a series of "ballistic strides where the body is repeatedly launched forward as a projectile" [71]. The body should lean forward approximately 45 degrees during acceleration and should quickly move upright to a less than 5-degree lean during maximal speed (with the lean coming from the ground up, not the waist up). Head should be relaxed with minimal movement, and eyes should be focused straight ahead.

Leg Action

During the **support phase,** the client's weight should be concentrated near the ball of the foot directly under the client; once the foot leaves the ground it remains dorsiflexed and should move directly toward the buttocks. Increasing sprinting speed should increase the height the foot moves toward the buttocks (the heel kick). The knee then extends to an approximately 90-degree position and then becomes nearly straight as the foot moves down and forward during flight. At foot strike, the foot should be placed directly under—or a very short distance in front of—the hips (i.e., center of gravity). Ground contact time should be minimal while allowing explosive leg movement.

Arm Action

Remaining relaxed, each elbow should be flexed to approximately 90 degrees; movement must be an aggressive front-to-back action originating from the shoulder with minimal frontal plane motion. Hands should rise to nose level during anterior arm swing and should pass the buttocks when moving posteriorly. Using aggressive hand and knee hammering or punching motions helps to improve leg action.

> During a sprint, support time should be kept brief while braking forces at ground contact are minimized and the backward velocity of the lower leg and foot at touchdown is maximized. Maximizing sprinting speed depends on a combination of optimal body posture, leg action, and arm action.

Speed Training Program Design

As with plyometric exercise prescription, research on program design for speed training is sparse and therefore practical experience must be the guide. Speed training exercise prescription uses typical program design variables to provide a safe and effective plan to improve a client's speed.

Mode

The *mode* of speed training is determined by the speed characteristics that the given drill is designed

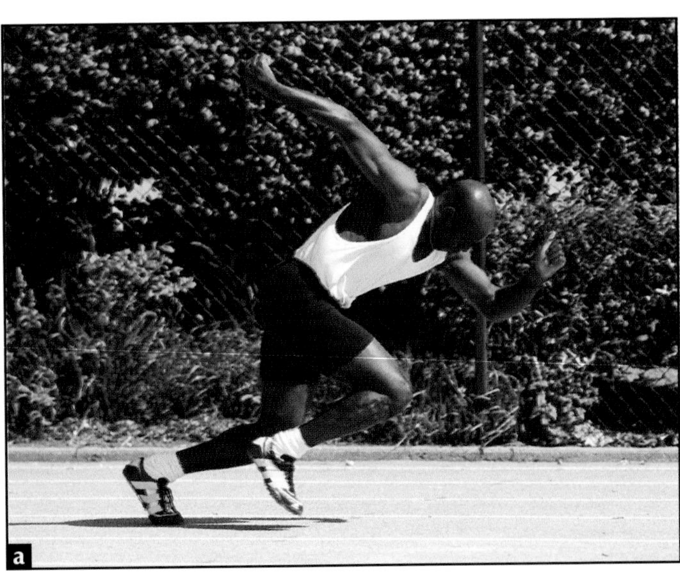

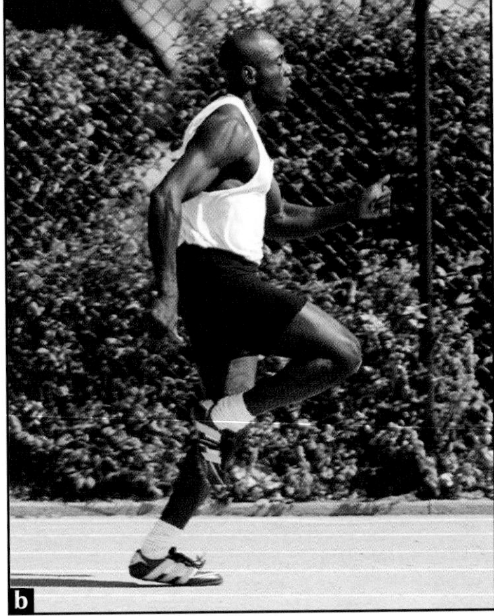

Figure 17.3 Proper sprinting technique. *(a)* At initial acceleration, the body should be leaning forward approximately 45 degrees, and *(b)* should then quickly move upright to a less than 5-degree lean.

to improve. Speed training focuses on three areas: form, stride frequency, and stride length. Improving sprinting technique may be accomplished in a number of ways, including sprint performance, stride analysis, and specific **form drills.** Drills designed to improve form are provided at the end of this chapter.

Within an analysis of running speed, stride frequency and stride length have an intimate relationship. In general, as both the **stride frequency** (the number of strides performed in a given amount of time) and **stride length** (the distance covered in one stride) increase, running speed improves. During the start, speed is highly dependent on stride length; as sprinting speed increases, frequency becomes the more important variable [61, 66, 67, 75, 87]. Of the two components, stride frequency is likely the more trainable, as stride length is highly dependent on body height and leg length [61, 62].

Stride frequency is typically increased through the use of **sprint-assisted training,** or running at speeds greater than a client is able to independently achieve [25]. The supramaximal speed forces the client to take more steps than he or she is accustomed to taking during a typical sprint. Assuming that stride length remains the same as during normal sprinting, increasing the frequency of strides will help the client run faster. There are a variety of methods by which to accomplish sprint-assisted training, including downgrade sprinting (3-7 degrees), high-speed towing, and use of a high-speed treadmill. Regardless of the method used, sprint-assisted training should not increase speed by more than 10% of the client's maximal speed.

Sprint-assisted training is an advanced technique that requires careful instruction and demonstration on the part of the personal trainer and clear understanding on the part of the client. Sprint-assisted training may cause a client to alter his or her technique, which will affect running without assistance. Further, a proper warm-up to each session should be considered mandatory.

Resisted sprinting is used to help a client increase stride length, as well as speed-strength, by increasing the client's ground force production during the support phase [26, 31, 39, 42, 47, 51, 55, 73], which is arguably the most important determinant of speed [76]. Again, while maintaining proper form, clients may use upgrade sprinting or sprinting while being resisted by a sled, elastic tubing, or a parachute [25]. Resisted sprinting should not increase external resistance by more than 10% [71].

As with most other speed training techniques, resisted sprinting targets clients wanting to improve speed strength. Adding resistance to a nonathletic client's gait, however, may also improve function. For example, attaching elastic tubing to provide resistance to a 70-year-old client during walking may improve his or her ability to walk up hills or may increase confidence during walking, thereby reducing the risk of injury from a possible fall. Providing resistance to a construction worker by having the individual push a weighted implement or sled may improve his or her ability to push a wheelbarrow filled with cement.

Although nearly all clients may perform form drills, sprint-assisted and -resisted training may be too advanced for some. A more general mode of speed training that most clients can easily perform is **interval sprinting.** Specifically, a client sprints (or runs or walks, depending on abilities) as fast as possible over a given distance or for a predetermined amount of time, then rests. Following the rest period, the client repeats the bout. In performing interval training, clients are able to maintain higher-intensity work periods (i.e., sprint/run/walk) by interspersing them with times of rest [33].

Intensity

Speed training *intensity* refers to the physical effort required during execution of a given drill, and is controlled both by the type of drill performed and by the distance covered. The intensity of speed training ranges from the low-level form drills to sprint-assisted and -resisted sprinting drills that apply significant stress to the body.

Frequency

Frequency, the number of speed training sessions per week, depends on the client's goals. As with other program variables, research is limited on the optimal frequency for speed training sessions; again, personal trainers must rely on practical experience when determining the appropriate frequency. For clients who are athletes participating in a sport, two to four speed sessions per week is common; nonathletic clients may benefit from one to two speed sessions per week.

Recovery

Because speed training drills involve maximal efforts to improve speed and anaerobic power, complete, adequate *recovery* (the time between repetitions and sets) is required to ensure maximal effort with each repetition [63, 83]. The time between repetitions is determined by a proper work-to-rest ratio (i.e., a range of 1:5 to 1:10) and is specific to the volume and type of drill being performed. That is, the higher the intensity of a drill, the more rest a client requires. Recovery for form training may be minimal, whereas rest between repetitions of downgrade running may last two to three minutes.

Volume

Speed training *volume* typically refers to the number of repetitions and sets performed during a given training session and is normally expressed as the distance covered. For example, a client beginning a speed training program may start with a 30-meter (33-yard) sprint but advance to 100 meters (109 yards) per repetition for the same drill. As with intensity, speed training volume should vary according to the client's goals.

Progression

Speed training must follow the principles of progressive overload—a systematic increase in training frequency, volume, and intensity through various combinations. Typically, as intensity increases, volume decreases. The program's intensity should progress from

1. low to moderate volume of low-intensity speed drills (e.g., stationary arm swing) to
2. low to moderate volumes of moderate intensity (e.g., butt kicker) to
3. low to moderate volumes of moderate to high intensity (e.g., downhill sprinting).

Warm-Up

As with any training program, the speed training session must begin with both general and specific warm-ups (refer to chapter 12 for a discussion of warm-up). The specific warm-up for speed training should consist of low-intensity, dynamic movements. Once mastered, many of the form drills provided at the end of this chapter may be incorporated into warm-up drills.

Speed Training Safety Considerations

While not inherently dangerous, speed training—like all modes of exercise—places the client at risk of injury. Injuries during speed training commonly occur because of insufficient strength or flexibility, inadequate instruction and supervision, or inappropriate training environment.

Pretraining Evaluation

To reduce the risk of injury during participation in a speed training program, the client must understand proper technique and possess a sufficient base of strength and flexibility. In addition, the client must be sufficiently prepared to participate in a speed training program. The following evaluative elements will help determine whether a client meets these conditions.

Physical Characteristics

As in the case of other forms of exercise, it is necessary to examine and review joint structure, posture, body type, and previous injuries before a client begins a speed training program. Previous injuries or abnormalities of the spine, lower extremities, and upper extremities may increase a client's risk of injury during participation in a speed training program. An area of concern is hamstring flexibility and strength; as the swing leg—the leg not on the training surface—transitions from an eccentric muscle action to concentric, the hamstring must be prepared to undergo extreme amounts of stretch (during the eccentric phase of the movement) followed by nearly instantaneous concentric muscle action. If this muscle is not prepared (through both strength and flexibility training), injury becomes likely.

Technique and Supervision

When a client will be performing speed training drills, the personal trainer must demonstrate proper technique—as previously described—to maximize the drill's effectiveness and to minimize the risk of injury. Posture and proper arm and leg actions are especially important characteristics for the personal trainer to watch. It is essential to monitor clients closely to ensure proper movement patterns and sprinting technique. Should the client not demonstrate correct technique, drill intensity must be lowered to allow successful completion of each drill. Common technique errors are listed for each drill at the end of this chapter.

Exercise Surface and Footwear

In addition to proper participant fitness, health, and technique, the area where the client performs speed training drills may significantly affect his or her safety. To prevent injuries, the landing surface used for speed training drills must possess adequate shock-absorbing properties, but must not be so absorbent as to significantly increase the transition between the eccentric and concentric phases of the SSC. Grass fields, suspended floors, and rubber mats are good surface choices [46]. Avoid excessively thick exercise mats (greater than or equal to six inches [15 centimeters]) because they may lengthen the amortization phase, thus not allowing efficient use of the stretch reflex. In addition, footwear with good ankle and arch support and a wide, nonslip sole is required [63, 83].

Combining Plyometrics and Speed Training With Other Forms of Exercise

Plyometrics and speed training are just parts of a client's overall training program. Many sports and activities use multiple energy systems or require other forms of exercise to properly prepare athletes for their competitions or to help clients reach their goals. A well-designed training program must address each energy system and training need.

Resistance, Plyometric, and Speed Training

Combining plyometric and speed training with resistance training requires careful consideration to optimize recovery while maximizing performance. The following list and table 17.7 provide appropriate guidelines for developing a program that combines these different, but complementary, modes of training:

- In general, clients should perform *either* lower body plyometric training, speed training, *or* lower body resistance training on a given day, but not more than one of these types of training on the same day.
- It is appropriate to combine lower body resistance training with upper body plyometrics, and upper body resistance training with lower body plyometrics.
- Performing heavy resistance training and plyometrics on the same day is not usually recommended [17, 42]. However, some athletes may benefit from **complex training**—a combination of resistance and plyometric training—by performing high-intensity resistance training followed by plyometrics. If an individual is engaging in this type of training, adequate recovery between the plyometrics and other high-intensity lower body training—including speed training—is essential.
- Traditional resistance training exercises may be combined with plyometric movements to further enhance gains in muscular power [85, 86]. For example, performing a squat jump with approximately 30% of one's 1RM squat as an external resistance further increases performance [85, 86]. This is an advanced form of complex training that should be performed only by clients with previous participation in high-intensity plyometric training programs.

Plyometric and Aerobic Exercise

Many sports and activities require both a power and an aerobic component. It is necessary to combine multiple types of training to best prepare clients for these types of sports. Because aerobic exercise may have a negative effect on power production during a given training session [17], it is advisable to perform plyometric exercise prior to the longer, aerobic endurance-type training. The design variables do not change and should complement each other

TABLE 17.7

Sample Schedule for Resistance, Plyometric, and Speed Training

Day	Resistance training	Plyometric training	Speed training
Monday	Upper body	Lower body	Rest
Tuesday	Lower body	Upper body	Rest
Wednesday	Rest	Rest	Technique and sprint-assisted drills
Thursday	Upper body	Lower body	Rest
Friday	Lower body	Upper body	Rest
Saturday	Rest	Rest	Technique and sprint-resisted drills

to most effectively train the athlete for competition or help a client meet his or her goals. Recent studies actually indicate that plyometrics may improve long-distance running [77]; therefore adding low-intensity bounding-type drills to non-running days may improve long-distance running performance.

Plyometric exercise should be incorporated into an overall training program, including both strength and aerobic exercise. Speed training may be combined with plyometric and resistance training, but this requires careful planning to optimize recovery while maximizing performance.

CONCLUSION

The ability to apply force quickly and provide an overload to the agonist muscles is the major goal of plyometric training, a benefit to most sporting activities and many occupations. Further, because the ability to move rapidly is needed in sport, speed training may be another important component to include for clients active in competitive and recreational sports. Necessary during performance of each of these forms of exercise is the proper application of force to the ground in a minimal amount of time. If the force used is insufficient or if it requires too long a time to generate, the ability to effectively accelerate, change direction, or overtake an opponent is lost.

In addition to improving the potential to succeed in sport, speed and especially plyometric training may improve function on the job or may reduce the risk of injury. Many occupations require employees to lift or move large objects, move quickly, or otherwise perform explosive movements. Using the plyometric and speed training principles outlined is an ideal method of improving the important speed-strength quality important to so many activities. In addition, the ability to decelerate efficiently and under control is indispensable to any attempt to reduce a client's risk of injury. Proper performance of plyometric drills helps clients learn how to decelerate when landing from a jump or when changing directions.

Plyometric training and speed training should not be considered ends in themselves, but as parts of an overall program (in addition to resistance, flexibility, and aerobic training and proper nutrition). Clients possessing adequate levels of strength perform plyometric and speed training drills more successfully. Further, combining these modes of exercise with others allows clients to optimize performance, regardless of sport or activity requirements.

Plyometric and Speed Drills

Lower-Body Plyometric Drills

Upper-Body Plyometric Drills

Speed Drills

Lower Body Plyometric Drills

Double-Leg Tuck Jump

Intensity level: Medium

Direction of jump: Vertical

Beginning position: Assume a comfortable upright stance with feet shoulder-width apart.

Arm action: Double arm

Preparatory movement: Begin with a countermovement.

Upward movement: Explosively jump up. Pull the knees to the chest and quickly grasp the knees with both hands and release before landing.

Downward movement: Land in the starting position and **immediately** repeat the jump.

Advanced variation: A way to increase the intensity of the double-leg tuck jump is to perform the jump with one leg only. This changes the drill's intensity from medium to high.

 **Common Errors**

- Amortization phase (i.e., time on the floor/ground) is too long.
- Clients do not jump and land in the same place; there is excessive lateral and anterior/posterior movement.

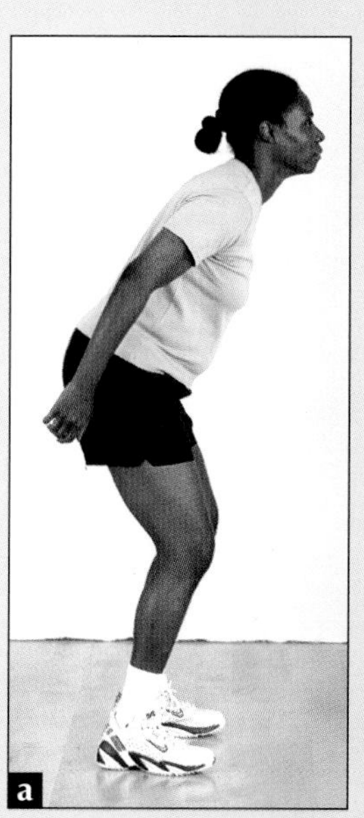
a

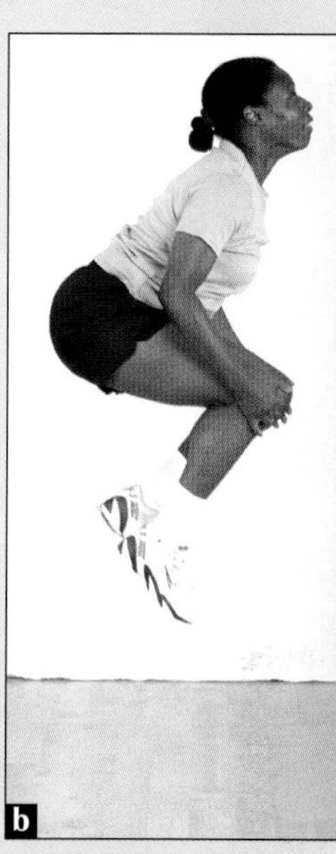
b

Split Squat Jump

Intensity level: Medium

Direction of jump: Vertical

Beginning position: Assume a lunge position with one leg forward (hip and knee joints in approximately 90 degrees of flexion) and the other behind the midline of the body.

Arm action: Double or none

Preparatory movement: Begin with a countermovement.

Upward movement: Explosively jump up, using the arms to assist as needed. Maximum height and power should be emphasized.

Downward movement: When landing, maintain the lunge position (same leg forward) and **immediately** repeat the jump.

Note: After completing a set, rest and switch front legs.

Advanced variation: While off the ground, switch the position of the legs so the front is in the back and the back is in the front. When landing, maintain the lunge position (opposite leg forward) and immediately repeat the jump.

 **Common Errors**

- The lunge position is too shallow.
- Amortization phase (i.e., time on the floor/ground) is too long.
- Clients do not jump and land in the same place; there is excessive lateral and anterior/posterior movement.

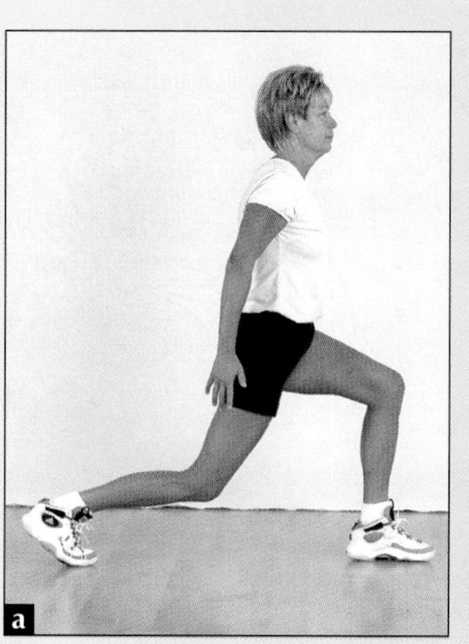
a

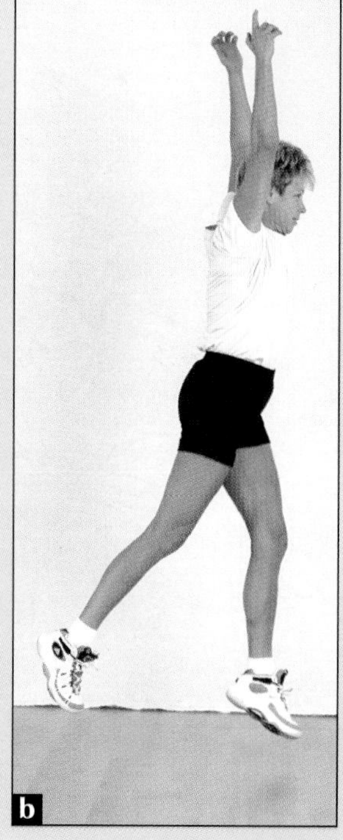
b

Standing Long Jump

Intensity level: Low

Direction of jump: Horizontal

Beginning position: Half-squat position with feet shoulder-width apart

Arm action: Double arm

Preparatory movement: Begin with a countermovement.

Upward movement: Explosively jump forward as far as possible with both feet. Use the arms to assist with the jump.

Downward movement: Land in the starting position and repeat jump. Allow complete rest between repetitions.

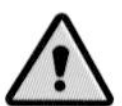 **Common Errors**

- Clients jump and land asynchronously; that is, feet neither leave nor contact the floor/ground at the same time.

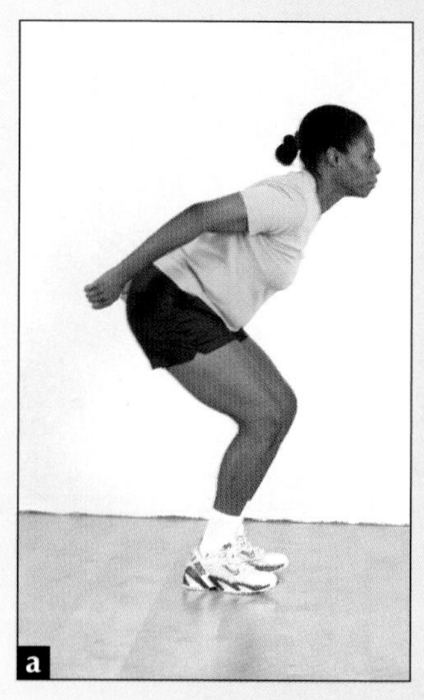

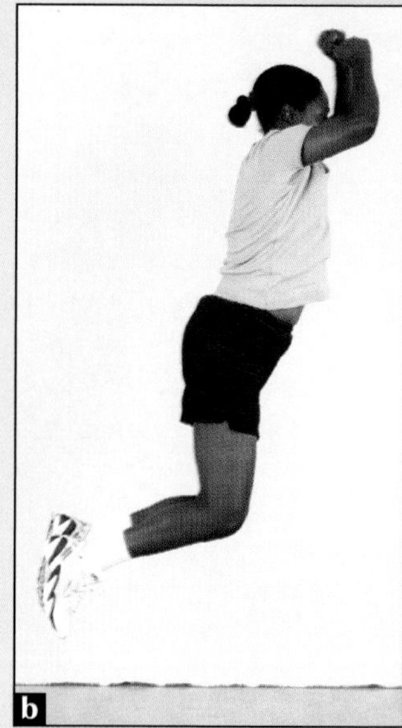

Double-Leg Vertical Jump

Intensity level: Low

Direction of jump: Vertical

Beginning position: Assume a comfortable upright stance with feet shoulder-width apart.

Arm action: Double arm

Preparatory movement: Begin with a countermovement.

Upward movement: Explosively jump up with both legs, using both arms to assist and reach for a target.

Downward movement: Land in the starting position and repeat the jump. Allow complete recovery between jumps.

Advanced variation: One can increase the intensity of the double-leg vertical jump by performing the jump with one leg only. This changes the drill's intensity from low to high.

 **Common Errors**

- Countermovement is too deep.
- Clients do not jump and land in the same place; there is excessive lateral and anterior/posterior movement.

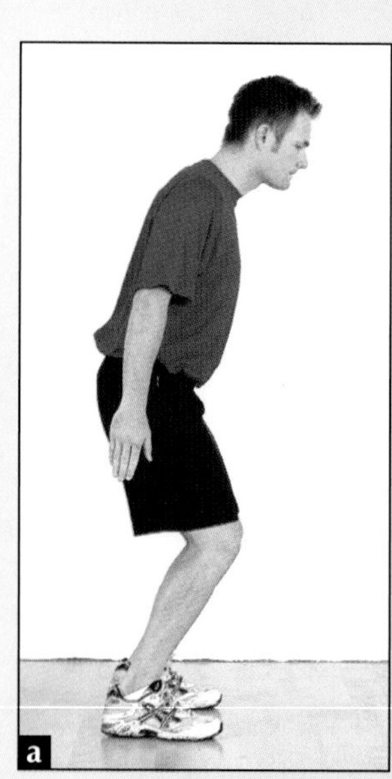

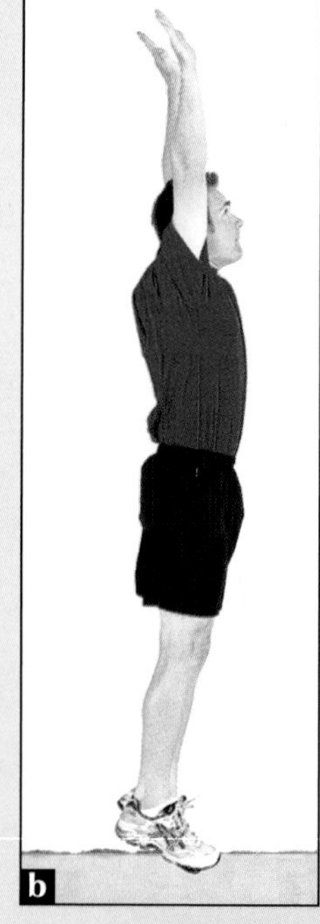

Double-Leg Hop

Intensity level: Medium

Direction of jump: Horizontal and vertical

Beginning position: Assume a comfortable upright stance with feet shoulder-width apart.

Arm action: Double arm

Preparatory movement: Begin with a countermovement.

Upward movement: Jump as far forward as possible.

Downward movement: Land in the beginning position and **immediately** repeat the hop.

Advanced variation: A way to increase the intensity of the double-leg hop is to perform the hop with one leg only. This changes the drill's intensity from medium to high.

 **Common Errors**

- Amortization phase (i.e., time on the floor/ground) between hops is too long.

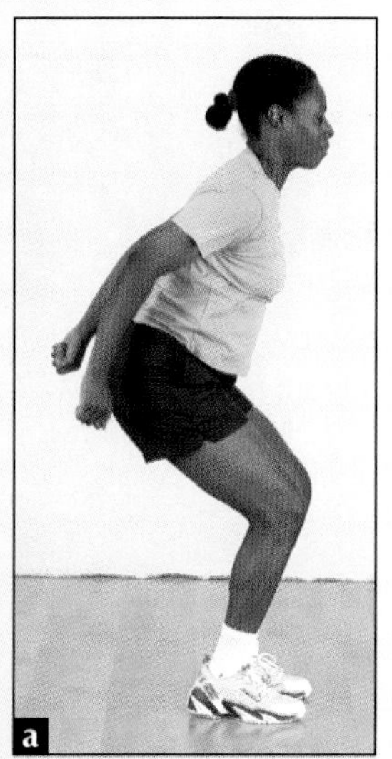

a

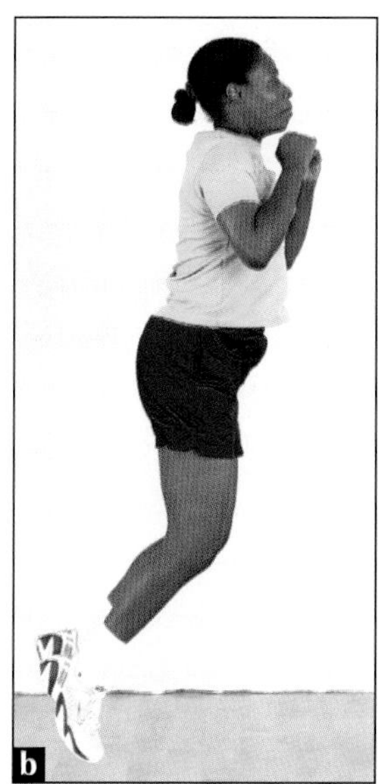

b

Front Barrier Hop

Intensity level: Medium

Direction of jump: Horizontal and vertical

Beginning position: Assume a comfortable upright stance facing a barrier, with feet shoulder-width apart.

Arm action: Double arm

Preparatory movement: Begin with a countermovement.

Upward movement: Jump over a barrier with both legs, using primarily hip and knee flexion to clear the barrier. Keep the knees and feet together without lateral deviation.

Downward movement: Land in the starting position and **immediately** repeat the jump over the next barrier.

Alternate variation: This drill may also be performed laterally. Stand to either side of the barrier; jump over the barrier with both legs. Land in the starting position and immediately repeat the jump to the starting side.

Advanced variations: A way to increase the intensity of barrier hops is to progressively increase the height of the barrier (e.g., from a cone to a hurdle) or to perform the hops with one leg only. This changes the drill's intensity from medium to high.

 **Common Errors**

- Amortization phase (i.e., time on the floor/ground) between hops is too long.
- Knees and feet separate in an effort to clear the barrier.

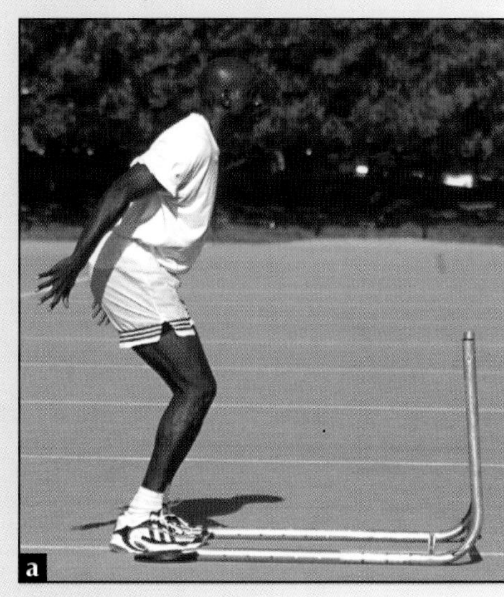

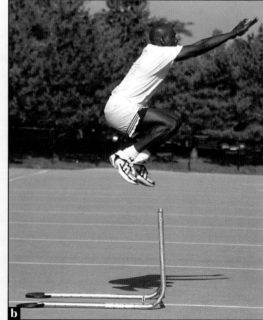

a

b

Skip

Intensity level: Low

Direction of jump: Horizontal and vertical

Beginning position: One leg is lifted to 90 degrees of hip and knee flexion.

Arm action: Reciprocal (as one leg is lifted, the opposite arm is lifted)

Preparatory movement: Begin with a countermovement.

Upward movement: Jump up and forward on one leg. The opposite leg should remain in the starting position until landing.

Downward movement: Land in the starting position with the same leg. Repeat the motion with the opposite leg.

Advanced variation: This drill may also be performed backward. Jump up and backward on one leg. Land in the starting position with the same leg. Repeat the motion with the opposite leg.

Common Errors

- Incoordination, that is, difficulty coordinating the transition from one leg to the other

a

b

c

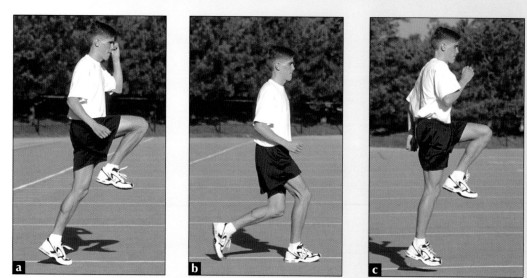

Alternate-Leg Bound—Double-Arm

Intensity level: Medium

Direction of jump: Horizontal and vertical

Beginning position: Assume a comfortable upright stance with feet shoulder-width apart.

Arm action: Single arm

Preparatory movement: Jog at a comfortable pace; begin the drill with the left foot forward.

Upward movement: Push off with the left foot as it contacts the ground. During push-off, bring the right leg forward by flexing the thigh to a position parallel with the ground and the knee at 90 degrees. During this flight phase of the drill, reach forward with both arms.

Downward movement: Land on the right leg and **immediately** repeat the sequence with the opposite leg upon landing.

Note: A bound is an exaggeration of the running gait; the goal is to cover as great a distance as possible during each stride.

a

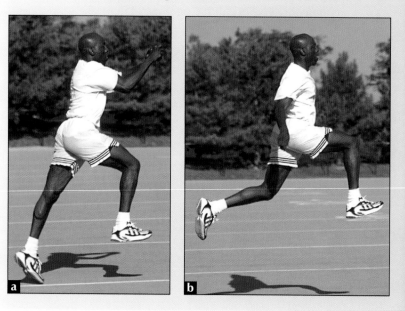
b

Alternate variation: Instead of reaching forward with both arms during the flight phase, the client may reach with a single arm while the opposite leg is in the flight phase.

Common Error:

- Clients do not have an appropriate balance between the horizontal and vertical components of the bound.

Jump to Box

Intensity level: Low

Equipment: Plyometric box, 6 to 42 inches (15 to 107 centimeters) high

Direction of jump: Vertical and slightly horizontal

Beginning position: Facing the plyometric box, assume a comfortable upright stance with feet shoulder-width apart.

Arm action: Double arm

Preparatory movement: Begin with a countermovement.

Upward movement: Jump onto the top of the box using both feet.

Downward movement: Land on both feet in a semisquat position; step down from the box and repeat.

Advanced variation: A way to increase the intensity of this jump is for the client to clasp the hands behind the head.

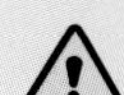 **Common Errors**

- Knees and feet separate in an effort to clear the barrier.
- Countermovement is too deep.
- Box is too tall for client's height or abilities.

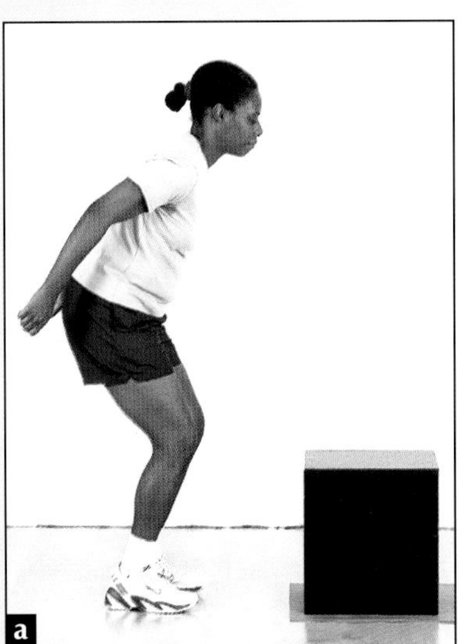

a

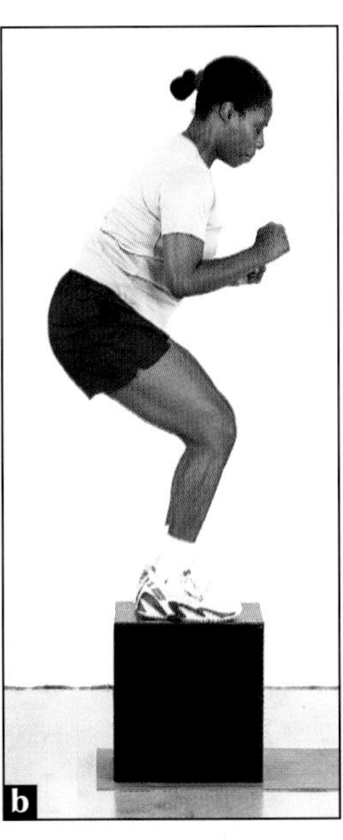

b

Jump From Box

Intensity level: Medium

Equipment: Plyometric box, 12 to 42 inches (30 to 107 centimeters) high

Direction of jump: Vertical

Beginning position: Assume a comfortable upright stance with feet shoulder-width apart on the plyometric box.

Arm action: None

Preparatory movement: Step from box.

Downward movement: Land on the floor with both feet quickly absorbing the impact upon touchdown. Step back onto box and repeat.

 **Common Errors**

- Clients land asynchronously; that is, feet do not contact the floor/ground at the same time.
- Box is too tall for client's height or abilities.

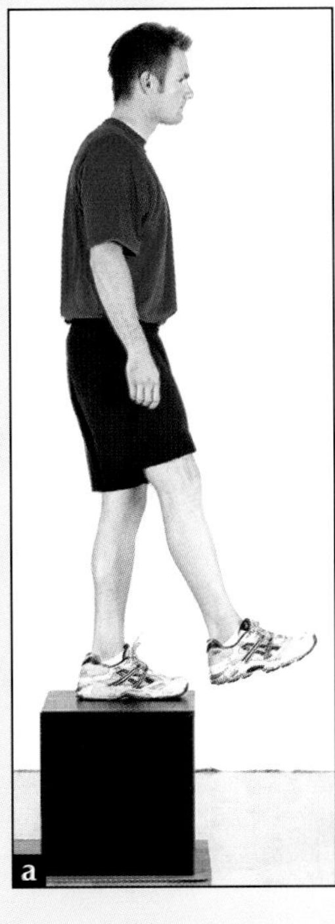

a

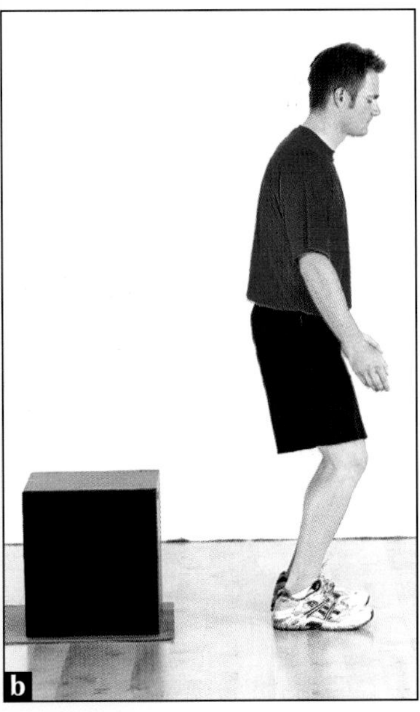

b

Depth Jump

Intensity level: High

Equipment: Plyometric box, 12 to 42 inches (30 to 107 centimeters) high

Direction of jump: Vertical

Beginning position: Assume a comfortable upright stance with feet shoulder-width apart on the plyometric box; toes should be near the edge of the box.

Arm action: Double arm

Preparatory movement: Step from box.

Downward movement: Land on the floor with both feet.

Upward movement: Upon landing, **immediately** jump up as high as possible.

Note: Time on the ground should be kept to a minimum.

Note: A way to vary the intensity is to increase the height of the box. Begin with height of 12 inches (30 centimeters).

 **Common Errors**

- Amortization phase (i.e., time on the floor/ground) is too long.
- Clients do not jump and land in the same place; there is excessive lateral and anterior/posterior movement after landing.
- Box is too tall for client's height or abilities.

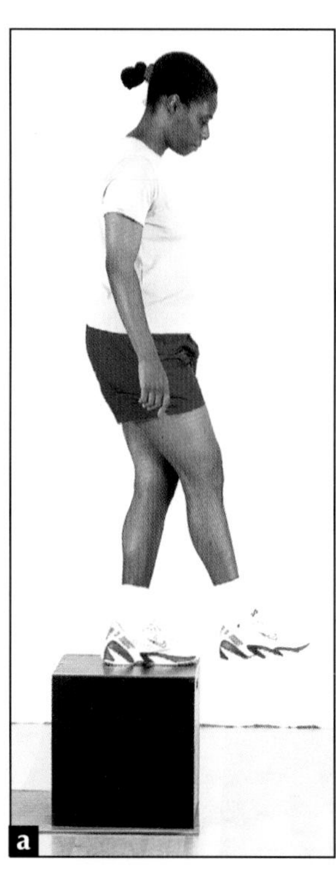

a

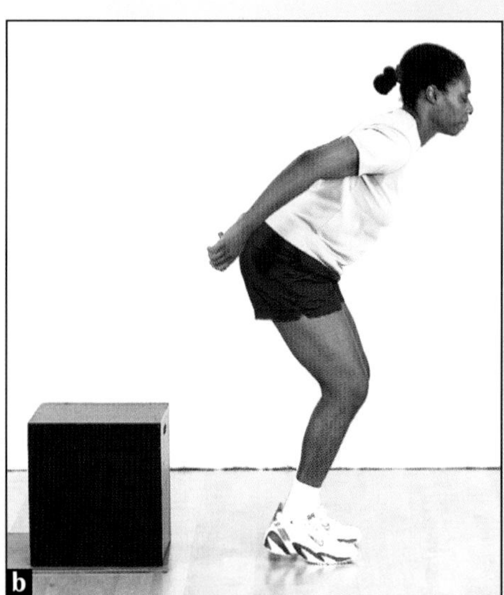

b

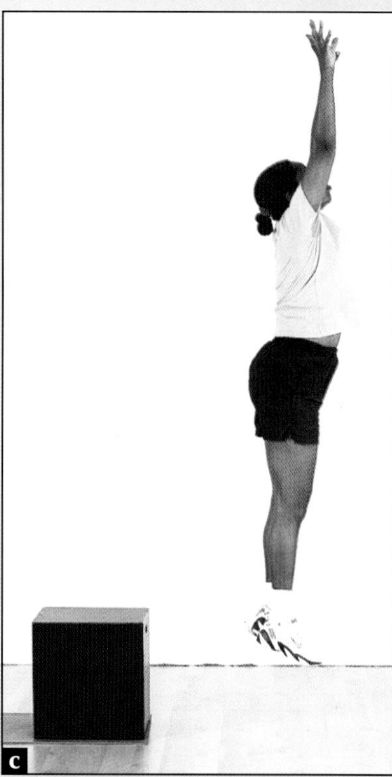

c

Upper Body Plyometric Drills

Chest Pass

Intensity level: Low

Equipment: Medicine or plyometric ball (weight 2-8 pounds [1-3.6 kilograms]); personal trainer or partner

Direction of throw: Forward

Beginning position: Assume a comfortable upright stance with feet shoulder-width apart; face the personal trainer or partner approximately 10 feet (three meters) away. Raise the ball to chest level with elbows flexed.

Preparatory movement: Begin with a countermovement. (With plyometric throws, a countermovement requires the performer to "cock" the arm(s), that is, move the arms slightly backward before the actual throw.)

Arm action: Using both arms, throw the ball to the personal trainer or partner by extending the elbows. When the personal trainer or partner returns the ball, catch it, return to the beginning position, and **immediately** repeat the movement.

Note: One can increase intensity by increasing the weight of the medicine ball. Begin with a 2-pound (1-kilogram) ball.

Common Errors

- Amortization phase (i.e., time ball is in hands) is too long.
- Ball is too heavy.

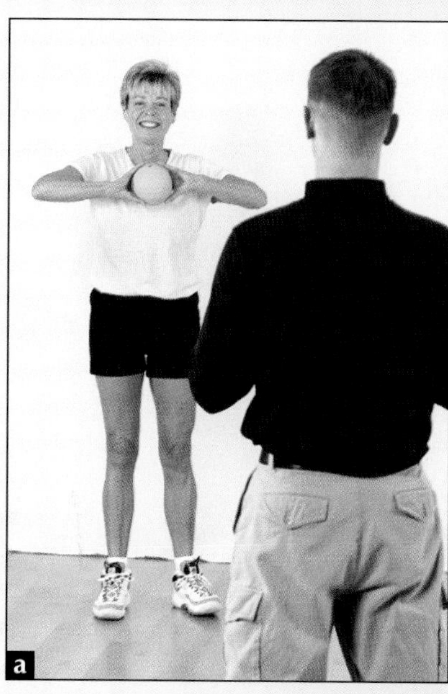

a

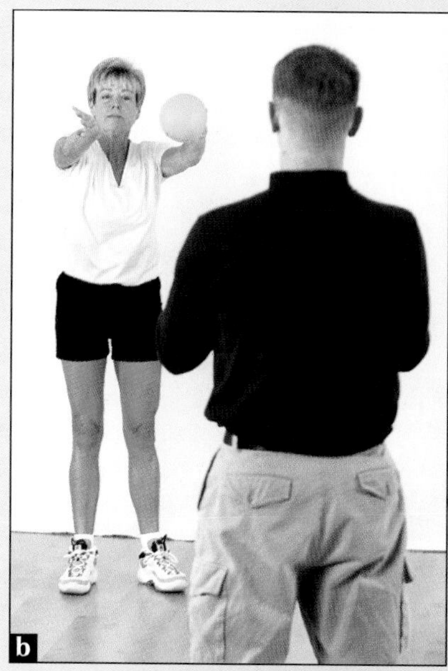

b

Depth Push-Up

Intensity level: Medium

Equipment: Medicine ball

Direction of movement: Vertical

Beginning position: Lie in a push-up position, with the hands on the medicine ball and elbows extended.

Preparatory movement: None

Downward movement: Quickly remove the hands from the medicine ball and drop down. Contact the ground with hands slightly more than shoulder-width apart and elbows slightly flexed. Allow the chest to almost touch the medicine ball.

Upward movement: **Immediately** and explosively push up by extending the elbows to full extension. Quickly place the palms on the medicine ball and repeat the exercise.

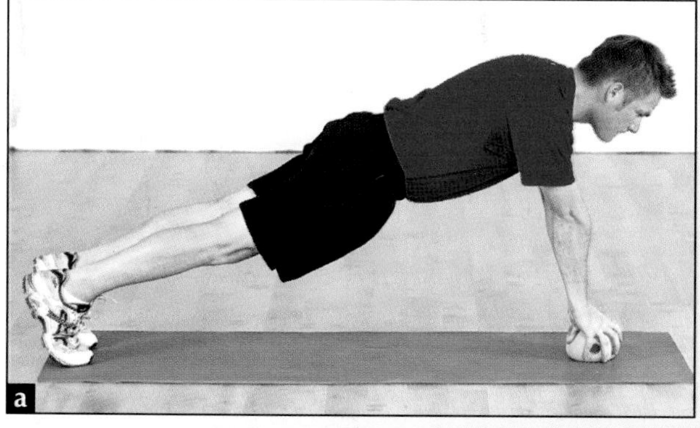

a

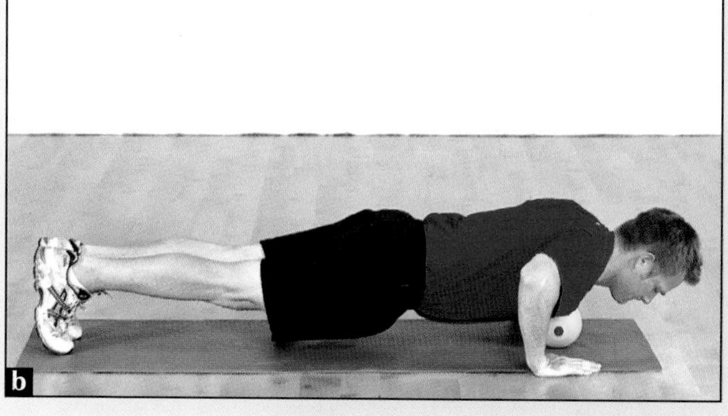

b

Note: When the upper body is at maximal height during the upward movement, the hands should be higher than the medicine ball.

Note: One can increase intensity by increasing the size of the medicine ball. Begin with a 5-pound (2.3-kilogram) ball.

Advanced variation: A way to increase the intensity of this drill is for the client to perform it as described with the feet placed on an elevated surface (e.g., a plyometric box).

 **Common Errors**

- Amortization phase (i.e., time hands are on the ground) is too long.
- Ball is too big, increasing the distance from the beginning position to the bottom of the downward movement.

45-Degree Sit-Up

Intensity level: Medium

Equipment: Medicine or plyometric ball; personal trainer or partner

Beginning position: Sit on the ground with the trunk approximately at a 45-degree angle to the ground. The personal trainer or partner should be in front with the medicine ball.

Preparatory movement: The personal trainer or partner throws the ball to outstretched hands.

Downward action: Once the partner throws the ball, catch it using both arms, allow some trunk extension, and **immediately** return the ball to the partner.

Note: One can increase the intensity by increasing the weight of the medicine ball. Begin with a 2-pound (1-kilogram) ball.

Note: The force used to return the ball to the personal trainer or partner should be predominantly derived from the abdominal muscles.

 **Common Errors**

- Eccentric phase (i.e., amount of trunk extension) is too long.
- Ball is too heavy.

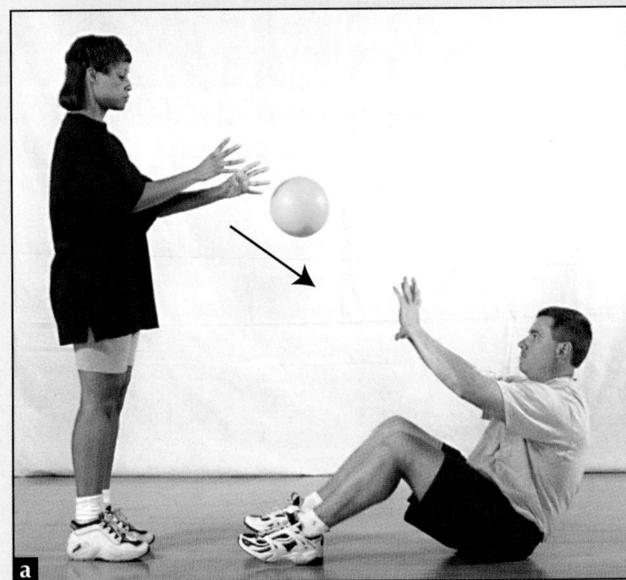
a

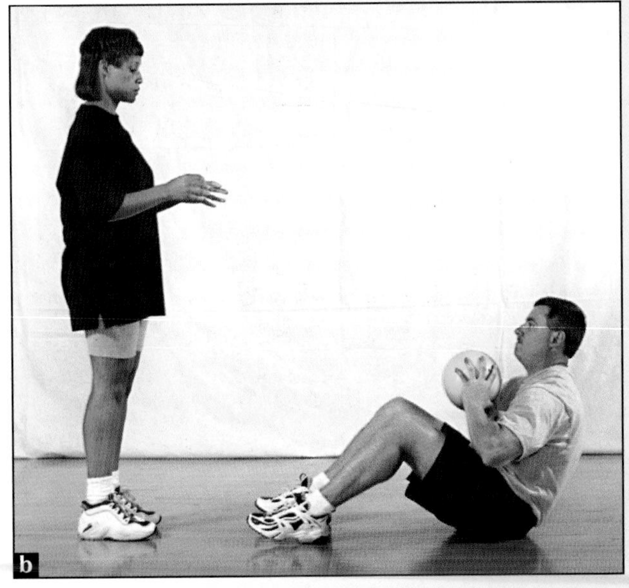
b

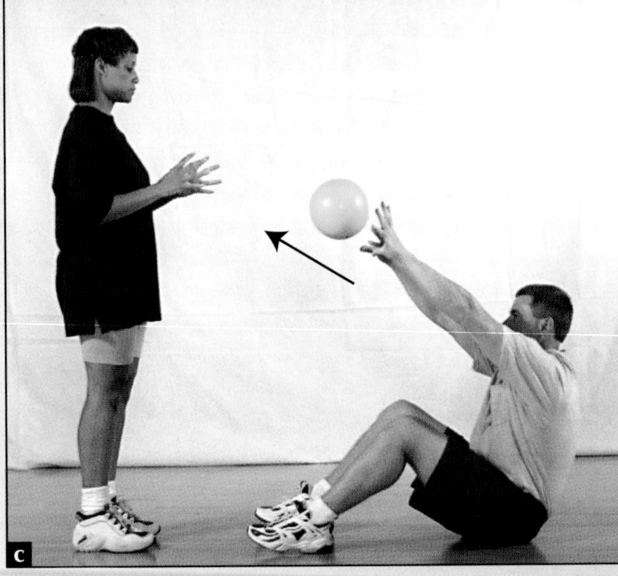
c

Speed Drills

Butt Kicker

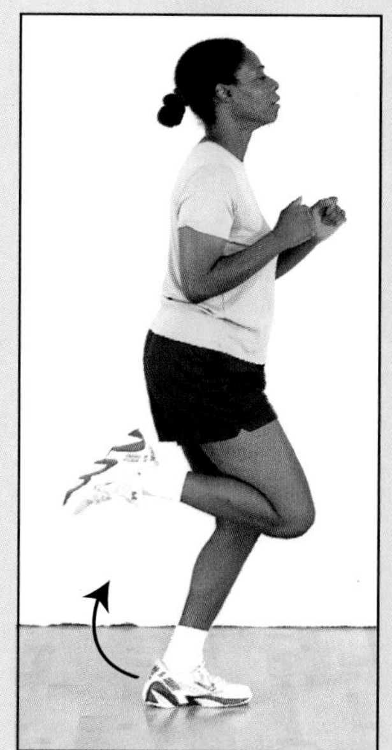

Intensity level: Low

Equipment: None

Beginning position: Assume a comfortable, upright stance with feet shoulder-width apart. Begin to jog.

Movement: Pull the heel toward the buttocks by swinging the lower leg back. Allow the heel to "bounce" off the buttocks.

Advanced variation: The wall slide is performed using this same technique, except that the heel of the recovery leg stays anterior to the buttocks. This variation improves knee lift during the flight phase of sprinting.

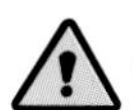 **Common Errors**

- Forcing the heel toward the buttocks; instead the client should "allow" the heel to elevate toward the buttocks.
- Excessive thigh motion; the thigh should not move too much, and the client should concentrate on moving at the knee versus the hip joint.

Stationary Arm Swing

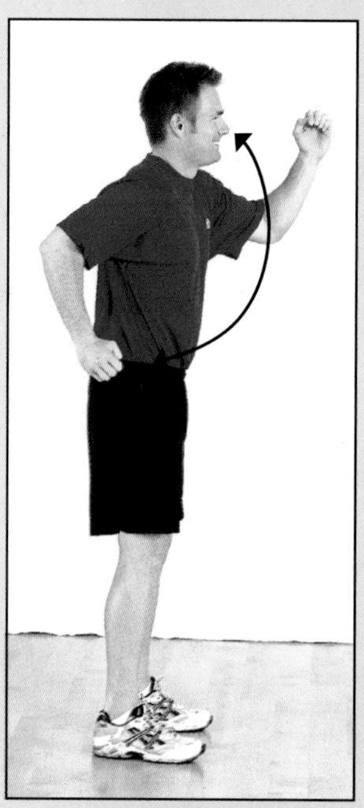

Intensity level: Low

Equipment: None

Beginning position: Assume a comfortable, upright stance with feet shoulder-width apart. Elbows should be in 90 degrees of flexion.

Movement: Maintaining elbows at 90 degrees and keeping hands relaxed, swing arms forward and back in a sprinting-type motion. The hands' arc of motion should be from nose level anteriorly to just past the hips posteriorly.

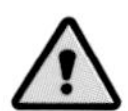 **Common Errors**

- Arms often cross the line of the body; client should maintain arm swing within the sagittal plane.
- Arm swing is often not forceful; be sure to maintain an aggressive hammering or punching motion.

Downhill Sprint

Intensity level: High

Equipment: A 3- to 7-degree downhill sprinting surface

Beginning position: At the top of the downhill area, assume a comfortable, upright stance with feet shoulder-width apart.

Movement: Maintaining correct posture and technique, sprint 30 to 50 meters (33 to 55 yards) downhill.

 **Common Errors**

- Excessive braking or deceleration; do not exceed a 7-degree slope, and decrease the slope if braking continues.
- Proper form is not maintained; decrease the slope until proper technique returns.

Partner-Assisted Towing

Intensity level: High

Equipment: 10 to 20 meters (11 to 22 yards) of rubber tubing; personal trainer or partner

Beginning position: Attach the tubing to both the client and the personal trainer or partner, with the personal trainer or partner in front. The personal trainer or partner moves approximately 5 meters (5.5 yards) ahead while the client maintains the beginning position.

Movement: Maintaining the beginning distance between them, the personal trainer or partner and client beginning sprinting simultaneously.

 **Common Errors**

- Insufficient assistance; be sure the personal trainer or partner is at least as fast as the client.
- Proper form is not maintained with increased speed; the personal trainer or partner should decrease the sprinting speed until proper technique returns.

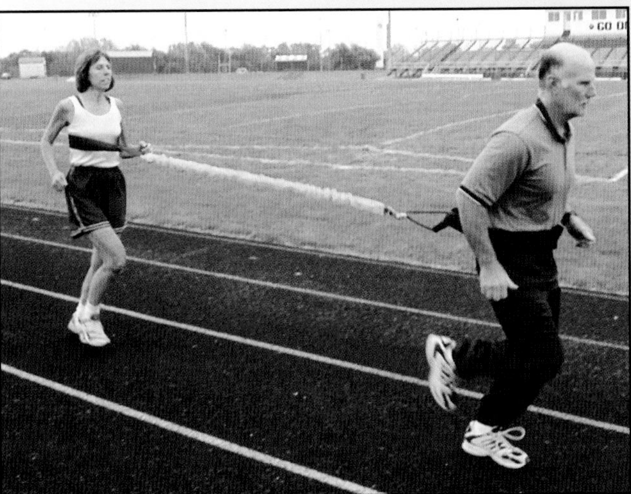

Uphill Sprint

Intensity level: High

Equipment: A 3- to 7-degree uphill sprinting surface

Beginning position: At the bottom of the downhill area, assume a comfortable, upright stance with feet shoulder-width apart.

Movement: Maintaining correct posture and technique, sprint 30 to 50 meters (33 to 55 yards) uphill.

Common Errors

- Sprinting speed slows more than 10%; do not exceed a 7-degree slope, and decrease the slope if slowdown continues.
- Proper form is not maintained; decrease the slope until proper technique returns.

Partner-Resisted Sprinting

Intensity level: High

Equipment: 10 to 20 meters (11 to 22 yards) of rubber tubing; personal trainer or partner

Beginning position: With the client in front, attach one end of the tubing to the client while the personal trainer or partner holds the other end. The client moves approximately five meters (5.5 yards) ahead while the personal trainer or partner maintains the beginning position.

Movement: Maintaining the beginning distance between them, the client begins sprinting while the personal trainer or partner resists.

 **Common Errors**

- Sprinting speed slows more than 10%; decrease the resistance until proper technique returns.
- Proper form is not maintained; the personal trainer or partner decreases the resistance until proper technique returns.

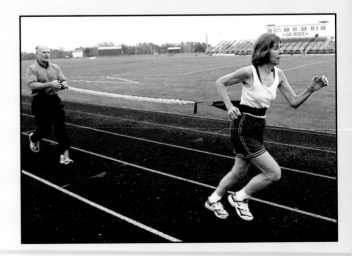

STUDY QUESTIONS

1. Which of the following exercises is best able to benefit from the advantages offered by the SSC?
   A. push press
   B. deadlift
   C. back squat
   D. front squat
2. Which of the following should be considered a requirement to participate in a plyometric training program?
   A. at least 18 years of age
   B. more than one year performing power exercises
   C. at least three months of general resistance training exercises
   D. less than 50 years of age
3. If a client is having difficulty performing a depth jump correctly—the amortization phase is too long—which of the following adjustments would be appropriate?
   A. discontinue the depth jump
   B. have the client try the jump using just one leg
   C. focus on "giving" with the landing
   D. decrease the height of the box
4. The personal trainer notices that a client takes short, choppy steps when sprinting. Which of the following types of training will help this client improve stride length?
   I. resisted sprinting
   II. assisted sprinting
   III. technique training
   IV. plyometric training
   A. I and III only
   B. II and IV only
   C. I, III, and IV only
   D. I, II, and III only

APPLIED KNOWLEDGE QUESTION

Fill in the chart to describe a sample plyometric training program based on the description and goals of the client.

A healthy, 35-year-old female who is a parttime aerobics instructor wants to begin a training program to compete in an aerobic fitness (sport aerobics) event. She has been resistance training since college and is familiar with how to perform plyometric drills. She is five feet, five inches (165 centimeters) tall, weighs 130 pounds (59 kilograms), and has a 195-pound (87-kilogram) 1RM back squat. During one of the weekly classes she teaches, she performs depth jumps and pushups off an aerobic step.

Mode	Intensity	Frequency	Volume	Activity-specific drills

REFERENCES

1. Allerheiligen, B., and R. Rogers. 1995. Plyometrics program design. *Strength and Conditioning* 17: 26-31.
2. Asmussen, E., and F. Bonde-Peterson. 1974. Storage of elastic energy in skeletal muscles in man. *Acta Physiologica Scandinavica* 91: 385-392.
3. Aura, O., and J.T. Vitasalo. 1989. Biomechanical characteristics of jumping. *International Journal of Sport Biomechanics* 5 (1): 89-97.
4. Berg, K., R.W. Latin, and T.R. Baechle. 1990. Physical and performance characteristics of NCAA division I football players. *Research Quarterly for Exercise and Sport* 61: 395-401.
5. Berg, K., R.W. Latin, and T.R. Baechle. 1992. Physical fitness of NCAA division I football players. *National Strength and Conditioning Journal* 14: 68-72.
6. Blattner, S., and L. Noble. 1979. Relative effects of isokinetic and plyometric training on vertical jumping performance. *Research Quarterly* 50 (4): 583-588.
7. Bobbert, M.F., K.G.M. Gerritsen, M.C.A Litjens, and A.J. Van Soest. 1996. Why is countermovement jump height greater than squat jump height? *Medicine and Science in Sports and Exercise* 28: 1402-1412.
8. Borkowski, J. 1990. Prevention of pre-season muscle soreness: Plyometric exercise (abstract). *Athletic Training* 25 (2): 122.
9. Bosco, C., A. Ito, P.V. Komi, P. Luhtanen, P. Rahkila, H. Rusko, and J.T. Vitasalo. 1982. Neuromuscular function and mechanical efficiency of human leg extensor muscles during jumping exercises. *Acta Physiologica Scandinavica* 114: 543-550.
10. Bosco, C., and P.V. Komi. 1979. Potentiation of the mechanical behavior of the human skeletal muscle through prestretching. *Acta Physiologica Scandinavica* 106: 467-472.
11. Bosco, C., P.V. Komi, and A. Ito. 1981. Pre-stretch potentiation of human skeletal muscle during ballistic movement. *Acta Physiologica Scandinavica* 111: 135-140.
12. Bosco, C., J.T. Vitasalo, P.V. Komi, and P. Luhtanen. 1982. Combined effect of elastic energy and myoelectrical potentiation during stretch shortening cycle exercise. *Acta Physiologica Scandinavica* 114: 557-565.
13. Brown, L.E., V.A. Ferrigno, and J.C. Santana. 2000. *Training for Speed, Agility, and Quickness.* Champaign, IL: Human Kinetics.
14. Cavagna, G.A. 1977. Storage and utilization of elastic energy in skeletal muscle. In: *Exercise and Sport Science Reviews,* vol. 5, R.S. Hutton, ed. Santa Barbara, CA: Journal Affiliates, pp. 80-129.
15. Cavagna, G.A., B. Dusman, and R. Margaria. 1968. Positive work done by a previously stretched muscle. *Journal of Applied Physiology* 24: 21-32.
16. Cavagna, G.A., F.P. Saibere, and R. Margaria. 1965. Effect of negative work on the amount of positive work performed by an isolated muscle. *Journal of Applied Physiology* 20: 157-158.
17. Chambers, C., T.D. Noakes, E.V. Lambert, and M.I. Lambert. 1998. Time course of recovery of vertical jump height and heart rate versus running speed after a 90-km foot race. *Journal of Sports Science* 16: 645-651.
18. Chu, D. 1983. Plyometrics: The link between strength and speed. *NSCA Journal* 5 (2): 20-21.
19. Chu, D. 1984. Plyometric exercise. *NSCA Journal* 5 (6): 56-59, 61-64.
20. Chu, D. 1998. *Jumping Into Plyometrics,* 2nd ed. Champaign, IL: Human Kinetics.
21. Chu, D., and F. Costello. 1985. Jumping into plyometrics. *NSCA Journal* 7 (3): 65.
22. Chu, D., and R. Korchemny. 1989. Sprinting stride actions: Analysis and evaluation. *NSCA Journal* 11 (6): 6-8, 82-85.
23. Chu, D., and R. Panariello. 1986. Jumping into plyometrics. *NSCA Journal* 8 (5): 73.
24. Chu, D., and L. Plummer. 1984. Jumping into plyometrics: The language of plyometrics. *NSCA Journal* 6 (5): 30-31.
25. Costello, F. 1985. Training for speed using resisted and assisted methods. *NSCA Journal* 7 (1): 74-75.
26. Dick, F.W. 1987. *Sprints and Relays.* London: British Amateur Athletic Board.
27. Dillman, C.J., G.S. Fleisig, and J.R. Andrews. 1993. Biomechanics of pitching with emphasis upon shoulder kinematics. *Journal of Orthopaedic and Sports Physical Therapy* 18 (2): 402-408.
28. Dintiman, G.B., R.D. Ward, and T. Tellez. 1998. *Sports Speed.* Champaign, IL: Human Kinetics.
29. Dursenev, L., and L. Raeysky. 1979. Strength training for jumpers. *Soviet Sports Review* 14 (2): 53-55.
30. Enoka, R.W. 1994. *Neuromechanical Basis of Kinesiology.* Champaign, IL: Human Kinetics.
31. Faccioni, A. 1994. Assisted and resisted methods for speed development (part II). *Modern Athlete Coach* 32 (3): 8-11.
32. Feltner, M., and J. Dapena. 1986. Dynamics of the shoulder and elbow joints of the throwing arm during a baseball pitch. *International Journal of Sport Biomechanics* 2: 235.
33. Fleck, S. 1983. Interval training: Physiological basis. *NSCA Journal* 5 (5): 40, 57-63.
34. Fleck, S., and W. Kraemer. 1997. *Designing Resistance Training Programs.* Champaign, IL: Human Kinetics.
35. Fleisig, G.S., S.W. Barrentine, N. Zheng, R.F. Escamilla, and J.R. Andrews. 1999. Kinematic and kinetic comparison of baseball pitching among various levels of development. *Journal of Biomechanics* 32 (12): 1371-1375.
36. Fowler, N.E., A. Lees, and T. Reilly. 1994. Spinal shrinkage in unloaded and loaded drop-jumping. *Ergonomics* 37: 133-139.
37. Fowler, N.E., A. Lees, and T. Reilly. 1997. Changes in stature following plyometric drop-jump and pendulum exercises. *Ergonomics* 40: 1279-1286.
38. Gambetta, V. 1978. Plyometric training. *Track and Field Quarterly Review* 80 (4): 56-57.
39. Gambetta, V., G. Winckler, J. Rogers, J. Orognen, L. Seagrave, and S. Jolly. 1989. Sprints and relays. In: *TAC Track and Field Coaching Manual,* 2nd ed., TAC Development Committees and V. Gambetta, eds. Champaign, IL: Leisure Press, pp. 55-70.
40. Guyton, A.C., and J.E. Hall. 1995. *Textbook of Medical Physiology,* 9th ed. Philadelphia: Saunders.
41. Harman, E.A., M.T. Rosenstein, P.N. Frykman, and R.M. Rosenstein. 1990. The effects of arms and countermovement on vertical jumping. *Medicine and Science in Sports and Exercise* 22: 825-833.
42. Harre, D., ed. 1982. *Principles of Sports Training.* Berlin: Sportverlag.
43. Hewett, T.E., T.N. Lindenfeld, J.V. Riccobene, and F.R. Noyes. 1999. The effect of neuromuscular training on the incidence of knee injury in female athletes. A prospective study. *American Journal of Sports Medicine* 27: 699-706.

44. Hewett, T.E, A.L. Stroupe, T.A. Nance, and F.R. Noyes. 1996. Plyometric training in female athletes. *American Journal of Sports Medicine* 24: 765-773.

45. Hill, A.V. 1970. *First and Last Experiments in Muscle Mechanics.* Cambridge: Cambridge University Press.

46. Holcomb, W.R., D.M. Kleiner, and D.A. Chu. 1998. Plyometrics: Considerations for safe and effective training. *Strength and Conditioning* 20 (3): 36-39.

47. Jarver, J., ed. 1990. *Sprints and Relays: Contemporary Theory, Technique and Training,* 3rd ed. Los Altos, CA: Tafnews Press.

48. Kaeding, C.C., and R. Whitehead. 1998. Musculoskeletal injuries in adolescents. *Primary Care* 25 (1): 211-23.

49. Kilani, H.A., S.S. Palmer, M.J. Adrian, and J.J. Gapsis. 1989. Block of the stretch reflex of vastus lateralis during vertical jump. *Human Movement Science* 8: 247-269.

50. Korchemny, R. 1985. Evaluation of sprinters. *NSCA Journal* 7 (4): 38-42.

51. Kozlov, I., and V. Muravyev. 1992. Muscles and the sprint. *Soviet Sports Review* 27 (6): 192-195.

52. Kraemer, W.J., S.A. Mazzetti, B.C. Nindl, L.A. Gotshalk, J.S. Volek, J.A. Bush, J.O. Marx, K. Dohi, A.L. Gomez, M. Miles, S.J. Fleck, R.U. Newton, and K. Häkkinen. 2001. Effect of resistance training on women's strength/power and occupational performances. *Medicine and Science in Sports and Exercise* 33 (6): 1011-1025.

53. LaChance, P. 1995. Plyometric exercise. *Strength and Conditioning* 17: 16-23.

54. Latin, R.W., K. Berg, and T.R. Baechle. 1994. Physical and performance characteristics of NCAA division I male basketball players. *Journal of Strength and Conditioning Research* 8: 214-218.

55. Lavrienko, A., J. Kravstev, and Z. Petrova. 1990. New approaches to sprint training. *Modern Athlete Coach* 28 (3): 3-5.

56. Lipp, E.J. 1998. Athletic epiphyseal injury in children and adolescents. *Orthopaedic Nursing* 17 (2): 17-22.

57. Luhtanen, P., and P. Komi. 1978. Mechanical factors influencing running speed. In: *Biomechanics VI-B,* E. Asmussen, ed. Baltimore: University Park Press, pp. 23-29.

58. Mach, G. 1985. The individual sprint events. In: *Athletes in Action: The Official International Amateur Athletic Federation Book on Track and Field Techniques.* London: Pelham Books, pp. 12-34.

59. Matavulj, D., M. Kukolj, D. Ugarkovic, J. Tihanyi, and S. Jaric. 2001. Effects of plyometric training on jumping performance in junior basketball players. *Journal of Sports Medicine and Physical Fitness* 41 (2): 159-164.

60. Matthews, P.B.C. 1990. The knee jerk: Still an enigma? *Canadian Journal of Physiology and Pharmacology* 68: 347-354.

61. Mero, A., P.V. Komi, and R.J. Gregor. 1992. Biomechanics of sprint running: A review. *Sports Medicine* 13 (6): 376-392.

62. Moravec, P., J. Ruzicka, P. Susanka, E. Dostal, M. Kodejs, and M. Nosek. 1988. The 1987 International Athletic Foundation/IAAF scientific project report: Time analysis of the 100 metres events at the II World Championships in athletics. *New Studies Athletics* 3 (3): 61-96.

63. National Strength and Conditioning Association. 1993. Position statement: Explosive/plyometric exercises. *NSCA Journal* 15 (3): 16.

64. Newton, R.U., W.J. Kraemer, and K. Häkkinen. 1999. Effects of ballistic training on preseason preparation of elite volleyball players. *Medicine and Science in Sports and Exercise* 31 (2): 323-330.

65. Newton, R.U., A.J. Murphy, B.J. Humphries, G.J. Wilson, W.J. Kraemer, and K. Häkkinen. 1997. Influence of load and stretch shortening cycle on the kinematics, kinetics and muscle activation that occurs during explosive upper-body movements. *European Journal of Applied Physiology* 75: 333-342.

66. Ozolin, E. 1986. Contemporary sprint technique (part 1). *Soviet Sports Review* 21 (3): 109-114.

67. Ozolin, E. 1986. Contemporary sprint technique (part 2). *Soviet Sports Review* 21 (4): 190-195.

68. Pappas, A.M., R.M. Zawacki, and T.J. Sullivan. 1985. Biomechanics of baseball pitching: A preliminary report. *American Journal of Sports Medicine* 13: 216-222.

69. Plattner, S., and L. Noble. 1979. Relative effects of isokinetic and plyometric training on vertical jumping performance. *Research Quarterly* 50 (4): 583-588.

70. Plisk, S.S. 1995. Theories, concepts and methodology of speed development as they relate to sports performance. Presented at the NSCA Certification Commission's Essential Principles of Strength Training and Conditioning Symposium, Phoenix, June.

71. Plisk, S.S. 2002. Personal communication, March 2002.

72. Radcliffe, J.C., and L.R. Osternig. 1995. Effects on performance of variable eccentric loads during depth jumps. *Journal of Sport Rehabilitation* 4: 31-41.

73. Romanova, N. 1990. The sprint: Nontraditional means of training (a review of scientific studies). *Soviet Sports Review* 25 (2): 99-102.

74. Sandler, R., and S. Robinovitch. 2001. An analysis of the effect of lower extremity strength on impact severity during a backward fall. *Journal of Biomechanical Engineering* 123 (6): 590-598.

75. Schmolinsky, G., ed. 2000. *Track and Field: The East German Textbook of Athletics.* Toronto: Sport Books.

76. Siff, M.C. 2000. *Supertraining,* 5th ed. Denver: Supertraining Institute.

77. Sinnett, A.M., K. Berg, R.W. Latin, and J.M. Noble. 2001. The relationship between field tests of anaerobic power and 10-km run performance. *Journal of Strength and Conditioning Research* 15 (4): 405-412.

78. Svantesson, U., G. Grimby, and R. Thomeé. 1994. Potentiation of concentric plantar flexion torque following eccentric and isometric muscle actions. *Acta Physiologica Scandinavica* 152: 287-293.

79. Verkhoshansky, Y. 1969. Perspectives in the improvement of speed-strength preparation of jumpers. *Yessis Review of Soviet Physical Education and Sports* 4 (2): 28-29.

80. Verkhoshansky, Y., and V. Tatyan. 1983. Speed-strength preparation of future champions. *Soviet Sports Review* 18 (4): 166-170.

81. Voight, M.L., P. Draovitch, and S. Tippett. 1995. Plyometrics. In: *Eccentric Muscle Training in Sports and Orthopaedics,* M. Albert, ed. New York: Churchill Livingstone, pp. 61-88.

82. Walshe, A.D., G.J. Wilson, and G.J.C. Ettema. 1998. Stretch-shorten cycle compared with isometric preload: Contributions to enhanced muscular performance. *Journal of Applied Physiology* 84: 97-106.

83. Wathen, D. 1993. Literature review: Plyometric exercise. *NSCA Journal* 15 (3): 17-19.

84. Wilk, K.E., M.L. Voight, M.A. Keirns, V. Gambetta, J.R. Andrews, and C.J. Dillman. 1993. Stretch-shortening drills for the upper extremities: Theory and clinical application. *Journal of Orthopaedic and Sports Physical Therapy* 17: 225-239.

85. Wilson, G.J., A.J. Murphy, and A. Giorgi. 1996. Weight and plyometric training: Effects on eccentric and concentric force production. *Canadian Journal of Applied Physiology* 21: 301-315.

86. Wilson, G.J., R.U. Newton, A.J. Murphy, and B.J. Humphries. 1993. The optimal training load for the development of dynamic athletic performance. *Medicine and Science in Sports and Exercise* 25: 1279-1286.

87. Wilt, F. 1968. Training for competitive running. In: *Exercise Physiology*, H.B. Falls, ed. New York: Academic Press, pp. 395-414.

88. Witzke, K.A., and C.M. Snow. 2000. Effects of plyometric jump training on bone mass in adolescent girls. *Medicine and Science in Sports and Exercise* 32 (6): 1051-1017.

PART V

Clients With Unique Needs

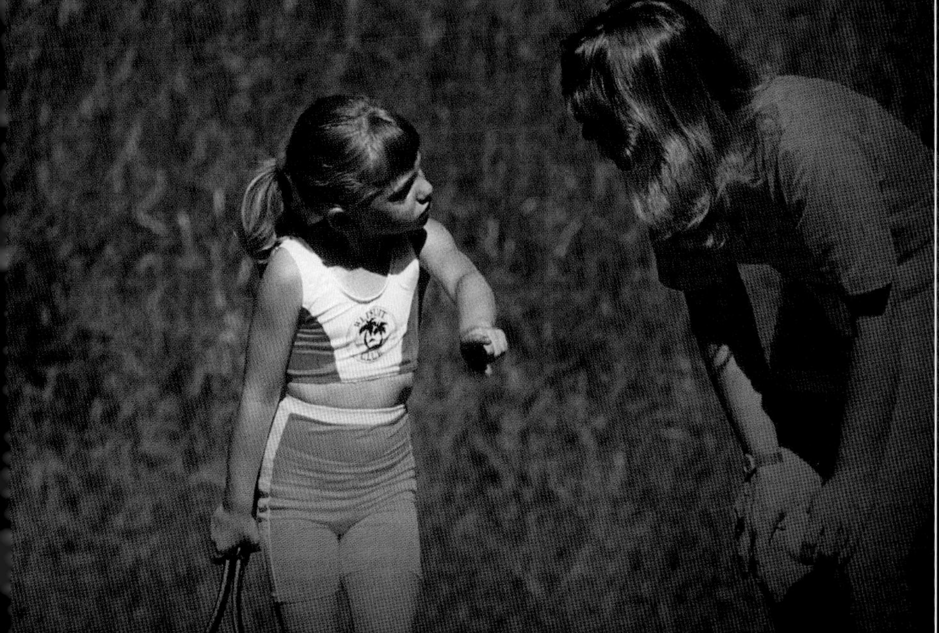

CHAPTER 18

Clients Who Are Pregnant, Older, or Preadolescent

Wayne L. Westcott | Avery D. Faigenbaum

After completing this chapter, you will be able to

- discuss exercise recommendations and precautions for pregnant women;
- explain the health benefits of senior exercise and outline exercise guidelines for older adults; and
- describe developmentally appropriate physical activity programs for preadolescents that demonstrate an understanding of age-specific needs and concerns.

The purpose of this chapter is to present general training considerations and specific exercise guidelines for three groups of people who typically need modified workouts to maximize their conditioning benefits and minimize their injury risk. Pregnant women, older adults, and preadolescent youth can safely perform aerobic endurance exercise for improved cardiovascular fitness, as well as resistance training for increased musculoskeletal fitness. However, because each of these special populations has particular characteristics, personal trainers must incorporate a number of recommendations into exercise programs for pregnant women, older adults, and preadolescent youth.

Pregnant Women

Women who are pregnant may seek out exercise programs for a number of reasons. They may feel self-conscious about their changing body, be concerned about having a healthy baby, want to stay in shape throughout their pregnancy, want to be able to handle the physical rigors of labor and delivery, or need additional social interactions and support during this new phase in their life. Pregnant women who exercise regularly may continue participating in appropriately adjusted sessions of physical activity, thereby maintaining cardiovascular and muscular fitness throughout pregnancy and postpartum [3,4]. Previously sedentary women may also benefit from regular exercise during pregnancy, although a program consistent with their physical capabilities should involve additional support, motivation, and professional guidance. In all cases, pregnant women should consult with their health care provider before initiating an exercise program or modifying a current program. In the presence of obstetric or medical complications, it may be necessary to alter the training program as determined by the client's obstetrician.

Recommendations with respect to exercise during pregnancy relate to three key concerns or potential adverse outcomes [4]:

1. Insufficient oxygen or energy substrates to the fetus
2. **Hyperthermia**-induced fetal distress or birth abnormalities
3. Increased uterine contractions

Fortunately, a properly designed fitness program should pose a very low risk for these problems in women with uncomplicated pregnancies.

Benefits of Exercise During Pregnancy

Most pregnant women who follow their physician's recommendations can attain maternal health and fitness benefits while subjecting the developing fetus to minimal risk [4]. The following are some of the benefits for pregnant women who engage in properly designed prenatal exercise programs [adapted from ACSM 2000, reference 4]:

- Improved cardiovascular and muscular fitness
- Facilitated recovery from labor
- Faster return to prepregnancy weight, strength, and flexibility levels
- Reduced postpartum belly
- Reduced back pain during pregnancy
- More energy reserve
- Fewer obstetric interventions
- Shorter active phase of labor and less pain
- Less weight gain
- Enhanced maternal psychological well-being that may reduce feelings of stress, anxiety, and depression often experienced during pregnancy
- Increased likelihood of adopting permanent healthy lifestyle habits

Participation in an exercise program may also be beneficial in the primary prevention of **gestational diabetes** [3]. The effects of regular exercise training on insulin secretion, insulin sensitivity, and glucose metabolism may improve glucose tolerance and thereby decrease the likelihood of a woman's developing gestational diabetes. Exercise training may also be beneficial in preventing or treating other conditions including physical discomforts, weakness, and lack of stamina [3, 4].

In the absence of either medical or obstetric complications, exercise during pregnancy appears to be associated with many of the physical and psychosocial health benefits typically observed in nonpregnant women.

Fetal Response to Exercise

Some research has revealed reduced birth weight in babies whose mothers performed high-intensity exercise throughout their pregnancy [18]. The lower birth weight was approximately 300 to 350 grams (10-12 ounces) and apparently resulted from a decreased amount of subcutaneous fat in the newborn. More moderate exercise sessions may therefore be advisable for pregnant women.

Vigorous exercise during pregnancy is associated with a 5 to 15 beat per minute increase in fetal heart rate, but there are no documented adverse fetal effects related to exercise-induced fetal heart rate changes [3]. With respect to preterm labor, the American College of Obstetricians and Gynecologists states that in the majority of healthy pregnant women without additional risk factors for preterm labor, exercise does not increase either baseline uterine activity or the incidence of preterm labor or delivery [3].

Accommodating Mechanical and Physiological Changes During Pregnancy

Medical and fitness organizations provide the following recommendations for accommodating the cardiovascular, respiratory, mechanical, metabolic, and thermoregulatory changes experienced during normal pregnancy [3, 4].

Cardiovascular Response

Since pregnancy alters the relationship between heart rate and oxygen consumption, personal trainers can use the **rating of perceived exertion** (RPE) scale to prescribe aerobic exercise intensity. Generally, an RPE rating on the original scale between 12 ("light" to "somewhat hard") and 16 ("hard" to "very hard") seems appropriate for aerobic conditioning during pregnancy. Of course, exercise programs need to be individually prescribed, and women may need to adjust the exercise intensity, duration, or both on any given day depending upon how they feel. (Refer to chapter 16 for more information on RPE scales.)

After the first trimester of pregnancy, the back-lying (supine) position results in restricted venous return of blood to the heart because of the increasingly larger uterus. This position reduces cardiac output and may cause **supine hypotensive syndrome**. Consequently, exercises performed on the back should be phased out of the client's training program before the second trimester. These include abdominal curls, bench presses, supine exercises on the stability ball, and stretching exercises with the back on the floor.

As an alternative, women can do curl-downs and splint their abdomens for safety and support (see figure 18.1). Additionally, women can perform abdominal exercises in the crawling or side-lying position (see figures 18.2 and 18.3) and upper and lower body resistance training exercises in the seated position. For example, instead of performing the barbell bench press exercise to enhance upper body strength, pregnant women can use the vertical chest press machine or perform wall push-ups or a rubber cord exercise in the seated position to strengthen the same muscle groups.

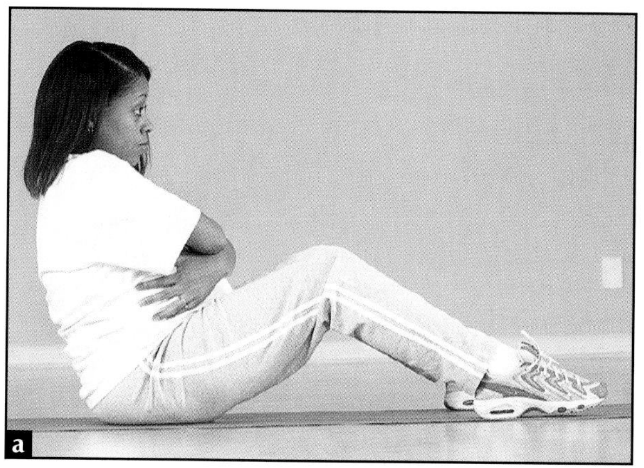

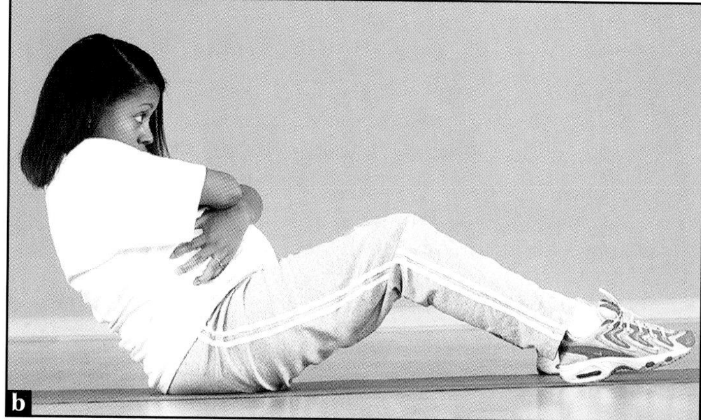

Figure 18.1 Curl-down exercise while splinting the abdomen, *(a)* beginning position and *(b)* final position.

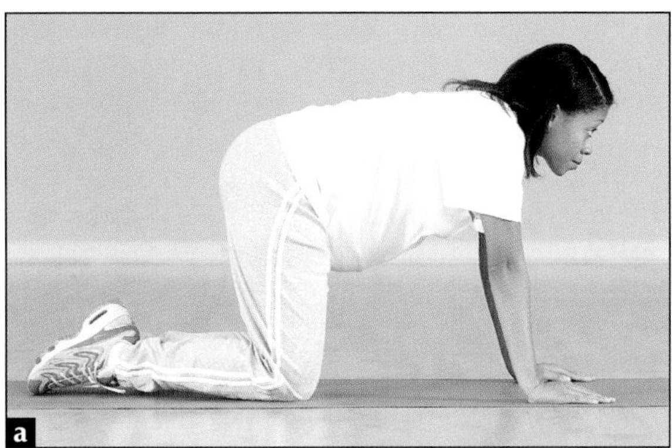

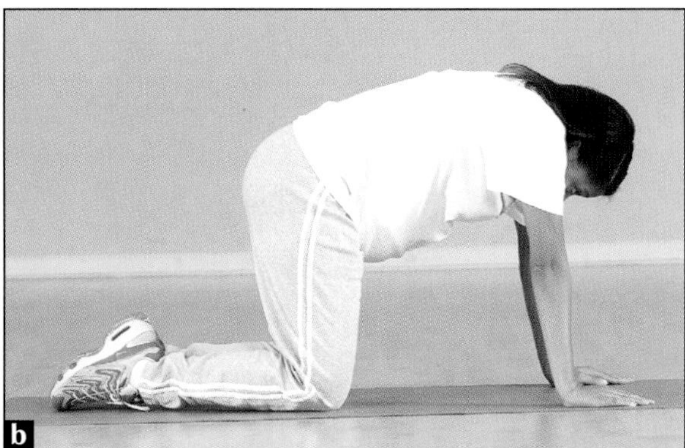

Figure 18.2 Abdominal exercise performed in crawling position, *(a)* beginning position and *(b)* final position.

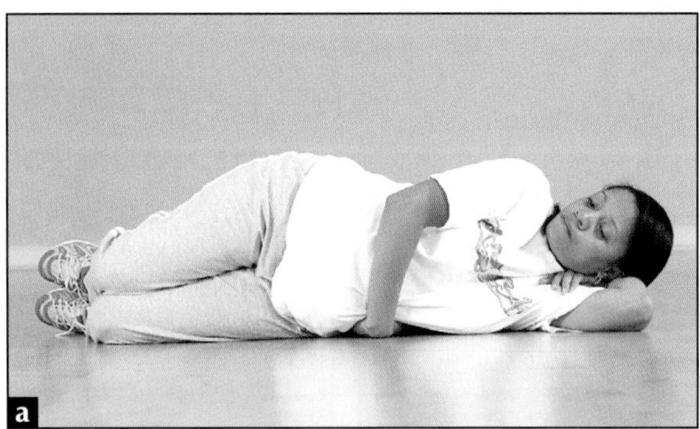

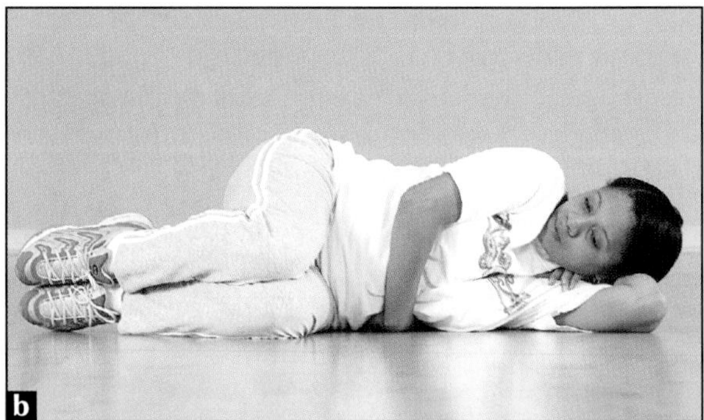

Figure 18.3 Abdominal exercise performed in side-lying position, *(a)* beginning position and *(b)* final position.

Because of changes in the center of gravity later in pregnancy, it also may be advisable for some pregnant women to use weight machines, which provide more stability and support than the corresponding free weight exercises (e.g., machine biceps curl rather than standing dumbbell curl). This recommendation may be particularly important for previously sedentary women who want to resistance train. Regardless of the type of equipment used, pregnant women should be cautioned to avoid the **Valsalva maneuver** while resistance training because breath-holding during exertion places excessive pressure on the abdominal contents and pelvic floor. A general resistance training recommendation is to exhale on exertion or in the "lifting" phase of every exercise repetition. (See chapter 13 for additional breathing guidelines.)

Exercises performed on the back should be phased out of the program before the second trimester of pregnancy.

Respiratory Response

Pregnant women may increase their minute ventilation by almost 50%, resulting in 10% to 20% more oxygen utilization at rest [3]. Consequently, less oxygen is available for aerobic activity. Additionally, as the pregnancy progresses, the enlarging uterus interferes with diaphragm movement, increasing the effort of breathing and decreasing both subjective workload and maximum exercise performance. Personal trainers should adjust pregnant women's exercise program accordingly to avoid training at high levels of fatigue or reaching physical exhaustion.

Mechanical Response

As the uterus and breasts become larger during pregnancy, a woman's center of mass changes. This may adversely affect her balance, body control, and movement mechanics in some physical activities. Consequently, exercises requiring balance and agility should be carefully prescribed, with special attention to activity selection during the third trimester of pregnancy.

Although any activity that presents the potential for falling or even mild abdominal trauma should be avoided, some activities designed to enhance physical balance may be beneficial for pregnant women. For example, personal trainers may include "centering" activities such as physical balance, deep abdominal breathing, and mental focus, that may help women achieve physical balance during pregnancy and help them become more aware of body movements during exercise [23]. Because of joint laxity during pregnancy, exercises should be performed slowly and in a controlled manner to avoid damage to the joints.

Pregnant women should avoid participating in activities such as downhill skiing, basketball, horseback riding, and vigorous racket sports that present a high risk of falling or abdominal trauma. They should also avoid scuba diving because of the risk of decompression sickness to the fetus [3].

Although it is important to strengthen all the major muscle groups, personal trainers should emphasize abdominal and pelvic floor strength because these muscles provide the basis for postural support and prepare a woman for delivery [23]. For example, strengthening the transverse abdominis, which is the deepest abdominal muscle located underneath the rectus abdominis and obliques, helps to support the lumbar spine and prepare a woman for the pushing stage of birth. The tranverse abdominis is strengthened by blowing air out through the mouth while compressing the abdomen. A good image of this activity is that of shortening the distance between the navel and the spine by "sucking in" the abdomen. This exercise can be performed in the seated position or the crawling position on hands and knees.

Pelvic floor exercises **(Kegels)** are another important element of resistance training during pregnancy. These exercises involve tightening and relaxing muscle groups in the pelvic region. With proper training, a woman can learn not only how to contract these muscles, but also how to relax them so that the baby can be delivered more easily [23]. Specific guidelines for performing Kegel exercises are beyond the scope of this chapter, but are available in most books on pregnancy.

Metabolic Response

The need for more oxygen during pregnancy is paralleled by the need for more energy substrate. Pregnant women typically use an extra 300 kilocalories per day to meet the increased metabolic requirements for **homeostasis** of their expanded life functions. During exercise, pregnant women also utilize carbohydrates at a higher rate than women who are not pregnant. The obvious indication is for pregnant clients to attain adequate intake of carbohydrate-rich foods through a balanced but expanded nutritional program. In addition, pregnant women should be sure to take in sufficient quantities of protein and water to sustain fetal growth and optimize training efficiency.

Thermoregulatory Response

Pregnancy elevates a woman's basal metabolic rate and heat production, which may be further increased by exercise. Exercise-associated rises in body temperature may be most likely in the first trimester of pregnancy. During this period, pregnant exercisers should be sure to facilitate heat dissipation through adequate hydration, appropriate clothing, and optimal environmental surroundings. If a client feels overheated or fatigued during an exercise session, the personal trainer should decrease the exercise intensity and begin the cool down. Severe headaches, dizziness, and disorientation are indications of potential serious conditions that require referral to a client's health care provider. Clearly, pregnant women should be made aware of safe exercise guidelines and should know when to reduce the exercise intensity or stop exercising.

Contraindications for Exercise

Women without obstetric or medical complications can continue to exercise during pregnancy and derive related health and fitness benefits [3]. However, certain conditions present contraindications to exercise. These include the following [adapted from the International Federation of Gynecology and Obstetrics 2002, reference 3]:

- Pregnancy-induced hypertension (preeclampsia)
- Ruptured membranes
- Premature labor during the current pregnancy
- Persistent bleeding after 12 weeks
- A cervix that dilates ahead of schedule (incompetent cervix)
- Significant heart disease or restrictive lung disease
- Multiple-birth pregnancy that creates a risk of premature labor
- A placenta that blocks the cervix after 26 weeks

There are also relative contraindications to exercise that should be evaluated by the client's physician before participation in an exercise program [adapted from International Federation of Gynecology and Obstetrics 2002, reference 3]:

- Poorly controlled type 1 diabetes, seizures, hypertension, or hyperthyroidism
- Extreme obesity
- Extremely low body weight (BMI < 12)
- History of a very sedentary lifestyle
- Unevaluated maternal cardiac arrhythmia
- Severe anemia
- Heavy smoking
- Chronic bronchitis
- Orthopedic limitations

Additionally, any of the following conditions is a reason to discontinue exercise and seek medical advice during pregnancy [reprinted from ACSM 2000, reference 4]:

- Any signs of bloody discharge from the vagina
- Any gush of fluid from the vagina
- Sudden swelling of the ankles, hands, or face
- Persistent, severe headaches; visual disturbance; or unexplained spell of fainting or dizziness
- Swelling, pain, or redness in the calf of one leg
- Elevation of pulse rate or blood pressure that persists after exercise
- Persistent contractions (6-8 per hour) that may suggest premature labor
- Unexplained abdominal pain
- Insufficient weight gain (less than 2 pounds [1 kilogram] per month during the last two trimesters)

Exercise Guidelines

The following exercise guidelines from the American College of Obstetricians and Gynecologists apply to pregnant women who do not have additional risk factors for adverse maternal or prenatal outcome [Adapted from International Federation of Gynecology and Obstetrics 2002, reference 3]:

- Perform 30 minutes or more of moderate exercise on most, if not all, days of the week.
- Avoid exercise in the supine position after the first trimester.
- Exercise should not continue past the point of fatigue and should never reach exhaustive levels.
- Non-weight-bearing activities such as cycling or swimming are favored for reducing injury risk and continuing the exercise program throughout pregnancy.
- Exercises that present potential for even mild abdominal trauma should be avoided, and activities that have high risk for loss of balance or for falling should be discontinued prior to the third trimester.
- Large increases in body temperature should be minimized through adequate hydration, appropriate clothing, and optimal environmental surroundings during exercise.

General Exercise Safety Guidelines for Pregnant Women

- Check with your health care provider before you begin exercising.
- Exercise at a comfortable level at which you can maintain a conversation.
- Do not exercise if you have a fever.
- See your health care provider if you experience bleeding, a large amount of discharge, or swelling in your face and hands.
- Avoid lying on your back after the third month.
- Avoid straining or stretching to the point of discomfort.
- Wear proper footwear, and dress in layers.
- Use equipment in good condition.
- Drink eight cups of water a day and avoid exercising in hot, humid conditions.
- Avoid fatigue and overtraining.

Adapted from Cowlin 2002 [23].

- Because many of the **physiologic** and **morphologic** changes of pregnancy persist four to six weeks postpartum, women should resume prepregnancy exercise programs gradually after giving birth.

Older Adults

Men and women 50 years of age and older, typically referred to as seniors, may begin sensible conditioning programs, including aerobic endurance training for improved cardiovascular fitness and resistance training for increased muscular fitness [2, 4]. However, various medical conditions common among older adults call for physician approval and appropriate modifications to the exercise protocols. These include cardiovascular disease, cancer, diabetes, osteoporosis, low back pain, arthritis, depression, obesity, and general frailty.

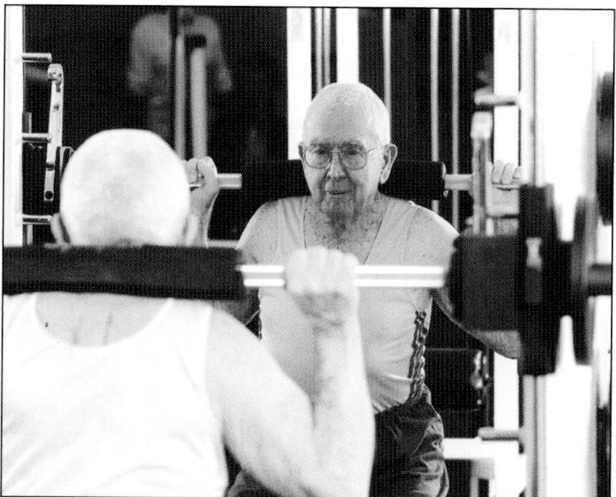

Figure 18.4 Recent research studies show that resistance training may reduce the risk of many diseases and debilitating conditions frequently experienced by older adults.

Health Benefits of Senior Exercise

This section briefly reviews the benefits of aerobic training for seniors but then focuses more intently on the lesser-known benefits of resistance training for seniors. Perhaps no other age group can experience more health benefits from exercise than those over 50 years old. Because the numerous health benefits associated with aerobic activity are better known, this section summarizes these relationships and then presents more detailed information on the equally important health benefits associated with resistance training.

Benefits of Aerobic Training

It is well established that aerobic endurance exercise such as walking, jogging, and cycling is effective for increasing calorie utilization and improving cardiovascular fitness [2, 4, 28]. In addition, reduced body weight associated with aerobic training may lessen the risk of high blood pressure, type 2 diabetes, and obesity [2, 4]. Other benefits of aerobic fitness include reduced risk of cardiovascular disease, stroke, osteoporosis, certain types of cancer, and psychological stress, as well as improved sleep, digestion, and elimination [7].

Benefits of Resistance Training

Although less well known, the health benefits of resistance exercise are equally impressive, especially for senior men and women. This section considers some recent research studies showing that resistance training may reduce the risk of many diseases and debilitating conditions frequently experienced by older adults.

Cardiovascular Disease There are two ways in which resistance training lowers the risk of cardiovascular disease. First, resistance training decreases resting blood pressure (systolic, diastolic, or both). Reductions in diastolic blood pressure average about 4% after several weeks of regular resistance exercise [49, 56, 63, 113]. Reductions in systolic blood pressure average about 3% over a similar training period [63], and two months of circuit resistance training may reduce systolic blood pressure by up to 7 mmHg (millimeters of mercury) [110]. In fact, some studies have shown that resistance training has been found to be as effective as aerobic exercise for reducing resting blood pressure [11, 92].

The second way in which resistance training benefits cardiovascular health is by improving blood lipid profiles. Although some studies have not shown significant changes in blood lipid levels [66, 67, 92], other research has revealed significantly decreased low-density lipoprotein cholesterol (LDL-cholesterol) in 40- to 55-year-old men [56]. Several researchers have reported improved blood lipid profiles following various programs of resistance training [13, 43, 96, 102], and other investigators have found that resistance training produces effects on blood lipids similar to those seen with aerobic exercise [8, 59, 92].

Coronary artery disease, the leading medical problem in the United States, is particularly prevalent among senior men and women. For most **postcoronary** patients, resistance training appears to be a safe and productive means for improving muscular fitness and physical performance, as well as for maintaining desirable body weight and positive self-concept in persons with cardiac problems. Numerous studies support resistance training for postcoronary patients [14, 32, 42, 46, 62, 95, 102, 105].

Colon Cancer Because a slow **gastrointestinal transit** speed appears to be associated with an increased risk of colon cancer [55], moving food more quickly through the gut should lessen the probability of this disease. Running [21] and resistance training [65] have both been shown to speed up gastrointestinal transit. Therefore, resistance training may be an effective means for addressing age-related gastrointestinal modality disorders, as well as for reducing the risk of colon cancer.

Type 2 Diabetes As our society becomes more sedentary, type 2 diabetes becomes more prevalent among men and women of all ages. Exercise promotes glucose utilization, and aerobic activity has traditionally been recommended for enhancing glucose uptake [22]. However, research on resistance training suggests that resistance exercise may be equally effective for enhancing glucose utilization [26, 75]. Resistance training has been shown to improve insulin response [24], improve glycemic control [27], and increase glucose utilization [55] in older men. In addition to stimulating more muscle glucose uptake [71], resistance training may be beneficial for preserving lean body mass [6] and addressing **muscle myopathy** [25], thereby lessening the severity and even reducing the risk of type 2 diabetes.

Osteoporosis Osteoporosis is a degenerative disease of the skeletal system resulting in a progressive loss of bone proteins and minerals. Several studies have shown that resistance training is effective for maintaining a strong and functional musculoskeletal system that resists deterioration and osteoporosis [7, 19, 68, 89, 93]. In fact, research with older men [74] and postmenopausal women [81, 98] indicates that bone loss can be changed to bone gain through regular resistance training. (See chapter 5 for further discussion.)

Low Back Pain Although not life threatening, low back pain is the most prevalent medical problem in the United States, affecting four out of every five adults during their lifetime. Research [60] has demonstrated a strong positive relationship between weak low back muscles and low back pain. Strengthening the low back (trunk extensor) muscles may alleviate or even eliminate low back pain in some patients [87].

With respect to prevention, strong low back muscles provide better musculoskeletal function, support, control, and shock absorption, which should reduce the risk of both low back injury and structural degeneration [77].

Arthritis Studies [72, 85] indicate that stronger muscles may improve joint function and reduce arthritic discomfort. In fact, researchers have found that resistance training actually eases the pain of osteoarthritis and rheumatoid arthritis [101].

Depression Depression in older individuals may be associated with decreased functionality. In one study [90], senior subjects experienced significant reductions in depression after 10 weeks of resistance training. Although more research is needed in this area, resistance training appears to be beneficial for enhancing self-confidence and counteracting depression in older adults.

Muscle Loss and Metabolic Rate Reduction In addition to reducing the risk of various degenerative diseases, resistance training offers even greater benefits for seniors with respect to replacing muscle tissue and recharging their metabolism. These are probably the most fundamental problems affecting men and women as they age. Adults lose about one-half pound (0.2 kilograms) of muscle per year during their 30s and 40s; this process of muscle loss is referred to as **sarcopenia** [28]. Even more disturbing, there is evidence that the rate of muscle loss may double to 1 pound (0.45 kilograms) per year in people past 50 years of age [81]. Figure 18.5 illustrates this insidious process, masked in most adults by their gradually increasing body weight due to progressively greater fat accumulation.

Although the average aging American adds about 10 pounds (4.5 kilograms) of body weight each decade of adult life, this actually represents approximately 5 to 10 pounds (2-4.5 kilograms) less muscle and 15 to 20 pounds (7-9 kilograms) more fat. Moreover, the loss of muscle may be partly responsible for the gain in fat. Researchers [28, 64] have found a 2% to 5% per decade reduction in resting metabolic rate attributed to decreased

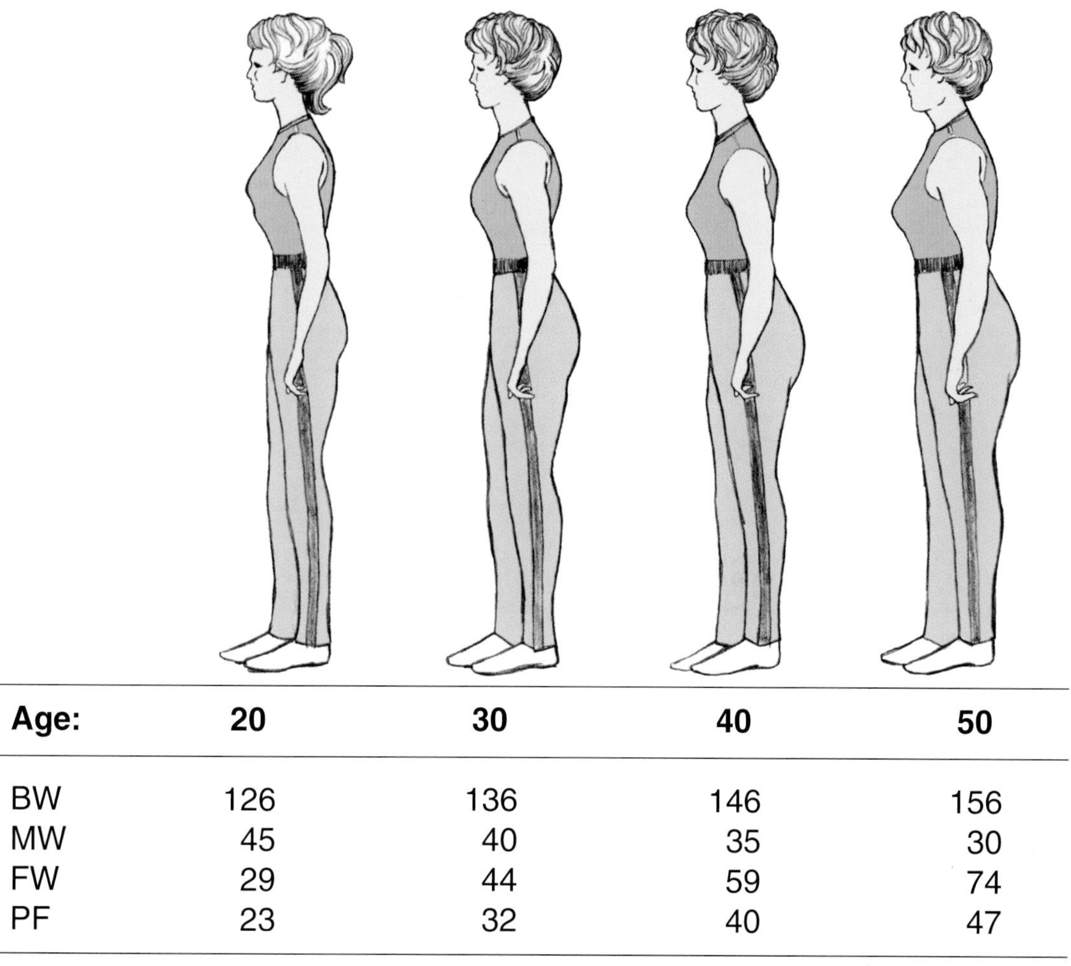

Age:	20	30	40	50
BW	126	136	146	156
MW	45	40	35	30
FW	29	44	59	74
PF	23	32	40	47

Abbreviations: BW, body weight; FW, fat weight; MW, muscle weight; PF, percent fat.

Figure 18.5 Body weight and body composition change throughout the life of an adult.
Reprinted from Westcott 1996.

amounts of muscle tissue. A slower resting metabolism means that some calories previously used by high-energy muscle tissue are no longer needed and are therefore stored as fat.

Clearly, it would be much more desirable for people to perform some basic resistance exercises to prevent muscle loss and metabolic slowdown. Resistance training can help maintain muscle tissue that enables physical activity and enhances energy utilization throughout the senior years. In fact, resistance training is the only type of exercise that can maintain muscle and metabolism as people age and should therefore be an essential component of every senior fitness program. Numerous studies [16, 38, 40, 45, 47, 53, 57, 73, 81, 84, 99, 110, 111] have shown significant increases in muscle mass following several weeks of standard strength training, and many [16, 54, 69, 84] have also demonstrated significant elevations in resting metabolic rate.

In addition to reducing the risks of various degenerative diseases, strength training offers even greater benefits for seniors with respect to replacing muscle tissue and recharging their metabolism.

Resistance Training Guidelines for Seniors

Generally speaking, seniors should perform resistance training two or three nonconsecutive days per week. Using both single- and multiple-joint movements, seniors may perform single or multiple sets for a variety of exercises that address at least the following major muscle groups: quadriceps, hamstrings, gluteals, pectoralis major, latissimus dorsi, deltoids, biceps, triceps, erector spinae, and rectus abdominis. Personal trainers should have seniors use controlled exercise speeds (typically four to six seconds per repetition) and full movement ranges

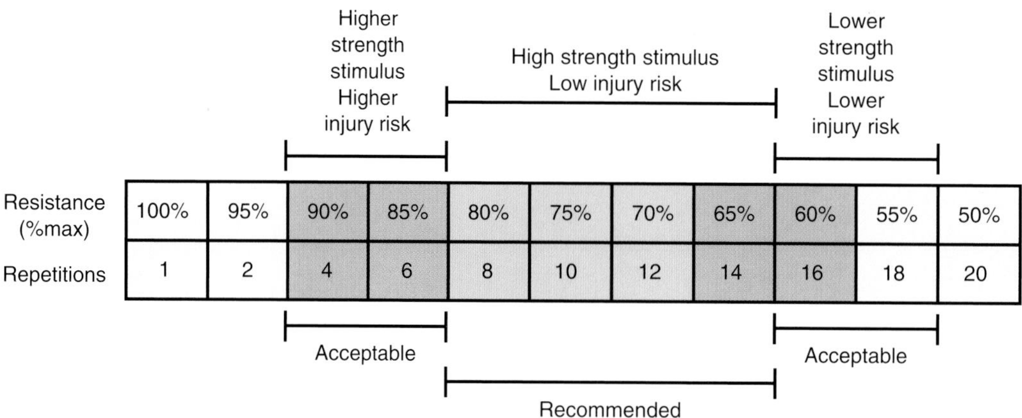

Figure 18.6 Resistance and repetition relationships for recommended resistance training protocols.
Reprinted from Westcott and Baechle 1999.

(excluding positions in which discomfort is experienced).

Seniors may train with a wide range of repetitions depending on their experience and physical condition. Beginners and less fit seniors may start with relatively light weight loads that permit many repetitions, whereas more advanced seniors may perform fewer repetitions with higher resistance [4]. As shown in figure 18.6, an acceptable resistance range may extend from 60% to 90% of maximum, with a corresponding repetition range of 4 to 16 repetitions [109].

The key to safe and successful senior resistance training experiences is competent instruction and careful supervision. With respect to teaching technique, we recommend the instructional model described below.

Instructional Model for Teaching Seniors

- Demonstrate exactly how the exercise is performed.
- Explain precisely each movement phase and the proper breathing pattern.
- Demonstrate the exercise again with emphasis on exhaling during the lifting phase and inhaling during the lowering phase.
- Have the client perform the exercise, with assistance if necessary.
- Provide positive reinforcement for correct technique with specific feedback and suggestions for improved performance.

From Westcott and Baechle 1999 [109].

Aerobic Endurance Training Guidelines for Seniors

Adults of all ages are advised to perform aerobic endurance exercise for cardiovascular health and fitness [4]. The recommended training frequency is two to five days per week, and the recommended exercise duration is 20 to 60 minutes per session. An exercise intensity of 60% to 90% of maximum heart rate is acceptable, but training at about 75% of maximum heart rate is generally prescribed [4]. Because maximum heart rate decreases as people age (approximately 10 heartbeats per decade), the relative exercise intensity should be essentially the same for young, middle, and older adults. Of course, seniors who have limited cardiovascular fitness must begin with shorter exercise duration and lower training intensity. For some older adults, this may be only 5 to 10 minutes of physical activity at approximately 40% of maximum heart rate.

Although the training protocol based on percentage of maximum heart rate is easy to monitor and generally appropriate for older adults, this method presents certain limitations. For example, a senior with perfectly normal heart function could have a maximum heart rate up to 30 beats per minute above or 30 beats per minute below that predicted by the formula 220 minus age [112]. Also, people taking certain medications, such as beta-blockers, have lower maximum heart rates due to the drug-induced **bradycardia.**

Consequently, assessing the exercise intensity in older adults by both their heart rate response and their personal effort level is advised. The latter may be best assessed by means of the Borg scale of perceived exertion, which provides a subjective assessment to complement heart rate monitoring [12]. (See figure 16.3.) Ideally, a healthy senior exercising at approximately 75% of maximum heart rate will report a perceived exertion rating of about 13 (range 12 to 14 on the original RPE scale). However, a healthy senior exerciser whose heart rate is *above* 75% of age-predicted maximum but who reports a *low level* of perceived exertion (e.g., 10-11) should probably not be advised to reduce the training intensity. On the other hand, a senior exerciser whose heart rate is *below* 75% of age-predicted maximum but who reports a *high level* of perceived exertion (e.g., 15-16) should definitely be advised to reduce the training intensity.

Another means of monitoring seniors' exercise effort is the talk test. Older adults who can talk in short to medium-length sentences while they are exercising are probably performing their aerobic activity at the appropriate level of intensity. If they have difficulty carrying on simple conversation during the activity, they are most likely exercising harder than necessary.

Screening and Program Design for Seniors

Resistance training is a vital physical activity for older adults. Aerobic endurance training is equally important for senior men and women to enhance heart health and help with weight management. Unfortunately, some mature individuals may have already experienced physical or mental conditions that make it difficult for them to participate in standard resistance and aerobic exercise programs. The first step in every case is to check with the client's personal physician for specific exercise guidelines and training modifications. With this information the personal trainer can design an individualized program that is safe and appropriate for the older adult. When training seniors, of course, the personal trainer must be especially observant for any exercise contraindications or undesirable responses. The personal trainer should keep careful and detailed records of senior clients' exercise sessions and fitness assessments. Such information provides important educational material for future program design and serves as a powerful motivational tool for older trainees.

Exercise Order

If seniors perform both resistance and aerobic exercise, they should begin with aerobic activity (including warm-up and cool-down phases), then do resistance training, and conclude with static stretches. If they do only resistance training, they should do 5 to 10 minutes of light aerobic activity followed by a few static stretches before and after the resistance exercises. In both exercise sequences, the less strenuous aerobic activity provides a warm-up for the more strenuous resistance exercise. Flexibility exercises should be performed after the resistance exercises to provide a relaxing conclusion to the training session.

Safety and Comfort

Certain conditions common to seniors can affect the comfort and safety of exercise. "Conditions Common to Older Adults and Suggested Adaptations" lists some of these conditions and the adjustments that clients or personal trainers can make to promote a safe exercise experience.

Conditions Common to Older Adults and Suggested Adaptations

Dry skin

- Clients can apply lotion to elbows, knees, and contact points before exercising.

Poor balance

- Clients should begin with weight-supporting machine exercises before progressing to weight-bearing free weight exercises.
- Clients should begin with weight-supporting aerobic endurance exercise such as stationary cycling before progressing to weight-bearing alternatives such as treadmill walking and stair climbing.
- Avoid hard-to-control exercises such as lunges or step-ups.
- Clients can perform exercises in a seated or lying position instead of standing.

(continued)

Conditions Common to Older Adults and Suggested Adaptations *(continued)*

Propensity for injuries	• Clients should train only in uncluttered facilities. • Clients should use controlled movement speeds. • Emphasize proper posture and exercise positioning.
Susceptibility to colds and flu	• Clients should drink plenty of fluids. • Clients should obtain ample rest and sleep. • Clients should shower or wash face and hands after exercise session.
Reduced flexibility	• Clients should warm up well prior to exercise. • Have the client perform appropriate stretching exercises at end of training session. • Avoid exercises that require extreme movement ranges such as lunges.
Reduced tolerance to heat and humidity	• Train in climate-controlled facilities whenever possible. • Schedule training sessions earlier in the day. • Clients should drink plenty of fluids. • Clients should wear lightweight and light-colored exercise attire.
Difficulties seeing and hearing	• Personal trainers should speak clearly and concisely with sufficient volume. • Use large-print materials and workout cards. • Give precise exercise demonstrations and manual assistance when necessary. • Frequently ask clients if they understand instructions.

Preadolescent Youth

Preadolescence refers to a period of time before the development of secondary sex characteristics (e.g., pubic hair and reproductive organs) and corresponds roughly to the ages 6 to 11 years in girls and 6 to 13 years in boys. Preadolescent youth should be encouraged to participate regularly in physical activities that promote cardiorespiratory and musculoskeletal health. Regular physical activity can improve aerobic fitness, muscle strength, bone mineral density, motor performance skills, body composition, and psychosocial well-being [17, 88]. The National Strength and Conditioning Association [30], the American College of Sports Medicine [4], the American Council on Exercise [34], and the National Association for Sports and Physical Education [79] support children's participation in physical activity programs that are consistent with the needs and abilities of the participants.

The promotion of physical activity among youth has become a major public health concern because childhood overweight and obesity continue to increase and the physical activity level of most boys and girls is down [103]. The percentage of overweight boys and girls has more than doubled during the past two decades [80], and many children who are overweight have one or more cardiovascular disease risk factors [39]. Daily participation in physical education classes continues to decline [103]; and on average, children and teenagers in the United States spend four hours a day using electronic media (e.g., watching television, playing video games, or using a computer) [61].

The negative health consequences of childhood obesity and physical inactivity include hypertension and the appearance of atherosclerosis and type 2 "adult-onset" diabetes in children and teenagers. Furthermore, since positive and negative behaviors established at a young age appear to track into adulthood, it is likely that inactive children and teens will become inactive adults [58, 100]. Health promotion programs for youth that involve physical activity could help to maintain the progress that has been made over the past few decades in reducing deaths from cardiovascular disease.

The key is to value the importance of physical activity and help children develop healthy habits and behavior patterns that persist into adulthood. Personal trainers who model and support participation in developmentally appropriate fitness activities that are safe, fun, and supported by cultural norms can have a powerful influence on a child's health and activity habits. Well-organized personal training sessions that give boys and girls the opportunity to experience the mere enjoyment of physical activity can have long-lasting effects on their health and well-being. *Healthy People 2010,* a statement on national health objectives, includes participation in physical activity as one of the nation's 10 leading health indicators [104].

Youth Fitness Guidelines

Because youth have different needs than adults and are active in different ways, adult exercise guidelines and training philosophies should not be imposed on children. Watching boys and girls on a playground supports the contention that the natural activity pattern of children is characterized by sporadic bursts of moderate- to vigorous-intensity activity with brief periods of low-intensity activity or rest as needed. While children often raise their heart rates into their target heart rate zone, they are intermittently active and often choose to exercise in an interval-type pattern characterized by haphazard increases and decreases in exercise intensity. Thus personal trainers should not expect preadolescents to exercise in the same manner as adults. Assuming that children are inactive simply because they do not perform continuous physical activity is inaccurate.

This does not mean that exercising continuously for 30 minutes or more within a predetermined target heart rate range (e.g., 70% to 85% predicted maximal heart rate) is not beneficial for children. Rather it means that this is not the most appropriate method for training preadolescents because they are concrete rather than abstract thinkers and do not see the benefit of prolonged periods of aerobic training. Further, because cardiorespiratory adaptations such as increasing aerobic capacity are less noticeable in children compared to older adults [83], prolonged periods of vigorous activity can decrease rather than increase motivation for future activity. As children enter their teenage years, some may want to adhere to the adult target heart rate model depending upon their needs, goals, and abilities.

While the absolute level of physical activity required to achieve and maintain fitness in youth has not yet been determined, the Children's Lifetime Physical Activity Model (C-LPAM) is a child-specific model that addresses the amount of physical activity necessary to produce health benefits associated with reduced morbidity and mortality [20]. The C-LPAM model, described in table 18.1, highlights the minimum activity recommendations and optimal functioning standards for children. Although the minimal recommendations for expending calories are similar between C-LPAM and the traditional adult model (i.e., 3-4 kcal · kg^{-1} · day^{-1}), the C-LPAM recommends that children alternate periods of physical activity with rest periods as needed. It is also suggested that children optimally expend 6 to 8 kcal · kg^{-1} · day^{-1}. So a girl who weighs 88 pounds (40 kilograms) should expend at least 120 kilocalories (40 kg × 3 kcals per kg) per day and optimally 280 kilocalories (40 kg × average of 7 kcals per kg) per day in physical activity.

TABLE 18.1

Children's Lifetime Physical Activity Model (C-LPAM)

The health standard: A minimum activity standard	
Frequency	Daily. Frequent activity sessions (three or more) each day.
Intensity	Moderate. Alternating bouts of activity with rest periods as needed, or moderate activity such as walking or riding a bike to school.
Time	Duration of activity necessary to expend at least 3 to 4 kcal · kg^{-1} · day^{-1}. Equal to caloric expenditure in 30 minutes or more of active play or moderate sustained activity that may be distributed over three or more activity sessions.

The optimal functioning standard: A goal for all children	
Frequency	Daily. Frequent activity sessions (three or more) each day.
Intensity	Moderate to vigorous. Alternating bouts of activity with rest periods as needed, or moderate activity such as walking or riding a bike to school.
Time	Duration of activity necessary to expend at least 6 to 8 kcal · kg^{-1} · day^{-1}. Equal to caloric expenditure in 60 minutes or more of active play or moderate sustained activity that may be distributed over three or more activity sessions.

Reprinted from Corbin, Pangrazi, and Welk 1994.

With support and encouragement, even sedentary children can perform relatively large volumes of physical activity by alternating moderate to vigorous physical activity with brief periods of rest and recovery. In addition to participation in structured programs (e.g., physical education classes and personal training sessions), playground games, recess, walking or biking to and from school, and physical chores around the home (e.g., doing yard work, sweeping floors) are lifestyle activities that are consistent with C-LPAM. Reducing time spent in sedentary pursuits such as television viewing or video games can considerably increase the amount of time children have available for physical activity [44].

Children can remain physically active for 30 minutes or more provided that the exercise intensity varies throughout the session and that children are given the opportunity to take a short break if needed. Instead of a 30-minute jogging workout, however, the personal trainer can create a circuit of 8 to 12 stations that includes jumping rope, stretching, body-weight exercises (e.g., jumping jacks, push-ups, and squats), medicine ball activities, balancing drills, and shuttle runs. As fitness levels improve, it becomes possible to decrease the rest period between stations and make the activities at each station more challenging.

With qualified instruction, enthusiastic leadership, and adherence to safety issues, children can safely enhance their fundamental movement abilities and be better prepared for successful and enjoyable participation in recreational activities and sport.

Resistance Training for Youth

For many years, youth fitness programs focused on aerobic activities such as jogging, swimming, dance, and tag games. However, over the past decade a compelling body of evidence has indicated that resistance training can be a safe, effective, and worthwhile method of conditioning for preadolescents provided that appropriate guidelines are followed [10, 37, 48]. Despite the traditional belief that resistance training was inappropriate or unsafe for children, qualified acceptance by medical and fitness organizations of youth resistance training is becoming universal [1, 4, 5, 30, 34].

Previously, the concern that resistance training could damage the epiphyseal plate of children or impede the statural growth of young weight trainers caused some people to recommend that children not participate in resistance training. In recent years, however, public health objectives have been initiated that aim to increase the number of children who regularly participate in physical activities that enhance and maintain muscular fitness [103]. Current observations indicate no evidence of decrease in stature in preadolescents who resistance train in supervised programs, and epiphyseal plate fractures have not been reported in any prospective youth resistance training study published to date. There is no scientific evidence to suggest that the risks associated with competently supervised and well-designed youth resistance training programs are greater than those of other recreational activities that children regularly participate in. However, accidents are possible if established training guidelines are not followed [41].

Muscle Strength Gains and Other Benefits

Many studies have convincingly shown that children can increase muscular strength above and beyond that accompanying growth and maturation by participating in a well-designed resistance training program [10, 30]. Strength gains of roughly 30% to 40% have been observed in children following short-term (8-12 weeks) resistance training programs. Various combinations of sets and repetitions and different training modalities—including child-sized weight machines, free weights (barbells and dumbbells), medicine balls, and body-weight exercises—have proven to be safe and effective methods of conditioning for apparently healthy children [33]. Children as young as age 6 have benefited from resistance training [36], and there is no evidence of any difference in muscular strength between preadolescent boys and girls [9].

Since children lack sufficient levels of circulating androgens to stimulate increases in muscle hypertrophy, it has been suggested that neural adaptations are primarily responsible for training-induced strength gains in preadolescents [82, 86]. Intrinsic muscle adaptations (i.e., changes in excitation-contraction coupling, myofibrillar packing density, and muscle fiber composition), as well as improvements in motor skill performance and the coordination of the involved muscle groups, could also contribute to gains in strength. Longer training periods and more precise measuring techniques (e.g., computerized imaging) may uncover the potential for training-induced muscle hypertrophy in preadolescent youth.

In addition to increasing muscle strength, regular participation in strength-building activities can positively influence several measurable indexes of health and fitness [29]. Reports indicate that appropriately prescribed youth resistance training programs may

- increase bone mineral density [76],
- improve body composition [35],
- enhance cardiorespiratory fitness [106],
- develop motor performance skills (e.g., vertical jump and sprint speed) [70], and
- lower elevated blood lipids [107].

It has recently been reported that youth with burn injuries [97], insulin-dependent diabetes mellitus [78], and obesity [94] can also benefit from participation in resistance training activities.

Preventing Sport-Related Injuries

Furthermore, since many sports have a significant strength or power component, it is attractive to assume that a stronger and more powerful child will perform better. Although more applied research regarding the effects of resistance training on youth sport performance is needed, it appears that young athletes who resistance train are more likely to experience success and less likely to drop out of sport due to frustration, embarrassment, failure, or injury than those who do not.

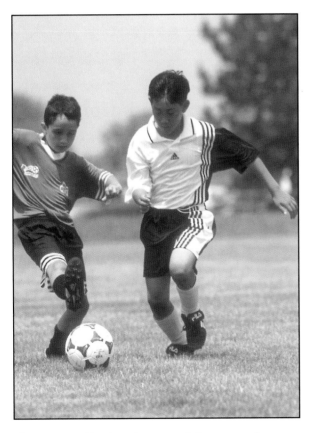

Figure 18.7 Youth resistance training may enhance sport performance and help prevent sport-related injuries.

Thus, aspiring young athletes who have been physically inactive for the past two to three months (e.g., no regular participation in recreational physical activities or sport) should be encouraged to participate in a "preseason" conditioning program (two to three times per week) that includes strength-building activities, aerobic conditioning, flexibility exercises, and agility drills. In some cases, youth may need to decrease the time they spend practicing sport-specific skills to allow time for preparatory conditioning.

Although the total elimination of youth sport injuries is an unrealistic goal, preseason conditioning programs have been shown to decrease sport-related injuries in high school athletes [15, 50, 51], and it is likely that a similar protective effect could be observed in preadolescent athletes. An estimated 50% of overuse injuries in youth sport could be prevented if more emphasis was placed on the development of fundamental fitness abilities (i.e., strength, power, aerobic endurance, and agility) than on sport-specific skills [91]. This concern may be particularly important for young female athletes, who appear to be particularly susceptible to knee injuries [52]. Although additional clinical trials are needed to determine the best method for reducing sport-related injuries, it seems prudent for inactive youth to participate in at least six to eight weeks of preparatory conditioning before sport participation.

Guidelines for Youth Resistance Training

The belief that resistance training is unsafe or inappropriate for children is not consistent with the needs of children and the documented benefits associated with this type of training. Guidelines from the National Strength and Conditioning Association suggest that youth resistance training can be a safe and worthwhile activity for preadolescents provided that the program is appropriately designed and competently supervised [30]. While there is no minimum age for participation in a youth resistance training program, all participants should have the emotional maturity to accept and follow directions and should understand the benefits and risks associated with this type of training.

It is important for youth to begin at a level that is commensurate with their physical abilities. Too often, the volume and intensity of training exceed a child's capabilities, and the prescribed rest periods are too short for an adequate recovery. This approach may undermine the enjoyment of the resistance training experience and may increase the risk of injury. When introducing preadolescents to resistance training activities, it is always better to underestimate their abilities than to overestimate their abilities and risk an injury. A weight that can be lifted for 10 to 15 repetitions appears to be a safe and effective training resistance for children to begin with when they are participating in an introductory resistance training program [31].

Youth Resistance Training Guidelines

- Qualified adults should provide supervision and instruction.
- The training environment should be safe and free of hazards.
- Resistance training should be preceded by 5- to 10-minute warm-up.
- Young people can perform one to three sets of 6 to 15 repetitions on single- and multijoint exercises, beginning with one set of 10 to 15 repetitions at the start of a program.
- Resistance should be increased gradually (e.g., about 5% to 10%) as strength improves.
- Two to three nonconsecutive training sessions per week is recommended.
- The resistance training program should be varied over time to optimize gains and prevent boredom.

Personal trainers working with a group of children should individually prescribe workloads and ask children to do the best they can within the allotted time period instead of setting one workload for all children in the group (e.g., 10 push-ups or 20 pounds [9 kilograms] on the chest press exercise). Personal trainers and children should work together to determine the workload that is most appropriate for each child's needs and abilities. Although some children may want to see how much weight they can lift during the first workout, their energy and enthusiasm should be redirected toward developing proper form and technique on a variety of exercises.

No matter how big or strong a child is, adult resistance training guidelines and training philosophies should not be imposed on young resistance-training clients. Parents, teachers, coaches, and personal trainers who work with children should not overlook the importance of having fun and developing a more positive attitude toward resistance training and all types of physical activity. Long-term adherence to any type of exercise program is more probable when children are internally driven to do their best and when they feel good about their performances.

Resistance training can be a safe, effective, and enjoyable method of conditioning for preadolescent boys and girls provided that qualified supervision is present and age-specific training guidelines are followed.

Teaching Preadolescent Youth

Although boys and girls should be aware of the potential health- and fitness-related benefits associated with regular physical activity, enthusiastic leadership, creative programming, and age-specific teaching strategies are more likely to get youth "turned on" to physical activity. If personal trainers display physical vitality, relate to children in a positive manner, understand how children think, and participate in activities with children, their efforts are likely to be worthwhile and long lasting.

Recommendations for Personal Trainers Who Train Children

- Provide close supervision and listen to each child's concerns.
- Speak to children using words they understand.
- Realize that children are active in different ways than adults.
- Design activities that ensure equal participation and enjoyment.
- Play down competition and focus on skill improvement, personal successes, and having fun.
- Remind children that it takes time to learn a new skill and get in shape.
- Offer a variety of activities and avoid regimentation.

CONCLUSION

Pregnant women, older adults, and preadolescent youth should be encouraged to participate regularly in physical activity programs that enhance and maintain cardiorespiratory and musculoskeletal fitness. Although the fundamental principles of exercise training are similar for individuals of all ages and abilities, there are unique considerations specific to each population. Personal trainers should understand and appreciate individual needs and concerns so that they can develop safe, effective, and enjoyable physical activity programs for pregnant women, older adults, and preadolescent youth.

STUDY QUESTIONS

1. Which of the following exercises would be used as a substitute for the bench press exercise for a pregnant woman who reached the end of her first trimester?
   A. close-grip bench press
   B. supine machine bench press
   C. dumbbell pullover
   D. vertical chest press
2. Which of the following describes how resistance training lowers the risk of *cardiovascular* disease in older adults?
   I. decreased diastolic blood pressure
   II. decreased serum LDL levels
   III. decreased gastrointestinal transit time
   IV. decreased glycogen utilization

   A. I and II only
   B. III and IV only
   C. I, II, and III only
   D. II, III, and IV only
3. Which of the following describes how the intensity of an aerobic exercise workout should be modified when a healthy senior exerciser reports an RPE of "10" on the original RPE scale but has an exercise heart rate of 80% of age-predicted heart rate max?
   A. maintain the same exercise intensity
   B. decrease the exercise intensity
   C. increase the exercise intensity
   D. stop the exercise session
4. Which of the following are appropriate recommendations for an 8-year-old female who wants to begin a resistance training program for the first time?
   A. Start with three sets of 20 repetitions using light weights.
   B. Avoid multijoint exercises as they place excessive strain on immature joints.
   C. Schedule at least one day of rest between exercise sessions.
   D. Tell her and her parents that she needs to wait two more years before beginning a resistance training program.

APPLIED KNOWLEDGE QUESTION

Fill in the chart to describe a *minimum* and *optimal* exercise program for a 9-year-old, 66-pound (30-kilogram) boy based on the C-LPAM activity standards.

	***Minimum* exercise program**	***Optimal* exercise program**
Number of activity sessions/day		
Intensity of the activity sessions (described by words)		
Intensity of the activity sessions (described by number of kcal $\times$ kg^{-1} $\times$ day^{-1})		
Intensity of the activity sessions (described by number of kilocalories per day)		
Approximate total duration of the activity sessions		
Examples of the activity sessions		

REFERENCES

1. American Academy of Pediatrics. 2001. Strength training by children and adolescents. *Pediatrics* 107: 1470-1472.
2. American Association of Cardiovascular and Pulmonary Rehabilitation. 1995. *Guidelines for Cardiac Rehabilitation Programs,* 2nd ed. Champaign, IL: Human Kinetics.
3. American College of Obstetricians and Gynecologists. 2002. Exercise during pregnancy and the postpartum period. *International Journal of Gynecology and Obstetrics* 77: 79-81.
4. American College of Sports Medicine. 2000. *ACSM's Guidelines for Exercise Testing and Prescription,* 6th ed. Philadelphia: Lippincott Williams & Wilkins.
5. American Orthopaedic Society for Sports Medicine. 1988. *Proceedings of the Conference on Strength Training and the Prepubescent.* Chicago: American Orthopaedic Society for Sports Medicine.
6. Ballor, D., V. Katch, M. Becque, and C. Marks. 1988. Resistance weight training during caloric restriction enhances lean body weight maintenance. *American Journal of Clinical Nutrition* 47: 19-25.
7. Bell, N., R. Godsen, and D. Henry. 1988. The effects of muscle-building exercise on vitamin D and mineral metabolism. *Journal of Bone Mineral Research* 3: 369-373.
8. Blessing, D., M. Stone, and R. Byrd. 1987. Blood lipid and hormonal changes from jogging and weight training of middle-aged men. *Journal of Applied Sports Science Research* 1: 25-29.
9. Blimkie, C. 1989. Age- and sex-associated variation in strength during childhood: Anthropometric, morphologic, neurological, biomechanical, endocrinologic, genetic and physical activity correlates. In: *Perspectives in Exercise Science and Sports,* C. Gisolfi and D. Lamb, eds. Indianapolis: Benchmark Press, pp. 99-163.
10. Blimkie, C. 1993. Resistance training during preadolescence. Issues and controversies. *Sports Medicine* 15: 389-407.
11. Blumenthal, J., W. Siegel, and M. Appelbaum. 1991. Failure of exercise to reduce blood pressure in patients with mild hypertension. *Journal of the American Medical Association* 266: 2098-2101.
12. Borg, G. 1998. *Borg's Perceived Exertion and Pain Scales.* Champaign, IL: Human Kinetics.
13. Boyden, T., R. Pamenter, S. Going, T. Lohman, M. Hall, L. Houtkooper, J. Bunt, C. Ritenbaugh, and M. Aickin. 1993. Resistance exercise training is associated with decreases in serum low-density lipoprotein cholesterol levels in premenopausal women. *Archives of Internal Medicine* 153: 97-100.
14. Butler, R., W. Baierwalter, and F. Rogers. 1987. The cardiovascular response to circuit weight training in patients with cardiac disease. *Journal of Cardiopulmonary Rehabilitation* 7: 402-409.
15. Cahill B., and E. Griffith. 1978. Effect of preseason conditioning on the incidence and severity of high school football knee injuries. *American Journal of Sports Medicine* 6: 180-184.
16. Campbell, W., M. Crim, V. Young, and W. Evans. 1994. Increased energy requirements and changes in body composition with resistance training in older adults. *American Journal of Clinical Nutrition* 60: 167-175.
17. Cheung, L., and J. Richmond, eds. 1995. *Child Health, Nutrition and Physical Activity.* Champaign, IL: Human Kinetics.

18. Clapp, J., and E. Capeless. 1990. Neonatal morphometrics after endurance exercise during pregnancy. *American Journal of Obstetrics and Gynecology* 163: 1805-1811.

19. Colletti, L., J. Edwards, L. Gordon, J. Shary, and N. Bell. 1989. The effects of muscle-building exercise on bone mineral density of the radius, spine and hip in young men. *Calcified Tissue International* 45: 12-14.

20. Corbin, C., R. Pangrazi, and G. Welk. 1994. Toward an understanding of appropriate physical activity levels of youth. *Physical Activity and Fitness Research Digest* 1 (8): 1-8.

21. Cordain, L., R. Latin, and J. Behnke. 1986. The effects of an aerobic running program on bowel transit time. *Journal of Sports Medicine* 26: 101-104.

22. Council on Exercise of the American Diabetes Association. 1990. Technical review: Exercise and NIDDM. *Diabetes Care* 13: 785-789.

23. Cowlin, A.F. 2002. *Women's Fitness Program Development.* Champaign, IL: Human Kinetics.

24. Craig, B., J. Everhart, and R. Brown. 1989. The influence of high-resistance training on glucose tolerance in young and elderly subjects. *Mechanisms of Aging and Development* 49: 147-157.

25. Durak, E. 1989. Exercise for specific populations: Diabetes mellitus. *Sports Training, Medicine and Rehabilitation* 1: 175-180.

26. Durak, E., L. Jovanovis-Peterson, and C. Peterson. 1990. Randomized crossover study of effect of resistance training on glycemic control, muscular strength, and cholesterol in Type I diabetic men. *Diabetes Care* 13: 1039-1042.

27. Eriksson, J., S. Taimela, K. Eriksson, S. Parvoinen, J. Peltonen, and U. Kujala. 1997. Resistance training in the treatment of non-insulin dependent diabetes mellitus. *International Journal of Sports Medicine* 18: 242-246.

28. Evans, W., and I. Rosenberg. 1992. *Biomarkers.* New York: Simon and Schuster.

29. Faigenbaum, A. 2001. Strength training and children's health. *Journal of Physical Education, Recreation and Dance* 72: 24-30.

30. Faigenbaum, A., W. Kraemer, B. Cahill, J. Chandler, J. Dziados, L. Elfrink, E. Forman, M. Gaudiose, L. Micheli, M. Nitka, and S. Roberts. 1996. Youth resistance training: Position statement paper and literature review. *Strength and Conditioning* 18: 62-75.

31. Faigenbaum, A., R. LaRosa Loud, J. O'Connell, S. Glover, J. O'Connell, and W. Westcott. 2001. Effects of different resistance training protocols on upper body strength and endurance development in children. *Journal of Strength and Conditioning Research* 15: 459-465.

32. Faigenbaum, A., G. Skrinar, W. Cesare, W. Kraemer, and H. Thomas. 1990. Physiologic and symptomatic responses of cardiac patients to resistance exercise. *Archives of Physical Medicine and Rehabilitation* 70: 395-398.

33. Faigenbaum, A., and W. Westcott. 2000. *Strength and Power for Young Athletes.* Champaign, IL: Human Kinetics.

34. Faigenbaum, A., and W. Westcott. 2001. *Youth Fitness.* San Diego: American Council on Exercise.

35. Faigenbaum, A., L. Zaichkowsky, W. Westcott, L. Micheli, and A. Fehlandt. 1993. The effects of a twice per week strength training program on children. *Pediatric Exercise Science* 5: 339-346.

36. Falk, B., and G. Mor. 1996. The effects of resistance and martial arts training in 6 to 8 year old boys. *Pediatric Exercise Science* 8: 48-56.

37. Falk, B., and G. Tenenbaum. 1996. The effectiveness of resistance training in children: A meta-analysis. *Sports Medicine* 22: 176-186.

38. Fiatarone, M., E. Marks, N. Ryan, C. Meredith, L. Lipsitz, and W. Evans. 1990. High-intensity strength training in nonagenarians. *Journal of the American Medical Association* 263: 3029-3034.

39. Freedman, D., W. Dietz, S. Srinivasan, and G. Berenson. 1999. The relationship of overweight to cardiovascular risk factors among children and adolescents: The Bogalusa heart study. *Pediatrics* 103: 1175-1182.

40. Frontera, W., C. Meredith, K. O'Reilly, H. Knuttgen, and W. Evans. 1988. Strength conditioning in older men: Skeletal muscle hypertrophy and improved function. *Journal of Applied Physiology* 64: 1038-1044.

41. George, D., K. Stakiw, and C. Wright 1989. Fatal accident with weight-lifting equipment: Implications for safety standards. *Canadian Medical Association Journal* 140: 925-926.

42. Ghilarducci, L., R. Holly, and E. Amsterdam. 1989. Effects of high resistance training in coronary heart disease. *American Journal of Cardiology* 64: 866-70.

43. Goldberg, L., L. Elliot, R. Schultz, and F. Kloste. 1984. Changes in lipid and lipoprotein levels after weight training. *Journal of the American Medical Association* 252: 504-506.

44. Gortmaker, S., A. Must, A. Sobol, K. Peterson, G. Colditz, and W. Dietz. 1996. Television viewing as a cause of increasing obesity among children in the United States, 1986-1990. *Archives of Pediatric and Adolescent Medicine* 150: 356-362.

45. Grimby, G., A. Aniansson, M. Hedberg, G. Henning, U. Granguard, and H. Kvist. 1992. Training can improve muscle strength and endurance in 78 to 84 year old men. *Journal of Applied Physiology* 73: 2517-2523.

46. Haennel, R., H. Quinney, and C. Kappogoda. 1991. Effects of hydraulic circuit training following coronary artery bypass surgery. *Medicine and Science in Sports and Exercise* 23: 158-165.

47. Hagerman, F., S. Walsh, R. Staron, R. Hikida, R. Gilders, T. Murray, K. Toma, and K. Ragg. 2000. Effects of high-intensity resistance training on untrained older men. I. Strength, cardiovascular, and metabolic responses. *Journals of Gerontology. Series A, Biological Sciences and Medical Sciences* 55: B336-346.

48. Hamill, B. 1994. Relative safety of weight lifting and weight training. *Journal of Strength and Conditioning Research* 8: 53-57.

49. Harris, K., and R. Holly. 1987. Physiological response to circuit weight training in borderline hypertensive subjects. *Medicine and Science in Sports and Exercise* 10: 246-252.

50. Heidt, R., L. Sweeterman, R. Carlonas, J. Traub, and F. Tekulve. 2000. Avoidance of soccer injuries with preseason conditioning. *American Journal of Sports Medicine* 28: 659-662.

51. Hejna, W., A. Rosenberg, D. Buturusis, and A. Krieger. 1982. The prevention of sports injuries in high school students through strength training. *National Strength Coaches Association Journal* 4: 28-31.

52. Hewett, T., A. Stroupe, T. Nance, and F. Noyes. 1996. Plyometric training in female athletes. *American Journal of Sports Medicine* 24: 765-773.

53. Hikida, R., R. Staron, F. Hagerman, S. Walsh, E. Kaiser, S. Shell, and S. Hervey. 2000. Effects of high-intensity resistance training on untrained older men. II. Muscle fiber characteristics and nucleo-cytoplasmic relationships. *Journals of Gerontology. Series A, Biological Sciences and Medical Sciences* 55: B347-354.

54. Hunter, G., C. Wetzstein, D. Fields, A. Brown, and M. Bamman. 2000. Resistance training increases total energy expenditure and free-living physical activity in older adults. *Journal of Applied Physiology* 89: 977-984.
55. Hurley, B. 1994. Does strength training improve health status? *Strength and Conditioning* 16: 7-13.
56. Hurley, B., J. Hagberg, A. Goldberg, D. Seals, A. Ehsani, R. Brennan, and J. Holloszy. 1988. Resistance training can reduce coronary risk factors without altering VO_2 max or percent body fat. *Medicine and Science in Sports and Exercise* 20: 150-154.
57. Ivey, F., S. Roth, R. Ferrell, B. Tracy, J. Lemmer, D. Hurlbut, G. Martel, E. Siegel, J. Fozard, E. Metter, J. Fleg, and B. Hurley. 2000. Effects of age, gender, and myostatin genotype on the hypertrophic responses to heavy resistance strength training. *Journals of Gerontology. Series A, Biological Sciences and Medical Sciences* 55: M641-648.
58. Janz, K., J. Dawson, and L. Mahoney. 2000. Tracking physical fitness and physical activity from childhood to adolescence: The Muscatine study. *Medicine and Science in Sports and Exercise* 32: 1250-1257.
59. Johnson, C., M. Stone, S. Lopez, J. Hebert, L. Kilgoe, and R. Byrd. 1982. Diet and exercise in middle-aged men. *Journal of the Dietetic Association* 81: 695-701.
60. Jones, A., M. Pollock, J. Graves, M. Fulton, W. Jones, M. MacMillan, D. Baldwin, and J. Cirulli. 1988. *Safe Specific Testing and Rehabilitative Exercise for Muscles of the Lumbar Spine.* Santa Barbara, CA: Sequoia Communications.
61. Kaiser Family Foundation. 1999, November. *Kids and Media the New Millennium* (monograph). Menlo Park, CA: Kaiser Family Foundation.
62. Kelemen, M., K. Stewart, R. Gillilan, C. Ewart, S. Valenti, J. Manley, and M. Kelemen. 1986. Circuit weight training in cardiac patients. *Journal of the American College of Cardiology* 7: 38-42.
63. Kelly, G. 1997. Dynamic resistance exercise and resting blood pressure in healthy adults: A meta-analysis. *Journal of Applied Physiology* 82: 1559-1565.
64. Keyes, A., H. Taylor, and F. Grande. 1973. Basal metabolism and age of adult man. *Metabolism* 22: 579-587.
65. Koffler, K., A. Menkes, R. Redmond, W. Whitehead, R. Pratley, and B. Hurley. 1992. Strength training accelerates gastrointestinal transit in middle-aged and older men. *Medicine and Science in Sports and Exercise* 24: 415-419.
66. Kokkinos, P., B. Hurley, M. Smutok, C. Farmer, C. Reece, R. Shulman, C. Charabogos, J. Patterson, S. Will, J. DeVane-Bell, and A. Goldberg. 1991. Strength training does not improve lipoprotein lipid profiles in men at risk for CHD. *Medicine and Science in Sports and Exercise* 23: 1134-1139.
67. Kokkinos, P., B. Hurley, P. Vaccaro, J. Patterson, L. Gardner, S. Ostrove, and A. Goldberg. 1998. Effects of low and high repetition resistive training on lipoprotein-lipid profiles. *Medicine and Science in Sports and Exercise* 20: 50-54.
68. Layne, J., and M. Nelson. 1999. The effects of progressive resistance training on bone density: A review. *Medicine and Science in Sports and Exercise* 31: 25-30.
69. Lemmer, J., F. Ivey, A. Ryan, G. Martel, D. Hurlbut, J. Metter, J. Fozard, J. Fleg, and B. Hurley. 2001. Effect of strength training on resting metabolic rate and physical activity. *Medicine and Science in Sports and Exercise* 33: 532-541.
70. Lillegard, W., E. Brown, D. Wilson, R. Henderson, and E. Lewis, 1997. Efficacy of strength training in prepubescent to early postpubescent males and females: Effects of gender and maturity. *Pediatric Rehabilitation* 1 (3): 147-157.
71. Lohmann, D., and F. Liebold. 1978. Diminished insulin response in highly trained athletes. *Metabolism* 27: 521-523.
72. Marks, R. 1993. The effects of isometric quadriceps strength training in mid-range for osteoarthritis of the knee. *Arthritis Care Research* 6: 52-56.
73. McCartney, N., A. Hicks, J. Martin, and C. Webber. 1996. A longitudinal trial of weight training in the elderly—continued improvements in year two. *Journals of Gerontology. Series A, Biological Sciences and Medical Sciences* 51: B425-B433.
74. Menkes, A., S. Mazel, R. Redmond, K. Koffler, C. Libanati, C. Gunberg, T. Zizic, J. Hagberg, R. Pratley, and B. Hurley. 1993. Strength training increases regional bone mineral density and bone remodeling in middle-aged and older men. *Journal of Applied Physiology* 74: 2478-2484.
75. Miller, W., W. Sherman, and J. Ivy. 1984. Effect of strength training on glucose tolerance and post glucose insulin response. *Medicine and Science in Sports and Exercise* 16: 539-543.
76. Morris, F., G. Naughton, J. Gibbs, J. Carlson, and J. Wark. 1997. Prospective ten-month exercise intervention in premenarcheal girls: Positive effects on bone and lean mass. *Journal of Bone and Mineral Research* 12: 1453-1462.
77. Morrow, J. 1997. Relationship of low back pain to exercise habits. Paper presented at the American College of Sports Medicine conference, Denver, May 31.
78. Mosher, P., M. Nash, A. Perry, A. LaPerriere, and R. Goldberg. 1998. Aerobic circuit exercise training: Effect on adolescents with well-controlled insulin dependent diabetes mellitus. *Archives of Physical Medicine and Rehabilitation* 79: 652-657.
79. National Association for Sport and Physical Education. 1998. *Physical Activity for Children: A Statement of Guidelines.* Reston, VA: NASPE.
80. National Center for Health Statistics. 2000. *Health, United States, 2000, with Adolescent Health Chartbook.* Retrieved October 11, 2002, from www.cdc.gov/nchs/data/hus/hus00.pdf.
81. Nelson, M., M. Fiatarone, C. Morganti, I. Trice, R. Greenberg, and W. Evans. 1994. Effects of high-intensity strength training on multiple risk factors for osteoporotic fractures. *Journal of the American Medical Association* 272: 1909-1914.
82. Ozmun, J., A. Mikesky, and P. Surburg. 1991. Neuromuscular adaptations during prepubescent strength training. *Medicine and Science in Sports and Exercise* 23: S31.
83. Payne, G., and J. Morrow. 1993. Exercise and VO_2 max in children: A meta-analysis. *Research Quarterly for Exercise and Sport* 64: 305-313.
84. Pratley, R., B. Nicklas, M. Rubin, J. Miller, A. Smith, M. Smith, B. Hurley, and A. Goldberg. 1994. Strength training increases resting metabolic rate and norepinephrine levels in healthy 50 to 65 year old men. *Journal of Applied Physiology* 76: 133-137.
85. Quirk, A., R. Newman, and K. Newman. 1985. An evaluation of interferential therapy, shortwave diathermy and exercise in the treatment of osteoarthritis of the knee. *Physiotherapy* 71: 55-57.
86. Ramsay, J., C. Blimkie, K. Smith, S. Garner, J. Macdougall, and D. Sale. 1990. Strength training effects in prepubescent boys. *Medicine and Science in Sports and Exercise* 22: 605-614.
87. Risch, S., N. Norvell, M. Polock, E. Risch, H. Langer, M. Fulton, M. Graves, and S. Leggett. 1993. Lumbar strengthening in chronic low back pain patients. *Spine* 18: 232-238.
88. Rowland, T. 1990. *Exercise and Children's Health.* Champaign, IL: Human Kinetics.

89. Ryan, A., M. Treuth, M. Rubin, J. Miller, B. Nicklas, D. Landis, R. Pratley, C. Libanati, C. Grundberg, and B. Hurley. 1994. Effects of strength training on bone mineral density: Hormonal and bone turnover relationships. *Journal of Applied Physiology* 77: 1678-1684.

90. Sing, N., K. Clements, and M. Fiatarone. 1997. A randomized controlled trial of progressive resistance training in depressed elders. *Journal of Gerontology* 52 A: M 27-M 35.

91. Smith, A., J. Andrish, and L. Micheli. 1993. The prevention of sports injuries of children and adolescents. *Medicine and Science in Sports and Exercise* 25 (Suppl 8): 1-7.

92. Smutok, M., C. Reece, P. Kokkinos, C. Farmer, P. Dawson, R. Shulman, J. De Vane-Bell, J. Patterson, C. Charabogos, A. Goldley, and B. Hurley. 1993. Aerobic vs. strength training for risk factor intervention in middle-aged men at high risk for coronary heart disease. *Metabolism* 42: 177-184.

93. Snow-Harter, C., M. Bouxsein, B. Lewis, D. Carter, and R. Marcus. 1992. Effects of resistance and endurance exercise on bone mineral status of young women. A randomized exercise intervention trial. *Journal of Bone Mineral Research* 7: 761-769.

94. Sothern, M., M. Loftin, J. Udall, R. Suskind, T. Ewing, S. Tang, and U. Blecker. 1999. Inclusion of resistance exercise in a multidisciplinary outpatient treatment program for preadolescent obese children. *Southern Medical Journal* 92: 585-592.

95. Stewart, K., M. Mason, and M. Kelemen. 1988. Three-year participation in circuit weight training improves muscular strength and self-efficacy in cardiac patients. *Journal of Cardiopulmonary Rehabilitation* 8: 292-296.

96. Stone, M., D. Blessing, R. Byrd, J. Tew, and D. Boatwright. 1982. Physiological effects of a short term resistance training program on middle-aged untrained men. *National Strength Coaches Association Journal* 4: 16-20.

97. Suman, O., R. Spies, M. Celis, R. Mlcak, and D. Herndon. 2001. Effects of a 12-wk resistance exercise program on skeletal muscle strength in children with burn injuries. *Journal of Applied Physiology* 91: 1168-1175.

98. Taunton, J., A. Martin, E. Rhodes, L. Wolski, M. Donnelly, and J. Elliot. 1997. Exercise for older women: Choosing the right prescription. *British Journal of Sports Medicine* 31: 5-10.

99. Trappe, S., D. Williamson, M. Godard, and P. Gallagher. 2001. Maintenance of whole muscle strength and size following resistance training in older men. *Medicine and Science in Sports and Exercise* 33: S147.

100. Trudeau, F., L. Laurencelle, J. Tremblay, M. Rajic, and R.J. Shephard. 1999. Daily primary school physical education: Effects on physical activity during adult life. *Medicine and Science in Sports and Exercise* 31: 111-117.

101. *Tufts University Diet and Nutrition Letter.* 1994. Never too late to build up your muscle. 12 (September): 6-7.

102. Ulrich, I., C. Reid, and R. Yeater. 1987. Increased HDL-cholesterol levels with a weight training program. *Southern Medical Journal* 80: 328-331.

103. United States Department of Health and Human Services. 1996. *Physical Activity and Health: A Report from the Surgeon General.* Atlanta: U.S. Department of Health and Human Services, Centers for Disease Control and Prevention, National Center for Chronic Disease Prevention and Health Promotion.

104. United States Department of Health and Human Services. 2000. *Healthy People 2010: Understanding and Improving Health.* Washington, DC: U.S. Department of Health and Human Services, Government Printing Office.

105. Vander, L., B. Franklin, D. Wrisley, and M. Rubenfire. 1986. Acute cardiovascular responses in cardiac patients: Implications for exercise training. *Annals of Sports Medicine* 2: 165-169.

106. Weltman, A., C. Janney, C. Rians, K. Strand, B. Berg, S. Tippit, J. Wise, B. Cahill, and F. Katch. 1986. The effects of hydraulic resistance strength training in pre-pubertal males. *Medicine and Science in Sports and Exercise* 18: 629-638.

107. Weltman, A., C. Janney, C. Rians, K. Strand, and F. Katch. 1987. Effects of hydraulic-resistance strength training on serum lipid levels in prepubertal boys. *American Journal of Diseases in Children* 141: 777-780.

108. Westcott, W. 1996. *Building Strength and Stamina.* Champaign, IL: Human Kinetics.

109. Westcott, W., and T. Baechle. 1999. *Strength Training for Seniors.* Champaign, IL: Human Kinetics.

110. Westcott, W., F. Dolan, and T. Cavicchi. 1996. Golf and strength training are compatible activities. *Strength and Conditioning* 18: 54-56.

111. Westcott, W., and J. Guy. 1996. A physical evolution: Sedentary adults see marked improvements in as little as two days a week. *IDEA Today* 14: 58-65.

112. Whaley, M.H., L.A. Kaminsky, G.B. Dwyer, L.H. Getchell, and J.A. Norton. 1992. Predictors of over- and underachievement of age-predicted maximal heart rate. *Medicine and Science in Sports and Exercise* 24 (10): 1173-1179.

113. Wilmore, J., R. Parr, P. Vodak, and T. Barstow. 1976. Strength, endurance, BMR and body composition changes with circuit weight training. *Medicine and Science in Sports and Exercise* 8: 59-60.

CHAPTER 19

Clients With Nutritional and Metabolic Concerns

Christine L. Vega | Carlos E. Jiménez

After completing this chapter, you will be able to

- delineate the scope of practice of the personal trainer when working with people who have nutritional and metabolic concerns;
- discuss the appropriate exercise prescription and program design for individuals who are obese, who are overweight, or who have hyperlipidemia, eating disorders, or diabetes;
- describe general nutritional guidelines for individuals with these nutritional and metabolic concerns; and
- discuss lifestyle change strategies (diet, exercise, and behavior changes) that will improve the health status of people with these nutritional and metabolic concerns.

Advances in technology, industrialization, and automation have decreased the need for rigorous physical work, allowed more leisure time, and greatly increased food availability. These advances, which are positive in some respects, in other respects have negatively affected the population's health. Along with other factors, these societal changes have led to an increased prevalence of obesity, hyperlipidemia, and diabetes, as well as a trend toward disordered eating and eating disorders.

Personal trainers are likely to encounter clients who have one or more of these nutritionally related conditions. A personal trainer should screen for these conditions as described in chapter 9 and obtain medical clearance when needed [15]. Clients who have the conditions described in this chapter should be referred to their physician for medical care and to a dietitian for medical nutrition therapy, as a personal trainer's role is limited to exercise program design and execution along with lifestyle change support. Personal trainers should not diagnose or prescribe care for their clients nor accept or train clients who have medical conditions that may exceed their level of knowledge and experience. Instead, personal trainers should refer such clients to a more appropriate health care professional [15].

Personal trainers are not to diagnose or prescribe care for their clients and should not accept or train clients who have medical conditions that may exceed their level of knowledge and experience. Such clients should be referred to an appropriate health care professional.

Overweight and Obesity

Obesity and overweight, in both children and adults, has become a "global epidemic" [35]. Recent surveys in the industrialized countries along with some of the developing countries have shown a growing proportion of children and adults who are overweight or obese [35]. While the prevalence of obesity in adults is 10% to 25% in most countries of western Europe, 20% to 25% in some countries in the Americas, and over 50% in some island nations of the western Pacific, the scope of the problem is even more alarming when the percentage of adults who are overweight (as opposed to obese only) is considered [35]. The most recent U.S. National Health and Nutrition Examination Survey (NHANES 1999-2000) showed that 30.5% of U.S. adults are obese and 64.5% of the adult population are overweight (which includes the obese percentage) [16].

These figures may increase even more in the future: National surveys in the United States have shown that the prevalence of obesity in childhood and adolescence has more than doubled since the early 1960s [30]. Increases in childhood obesity may lead to even greater numbers for adult obesity.

This is a public health problem of significant concern, as the condition of being overweight or obese raises the risk of morbidity from hypertension; hyperlipidemia; type 2 diabetes; **coronary heart disease** (CHD); stroke; gallbladder disease; osteoarthritis; **sleep apnea** and respiratory problems; and endometrial, breast, prostrate, and colon cancers [21, 35]. Further, higher body weights are also associated with increases in all-cause mortality. Overweight and obesity have been designated as the second leading cause of preventable death in the United States [21, 22].

Definitions of Overweight and Obesity and Important Differences

Overweight is defined as a **body mass index (BMI)** of 25 to 29.9 kg/m^2, and obesity as a BMI of ≥30 kg/m^2 [21]. The BMI describes relative weight for height and is significantly correlated with total body fat content. The use of the BMI has limitations with individuals who are very muscular (overestimates body fat) and with persons such as those of advanced age who have lost muscle mass (underestimates body fat) [22]. The BMI should be used to assess overweight and obesity in addition to monitoring changes in body weight [21, 22, 35].

The BMI is calculated as weight (kg) ÷ height squared (m^2). To estimate BMI using pounds and inches, one uses: [weight (pounds) ÷ height squared ($inches^2$)] × 703. See table 19.1 for the NHLBI agreed-on weight classifications by BMI. See "Calculating BMI" on the next page for examples of how to calculate BMI using non-metric and metric units.

To select appropriate prevention strategies and design effective exercise programs, the personal trainer must understand the complex and important differences between overweight and obesity [10]:

- People who are obese have a significantly greater excess of weight, particularly adipose tissue mass, than those who are overweight. Additionally, the percentage of adipose tissue as opposed to fat-free tissue is higher in persons who are obese. This means that people who are obese have significantly increased their fat stores without a concomitant increase in muscle mass [10].

TABLE 19.1

Classification of Overweight and Obesity by BMI

	Obesity class	BMI (kg/m^2)
Underweight		<18.5
Normal		18.5-24.9
Overweight		25.0-29.9
Obesity	I	30.0-34.9
	II	35.0-39.9
Extreme obesity	III	≥40.0

Data from National Institutes of Health and National Heart, Lung, and Blood Institute 1998.

Calculating BMI

Non-Metric Conversion

To calculate BMI using non-metric units, use this formula:

$$[\text{weight (pounds)} \div \text{height squared (in.}^2)] \times 703 \quad \textbf{(19.1)}$$

For example, a person who weighs 164 pounds and is 68 inches (or 5 feet 8 inches) tall has a BMI of 25:

$$[164 \div 68^2] \times 703 = 25$$

Metric Conversion

To calculate BMI using metric units, use this formula :

$$\text{weight (kilograms)} \div \text{height squared (m}^2) \quad \textbf{(19.2)}$$

For example, a person who weighs 78.93 kilograms and is 177 centimeters (1.77 meters) tall has a BMI of 25:

$$78.93 \div 1.77^2 = 25$$

Remember that 100 centimeters = 1 meter.

- In general, persons who are obese are more likely to have had a larger positive energy balance over a longer period of time than those who are overweight. Contribution to the positive energy balance is not only from a decrease in physical activity, but also from an increase in food consumption [10]. **Energy balance** occurs when an individual is consuming as many calories as he or she expends, resulting in no change of body weight. A **positive energy balance**, or consuming more calories than are expended, will result in an increase in body weight; a **negative energy balance**, or the consumption of less calories than are expended, will result in a decrease in body weight.
- On the average, persons who are obese have a higher resting metabolic rate and expend more energy on activities than those who are overweight or normal weight. The reason is that moving a heavy mass around requires more energy [10].

A review of these differences and their implications would seem to indicate that a sedentary lifestyle or a low level of habitual activity appears to be the mechanism for a large proportion of adult overweight cases [9, 10]. In other words, it is possible for an individual to become overweight by simply decreasing his or her activity level without consuming more food each day.

It is for this population—those who are overweight—that early intervention with an exercise program and increased physical activity are important. Hopefully, overweight individuals can be encouraged and convinced to start working with a personal trainer before they become obese. A return to previous activity levels or beyond would at least prevent a progression to obesity and possibly achieve significant weight loss, affording people the hope of returning to a normal weight classification without having to resort to moderate or severe caloric restriction.

Alternatively, individuals with severe obesity (e.g., BMIs of 35 or 40 or more) have likely sustained a positive energy balance for long periods of time, that is, at least a few years. In most cases, this condition is achieved with an increase in energy intakes (increased consumption of food) and a decrease in energy expenditure (physical activity) [10]. Therefore, it seems that in the case of people who are severely obese, inactivity is an important factor, but it is also coupled with increased consumption. Consequently, persons who are obese must have a strong emphasis on both cutting caloric intake and increasing activity.

Clients who are overweight may benefit simply by increasing physical activity along with some minor changes in their diets. Those who are obese should concentrate on both reducing caloric intake and increasing physical activity.

Causes and Correlates of Overweight and Obesity

No one theory completely answers the question of how and why obesity occurs. Although a positive energy balance due to the increased availability of calorie-rich food coupled with a sedentary lifestyle is a major factor in the worldwide increase in obesity, there are still other factors to consider [35]. Obesity is a complex multifactorial chronic disease that develops from an interaction of genetic, environmental, social, behavioral, metabolic, and possibly racial influences [21, 22].

These factors combine in a variety of ways in each individual to bring about the obese state. For example, environmental factors can include food availability, socioeconomic status, and lack of access to exercise facilities such as a gym or a track. Behavioral factors include eating patterns determined by individual preferences and ethnic backgrounds, including overeating or binge eating and activity patterns. Genetic and metabolic factors can include differences in resting metabolic rate, levels of lipoprotein lipase and other enzymes, sympathetic nervous system activity, and dietary-induced thermogenesis. Some of these variables serve as true predictors of body fat gain, allowing them to be considered risk factors. In other cases, researchers do not know whether the relationship is causal or whether the correlate is secondary to being obese. In most cases, the associations are, in fact, secondary and are a result of obesity [10].

Fat Distribution

It is important not only to note whether a client falls into the overweight or obese category, but to also discern the pattern of fat distribution. There are two types of fat distribution, android **obesity** and **gynoid obesity.** Gynoid obesity (pear-shaped body) denotes the condition in which high amounts of body fat have been deposited in the hip and thigh areas. Android obesity (apple shape) is characterized by high amounts of body fat in the trunk and abdominal areas. It is this presence of excess fat in the abdomen, out of proportion to total body fat, that acts as an independent predictor of disease risk for type 2 diabetes, hypertension, and CVD [21, 22].

Measuring Abdominal Fat

There is a positive correlation between the abdominal fat content and the waist circumference measurement [21, 22, 35]. The personal trainer can use this clinically acceptable measurement to assess the client's abdominal fat content before and during a weight loss program [21, 22]. Proper measurement of the waist circumference is demonstrated in chapter 11, page 226. Refer to the sex-specific cutoffs in "Assessing Abdominal Fat in Clients Who Are Overweight or Obese" on the next page to identify those individuals at increased relative risk for the development of type 2 diabetes, dyslipidemia, hypertension, and CVD in most adults with a BMI of 25 to 34.9 kg/m^2 [21, 22]. Please note that these waist circumference limits are not useful in terms of incremental risk prediction in patients with a BMI ≥ 35 kg/m^2, as these individuals will automatically exceed the cutoff points because of their higher weights.

Skinfold measurements of persons who are obese are very difficult; correctly placing the calipers requires a good deal of experience. Additionally, the process can be demeaning to a client who is obese because of the size of the skinfold. Because of the high acceptability of the BMI and waist circumference measurements, personal trainers are encouraged to use these measurements for both the initial assessment and follow-up measurements. In fact, the demonstration of the loss of inches can have more meaning to a client. Circumference measurements can also be made of other parts of the body—for instance, the hips, arms, and thighs—to track progress in terms of weight loss.

Controlling Cardiovascular Risk Factors

Table 19.2 adds the disease risk of increased abdominal fat to the disease risk of BMI [21, 22]. As is evident, the increased abdominal fat distribution moves an individual in the overweight or Class I obesity category to an even higher disease risk category. The categories in the table indicate *relative risk, not absolute risk* [21, 22]. In other words, the comparison of risk is being made relative to a normal weight. This is in contrast to the calculation of absolute risk for disease, which is determined by a summation of risk factors [21, 22].

Personal trainers working with clients who are overweight should give as much emphasis to the control of cardiovascular risk factors as they do to weight loss in their clients' overall programs [22]. In

Assessing Abdominal Fat in Clients Who Are Overweight or Obese

- Use waist circumference and BMI measures, in lieu of or in addition to skinfold measures.
- Conduct the assessment in a private setting and assure the client that no one else will see the results.
- Conduct the assessment in a matter-of-fact, yet sensitive manner. Avoid uncomfortable humor.
- If the client is too embarrassed for someone to measure his or her waist, allow the client to conduct the measurement him- or herself after having received instruction.
- Tell the client beforehand to wear thin clothing, and allow the client to keep all clothes on during the measurement if the client is too uncomfortable to remove clothing. Although measurement will not be accurate, it will provide a starting point and avoid embarrassment.
- The following cutoffs indicate an increased risk for type 2 diabetes, dyslipidemia, hypertension, and CVD in individuals with a BMI between 25 and 34.9 kg/m^2 [21, 22]:

  Men: >102 centimeters (>40 inches)

  Women: >88 centimeters (>35 inches)

TABLE 19.2

Classification of Overweight and Obesity by Body Mass Index (BMI), Waist Circumference, and Associated Disease Risks

	BMI (kg/m^2)	Obesity class	Disease risk* relative to normal weight and waist circumference: Men ≤102 cm (≤40 in) Women ≤88 cm (≤35 in)	Men >102 cm (>40 in) Women >88 cm (>35 in)
Underweight	<18.5		–	–
Normal**	18.5-24.9		–	–
Overweight	25.0-29.9		Increased	High
Obesity	30.0-34.9	I	High	Very high
	35.0-39.9	II	Very high	Very high
Extreme obesity	≥40.0	III	Extremely high	Extremely high

*Disease risk for type 2 diabetes, hypertension, and coronary heart disease.

**Increased waist circumference can also be a marker for increased risk even in persons of normal weight.

Reprinted from National Institutes of Health and National Heart, Lung, and Blood Institute, 1998.

other words, the client must understand that an increase in physical activity along with the cessation of smoking and the consumption of a heart healthy diet, with or without weight loss, will significantly improve his or her health status. In fact, even if clients do not change any of their other health habits but improve fitness to a moderate or high level, they will experience lower adjusted premature death rates from CVD and all-cause mortality [8]. This allows one to measure the success of the client's program not only in weight loss, but also in positive behavior changes.

An increase in physical activity along with the cessation of smoking and the consumption of a heart healthy diet, with or without weight loss, will significantly improve a client's health status.

Benefits of Exercise in a Weight Reduction Program

The inclusion of physical activity in a weight reduction program provides physiological and psychological benefits. Although the exact mechanism by which physical activity affects weight loss and the degree to which it affects weight loss are not yet completely understood, exercise should be included in a weight loss program to ensure a better chance of success. A review of the literature showed that adults with obesity who participated in physical activity did realize modest weight loss and a lowering of the risk factors for CVD [21].

It seems that some of the physiological benefits of exercise may not have as great an effect on weight loss as previously thought. For example, a person with obesity who is out of shape is often unable to perform exercise of sufficient duration or sufficient intensity to expend enough calories to significantly affect the targeted daily caloric deficit. Hence, although the exercise session is important, a decrease in calories consumed would have even a greater effect on weight loss. Still, an exercise program is important for its positive effects on lowering the risk factors for CVD along with the other general physiological and psychological benefits listed in table 19.3 [6, 21].

While the area of the psychological and emotional benefits of exercise and their effects on increased motivation, commitment, and psychological resources deserves further research, the combination of the existing studies and experiential data indicates that these benefits do occur. The possible psychological outcomes of an exercise program that promote these increases in motivation and commitment are increased well-being and mood, improved body image, improved self-esteem and self-efficacy, and improved coping abilities [6]. For example, the improved well-being and enhanced self-esteem produced by physical activity may generalize to other areas of life and lead to improved dietary adherence. In other words, the client feels more productive and in control of his or her life and is therefore better able and willing to make the proper choices of food and portion sizes. Figure 19.1

TABLE 19.3

Benefits of Exercise in a Weight Loss Program
Increases energy expenditure
Reduces the risk of heart disease more than what can be achieved by weight loss alone
May help reduce body fat and prevent the decrease in muscle mass that often occurs during weight loss
May decrease abdominal fat
Decreases insulin resistance
May contribute to better dietary compliance, including reduced caloric intake
May not prevent the decline in RMR associated with a low-calorie diet, but may minimize the decrease
Improves mood and general well-being
Improves body image
Increases self-esteem and self-efficacy
Serves as a coping strategy

Compiled from National Institutes of Health and National Heart, Lung, and Blood Institute 2000; and Baker and Brownwell, 2000.

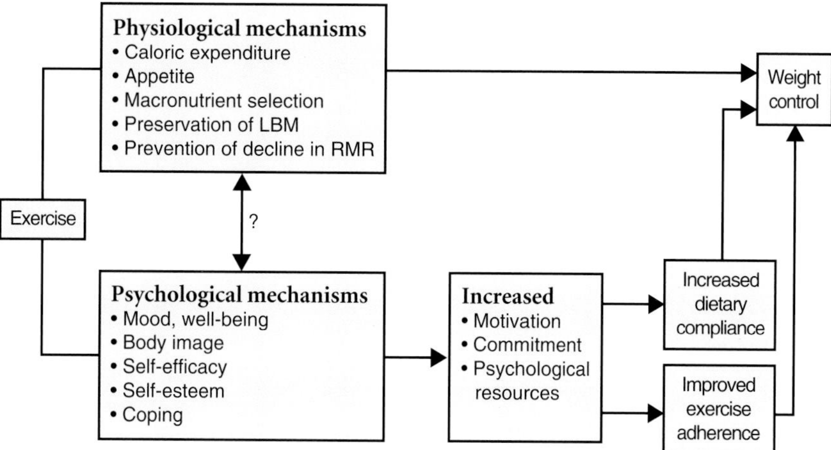

Figure 19.1 Proposed mechanisms and potential pathways linking exercise and weight control. LBM = lean body mass; RMR = resting metabolic rate.
Reprinted from Baker and Brownwell 2000.

[6] provides an overview of the proposed mechanisms and potential pathways that link exercise to success in weight control.

Although the results of the research supporting the benefit of physical activity during the weight loss phase of a weight management program are mixed, strong evidence supports the role of physical activity as a necessary factor for long-term weight maintenance [28]. Regular physical activity not only helps to improve weight loss and physical fitness during the weight loss phase of a weight management program, but is also needed to ensure that the client maintains his or her target weight over time. One of the main goals of the personal trainer should be to help clients establish the habit of frequent exercise.

While physical activity may or may not help a client to lose weight, it reduces many obesity-related risk factors and is critical for long-term weight maintenance.

Lifestyle Change Program for Obesity

In general, the most successful weight management programs consist of a combination of diet modification, increased physical activity, and lifestyle change [21, 22]. Personal trainers work with their clients to not only increase physical activity levels but also to provide lifestyle change support.

Diet Modification and the Low-Calorie Diet

The majority of clients who are overweight or obese need to make adjustments in their diets in order to achieve a caloric deficit resulting in weight loss. Personal trainers should refer these clients to a dietitian. The dietitian will most likely evaluate the client's diet, design an appropriate calorie-reduced yet nutrient-dense diet, offer follow-up to make adjustments in the diet, answer questions and concerns, and solve any problems. Referral to a dietitian is very highly recommended for clients who are obese and who have high cholesterol levels and is necessary for clients with diabetes. (Diabetes is managed by a physician and normally in conjunction with a dietitian.)

To be effective, the diet must be designed in accordance with the client's cultural and ethnic background, should include the client's food preferences, should take into account the availability and cost of the food in the diet, should contain a composition of foods that will decrease the risk of other nutritionally related cardiovascular risk factors such as hyperlipidemia and high blood pressure, and should fit into the client's particular lifestyle [22]. Additionally, the diet should ensure that all of the recommended dietary allowances are met, which may require the use of a dietary or vitamin supplement for those who are eating in the lower calorie ranges [22]. Once the diet is individualized to the client's needs and likes, the personal trainer can be of great help in supporting and motivating the client to adhere to the diet.

Most weight loss in the persons who are obese occurs primarily because of decreased caloric intake. The NHLBI Guidelines recommend that a diet be individually planned to help create a deficit of 500 to 1,000 calories per day in order to facilitate a weight loss of 1 to 2 pounds (0.45-0.9 kilograms) per week. This moderate reduction in calories is recommended in order to achieve a slow yet progressive weight loss. Excess weight will gradually decrease with this level of caloric intake. (The target amount also depends on the amount of exercise the client performs on a daily basis. In other words, if the client expends 250 calories a day in an exercise session, the diet may have to be reduced by only 250 to 750 calories per day and still produce the 1- to 2-pound weight loss per week. This smaller decrease in caloric restriction may make it easier for the client to stick to the diet.)

The exact calorie load for each individual is determined through use of the calorie calculation formulas found on page 127 of chapter 7 and trial-and-error adjustments. It is recommended that caloric intake be reduced only to the level required to maintain weight at a desired level.

In general, women should consume diets containing not less than 1,000 to 1,200 kilocalories (kcal)/day, and men should consume a diet no lower than 1,200 kcal/day to 1,600 kcal/day [22]. The higher intake of 1,200 to 1,600 kcal/day may also be appropriate for women who weigh 165 pounds (75 kilograms) or more or for women who exercise regularly [22]. If a client consumes a 1,600 kcal/day diet and does not lose weight, it may be advisable to try the 1,200 kcal/day diet. On the other hand, if a client gets hungry on the lower-calorie diet or is without sufficient energy to make it through the day or to engage in physical activity, then he or she may need to consume an additional 100 to 200 kcal/day [22].

Additionally, more lean body tissue will be spared if the client consumes a **low-calorie diet (LCD)** in comparison to the great losses that occur with the **very low calorie diets (VLCDs),** which consist of less than 800 kcal/day. The use of a VLCD is to be carried out only by physicians with specialized training and experience, as the diet requires special monitoring and supplementation and should be used only in limited circumstances with specific individuals [24]. In actuality, clinical trials have demonstrated that LCDs have the same success rates as VLCDs in promoting weight loss after one year [34].

Refer to table 19.4 for the general dietary guidelines for an LCD diet as outlined in the Low-Calorie Step I Diet recommended by NHLBI. This diet also contains the nutrient composition that will decrease other risk factors for CVD such as high blood cholesterol levels and hypertension.

An initial and reasonable goal of a weight loss program is a 10% reduction in body weight. A reasonable time to achieve this goal is six months [22]. After six months, the personal trainer along with the dietitian and physician can set new goals. Even if the client only reaches this initial 10% reduction and maintains it, he or she has accomplished a significant decrease in the severity of the obesity-associated risk factors [21, 22].

An initial and reasonable goal of a weight loss program is a 10% reduction in body weight. A reasonable time to achieve this goal is six months. After six months, the personal trainer along with the dietitian and physician can set new goals.

Many clients may find it difficult to lose weight after the first six months because of a decrease in their resting metabolic rates and the increased challenge over time of sticking to the diet and exercise regime. Additionally, their energy requirements decrease as their weight decreases (less mass to move around means less workload). Thus an even larger increase in the dietary goals (may need to decrease calories even more) and physical activity goals (may need to increase activity levels even higher) is needed in order to create an energy deficit at the lower weight [22].

After the initial weight goal of a 10% reduction in body weight has been achieved, the personal trainer and client can set new goals for weight loss, if appropriate. The benefits of achieving a moderate weight loss over a long period of time far outweigh the benefits of losing a great deal of weight quickly only to gain most of it back. This situation of weight regain, especially when repeated a number of times, undermines the benefits of participating in a weight loss program in terms of time spent, financial costs, health detriments, and especially a possible decrease in self-esteem [22].

The benefits of achieving a moderate weight loss over a long period of time far outweigh the benefits of losing a great deal of weight quickly only to gain most of it back.

Although it is not within the scope of practice for personal trainers to offer dietary prescription and counseling to their clients, personal trainers can support their clients' efforts by offering nutrition education or orientation. Topics may include low-calorie food choices (see the "Lower-Fat and Lower-Calorie Eating Strategies" on page 492), low-fat food preparation techniques, food label reading, holiday eating strategies, the importance of adequate hydration, ways to include more fruits and vegetables in the diet, and so on.

TABLE 19.4

Low-Calorie Step I Diet

Nutrient	Recommended daily intake
Calories[1]	Approximately a 500 to 1,000 kcal reduction from usual intake
Total fat[2]	30% or less of total calories
Saturated fatty acids[3]	8%-10% of total calories
Monounsaturated fatty acids	Up to 15% of total calories
Polyunsaturated fatty acids	Up to 10% of total calories
Cholesterol[3]	<300 mg
Protein[4]	Approximately 15% of total calories
Carbohydrate [5]	55% or more of total calories
Sodium	No more than 100 mmol (approximately 2.4 g of sodium) or approximately 6 g of sodium chloride
Calcium[6]	1,000 to 1,500 mg
Fiber[5]	20 to 30 g

[1]A reduction in calories of 500 to 1,000 kcal/day will help achieve a weight loss of 1 to 2 pounds/week. Alcohol provides unneeded calories and displaces more nutritious foods. Alcohol consumption not only increases the number of calories in a diet but has been associated with obesity in epidemiologic studies as well as in experimental studies. The impact of alcohol calories on a person's overall caloric intake needs to be assessed and appropriately controlled.

[2]Fat-modified foods may provide a helpful strategy for lowering total fat intake but will only be effective if they are also low in calories and if there is no compensation by calories from other foods.

[3]Patients with high blood cholesterol levels may need to use the Step II diet to achieve further reductions in LDL-cholesterol levels; in the Step II diet, saturated fats are reduced to less than 7% of total calories, and cholesterol levels to less than 200 mg/day. All of the other nutrients are the same as in Step I.

[4]Protein should be derived from plant sources and lean sources of animal protein.

[5]Complex carbohydrates from different vegetables, fruits, and whole grains are good sources of vitamins, minerals, and fiber. A diet rich in soluble fiber, including oat bran, legumes, barley, and most fruits and vegetables, may be effective in reducing blood cholesterol levels. A diet high in all types of fiber may also aid in weight management by promoting satiety at lower levels of calorie and fat intake. Some authorities recommend 20 to 30 grams of fiber daily, with an upper limit of 35 grams.

[6]During weight loss, attention should be given to maintaining an adequate intake of vitamins and minerals. Maintenance of the recommended calcium intake of 1,000 to 1,500 mg/day is especially important for women who may be at risk of osteoporosis.

Reprinted from National Institutes of Health and National Heart, Lung, and Blood Institute 2000.

It is not within the scope of practice for personal trainers to offer dietary prescription and counseling to their clients, but they can support clients' efforts by offering nutrition education.

Physical Activity

Moderate levels of physical activity for 30 to 45 minutes, three to five days per week, are recommended for clients who are overweight or obese and who are beginning an exercise program [21, 22]. A moderate level of physical activity is defined as the amount of activity that uses approximately 150 calories a day, with a total of approximately 1,000 calories per week [21, 22]. In fact, the Centers for Disease Control and Prevention, the American College of Sports Medicine, the Surgeon General, and the National Institutes of Health (NIH)/NHLBI make the following general recommendation as expressed in the NHLBI *Practical Guide:* "All adults should set a long term goal to accumulate at least 30 minutes or more of moderate-intensity physical activity on most, and preferably all, days of the week" [22, 26, 31]. Examples of moderate amounts of physical activity are found in table 19.5.

Lower-Fat and Lower-Calorie Eating Strategies

Personal trainers can encourage their clients to use some of the following dietary strategies to cut down on both caloric and fat intake:

- Eat red meat no more than three times per week and consume smaller portions.*
- Trim all visible fat from meat, poultry, and fish.*
- Remove the skin from chicken and turkey.*
- Eat low-fat meat such as the white meat of chicken and turkey and the low-fat cuts of pork and beef.*
- Broil, boil, poach, or bake instead of frying food.*
- Eat more meatless meals.*
- Eat cheese no more than three times per week.*
- Avoid bologna, salami, and other high-fat luncheon meats.*
- Use margarine, oil, butter, cream, cream cheese, and sour cream sparingly.*
- Drink skim milk and eat nonfat or low-fat yogurt.*
- Replace mayonnaise and salad dressings with lower-fat versions.
- Avoid gravies and other high-fat sauces.*
- Choose low-fat recipes.*
- Avoid high-fat snacks like chips* and nuts.
- Eat minimal or occasional sweets such as cakes, cookies, and candy.
- Practice portion control.
- Restrict soda intake.
- Eat only to mild fullness; do not push beyond.
- Replace desserts with fresh fruit.
- Eat only when hungry.

*Indicates dietary measures that will decrease saturated fat and cholesterol intakes.

Adapted from Vega 2001.

It is important to consider the concept of progression when designing a physical activity program for a client. Many clients who are obese may not be able to start with a moderate-level activity program. For these clients, the initial activities may have to be low in intensity or even simply a matter of focusing on increasing the tasks of daily living. For example, clients might

- take a walk after lunch,
- walk to a coworker's desk or office instead of using the phone,
- use stairs instead of an elevator or escalator,
- walk to pick up lunch instead of ordering a delivery,
- get off the bus or subway at least one stop early and walk the remainder of the way,
- park in a space at the mall that is farther from the entrance and requires more walking,
- walk to the neighborhood mini-mart to pick up milk instead of driving the block or two,
- walk the dog,
- do yard work, or
- play actively with children or grandchildren.

A well-designed, progressive program avoids the incidence of injury in addition to making the beginning exercise sessions comfortable and tolerable. Many people with obesity, because of their sedentary lifestyles, have very low functional capacities. What may seem like a moderate intensity or a moderate amount of physical activity to a personal trainer may actually be a great challenge to

TABLE 19.5

Examples of Moderate Amounts of Physical Activity

Common chores	Sporting activities	
Washing or waxing a car for 45-60 minutes	Playing volleyball for 45-60 minutes	Less vigorous, more time* ↑
Washing windows or floors for 45-60 minutes	Playing touch football for 45 minutes	
Gardening for 30-45 minutes	Walking 1-3/4 miles in 35 minutes (20 min/mile)	
Wheeling self in wheelchair for 30-40 minutes	Basketball (shooting baskets) for 30 minutes	
Pushing a stroller 1-1/2 miles in 30 minutes	Bicycling 5 miles in 30 minutes	
Raking leaves for 30 minutes	Dancing fast (social) for 30 minutes	
Walking 2 miles in 30 minutes (15 min/mile)	Water aerobics for 30 minutes	
Shoveling snow for 15 minutes	Swimming laps for 20 minutes	
Stairwalking for 15 minutes	Basketball (playing a game) for 15-20 minutes	
	Jumping rope for 15 minutes	
	Running 1-1/2 miles in 15 minutes (10 min/mile)	↓ More vigorous, less time

Note: A moderate amount of physical activity is roughly equivalent to physical activity that uses approximately 150 calories of energy per day, or 1,000 calories per week.

*Some activities can be performed at various intensities; the suggested durations correspond to expected intensity of effort.

Reprinted from National Institutes of Health and National Heart, Lung, and Blood Institute 2000.

obese clients. Working out at a high intensity, relative to their fitness level, or for an extended period of time may cause labored breathing and muscle soreness to which they are not accustomed. These uncomfortable sensations may demotivate a client from continuing with the program. Therefore, it is best to start at a lower demand. Low-level interval training programs (bouts of activity interspersed with rest periods) are also appropriate for a client in the early training stages.

A well-designed, progressive program avoids the incidence of injury in addition to making the initial exercise sessions comfortable and tolerable for the client who is overweight or obese.

As the client loses weight and increases his or her functional capacity, exercise of increased intensity and increased duration can be programmed. Although longer sessions of moderate-intensity activities (such as fitness walking) can involve the same amount of activity and caloric expenditure as shorter sessions of higher-intensity exercises (such as running), it is best to go with the longer-duration, lower-intensity exercise (at least at the start of the program) in order to avoid injury and promote adherence to the program. Examples of appropriate exercises include fitness walking, fitness swimming, aqua fitness classes, cycling in and out of doors, rowing, hiking, square dancing, and aerobic dance in addition to resistance and flexibility training.

Although longer sessions of moderate-intensity activities (such as fitness walking) can entail the same amount of activity and caloric expenditure as shorter sessions of higher-intensity exercises (such as running), for clients who are overweight or obese it is best to go with the longer-duration, lower-intensity exercise (at least at the start of the program) in order to avoid injury and promote adherence to the program.

Although a caloric expenditure of 150 calories per day from physical activity is recommended by the NHLBI, this amount can be increased as the client adapts to the program. The increase in exercise duration, intensity, or both will result in expenditure of even more calories. In fact, the American College of Sports Medicine recommends a higher total caloric expenditure of 1,000 to 2,000 kcal/week or 300 to 500 kcal/day in order to facilitate weight loss. Obviously, clients should start with moderate levels of activity and progress toward the 2,000-kcal recommendation over time [2, 3].

An additional 100 to 200 kcal/day spent in common chores and recreational activities will promote an even larger caloric deficit with a concomitant increase in fat loss, functional capacity, and lean body mass [22]. All of this increased activity along with programmed exercise sessions will add up and contribute to the caloric deficit needed to ensure weight loss and subsequent weight maintenance.

Lifestyle Change Support

Lifestyle change support consists of various strategies that can help clients adhere to their physical activity and diet programs. Lifestyle change support helps clients identify the obstacles that are keeping them from following the program and then uses a problem-solving approach to design and implement strategies to overcome these obstacles. It is not easy for anyone to change well-established behaviors and to overcome the obstacles to those changes. Specifically, the techniques of self-monitoring, rewards, goal setting, stimulus control, and dietary behavior changes may help clients stick to their weight loss or weight maintenance program [22].

Self-Monitoring The practice of a client's taking note of his or her activity and diet behaviors and recording them is referred to as self-monitoring. Recording food and calorie intake, bouts of exercise and physical activity, moods when eating, where a food was eaten, weight lost or gained, and so forth can provide valuable information for both the personal trainer and the client. Further, in some cases, just self-monitoring a behavior can bring about positive changes as the client becomes keenly aware of what he or she is doing and can make immediate changes [22]. The personal trainer can provide clients with specific self-monitoring forms such as the one found in "Small Steps . . . Big Changes® Diet and Activity Diary" on the next page. Self-monitoring can help the client and personal trainer

- identify behaviors that put the success of the program at risk,
- identify obstacles to engaging in physical activity or eating healthfully,
- chart progress, and
- provide a track history to both motivate the client and serve as a basis for the reward system.

As an example of identifying risky behaviors, a diet history form that notes the food consumed, time of food consumption, site of food consumption, and even the mood of the client at the time may bring forth the fact that the client tends to eat high-calorie snacks, in relatively large amounts, when sitting in front of the television. The client could be advised to prepare a bowl of cut, crisp fresh vegetables or a controlled amount of unbuttered popcorn to consume during a show. Or, the client may detect on his or her form that upon arrival home from work, he or she makes a trip directly to the refrigerator to eat whatever is available. The client could solve this problem by eating a piece of fruit on the way home in order to wait until the planned dinner is prepared and on the table.

Self-monitoring of exercise behaviors also helps identify obstacles to engaging in the prescribed amount of physical activity. For example, the client and personal trainer may have agreed that they would meet twice a week for a weight training session and that the client would engage in a 30- to 45-minute walk on alternate days. Inspection of the exercise self-monitoring form may bring to light that the client did exercise on the days planned for an early morning walk before work. Conversely, when the client planned to walk in the afternoon, he or she never got around to it because of work constraints and finally just being too tired to exercise upon arrival at home. This client would need to plan his or her exercise sessions in the morning.

Rewards Rewards can be used to encourage and acknowledge attainment of the client's behavioral goals or specific outcomes. An effective reward is something that is desirable to the client, awarded to the client on a timely basis, and contingent on meeting the goal [22].

Small Steps . . . Big Changes®
Diet and Activity Diary

Name: ________________________ Day and date: ____________

Time	Food eaten or activity performed	Time spent eating or doing activity	Place	Thoughts or feelings

Food

1. Record the time at which you ate a snack or meal. Also record the amount of time you spent eating.
2. List the foods that you ate and the amount that you ate.
3. Record where you were when you ate and whether or not you had any feelings and/or thoughts (positive, negative, or neutral).

Exercise/Activity

1. Record any formal exercise in which you participated (i.e., walking, aerobics class, biking, resistance training, aqua exercise, etc.).
2. Also record the time of day, the amount of time you spent exercising, and any accompanying feelings and/or thoughts (positive, negative, or neutral).
3. Record any other physical activities in which you engaged along with the time performed and time spent (i.e., walking up stairs, sweeping, mopping, yard work, washing windows, etc.).

Rewards can be big or small, tangible or intangible, awarded by the client's family or the client to him- or herself, or awarded to the client by the personal trainer. Tangible rewards include some sort of an item, a new blouse, an exercise outfit, a new book, and so on. Intangible rewards usually include some pleasant use of time such as time off to go fishing, an afternoon at the mall, quiet time to read a book, or a weekend getaway to an country inn. Usually, small rewards are given for the attainment of steps within a goal or a short-term goal, while bigger awards are granted for attaining a long-term goal such as the target 10% reduction of body weight within a six-month period.

Goal Setting Goal setting is covered in chapter 8. When one is working with clients who are overweight or obese, it is especially important to set goals that are realistic and to set short-term goals within long-term goals. For example, a client may have the goal of losing 20 pounds (9 kilograms) over a six-month period. Breaking this down to 3 to 4 pounds (1.3-1.8 kilograms) per month enables the client to celebrate the attainment of each goal. Fortunately, if the client does not achieve the whole weight goal in the first six months but has achieved some of the smaller goals, the client will most likely still feel motivated to continue the program [32].

However, focusing only on weight loss goals as opposed to behavior change can set clients up for failure. Using behavior change goals in addition to weight loss goals will help clients stick with the program when they experience plateaus in weight loss. For example, a goal may be to walk 40 minutes at least four times per week. If the client meets this goal, he or she is successful, regardless of the amount of weight lost.

Goal setting is to be used in conjunction with self-monitoring and rewards. Additionally, the client can commit to a self-contract. In a self-contract, the client usually outlines a desired goal or behavior (e.g., to lose 1/2 pound [0.2 kilograms] per week for a total of 2 pounds [0.9 kilograms] per month, to walk 30 minutes at least four times per week). The client will also decide on the reward for achievement of the goal. The Activity/Exercise Contract on the next page is an example of a self-contract.

Stimulus Control Stimulus control consists of identifying the social or environmental cues that seem to trigger undesired eating patterns or nonparticipation in physical activity and then modifying those cues [22]. Sometimes the term "environmental trigger" is used in place of "stimulus," as triggering is exactly what happens. Something in the environment sets off an unwanted behavior, and the client starts engaging in unwanted eating patterns. For example, a client may find that he or she always eats popcorn and drinks a soda at a movie despite not being hungry, overeats at a buffet, overeats while working at his or her desk, or tends to have rich desserts when out with a particular friend.

Using the self-monitoring strategy, reflection, or both, the client may be able to identify these cues in the environment and problem solve ways to manage the situation. For example, if a client eats popcorn at the movies even when not hungry, the client could either eat a smaller meal before going to the movies or eat a salad and then go to the movies and eat popcorn. If a client eats large amounts at a buffet, a solution could be to go only to restaurants where food is served from a menu. Clients who unwittingly overeat while working at their desks may be advised to make a rule only to eat a snack away from the desk. Clients who tend to overeat or overdrink when they go out to eat with a particular friend may need to decide to meet the friend for a nonfood activity like shopping or going to the movies. The problem-solving step either seeks to eliminate the cue or to manage it in a way that avoids overeating.

Food Consumption Behavior Changes Food consumption behavior changes may also help the client eat less without feeling deprived [22]. Some clients should be encouraged to slow the rate of eating. Eating too fast does not allow the body time to identify the satiety signals that develop before the end of a meal. Clients can also use smaller plates in order to make portion sizes appear bigger. The use of smaller plates is also recommended at buffets to prevent placing large amounts of food on the plate. Some clients do best by eating only three meals a day in order to avoid eating too many snacks, while others do better with four to six small meals, as they tend to overeat at a meal when they eat only three times per day. Clients who tend to skip or delay meals and overeat later because they are overly hungry must consider tightly scheduling their meals to avoid this problem. As every client is an individual, there is no recipe for eating patterns that will work best for each client. Through trial and error, the personal trainer and client will find what works best for that client.

Exercise Concerns of Clients Who Are Overweight or Obese

There are a number of physiological and biomechanical concerns to consider when one is work-

Activity/Exercise Contract

I, ______________________________, will incorporate the following activity/exercise into my daily/weekly schedule for the week of ______________________________.

Extra physical activities* I will incorporate into my daily routine:

Activity	Where	When	Number of times performed	Duration

Formal exercise sessions** in which I will participate:

Name of exercise/ program	Where	When	Duration	Times per week

*Examples include taking the stairs at work and taking a 10-minute walk at lunch.

**Examples include a session with a personal trainer, a 30-minute walk, an aerobics class, or lap swimming.

If I fulfill this one-week contract, I will reward myself by:

____

____

Signature: ______________________________ Date: ______________

ing with individuals who are overweight or obese. Storlie and Franklin [29] list the following concerns, which may affect the exercise program design, exercise selection, and instruction of the client: heat intolerance, movement restriction and limited mobility, weight-bearing stress, posture problems and low back pain, balance concerns, and hyperpnea and dyspnea.

Heat Intolerance

Heat intolerance is a result of the added insulation of excess fat. Compared to persons of normal weight, it is harder for individuals with obesity to thermoregulate, especially under hot and humid conditions [29]. The personal trainer should encourage clients to wear cotton clothes, preferably shorts and a T-shirt, in moderate and hot temperatures. (Wearing shorts may be embarrassing to some clients, although they can cover up with a long T-shirt worn over bicycle pants or basketball-length shorts. If the client does not want to wear shorts, then the personal trainer should encourage lightweight, loose-fitting cotton pants.) On particularly hot or humid days, the personal trainer should consider any of the following modifications: lowering the intensity of the workout in order to avoid discomfort and a possible heat emergency; training in a temperature-controlled environment; swimming or performing aqua exercise for the cardiovascular training component of the workout; conducting the resistance training in the pool; and water walking and jogging in the pool. Personal trainers must ensure that the client drinks enough cool water before, during, and after the exercise session. (See chapter 7 for recommendations.)

Movement Restriction and Limited Mobility

In people who are obese, movement restriction or limited mobility due to the excess fat mass may require the modification of various exercises [29]. For example, excess fat on the thigh and calf may make it difficult for a client to perform a quadriceps stretch with the leg held behind and the foot pressed into the buttock. For a more suitable quadriceps stretch, one could have the client lower the back knee and press the hips forward from a calf stretch. Alternatively, the client could perform an active stretch of the quadriceps by using the hamstring muscles to bend the knee as far back as the fat mass allows while performing a pelvic tilt to put the hip into extension (see figure 19.2). Although these modifications would not allow a full stretch of the quadriceps, they would provide some flexibility training benefit.

As another example, a client may be unable to reach his or her leg (because of the restriction imposed by the abdominal fat mass) in order to move it toward the chest during a back-lying hamstring stretch. In this case, the client could be given a towel to wrap around the back of the thigh to perform the assisted passive stretch (see figure 19.3), or simply be instructed to perform an active stretch of the hamstrings by using the hip flexors to put the leg into the stretch position. The personal trainer needs to observe the client performing various stretches and exercises in order to make the modifications specific to the client's limitations (see figure 19.4).

Weight-Bearing Stress

Weight-bearing stress on the joints is definitely a concern for people who are overweight or obese, especially those who have osteoarthritis or musculoskeletal injuries [29]. Low-impact activities, not necessarily low in intensity, will prevent some of this stress. For example, fitness walking provides less stress to the joints than jogging or running. Other low-impact activities include indoor and outdoor cycling; swimming; aqua aerobics; shallow-water walking, jogging, and aerobics; deep-water run-

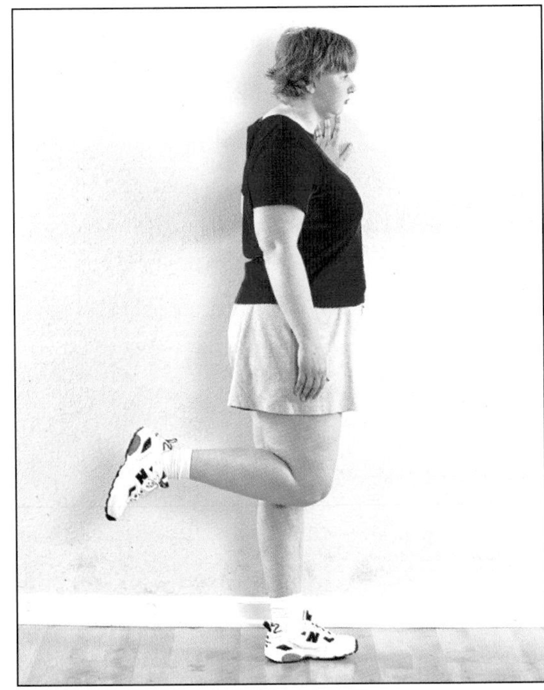

Figure 19.2 In the modified quadriceps stretch, the client performs an active stretch by flexing the right knee as much as possible and "rocking" or pressing the right hip forward while maintaining an erect posture.

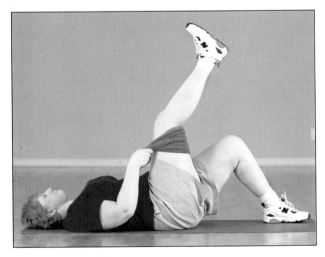

Figure 19.3 In the modified hamstrings stretch, the client pulls the right leg toward the chest with the help of a towel while trying to extend (not hyperextend) the knee.

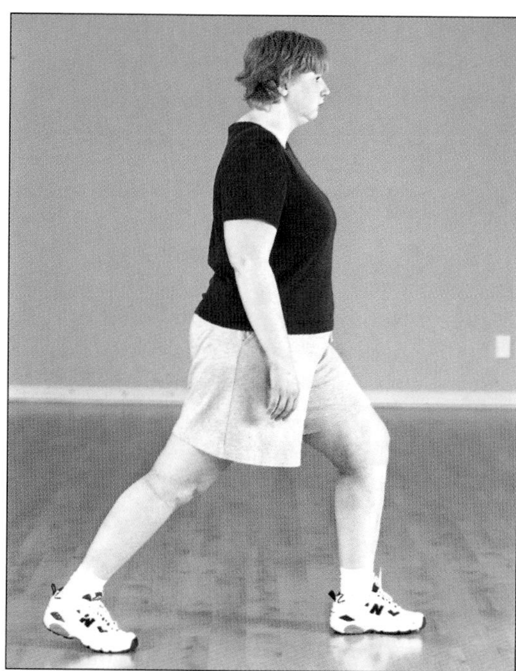

Figure 19.4 In the modified hip flexors stretch, the client takes a lunge stance with the ball of the right (rear) foot on the floor. The client then "rocks" or presses the right hip forward to actively stretch the hip flexors. The rear knee can have a slight or significant degree of flexion.

ning; hiking; and rowing (not advised if the client has a movement restriction due to the fat mass). Activities that require sustained single-limb support (standing on one leg for an extended period of time while performing exercises with the other leg) can also impose an excessive weight-bearing stress on the involved joints, especially the hips. Many traditional aerobics classes and balance activities include such standing legwork. A way to avoid this situation is to alternate the supporting leg frequently when performing these exercises.

Posture Problems and Low Back Pain

Because of the stress of the abdominal fat mass on the spine and often inadequate strength of the muscles of the abdominal wall, posture problems and low back pain are not uncommon in persons who are obese. This situation may cause lordosis of the lower spine, with or without an accommodating kyphosis of the upper spine, along with other possible postural changes. Further, the hip flexors in persons with obesity can be quite strong owing to the repeated load of moving a large mass around; this further contributes to the muscular imbalance caused by weaker abdominal muscles. Therefore, the personal trainer must include a variety of exercises to strengthen the abdominal muscles along with flexibility exercises for the hip flexors (e.g., iliopsoas) in the training program. Because of the larger fat mass and weaker abdominal muscles, some of the abdominal exercises may have to be modified. Further, attention must be given to exercises to strengthen the muscles of the upper back and increase the flexibility of the chest muscles. Clients with significant or chronic low back pain should be referred to an orthopedist for an evaluation. The physician may refer the client to a physical therapist for a back education and rehabilitation program in addition to the personal training sessions.

Balance Concerns

Clients who are obese may have little experience in movement and sport and may not have had the chance to develop good balance [29]. Unfortunately, when clients do start to fall because of lack of balance in a movement, the excess weight, lack of experience in proprioceptive adjustments, and lack of adequate strength can contribute to a greater difficulty in righting themselves. Therefore, the personal trainer should include balance training, but on a progressive basis, and needs to observe, correct, and spot the client during the various exercises that require good balance.

Hyperpnea and Dyspnea

Hyperpnea and **dyspnea** during exercise can be both uncomfortable and a source of anxiety to clients who are obese [29]. Although some hyperpnea (increased respiratory rate) or dyspnea (labored or difficult breathing) is expected during an exercise session, persons with obesity may experience more because of their low functional capacity. This condition can be disquieting and uncomfortable enough to cause them to give up on the exercise training due to fear. The personal trainer can avoid problems in this area by ensuring that clients are working at the appropriate exercise intensity through use of a **Rating of Perceived Exertion Scale** (see chapter 16). The use of modified interval training, especially at the beginning of an exercise program, is highly recommended, as the rest intervals (active or inactive) will allow clients to bring their breathing into better control. With time, the work intervals can be increased and the rest intervals can be decreased.

Exercise Prescription and Program Design for Clients Who Are Overweight or Obese

The components of a well-rounded exercise program for those who are obese or overweight include aerobic conditioning, resistance training, and flexibility training (table 19.6). The personal trainer and client must first come to an agreement regarding how many days a week they will schedule and the content of the workout sessions. For example, they could decide that the personal training sessions will consist of all three of the components or only a warm-up followed by a resistance and flexibility training program. This would mean that the client would perform aerobic conditioning on alternate days from the personal training session days, before the personal training sessions, or both. The initial sessions should contain the aerobic conditioning phase so that the personal trainer can supervise, instruct, motivate, and ensure that the client is working both correctly and efficiently on the cardiovascular training program. If the client has any difficulty complying with the cardiovascular program, then this component should remain within the personal training session.

Aerobic Conditioning

A typical exercise prescription for a person who is overweight or obese calls for five days of participation in an aerobic conditioning program to ensure that the client expends the maximal calories possible during the week and establishes a regular physical activity habit. Some clients may not be able to start with the full cardiovascular component of the exercise program. In this case the beginning sessions need to be low in intensity, and the client would also be asked to work at increasing daily living activities as described earlier. Even when the client does achieve a full workout, it is important to encourage the daily activity levels so that the client expends more calories, thereby enhancing weight loss.

Some individuals will be so out of shape that they will not be able to walk one lap of a track, or even less, without stopping to rest. In such a situation, the personal trainer should consider an interval train-

TABLE 19.6

Exercise Prescription for Clients Who Are Obese

Mode	Intensity/frequency/duration	Guidelines/concerns
Aerobic conditioning	• 5 days/week (or daily) • Can begin with 2 daily sessions of 20-30 min each • Eventual goal: 40-60 minutes/day • 40 or 50-70% $\dot{V}O_2max$ • Can intersperse short aerobic exercise intervals with rest or resistance training	• Use low-impact activities • Take appropriate precautions due to increased risk of orthopedic injury, cardiovascular disease, and hyperthermia • Initially emphasize increasing duration rather than increasing intensity to optimize caloric expenditure • Modify equipment as necessary (e.g., wide seats on cycle ergometers and rowers)
Resistance training	• 2-3 days/week on non-consecutive days • 1-3 sets, 10-15 repetitions/set • Up to 8-10 exercises • Gradual load increases	• Can begin with body-weight exercises • Can intersperse with aerobic exercise • Modify equipment as necessary (e.g., larger-framed machines) • Can complement aerobic conditioning (i.e., to maintain or gain lean body weight)
Flexibility training	• Daily or at least 5 sessions/week • Hold static stretches for 10-30 seconds	

Adapted from ACSM 2003.

ing program. For example, the client would walk one-half of the track, stop to do a body-weight calisthenic or exercise with a band, walk another half of a lap, stop to perform another exercise for 10 to 20 repetitions, and so on until the client has walked a mile. With time, the client would increase the length of the walk intervals until he or she can walk half a mile before stopping to do half of the resistance exercises, and then complete the next half-mile before performing the last half of the resistance exercises. Eventually the client will be able to walk a mile or two without stopping before doing the resistance training exercises.

Resistance Training

Resistance training may be responsible for enhancing cardiovascular health by mitigating several of the risk factors associated with CVD. The benefit of including resistance training in an exercise program for persons with obesity cannot be overlooked. The design of the resistance training program will depend on the available equipment along with the abilities and limitations of the client. It is recommended that the personal trainer check with the client for any orthopedic problems such as hip, back, or knee injuries and modify the program and specific exercises accordingly. Clients can start with body-weight exercises (see figure 19.5 for example) and move on to machines or light free

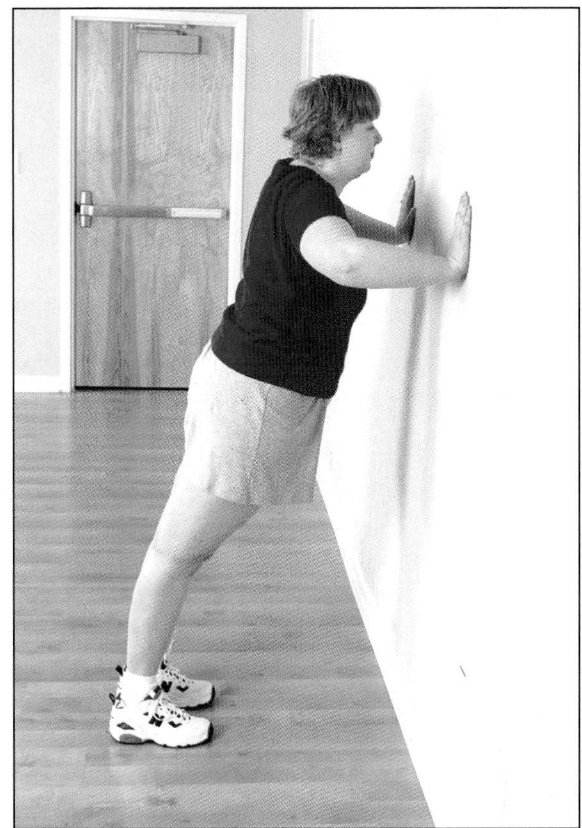

Figure 19.5 The wall push-up can be used for clients who cannot perform the standard push-up (i.e, on the floor).

Program Modifications and Motivational Strategies for Clients Who Are Obese

- Avoid being judgmental about or to your client.
- Get the client to focus on lifestyle change (activity and diet) as opposed to measuring success in pounds lost.
- Modify standard exercise training methods for persons with obesity in order to provide a safe and effective exercise program.
- Use progression—start with activities of daily living (if necessary), move to low-, then to moderate-intensity activities.
- Use interval training for individuals who are unfit.
- Establish a regular workout schedule.
- Incorporate lifestyle change strategies such as goal setting, feedback and praise, self-monitoring, and self-contracting.
- Promote the increase of everyday activities to burn extra calories.

weights. The personal trainer must keep in mind that the client has a built-in workload with the excess body weight.

People who are obese are often quite strong in the lower body because of the adaptations the body makes to carrying the excess body weight. Hence, upper body strength should also be well addressed in a training session. Still, as the major goals of the resistance training session are to expend calories and increase muscle mass, emphasis should be on the core exercises, and the client should not spend a great deal of time on the smaller muscle groups. In general, one should follow the guidelines for resistance training presented in chapters 13 and 15.

Flexibility Training

Although stretching exercises typically do not result in large expenditures of energy, they are important to prevent injury and maintain range of motion around the joints. Light stretching can be included in the warm-up, while more intense stretches would be included at the end of an exercise session or after various resistance training exercises in order to develop flexibility. This timing ensures that the muscles are well warmed and thus more pliable. Stretches should be performed for all the major muscle groups.

Stretches are to be modified in accordance with the client's structural and physiological limitations. See page 498 for examples of modifications. The personal trainer must be cognizant of the limited range of motion of clients who are overweight or obese. For instance, in a sitting toe touch, the client may only be able to reach just below the knees. The goal would not be to actually reach the toes. Instead, the goal would be to stretch until light tension is felt.

Eating Disorders

There is tremendous pressure in our society to be thin. Thin is in, and many of our young girls and women—and even some boys and men—are compromising their health to try to get there.

About 1% to 5% of adolescents and young adult women have eating disorders [20]. Although cases have been reported in all social and racial groups, there seems to be a predominance in Caucasian upper middle and middle classes. Clinical samples have shown that only 5% to 10% of individuals with eating disorders are males [20]. Given the current social and cultural environment, this number may increase in the future.

Personal trainers not only have a responsibility to educate clients about the risks of engaging in disordered eating, they also must be sure not to promote unnecessary or risky behaviors to lose weight and not to set unrealistic goals that may push a client into disordered eating patterns. Although a personal trainer would not be the sole cause of a client's eating disorder (the client would have to be already susceptible), an inappropriate comment or goal can serve as a trigger for someone to engage in disordered eating practices and possibly end up with an eating disorder.

> Personal trainers have a responsibility to educate their clients about the risks of engaging in disordered eating. They also must be sure not to promote unnecessary or risky behaviors to lose weight and not to set unrealistic goals that may push a client into disordered eating patterns.

Personal trainers need to orient their clients to the genetically determined differences in body types and the differences in body composition between men and women. Personal trainers need to be sure that they help each client set a goal that is realistic and in accordance with the client's genetic makeup, which has a significant effect on both the client's metabolism and body type. According to Dr. Carol Otis, "your ideal body weight is the range where you feel healthy and fit, have no signs of an eating disorder to maintain that weight, and have healthy, functioning immune and reproductive systems" [25].

Disordered Eating

The development of an eating disorder usually passes through the stages of dieting, disordered eating, and finally a full-blown eating disorder. Clients may start out by dieting to lose weight and become frustrated when the weight loss does not seem fast enough or significant, or both. This frustration, even desperation, causes them to restrict their diet even further. When this does not work, in their viewpoint, they start to experiment with even more dangerous disordered eating practices such as the use of diuretics (a medication that increases the rate of urination, hence increases water loss), diet pills, self-induced vomiting, food faddism (eating only one or few specific foods or following fad diets such as the pineapple diet or the grapefruit diet), fasting, using saunas to sweat weight off, spitting out food that has been chewed, and using laxatives or even enemas [25]. Unfortunately, these practices do not work. Although there may be a loss of weight according to the scale, the lost poundage can be attributed to water loss and probably lean tissue as opposed to fat.

There is a wide range in the frequency of disordered eating practices. Some may engage infrequently in one of the techniques mentioned, while others may do so several times a day. Engaging in these disordered eating practices is the first step toward developing the eating disorders of anorexia nervosa and bulimia.

The key to preventing the development of an eating disorder is for the personal trainer, client, or both to recognize this common and complex condition. The personal trainer may be able to pick up on some of the disordered eating practices just by talking with the client about his or her diet or by having a client fill out a self-monitoring form for a few days to a week. Although many of the disordered eating practices may not be identifiable on the monitoring form, at least the types of foods consumed could be noticed. The main point is that if the personal trainer offers good education, appropriate goal setting, and support, perhaps the client can be convinced to return to healthy eating before developing a full-blown eating disorder.

If a personal trainer suspects a client has an eating disorder, the personal trainer may ask the client these questions [19]:

- Do you feel fat even though people tell you you're thin?
- Do you get anxious if you can't exercise?
- Do you worry about what you will eat?
- If you gain weight, do you get anxious or depressed?
- Do you feel guilty when you eat?
- Would you rather eat by yourself than with family or friends?
- Do you avoid talking about your fear of being fat, because you feel that no one understands how you feel?
- Do you have a secret stash of food?
- When you eat, are you afraid that you won't be able to stop?
- Do you get anxious when people urge you to eat?
- Do you sometimes think that your eating or exercising is not normal?

The concern is that individuals engaging in disordered eating practices can experience both the short- and long-term medical and psychological conditions characteristic of persons with anorexia and bulimia. These complications include depression, low self-esteem, stomach and digestive problems, menstrual irregularities, and heart problems and may even result in death by heart failure or suicide [25]. The earlier an individual seeks help, the better chance he or she has at preventing and treating an eating disorder.

Anorexia Nervosa

Anorexia nervosa is characterized by extreme weight loss, a refusal to maintain body weight, an intense fear of gaining weight or becoming fat although the individual is underweight, distorted body image, and **amenorrhea** (loss of menses for at least three consecutive menstrual cycles) [5]. The weight loss is usually facilitated through the restriction of food intake in conjunction with excessive exercise and may include the aforementioned disordered eating practices. The psychological and emotional problems associated with anorexia may include low self-esteem and a distorted body image among others. Further, the condition of any extremely malnourished person may lead to symptoms of apathy, confusion, social isolation, and nonresponsiveness [20].

The two specific types of anorexia are the *restricting type* and the *binge eating/purging type* [20]. An individual with the restricting type of anorexia does not regularly engage in binge eating or purging behaviors such as self-induced vomiting or the misuse of laxatives, diuretics, or enemas during an episode, although he or she does severely restrict food intake in terms of the type and amount of food [20]. This is the most common type of anorexia. Alternatively, individuals with the binge eating/purging type of anorexia nervosa regularly engage in binge eating followed by purging behaviors [20].

Personal trainers can refer to table 19.7 for the warning signs of anorexia. If a personal trainer notes these signs in a client, it becomes important to refer the client to his or her physician for a comprehensive treatment plan, which usually includes medical, dietary, and psychological or spiritual counseling from a team of professionals (physician, dietitian, psychologist, or religious or spiritual counselor). It may be hard for individuals with anorexia to acknowledge they have a problem. Therefore, the personal trainer should share this list with the client in the hopes of getting the person to seek help.

TABLE 19.7

Warning Signs for Anorexia

Warning Signs for Anorexia
Dramatic loss of weight (up to 15% or more below expected weight range)
Denial; feelings of being fat even when thin; obsession with weight, diet, and appearance
Use of food rituals or avoidance of social situations involving food
Obsession with exercise; hyperactivity
Sensitivity to cold
Use of layers of baggy clothing to disguise weight loss
Fatigue (in later stages)
Decline in work, school, or athletic performance
Growth of baby-fine hair over face and body, called lanugo hair
Yellow tint to skin, palms, and soles of feet (from high levels of carotene)
Hair loss, dry hair, dry skin, brittle nails
Loss of muscle mass and tone
No menstrual periods (amenorrhea)
Slow pulse at rest, light-headedness on standing up quickly
Constipation

Reprinted from Otis and Goldingay 2000.

Bulimia Nervosa

Bulimia is a complicated disorder that consists of recurring episodes of binge eating followed by purging behaviors. During the bingeing phase the person eats large amounts of food over a short period of time. The purging behaviors may include self-induced vomiting; taking laxatives, diuretics, or enemas; and exercising excessively and obsessively in order to burn calories [20, 25]. Whereas an individual with anorexia exhibits strict control of food intake, the individual with bulimia is experiencing a loss of control [20, 25].

The diagnosis of bulimia comes when the binge eating and purging behaviors occur on an average of at least twice a week for at least three months. The bingeing phase consists of eating large amounts of food within any two-hour span and a feeling of lack of control to stop eating, lack of control over what or how much to eat, or both. Further criteria for the diagnosis of bulimia include the use of one or more purging methods or compensatory behaviors such as excessive exercise or fasting, and overconcern with body shape or weight [5]. Even if the bingeing and purging behaviors are occurring with less frequency than just described, emphasis should be on prevention and breaking the cycle. Early detection and help in this condition to break the cycle will prevent further or permanent damage to the body, mind, and spirit.

It is not easy to recognize bulimia in women. In fact, the condition often goes undetected. Individuals with bulimia often try to hide the condition from their family and friends. People with bulimia can be of normal weight or slightly overweight, come from diverse backgrounds, and practice many types of eating behaviors. They frequently have weight fluctuations greater than 10 pounds (4.5 kilograms) due to alternative binges and fasts [20]. It is important for personal trainers to be familiar with the signs, effects, and behaviors associated with bulimia so they may be able to identify the condition in a client and refer him or her for help. The warning signs of bulimia are listed in table 19.8.

Female Athlete Triad

Eating disorders can result in the female athlete triad, composed of the following interrelated disorders [1]:

TABLE 19.8

Warning Signs for Bulimia

Warning Signs for Bulimia
Self-induced vomiting (at least 2 times a week for at least 3 months)
Laxative, diuretics, or enema use
Excessive exercise
Overconcern of body shape
Weight fluctuations of more than 10 pounds (4.5 kg)
Traces of odor of vomit on the breath
Scabs or scars on knuckles
Swollen, persistently puffy face and cheeks
Broken blood vessels in the face and eyes
Sore throat and dental problems
Abdominal symptoms
Rapid weight changes of 2 to 5 pounds (0.9-2.5 kg) overnight
Erratic performance in work, sport, and academics
Irregular or absent menstrual periods
Lacerations of the oral cavity
Diarrhea
Constipation
Fatigue
Electrolyte disturbances
Heart irregularities
Ruptures in the stomach

Adapted from Otis and Goldingay 2000.

- Disordered eating
- Amenorrhea
- Osteoporosis

The label includes the word "athlete" because this condition was first discovered in young female athletes. In actuality, the condition affects a wide range of women with different levels of activity, not just athletes [1]. It is not the participation in exercise or sport that causes the triad, but the misguided goal of girls and women to become unrealistically thin, consequent to their thinking that this will improve sport performance or appearance [25].

The woman starts with disordered eating practices and consequently puts her body into an energy deficit, which results in amenorrhea over time. Amenorrhea (loss of menses) is a serious medical problem as the woman is now deficient in the hormones necessary for bone density accruement, which normally occurs from birth through the age of 30. Unfortunately, this condition leads to a lack of normal bone formation and irreversible loss in bone mass, resulting in osteoporosis and its subsequent complications [1, 27]. Personal trainers should be alert to women who exhibit signs of the female athlete triad and refer such clients to a health care professional for evaluation.

The female athlete triad often begins with disordered eating, which leads to amenorrhea, which leads to osteoporosis. It occurs in a wide range of women, not just athletes.

Exercise Prescription and Program Design for Clients Recovering From an Eating Disorder

Clients with a diagnosed eating disorder should receive clearance from their physician before returning to an exercise program. An exercise program can be beneficial, both physically and emotionally, but the program must be designed so that it is safe and does not prompt a return to the use of exercise as a purging technique. The physician must determine whether and when it is medically safe for the client to start exercise.

When resuming a client's exercise program, the personal trainer needs to reassess the client. Some clients may have stress fractures due to the osteoporosis and will have to find alternative forms of exercise until healing occurs, such as swimming or deep-water aqua exercise, in which there is no impact. Yoga and Pilates classes could also be considered. Clients who have experienced complications of the eating disorder (abnormal electrolytes, an irregular heartbeat, having passed out at any time) will not be able to exercise until the problem is corrected or alleviated. Once a client with the triad returns to exercise, it is important to monitor the heart rate and blood pressure.

An exercise program should de-emphasize weight loss and emphasize exercise with a low energy demand [2]. A return to high caloric expenditure exercise should be delayed until the client is

Program Design for Clients Recovering From an Eating Disorder

- Require the client recovering from an eating disorder to see a physician for a complete medical exam before returning to or continuing an exercise program.
- Do not prescribe a vigorous exercise program.
- Help the client to engage in a well-rounded program of aerobic conditioning, resistance training, and flexibility exercise.
- Ensure adequate hydration and rehydration.
- Encourage the client to ingest an adequate dietary intake.
- Encourage the client to consume 200 to 400 kcal of complex carbohydrates during the first 30 to 90 minutes following an exercise session.
- Schedule exercise sessions so that the client does not exercise every day and takes two to three days off a week.
- Check the client's blood pressure and pulse.
- Do not allow impact exercise if the client has a stress fracture.
- Maintain regular communication with the client's physician, dietitian, and other health care professionals.
- If a client experiences any of the following signs or symptoms, he or she should seek medical clearance before continuing the exercise program: light-headedness, irregular heartbeats, nausea, injuries, abnormal blood pressure levels or pulse.

cleared by his or her physician. Resistance exercise should be included in order to preserve lean body mass, although its effectiveness will be severely compromised if the client does not consume adequate calories and nutrients.

The personal trainer may encounter an individual who has an eating disorder but refuses to see a physician. Although the personal trainer, as one of very few people who may be in touch with the client, may be tempted to continue to train the client, he or she should require a medical release before continuing training. Should the client refuse to see a physician, the personal trainer cannot train the client.

Hyperlipidemia

Cardiovascular disease is the leading cause of death in the industrialized nations and is responsible for more than 1 million deaths a year in the United States. Blood lipid disorders are risk factors that play a significant role in the process of arteriosclerosis resulting in the clinical syndromes of coronary heart disease, angina pectoris, myocardial infarction, sudden cardiac death, and chronic heart failure.

Blood lipid disorders include hyperlipidemia and dyslipidemia. **Hyperlipidemia** is a general term for elevated concentrations of any or all of the lipids (fats) in the blood, such as cholesterol, **triglycerides,** and lipoproteins. This term usually indicates high levels of **low-density lipoproteins (LDLs)** and **very low density lipoproteins (VLDLs)**. The term **dyslipidemia** refers to abnormal lipid (fat) levels in the blood, lipoprotein composition or both.

In 2001, the NIH released the National Cholesterol Education Program Adult Treatment Panel III guidelines for the detection, evaluation, and treatment of cholesterol [23]. The new guidelines set lower LDLs goals, raise **high-density lipoproteins (HDLs)** goals, and also lower the triglyceride classification cut points. Refer to table 19.9 for this information.

These guidelines also recommend **therapeutic lifestyle change** or **TLC** as the first line of therapy for the majority of the disorders. Therapeutic lifestyle change includes diet, physical activity, and weight loss. Drug therapy may be necessary for higher-risk individuals or those who do not respond well to TLC. Personal trainers should become familiar with these and future NIH guidelines in order to be able to design an effective physical activity program and promote the other necessary lifestyle changes prescribed by the client's physician to improve the lipid profile and other risk factors for CVD.

Possible Causes of Hyperlipidemia

Substantial amounts of research have shown that an elevated **LDL** level is a major cause of coronary heart disease (CHD) [23]. Furthermore, clinical trials provide strong evidence that LDL-lowering therapy reduces risk for CHD. Hence, the **ATP III** guidelines identify elevated LDLs as the primary target of cholesterol-lowering therapy [23]. The goal for the majority of adults who do not have diabetes or CVD is <130 mg/dL, while the goal for those who do have diabetes or CVD is <100 mg/dL.

The ATP III has also designated low HDLs, defined as a level <40 mg/dL, as a strong independent predictor of CHD. The possible causes of low HDL levels, which are also correlated to insulin resistance, include elevated triglycerides, overweight and obesity, physical inactivity, and type 2 diabetes. Other causes include cigarette smoking, high carbohydrate intakes (especially simple sugars), and certain drugs (e.g., beta-blockers, anabolic steroids, progestational agents). Therapy to increase low HDL levels is twofold. The goal is to focus on lowering LDL levels with the diet, drug therapy, or both and to increase physical activity and weight loss for those who have the metabolic syndrome (as diagnosed by a physician when a client has three or more of the risk determinants listed on page 511 along with its increased risk of CVD and diabetes) [23].

Elevated triglycerides are an additional concern as they have been shown to be an independent CHD risk factor [23]. The following are factors that can raise triglycerides to higher-than-normal levels in the general population: obesity and overweight; lack of physical activity; cigarette smoking; excess alcohol intake; high-carbohydrate diets; and several diseases including type 2 diabetes, chronic renal failure, nephritic syndrome along with certain drugs, and genetic disorders. (The personal trainer who is aware of some of these causes can encourage clients to make changes in their habits such as consuming less alcohol, eating less sweets and high-carbohydrate foods, and stopping smoking in addition to following the overall TLC program.)

Table 19.10 offers a review of the possible causes and treatment of unfavorable levels of LDL, HDL, and triglyceride levels.

TABLE 19.9

ATP III Classification of LDLs, HDLs, Total Cholesterol, and Triglycerides (mg/dL)

Low-density lipoproteins (LDLs)	
<100	Optimal
100-129	Near optimal/above optimal
130-159	Borderline high
160-189	High
≥190	Very high
High-density lipoproteins (HDLs)	
<40	Low
≥60	High
Total cholesterol	
<200	Desirable
200-239	Borderline high
≥240	High
Triglycerides	
<150	Normal
150-199	Borderline high
200-499	High
≥500	Very high

Reprinted from National Institutes of Health and National Heart, Lung, and Blood Institute 2001.

Because diet and weight loss play a major role in lowering LDL and triglyceride levels, clients with hyperlipidemia should see a registered dietitian in addition to visiting their physician regularly. The dietitian will provide the client with **medical nutrition therapy**, the term for the nutritional intervention and guidance provided by a registered dietitian. Medical nutrition therapy for blood lipid disorders is a process that includes assessing the client's current diet, using the ATP III guidelines to design a diet to lower LDL and triglyceride levels in addition to controlling weight, and offering behavior modification strategies to ensure that the client can adhere to the diet. Follow-up sessions are important to ensure the success of the diet program.

The personal trainer can play an effective role in the implementation and success of a TLC program. As mentioned earlier, the multifaceted approach consists of diet, increased physical activity, and weight loss. The personal trainer will be the one to facilitate the exercise program with its positive effects on increasing HDLs, lowering triglycerides, and promoting weight loss. Additionally, the personal trainer can serve a supportive role in motivating the client to adhere to the TLC diet prescribed by the physician with subsequent dietary counseling from a registered dietitian.

TLC Diet

The *major emphasis and most important* phase of TLC for high LDL levels is the consumption of an anti-atherogenic diet [23]. The term anti-atherogenic diet or TLC diet is referred to as a "heart healthy diet" in the lay literature as it tends to lower cholesterol

TABLE 19.10

Possible Causes and Treatment Strategies of Unfavorable Lipid Levels

Lipid	Possible etiology (possible causes)	Possible treatment strategies*
High LDL levels	Abdominal obesity Sedentary lifestyle Overweight and obesity Atherogenic diet** Insulin resistance Glucose intolerance Genetic predisposition Genetic disorders Other diseases, such as hypothyroidism, obstructive liver disease, chronic renal failure Certain drugs (e.g., progestins, anabolic steroids, and corticosteroids)	Weight reduction TLC diet including control of saturated fat and cholesterol intake Reduce calorie consumption where appropriate Increase consumption of (soluble) fiber (10-25 g/day) Increase physical activity Drug therapy Control of other risk factors (such as smoking, hypertension, etc.)
Low HDL levels	Overweight and obesity Sedentary lifestyle Elevated trigycerides Insulin resistance Type 2 diabetes Cigarette smoking High carbohydrate intake (>60% of kcals) Certain drugs (e.g., beta-blockers, anabolic steroids, progestational agents)	Control of LDL level Weight reduction Physical activity Smoking cessation TLC diet, including control of caloric and carbohydrate intake Drug therapy
Triglycerides	Overweight and obesity Sedentary lifestyle Cigarette smoking Excessive alcohol intake High carbohydrate intake (>60% of kcals) Insulin resistance Other diseases, such as type 2 diabetes, chronic renal failure, nephritic syndrome Certain drugs (e.g., corticosteroids, estrogens, retinoids, higher doses of beta-adrenergic blocking agents) Genetic disorders	Control of LDL level Physical activity Weight reduction TLC diet including control of caloric and carbohydrate intake Restriction of excessive alcohol intake Drug therapy Very low fat diets for clients with *very high triglyceride levels* (≥500 mg/dL)

*The client's physician will decide on each client's specific treatment strategy in accordance with each client's specific condition and its severity.

**An atherogenic diet is high in fat, high in saturated fats, high in cholesterol, high in trans fatty acids, high in calories, low in fruits and vegetables or any combination of the aforementioned.

Data from National Institutes of Health and National Heart, Lung, and Blood Institute 2001.

levels, especially if combined with physical activity and weight loss.

The mainstay of the TLC diet is the limited intake of saturated fats (<7% of total calories) and cholesterol (<200 milligrams per day). Table 19.11 shows the overall composition of the diet.

In practical terms, the recommendations in table 19.11 translate to eating a diet that is low in overall fat intake and in saturated fat; low in cholesterol; adequate in nutrients; and high in fruits, vegetables, and whole grains.

TABLE 19.11

Nutrient Composition of the TLC Diet

Nutrient	Recommended intake
Saturated fat*	<7% of total calories
Polyunsaturated fat	Up to 10% of total calories
Monounsaturated fat	Up to 20% of total calories
Total fat	25%-35% of total calories
Carbohydrate**	50%-60% of total calories
Fiber	20-30 g/day
Protein	Approximately 15% of total calories
Cholesterol	<200 mg/day
Total calories	Balance energy intake and expenditure to maintain desirable body weight and prevent weight gain***

*Trans fatty acids are another LDL-raising fat that should be kept at a low intake.

**Carbohydrate should be derived predominantly from foods rich in complex carbohydrates including grains, especially whole grains, fruits, and vegetables.

***Daily energy expenditure should include at least moderate physical activity (contributing approximately 200 kcal per day).

Reprinted from National Institutes of Health and National Heart, Lung, and Blood Institute 2001.

TLC Physical Activity: Exercise Prescription and Program Design for Clients with Hyperlipidemia

Physical inactivity is targeted for therapy by the ATP III guidelines as a major, underlying risk factor for CHD. Regular physical activity lowers risk by reducing VLDL levels with a subsequent decrease in triglycerides, raising HDLs, and in some individuals, lowering LDL levels [21]. Other risk factors for CHD are also mitigated by physical activity, as it can also play a significant role in lowering blood pressure, reducing insulin resistance, and improving cardiovascular function. It is for these reasons that the ATP III recommends that regular physical activity become a routine component in the management of high serum cholesterol [21, 26].

Although a single session of aerobic exercise produces beneficial lipoprotein changes, it is necessary to participate in a regular, long-term exercise program of at least a year and to continue thereafter in order to attain and sustain lasting results [7, 18]. Furthermore, programs should involve a relatively high frequency of exercise sessions per week, as acute exercise has been shown to improve both insulin action and lipid profiles for up to 48 to 72 hours after each exercise session [13]. The target exercise guidelines for improving lipid levels are listed in table 19.12.

Although the evidence is not conclusive, resistance training may have a positive effect on the lipid profile and other concomitant risk factors for CHD such as diabetes mellitus, obesity, and overweight [12, 27]. A resistance training program would follow the recommendations found in chapter 15. In light of these benefits, it is prudent for the personal trainer to provide clients with a well-rounded exercise program that includes aerobic, resistance, and flexibility training components.

TLC Weight Loss

Weight loss in conjunction with an exercise and diet program can bring about even larger decreases in LDLs, increase HDLs, and reduce total cholesterol [23]. The personal trainer must educate clients about the importance of weight loss management of hyperlipidemia. Information on safe weight loss is included at the beginning of this chapter.

TABLE 19.12

Exercise Prescription for Clients With Hyperlipidemia

Mode	Intensity/frequency/duration	Guidelines/concerns
Aerobic conditioning	• 3-7 days/week (preferably at least 5 days/week) • Can begin with 2 daily sessions of 20-30 min each • Eventual goal: 40-60 minutes/day • 40-70% of functional capacity (either % of $\dot{V}O_2max$ or % of peak $\dot{V}O_2$) • Can monitor intensity via RPE (11-16 on a 6-20 scale)	• Obesity may limit exercise type • Initially emphasize increasing duration rather than increasing intensity to optimize caloric expenditure

Adapted from ACSM 2003.

Metabolic Syndrome

Many persons have a cluster of major cardiac risk factors and abdominal obesity that constitute a condition called the **metabolic syndrome**. This syndrome has also been referred to as syndrome X, dyslipidemic hypertension, and insulin resistance syndrome. People with the metabolic syndrome are at increased risk for developing diabetes mellitus and CVD, as well as increased mortality from CVD and other illnesses. The *Third Report of the Expert Panel on Detection, Evaluation, and Treatment of High Blood Cholesterol in Adults (Adult Treatment Panel III) Executive Summary* [23] recently provided a consensus definition of this syndrome. Persons having three or more of the following criteria were defined as having the metabolic syndrome [17]:

1. Abdominal obesity: waist circumference >102 centimeters (>40 inches) in men and >88 centimeters (>35 inches) in women
2. Hypertriglyceridemia: ≥150 mg/dL (1.69 $mmol \cdot L^{-1}$)
3. Reduced HDL-cholesterol: <40 mg/dL (1.04 $mmol \cdot L^{-1}$) in men and <50 mg/dL (1.29 $mmol \cdot L^{-1}$) in women
4. Elevated blood pressure: ≥130/85 mmHg
5. Elevated fasting glucose:≥110 mg/dL (≥6.1 $mmol \cdot L^{-1}$)

The overall prevalence of the metabolic syndrome is approximately 22%, and it increases with age [21]. Poor blood glucose regulation, due to insulin resistance, has been proposed as the underlying cause of this syndrome. Insulin is an important hormone that stimulates the cells of the body to take in glucose from the blood. Insulin does this by binding with specific receptor sites on the cells' surfaces. People with the metabolic syndrome typically have **hyperinsulinemia,** which means high levels of insulin in the blood. Insulin levels appear to be high because of insulin resistance, which means that the cells are not responding appropriately to insulin. Insulin receptors become less numerous and less sensitive to insulin, so the insulin stays in the blood rather than binding to the cells. Meanwhile, blood glucose levels remain high as well, since the receptors are not letting insulin help the glucose get into the cells.

People with metabolic syndrome often have the "apple-shaped" or android body type, which is characterized by high amounts of fat in the trunk and abdomen. Researchers have found that abdominal fat cells deposit high amounts of triglycerides into the bloodstream. The nearby liver then takes up this fat and produces very low density lipoprotein (VLDL) molecules, which transport triglycerides to the cells of the body. Upon losing the triglycerides, VLDLs convert into low density lipoproteins (LDLs). It is the LDL molecule that carries large amounts of cholesterol and deposits the cholesterol around the body. Therefore, high levels of LDLs are associated with an increased risk of coronary heart disease and stroke due to the progression of atherosclerosis. The elevation in triglycerides is also believed to disrupt blood glucose regulation. The resulting rise in insulin levels may, in turn, stimulate sympathetic nervous system regulation, which increases blood pressure. The combination of these conditions results in the following unhealthy "total package" called the metabolic syndrome: high blood glucose, high blood lipids, hypertension, and abdominal obesity.

Like coronary heart disease, the metabolic syndrome usually develops slowly and even several years before the affected individual meets the criteria for medical intervention. Unfortunately, people with abnormal levels of glucose, blood pressure, fat, and blood lipids are at high risk for developing heart disease and strokes. People with abdominal obesity or a family history of diabetes should be especially vigilant for the early signs of metabolic syndrome development.

The metabolic syndrome has both a genetic and a behavioral component. Family history increases one's risk for developing this syndrome in addition to cigarette smoking, a sedentary lifestyle, alcohol consumption, a poor diet, and stress. Early intervention that includes weight loss through dietary modification and enhanced physical activity can significantly delay or prevent the development of this syndrome.

Early intervention that includes weight loss through dietary modification and enhanced physical activity can significantly delay or prevent the development of the metabolic syndrome.

Exercise is the first line of treatment for the metabolic syndrome because it influences all components of this disorder. Regular physical activity helps reduce excess body fat. Exercise also improves the sensitivity of the cells to insulin, thus normalizing blood insulin levels and decreasing blood glucose levels. Exercise also helps to decrease blood pressure, in addition to increasing HDL-cholesterol levels. Personal trainers should be sure to work in conjunction with the client's physician and a registered dietitian in order to ensure the client's success in dealing with the various conditions of the metabolic syndrome.

Diabetes Mellitus

Diabetes mellitus refers to a group of metabolic diseases that are characterized by an excessively high (or uncontrolled) blood glucose level. Some of the signs and symptoms of diabetes include

- increased frequency of urination,
- increased thirst,
- increased appetite, and
- general weakness.

The diagnosis of diabetes mellitus is based on two fasting glucose levels of 126 mg/dL or higher. Other options for diagnosis include two 2-hour **postprandial** (i.e., after a meal) plasma glucose measurements of 200 mg/dL or higher after a glucose load of 75 grams or two casual glucose readings of 200 mg/dL. Chronic uncontrolled diabetes is associated with long-term damage to various body organs including the eyes, kidneys, nerves, heart, and blood vessels. Diabetes is the leading cause of blindness, renal failure, and lower extremity amputations.

Types of Diabetes

The major types of diabetes mellitus are type 1, type 2, and gestational. **Type 1 diabetes mellitus,** formerly known as "insulin-dependent diabetes mellitus" (IDDM), is associated with pancreatic beta cell destruction by an autoimmune process, usually leading to absolute insulin deficiency. Approximately 10% of patients with diabetes have type 1, and most of these people develop the disease before the age of 25. Exogenous insulin by either injection or pump is required for survival. People with uncontrolled or newly diagnosed type 1 diabetes are prone to developing diabetic ketoacidosis. Diabetic ketoacidosis is a metabolic acidosis caused by the accumulation of **ketones** due to severely depressed insulin levels. The initial symptoms are frequent urination, nausea, vomiting, abdominal pain, and lethargy. Untreated individuals may progress to coma.

Type 2 diabetes mellitus, was formerly referred to as non-insulin-dependent diabetes mellitus (NIDDM) and is characterized by insulin resistance in peripheral tissues and an insulin secretory deficit of the pancreatic beta cells. This is the most common form of diabetes mellitus (composing about 90% of cases of diabetes) and is highly associated with a family history of diabetes, older age, obesity, and lack of exercise. The treatment for type 2 diabetes usually includes diet modification, weight control, regular exercises, and oral hypoglycemic agents.

Gestational diabetes mellitus is a condition in which the glucose level is elevated and other diabetic symptoms appear during pregnancy in women who have not previously been diagnosed with diabetes. Gestational diabetes is not caused by a lack of insulin, but by insulin resistance. All diabetic symptoms usually disappear following delivery, but affected mothers are at increased risk of developing type 2 diabetes mellitus later in life. Approximately 2% to 5% of all pregnant women in the United States are diagnosed with gestational diabetes. Treatment for gestational diabetes includes special diet, exercise, and insulin injections.

Exercise Prescription and Program Design for Clients With Diabetes Mellitus

Exercise is an essential component of diabetic management. In both types of diabetes mellitus, exercise can increase insulin sensitivity and glucose utilization, thus lowering blood glucose levels. In addition, regular physical activity reduces other risk factors related to CVD such as hypertension, dyslipidemia, and obesity. Although exercise is highly beneficial for clients with diabetes, there are some potential complications, such as **hypoglycemia** (blood glucose level of 65 mg/dL or lower), that the personal trainer needs to keep in mind when designing and supervising an exercise program [11].

Before beginning an exercise program, clients with diabetes should have a medical evaluation to assess their glycemic control and to screen for any complications that may be exacerbated by exercise. Stress cardiac testing performed by a medical professional is also generally recommended for all clients with diabetes who are planning to engage in moderate-intensity exercise and are considered at risk for heart disease. This group includes clients who are older than 35 years, those with type 2 diabetes of more than 10 years' duration, those with type 1 diabetes of more than 15 years' duration, and those with evidence of microvascular disease (retinopathy or nephropathy) [11].

Individuals exhibiting organ damage from longstanding diabetes need to be careful and to abstain from certain exacerbating physical activities. For example, individuals with peripheral neuropathy are at an increased risk of ulceration and infection of the feet because of lack of sensation and decreased healing reaction. Therefore, in this condition, low-impact exercises, such as swimming and biking, may be preferable to walking and jogging. Also proper footwear—shoes that are comfortable and well fitted—is essential to prevent blisters and other foot injuries. Any dizziness, weakness, or shortness of breath should alert the personal trainer to the possibility of cardiac disease and the need for a medical evaluation. Contraindications to exercise for persons with diabetes are listed in table 19.13.

Glycemic Control

The principal risk of exercise among those who have diabetes is hypoglycemia (blood glucose level of 65 mg/dL or lower). This is of greater concern for patients who have type 1 diabetes than for those who have type 2.

Factors that predispose to hypoglycemia during exercise include

- increased exercise intensity,
- longer exercise time,
- inadequate caloric intake prior to exercise,
- excessive insulin dose,
- insulin injection into exercising muscle, and
- colder environmental temperatures.

The mechanism for exercise-induced hypoglycemia is related to the fact that exercise enhances the absorption of exogenous insulin, increases the

TABLE 19.13

Contraindications to Exercise for Clients With Diabetes
Blood glucose >250 mg/dL and ketones in urine for type 1 diabetes
Blood glucose >300 mg/dL without ketones
Clients with proliferative retinopathy should avoid strenuous high-intensity activities
Severe kidney disease
Clients with a loss of protective sensation in the feet (peripheral neuropathy) should avoid outdoor walking and jogging. Swimming or biking is recommended.
Acute illness, infection, or fever
Evidence of underlying cardiovascular disease that has not been medically evaluated

muscle uptake of glucose, and impairs the mobilization of glucose in blood. Signs of hypoglycemia include apparent loss of concentration, shaking or shivering, sweating, tachycardia, and loss of consciousness. See table 19.14 for a comprehensive list of the signs and symptoms of hypoglycemia.

TABLE 19.14

Signs and Symptoms of Hypoglycemia
Sweating
Hunger
Palpitations
Headache
Tachycardia
Anxiety
Tremor
Dizziness
Blurred vision
Confusion
Convulsion
Syncope
Coma

Personal trainers working with clients who have diabetes should know how to recognize the signs of hypoglycemia and be able to manage hypoglycemia cases with glucose or fructose foods and drinks when affected individuals are unable to treat themselves. See table 19.15 for a recommended response to hypoglycemia. Clients with diabetes should always wear a medical alert identification bracelet where it can be seen easily in case of a hypoglycemic reaction [14].

Blood glucose measurements using portable glucose monitors are an essential part of the exercise prescription. Clients should monitor their blood sugar before and after exercise, and during prolonged exercise every 30 minutes. According to the American Diabetes Association, people with diabetes should not exercise if their glucose level is greater than 300 mg/dL or greater than 250 mg/dL with urinary ketones [4]. Exercising at these levels can worsen the hyperglycemia and promote ketosis and acidosis. On the other hand, individuals with pre-exercise glucose levels below 100 mg/dL are at risk of developing hypoglycemia during or after exercise; therefore they should ingest a carbohydrate snack before exercise.

Adjustment of medication dosage, either insulin or oral hypoglycemic drugs, as well as proper timing of meals, is the key for maintaining good glycemic control during physical activity. Exercise should be generally scheduled one to two hours after a meal, or when the hypoglycemic medication is not at its peak activity. After exercise, carbohydrate stores

TABLE 19.15

Responding to a Client Who Has Hypoglycemia
Consider dialing 911.
Immediate treatment with carbohydrate is essential.
Measure blood glucose level with glucose monitor device (if available).
If the blood glucose level is below 70 mg/dL or the client is known to have diabetes and is having signs or symptoms of hypoglycemia, provide 15 g of carbohydrate, which is equivalent to: • about 3 or 4 glucose tablets • 1/2 cup of regular soft drink or fruit juice • about 6 saltine crackers • 1 tablespoon of sugar or honey
Wait about 15 minutes and remeasure glucose level. If the level remains under 70 mg/dL, provide with another 15 g of carbohydrate. Repeat testing and giving food or tablets until blood glucose level rises above 70 mg/dL.

should be replenished according to the duration and intensity of the activity. The client's physician will direct the patient's insulin use. This is normally done in conjunction with a dietitian to ensure that a hypoglycemic event does not occur. The personal trainer is in no way to give advice to the client about the use of insulin or the timing of meals. Should the client experience regular episodes of lack of blood glucose control, the client should be sent back to his or her physician for care.

Finally, each client with diabetes has his or her own metabolic response to exercise. No general guideline can take the place of intelligent self-observation and regular glucose monitoring in developing an individualized plan to facilitate safe, enjoyable exercise. Guidelines for aerobic conditioning and resistance exercise are shown in table 19.16.

Aerobic Conditioning

Exercise prescription for clients with diabetes should include aerobic physical activity with a minimum frequency of four to six days a week, for 20 to 60 minutes at 40% to 70% of $\dot{V}O_2max$ [2, 3]. People who are unconditioned can perform exercise at a lower intensity level for a longer duration, at least until they achieve a higher level of fitness. Exercise sessions should begin with a low-intensity warm-up and stretching of the muscle to be exercised and should conclude with a cool-down period. These activities ease the cardiovascular transition between rest and exercise and help prevent muscle and joint injuries. Clients should also be instructed to work to voluntary fatigue, not to exhaustion.

Resistance Training

The recommendation for resistance training is two to three days a week, with sessions including at least one set of each of 8 to 10 different exercises using the major muscle groups. Each set should consist of 8 to 12 repetitions, with the amount of weight increased when the individual can complete 12 or more repetitions. For clients with diabetes who are older than 50 or who have other health conditions such as hypertension, more repetitions (12 to 15) at a lower weight may be more suitable [2, 27].

TABLE 19.16

Exercise Prescription for Clients With Diabetes

Mode	Intensity/frequency/duration	Guidelines/concerns
Aerobic conditioning	• 4-6 days/week (or daily) • Eventual goal: 20-60 minutes/day • 40-70% $\dot{V}O_2max$ • Monitor intensity via RPE, especially if the client is taking a heart rate-altering medication	• A snack may be needed before exercise • Monitor blood glucose before and after exercise • Include a 5-10 minute warm-up and cool-down period
Resistance training	• 2-3 nonconsecutive days/week • 1-3 sets, 10-15 repetitions/set (or more, with a lower weight, for more untrained or older clients) • Up to 8-10 exercises	• Can begin with body weight exercises and progress to free weights and resistance machines • Clients with well-controlled diabetes can progress to strength training (i.e., higher loads, fewer repetitions)
Flexibility training	• Minimum of 2-3 sessions/week • Hold static stretches for 10-30 seconds	

Adapted from ACSM 2003.

CONCLUSION

Personal trainers play a valuable role in helping clients with obesity, eating disorders, hyperlipidemia, and diabetes to achieve fitness and health goals through adherence to a healthy diet and a well-designed exercise program. Personal trainers should strongly consider the value of working in conjunction with the client's physician and with a dietitian in order to ensure the client's success. In so doing, a personal trainer can play a significant role in the client's health care team.

STUDY QUESTIONS

1. Based on his calculated BMI, which of the following is the disease risk of a client who is male; 5 feet, 9 inches tall (175 centimeters); weighs 198 pounds (90 kilograms); and has a waist circumference of 41 inches (104 centimeters)?
   A. no risk
   B. increased
   C. high
   D. very high
2. All of the following are dietary modifications or goals that can apply to all clients who are overweight or obese EXCEPT:
   A. set a weight loss goal of 10% of body weight over the first six months
   B. change food selections that will decrease caloric and fat intake
   C. aim for a 1 to 2 pound (0.45-0.9 kilogram) weight loss per week
   D. follow a 1,200 kcal/day food plan
3. Which of the following is an undesirable blood lipid level?
   I. total cholesterol: 250 mg/dL
   II. triglycerides: 200 mg/dL
   III. LDLs: 100 mg/dL
   IV. HDLs: 50 mg/dL

   A. I only
   B. I and II only
   C. II and III only
   D. III and IV only
4. Which of the following describes a difference between type 1 and type 2 diabetes?
   A. only clients with type 1 diabetes can have gestational diabetes
   B. clients with type 1 diabetes are more prevalent
   C. clients with type 2 diabetes can produce insulin
   D. only clients with type 2 diabetes can receive exogenous insulin

APPLIED KNOWLEDGE QUESTION

Provide dietary modifications, exercise program guidelines, and lifestyle change support suggestions for a client who is obese.

REFERENCES

1. American College of Sports Medicine. 1997. Position stand: Female athlete triad. *Medicine and Science in Sports and Exercise* 29: i-ix.
2. American College of Sports Medicine. 2000. *ACSM's Guidelines for Exercise Testing and Prescription*. Philadelphia: Lippincott Williams & Wilkins.

3. American College of Sports Medicine. 2001. *ACSM's Resource Manual for Guidelines for Exercise Testing and Prescription.* Philadelphia: Lippincott Williams & Wilkins.
4. American Diabetes Association. 2002. Position statement: Diabetes mellitus and exercise. *Diabetes Care* 25 (Suppl 1): S64. http://www.diabetes.org.
5. American Psychiatric Association. 1994. *Diagnostic and Statistical Manual of Mental Disorders* [DSMV IV], 4th ed. Washington, DC: APA.
6. Baker, C., and K.D. Brownwell. 2000. Physical activity and maintenance of weight loss: Physiological and psychological mechanisms. In: *Physical Activity and Obesity,* C. Bouchard, ed. Champaign, IL: Human Kinetics, pp. 311-328.
7. Berg, A., I. Frey, M.W. Baumstark, H. Halle, and J. Keul. 1994. Physical activity and lipoprotein lipid disorders. *Sports Medicine* 17 (1): 6-21.
8. Blair, S.N., J.B. Kampert, H.W. Kohl, C.E. Barlow, C.A. Macera, R.S. Paffenbarger, and L.W. Gibbons. 1996. Influences of cardiorespiratory fitness and other precursors on cardiovascular disease and all-cause mortality in men and women. *Journal of the American Medical Association* 276 (3): 205-210.
9. Blair, S., and M.Z. Nichaman. 2002. The public health problem of increasing prevalence rates of obesity and what should be done about it. *Mayo Clinic Proceedings* 77: 109-113.
10. Bouchard, C. 2000. Introduction. In: *Physical Activity and Obesity,* C. Bouchard, ed. Champaign, IL: Human Kinetics, pp. 3-19.
11. Colberg, S.R., and D.P. Swain. 2000. Exercise and diabetic control. *Physician and Sportsmedicine* 28 (4): 63-81.
12. Conley, M.S., and R. Rozenek. 2001. National Strength and Conditioning Association position statement: Health aspects of resistance exercise and training. *Strength and Conditioning Journal* 23 (6): 9-23.
13. Despres, J.P., and B. Lamarche. 2000. Physical activity and the metabolic complications of obesity. In: *Physical Activity and Obesity,* C. Bouchard, ed. Champaign, IL: Human Kinetics, pp. 329-354.
14. Drazin, M.B. 2002. Type 1 diabetes and sports participation. *Physician and Sports Medicine* 28 (12): 49-66.
15. Eickhoff-Shemek, J. 2002. Scope of practice. *ACSM's Health and Fitness Journal* 6 (5): 28-31.
16. Flegal, K.M., M.D. Carroll, C.L. Ogden, and C.L. Johnson. 2002. Prevalence and trends in obesity among US adults, 1999-2000. *Journal of the American Medical Association* 288: 1723-1727.
17. Ford, E.S., W.H. Giles, and W.H. Dietz. 2002. Prevalence of the metabolic syndrome among US adults: Findings from the Third National Health and Nutrition Examination Survey. *Journal of the American Medical Association* 287: 356-359.
18. Kokkinos, P.F., and B. Fernhall. 1999. Physical activity and high density lipoprotein cholesterol levels. *Sports Medicine* 28:307-314.
19. B. Ludovise, B. 1992. Eating disorders: Toll on the body. *Los Angeles Times* December 6.
20. Magrann, S., and S. Radford Keagy. 2001. *Weight Control and Eating Disorders.* Eureka, CA: Nutrition Dimension.
21. National Institutes of Health and National Heart, Lung, and Blood Institute. 1998. *Clinical Guidelines on the Identification, Evaluation, and Treatment of Overweight and Obesity in Adults Executive Summary.* NIH Pub. No. 98-4083. Retrieved January 13, 2003, from www.nhlbi.nih.gov/guidelines/obesity/ob_gdlns.pdf.
22. National Institutes of Health and National Heart, Lung, and Blood Institute. 2000. *The Practical Guide: Identification, Evaluation, and Treatment of Overweight and Obesity in Adults.* NIH Pub. No. 00-4084. Retrieved November 21, 2002, from www.nhlbi.nih.gov/guidelines/obesity/prctgd_c.pdf.
23. National Institutes of Health and National Heart, Lung, and Blood Institute. 2001. *Third Report of the Expert Panel on Detection, Evaluation, and Treatment of High Blood Cholesterol in Adults (Adult Treatment Panel III) Executive Summary.* NIH Pub. No. 01-3670. Retrieved November 21, 2002, from http://www.nhlbi.nih.gov/guidelines/cholesterol/atp3xsum.pdf.
24. National Task Force on the Prevention and Treatment of Obesity, National Institutes of Health. 1993. Very low-calorie diets. *Journal of the American Medical Association* 270: 967-974.
25. Otis, C., and R. Goldingay. 2000. *The Athletic Woman's Survival Guide.* Champaign, IL: Human Kinetics.
26. Pate, R.R., M. Pratt, S.N. Blair, W.L. Haskell, C.A. Macera, C. Bouchard, D. Buchner, W. Ettinger, G.W. Heath, A.C. King. 1995. Physical activity and public health: A recommendation from the Centers for Disease Control and Prevention and the American College of Sports Medicine. *Journal of the American Medical Association* 273: 402-407.
27. Pollock, M.L., B.A. Franklin, G.J. Balady, B.L. Chaitman, J.L. Fleg, B. Fletcher, M. Limacher, I. Piña, R.A. Stein, M. Williams, and T. Bazzarre. 2000. AHA Science Advisory. Resistance exercise in individuals with and without cardiovascular disease: Benefits, rationale, safety, and prescription. *Circulation* 101 (7): 828-833.
28. Pronk, N.P., and R.R. Wing. 1994. Physical activity and long-term maintenance of weight loss. *Obesity Research* 2: 587-599.
29. Storlie, J., and H.A. Jordan, eds. 1984. *Behavioral Management of Obesity.* Champaign, IL: Human Kinetics.
30. Troiano, R.P., K.M. Flegal, R.J. Kuczmarski, S.M. Campbell, and C.L. Johnson. 1995. Overweight prevalence and trends for children and adolescents. The National Health and Nutrition Examination Surveys, 1963 to 1991. *Archives of Pediatrics and Adolescent Medicine* 149: 1085-1091.
31. U.S. Department of Health and Human Services. 1996. Historical background, terminology, evolution of recommendations, and measurement, Appendix B, NIH consensus conference statement, p. 47. In: *Physical Activity and Health: A Report of the Surgeon General.* Atlanta: U.S. Department of Health and Human Services, Centers for Disease Control and Prevention, National Center for Chronic Disease Prevention and Health Promotion.
32. Vega, C.L. 1991. Taking small steps . . . to big changes. *IDEA Today* 2: 20-22.
33. Vega, C.L. 2001. Nutrition. In *Aquatic Fitness Instructor Fitness Manual.* Nokomis, FL: Aquatic Exercise Association.
34. Wadden, T.A., G.D. Forester, and K.A. Letizia. 1994. One-year behavioral treatment of obesity: Comparison of moderate and severe caloric restriction and the effects of weight maintenance therapy. *Journal of Consulting and Clinical Psychology* 621: 165-171.
35. World Health Organization. 1998. *Obesity: Preventing and Managing the Global Epidemic.* Report of a WHO Consultation on Obesity. Geneva: World Health Organization.

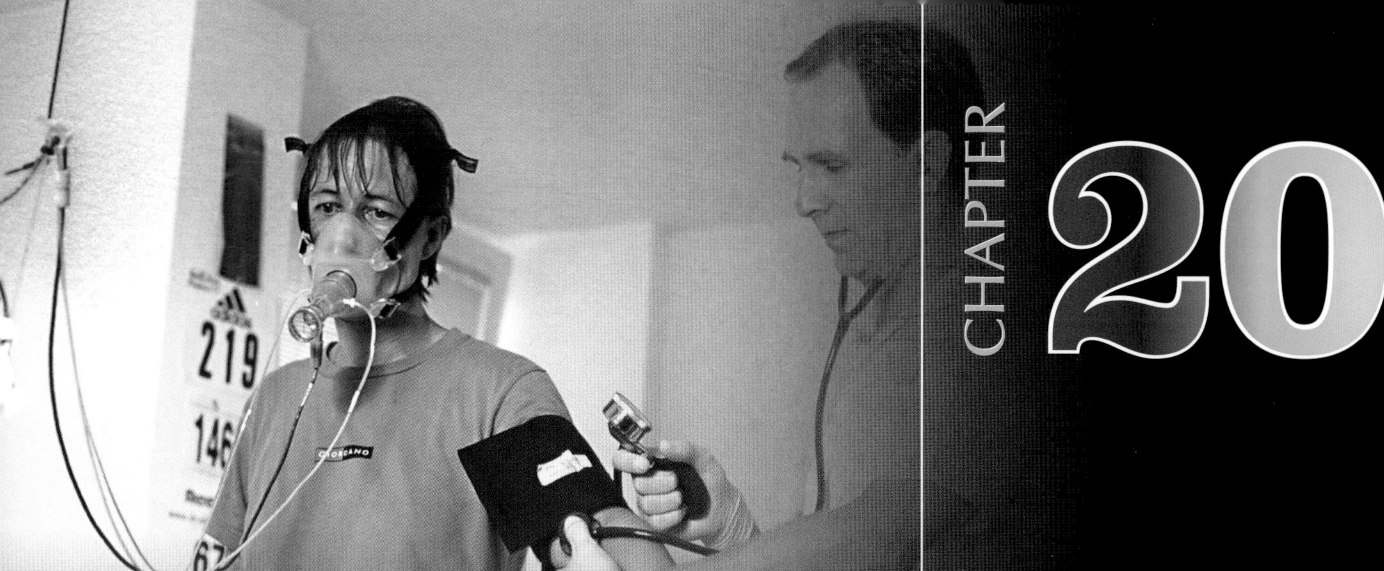

CHAPTER 20

Clients With Cardiovascular and Respiratory Conditions

Robert Watine

After completing this chapter, you will be able to

- understand the pathophysiology and risk factors for hypertension, myocardial infarction, cerebrovascular accident, peripheral vascular disease, asthma, and exercise-induced asthma;
- understand the stages of the various diseases and how exercise can be used to enhance the client's quality of life; and
- know when it is appropriate to refer a client to a medical professional.

Cardiovascular and respiratory diseases present a challenge not only to the traditional health care provider, but also to the personal trainer. Hypertension is a major risk factor for cardiovascular disease, with myocardial infarctions (heart attacks) and cerebrovascular accidents (strokes) the most common cardiovascular diseases that personal trainers will encounter. In addition, this chapter includes information about training clients with peripheral vascular disease, as such clients can benefit a great deal from light-intensity aerobic conditioning.

Respiratory disease in general is a topic well beyond the scope of this chapter. However, the chapter does address asthma and exercise-induced asthma, both of which are commonly seen in personal training clients. The rehabilitation and training programs of the chronic lung patient need to be overseen by a respiratory rehabilitation specialist, whose level of training is beyond that of a personal trainer.

To properly guide, educate, and train cardiovascular and respiratory patients, the personal trainer must understand the pathophysiology of the disease and be able to recognize the early signs of inadequate blood circulation and labored breathing during training. This said, personal trainers can have a dramatic positive impact on the quality of life for their clients, as long as they pay careful attention to their clients. Additionally, it is important for the personal trainer to approach the exercise regimen as part of a team, with the physician as the leader. Any client who has a medical condition or disease should receive clearance from his or her physician. Of course, liability waivers should be signed by all parties to provide as much protection as possible should issues of liability ever arise (see chapter 25).

Hypertension

Hypertension is a disease of not just the old, but of the young also [25, 26, 27]. Over 50 million Americans age 6 and above have this disease, defined by a systolic reading of 140+ mmHg (millimeters of mercury) and/or a diastolic reading of 90+ mmHg [2]. Hypertension is an idiopathic disease, which means that it occurs without a known etiology (cause). This is why hypertension is considered the "silent killer." No person, not even a doctor, can look at 10 people in a room and pick out who has the disease and who does not. Ninety percent of cases are idiopathic. It is the other 10% that are curable because they are due to secondary causes, that is, other diseases.

Those secondary causes include hyperthyroidism, pheochromocytoma, hypercortisolism, hyperaldosteronism, and renal artery stenosis. Each of these diseases has subclassifications that are tangential to this discussion. However, the important point is twofold: (1) anyone under the age of 35 with hypertension needs to be aggressively evaluated for one of these diagnoses (to be performed by a doctor); and (2) any client observed to be hypertensive must be referred to a doctor for further evaluation and treatment. It has been found that those newly diagnosed with hypertension who are under 35 years have a greater incidence of the secondary causes.

Elevated blood pressure puts an individual at risk for a heart attack, stroke, or both. Mildly elevated blood pressure (over time) can lead to kidney disease and generalized vascular disease. People cannot determine how high their blood pressure is based on how they feel. If a person truly were to perceive his or her blood pressure to be high, it would most likely be in the range of a hypertensive crisis with associated chest pains, visual blurring, neurologic deficits, or some combination of these.

Blood pressure risk stratification is shown in table 20.1. The stages are stratified into three risk groups: A, B, and C. The groups are based on the presence of major risk factors (e.g., smoking, dyslipidemia, diabetes mellitus, age greater than 60, men and postmenopausal women, and a family history), as well as target organ damage (TOD) and clinical cardiovascular disease (CCD). Any client with Stage 1 or greater readings should not begin an exercise program until a physician has his or her pressure controlled and has cleared the person for exercise [4, 6].

Target organ damage includes cardiac, brain, kidney, peripheral vascular, and retinal disease. Target organ cardiac disease refers to left ventricular thickening or hypertrophy due to untreated or inadequately treated hypertension, a history of exertional chest pain or angina, history of having had a heart attack, having had reperfusion surgery (i.e., coronary bypass, stenting, or balloon angioplasty), and overall cardiac dysfunction (failure). Stroke and peripheral vascular disease have pathophysiology similar to coronary artery disease. Kidney disease results in glomerular dysfunction, leading to the kidneys' inability to cleanse the blood, as well as affecting blood flow to and from the kidney, which can lead to hypertension as well. Retinal disease is a function of hemorrhages from high blood pressure,

TABLE 20.1

The JNC VI Guide to Prevention and Treatment of Hypertension Recommendations

Blood pressure stages (systolic/diastolic in mmHg)	Risk group A No major risk factors* No TOD/CCD**	Risk group B At least one major risk factor (not including diabetes) No TOD/CCD	Risk group C TOD/CCD and/or diabetes, with or without other risk factors
High normal (130-139/85-89)	Lifestyle modification	Lifestyle modification	Drug therapy for those with heart failure, renal insufficiency, or diabetes Lifestyle modification
Stage 1 (140-159/90-99)	Lifestyle modification (up to 12 months)	Lifestyle modification (up to six months) For patients with multiple risk factors, clinicians should consider drugs as initial therapy plus lifestyle modification	Drug therapy Lifestyle modification
Stages 2 and 3 (≥160/≥100)	Drug therapy Lifestyle modification	Drug therapy Lifestyle modification	Drug therapy Lifestyle modification
Goal blood pressure values			
<140/90 mmHg		People with uncomplicated hypertension, risk group A, risk group B, risk group C (except as specified below)	
<130/85 mmHg		People with diabetes, renal failure, heart failure	
<125/75 mmHg		People with renal failure with proteinuria	

*Risk factors: smoking, dyslipidemia, diabetes mellitus, age greater than 60, men and postmenopausal women, and a family history.

**TOD/CCD = target organ damage/clinical cardiovascular disease. TOD/CCD includes heart diseases (e.g., left ventricular hypertrophy, angina/prior heart attack, prior coronary artery bypass graft, heart failure), stroke, nephropathy, peripheral arterial disease, hypertensive retinopathy.

Adapted from the NIH 1997.

thereby affecting eyesight with the potential for the development of blindness.

A client with high normal readings in Group A (no major risk factors; no TOD or CCD) is treated with lifestyle modification. The same applies to Group B (at least one major risk factor, not including diabetes; no TOD or CCD). Group C has TOD/CCD, diabetes, or both, with or without other risk factors, thereby necessitating physician intervention for treatment and clearance.

Clients with Stage 1 or greater readings (≤140/≤90) should not be trained until their blood pressure is controlled and a physician has cleared them for exercise.

Management of Hypertension

Lifestyle modification for clients with hypertension includes the nonpharmacologic interventions, for example proper exercise, weight loss, and dietary changes. General lifestyle changes include adequate amount of sleep, reduction in daily sodium intake to 1 teaspoon of salt daily, adequate potassium intake, weight loss if needed, limiting alcohol intake, increasing aerobic activity to 30 to 45 minutes four or more days per week, reducing dietary saturated fat and cholesterol, and the cessation of smoking.

The DASH diet has received a great deal of favorable publicity for lowering blood pressure. It entails reducing saturated fats, cholesterol, and total fat intake. Emphasis is on more fruits, vegetables, and low-fat dairy products; more whole grain products, fish, poultry, and nuts; reduction in red meat, sweets, and sugar-containing beverages; and an increase in foods rich in magnesium, potassium, calcium, protein, and fiber.

Clients with hypertension will be taking one or more of a multitude of medications. The classes of medications include **beta-blockers, calcium channel blockers, ACE (angiotensin converting enzyme) inhibitors, ARBs (angiotensin receptor blockers), diuretics,** and **alpha-blockers.** The exact mechanisms of action of these medications are beyond the scope of this chapter except for the fact that they all lower blood pressure. Diuretics cause volume depletion. However, the personal trainer should never restrict the client's use of fluids or worry about their use of electrolyte solutions. Alpha-, beta-, and calcium channel blockers cause vasodilation with the potential for blood pooling. Angiotensin converting enzyme inhibitors and the ARBs exert their effects on the kidneys' vasculature. These medications can cause blood pooling, which necessitates a longer period for cool-down, especially after treadmill walking, jogging, and circuit weight training. Additionally, beta-blockers not only slow the heart rate, but also prevent the heart rate from elevating as a normal response to exercise. This makes it difficult to follow heart rate as a measure of intensity and necessitates use of the rating of perceived exertion (RPE) scale.

Safety Considerations for Clients With Hypertension

What is most promising for the client and exciting for the personal trainer is that the client with *controlled* hypertension can exercise with limited restrictions. Simple precautions need only to be maintained to allow for the application of all modalities. There are numerous benefits of exercise to the body, but from a specific cardiovascular perspective and its relationship to hypertension, several studies have shown significant reductions in resting blood pressure after long-term exercise. A review of the literature by meta-analysis revealed approximate decreases in systolic and diastolic pressures of 4.5/3.8 mmHg and 4.7/3.1 mmHg, respectively, due to long-term resistance and aerobic training [7, 9, 12, 13, 14, 15, 16, 17, 18]. The questions now to be raised are as follows:

1. At what intensity level can a client be placed in order to cause the desired response?
2. Are any exercises contraindicated?
3. What exercises can be given to the client?

Clients with *controlled* hypertension can exercise with limited restrictions.

Intensity

Since it has been shown that a positive training adaptation to exercise, that is, lowered resting blood pressure, can be reached by training at intensities of 40% to 50% maximal oxygen uptake [5, 24], the personal trainer can design a program that will cause the adaptation without increasing the risk for the client. According to research, low-intensity exercise appears to be a more effective stimulus than moderate-intensity exercise training in reducing resting blood pressure and blood pressure responses to stress.

This is important because often a client comes with medical clearance for exercise but the personal trainer believes that the client is not in "condition" to embark on a strenuous program. The personal trainer can now feel secure in beginning a low-intensity program with such a client because the training will be at a level that will not unduly stress the physiology or cause an increased risk of an acute cardiac or neurologic event (figure 20.1) [5].

Contraindications

As for which exercises are contraindicated, these include any type of activity that would increase intrathoracic pressure, thereby decreasing blood flow return to the heart, with a corresponding decrease in cardiac output. Essentially this means any exercise with an associated prolonged Valsalva maneuver (greater than one to two seconds). The burden is on the personal trainer to be certain not only that the client is performing the exercise in a technically

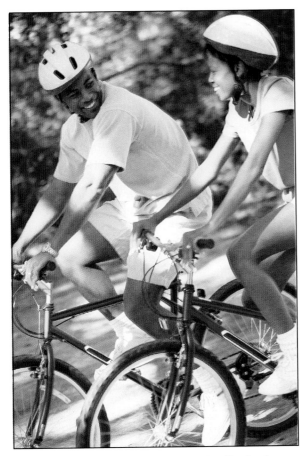

Figure 20.1 Low-intensity exercise is effective in reducing resting blood pressure.

correct manner, but also that he or she is breathing properly (see chapter 13 for more breathing guidelines).

Safe Exercises

Clients with controlled hypertension may participate in many types of training including, but not limited to, the use of free weights, weight machines, body weight, elastic bands [3]; aerobic exercise (walking, jogging, swimming); and circuit weight training. Essentially all exercises are permissible. If a client with hypertension has a comorbid condition, however, the choice of exercise may be altered or restricted [30].

Comorbid conditions include the following:

1. Musculoskeletal conditions or diseases: degenerative joint diseases, rheumatologic diseases
2. Neurologic disorders: strokes, myasthenia gravis, muscular dystrophy
3. Vascular diseases: carotid artery disease, cardiac conditions, aneurysms

Exercise Guidelines for Clients With Hypertension

If the blood pressure is Stage 1, it is imperative to cancel the exercise session and advise the client to speak with his or her doctor. If the client is typically **normotensive**, reschedule the session and recheck before the next exercise session as previously discussed.

Aerobic Conditioning

The goals of an aerobic program are to increase the $\dot{V}O_2$max as well as the ventilatory threshold (which will increase the time before "shortness of breath" is perceived) [28]. Additionally, the client will see an increase in both maximal workload and endurance levels. Caloric expenditure will be greater, and this will facilitate greater weight reduction (if needed). Finally, a low- to moderate-intensity program will achieve the goal of lowered blood pressure, that is, lifestyle modification [21].

It is advised that the intensity level begin at 40% to 50% $\dot{V}O_2$max, ultimately attaining 50% to 85% $\dot{V}O_2$max [2]. The RPE initially should be 8 to 10 (on the 6-20 scale), with a goal range of 11 to 13 (on the 6-20 scale). Each session should last between 15 and 30 minutes with a target of 30 to 60 minutes, and the frequency should be three to seven days per week. The weekly caloric expenditure will be between 700 and 2,000 kilocalories.

The time necessary to achieve these goals is four to six months. However, as in all cases, each program must be individualized.

Resistance Training

As for the remainder of the program, it should include some form of resistance exercise [19]. To maintain consistency, clients should begin with a repetition range from 16 to 20 per set. This would yield about 50% to 60% of the 1RM, thereby keeping the client within the same guidelines for aerobic intensity [2].

The rest interval initially should be two to three minutes (or longer) to allow the client to fully recover between sets. This will allow for physiologic compensation from the exercise, necessary especially in view of the potential use of prescription medications for hypertension control [20]. The client can do as few as one set per exercise, with a maximum of three per exercise, at the beginning of the program. As for the types of exercise performed, large-muscle, multijoint movements are the safest choice at the beginning.

Over time (i.e., four to six months), the number of repetitions can decrease to the 8- to 12-repetition range. Exercise frequency should be two to three times a week, with a duration between 30 and 60 minutes per session.

Goals for Clients With Hypertension

- Increase $\dot{V}O_2$max and ventilatory threshold.
- Increase maximal work and endurance.
- Increase caloric expenditure.
- Control blood pressure.
- Increase muscular endurance.

Myocardial Infarction, Stroke, and Peripheral Vascular Disease

Myocardial infarction (MI), stroke, and **peripheral vascular disease** (PVD) all have very serious ramifications for a client's physiology as well as his or her psychology [22, 23]. Physiologically, known disease is present, and thus also are true deficiencies or deficits in their body. Beyond the physiologic effect there are true psychological problems whether the client realizes them consciously or not. These can manifest themselves in many ways, from a fear of exercise (i.e., fear of the precipitation of another acute event) to the other end of the spectrum of fearlessness on the part of the client. The attitude of "I'll show you, I can beat this thing, I'll just push through the barriers" must also be considered with the client. Thus the personal trainer must actively listen to the client and pay attention to the messages that are being relayed via nonverbal cues and innuendo.

Pathophysiology

The pathophysiology is essentially the same for all three diseases, since they represent the end result of vascular occlusive diseases at various levels of the body, that is, the heart, the brain, or the generalized vascular system [11].

An atheromatous (lipid/cholesterol) plaque forms within the lumen of a blood vessel. Focal inflammation around the area of the plaque occurs, leading to its instability. Over time, a collagen cap develops to stabilize the area, with a subsequent overlaying by smooth muscle cells (the normal inside lining of the blood vessel) (figure 20.2). Depending on the timeline, the outcomes can be very different.

If the collagen cap and smooth muscles grow to a point of stability, the diameter of the blood vessel is dramatically reduced. This results in decreased blood flow with the potential for eddy currents to develop, as well as sludging of the circulation and the development of a thrombus that can either occlude the lumen or break off and flow downstream to occlude a more distal site.

While the collagen cap is still soft and unstable, it can rupture (figure 20.3) and then release all the material within the cap to flow downstream and cause sudden occlusive disease. The situation of the "mature" collagen cap as described in the preceding paragraph makes it more difficult for a rupture to occur and thus is more stable, allowing the body to dissolve the thrombus and thereby prevent it from reaching critical mass. A homeostatic mechanism with antithrombin III provides this protection. The collagen cap rupture is more dangerous, since a sudden release of the intracap material is sent flowing distally to cause a sudden event, that is, acute MI or **cerebrovascular accident** (CVA). The problems associated with the stable collagen cap are more typical of the peripheral circulation, but can also be seen in the coronary arteries, as in **angina** (chest pain).

Risk Factors

Risk factors include hypertension, hypercholesterolemia, diabetes, smoking, obesity, and family history. High blood pressure increases the systemic vascular resistance, which increases the intracardiac pressure within the left ventricle to allow for systole to occur. During systole there is a compression of the cardiac vessels that feed the heart. When the pressure exceeds a certain threshold, there is a decrease in or a lack of flow to the interior of the heart, and thus chest pain occurs. Of course, with corresponding high cholesterol and cap formation, a rupture can occur, causing the same end result. This also can take place in the coronary arteries.

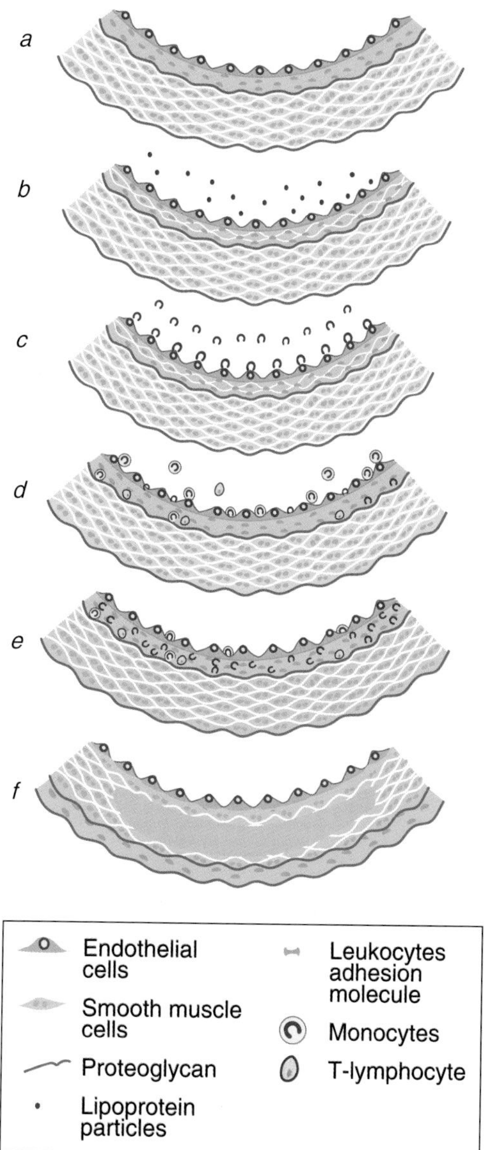

Figure 20.2 Development of a collagen cap. A normal artery *(a)* with the inner-most layer of endothelial cells. As plaque (lipoprotein molecules) accumulates *(b-e)*, a cap or layer of collagen is eventually created and covered by a layer of smooth muscle cells (fibers) *(f)*.
Reprinted from Fauci, Braunwald, Isselbacher, et al. 1998.

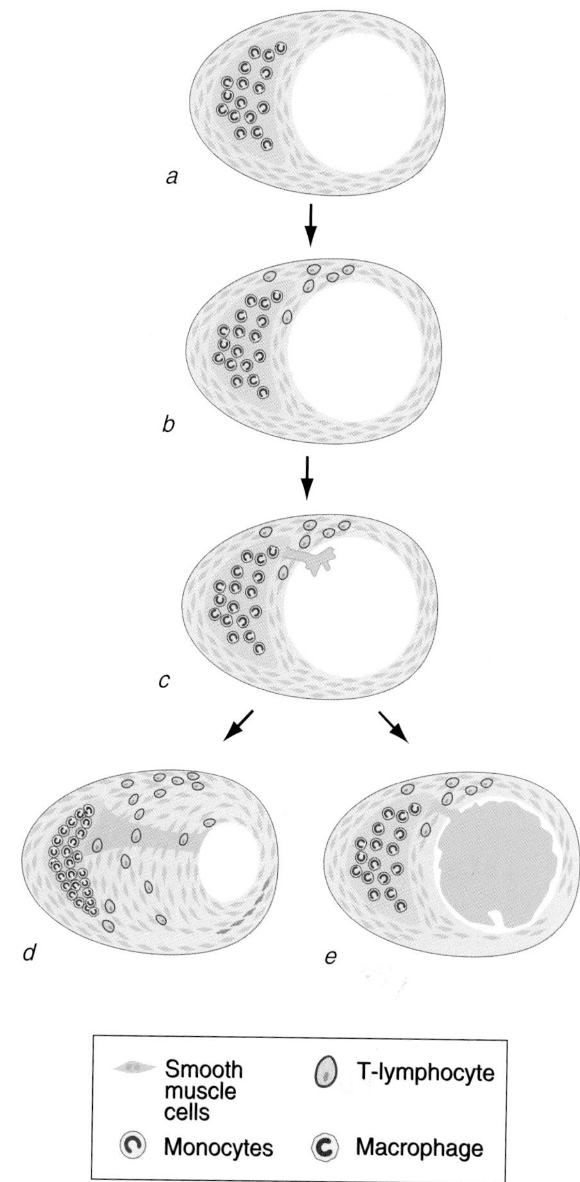

Figure 20.3 Rupture of immature collagen cap. If a normal artery *(a)* begins to develop a collagen cap *(b)*, but ruptures *(c)*, the artery can become partially *(d)* or fully *(e)* occluded.
Reprinted from Fauci, Braunwald, Isselbacher, et al. 1998

Diabetes exerts an acceleration effect on the process of vascular disease and thus has an independent effect on the pathophysiology of heart attacks. Nicotine (i.e., smoking) increases systemic vascular resistance, that is, blood pressure, causing an effect similar to that described in the previous section. People who are obese require more blood vessels to feed the adipose tissue. This effectively increases the cardiac workload, affecting the circulatory efficiency of the heart's pumping action. Over time, this can lead to the development of one of the various types of cardiomyopathy and heart failure.

As for family history, anyone who has a first-degree relative (parent or sibling) with known cardiac disease diagnosed before the age of 55 (male relative) or 65 (female relative) has an increased risk [1].

Myocardial Infarction

When an MI occurs, cardiac muscle potentially dies. Medical professionals intervene to try to salvage some of the damaged tissue or even reverse the entire process altogether. The personal trainer, however, will be working with a client who has had a heart attack, has gone through cardiac rehabilitation, and has been discharged from the physician to continue with an exercise program. This places the personal trainer in a most opportune position to get the most recent test data on the new client—exercise stress test results, echocardiogram results, and a letter of clearance and recommendations from the cardiologist.

These reports give the personal trainer the needed information regarding where the doctor left off, and thus where the personal trainer can begin (i.e., intensity level, among other parameters). The stress test provides the maximal oxygen uptake to enable one to determine the intensity level.

It also becomes important to recognize that there is a subpopulation of clients who have underlying coronary artery disease without associated chest pain during activity. These individuals are at risk for sudden death since they will exercise to the point of coronary artery spasm, acute heart attack, with a sudden stoppage of beating of the heart. Again, the stress test can reveal whether an individual is in this subclass. The personal trainer should not train these clients. These clients should exercise in a medically monitored setting.

Personal trainers should not train clients who are post-MI and have existing coronary artery disease without associated chest pain. Such clients must be medically monitored while exercising.

Exercise Guidelines for Clients Post-Myocardial Infarction

Post-MI clients are not to be trained until they have received clearance from their cardiologist, cardiovascular surgeon, or both [10]. At that point, the medical professional must be able to provide an intensity level and training range for the personal trainer to work with. The medical professional should provide a metabolic equivalent (MET) level or $\dot{V}O_2max$ for the personal trainer to use as a baseline for design of a program. The program should also be sent to the doctor for his or her approval, or at the very least to be placed in the client's medical file.

What is most important is for the personal trainer to be cognizant of and monitor for abnormal signs and symptoms. Some of these signs and symptoms are chest pain, palpitations, shortness of breath, diaphoresis, nausea, neck pain, arm pain (left or right), back pain, and a sense of impending doom.

One caveat is that many post-MI clients have comorbid diseases, such as diabetes and PVD. Peripheral vascular disease is discussed later in this chapter, and programming for clients with diabetes is addressed in chapter 19.

Exercise Program Components for Clients Post-Myocardial Infarction

Once the client has been cleared by the physician(s), the goals are to increase $\dot{V}O_2max$, decrease blood pressure, and reduce the risk for further coronary artery disease events. The training intensity for aerobic conditioning typically begins at 40% of $\dot{V}O_2max$ or an RPE of 9 to 11 (on the 6-20 scale). Sessions last between 15 and 40 minutes and take place three to four times per week. Additional time is devoted to warm-up and cool-down periods. There is not a definite timeline for goal achievement, since the aim is to prevent further events as well as strengthen the heart muscle. Follow-up exercise stress tests provide the necessary documentation regarding those endpoints, of course to be performed by a cardiologist.

Since many post-MI patients become fearful of simple activities of daily living, the goals are to rebuild their confidence to perform such tasks. Examples are lifting a milk carton, pouring from a bottle of orange juice, holding a handbag, or even pushing a grocery cart.

By performing resistance exercises, the client can receive immediate feedback as to his or her strength capabilities. This is more of a psychological boost than a reflection of actual strength increase. Programs should begin at 20 reps, one to three sets, two to three days per week. The personal trainer and the physician need to discuss the actual goals. The client is to be instructed to never perform a Valsalva maneuver.

Clients who have had a myocardial infarction should never perform a Valsalva maneuver.

Cerebrovascular Accident

The client who has had a stroke, or **cerebrovascular accident,** has considerations other than the occlusive nature of the disease. Such clients typically have neurologic deficits and are often best served in a setting monitored by health care professionals.

Goals for Clients Who Have Had a Myocardial Infarction

- Increase aerobic capacity.
- Decrease blood pressure.
- Reduce risk of coronary artery disease.
- Increase ability to perform leisure, occupational, and daily living activities.
- Increase muscle strength and endurance.

However, if a client has no neurological deficit and is released by his or her physician to exercise in an unmonitored setting, the personal trainer can follow the program design guidelines provided here and can help the client strive for improvements.

Exercise Guidelines for Post-Cerebrovascular Accident Clients

The post-CVA client faces many different challenges, all depending on which area of the brain has been affected. A good many individuals after CVA have difficulty with simple daily tasks because of a loss of motor function, often in the arm, leg, face, or mouth.Others have trouble hearing, speaking, or understanding spatial arrangements—or they may even ignore one side of their body. The discussion here is limited to the client who has experienced a left brain CVA, resulting in motor deficits of the right arm, leg, or both.

There is no question whatsoever that a properly instituted exercise program can significantly improve the life of people who have had a CVA. The program, however, must begin where the post-CVA rehabilitation left off. Therefore the personal trainer needs to have close contact with the rehabilitation team in order to ascertain the direction of the post-rehabilitation training and the establishment of goals.

Exercise can significantly improve the life of an individual who has had a stroke. Personal trainers may train post-CVA clients who have no neurological deficit and are released by their physicians to exercise in an unmonitored setting.

Exercise Program Components for Post-Cerebrovascular Accident Clients

Ergometers need to be the mainstay of aerobic conditioning for the post-CVA client. This is in contrast to the situation with the post-MI client, who can utilize a treadmill (figure 20.4). With compromised limb function, not only is strength obviously affected, but so too is the client's balance. The exercise intensity can begin as low as 30% peak $\dot{V}O_2$, since these clients become deconditioned rapidly after the CVA. Interestingly, this is why $\dot{V}O_2max$ is undefined in patients after a CVA. They become so deconditioned that the $\dot{V}O_2max$ cannot be determined, giving rise to the term peak $\dot{V}O_2$. Post-CVA clients may eventually exercise at 40% to 70% peak $\dot{V}O_2$. Meanwhile, any activity will improve their capacity. The sessions can last between 5 and 60 minutes, depending on the individual, and the frequency is typically at least three times per week.

Not only will resistance training help to improve the overall sense of well-being; it will also help develop new neurologic pathways to the affected limbs via the recruiting of dormant channels. Additionally, resistance training of the healthy limb will have a crossover effect on the compromised limb. Regarding the amount of weight to be utilized, a

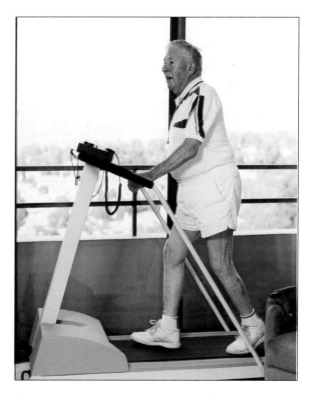

Figure 20.4 Post-MI clients frequently incorporate treadmill walking in their exercise program.

1-repetition maximum cannot be determined; therefore slow and judicious evaluation of the client for starting poundages is a responsibility of the personal trainer. Nonetheless, the personal trainer should eventually encourage the client to strive for three sets of 8 to 12 repetitions, two to three days per week.

The purpose of flexibility training should be obvious in clients in this group. This type of activity will help to maintain mobility in the healthy limbs and hopefully improve the range of motion in an affected limb as well. Too often the post-CVA patient experiences joint contractures as a result of the lack of motion around the joint. The joint can be considered frozen, but over time, bone remodeling by osteoclasts and osteoblasts will occur until the joint becomes calcified. Early range of motion training may prevent this from happening. Range of motion exercises should be performed before and after each training session (for as little as five minutes), as well as on nontraining days.

Coordination and balance exercises can also be added to the program. Standing on one foot, finger-to-nose activity, and finger-to-moving-target activity are just a few examples. This is where the personal trainer can get creative in the design of a truly individualized program.

Goals for Clients Following Cerebrovascular Accident (Stroke)

- Increase daily living activities.
- Increase strength for both involved and uninvolved limbs.
- Increase range of motion of the involved side.
- Prevent joint contractures.

Peripheral Vascular Disease

A client with PVD presents a real challenge; but clients in this group have the potential to make very impressive gains in their capacity. Essentially, people with PVD have pain upon walking. Typically they cannot walk for more than two to five minutes without having to stop and rest because of the searing pain in their calves. The goal is to increase the length of their activity to improve quality of life, and possibly avoid the need for surgical intervention.

Pharmacologic considerations for PVD are essentially the same as for persons with hypertension. The only notable addition is the use of physician-prescribed nitrates, that is, nitroglycerin, for chest pain. Nitroglycerin tablets or spray is applied under the tongue. If the medication is working, there will be a bitter taste and a soon-to-follow headache. If the client is experiencing anything suggestive of cardiac compromise (i.e., chest pain, ache, shortness of breath, etc.), he or she must stop immediately, sit down or even lie flat, and use the nitroglycerin as prescribed while someone calls 911. It is best if another person is available to either make the call or stay with the client; otherwise, the personal trainer must first call 911.

Exercise Guidelines for Clients With Peripheral Vascular Disease

Since the pathophysiology of PVD is present throughout the body, the personal trainer must be aware that exercise in a client with PVD may cause a cardiac event. Therefore, it is preferable for the client with PVD to be cleared from a cardiac viewpoint by an exercise stress test before embarking on a training program. For the same reasons as in cardiac and stroke patients, aggressive lifestyle changes must occur along with hyperlipidemia management.

Exercise Program Components for Clients With Peripheral Vascular Disease

The reason the client needs aerobic conditioning is straightforward—to be able to walk greater distances pain free. The claudication or calf pain with walking is the rate-limiting factor. The pain is incapacitating. The client will not say that it hurts a little; it will hurt a lot. Clients will not be able to "walk through" the pain; rather they will need to stop, sit down, and rest. Some may be able to walk for only a minute before needing to stop. Therefore, program design becomes simple—walk until it hurts, stop, then do it again, and so on. The duration for walking should be between 10 and 30 minutes. The goal is to lengthen the time walking and shorten the rest interval until the exercise becomes one long continuous activity.

As for resistance training, including repetition ranges, sets and rest periods, the same recommendations apply to clients with PVD as to clients who are hypertensive.

Goals for Clients With Peripheral Vascular Disease

- Improve pain response; be active for increasingly longer periods.
- Reduce risk of coronary artery disease.
- Improve gait.
- Increase daily living activities.
- Increase work potential.
- Improve quality of life.

Finally, any discussion of the client with angina pectoris has been intentionally omitted from this chapter, since clients in this group are felt to be at too high a risk for the personal trainer who is functioning in the typical health club or home gym setting. Such clients should be trained and thus monitored at a medical facility by the appropriately trained personnel with the necessary emergency back-up support systems.

Chronic Obstructive Pulmonary Disease

Training individuals with **chronic obstructive pulmonary disease** (COPD) [8], which often includes elements of asthma, chronic bronchitis, and emphysema, is beyond the scope of this chapter and beyond the scope of the personal trainer. People with emphysema are often older and often have been smoking for many years. They typically have accompanying diseases, such as cardiovascular problems. Although the specifics of the pulmonary problem in emphysema are little different from those in a patient with asthma, training a client with emphysema necessitates as much attention to the other illnesses, if not more. People with COPD often exercise as part of a pulmonary rehabilitation program and are not likely to work with a personal trainer.

Patients with COPD should exercise in a formal pulmonary and respiratory rehabilitation facility and not under the direction of a personal trainer.

Asthma

By definition, asthma is reversible airway disease with associated hyperreactivity, characterized by the ease of developing bronchospasm, constriction, or both. A very common subset of asthma is **exercise-induced asthma** (EIA) [29]. Compared to the more common variety, exercise-induced asthma is usually self-limited, rarely results in hospitalization, begins 15 to 20 minutes (or as early as five minutes in some cases) into an exercise session, and has associated coughing, wheezing, or both. In addition, if left untreated the client will recover and become symptom free within 10 to 30 minutes after cessation of exercise. The adult client, in contrast to a child, notices the onset of symptoms later in the exercise session, and the symptoms will last longer once started.

The two types of asthma clients experience similar symptomatology, the difference lying in the fact that the typical asthma client has symptoms during periods of rest or nonexercise. It is also important to realize that there are more severe forms of asthma necessitating the use of medications beyond inhaled bronchodilators. These medications can include inhaled and oral steroids. Some people who have asthma experience emergencies due to acute mucus plugging of the airways (i.e., status asthmaticus); however, these people are under the care of a pulmonary doctor who is supervising the rehabilitation program.

In both asthma and EIA, the bronchospasm has an early and a late phase. The early phase is the result of bronchoconstriction, which responds favorably to inhaled bronchodilators. Prevention can be achieved by using a bronchodilator 15 to 20 minutes prior to the start of the exercise. The late phase is delayed in onset by one to six hours and is due to airway edema. It is best controlled with inhaled steroids. Clients with this late-phase component are best treated two to three hours after exercise.

Exercise Guidelines for Clients With Asthma

In working with clients who have asthma, the best way to monitor intensity is through RPE and the sense of shortness of breath. This is necessary because many clients are unable to achieve a "training" heart rate but will objectively show physiological gains. Clients who are taking systemic glucocorticoids (steroids) may have muscular disease of the respiratory muscles, which can make breathing under stress more of a challenge.

Asthmatic clients do better with mid- to late-morning exercise sessions because of the natural daytime release of cortisol from the adrenal glands. They should avoid temperature extremes, since the ambient or inhaled air can precipitate bronchospasm. High humidity can have a similar effect. It is important to remember that the shortness of breath associated with the asthmatic client can lead to rather significant anxiety and depression, as well as fear over exercise.

In the client with asthma, exercise intensity should be monitored with ratings of perceived exertion and sense of shortness of breath. Many clients with asthma are unable to achieve a training heart rate but will still exhibit physiological improvements.

Exercise Program Components for Clients With Asthma

Large-muscle aerobic activity (i.e., walking, cycling and swimming) helps to improve $\dot{V}O_2max$ and thus aerobic capacity and endurance. There will be an associated increase in lactate and ventilatory thresholds, and a desensitization to **dyspnea** (shortness of breath) will occur. With a decrease in shortness of breath, an increase in activities of daily living can result as well.

An RPE of 11 to 13 (on the 6-20 scale) should be maintained, with continuous monitoring for dyspnea. Sessions should occur one to two times daily, three to seven days per week. Each session should last 30 minutes, although in the beginning clients may be able to perform for only 5 to 10 minutes. The emphasis is on the progression of duration versus intensity in order to desensitize the client to the dyspnea.

A general resistance training program is recommended. There are several objectives: to increase the maximal number of repetitions (to desensitize to shortness of breath), increase the amount of training volume, and increase lean body mass. The initial program should use lighter loads for more repetitions (≤16), two to three days per week.

A general flexibility program for the client with asthma should be followed.

CONCLUSION

Working with clients who have cardiovascular and respiratory conditions poses unique challenges. The guidelines in this chapter have been presented with the idea of simplifying topics that can be very complex. The personal trainer must keep the need for finesse and true individualization of a program at the forefront during program design. It is always best to err on the side of conservativism. If in doubt, it is best to begin the program at a lower intensity than has been indicated. This way the client (who may already be fearful of exercise) has much room for improvement without the risk of injury or exacerbation of the underlying disease. With goals that are easy to attain, reaching goals will help clients psychologically to want to continue to train while limiting the risk of adverse effects.

STUDY QUESTIONS

1. A 44-year-old-male with history of high blood pressure (144/92) has never exercised before but would like to start an exercise program. His physician cleared him to participate. Which of the following is an example of the most appropriate beginning exercise intensity for this client?
   A. treadmill walking at an RPE of 14
   B. back squat at 75% of 1RM for 10 repetitions
   C. elliptical trainer at 65% $\dot{V}O_2$ max
   D. dumbbell bench press at 50% 1RM for 16 repetitions
2. A 52-year-old-client had a heart attack three months ago and was recently cleared by his physician to begin a low intensity exercise program. Which of the following combinations of exercise, intensity, and duration are most appropriate for this client?

	Mode	Intensity	Duration
A.	stationary bicycle	RPE of 12	15 minutes
B.	treadmill walking	40% $\dot{V}O_2$ max	20 minutes
C.	stair stepper	70% HRmax	25 minutes
D.	elliptical trainer	RPE of 8	10 minutes

3. A 63-year-old client with peripheral vascular disease describes significant pain when walking for 5 minutes or more. Which of the following programs would best help her increase the amount of time she is able to walk pain free?
   A. Have the client "walk through" the pain for 2 minutes after the pain begins.
   B. Decrease the duration to 2 minutes at the same intensity.
   C. Have the client take a short rest break once the pain begins, then continue walking until the pain returns.
   D. For now, discontinue walking as a form of exercise since it is too painful.

4. A client with exercise-induced asthma has been performing primarily resistance training exercises for the past year. She now requests help in improving her "stamina." Which of the following methods of monitoring aerobic intensity should be used for this client?
   I. target heart rate
   II. sense of dyspnea
   III. METs
   IV. RPE

   A. I and III only
   B. II and IV only
   C. I, II, and III only
   D. II, III, and IV only

APPLIED KNOWLEDGE QUESTION

Fill in the chart to describe recommendations for a *beginning* exercise program and any exercise-related concerns that a personal trainer should be aware of with clients who have these conditions.

	Beginning exercise program				Exercise concerns
	Mode	Intensity	Frequency	Duration	
Hypertension					
MI					
Stroke					
PVD					
Asthma					

REFERENCES

1. American College of Sports Medicine. 2000. *ACSM's Guidelines for Exercise Testing and Prescription*, 6th ed. Philadelphia: Lippincott Williams & Williams.
2. American College of Sports Medicine. 2003. *Exercise Management for Persons With Chronic Diseases and Disabilities*, 2nd ed. Champaign, IL: Human Kinetics.
3. American Heart Association. 1995. *Heart and Stroke Facts: 1995 Statistical Supplement*. Dallas: AHA.
4. Arakawa, K. 1996. Effect of exercise on hypertension and associated complications. *Hypertension Research* 19 (Suppl 1): S87-S91.
5. Arakawa, K. 1999. Exercise, a measure to lower blood pressure and reduce other risks. *Clinical and Experimental Hypertension* 21 (5-6): 797-803.
6. Blumenthal, J.A., E.T. Thyrum, E.D. Gullette, A. Sherwood, and R. Waugh. 1995. Do exercise and weight loss reduce blood pressure in patients with mild hypertension? *North Carolina Medical Journal* 56 (2): 92-95.
7. Borhani, N.O. 1996. Significance of physical activity for prevention and control of hypertension. *Journal of Human Hypertension* 10 (Suppl 2): S7-S11.
8. CIBA-GEIGY Corporation. 1991. *Hazards of Smoking: A Patient Guide to COPD and Lung Cancer*. Peapack, NJ: Tim Peters and Company.
9. Conley, M., and R. Rozeneck. 2001. Health aspects of resistance exercise and training: NSCA position statement. *Strength and Conditioning Journal* 23 (6): 9-23.
10. Engstrom, G., B. Hedblad, and L. Janzon. 1999. Hypertensive men who exercise regularly have lower rate of cardiovascular mortality. *Journal of Hypertension* 17 (6): 737-742.
11. Fauci, A.S., E. Braunwald, K.J. Isselbacher, et al., eds. 1998. Disorders of the cardiovascular system. In: *Harrison's Principles of Internal Medicine*, 14th ed. New York: McGraw Hill, pp. 1345-1352
12. Hagberg, J.M., A.A. Ehsoni, and D. Goldring. 1984. Effect of weight training on blood pressure and haemodynamics in hypertensive adolescents. *Journal of Pediatrics* 104: 147-151.
13. Hagberg, J.M., J.J. Park, and M.D. Brown. 2000. The role of exercise training in the treatment of hypertension: An update. *Sports Medicine* 30 (3): 193-206.
14. Halbert, J.A., C.A. Silagy, R.T. Withers, P.A. Hamdorf, and G.R. Andrews. 1997. The effectiveness of exercise in lowering blood pressure: A meta-analysis of randomized controlled trials of 4 weeks or longer. *Journal of Human Hypertension* 11 (10): 641-649.
15. Harris, K.A., and R.G. Holly. 1987. Physiological responses to circuit weight training in borderline hypertensive subjects. *Medicine and Science in Sports and Exercise* 19: 246-252.
16. Kelley, G. 1997. Dynamic resistance exercise and resting blood pressure in adults: A meta-analysis. *Journal of Applied Physiology* 82 (5): 1559-1565.
17. Kelley, G.A., and K.A. Kelley. 2000. Progressive resistance exercise and resting blood pressure: A meta-analysis of randomized controlled trials. *Hypertension* 35 (3): 838-843.
18. Kokkinos, P.F., and V. Papademetriou. 2000. Exercise and hypertension. *Coronary Artery Disease* 11 (2): 99-102.
19. Majahalme, S., V. Turjanmaa, M. Tuomisto, H. Kautiainen, and A. Uusitalo. 1997. Intra-arterial blood pressure during exercise and left ventricular indices in normotension and borderline and mild hypertension. *Blood Pressure* 6 (1): 5-12.
20. Manolas, J. 1997. Patterns of diastolic abnormalities during isometric stress in patients with systemic hypertension. *Cardiology* 88 (1): 36-47.
21. Mughal, M.A., I.A. Alvi, I.A. Akhund, and A.K. Ansari. 2001. The effect of aerobic exercise training on resting blood pressure in hypertensive patients. *Journal of the Pakistan Medical Association* 51 (6): 222-226.
22. Papademetriou, V., and P.F. Kokkinos. 1996. The role of exercise in the control of hypertension and cardiovascular risk. *Current Opinion in Nephrology and Hypertension* 5 (5): 459-462.
23. Roberts, S. 1992. Resistance training: Guidelines for individuals with heart disease. *Conditioning Instructor* 2 (3): 4-6.
24. Rogers, M.W., M.M. Probst, J.J. Gruber, R. Berger, and J.B. Boone. 1996. Differential effects of exercise training intensity on blood pressure and cardiovascular responses to stress in borderline hypertensive humans. *Journal of Hypertension* 14 (11): 1369-1375.
25. Roos, R.J. 1997. The Surgeon General's report: A prime source for exercise advocates. *Physician and Sportsmedicine* 25 (4): 122-131.
26. Sallis, R.E., ed. 1997. *Essentials of Sports Medicine*. St. Louis: Mosby-Year Book.
27. Sallis, R.E., M. Allen, and F. Massimino, eds. 1997. *Sports Medicine Review*. St. Louis: Mosby Year Book.
28. Seals, D.R., H.G. Silverman, M.J. Reiling, and K.P. Davy. 1997. Effect of regular aerobic exercise on elevated blood pressure in postmenopausal women. *American Journal of Cardiology* 80 (1): 49-55.
29. Storms, W., and D.M. Joyner. 1997. Update on exercise-induced asthma. *Physician and Sportsmedicine* 25 (3): 45-55.
30. Tulio, S., S. Egle, and G. Greily. 1995. Blood pressure response to exercise of obese and lean hypertensive and normotensive male adolescents. *Journal of Human Hypertension* 9 (12): 953-958.

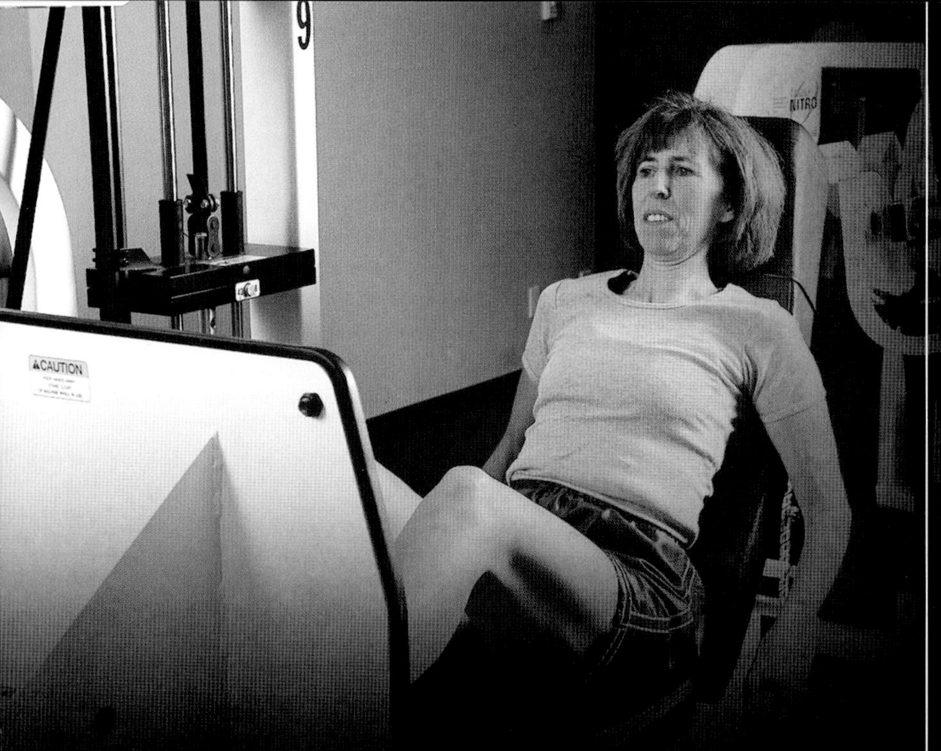

CHAPTER 21

Clients With Orthopedic, Injury, and Rehabilitation Concerns

David H. Potach | Todd Ellenbecker

After completing this chapter, you will be able to

- understand the timing and events of tissue healing;
- recognize the types of injuries that clients sustain;
- explain the goals of each phase of tissue healing; and
- describe the personal trainer's role in relation to specific orthopedic, injury, and rehabilitation concerns.

As the personal training profession continues to gain acceptance by both potential clients and health care professionals, the personal trainer's role will expand to allow more active participation in the training of persons who have been recently injured or have orthopedic dysfunctions. In combination with health insurance coverage limitations of clients recovering from injury or surgery, personal trainers' distinct exercise knowledge and their regular contact with the general exercising public place them in a unique position to help improve function in clients restricted by disease or injury. To fulfill this role, the personal trainer must understand not only the different types of injury but also the physiological healing process; knowledge of both is essential in helping to hasten recovery from injury and improving overall client function.

This chapter is not intended to provide the reader with rehabilitation protocols for specific injuries, nor is it designed to take the place of medical advice given by health care professionals. Rather, it is designed to explain the physiological events that accompany orthopedic-related injury and disease processes, thereby putting the personal trainer in an ideal position to improve outcomes. The information contained in this chapter should ultimately be used as an adjunct to communication with other health care professionals to maximize client function.

Tissue Healing Following Injury

To better understand the role of the personal trainer in working with clients following injury or surgery, it is necessary to review the general phases of tissue healing after musculoskeletal injury. The severity and rate of the events occurring within each phase are different for each tissue type and for various types of injury and surgeries, but all tissues follow the same basic pattern of healing (see "Goals During Tissue Healing" on the next page).

Inflammation Phase

Inflammation is the body's initial reaction to injury and is necessary in order for normal healing to occur. During the inflammatory phase, several events contribute to both tissue healing and an initial decrease in function. After tissues are damaged, several chemical mediators, including histamine and bradykinin, are released. These substances increase blood flow and capillary permeability, causing **edema**—the escape of fluid into the surrounding tissues—inhibiting contractile tissue function and significantly limiting the injured client's activity level. In addition, the inflammatory substances may noxiously stimulate sensory nerve fibers, causing pain that may contribute to decreased function. This phase typically lasts two to three days following an acute injury but may last longer with a compromised blood supply, more severe structural damage, and following surgery. Although the inflammatory phase is critical to tissue healing, if it does not end within a reasonable amount of time, further healing may not occur, thereby delaying the rehabilitation process.

The goal during the inflammatory phase is to prepare for the new tissue formation that occurs during the subsequent phases of tissue healing. A healthy environment for new tissue regeneration and formation is essential to prevent prolonged inflammation and disruption of the production of new blood vessels and collagen. To achieve these goals, *relative rest* and *passive modalities,* including ice, compression, and elevation, are the primary treatment options. While a rapid return to pre-injury activity is important, the damaged tissue requires rest to protect it from additional injury. Therefore, active treatment—including exercise—to the injured area is not recommended during this phase.

Repair Phase

Though the inflammatory phase may continue, tissue **repair** begins within three to five days following injury and may last up to two months. This phase of healing allows for the replacement of tissues that are not viable following injury or surgery. In an attempt to improve tissue integrity, the damaged tissue is regenerated (i.e., scar tissue is formed). New capillaries and connective tissue form in the area, and collagen fibers—the structural component of the new tissue—are randomly laid down to serve as the framework on which the repair takes place. Collagen fibers are strongest when they are parallel and lie longitudinally to the primary line of stress, yet many of the new fibers are laid down transversely. This alignment does not allow optimal strength of the new tissue and therefore limits its ability to transmit force.

The goals during the repair phase are to prevent excessive muscle atrophy and joint degeneration of the injured area, promote collagen synthesis, and avoid disruption of the newly formed collagen fibers. These cautions must be balanced with

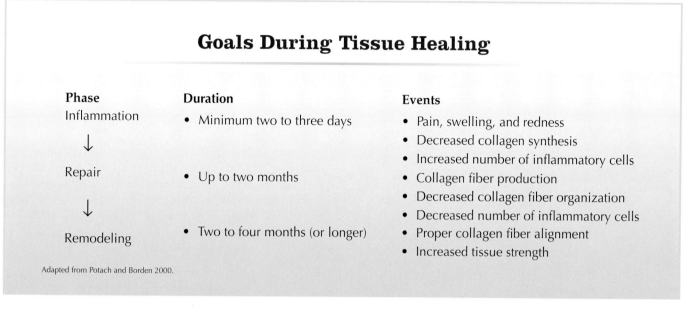

Goals During Tissue Healing

Phase	Duration	Events
Inflammation	• Minimum two to three days	• Pain, swelling, and redness • Decreased collagen synthesis • Increased number of inflammatory cells
↓		
Repair	• Up to two months	• Collagen fiber production • Decreased collagen fiber organization • Decreased number of inflammatory cells
↓		
Remodeling	• Two to four months (or longer)	• Proper collagen fiber alignment • Increased tissue strength

Adapted from Potach and Borden 2000.

the gradual introduction of low-load stresses to promote increased collagen synthesis and prevent loss of joint motion. To protect the new, relatively weak collagen fibers, resistive exercises affecting the damaged tissue should be avoided. Specific exercises should be used during the repair phase *only* after consultation with the client's physician or physical therapist. Submaximal isometric exercise may be performed, provided that it is pain free and otherwise indicated. Submaximal isometric exercise allows strength gains to occur with an intensity low enough that the newly formed collagen fibers are not disrupted.

Remodeling Phase

The weakened tissue produced during repair is strengthened during the **remodeling** phase of healing. Production of collagen fibers has now decreased significantly, allowing the newly formed tissue the opportunity to improve its structure, strength, and function. With increased loading, the collagen fibers of the newly formed scar tissue begin to hypertrophy and align themselves along the lines of stress [31], increasing the strength of the newly formed tissue and allowing for the injured client's return to function. Although strength of the collagen fibers improves significantly, the new tissue will likely never be as strong as the tissue it has replaced [1, 16, 28, 29]. Tissue remodeling can last up to two to four months (or longer) after injury [47].

Optimizing tissue function is the primary goal during this final phase of healing. Clients improve function by continuing the exercises performed during the repair phase and by adding more advanced, activity-specific exercises that allow progressive stresses to be applied to the injured tissue. Progressive tissue loading allows improved collagen fiber alignment and fiber hypertrophy. Ultimately, rehabilitation and reconditioning exercises must be functional to facilitate a return to activity. Strengthening should transition from general exercises to activity-specific exercises designed to replicate movements common in given sports and activities.

All injured structures follow the same general phases of healing: inflammation, repair, and remodeling. Characteristic events define and separate each phase from the others.

Injury Classification

There are several ways to classify injuries to the body. One is by the type of injury (i.e., sudden or gradual onset), and the second is by type of tissue (e.g., bone, muscle) damaged. **Macrotrauma** is a specific, sudden episode of overload injury to a given tissue, resulting in disrupted tissue integrity. **Microtrauma,** or overuse injury, results from repeated, abnormal stress applied to a tissue by continuous training or training with too little recovery time. Overuse injuries may be due to training errors (e.g., poor program design), suboptimal training surfaces (e.g., too hard or uneven), faulty biomechanics or technique during performance, insufficient motor control, decreased flexibility, or skeletal malalignment and predisposition [30]. Table 21.1 covers common macro- and microtraumatic injuries to muscle, tendon, bone, and joint.

Orthopedic Concerns and the Personal Trainer

Personal trainers need to have a basic familiarity with exercise strategies for common muscle, bone, and joint injuries and surgeries. For each type of orthopedic injury with its particular pathophysiology, each surgical procedure, and each disease process, exercise and movement guidelines include indications, contraindications, and precautions.

An **indication** is an activity that will benefit the injured client [60]. For example, a client who recently had a knee replacement must maintain upper extremity function, so the personal trainer may design a program that allows the client to continue performing upper extremity strength training exercises during rehabilitation of the knee. A **contraindication** is an activity or practice that is inadvisable or prohibited because of the given injury [60]. For example, during the rehabilitation from reconstruction of the knee's anterior cruciate ligament, a client must protect the anterior cruciate ligament graft.

TABLE 21.1

Common Injuries to Muscles, Tendons, Bones, and Joints

Injury	Definition
Muscle contusion	An area of excess accumulation of blood and fluid in the tissues surrounding the injured muscle [4, 7, 78]; may severely limit movement of the injured muscle.
Muscle strain	Tear to the fibers of the muscle; assigned grades or degrees [4, 78]: • A *first-degree* strain is a partial tear of individual fibers and is characterized by strong but painful muscle activity. • A *second-degree* strain is also a partial tear, differentiated from the first-degree strain by weak, painful muscle activity. • A *third-degree* muscle strain is a complete tear of the fibers and is manifested by very weak but painless muscle activity.
Tendinitis	Inflammation of a tendon [32]; if the cause of the inflammation is left uncorrected or if the client returns to full activity before the tendon has had a chance to regain its full strength [26, 30], further breakdown and structural degeneration of the injured tendon will occur.
Tendinopathy	The progression of tendinitis, resulting in abnormal tendinous tissue.
Bone fracture	Skeletal fractures that can result from a direct blow to a bone and can be given a variety of classifications (e.g., closed, open, avulsed, incomplete). The most common overuse—microtraumatic—injury to bone is a stress fracture, and although body type and structure play a large role [31], it is often the result of excessive training volume on hard training surfaces [24, 66].
Joint dislocation	Complete displacement of the joint surfaces.
Joint subluxation	Partial displacement of the joint surfaces.
Joint sprain	Ligamentous trauma—injury to the structures that connect bones and help maintain joint stability—is termed a sprain and is assigned one of three classifications: • A *first degree* sprain is a partial tear of the ligament without increased joint instability. • A *second degree* sprain is a partial tear with minor joint instability. • A *third degree* sprain is a complete tear with full joint instability.

Therefore, the final 30 degrees of the leg extension exercise is contraindicated as it can place the graft in a compromised position. A **precaution** is an activity that may be performed under supervision of a qualified personal trainer and according to client limitations and symptom reproduction [60]. For example, while typically not advised, a client with anterior shoulder instability may perform the bench press provided that he or she avoids excessive shoulder horizontal abduction (i.e., the client's upper arms stay above parallel to the client's body) and uses proper weight increases. It is not the personal trainer's responsibility to determine movement or exercise restrictions. Rather, to identify appropriate contraindications and precautions, the personal trainer must communicate with the client's physical therapist or physician.

It is not the personal trainer's responsibility to determine movement or exercise restrictions. These should be determined through consultation with the client's physician or physical therapist.

It would be impossible for this chapter to give an in-depth description of every injury, surgical procedure, or disease process, and it is also difficult to provide all of the possible exercise and movement guidelines. The sections that follow offer both general descriptions for common diagnoses and surgeries, and guidelines to use when designing exercise programs for these postsurgical clients. It is imperative that the personal trainer contact both the client's surgeon (for a surgical description) and physical therapist (for a list of movement and exercise guidelines) prior to beginning an exercise program.

Because of the many different surgical procedures currently used, designing exercise programs for clients following surgery can be a challenging prospect. Typically these clients have undergone some form of formal rehabilitation or have been instructed in a home exercise program following their surgical procedure. Unfortunately, rehabilitation exercise programs often fail to allow the client's return to full function, whether due to lack of insurance coverage or to lack of compliance. This places the personal trainer in an ideal position to improve function through the use of both traditional and nontraditional exercise programs. Before designing these programs, however, it is important that the personal trainer not only generally understand the surgical procedure but also understand and abide by the contraindications and precautions brought about by the surgery.

The information in the remaining sections of this chapter should not be considered a substitute for injury or postsurgical protocols. Nor should it replace the guidance of health care providers. Rather, discussion of each injury, surgical procedure, or disease is intended to improve the personal trainer's base of knowledge, thereby improving communication with health care providers and ultimately improving client function in a safe, efficient manner.

Low Back

As one of the leading causes of pain and disability [8], low back pain has become a significant concern not only for health care providers, but also for personal trainers hired by clients with this diagnosis. Unfortunately, low back pain is a catch-all term involving several different diagnoses, including, but not limited to, disc dysfunction, muscle strain, lumbar spinal stenosis, and spondylolisthesis. Each of these diagnoses presents differently and each requires a different treatment approach. For example, persons with disc herniation typically respond best to exercises involving lumbosacral extension [58], while those diagnosed with lumbar spinal stenosis tend to favor flexion [12]. The aim of this section, then, is to provide the personal trainer with appropriate and inappropriate movements and exercises for clients with given diagnoses. Figure 21.1 shows the basic anatomy of the lumbosacral spine and will be referred to throughout this section.

Lumbar Disc Injury

In all sections of the vertebral column, the bodies of each vertebra are connected to each other by intervertebral discs (figure 21.2). These discs are designed to absorb shock and stabilize the vertebral column by preventing excessive shear. Each disc has essentially two layers; the **annulus fibrosus** is the tough outer layer that surrounds the **nucleus pulposus,** the gelatinous inner layer [59]. In the lumbar region of the back, the annulus fibrosus is reinforced anteriorly by the strong anterior longitudinal ligament; because the posterior longitudinal ligament narrows in the lumbar region, the support it is able to provide the posterior aspects of the intervertebral discs is limited. This limited posterior support is one cause of posterolateral disc herniations, the most common type of disc herniation.

When an intervertebral disc herniates, part of the nucleus pulposus makes its way through the outer annulus fibrosus, resulting in inflammation; this inflammation subsequently irritates the spinal

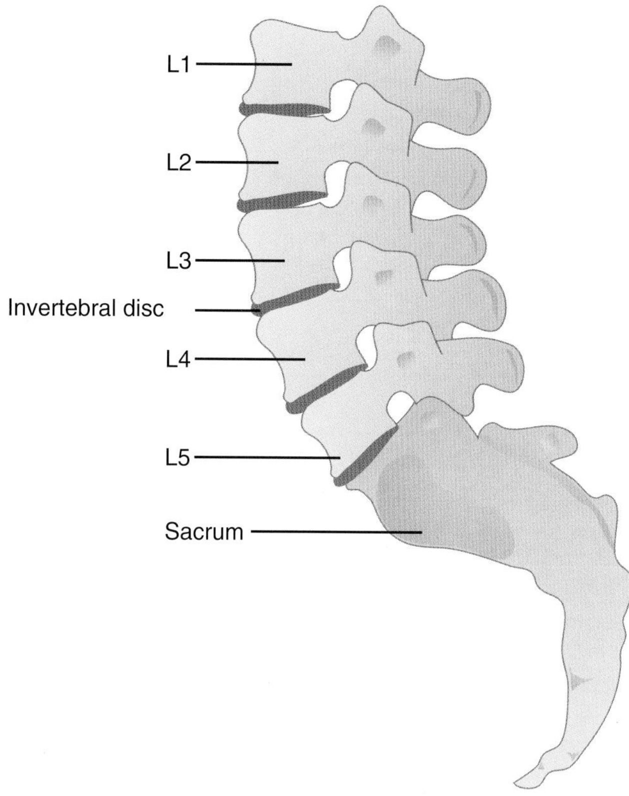

Figure 21.1 Lumbar spine anatomy.

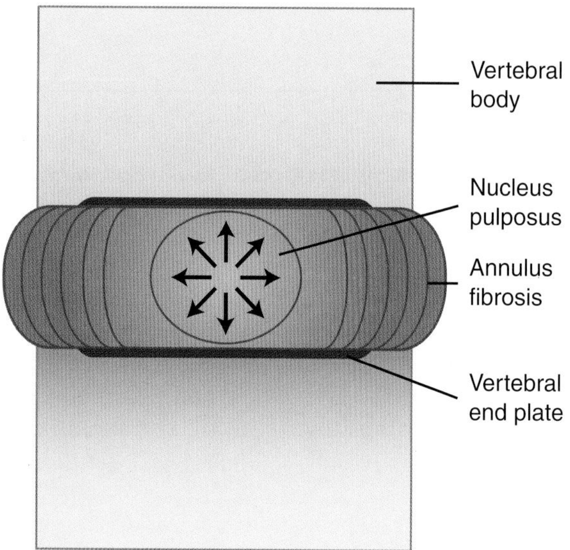

Figure 21.2 The three components of the intervertebral disc—the vertebral body, nucleus pulposus, annulus fibrosus, and vertebral endplate.
Reprinted from Porterfield and DeRosa 1998.

nerve roots [61]. The irritation can manifest itself in several ways. The client may feel pain in the back; or changes may occur in the lower extremities, including pain, abnormal sensation, and weakness. In addition to the weak posterior mechanical restraints to disc herniation, position is a significant contributor to lumbar disc dysfunction and injury. Excessive flexion (i.e., forward bending) tends to push the disc's nuclear material posteriorly, encouraging it to move beyond its normal confines toward the spinal canal and nerve roots. When a client has a herniated disc, he or she should seek treatment from a physician whose treatment plan may include therapeutic exercise as prescribed by a physical therapist.

Movement and Exercise Guidelines

For the reasons just outlined, clients with herniated lumbar discs are generally encouraged to avoid lumbar flexion in favor of extension to prevent the posterior protrusion of the disc material [74]. Therefore, they should avoid exercises involving significant lumbar flexion. Resistance training contraindications may include full sit-ups, while precautions may include the squat, all rowing movements (e.g., seated row, bent-over row), and the deadlift. Aerobic exercise precautions may include bicycle riding (due to possible increased flexion with forward lean), use of the rowing ergometer, and flexion-based movements in aerobic dance. Flexibility is important with clients who have a herniated disk, but stretching exercises involving flexion should be used with caution; contraindicated flexibility exercises include hamstring stretches emphasizing lumbar flexion (e.g., standing toe touch) and other stretches requiring similar movements in the lumbar spine. Precautions may include gluteal, hip adductor, and upper back stretches.

Muscle Strain

As previously discussed, muscle strains are tears to muscle fibers. Strains to the muscles of the lumbosacral spine are quite common and may have a variety of causes, including direct trauma and overuse. Traumatic muscle strains require the affected muscle(s) to complete the various phases of tissue healing with guidance from the client's health care practitioners. An overuse injury, on the other hand, requires the client to correct any improper posture and movement patterns. Retraining muscles to function in their designed manner will enable the muscles to work more efficiently, thereby decreasing the abnormal stresses the affected muscle(s) experience.

Movement and Exercise Guidelines

Movement and exercise restriction following muscle strain is highly dependent on the muscle that has been strained. Once a physician or physical therapist has determined which muscle has been strained, exercises and movements that rely on that muscle should be avoided. For example, if the erector spinae muscles have been strained, lumbar extension exercises (e.g., hyperextension) and exercises requiring static maintenance of the normal lumbar lordosis (e.g., bent-over barbell row, use of elliptical trainer) should be avoided during the early phases of tissue healing; these and similar exercises may be included in exercise programming during the remodeling phase.

Spondylolysis and Spondylolisthesis

Spondylolysis is a defect, or fracture, of the pars interarticularis region of a lumbar vertebra (an arched area of the vertebra that connects the superior and inferior facet joints—see figure 21.1) [24, 39, 40, 41, 43]; spondylolisthesis is the possible progression of spondylolysis, a forward slippage of one vertebral body on another [46, 64]. While causes vary, spondylolysis and spondylolisthesis commonly occur following lumbar extension injuries or in persons participating in activities requiring lumbar extension (e.g., divers and football linemen). Clients with spondylolysis and spondylolisthesis typically describe low back pain and possible lower extremity radicular pain, paresthesia, or muscle weakness. Complaints most often increase with lumbar extension and improve with flexion.

Movement and Exercise Guidelines

Like clients with lumbar spinal stenosis, clients with spondylolysis or spondylolisthesis should focus on strengthening the muscles surrounding the spine and should avoid exercises involving lumbar extension. Most abdominal exercises are appropriate, especially crunches and exercises for the obliques and transverse abdominis, as are stabilization-type exercises such as those performed on stability balls (see chapter 12 for examples of these exercises). In contrast to the situation with lumbar spinal stenosis, walking and other forms of standing cardiovascular exercise should not be considered contraindications for clients with spondylolysis or spondylolisthesis. Rather, it is well to encourage these modes of exercise, though they may require modification to adapt to each client's needs. For example, if a client is unable to perform on a stair stepper for more than 10 minutes because of increased low back pain, exercise duration should be kept under that level and then gradually increased as tolerated by the client. Table 21.2 provides a movement guide for clients with low back pain.

TABLE 21.2

Low Back Pain Movement and Exercise Guidelines

Diagnosis	Movement contraindications	Exercise contraindications	Exercise indications
Disc injury	Lumbar flexion Lumbar rotation	Sit-up Knee to chest stretch Spinal twist	Passive lumbar extension stretches Isometric abdominal and extensor strengthening, progressing to lumbar stabilization program
Muscle strain	Passive lumbar flexion *(during inflammatory phase)* Active lumbar extension *(during inflammatory phase)*	Knee to chest stretch	None during inflammatory phase, progressing to gentle flexion stretching, followed by extension strengthening
Spondylolysis and spondylolisthesis	Lumbar extension	Squat Shoulder press Push press	Knee to chest stretch Abdominal crunch

Low back pain is one of the leading causes of pain and disability. Low back pain is a catch-all term involving several different diagnoses, including, but not limited to, disc dysfunction, muscle strain, lumbar spinal stenosis, and spondylolisthesis. Each of these diagnoses requires a different exercise strategy.

Shoulder

Because of the inherent mobility of the shoulder and the need for dynamic muscular stability for proper function, the shoulder is an area where specific exercises following injury and postoperatively can have a tremendous influence in the client's overall function. The following sections present an overview of each injury or surgical procedure, followed by specific exercise indications and contraindications. Included are estimates of the general time frames during which exercise can be most appropriately used.

Impingement Syndrome

Impingement syndrome is a "pinching" of the supraspinatus, the long head of the biceps tendon, or **subacromial bursa** under the acromial arch (figure 21.3). Impingement has many contributory factors; some are changeable with conservative treatment, and other factors require surgical intervention (e.g., subacromial decompression). Causative factors that may necessitate surgery include anatomic or bony abnormalities (e.g., acromion that is "hooked" to compress the subacromial structures). Factors that may be altered include muscle imbalances, poor posture and scapular control, and improper exercise technique or overuse of the shoulder, typically overhead (e.g., baseball pitchers, swimmers).

Physical therapists, after reducing inflammation, focus on education and exercises to improve muscular imbalance, range of motion (if limited), scapular control, and posture. Once formal physical therapy has ended, personal trainers have the important job of continuing the exercises performed during rehabilitation. Once rotator cuff strength and scapular stability have returned, often as the client notes significantly decreased or absent shoulder pain, personal trainers gradually add typical resistance training exercises.

The **rotator cuff** muscles function to position the humeral head in the shallow glenoid, thereby resisting the upward migration of the humeral head into the acromion. Further, muscles attaching to the scapula—primarily the upper and lower trapezius, serratus anterior, and levator scapula muscles—must function properly to rotate the scapula during overhead movements. When any of these muscles become weak or fail to function properly, impingement may occur.

Movement and Exercise Guidelines

Figures 21.4 to 21.8 contain a series of rotator cuff exercises that elicit high levels of rotator cuff activation while minimizing compensation from other muscle groups [5, 11, 70]. These exercises are a staple of nonoperative and postoperative shoulder rehabilitation programs [17] and are indicated in postrehabilitation training programs to continue rotator cuff strengthening and maintain proper muscular balance. Because the rotator cuff muscles function in a primarily endurance role, these exercises are typically performed with light weights (seldom more than 4 pounds [1.8 kilograms]) and high repetitions (sets of 15 to 20 repetitions). The exercises are chosen for their muscle activation characteristics, as well as the positioning of the shoulder in safe, neutral environments below 90 degrees of elevation and with the arm in a forward position relative to the body (anterior to the frontal plane). These positions minimize rotator cuff impingement and allow for pain-free exercise in most individuals.

Clients who have had impingement syndrome should concentrate on continued rotator cuff and scapular exercises. Multiple types of rowing exercise targeting the rhomboids and middle and lower trapezius are recommended. Overhead pressing

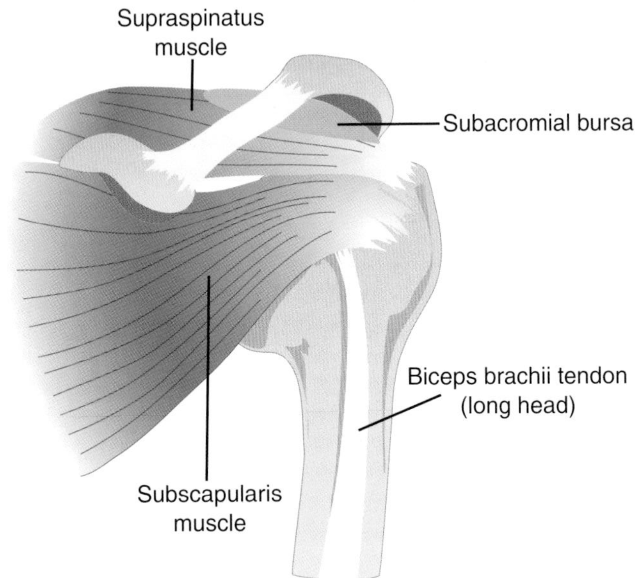

Figure 21.3 Anterior aspect of the shoulder.

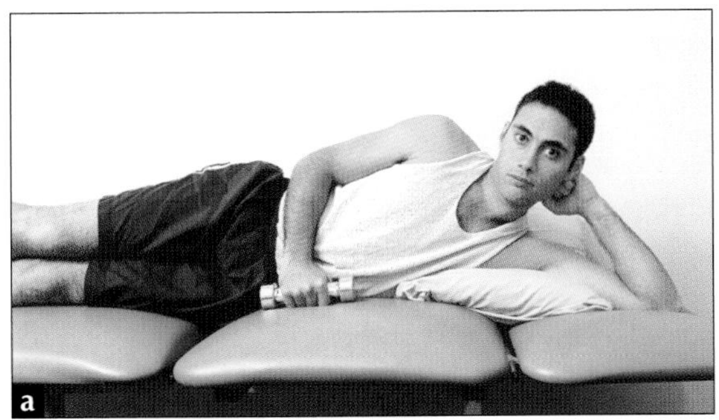

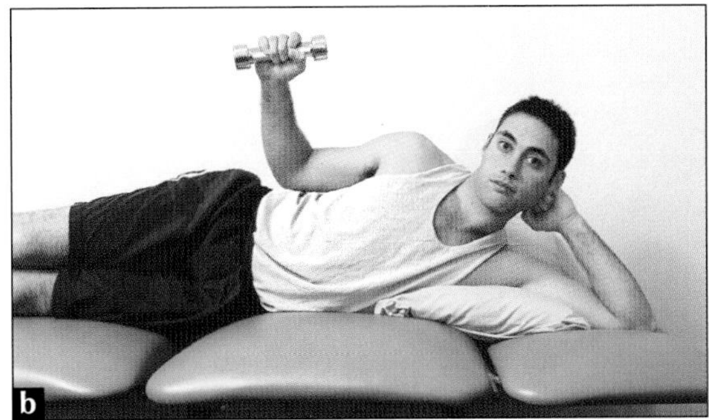

Figure 21.4 Side-lying external rotation: *(a)* beginning position; *(b)* end position.

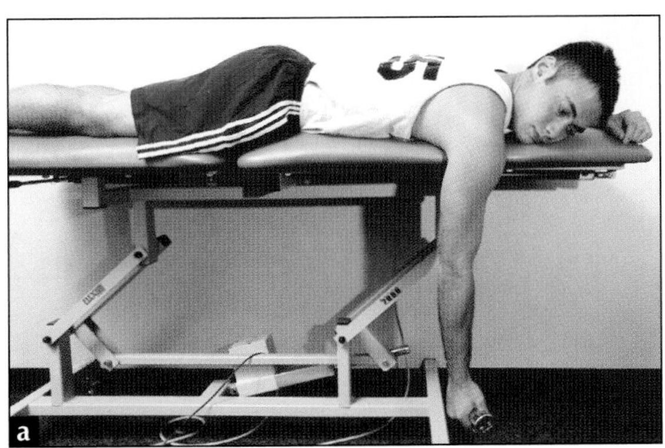

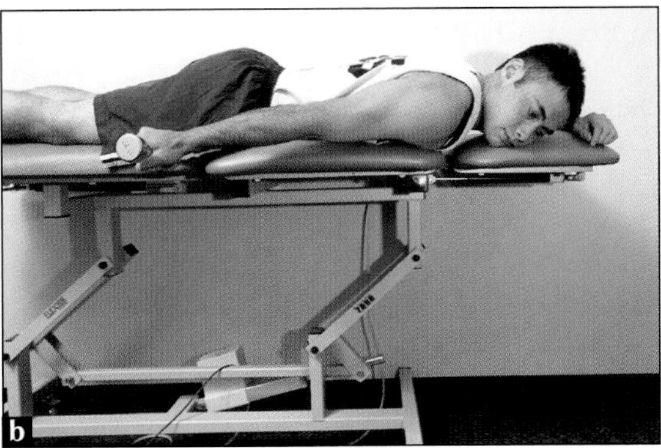

Figure 21.5 Prone shoulder extension: *(a)* beginning position; *(b)* end position.

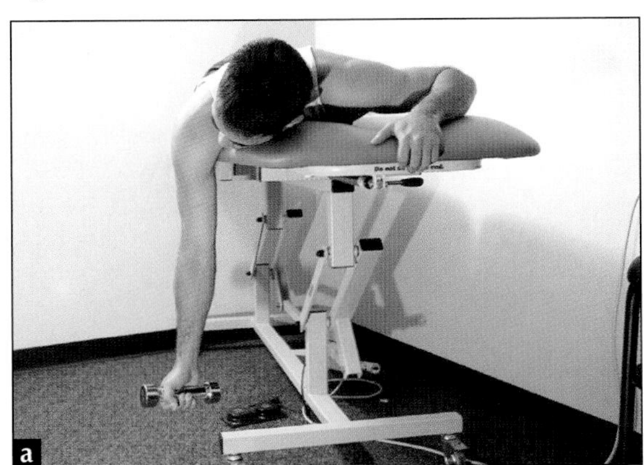

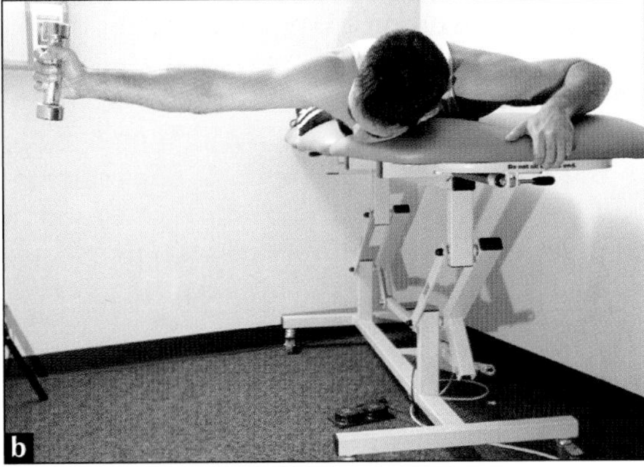

Figure 21.6 Prone horizontal abduction: *(a)* beginning position; *(b)* end position.

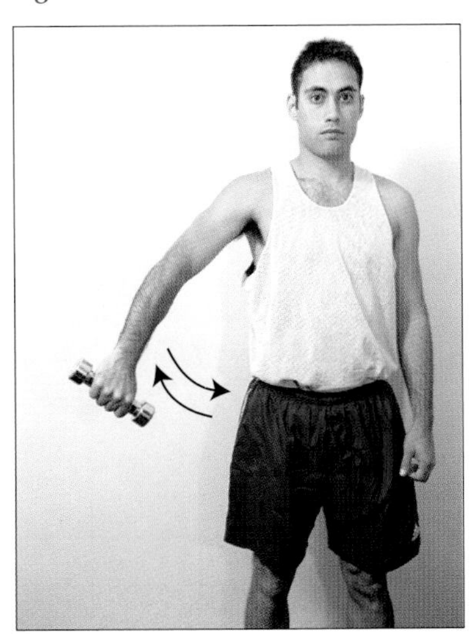

Figure 21.7 Standing empty can.

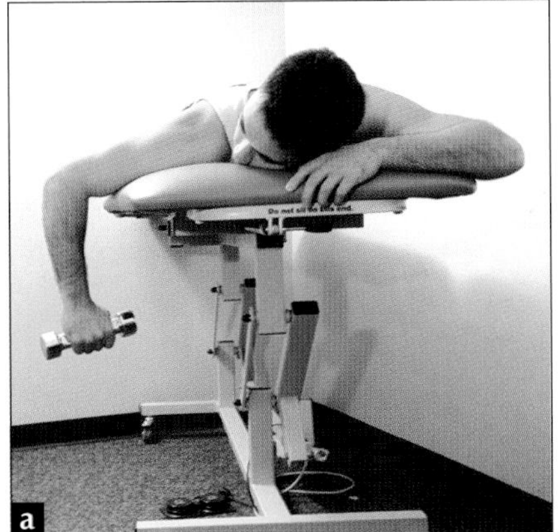

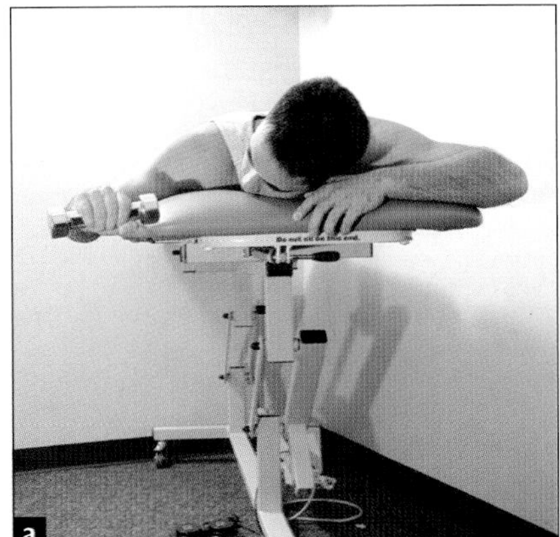

Figure 21.8 Prone 90 degree/90 degree external rotation: *(a)* beginning position; *(b)* end position.

exercises (e.g., shoulder press) and all forms of the bench press exercise should be used cautiously; decline bench press stresses this area the least and may therefore be an appropriate exercise choice in reintroduction of the bench press. The upright row should also be used with caution, as rowing too high (elbows up too high) may aggravate impingement-type pain. It is safe to apply exercises such as the lat pulldown by having the client pull the bar in front to the chest, rather than behind the neck, as described in chapter 13.

Some cardiovascular exercises may also pose problems for the client recovering from shoulder impingement. Use of a VersaClimber® should be considered a contraindication as it places the shoulder in prime position to be impinged (i.e., overhead), especially if strength of the rotator cuff muscles and scapular stabilizers has yet to return. Caution must be used with racket sports; again, placing the arm overhead, as with a tennis serve or racquetball smash, increases the likelihood of impinging structures within the shoulder.

Anterior Instability

In anterior shoulder (glenohumeral joint) instability, the head of the humerus moves too far forward, resulting in possible injury or dislocation [32]. Management of individuals with this condition is one of the greatest challenges facing medical professionals in the orthopedic sports medicine area today. Because posterior instability occurs less frequently, the discussion here is limited to management of anterior instability.

Research has shown that, following an anterior dislocation of the shoulder, redislocation can occur in as many as 90% of young, active individuals while only 30% to 50% of middle-aged individuals redislocate their shoulders. In recent years tremendous advances have been made in rehabilitative and surgical methodology to treat people with shoulder instability. Surgical management of shoulder instability has progressed to include procedures using primarily arthroscopy, as well as high tech instruments that literally shrink the joint capsule (thermal capsulorraphy) to assist in stabilizing the humeral head within the glenoid.

Movement and Exercise Guidelines

Exercise indications for instability (i.e., rotator cuff and scapular strengthening) are similar to those for impingement, since ultimately the rotator cuff is the primary dynamic stabilizer of the glenohumeral joint. Exercises included in figures 21.4 through 21.8, as well as the contraindications listed in table 21.3, must be closely followed. Movements that involve greater than 90 degrees of elevation, placing the hands and arms behind the plane of the shoulder (i.e., approximately 90° anterior to the frontal plane), are dangerous as they may lead to a redislocation. These criteria for shoulder exercises have led to the use of a **safe zone** that describes the position below 90 degrees of elevation of the shoulder and arms anterior to the frontal plane of the body (figure 21.9) [18].

Clients with unstable shoulders may choose either a conservative, exercise-based approach or

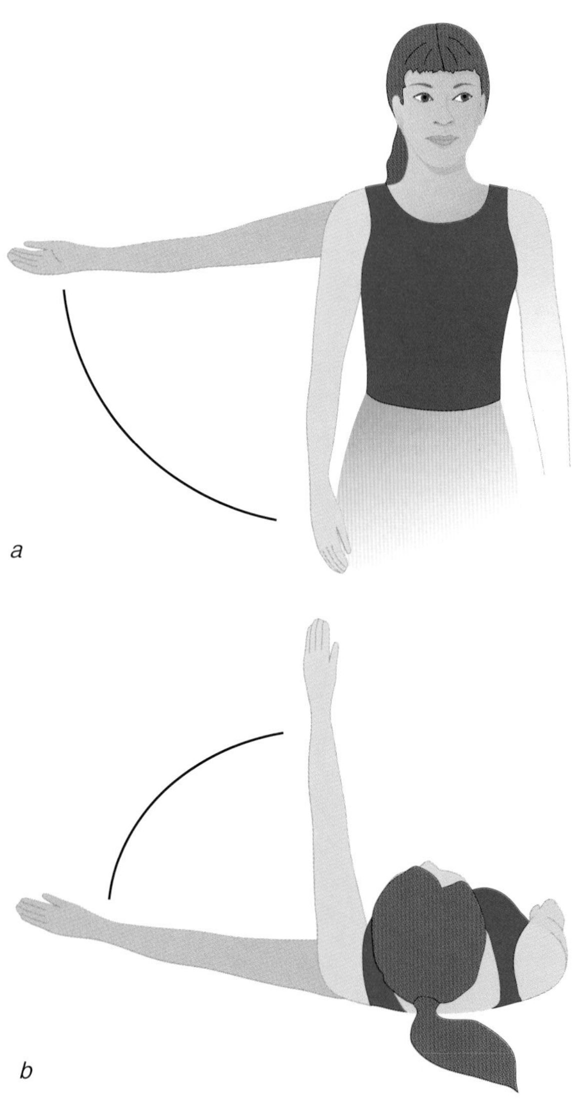

Figure 21.9 Safe zone exercise positions. Positions should be *(a)* below shoulder level and *(b)* in front of the body's frontal plane.

Adapted with permission of IDEA Health & Fitness Association, (800) 999-IDEA, www.IDEAfit.com.

may choose surgery as a remedy for instability. Individuals with unstable shoulders—both conservatively and surgically treated—frequently wish to return to traditional strength training or aerobic conditioning activities, or both. It is imperative that exercise modifications be followed to protect the structures that were repaired during the surgical procedures. Following these exercise modifications may prove to be a permanent part of that individual's lifting program, to ensure that shoulder stability is not compromised (figure 21.10) [32].

Once a client has completed treatment for an unstable shoulder, most aerobic training activities are generally safe to perform, with the exception of some aerobic dance steps, swimming (specifically the freestyle, backstroke, and butterfly), and some racket sport activities. Flexibility exercises that place the shoulder in a position outside the aforementioned safe zone are contraindicated (e.g., the hands-behind-back stretch and the behind-neck stretch, page 278) because of the adverse stresses placed across an already unstable shoulder joint. Table 21.3 provides a movement guide for clients experiencing shoulder dysfunction.

Rotator Cuff Debridement and Subacromial Decompression

Debridement of the rotator cuff and subacromial decompression are typically performed via arthroscopy when impingement or damage to the rotator cuff tendons does not respond to conservative treatment. **Debridement** involves scraping away at the edge of the tear until a clean, bleeding surface of tendon is achieved. This allows for greater healing of the partially torn tendon. Subacromial decompression (SAD) involves scraping or shaving away the bone on the anterior and inferior surfaces of the acromion to decrease the stress or impingement of the rotator cuff tendons between the acromion and head of the humerus. The shaved bone often takes 12 weeks or more to heal, creating significant amounts of pain for the individual following the procedure.

Range of motion and gentle progression of exercise in physical therapy commonly begin immediately following both surgical procedures. Typically, by four to six weeks after surgery, clients can perform rotator cuff exercises in a pain-free manner, and by six to eight weeks following surgery the individual is discharged from formal physical therapy.

Movement and Exercise Guidelines

Clients discharged from formal physical therapy should continue the rotator cuff and scapular strengthening exercises previously discussed. Contraindications for individuals after these surgical procedures include the use of high-resistance and low-repetition upper extremity strength training, as well as exercises using positions outside the safe zone (figure 21.9).

Examples of contraindicated exercises are the full range of motion shoulder press, bench press, pec deck, and behind-the-neck lat pulldown. Recommended modifications of these traditional exercises are presented in table 21.4 for clients following shoulder injury or shoulder surgery. Additional information regarding the modification of traditional exercises after shoulder injury or surgery can be found in Gross et al. [32]. In addition, throwing activities, racket sports, and swimming should be avoided, especially soon after surgery. None of these activities is specifically contraindicated once rehabilitation and recovery from surgery are complete, but one must exercise caution when introducing these activities to postsurgical clients. Aerobic conditioning exercises that are indicated include those on the bicycle, elliptical trainer, and stair stepper.

Rotator Cuff Repair

A rotator cuff repair is typically carried out when damage to the rotator cuff tendons—most often the tendon of the supraspinatus muscle—includes a tear that is "full thickness," meaning that the rotator cuff is not merely frayed but has a tear that goes through its entirety. These tears cause significantly altered joint mechanics [57] and are traditionally repaired using either sutures or suture anchors (fasteners that help reattach the torn tendon to its insertion), most often involving an open incision, in addition to arthroscopy.

Due to the additional open incision and greater extent of damage to the rotator cuff tendons, greater periods of immobilization in a sling are used following a rotator cuff repair. The exact amount of time spent in a sling without movement (commonly ranging from two days to six weeks) is determined by the surgeon and is dictated by factors such as individual's age, tissue quality, and presence of additional injuries found at the time of surgery.

Movement and Exercise Guidelines

Overzealous client activity and inappropriate exercise introduction can lead to failure of the rotator

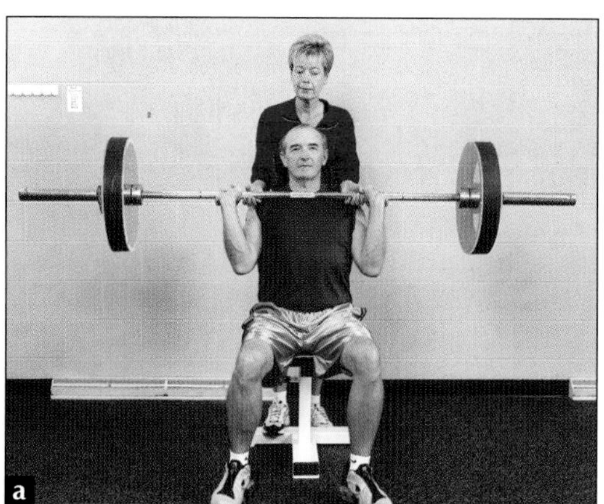

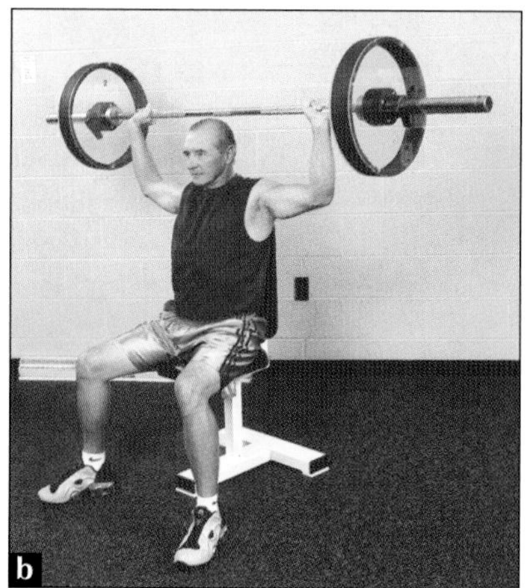

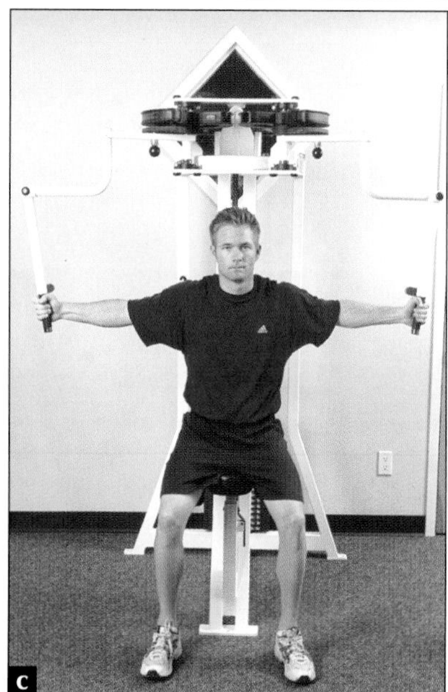

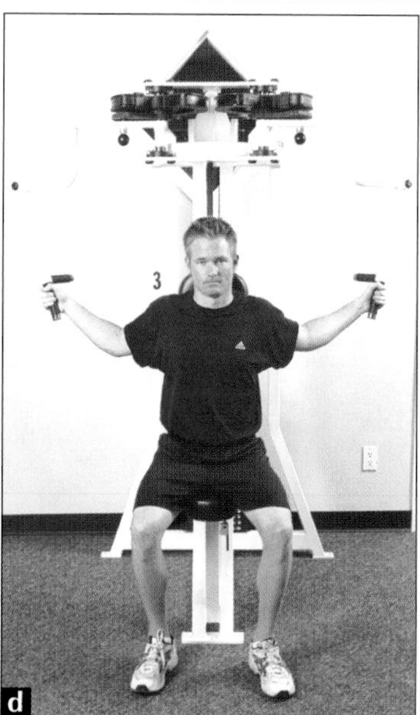

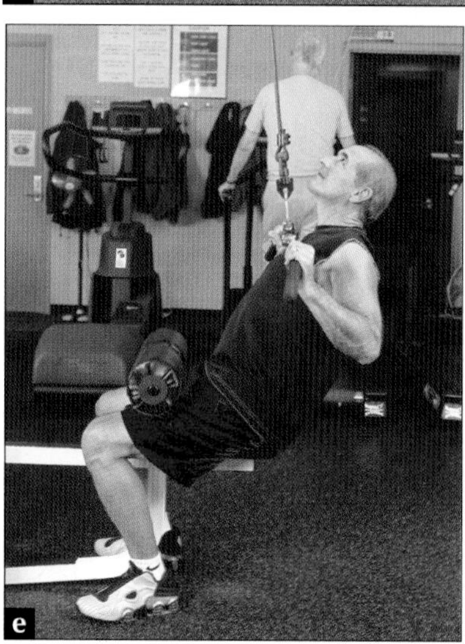

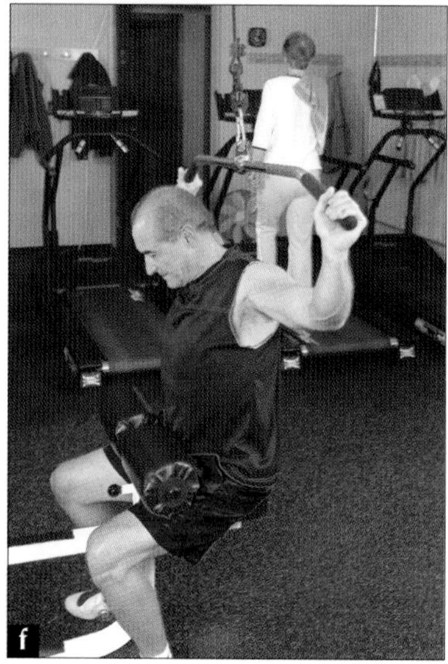

Figure 21.10 Exercise modification and anterior capsule stress. The photos in the left-hand column show exercises being performed correctly, so as to not stress the anterior capsule. Harmful anterior capsule stress results from these exercises being performed incorrectly, as shown in the right-hand column. *(a)* Correct technique: front-of-face shoulder press. *(b)* Incorrect technique: behind-the-neck shoulder press. *(c)* Correct technique: pec deck. *(d)* Incorrect technique: excessive horizontal abduction with pec deck. *(e)* Correct technique: front-of-face lat pulldown. *(f)* Incorrect technique: behind-the-neck lat pulldown.

TABLE 21.3

Shoulder Movement and Exercise Guidelines

Diagnosis	Movement contraindications*	Exercise contraindications*	Exercise indications
Impingement syndrome	Overhead with internally rotated shoulder	Shoulder press Lateral dumbbell raise with internally rotated shoulder Upright row above shoulder level Incline bench press	Rotator cuff strengthening exercises Bench press Lateral dumbbell raise with externally rotated shoulder
Anterior instability	External rotation with >90° abduction Horizontal abduction	Bench press Pec deck Shoulder press Behind-the-neck lat pulldown	Rotator cuff strengthening exercises Lateral and front dumbbell raises Upright row
Rotator cuff debridement and subacromial decompression	Resisted overhead movements	Shoulder press Upright row above shoulder level	Rotator cuff strengthening exercises (beginning one month after surgery) Front dumbbell raise
Rotator cuff repair	Resisted overhead movements	Shoulder press Upright row above shoulder level	Rotator cuff strengthening exercises (beginning six weeks after surgery) Front dumbbell raise

*Consult with a medical professional to determine when or if these movements are no longer contraindicated for a specific client.

cuff repair and disastrous results [14]. Exercise for the scapular muscles and rotator cuff (figures 21.4 through 21.8) are also applied for these clients, but often not for four to six weeks following surgery. Individuals are often discharged from formal physical therapy three to four months after the rotator cuff repair. The exercises in figures 21.4 through 21.8 receive continued emphasis in the post-rehabilitation programming, to ensure continued activation of the rotator cuff musculature.

Contraindicated exercises for these clients are also listed in table 21.3. Overhead lifting and exercises such as push-ups and bench presses place the shoulder in a position of stress and can result in overload to the rotator cuff. Aerobic endurance activities that cause discomfort or pain (e.g., swimming, VersaClimber) should be limited. Typically, aerobic endurance training using lower body exercises such as walking, running, and stair stepping is well tolerated and safe for inclusion during shoulder rehabilitation. Additionally, one complication following rotator cuff surgery is loss of range of motion, the extent dependent on the amount of immobilization used after the surgery. The range of motion loss usually includes the patterns of external rotation, internal rotation, and abduction. This finding further complicates the performance of traditional exercises, such as those that place the shoulder behind the head or body.

Several of the types of shoulder conditions discussed in this section preclude performance of standard upper extremity strength training exercises. Responsible intervention by a personal trainer should include screening of individuals who may be at risk for the performance of these exercises. See "Conditions Requiring Shoulder Exercise Modification" on the next page. Application of rotator cuff and scapular exercises as a "core" aspect of any upper extremity training program is recommended because of the important role these muscles play in providing movement and stabilization of the shoulder complex.

TABLE 21.4

Shoulder Exercise Modifications

Exercise	Modification
Shoulder press	When lowering the barbell, allow the bar to pass in front of the client's head in order to minimize anterior shoulder stress.
Bench press	When lowering the bar, clients with shoulder dysfunction should not allow the bar to touch the chest at its lowest point in order to minimize anterior shoulder stress. Keep the upper arms near the body to limit horizontal abduction and decrease shoulder stress. Using a reverse (supinated) grip reduces shoulder joint stress as well.
Pec deck	During the eccentric phase, clients with shoulder dysfunction should not allow the pads to pass behind the body at their most posterior position in order to minimize anterior shoulder stress.
Lat pulldown	When pulling down the bar, allow the bar to pass in front of the client's head in order to minimize anterior shoulder stress. Use a reverse (supinated) grip to reduce shoulder joint stress.

Conditions Requiring Shoulder Exercise Modification

Exercise for clients with the following conditions is not contraindicated. Each condition, however, requires specific modifications to allow exercise participation.

- Rotator cuff repair
- Rotator cuff tendinitis
- Glenohumeral joint instability (prior dislocation or subluxation)
- Acromioclaviular joint injury (separation)
- Glenohumeral joint osteoarthritis

Knee

As with the shoulder, a variety of injuries and surgical procedures exist for the knee joint; anterior knee pain and three common surgical procedures are described here. Again, we do not give detailed descriptions of injury pathophysiologies and surgical procedures. Rather we overview these procedures, discuss general postoperative rehabilitation, and outline exercise indications and contraindications after discharge from formal physical therapy.

Anterior Knee Pain

Anterior knee pain, a common malady for personal training clients, can include a variety of diagnoses (e.g., chondromalacia, iliotibial band friction syndrome, irritated plica, patellar tendinitis). Clients with anterior knee pain commonly describe pain with prolonged sitting and when walking up and down stairs. Frequent causes of these diagnoses include overuse (particularly with running), biomechanical faults, and muscular imbalance. While each specific anterior knee pain diagnosis requires an individualized approach, all diagnoses have several treatment commonalities to address these precipitating factors. Rehabilitation focuses on reducing inflammation and optimizing tissue function.

Movement and Exercise Guidelines

Overuse is a common cause of anterior knee pain and often occurs with running, jumping, and bicycling. Education on proper running surfaces (concrete vs. asphalt vs. treadmill) and on the benefits of cross-training is quite important in addressing overuse. Biomechanical faults leading to anterior knee pain are often due to patellofemoral malalignment, including improper patellar positioning (either too high [i.e., superior] or too low), tightness of surrounding tissues (e.g., lateral retinaculum, iliotibial band), or altered foot biomechanics (e.g., excessive or improper pronation or supination).

Muscular imbalances surrounding anterior knee pain commonly have to do with the relationship between the vastus lateralis and a portion of the vastus medialis, the **vastus medialis obliquus (VMO)**. The common belief is that the vastus lateralis overpowers the VMO and pulls excessively on the patella, causing the patella to move laterally when the quadriceps muscles are active. Although it is possible that such an imbalance exists, its treatment is rather controversial. It would seem logical to strengthen the VMO to improve this balance, but research has yet to demonstrate that preferential VMO recruitment is possible.

Because the quadriceps muscles help clients walk up stairs and assist deceleration of the body during walking on level surfaces and down steps, general quadriceps strengthening does improve patellofemoral function and reduces anterior knee pain. Care must be taken, however, to use exercises that do not adversely stress the patellofemoral joint. No exercises are explicitly contraindicated for clients experiencing anterior knee pain, but some exercises require caution. Deep squats, and other closed kinetic chain exercises requiring knee flexion of more than 90 degrees, must be prescribed with caution as these increase compression between the patella and femur. Aerobic endurance activities such as high-impact aerobic dance or step aerobics, and aerobic endurance training that places the knee in positions such as a deep lunging or squatting position, would be contraindicated. Typically, cycling and water-based aerobic training activities are recommended to minimize impact and trauma to the knee joint and maintain an individual's aerobic condition during training.

Anterior Cruciate Ligament Reconstruction

Exercises following **anterior cruciate ligament (ACL)** reconstruction are an extremely important part of a person's return to function. The function of the ACL, in concert with other anatomical structures, is to control knee motion and provide proprioceptive feedback [9, 42, 76]. The ACL primarily limits anterior tibial translation [3, 78] and rotation relative to the femur [38, 48]. Because of these important functions, reconstruction is a common treatment choice for joint laxity and possible functional instability, especially with active, competitive people and those with high-demand occupations (e.g., firefighter, construction).

Advances in surgical technique and more aggressive and accelerated postoperative rehabilitation programs have allowed individuals to return to functional activities sooner and with fewer complications than in the past [63]. The most common ACL reconstruction technique uses the central third of the patellar tendon as the graft source, though use of a semitendinosus and gracilis graft is increasing in popularity. There is conflicting evidence as to the relative strength of each graft [2, 6, 22, 75], and each has its own set of advantages and disadvantages.

Movement and Exercise Guidelines

For the most part, rehabilitation and post-rehabilitation contraindications and precautions are the same for the two types of grafts. The primary difference between the grafts is the ability to use the hamstring muscles; semitendinosus/gracilis grafts preclude immediate postoperative active or resistive knee flexion exercise until four to six weeks following surgery (regardless of the type of graft used). At discharge from physical therapy (as early as three to four months after surgery), individuals should have full range of motion of their postoperative knee and good quadriceps function and general lower extremity strength.

During rehabilitation, both open and closed kinetic chain exercises are important parts of the overall program. **Open kinetic chain** exercises are exercises that have the distal aspect of the extremity terminating free in space [19, 66]. Examples of open kinetic chain exercises include the straight leg raise; leg curl; and hip flexion, extension, abduction, and adduction. **Closed kinetic chain** exercises are those that occur with the distal part of the extremity fixed to an object that is either stationary or moving [66]. Closed kinetic chain exercises include the leg press, squat, multidirection lunges, step-ups, and unilateral stance activities. Translation of the tibia relative to the femur is minimized because of the weight bearing and muscular co-contraction (quadriceps and hamstring muscles) during closed kinetic chain exercises; further, these exercises allow multiple joints and muscle groups to be trained simultaneously.

Post-rehabilitation exercises should use a combination of open and closed kinetic chain exercise. The open kinetic chain leg extension exercise should be

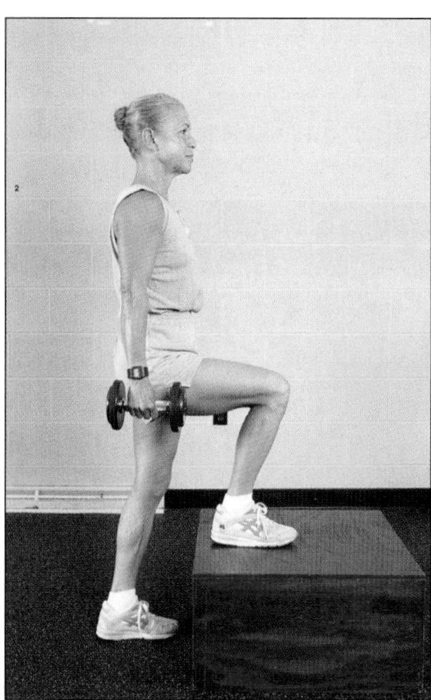

Figure 21.11 A closed kinetic chain exercise: The step-up.

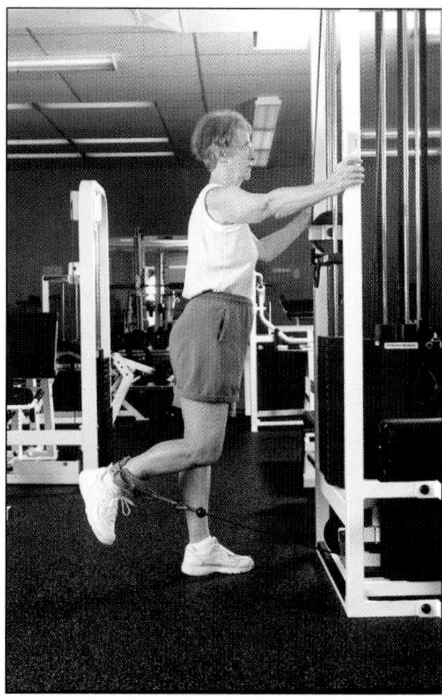

Figure 21.12 An open kinetic chain exercise: The standing leg curl.

used with caution; research has shown that the greatest amount of anterior tibial translation—hence the greatest stress on the ACL graft—occurs in the final 30 degrees of leg extension performed in an open kinetic chain [73]. Therefore, open kinetic chain leg extension exercises should be performed using a range of motion from 90 degrees of knee flexion to only 45 degrees of knee extension to decrease stresses placed on the ACL graft. Clients should adhere to this important modification, at a minimum, for the first six months to one year after surgery to protect the maturing graft and minimize damaging stress application.

Recent research [54] has shown that ACL reconstruction individuals who perform bilateral closed kinetic chain exercise shield weight bearing away from the injured limb for up to a year following surgery, placing a greater percentage of weight bearing on the uninvolved or uninjured limb. They do this subconsciously and without volition. Therefore, reliance on only bilateral closed kinetic chain exercise activities for individuals following ACL reconstruction may result in inadequate training stimulus to the injured limb and suboptimal loading paradigms. Use of unilateral stance and exercise patterns such as single-leg squats and step-ups helps to ensure that this training compensation does not occur.

To summarize from the information presented, specific contraindications for exercise following ACL reconstruction include full range of motion open kinetic chain leg extension exercise, as well as closed kinetic chain exercise using greater than 90 degrees of knee flexion. For those ACL reconstructions using a semitendinosus/gracilis graft, active and resistive hamstring exercise is contraindicated for the first four to six weeks; this becomes a precaution for the personal trainer during post-rehabilitation strength training and conditioning. Further, because both the patella and patellar tendon have become weakened with the patellar tendon graft, caution is warranted when using activities that rely on significant quadriceps use (e.g., full squats and lunges, stair stepper using deep step movements). Bicycles, elliptical trainers, stair steppers using shallow steps, and swimming are all appropriate following ACL reconstruction, regardless of the type of graft used.

Total Knee Arthroplasty

Years of repetitive loading to the human knee can result in degeneration and degradation of the joint surfaces of the distal femur and proximal tibia. Often this degeneration is specifically located on either the medial or the lateral side of the knee joint, based on wear patterns and more specifically the individual's lower extremity alignment. People who are excessively bow-legged *(genu varum)*, knock-kneed *(genu valgum)*, or who have had serious injury to the knee (such as extensive fractures through the joint, meniscal pathology, or instability of the knee due to unrepaired or failed repair of ligamentous structures), are often candidates for a total knee replacement.

Total knee arthroplasty (TKA) requires extensive exposure of the joint with a large central incision. Prosthetic components are selected and inserted to cover the worn areas at the ends of both the femur and tibia. Rehabilitation begins immediately with a range of motion focus. Individuals perform open and closed kinetic chain exercises initially in the hospital and at home prior to formal outpatient physical therapy.

Movement and Exercise Guidelines

Following discharge from physical therapy, clients often have 100 degrees to 120 degrees of knee flexion and nearly complete knee extension. Indications for exercise include cycling, swimming, and endurance-based activities that minimize joint impact loading and improve muscular and cardiovascular function and fitness levels. Specific exercises such as leg press, multidirection hip strengthening, calf raises, and knee flexion and extension exercises using a low resistance and high repetition format are recommended.

Again, closed kinetic chain exercises that place the knee in greater than 100 degrees of flexion are risky and impose added stresses on the knee. Further, because kneeling is contraindicated for clients following TKA, it is necessary for them to avoid exercises requiring that position (e.g., kneeling lat pulldown, bent-over dumbbell row using a bench) or exercises that may cause them to kneel inadvertently (e.g., lunges performed too deeply) (figure 21.13). Exercises using less than 90 degrees knee flexion postures are recommended in both open and closed kinetic chain exercises. Table 21.5 provides movement guidelines for clients experiencing knee pain.

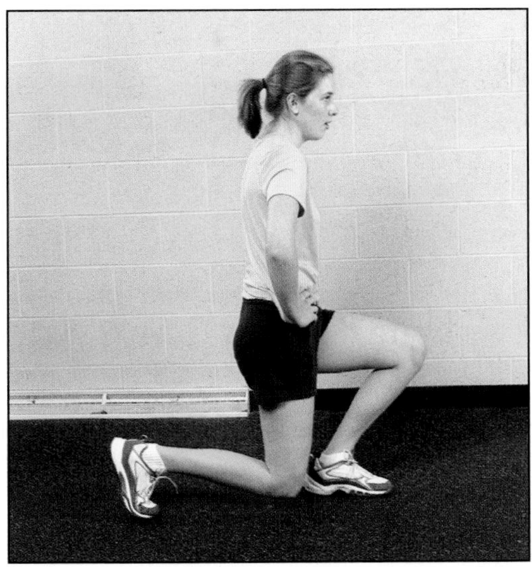

Figure 21.13 Clients who have undergone total knee arthroplasty should avoid excessive knee flexion, such as in a deep lunge as shown here.

Each of the knee joint's structures requires a specific type of exercise to return the client to full function after injury or surgery; with anterior knee pain, for example, the focus is on reducing inflammation, whereas after total knee arthroplasty the emphasis is on range of motion. Quadriceps strengthening is a common goal in nearly all knee injury rehabilitation and is a key to returning more normal function after injury.

Hip

Though hip dysfunction does occur, in comparison to injuries to the knee and shoulder joints there are relatively few hip injuries and surgical procedures personal trainers will encounter. This paucity of hip pathology is primarily due to the inherent stability of the hip; although it is the same type of joint as the shoulder, the hip has a much deeper acetabulum, or socket, which provides a much more stable articulation. This stability precludes many of the abnormal wear patterns and eliminates many of the traumas the other joints experience, resulting in fewer surgical procedures. Despite its generally good fit, however, the hip joint can experience injury and may be poorly aligned, with osteoarthritis and pain the result.

Total Hip Arthroplasty

Commonly termed a hip replacement, total hip arthroplasty (THA) is the surgical treatment of choice if nonsurgical intervention (e.g., pharmaceutical and physical therapies) for hip osteoarthritis fails. More than 100,000 prosthetic hips are implanted each year, primarily to relieve osteoarthritic pain, with pain relief typically lasting more than 15 years. There are two primary prostheses: cemented and uncemented. A variety of techniques (i.e., posterior, anterolateral, and transtrochanteric) are used during THA. Each has special movement and exercise indications and contraindications.

Cemented prostheses involve affixing the femoral and acetabular components with bone cement,

TABLE 21.5

Knee Movement and Exercise Guidelines

Diagnosis	Movement contraindications	Exercise contraindications	Exercise indications
Anterior knee pain*	Closed chain knee movements with >90° knee flexion Open chain knee movements 0-30° knee flexion	Full squat Full lunge End range of leg extension Stair stepper with large steps	1/4 to 1/2 squat and leg press Partial lunge Leg curl Stair stepper with short, choppy steps
Anterior cruciate ligament reconstruction	Open chain knee movements <45° knee flexion	End range of leg extension	3/4 squat and leg press Step-up Leg curl Stiff-leg deadlift Elliptical trainer
Total knee arthroplasty	Closed chain knee movements with >100° knee flexion Kneeling	Full squat Full lunge	1/4 to 1/2 squat and leg press Partial lunge Leg extension and leg curl Stationary bicycle Water aerobics/Swimming

*Although these movement and exercise contraindications are commonly used, it should be remembered that individual clients react to anterior knee pain differently; therefore, for those clients with this general diagnosis, the ranges of motion and exercises provided should be considered relative. Exercises and movements that cause anterior knee pain become absolute contraindications and should be eliminated from the client's exercise program.

whereas uncemented prostheses allow direct attachment of the prosthetic components to the bone. Each type of prosthesis has its advantages and disadvantages; one of the primary differences, however, is weight-bearing restriction following surgery. Cemented prostheses allow immediate postoperative weight bearing while uncemented prostheses require weight-bearing restrictions anywhere from 6 to 12 weeks.

Like the options for prosthesis, each surgical approach has distinct advantages and disadvantages. Most importantly for the personal trainer are the movement restrictions following each method. Each technique approaches the hip joint from a different angle, thereby decreasing the strength of the hip joint's capsule at the point of entry. For example, the posterior approach—the most common approach in the United States—weakens the posterior aspect of the joint capsule, leaving the hip at increased risk of dislocation. Individuals typically adhere to the restrictions for a minimum of six weeks, though these depend on the surgeon protocols.

Total hip arthroplasty movement restrictions include the following:

- No hip flexion greater than 90°
- No hip adduction past neutral
- No hip internal rotation

Formal physical therapy following THA is not prescribed as often as for the previously discussed surgical procedures. Postoperatively, individuals should progress to hip and lower extremity strengthening exercises (per surgeon protocol) and should concentrate on improving their patterns of gait.

Movement and Exercise Guidelines

When working with clients who have undergone THA, personal trainers should contact the surgeon who performed the procedure to discuss any con-

TABLE 21.6

Hip Movement and Exercise Guidelines

Diagnosis	Movement contraindications	Exercise contraindications	Exercise indications
Total hip arthroplasty (THA)	Hip flexion greater than 90° Hip adduction past neutral Hip internal rotation	Resisted hip flexion (e.g., four-way hip machine) Full sit-up Hip adduction machine	1/2 squat or leg press Stair stepper Elliptical trainer

tinued movement restrictions. When prescribing exercise, the personal trainer should avoid high-impact activities (e.g., running, step aerobics, plyometrics). Lower-impact activities (e.g., swimming, walking, stair stepping, use of elliptical trainer) are indicated following surgery to improve functions following THA. Weight training is not contraindicated after THA, but some specific exercises should be modified in accordance with the physical abilities and limitations of the client. Consulting with the surgeon should be considered mandatory when one is in doubt about movement and exercise choices. Table 21.6 provides a list of exercise indications and contraindications following THA.

Arthritis

Arthritis is a general term encompassing several different diseases. The two primary arthritis classifications are osteoarthritis and rheumatoid arthritis. Although both terms refer to the joint, these are two quite different diseases. **Osteoarthritis (OA)**, commonly referred to as degenerative joint disease, is the progressive destruction of a joint's articular cartilage—the cartilage covering the surface of the given joint. **Rheumatoid arthritis (RA)**, on the other hand, is a systemic inflammatory disease affecting not only the joint surface, but also connective tissue (e.g., joint capsules and ligaments). In the paragraphs that follow we discuss each form of arthritis and appropriate exercise choices.

Osteoarthritis

Osteoarthritis (OA) is a degenerative joint condition characterized by deterioration of the cartilaginous weight-bearing surfaces of articular joints, sclerotic changes in subchondral bone, and proliferation of new bone at the margins of joints [69]. The proliferation of new bone, which often manifests itself as spurs or osteophytes, can interfere with normal joint function and cause both pain and limitation in range of motion. Osteoarthritis is present in 15% of adult females and 11% of adult males, and some form of OA is present in some manner in the majority of people age 55 and older [71].

The proposed pathophysiology of OA includes mechanical stresses that result in microfractures. This microfracturing leads to altered metabolism of chondrocytes, which then leads to a loss of cartilage, altered joint structure, and osteophyte production [15]. Loss of cartilage at the joint leads to bone-on-bone contact, thereby causing inflammation.

Oral viscosupplementation—the use of dietary supplements to improve joint function— is currently recommended by physicians for nearly all forms of OA. The common oral, over-the-counter supplements chondroitin sulfate and glucosamine have received favorable recommendations for treatment of OA in weight-bearing joints [15]. Further research needs to be done to bring about better understanding of both the mechanism and the stage at which these supplements are most beneficial to individuals with OA.

Movement and Exercise Guidelines

Exercise indications for individuals with OA include low-resistance, high-repetition programs of exercise that minimize loading of articular surfaces. One application that is particularly helpful in clients with OA is aquatic exercise. The naturally buoyant properties of water allow individuals to exercise with significantly less joint loading than with other forms of activity [68]. Additional indications for exercise are the inclusion of cardiovascular training activities with limited weight bearing such as biking, use of the elliptical trainer, and swimming to protect the joint surfaces and minimize impact loading. Weight management, as well as muscular endurance gained via cardiovascular exercise, is of great benefit to the client with OA (table 21.7).

TABLE 21.7

Osteoarthritis Movement and Exercise Guidelines

Movement contraindications	Exercise contraindications	Exercise indications
High-impact activities	Running, jogging, snow skiing	Bicycle Stair stepper Elliptical trainer Water aerobics/Swimming

Resistance exercise programs using predominantly open kinetic chain exercises in the upper extremity are recommended. Closed kinetic chain exercises such as push-ups are contraindicated due to the compressive nature of the exercise at the glenohumeral joint. In the lower extremity, open kinetic chain exercises are typically indicated with the exception of full range of motion leg extension exercises for the individual with patellofemoral OA. As discussed previously, modifications for this open kinetic chain leg extension exercise would include partial range of motion arcs either from 90 degrees to 45 degrees or from 0 degrees to 30 degrees of knee motion, where patellofemoral compressive forces are the least damaging [49].

Clients can perform lightweight closed kinetic chain exercises for the lower extremities based on the presence of pain and the individual's general tolerance. Inclusion of balance training to enhance proprioception and motor control for the client with OA is another recommendation. This is particularly effective for training older individuals, who frequently have problems with balance.

Rheumatoid Arthritis

Rheumatoid arthritis (RA) is an inflammatory, autoimmune disease affecting many joints and often several body systems. Though it may be caused by a bacterial or viral precipitant, the etiology of RA is as of yet unknown. The most likely cause is the aberrant regulation of T-cells leading to the inflammation and destruction of joints [10, 13, 20, 56].

Rheumatoid arthritis involves the inflammation and proliferation of a joint's synovial lining. This proliferation, or thickening, increases joint pressure and, in concert with rheumatoid pannus (a tissue that dissolves collagen), leads to poor joint nutrition, joint swelling, and muscular inhibition. The inflammatory process, swelling, and lack of nutrition weaken the joint capsule and its ligamentous restraints; further, the joint surfaces (i.e., articular cartilage) deteriorate from the same causes. All of this can result in a hypermobile—or *loose*—and potentially unstable joint. A personal trainer who suspects that a client has an unstable joint should refer the client to his or her physician or physical therapist for further evaluation and exercise programming. These changes are painful and typically cause a person with RA to limit movements to avoid pain, resulting in disuse atrophy [62, 72]. The immobility contributes to continued cartilage degeneration, increasing the pain and further weakening the joint surface structure [33]. So, from the primary joint deterioration, the secondary impairments of RA include decreased strength, aerobic endurance, and flexibility [10, 51].

Presentation of RA is variable, with cycles of **exacerbation** (flare-ups with increased pain, swelling, and stiffness) and **remission** (periods of relative comfort with no outward signs of inflammation). During RA exacerbation, clients typically describe warm, swollen joints and morning stiffness. In addition to these disease cycles, RA is considered progressive. Manifestations may include osteoporosis, muscle atrophy, periarticular nodules, joint deformity, and eventual joint ankylosis.

Areas commonly affected by RA include the neck, shoulders, and wrists and hands. The upper and midcervical regions of the neck are common sites of inflammation, resulting in the aforementioned tissue degeneration [52, 45]. Degeneration or rupture of the ligaments supporting the first two cervical vertebrae may result in a life-threatening situation. For this reason, neck-specific exercises should be considered contraindicated or should be used only under supervision of a health care professional.

In addition to joints, RA affects muscles and bursae. Degeneration of the shoulder joints and associated structures (e.g., rotator cuff muscles and tendons) may lead to joint laxity resulting in abnormal movement patterns, possibly leading to an unstable shoulder joint. Rotator cuff tears occur in 30% to 40% of those with RA [26, 27, 53]. Ligamentous and capsular degeneration may result in unstable wrist joints; further, the joints of the fingers and thumb commonly swell, causing the client to lose grip strength.

Movement and Exercise Guidelines

As in OA, the pathology of RA cannot be prevented once started. However, it may be possible to slow the debilitating effects of RA's secondary impairments (i.e., decreased strength, aerobic endurance, and flexibility). Exercise goals for clients with RA focus on improving function during daily activities, improving general health, and providing protection to the affected joints. Maintaining muscular strength, aerobic endurance, joint and musculotendinous flexibility, functional balance, and body composition addresses these goals; and these are areas that personal trainers are well equipped to deal with.

Properly designed exercise programs that address these goals do not increase pain and may actually decrease the client's pain [50, 67]. Resistance training is indicated for clients with RA. Both isometric and dynamic resistance training modes are appropriate [33, 34, 36, 55, 72], with isometric resistance training appropriate during periods of exacerbation [62]. Further, and perhaps surprisingly, vigorous aerobic endurance exercise is not contraindicated. In fact, clients with RA not only tolerate high-intensity exercise; this type of exercise may actually be anti-inflammatory and pain relieving [21, 35, 37, 44, 50, 72]. A client who is experiencing joint inflammation, however, should avoid vigorous aerobic endurance exercise. Flexibility training is another form of exercise appropriate for clients with RA [51]. While the personal trainer should emphasize not overstretching loose or unstable joints, clients with RA should perform flexibility exercises to maintain adequate joint movement [51, 55]. They should perform stretching every day and can do so in a pain-free range during flare-ups.

The commonly affected areas (i.e., cervical spine, shoulders, and wrists) require modification of exercise programming. Exercises involving the cervical spine should be avoided (e.g., stretching and manually resisted neck strengthening exercises), as should exercises that place the shoulder in an impingement-prone position (e.g., upright row) or in a position outside the safe zone shown in figure 21.9 (e.g., behind-the-neck shoulder press). A last guideline is for exercises involving the wrists and hands; because the hands and wrists are affected, clients with RA may need to have the diameter of the bar, dumbbell, or handle increased in an attempt to offset their weakened grip. For example, if a client has difficulty performing a dumbbell biceps curl, tape or padding may be applied to the dumbbell handle to "build up" the grip's diameter, thereby improving the client's ability to maintain his or her grasp on the dumbbell.

Because of the periods of changing pain and functional impairment, selection of exercises and intensities for clients with RA must be according to individual tolerances. Clients must be aware of the occurrence of periods of exacerbation and should adjust activity and exercise accordingly; specifically, "If a joint is inflamed, it rests" [10, 51]. Table 21.8 provides a list of appropriate and inappropriate exercises for clients diagnosed with RA.

Although the pathophysiology is quite different for each, clients with osteoarthritis or rheumatoid arthritis benefit from performing strengthening and aerobic exercise. The difference between the two is the body's response to activity. Exercise should not increase joint pain for either group. Particular care must be given to the client with rheumatoid arthritis during periods of exacerbation.

TABLE 21.8

Rheumatoid Arthritis Movement and Exercise Guidelines

Movement contraindications	Exercise contraindications	Exercise indications
High-impact cardiovascular exercise Neck flexibility or strengthening in clients with history of neck instability Movements outside the safe zone	Running, jogging Upper trapezius stretch Manually resisted neck strengthening Behind-the-neck shoulder press	Moderate intensity (60-80% maximal heart rate) [52] aerobic endurance exercise (e.g., stationary bicycle, elliptical trainer, stair stepper) Range of motion and flexibility exercises Isometric exercise (for the unstable joint) Water aerobics Stationary bicycling

CONCLUSION

Personal trainers work with a wide variety of clients, many of whom have experienced injury or have undergone surgery necessitating a modified approach to exercise prescription. When designing exercise programs for this population, it is important to understand the basic types of injury and the stages of healing that all musculoskeletal tissues follow. In concert with communication between the personal trainer and other health care practitioners, familiarity with these stages of healing and with individual injury, surgical procedures, and disease processes will assist personal trainers in using safe and appropriate programs of exercise for their clients.

STUDY QUESTIONS

1. Which of the following exercises should a client diagnosed with advanced spondylolisthesis avoid?
   A. full sit-up
   B. abdominal crunch
   C. reverse hyperextension
   D. stability ball abdominal crunch
2. An electrician describes shoulder pain following a fall from a ladder. His physician has diagnosed him with impingement syndrome, but he has been cleared to perform any exercises. Which of the following exercises is the MOST appropriate for this client?
   A. upright row
   B. shoulder press
   C. decline bench press
   D. incline dumbbell fly
3. Which of the following describes a recommended technique guideline for performing exercises to strengthen the rotator cuff muscles?
   A. only position the upper arm parallel to the torso
   B. do not move the upper arm anterior to the frontal plane
   C. do not raise the upper arm higher than 90 degrees of elevation
   D. involve the trapezius muscle when the rotator cuff muscles become fatigued
4. A client had her ACL reconstructed and, three months later, she describes chronically decreased quadriceps strength. To reach the goal of returning to play beach volleyball, this client wants to begin a resistance training program. Which of the following exercises should be avoided?
   A. full range of motion leg extension
   B. full range of motion leg curl
   C. 3/4 back squat
   D. step-up

APPLIED KNOWLEDGE QUESTION

A 50-year-old female client was diagnosed with rheumatoid arthritis 5 year ago. She describes a history of left shoulder subluxations but is otherwise healthy. Her physician released her to be involved with an exercise program; her goals are to improve aerobic conditioning and overall function. Describe an appropriate beginning exercise program for this client.

Three months after beginning, the client describes an overall improvement, but states that her wrists have been more sore than usual and she is experiencing a flare-up. How should the above program be modified?

REFERENCES

1. Amadio, P.C. 1992. Tendon and ligament. In: *Wound Healing: Biochemical and Clinical Aspects,* I.K. Cohen, R.F. Diegelmann, and W.J. Lindblad, eds. Philadelphia: Saunders, p. 384.
2. Anderson, A.F., R.B. Snyder, and A.B. Lipscomb Jr. 2001. Anterior cruciate ligament reconstruction. A prospective randomized study of three surgical methods. *American Journal of Sports Medicine* 29 (3): 272-279.
3. Andersson, C., M. Odensten, and J. Gillquist. 1991. Knee function after surgical or nonsurgical treatment of acute rupture of the anterior cruciate ligament: A randomized study with a long-term follow-up period. *Clinical Orthopaedics and Related Research* 264 (March): 255-263.
4. Arrington, E.D., and M.D. Miller. 1995. Skeletal muscle injuries. *Orthopedic Clinics of North America* 26 (3): 411-422.
5. Ballantyne, B.T., S.J. O'Hare, J.L. Paschall, M.M. Pavia-Smith, A.M. Pitz, J.F. Gillon, and G.L. Soderberg. 1993. Electromyographic activity of selected shoulder muscles in commonly used therapeutic exercises. *Physical Therapy* 73: 668-682.
6. Barrett, G.R., F.K. Noojin, C.W. Hartzog, and C.R. Nash. 2002. Reconstruction of the anterior cruciate ligament in females: A comparison of hamstring versus patellar tendon autograft. *Arthroscopy* 18 (1): 46-54.
7. Beiner, J.M., and P. Jokl. 2001. Muscle contusion injuries: Current treatment options. *Journal of the American Academy of Orthopaedic Surgeons* 9 (4): 227-237.
8. Berkowitz, M., and C. Greene. 1989. Disability expenditures. *American Rehabilitation* 15 (1): 7.
9. Biedert, R.M., E. Stauffer, and N.F. Friederich. 1992. Occurrence of free nerve endings in the soft tissue of the knee joint. A histologic investigation. *American Journal of Sports Medicine* 20 (4, July-August): 430-433.
10. Bilek, L. Personal communication, 31 October, 2002.
11. Blackburn, T.A., W.E. McLeod, B. White, and L. Wofford. 1990. EMG analysis of posterior rotator cuff exercises. *Athletic Training* 25: 40-45.
12. Bodack, M.P., and M. Monteiro. 2001. Therapeutic exercise in the treatment of patients with lumbar spinal stenosis. *Clinical Orthopaedics and Related Research* 384 (March): 144-152.
13. Breedveld, F.C. 1998. New insights in the pathogenesis of rheumatoid arthritis. *The Journal of Rheumatology* (Suppl) 53: 3-7.
14. Burkhart, S.S., D.L. Diaz Pagan, M.A. Wirth, and K.A. Athanasiou. 1997. Cyclic loading of anchor-based rotator cuff repairs. *Arthroscopy* 13 (2): 720-824.
15. Carfagno, D., and T.S. Ellenbecker. 2002. Osteoarthritis of the glenohumeral joint: Nonsurgical treatment options. *Physician and Sportsmedicine* 30 (4, April): 19-32.
16. Curwin, S., and W. Stanish. 1984. *Tendinitis: Its Etiology and Treatment.* Lexington, MA: Collamore Press.
17. Ellenbecker, T.S. 1995. Rehabilitation of shoulder and elbow injuries in tennis players. *Clinics in Sports Medicine* 14 (1): 87-110.
18. Ellenbecker, T.S. 2000. Postrehabilitation: Shoulder conditioning for tennis. *IDEA Personal Trainer* (March): 18-27.
19. Ellenbecker, T.S., and G.J. Davies. 2001. *Closed Kinetic Chain Rehabilitation.* Champaign, IL: Human Kinetics.
20. Feldmann, M., F.M. Brennan, and R.N. Maini. 1996. Rheumatoid arthritis. *Cell* 85 (3): 307-310.
21. Feldmann, S.V. 1996. *Exercise for the Person with Rheumatoid Arthritis. Rehabilitation of Persons with Rheumatoid Arthritis.* Gaithersburg, MD: Aspen.
22. Feller, J.A., K.E. Webster, and B. Gavin. 2001. Early post-operative morbidity following anterior cruciate ligament reconstruction: Patellar tendon versus hamstring graft. *Knee Surgery, Sports Traumatology, Arthroscopy: Official Journal of the ESSKA* 9 (5, September): 260-266.
23. Fredericson, M., A. Bergman, K. Hoffman, and M. Dillingham. 1995. Tibial stress fractures in runners. *American Journal of Sports Medicine* 23: 472-481.
24. Fredrickson, B.E., D. Baker, W.J. McHolick, H.A. Yaun, and J.P. Lubicky. 1984. The natural history of spondylolysis and spondylolisthesis. *The Journal of Bone and Joint Surgery* 66A: 699-707.
25. Frey, C.C., and M.J. Shereff. 1988. Tendon injuries about the ankle in athletes. *Clinics in Sports Medicine* 7: 103-118.
26. Friedman, R.J. 1990. Total shoulder arthroplasty in rheumatoid arthritis. In: *Shoulder Reconstruction.* Philadelphia: Saunders, p. 158.
27. Friedman, R.J., T.S. Thornhill, W.H. Thomas, and C.B. Sledge. 1979. Nonconstrained total shoulder replacement in patients who have rheumatoid arthritis and class IV function. *Journal of Bone and Joint Surgery* 71A: 494.
28. Galin, J.I., I.M. Goldstein, and R. Snyderman. 1988. *Inflammation: Basic Principles and Clinical Correlates.* New York: Raven Press.
29. Gelberman, R., V. Goldberg, K.N. An, et al. 1988. Tendinitis. In: *Injury and Repair of the Musculoskeletal Soft Tissue,* S.L.-Y. Woo and J.A. Buckwalter, eds. Park Ridge, IL: American Academy of Orthopaedic Surgeons, p. 5.
30. Giladi, M., C. Milgrom, A. Simkin, and Y. Danon. 1991. Stress fractures: Identifiable risk factors. *American Journal of Sports Medicine* 19 (6): 647-652.
31. Gross, M.T. 1992. Chronic tendinitis: Pathomechanics of injury, factors affecting the healing response, and treatment. *The Journal of Orthopaedic and Sports Physical Therapy* 16 (6): 248-261.
32. Gross, M.L., S.L. Brenner, I. Esformes, and J.J. Sonzogni. 1993. Anterior shoulder instability in weight lifters. *American Journal of Sports Medicine* 21 (4): 599-603.
33. Hakkinen, A., K. Hakkinen, and P. Hannonen. 1994. Effects of strength training on neuromuscular function and disease activity in patients with recent-onset inflammatory arthritis. *Scandinavian Journal of Rheumatology* 23 (5): 237-242.
34. Hakkinen, A., T. Sokka, A. Kotaniemi, H. Kautiainen, I. Jappinen, L. Laitinen, and P. Hannonen. 1999. Dynamic strength training in patients with early rheumatoid arthritis increases muscle strength but not bone density. *Journal of Rheumatology* 26: 1257-1263.
35. Hakkinen, A., T. Sokka, A. Kotaniemi, and P. Hannonen. 2001. A randomized two-year study of the effects of dynamic strength training on muscle strength, disease activity, functional capacity, and bone mineral density in early rheumatoid arthritis. *Arthritis and Rheumatism* 44 (3): 515-522.
36. Harkcom, T.M., R.M. Lampman, B.F. Banwell, and C.W. Castor. 1985. Therapeutic value of graded aerobic exercise training in rheumatoid arthritis. *Arthritis and Rheumatism* 28 (1): 32-39.
37. Hazes, J.M., and C.H.M. van den Ende. 1996. How vigorously should we exercise our rheumatoid arthritis patients? *Annals of Rheumatic Diseases* 55: 861-862.
38. Hefzy, M.S., and E.S. Grood. 1983. An analytical technique for modeling knee joint stiffness—Part II: Ligamentous geometric nonlinearities. *Journal of Biomechanical Engineering* 105 (2, May): 145-153.

39. Hensinger, R.N. 1989. Spondylolysis and spondylolisthesis in children and adolescents. *Journal of Bone and Joint Surgery* 71A: 1098-1107.

40. Hoshina, H. 1980. Spondylolysis in athletes. *The Physician and Sportsmedicine* 8 (9): 75-79.

41. Jackson, D.W., L.L. Wiltse, R.D. Dingeman, and M. Hayes. 1981. Stress reactions involving the pars interarticularis in young athletes. *American Journal of Sports Medicine* 9: 304-312.

42. Johansson, H., P. Sjolander, and P. Sojka. 1991. Receptors in the knee joint ligaments and their role in the biomechanics of the joint. *Critical Reviews in Biomedical Engineering*18 (5): 341-368.

43. Johnson, R.J. 1993. Low back pain in sports—managing spondylolysis in young patients. *The Physician and Sportsmedicine* 21 (4): 53-59.

44. Komatireddy, G.R., R.W. Leitch, K. Cella, G. Browning, and M. Minor. 1997. Efficacy of low load resistive muscle training in patients with rheumatoid arthritis functional class II and III. *Journal of Rheumatology* 24 (8): 1531-1539.

45. Kramer, J., F. Jolesz, and J. Kleefield. 1991. Rheumatoid arthritis of the cervical spine. *Rheumatic Diseases Clinics of North America* 17: 757.

46. Kraus, D.R., and D. Shapiro. 1989. The symptomatic lumbar spine in the athlete. *Clinics in Sports Medicine* 8: 59-69.

47. Leadbetter, W.B. 1992. Cell-matrix response in tendon injury. *Clinics in Sports Medicine* 11 (3): 533-578.

48. Markolf, K.L., D.C. Wascher, and G.A. Finerman. 1993. Direct in vitro measurement of forces in the cruciate ligaments. Part II: The effect of section of the posterolateral structures. *Journal of Bone and Joint Surgery* 75 (3, March): 387-394.

49. McConnell, J. 2000. Patellofemoral joint complications and considerations. In: *Knee Ligament Rehabilitation,* 2nd ed., T.S. Ellenbecker, ed. Philadelphia: Churchill Livingstone.

50. Minor, M.A., J.E. Hewett, R.R. Webel, S.K. Anderson, and D.R. Kay. 1989. Efficacy of physical conditioning exercises in patients with rheumatoid arthritis and osteoarthritis. *Arthritis and Rheumatism* 32: 1396-1405.

51. Minor, M.A., and D.R. Kay. 2003. Arthritis. In: *ACSM's Exercise Management for Persons with Chronic Diseases and Disabilities,* 2nd ed., J.L. Durstine and G.E. Moore, eds. Champaign, IL: Human Kinetics.

52. Moncur, D., and H.J. Williams. 1988. Cervical spine management in patients with rheumatoid arthritis. *Physical Therapy* 68: 509.

53. Neer, C.S., K.C. Weston, and F.J. Stanton. 1982. Recent experience in total shoulder replacement. *Journal of Bone and Joint Surgery* 64A: 319.

54. Neitzel, J.A., T. Kernozek, G.J. Davies. 2002. Loading response following ACL reconstruction during parallel squat exercise. *Clinical Biomechanics* 17: 551-554.

55. Nieman, D.C. 2000. Exercise soothes arthritis joint effects. *ACSM's Health and Fitness Journal* 4: 20-27.

56. Panayi, G.S. 1997. T-cell-dependent pathways in rheumatoid arthritis. *Current Opinion in Rheumatology* 9 (3): 236-240.

57. Parsons, I.M., M. Apreleva, F.H. Fu, and S.L. Woo. 2002. The effect of rotator cuff tears on reaction forces at the glenohumeral joint. *Journal of Orthopaedic Research* 20 (3, May): 439-446.

58. Petersen, T., P. Kryger, C. Ekdahl, S. Olsen, and S. Jacobsen. 2002. The effect of McKenzie therapy as compared with that of intensive strengthening training for the treatment of patients with subacute or chronic low back pain: A randomized controlled trial. *Spine* 27 (16, August 15): 1702-1709.

59. Porterfield, J.A., and C. DeRosa. 1998. Mechanical low back pain. In: *Perspectives in Functional Anatomy,* 2nd ed. Philadelphia: Saunders.

60. Potach, D.H., and R. Borden. 2000. Rehabilitation and reconditioning. In: *Essentials of Strength Training and Conditioning,* 2nd ed., T.R. Baechle and R.W. Earle, eds. Champaign, IL: Human Kinetics.

61. Saal, J. 1995. The role of inflammation in lumbar pain. *Spine* 20: 1821-1827.

62. Semble, E.L., R.F. Loeser, and C.M. Wise. 1990. Therapeutic exercise for rheumatoid arthritis and osteoarthritis. *Seminars in Arthritis and Rheumatism* 20: 32-40.

63. Shelbourne, K.D., and R.V. Trumper. 2000. Anterior cruciate ligament reconstruction: Evolution of rehabilitation. In: *Knee Ligament Rehabilitation,* 2nd ed., T.S. Ellenbecker, ed. Philadelphia: Churchill Livingstone.

64. Standaert, C.J. 2002. Spondylolysis in the adolescent athlete. *Clinical Journal of Sport Medicine* 12 (2, March): 119-122.

65. Stanski, C., J. McMaster, and P. Scranton. 1978. On the nature of stress fractures. *American Journal of Sports Medicine* 6: 391-396.

66. Steindler, A. 1955. *Kinesiology of the Human Body Under Normal and Pathological Conditions.* Springfield, IL: Charles C Thomas.

67. Stenstrom, C. 1994. Therapeutic exercise in rheumatoid arthritis. *Arthritis Care Research* 7: 190-197.

68. Thein, J.M., and L. Thein-Brody. 2000. Aquatic therapy. In: *Knee Ligament Rehabilitation,* 2nd ed., T.S. Ellenbecker, ed. Philadelphia: Churchill Livingstone.

69. Timm, K.E. 1994. The knee. In: *Clinical Orthopaedic Physical Therapy,* J.K. Richardson and Z.A. Iglarish, eds. Philadelphia: Saunders.

70. Townsend, H., F.W. Jobe, M. Pink, and J. Perry 1991. Electromyographic analysis of the glenohumeral muscles during a baseball rehabilitation program. *American Journal of Sports Medicine* 19: 264-272.

71. Turco, V.J. and A.J. Spinella 1985. Anterolateral dislocation of the head of the fibula in sports. *American Journal of Sports Medicine* 13(4): 209-215.

72. van den Ende, C.H.M., J.M.W. Hazes, S. le Cessie, W.J. Mulder, D.G. Belfor, F.C. Breedveld, and B.A. Dijkmans. 1996. Comparison of high and low intensity training in well controlled rheumatoid arthritis. Results of a randomized clinical trial. *Annals of Rheumatic Diseases* 55: 798-805.

73. Wilk, K.E., and J.R. Andrews. 1990. The effects of pad placement and angular velocity on tibial displacement during isokinetic exercise. *The Journal of Orthopaedic and Sports Physical Therapy* 17 (1): 24-30.

74. Williams, M.M., J.A. Hawley, R.A. McKenzie, and P.M. van Wijmen. 1991. A comparison of the effects of two sitting postures on back and referred pain. *Spine* 16 (10, October): 1185-1191.

75. Witvrouw, E., J. Bellemans, R. Verdonk, D. Cambier, P. Coorevits, and F. Almqvist. 2001. Patellar tendon vs. doubled semitendinosus and gracilis tendon for anterior cruciate ligament reconstruction. *International Orthopaedics* 25 (5): 308-311.

76. Yahia, L.H., and N. Newman. 1991. Mechanoreceptors in the canine anterior cruciate ligaments. *Anatomischer Anzeiger* 173 (4): 233-238.

77. Young, J.L., E.R. Laskowski, and M.G. Rock. 1993. Thigh injuries in athletes. *Mayo Clinic Proceedings* 68 (11, November): 1099-1106.

78. Zavatsky, A.B., and J.J. O'Connor. 1993. Ligament forces at the knee during isometric quadriceps contractions. *Proceedings of the Institution of Mechanical Engineers H, Journal of Engineering in Medicine* 207 (1): 7-18.

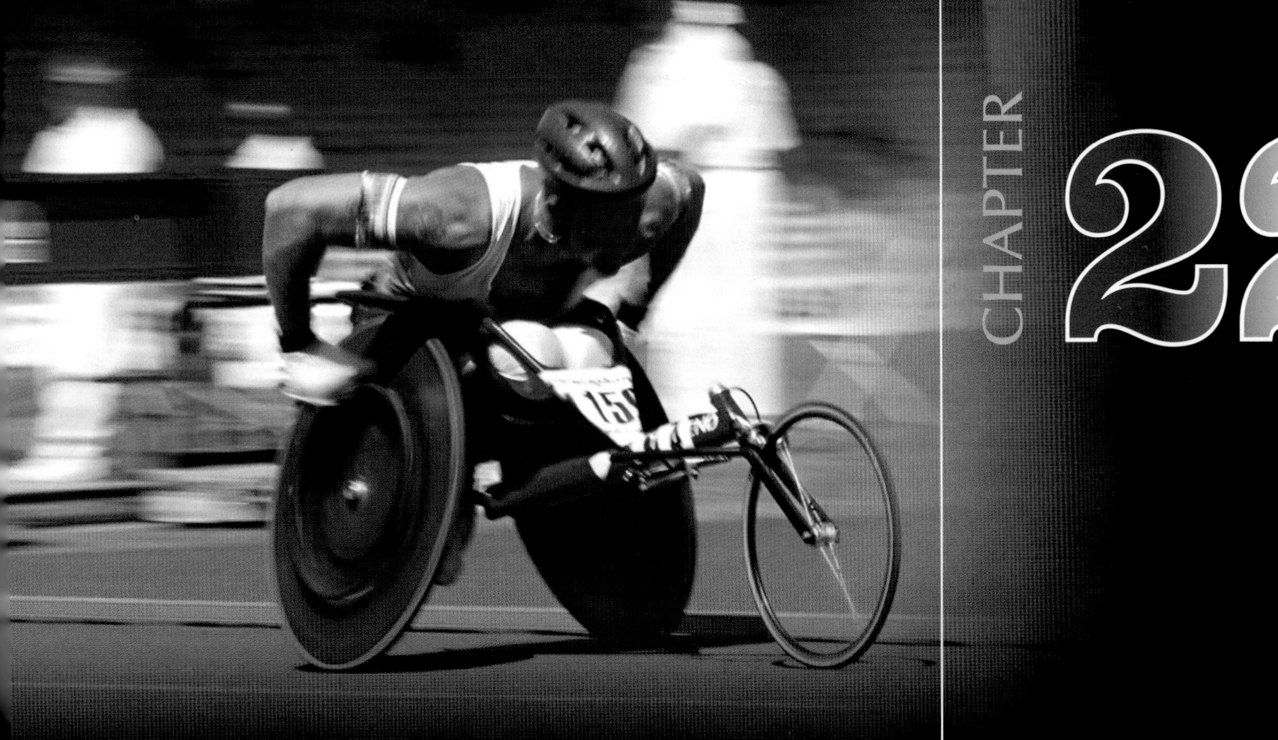

CHAPTER 22

Clients With Spinal Cord Injury, Multiple Sclerosis, Epilepsy, and Cerebral Palsy

Tom LaFontaine

After completing this chapter, you will be able to

- understand the basic etiology and epidemiology of spinal cord injury, multiple sclerosis, epilepsy, and cerebral palsy;
- recognize the physiological, functional, and health-related impairments caused or exacerbated by spinal cord injury, multiple sclerosis, epilepsy, and cerebral palsy;
- understand the basic physiological responses to exercise among clients with these disorders compared to others;
- recognize abnormal physiological responses to exercise in clients with these disorders,
- take necessary precautions in planning and implementing exercise and physical activity programs for clients with these disorders; and
- understand the potential functional and health benefits of regular exercise in clients with these disorders.

The many benefits of regular exercise have been well defined in apparently healthy populations. In recent years, studies have demonstrated that persons with various chronic diseases and disabilities also derive significant health and fitness benefits from a regular, systematic exercise program. This chapter presents information on four chronic neuromuscular disorders: spinal cord injury, multiple sclerosis, epilepsy, and cerebral palsy. The chapter addresses the epidemiology and pathology of these diseases and disabilities, as well as the exercise responses, documented benefits of exercise, and exercise testing and training guidelines in these client populations.

Spinal Cord Injury

Spinal cord injury (SCI) results in the impairment or loss of motor function, sensory function, or both in the trunk or limbs due to irreversible damage to neural tissues within the spinal canal [27]. The various grades of SCI may be classified as either complete or incomplete. In the complete form of paralysis, if the injury occurs between the highest thoracic (T-1) and highest cervical (C-1) segments of the spine, impairment of the arms, trunk, legs, and pelvic organs occurs (**quadriplegia,** also called **tetraplegia**). Injury to thoracic segments T-2 to T-12 causes impairment in the trunk, legs, and/or pelvic organs (**paraplegia**). Paraplegia is also the result of irreversible SCI of the lumbosacral (cauda equina) segments of the spine.

In general, the higher the injury level, the more extensive the resulting deficits. If the SCI is incomplete, the injury to the spinal cord has been only partial. In comparison to the person with complete SCI, the person with incomplete SCI may have some sensation or motor function at least partially intact below the level of the injury. In these cases it is best to ask for a physician's statement regarding what muscle and sensory function remains for the individual.

Clinical Manifestations

Clinical manifestations of the acute phase of SCI are many and varied. There is an increased incidence of thromboembolic events and dysrhythmias [62]. Disruption of the autonomic nervous system leads to reduced vascular tone and unbalanced hyperactivity of the vagal system. Individuals with high lesions, T-3/T-4 and above, are prone to symptomatic **bradycardia** (low heart rate), primary cardiac arrest, and serious cardiac conduction disturbances.

More relevant to the personal trainer are clinical manifestations associated with the chronic stage of SCI. Of particular importance are potential cardiovascular problems and events. Table 22.1 lists common cardiovascular problems observed in persons with chronic SCI.

TABLE 22.1

Common Cardiovascular Manifestations of Chronic Spinal Cord Injury
Orthostatic hypotension (i.e., baroreceptor insufficiency)
Autonomic dysreflexia (described in text)
Impaired transmission of cardiogenic pain (T-4 lesion and above)
Loss of reflex cardiac acceleration (T-1 through T-4 and above)
Quadriplegic cardiac atrophy (loss of left ventricular mass)
Atrial fibrillation and other cardiac conduction disorders
Congestive heart failure
Pseudomyocardial infarction (abnormal ST wave changes)
Sudden death due to asystole
Atherosclerosis and its manifestations of angina pectoris and myocardial infarction

A relatively common manifestation of SCI that the personal trainer needs to be aware of is **autonomic dysreflexia** (AD). Spinal cord injury disrupts normal neural regulation of arterial blood pressure, particularly in persons with tetraplegia and lesions above the T-6 level [62]. Autonomic dysreflexia results from noxious stimuli such as a distended bladder or bowel, constricted clothing, and infections that cause heightened sympathetic nervous system activity resulting in the sudden onset of hypertension. Tables 22.2 and 22.3 list typical clinical manifestations and precipitators of AD [62].

Autonomic dysreflexia can be a life-threatening condition. To prevent AD, the personal trainer should ask clients with SCI each session if they have symptoms such as a headache, blurred vision,

TABLE 22.2

Signs and Symptoms of Autonomic Dysreflexia
Sudden systolic blood pressure increase of >20 to 40 mmHg
Pounding headache
Profuse sweating and flushing of skin above level of injury, particularly of the head, neck, and shoulders
Piloerection ("goose bumps")
Blurred vision with spots in visual fields
Nasal congestion
Feelings of anxiety
Cardiac dysrhythmias—atrial fibrillation, premature ventricular depolarizations, conduction abnormalities

TABLE 22.3

Common Precipitators of Autonomic Dysreflexia
Bladder distension, urinary tract infection, bladder or kidney stones
Epididymis or scrotal compression
Bowel distension or impaction
Gallstones
Gastric ulcers, gastritis, gastric/colonic irritation, appendicitis
Menstruation, vaginitis, pregnancy
Intercourse/ejaculation
Deep vein thrombosis and pulmonary emboli
Temperature fluctuations
Pressure sores, in-grown toenail, sunburn, burn, blisters, insect bites
Constrictive clothing, shoes, appliances
Pain, fracture, other trauma
Any pain or irritating stimuli below injury level

goose bumps, and anxiety; check blood pressure before the session; and be sure clients have emptied their bowel and bladder before beginning the session. One should look for untreated high blood pressure at rest or sustained high blood pressure during recovery from exercise. Diastolic blood pressure should be back to baseline by 15 minutes. In athletes, an increase in usual systolic blood pressure of 20 to 40 mm Hg (millimeters of mercury) or greater could suggest "boosting."

Autonomic dysreflexia can be life-threatening. The personal trainer should look for signs of high blood pressure or boosting.

The personal trainer needs to be alert to sudden increases in blood pressure that could reflect AD. In addition, some athletic clients with SCI attempt to take advantage of this phenomenon by inducing it ("boosting") prior to competition. This practice has potentially hazardous consequences and must be discouraged. Clients with SCI generally demonstrate higher heart rates and lower blood pressures compared to others. To "boost" or maximize circulation during performance, some athletic clients with SCI attempt to increase their blood pressure by invoking AD through maneuvers such as holding their urine to distend their bladder or pinching themselves hard enough to cause a reflex response. One study showed that this practice can increase performance in track wheelchair and swimming events by 9.7% [58].

Preventing Injuries in Clients With Spinal Cord Injury

The most common exercise-induced injuries among persons with SCI occur at the shoulders, wrists, and elbows and are often overuse injuries. Among athletes in the National Wheelchair Athletic Association, 57% of reported injuries were to the shoulders and elbows [23]. Carpal tunnel syndrome (CTS) is also common among wheelchair athletes, with 23% reporting CTS in one study [6]. An excellent overview of medical and injury concerns in physically challenged athletes [67] emphasizes that although these types of injuries can be expected, many are preventable with adequate conditioning and training techniques, proper protective equipment, and excellent client-personal trainer communication. For example, stretching the anterior shoulder musculature and strengthening the posterior musculature can reduce shoulder injury and pain significantly [12].

Shoulder, wrist, and elbow overuse injuries are common in persons with SCI. These injuries may be prevented through an exercise program designed to stretch the anterior and strengthen the posterior muscle groups of the shoulder girdle.

Personal trainers working with persons with SCI need to be cognizant of these and other potential injuries in this population. Adhering to appropriate exercise technique and exercise physiology principles regarding intensity, duration, frequency, balance in exercise choice, and, in particular, progression and rest/recovery is essential to injury prevention and optimal physiological adaptation in this population.

Exercise Concerns in the Spinal Cord Injury Population

In addition to higher heart rate and lower blood pressure compared to others, several special concerns need to be addressed in the exercising SCI population, including temperature regulation and venous return. The personal trainer working with persons with SCI needs to be alert to potential adverse consequences of exercise in this population.

Temperature Regulation

Disorders of temperature regulation can be expected in persons with SCI, particularly those with lesions at T-6 or above. In extreme hot or cold environments, SCI clients with lesions at or above T-6 are unable to adequately thermoregulate through sweating or shivering [77]. Adaptations that may be necessary for clients competing in these thermally challenging environments include wearing a wet suit in a cool pool or being splashed with cool water during track racing in hot, humid environments. Hot whirlpools and similar extreme temperature environments should be avoided. It is important to beware of freezer burn from cold packs or burns from heat packs.

Persons with SCI, particularly those with high lesions, are unable to increase skin blood flow in paralyzed areas; this impairs the ability to dissipate metabolic heat and places them at increased risk for heat-related injuries. The phenomenon also exposes them to increased risk for cold-related injuries.

It is crucial that persons with SCI who are exercising maintain adequate hydration and adapt gradually to environmental changes. Dehydration contributes greatly to the risk of hyper- or hypothermia. The personal trainer needs to pay special attention to ensuring good nutrition and fluid intake practices among clients with SCI. Measures the personal trainer can take to enhance exercise comfort in these clients include maintaining as constant an exercise environment as possible; having clients wear loose-fitting, lightweight, and breathable materials (capilene, polypropylene, etc.); and ensuring access to cool water or sport drinks.

Venous Return

Persons with SCI have poor venous return, particularly in the seated or upright posture, due to lower limb venous pooling secondary to lack of sympathetic tone and absence of the venous "muscle pump." This not only limits the degree of cardiovascular trainability but also can result in hypotension during exercise, with symptoms of light-headedness and faintness and inability to maintain stroke volume and cardiac output. Studies suggest that training persons with SCI in the supine posture may minimize this problem and improve the effectiveness of upper body arm exercise [29, 46]. The use of gradient-style compression hosiery may be helpful as well to prevent swelling into the lower extremities.

Persons with SCI have poor venous return due to autonomic nervous system impairment and absence of the venous "muscle pump." Therefore they are at increased risk of hypotension (low blood pressure) during exercise. The personal trainer needs to be alert to symptoms of dizziness, light-headedness, and a sensation of fainting due to inadequate cerebral perfusion or blood flow.

General Health Issues of Persons With Spinal Cord Injury

Persons with SCI are at risk for several metabolic disturbances. As a consequence of relative inactivity, decreased muscle mass, and increased adiposity, a high percentage of persons with SCI have abnormalities in oral carbohydrate processing resulting in insulin resistance and hyperinsulinemia [2]. Persons with SCI also have frequencies of dyslipidemia, hypertension, and CVD that are slightly greater than in the non-SCI population [62].

A frequent consequence of tetraplegia is atrophy of cardiac muscle. This can result in cardiac dysfunction, further impairing exercise tolerance and increasing the risk for congestive heart failure. Such atrophy is probably related to neuromuscular dysfunction and inactivity that could possibly be lessened by electrical stimulation of paralyzed leg muscles and arm exercises [53].

Although the person with SCI may not perceive ischemic cardiac pain, other signs and symptoms such as unusual shortness of breath, excessive sweating, fatigue, light-headedness or sensation of fainting, and palpitations may occur. An exercise session should not be started, or should be terminated, if any of these symptoms are present, and medical follow-up should occur as soon as possible. In clients with suspected or known coronary heart disease, a physician-supervised clinical diagnostic exercise test should take place before the client starts a vigorous exercise program.

Exercise Testing and Training of Clients With Spinal Cord Injury

Persons with SCI can respond to exercise training in much the same way others do. However, problems associated with wheelchair use such as access to facilities, equipment, sidewalks, trails, and so on often make it challenging for people with SCI to engage in regular exercise. The personal trainer needs to be cognizant of these types of problems. In addition, a sound basic understanding of the acute and chronic responses to exercise in this population is critical to the implementation of a safe and effective exercise program.

The major pathophysiologic problems limiting the ability of persons with SCI to engage in and adapt to exercise training are (1) extensive skeletal muscle paralysis and (2) sympathetic autonomic nervous system impairment. These impairments in function reduce the capacity to support high rates of breathing frequency, heart rate, cardiac output, and metabolism. These factors, combined with the relatively sedentary lifestyle imposed by the neuromuscular disorder, result in markedly reduced cardiorespiratory and residual musculoskeletal fitness.

In a "sedentary lifestyle—loss of fitness model" that has been proposed for persons with SCI, impaired autonomic nervous system function and restricted physical activity lead to physical deconditioning and loss of musculoskeletal and cardiorespiratory fitness [16]. Most persons with SCI have a markedly reduced physical fitness compared to apparently healthy age- and gender-matched peers. The sedentary lifestyle—loss of fitness model is useful for understanding the basis for this phenomenon and provides a clear recognition of the need for implementing exercise programs in clients with SCI.

Exercise Testing

The most common mode of exercise testing for persons with SCI is the arm crank ergometer. Because of the high risk of cardiovascular impairment in this group, maximal exercise testing should be administered *only* in medical settings. However, with proper screening and medical clearance, the competent personal trainer can safely administer submaximal cardiorespiratory fitness testing. Although beyond the scope of this discussion, protocols and norms for standardized arm ergometry testing in persons with SCI have been developed [15, 39].

A field test has been developed whereby the $\dot{V}O_2$ peak of a person with paraplegia may be predicted from a 12-minute wheelchair propulsion distance test [30]. However, this test requires significant skill, motivation, and a basic level of fitness on the part of the wheelchair user. There also is significant interindividual variability. In addition, these tests typically require a maximal effort that would be beyond the scope of practice of the personal trainer. Wheelchair ergometers also have been developed for exercise testing of persons with SCI, but the availability and practicality of these instruments are very limited.

> Maximal exercise testing of clients with SCI should be administered only in medical settings with appropriate professional and physician supervision.

Physical Activity and Fitness Levels in Persons With Spinal Cord Injury

The reduction in physical fitness in persons with SCI is due in part to the sedentary lifestyle imposed by the condition [16] but also may be related to the level of injury and degree of neuromuscular impairment. Several studies in the 1980s showed that there were few differences in physical performance, cardiorespiratory fitness, or muscular strength among persons with SCI who had lesions below T-6 when classified by the specific site (T-7, T-8, L-1, etc.) of SCI [39, 40, 75]. However, those with lesions above T-6 (persons with tetraplegia) had markedly reduced cardiorespiratory fitness (as measured by $\dot{V}$O2 peak and muscle strength) compared to persons with lesions below T-6 [36].

Other researchers, however, have suggested that a significant proportion of variation in physical fitness could be attributed to neuromuscular impairment as defined by lesion level [5]. One group reported that 46% of the variation in $\dot{V}O_2$ peak could be explained by the level of injury, suggesting a moderate to strong relationship between neurological disruption and cardiorespiratory fitness [5].

As with other populations, there is a strong relationship between physical activity levels and both $\dot{V}O_2$ peak and upper body muscle strength and endurance in persons with SCI (figure 22.1); the greater the daily physical activity level, the greater the $\dot{V}O_2$ peak and muscle strength and endurance [19, 21]. Research evidence has also shown that physically active persons with SCI have 13% to 23% and 16% to 22% greater maximal cardiac outputs and stroke volumes, respectively, than their sedentary counterparts [17, 18]. Thus, although there is controversy about the causes of the decreased cardiorespiratory and musculoskeletal fitness in persons with SCI, there appears to be a strong positive relationship between habitual physical activity levels and $\dot{V}O_2$ peak, muscular strength, and other measures of physical fitness.

Particularly in people with tetraplegia, it is difficult to engage enough muscle mass to adequately

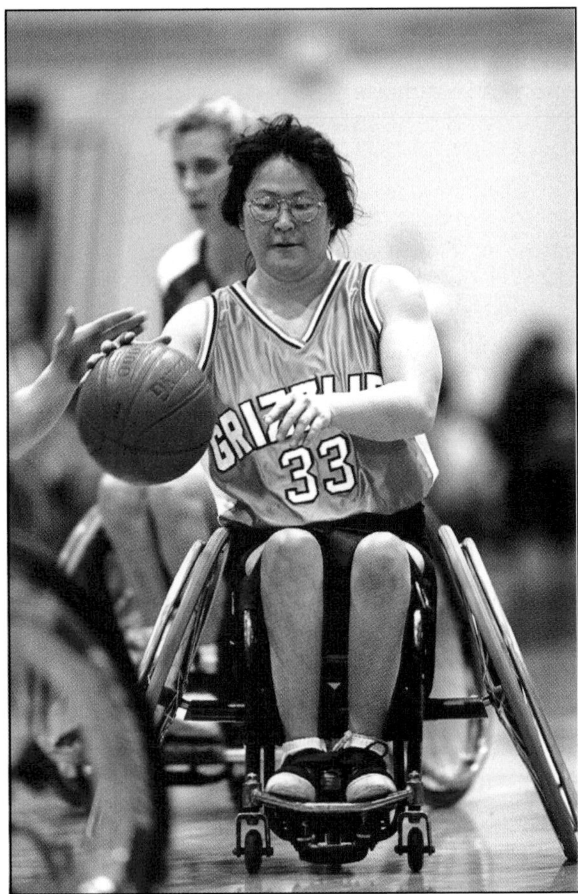

Figure 22.1 Regular physical activity can have dramatic effects on the aerobic and muscular fitness of individuals with SCI.

stress the central circulation or the heart. For example, most of the cardiorespiratory improvements with arm crank training seen in persons with tetraplegia are peripheral (increased mitochondria density, aerobic enzymes, myoglobin, and capillary density) [26]. In deconditioned persons with tetraplegia, however, the stimulus of upper body aerobic exercise may be sufficient to modestly improve maximal cardiac output and stroke volume [25].

Tetraplegia presents unique problems for cardiorespiratory training. Particularly in the upright posture, the hemodynamic responses to arm crank ergometry are markedly reduced. Peak heart rate is usually no greater than 120 to 130 beats per minute; and cardiac output, stroke volume, and blood pressure are subnormal for given levels of oxygen uptake [28]. Persons with SCI, particularly those with tetraplegia, have excessive lower limb and trunk venous pooling during exercise due to autonomic impairment and lack of lower limb and trunk muscle venous pump. In addition, upper body peripheral vasodilation during exercise is not compensated adequately by concomitant lower limb vasoconstriction [26]. This reduces central circulatory volume and thereby limits hemodynamic responses to exercise. This dysfunctional syndrome has been referred to as "hypokinetic circulation" [20, 32, 33].

Forced vital capacity is reduced by 50% in persons with high tetraplegia [44]. A recent study demonstrated that resistive inspiratory muscle training (RIMT) can improve pulmonary function in persons with tetraplegia [43]. Thus RIMT may be of benefit and should be considered by the personal trainer who is planning an exercise training program for these clients (readers may refer to Liaw et al. [43] for more information on RIMT).

Exercise Prescription

In general, the FITT (frequency, intensity, time or duration, and type) principle is as applicable in persons with SCI as with others. Initially, for cardiovascular training, intensity of 40% to 60% of maximal oxygen uptake, duration of 10 to 20 minutes, and frequency of three days per week or every other day are recommended. For resistance training, a suitable starting program is 8 to 12 exercises at 40% to 70% of 1-repetition maximum (1RM), performed for two to three sets of 8 to 12 repetitions with one to two minutes of rest between sets. The program should adhere to the principles of gradual progression, specificity, and overload as for persons in other groups. See chapters 12 to 16 for general exercise technique and prescription.

People with SCI should eventually strive for a minimum of 30 minutes or more of physical activity on most days of the week. Goals for persons with SCI are no different than for others: increase functional capacity, improve health risk factors, enhance self-image and confidence, and so on. Clients with SCI are prone to **spasticity** (exaggerated muscle tone and reflexes), which can impair the ability to exercise. A gradual warm-up with a systematic, progressive increase in intensity and slow-paced muscle contractions during resistance training, for example, can limit spasticity. Excessive, frequent spasticity warrants medical follow-up for possible adjustment in medical therapy. "Exercise Guidelines for Persons With Spinal Cord Injury" on page 564 presents guidelines for personal trainers to follow in planning aerobic, flexibility, and resistance exercise for persons with SCI.

In conclusion, it is clear that persons with SCI can benefit from a systematic and progressive comprehensive exercise program. Several publications provide more information on exercise for persons with SCI [3, 4, 42, 45, 76].

Multiple Sclerosis

Multiple sclerosis (MS) is an immune-mediated (autoimmune) disorder that occurs in genetically susceptible persons. Although the etiology of MS is uncertain, recent evidence suggests a viral origin such as Epstein-Barr virus [1]. Multiple sclerosis is characterized by inflammation and progressive degeneration of the myelin sheath involving predominantly nerves of the eye, brain, periventricular gray matter, cerebellum, brain stem, and spinal cord [54].

Early symptoms of MS (sensory disturbances, fatigue and weakness, ipsilateral optical neuritis, gait ataxia, neurogenic bowel and bladder, and trunk and limb paresthesia evoked by neck flexion) are thought to be the result of axonal demyelination leading to a slowing or blockade of nerve conduction [54]. Multiple sclerosis typically begins in early adulthood (ages 20 to 40 years) and has a variable clinical course and prognosis. Eighty percent of individuals have the relapsing-remitting type of MS while 20% have chronic (primary) progressive MS [54]. The relapsing-remitting type can be further classified into benign, classical relapsing-remitting, and chronic-relapsing. Table 22.4 describes the clinical classifications of MS [64].

Multiple sclerosis is a devastating and potentially debilitating disease. Although there is no known

Exercise Guidelines for Persons With Spinal Cord Injury

- Incorporate exercise that will restore or enhance balance around functional joints; in particular, strengthen muscle groups of the posterior shoulder and upper back areas, and stretch muscles of the anterior shoulder and chest areas.
- A conventional resistance training program of three sets of 8 to 12 repetitions performed for all functional muscle groups, two to three days per week, is recommended. Clients may also benefit, however, from a program of a single set to fatigue of 8 to 12 repetitions using 8 to 12 exercises, two to three days per week.
- As with all resistance exercise programs, full range of motion, proper exercise technique, avoidance of breath-holding, and controlled movement should be emphasized.
- Due to risk of shoulder, elbow, and wrist overuse injuries, caution in choice, intensity, and volume of exercise is necessary.
- Persons with SCI often have spasticity and may need to refrain from resistance training if the spasticity is severe (referral to medical team may be indicated) [27].
- Any exercise that triggers abnormal muscle tone must be stopped and avoided [27].
- In youth with SCI, precautions for resistance training include not overloading growing bones, as well as possibly limiting resistance training and emphasizing flexibility and aerobic training during periods of rapid growth [27].
- Standard guidelines for flexibility training apply, with particular attention paid to the shoulders, wrists, arms, trunk, and lower limbs (see chapter 12 on flexibility training).
- Aerobic exercise should begin at a moderate level and progress gradually in duration, frequency, and intensity with a goal of 30 minutes four or more days per week.
- Cardiovascular training modes may include arm cranking; wheelchair ergometry; wheelchair propulsion on a treadmill or rollers (in highly skilled clients in wheelchairs) or on accessible sidewalks, indoor or outdoor tracks, or trail surfaces; swimming; sports such as wheelchair basketball; ambulation with crutches and braces; arm-powered cycling; and FES or facilitated support treadmill walking (generally in research and rehabilitative settings).
- Persons with SCI should be supervised during exercise and likely will need assistance with equipment adjustments, transfers, and so on.
- Most persons with SCI have their own bladder/bowel program and should empty both prior to exercise.
- Blood pressure should be monitored regularly at rest and frequently with exercise to avoid exercise-induced hypotension, particularly with exercise in the upright posture.
- Supine arm cranking may be preferred in clients with tetraplegia if equipment can be modified for this purpose.
- Avoid exercise within two to three hours after a meal. Digestion can impair the ability to shunt blood to the working muscles during exercise, creating competition between a limited cardiac output and blood flow, which can result in gastrointestinal disturbances during exercise.
- Because of loss of muscle function, loss of trunk control and balance, and loss of sensation in paralyzed areas, special equipment such as additional padding on equipment, gloves, elastic bandages, seat belts, and Velcro® straps may be necessary.
- The client should avoid prolonged sitting and abrasions, particularly of the weight-bearing areas of the hip, ischium, sacrum, and coccyx, because of the risk of pressure sores, which do not heal easily.
- The client should avoid exercise during an illness such as cold, flu, bladder infection, constipation, and fever and should limit aerobic and resistance training during periods of increased spasticity (mild stretching may reduce spasticity but should be implemented by a personal trainer only with guidance and instruction from the client's personal physician).
- Be aware of the client's regular medications and their side effects.

TABLE 22.4

Clinical Classifications and Characteristics of Multiple Sclerosis

Clinical classification	Clinical characteristics and course of disease
Benign (10-15%)	Few and mild exacerbations, complete or nearly complete remissions, and minimal or no disability.
Classical relapsing-remitting (25-30%)	Frequent exacerbations but often with long periods of stability. However, there often are frequent relapses in the first two years.
Chronic-relapsing (40-45%)	Fewer periods of remission and stability, often some permanent motor or sensory deficits.
Chronic (primary) progressive (15-20%)	Insidious onset, gradual but steady worsening of symptoms with no periods of remission—poor prognosis often leading rapidly to quadriparesis; cognitive decline; visual loss; loss of bowel, bladder, and sexual function.

cure, early diagnosis and treatment including rehabilitation, medical therapy, and exercise can improve the quality of life, functional status, and long-term outcomes in many persons with MS [60, 69].

Medical Management of Multiple Sclerosis

Essentially there are four aspects to the treatment of MS. The first involves education of the individual and family regarding the disease process, its progression, prognosis, and ways in which the disease can be managed. This aspect is primarily the responsibility of the client's physician and health care team. However, a knowledgeable personal trainer can reinforce the information and recommendations.

The second aspect of MS treatment involves the management of symptoms and secondary complications such as **dystonic spasms** (brief, recurring, painful posturing of one or more limbs), general spasticity, ataxia, incoordination, depression, other emotional disturbances, bladder and bowel dysfunction, and related pain syndromes.

The third aspect of treatment concerns the management of the disease process. Persons with MS will be on medication for (1) managing the inflammation associated with the disease process and (2) modifying the disease process. Medical treatment for MS is very complex, and most individuals are under the care of a neurologist for this purpose. The personal trainer needs to be aware of medications that the person with MS may be taking and should seek the assistance of the client's medical team and resources such as the *Physician's Desk Reference* (PDR) in order to ensure the safety and efficacy of exercise therapy.

The fourth aspect of therapy for MS involves exercise. Persons with MS are generally sedentary, often because of the difficulties with movement and the associated fatigue and weakness. According to one study, an aerobic exercise program can increase cardiorespiratory fitness by as much as 22% [59]. Another researcher showed that aerobic training in persons with MS may result in an increased aerobic capacity of 30%, but emphasized that the individual response to the same program over several weeks to months may vary by 2% to 54% [63]. Exercise and behavioral therapy have been recommended as a management strategy for persons with MS who experience persistent fatigue [9]. Regular stretching is essential to maintaining joint range of motion and tissue elasticity. Resistance training can increase muscle strength and endurance and prevent muscle atrophy. Exercise modalities such as tai chi and yoga also may be beneficial (figure 22.2).

Exercise Testing and Training of Clients With Multiple Sclerosis

The benefits of aerobic exercise for clients with MS seem clear. Aerobic exercise training in persons with MS can improve $\dot{V}O_2$ peak, upper and lower body strength, body composition, and risk factors for CVD [48, 65, 69, 70]. After 15 weeks of aerobic training, a group of persons with MS showed

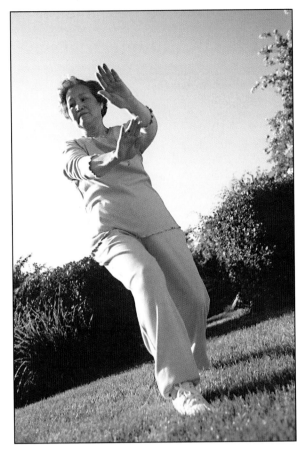

Figure 22.2 Clients with multiple sclerosis can benefit greatly from regular exercise.

significantly improved anger, depression, and fatigue (on the Profile of Mood States) and an improved total score on the Sickness Impact Profile, as well as on a number of its components (physical dimensions scale, social interaction, emotional behavior, and recreational pursuits) [59]. In addition, exercise training can enhance general well-being while offsetting some of the typical psychological difficulties including fatigue, stress, and depression common in persons with MS [69].

Many persons with MS experience heat sensitivity that is often associated with a transient increase in clinical signs and symptoms. This may preclude or deter persons with MS from participation in a regular exercise program in which metabolic heat is increased. Several studies have yielded positive results in this area, although, as with most studies on people with MS, few if any have included subjects over 55 years of age. Applying a precooling procedure (cool shower or whirlpool, cool wet neck wraps or cooling collars, or cool water sprays before and during exercise) to thermosensitive persons with MS prior to exercise may result in lower rectal temperature, heart rate, and perceived exertion than in exercisers who do not receive cooling treatment [74]. And, although persons with MS are prone to heat intolerance, with the proper precautions, warm water aquatic therapy may benefit some without aggravating fatigue or increasing risk for heat-related problems [61].

Persons with MS are prone to heat intolerance. Methods to precool the client and to ensure a cool, comfortable environment for exercise can enhance the physiological benefits and increase adherence. Proper hydration is critical to maintaining temperature balance during exercise in persons with MS.

Exercise Testing

Exercise testing of persons with MS should be administered with extreme caution. Persons with MS who have or who are at risk for CVD must be screened and administered a clinical exercise test with professional and physician supervision in order to rule out ischemia and coronary heart disease prior to starting an exercise program. However, with proper medical clearance, the personal trainer can safely administer a submaximal aerobic exercise test to establish a baseline for future comparisons. Because of incoordination and possible spasticity, leg or arm ergometry is the preferred modality. Flexibility tests such as the sit and reach can be safely administered with careful attention to technique. Little is known about the safety or efficacy of maximal 1RM or other forms of isotonic muscle strength or endurance testing for people with MS. The recommendation would be to use caution in administering maximal strength or muscular endurance testing to fatigue, but data to support the risks of these procedures, as well as the safety and efficacy, are limited.

Thus little research exists that would allow one to systematically assess the safety and efficacy of resistance training in persons with MS. Field experience suggests that a standard progressive resistance training program of 8 to 12 exercises, performed at 40% to 60% 1RM load for one to three sets of 8 to 12 repetitions, results in beneficial outcomes in persons with MS with little or no risk. Progression may need to occur at about 50% of the rate for persons without the disorder (i.e., increase loads every three to four instead of one to two weeks).

Aerobic Conditioning

In the past, exercise training was not recommended for persons with MS because it was believed that exercise increased MS-associated fatigue. Exercise programs for people with MS should be carefully designed to adequately stimulate cardiorespiratory and musculoskeletal function in accordance with the principles of overload and progressive resistance. However, the overload must be presented gradually in order not to cause or exacerbate fatigue, nerve conduction block, or both.

The response of persons with MS to submaximal aerobic exercise appears to vary depending on the stage and severity of the disease process. In two studies, heart rate, ventilation, and oxygen uptake were higher and net energy expenditure was two to three times greater during submaximal treadmill walking in persons with MS than in age- and gender-matched peers [56, 57]. However, a more recent study in moderately impaired persons with MS did not show a significant difference from age- and gender-matched controls in net energy expenditure at similar submaximal workloads [71]. This research illustrates the need to carefully prescribe aerobic exercise intensity to ensure a light to moderate workload. The recommended aerobic intensity is 40% to 70% of $\dot{V}O_2$ peak or heart rate reserve (HRR). In most persons with MS, initiating exercise at 40% to 50% of $\dot{V}O_2$ or HRR is advised, with progression over three to six months to 50% to 70% as the client adapts.

Clients with MS are prone to fatigue that can be disabling. Precautions must be taken to provide a systematic program that starts at the lower end of traditional recommendations and progresses at a rate that is 50% slower than for apparently healthy adults. For more information, readers may refer to published recommendations for physical activity in persons with MS [55].

Exercise to exhaustion in clients with MS should be avoided. Persistent fatigue lasting more than two days should be a warning sign that an exercise program is excessive.

Precautions and guidelines for exercise testing and training of persons with MS are presented on page 568.

Epilepsy

Epilepsy is defined medically as two or more unprovoked, recurring seizures [37]. A **seizure** is an uncontrolled, paroxysmal electrical discharge within any part of the brain that causes physical or mental symptoms and may or may not be associated with convulsions. Seizures result in involuntary alteration in movement, sensation, perception, cognitive behavior, and/or loss of consciousness (LOC). Table 22.5 defines classifications of seizures with characteristic signs and symptoms [10, 11].

Status epilepticus is defined as a seizure lasting more than 30 minutes or a seizure that occurs so frequently that consciousness is not restored [37]. Status epilepticus is a medical emergency, necessitating activation of emergency protocols including calling 911 or other local emergency number and transporting to a hospital emergency department.

It is important that the personal trainer understand and recognize common **precipitants** (causes or triggers) in clients with idiopathic or secondary seizures. Table 22.6 summarizes some known precipitants and recommendations for exercise session modification.

Anecdotal reports have suggested that physical activity may be a precipitant of seizure [41, 55, 66]. However, systematic studies have shown that physical activity and sport have no adverse effects on seizure occurrence in the majority of clients with epilepsy and, in fact, may contribute to better seizure control [50, 51]. As a cautionary note for the personal trainer working with clients who have epilepsy, however, these studies do suggest that exercise may be a seizure precipitant in approximately 10% of these individuals. This is particularly apparent in clients with seizures secondary to trauma, infections, or stroke.

In many persons with epilepsy, regular aerobic exercise may contribute to improved seizure control. However, in 10% of individuals, vigorous exercise may be a seizure precipitant.

Many persons with epilepsy unnecessarily avoid physical activity and sport because of fear of seizure induction, seizure-related injury, or both. In general, studies suggest that persons with epilepsy are less active than the general population, but the results are equivocal. A Norwegian research group, for example, found no difference in physical activity levels among persons with epilepsy and the general population [51]. The consensus of experts is that not only should exercise and sport participation in persons with epilepsy *not* be restricted; in fact, it should be encouraged [31, 68]. The personal trainer needs to be aware of these issues and gently encourage clients with epilepsy to increase their physical activity levels.

Precautions and Guidelines for Exercise Testing and Training of Persons With Multiple Sclerosis

- Complex skill-oriented exercises should be avoided in most persons with MS, partly because of the loss of proprioception or ability to perceive muscle and joint position in space.
- The energy cost of walking may be two to three times higher than normal for a person with MS, particularly those with advanced disease; thus adjustments in workloads to maintain a 60% to 75% maximal heart rate are necessary.
- Persons with MS are thermosensitive and therefore at increased risk for both heat- and cold-related injuries; this emphasizes the need to ensure adequate hydration and to have persons with MS exercise in thermoneutral environments. In addition, dehydration during exercise could be exacerbated in persons with MS who have bladder dysfunction (incontinence and/or sense of urgent need to urinate) and sometimes limit their fluid intake.
- It is important to be cautious with large-muscle lower limb exercise, since muscle spasticity may be particularly predominant in the hip abductors/adductors.
- Sensory loss may preclude certain exercises such as free weights because of a client's inability to grasp the bars effectively, and may necessitate modification in other forms of exercise.
- Strapping may be necessary if more severe spasticity is present.
- Some evidence suggests that morning may be the preferred time for exercise when circadian body temperature is at its lowest.
- Recumbent bicycling may be preferred over upright cycling in clients with balance problems.
- Imbalances between agonist and antagonist muscles are common.
- Muscle weakness tends to be greatest in the lower limb and trunk muscles.
- Neuromuscular problems such as foot drop may be present in more advanced cases.
- Some clients may have cognitive deficits and are prone to depression; caution is warranted in education of these individuals, and constant reinforcement to enhance compliance is generally needed in clients with MS.
- The variable nature of MS symptoms and progression requires that the personal trainer adjust the exercise program on a daily basis.
- It is advisable to monitor heart rate before, during, and after aerobic exercise in order to ensure the appropriate metabolic intensity and stimulus.
- Regular follow-ups to monitor progress are highly recommended with persons who have MS in order to facilitate compliance and to adjust the exercise prescription appropriately.
- In the case of an exacerbation, exercise should be discontinued until complete remission.
- Since some individuals with MS have cognitive impairments, it may be necessary to provide information and instruction in both written and diagram formats. Frequent reminders of exercises, technique, and proper use of equipment may be necessary.
- If the client has incoordination in either the upper or the lower limbs, the use of a synchronized leg and arm ergometer may improve exercise performance by allowing the arms or legs to assist the weaker limbs.
- Finally, the personal trainer should maintain regular contact with the client's physician.

Medical Management of Seizures

Medical management of seizures is completely effective in approximately 75% of cases [38]. The choice of medication is determined by the client's physician based on the type of seizure and the client's tolerance of side effects. The personal trainer needs to be aware of the medications a client may be on and consult a reference such as PDR for descriptions of the medications and their side effects.

TABLE 22.5

Classification and Common Signs and Symptoms of Seizure Disorders and Approximate Percentage of Cases

Type of seizure	Signs and symptoms
Partial seizures (60%)	
Simple (15-20%)	Motor, cognitive, sensory, autonomic effects with no loss of consciousness (LOC)
Complex (35-40%)	Partial or complete LOC, often preceded by aura associated with no memory of event and usually no motor involvement
Evolving to generalized (40-45%)	Involves both hemispheres with complete LOC with bilateral involvement
Generalized seizures (40%)	
Absence (petit mal)	Staring or eye flickering, some body involvement possible, no convulsions, no post-ictal (i.e., immediately after the seizure) symptoms
Myoclonic	Symmetric jerking of limbs
Clonic	Rapid, repetitive motor activity
Tonic	Involuntary rigidity
Tonic-clonic (grand mal)	Rigidity followed by flexion actions often with labored breathing, tongue biting, cyanosis, incontinence, post-ictal confusion, fatigue, stupor
Atonic	Paroxysmal loss of postural tone

TABLE 22.6

Precipitants of Seizures and Exercise Modifications

Common precipitants of seizures	Suggested exercise modifications
Emotional stress	Modify intensity to lower level.
Hyperventilation	Teach breathing techniques and control.
Menstruation	Modify intensity to lower level.
Sleep deprivation	Avoid exercise.
Fever	Avoid exercise.
Photic stimulation (strobe lights, TV, etc.)	Avoid situations during exercise.
Alcohol excess or withdrawal	Modify intensity to lower level.

Exercise Testing and Training of Clients With Epilepsy

Most persons with epilepsy, unfortunately, live sedentary lives and therefore generally have low physical fitness. This appears to be the case despite the fact that in most cases physical exercise and other leisure pursuits are not precipitators of seizures and do not increase the risk of seizure-related injuries [47, 52]. In fact in the Norwegian study mentioned earlier, 36% of persons with epilepsy indicated that regular exercise contributed to better seizure control [51].

However, studies do suggest that exercise may precipitate seizures in a small percentage (~10%) of persons with epilepsy, particularly those with seizures secondary to infection, trauma, or stroke. Persons with epilepsy whose fitness level is low may be more prone to exercise-induced seizures [51]. The personal trainer needs to be aware of the type of seizure disorder a client has and be alert to signs and symptoms suggestive of a seizure. Many persons with epilepsy have an aura prior to a seizure. The personal trainer should know his or her client and be able to recognize signs and symptoms that suggest an impending seizure.

Persons with epilepsy who have low fitness levels and history of a sedentary lifestyle may be particularly prone to exercise-induced seizures.

In general, there are no contraindications or restrictions to exercise in persons with epilepsy. In fact, sport and regular exercise should be encouraged with minimal restrictions assuming that seizure management is optimal.

In the context of good seizure management, persons with epilepsy should be strongly encouraged to participate in regular physical activity.

The personal trainer can apply the same exercise principles for persons with epilepsy as are recommended for apparently healthy populations. A gradual and progressive approach to physical activity and weight control is recommended. With proper medical clearance and adherence to standard guidelines, it is safe to administer submaximal exercise testing to establish baseline cardiorespiratory fitness, muscle strength and endurance, flexibility, and body composition. With regard to weight control, it is important to note that even a modest weight loss of 10 pounds (4.5 kilograms) may affect the biological availability of antiseizure medications and thus increase the risk of side effects.

Finally, the personal trainer should know first aid for seizure, particularly the tonic-clonic (grand mal) type. "First Aid for Seizures" describes basic first aid steps to take during a seizure and the **post-ictal state** (the period immediately after the seizure).

A weight loss of 10 pounds (4.5 kilograms) can increase the bioavailability of antiseizure medications and thus increase the risk of side effects.

First Aid for Seizures

1. Keep client prone—lying facedown if possible.
2. Remove eyeglasses and other items that may break and cause injury.
3. Loosen any tight clothing, particularly around the neck.
4. Do *not* restrain the client.
5. Keep objects out of client's path.
6. Do *not* place anything in the client's mouth.
7. After the seizure, turn the client to his or her side in recovery position (refer to CPR guidelines) to prevent aspiration.
8. Observe the client until he or she is fully awake.
9. Alert the client's physician and family.
10. The client may be able to return to exercise, but evaluate this with the client's physician on a case-by-case basis.

Cerebral Palsy

Cerebral palsy (CP) is a term used to describe a group of chronic musculoskeletal deficits causing impaired body movement and muscle coordination. It is caused by damage to one or more areas of the brain occurring during fetal development, or during or shortly after the birthing process, or in early infancy [73]. Cerebral palsy is characterized by limitation in the ability to move, control balance and coordination, and maintain posture due to damage to the motor areas of the brain that control muscle function and spinal reflexes. It is not a progressive disease, as the brain damage does not worsen. However, secondary conditions such as spasticity can and often do worsen if not well managed, leading to further loss of joint motion and mobility and potential **contractures** (permanent shortening of muscles and tendons). See

Definitions of Cerebral Palsy–Related Terms

apraxia—Inability to perform coordinated voluntary gross and fine motor skills.

ataxia—Uncoordinated, voluntary movements; clients with ataxia often have a wide-based gait with genu recurvatum or "hyperextended knee" and may exhibit mild intention tremors.

athetosis—Slow, writhing, contortion-like motions of the appendicular musculature.

chorea—State of excessive, spontaneous movements, irregularly timed, that are nonrepetitive and abrupt; client is unable to maintain voluntary muscle contractions.

dyskinesis—Impairment of voluntary movement resulting in incomplete movements.

dystonia—Sustained muscle contractions that result in twisting and repetitive movements or abnormal posture.

myoclonus—Shocklike synchronous or asynchronous contractions of a portion of a muscle, an entire muscle, or a group of muscles.

spasticity—A state of increased tonus of a muscle characterized by heightened deep tendon reflexes.

"Definitions of Cerebral Palsy–Related Terms" for definitions of related terms.

Characteristic signs and symptoms of CP include muscle tightness, spasticity, involuntary muscle movement, gait disturbances, muscle weakness, incoordination, and speech and swallowing impairments. Other signs and symptoms that may be noted are deficiencies in sensation and perception, impaired vision and/or hearing, seizures, cognitive dysfunction and learning deficiencies, and breathing difficulty secondary to postural deformities.

Medically, CP can be classified by the specific type of muscle abnormalities noted. In addition, the type of muscle abnormality suggests the site of brain injury:

- A client with marked spasticity likely has had damage within the motor cortex of the cerebrum [7, 24].
- Athetosis suggests midbrain damage.
- Ataxia suggests damage to the cerebellum.
- Dyskinesis suggests damage to the basal ganglia.

In mixed forms, which also exist, damage has occurred to multiple areas [7, 24].

The Cerebral Palsy International Sports and Recreation Association functional classifications are often used to differentiate various forms of CP and are presented in table 22.7 [7]. Although originally designed for sport participation, this classification system is a useful tool that can give the personal trainer insight into the range of functional abilities of persons with CP.

Cerebral palsy is an irreversible condition, and medical and rehabilitative therapy focuses on controlling spasticity and athetosis and improving function and neuromuscular coordination.

Although CP cannot be corrected, it can be managed to prevent complications and further loss of function and independence. Medical therapy focuses on reducing spasticity if present and on improving nerve and muscle coordination. Physical therapy and rehabilitation are essential for optimizing growth and development, preventing disability, and minimizing muscle and locomotor dysfunction. An ongoing exercise program can greatly assist persons with CP in becoming and remaining independent, productive members of society.

Medical Management of Cerebral Palsy

The medical management of CP mostly involves managing the secondary complications of the

TABLE 22.7

Cerebral Palsy International Sports and Recreation Association Functional Classifications

CP1: Severe spastic or athetoid tetraplegia—is unable to propel a manual wheelchair with nonfunctional lower limbs; has very poor to no trunk stability, severely decreased function in the upper limbs
CP2: Moderate to severe spastic or athetoid tetraplegia—is able to propel a manual wheelchair slowly and inefficiently; has differential functional abilities between lower and upper limbs with fair trunk stability
CP3: Moderate spastic tetraplegia or severe spastic hemiplegia (weakness and loss of neuromuscular function on one side of the body)—is able to propel a manual wheelchair independently; may ambulate with assistance; has moderate spasticity in lower limbs, fair dynamic trunk stability, and moderate limitations of function in the dominant arm
CP4: Moderate to severe spastic diplegia (weakness and loss of neuromuscular function on both sides of the body)—ambulates with aids for short distances; has moderate to severe involvement of the lower limbs, good dynamic trunk stability, minimal to near-normal function of the upper limbs at rest
CP5: Moderate spastic diplegia—ambulates well with assistive devices; has minimal to moderate spasticity in one or both lower limbs but is able to run some
CP6: Moderate athetosis or ataxia—ambulates without assistive devices; lower limb functioning improves from walking to running or cycling; has poor static and dynamic trunk stability; has good upper limb range of motion and strength; has poor throwing, grasp, and release
CP7: True ambulatory hemiplegia—has mild to moderately affected upper limb and minimal to mildly affected lower limb
CP8: Minimally affected diplegia, hemiplegia, athetosis, or monoplegia (weakness and loss of neuromuscular function in one limb)

Adapted from Cerebral Palsy International Sports and Recreation Association 1991.

irreversible lesion. Seizures or seizure tendencies occur in 60% of persons with CP. Thus persons with CP may be on antiseizure medications, antispasmodic medications, and muscle relaxants. In addition, many persons with CP have other secondary complications including joint pain, hip and back deformities, bladder/bowel dysfunction, and gastroesophageal reflux for which they may be on medications. Finally, persons with CP, in general, are sedentary and thus prone to several risk factors for CVD.

Exercise Testing and Training of Clients With Cerebral Palsy

Little research has examined the exercise responses and effects of exercise training in persons with CP. Historically, few persons with CP have participated in formal or informal physical activity programs. However, a recent survey of women with CP reported that a significant proportion of independent women with CP did engage in daily exercise (43% of respondents indicated that they had done range of motion exercise or aerobic exercise in the past week) [72]. Exercise testing and training of persons with CP are complicated by the deformities, athetosis, ataxia, incoordination, and spasticity often associated with this disorder. However, there is no pathological basis for expecting persons with CP not to benefit from regular physical activity, which should be encouraged. Research in this area is increasing, and what is available clearly suggests that persons with CP can expect to derive benefits from a regular program of physical activity that are similar to those for people who do not have the disorder. Table 22.8 summarizes some of the findings from research concerning the trainability of persons with CP.

Persons with CP can expect a systematic program of physical exercise to yield health and fitness benefits similar to those obtained by persons without CP.

TABLE 22.8

Selected Outcomes of Exercise Research in Persons With Cerebral Palsy

Improved capacity to perform activities of daily life [24]
Improved sense of wellness and body image [24]
Apparent lessening of severity of symptoms such as spasticity and athetosis [24]
Improved peak oxygen uptake, ventilatory threshold, work rates at submaximal heart rates, range of motion, and coordination/skill of movement [24]
Increased muscle strength and endurance including hypertrophy [13, 14]
Increased skeletal bone mineral density of the femoral neck [8]
Improved ventilatory capacities in children ages 5 to 7 [35]
Higher gait velocity following resistance with improved symmetry in muscle strength [13]
Improved water orientation skills and self-concept after swimming exercise in kindergarten children [34]

All persons with CP should be screened properly for musculoskeletal abnormalities, CVD, and risk factors for chronic diseases such as atherosclerosis, diabetes, arthritis, and hypertension. High-risk clients with two or more risk factors for CVD (hypertension, dyslipidemia, tobacco use, sedentary lifestyle, age greater than 40, obesity, diabetes) or with symptoms (chest pain, dyspnea, increasing weakness or fatigue, palpitations) should undergo a clinical examination, including an electrocardiographically monitored graded exercise test supervised by a professional team including a physician. The client must obtain medical clearance before starting a moderate-intensity exercise program. Standardized submaximal fitness testing may then be recommended in persons with CP who are at low risk and in those at risk who have been properly screened and cleared medically. The competent personal trainer should be able to administer submaximal testing under these conditions.

In ambulatory persons with CP, the leg ergometer and the arm and leg ergometer are preferred modalities for exercise testing. The treadmill may be used in persons with CP who have good balance and coordination. Because of spasticity or athetosis, the client's feet may need to be strapped to the pedals, and sufficient practice is necessary to ensure good performance. In nonambulatory persons with CP, the arm crank ergometer and wheelchair ergometer, if available, are the preferred modalities for submaximal testing. Clients should wear gloves to prevent skin abrasions, particularly if they use a wheelchair. To assess aerobic endurance, the 6- to 12-minute walk or wheelchair push may be appropriate. These tests, however, assume maximal effort, as the objective is for clients to travel "as much distance as they can" in the timed period. Therefore, this test should be administered only to low-risk and properly screened clients.

Common tests of flexibility and muscle function such as the sit and reach and 1RM can be safely administered. Finally, skinfold thickness measurements can be taken at several sites, preferably on noninvolved body parts, and totaled for a score to establish a baseline for assessing changes in body composition. Although valid equations for predicting body fat percentage from skinfold measurements are limited in this population, the total thickness of seven to eight sites can be used for monitoring progress.

Although research guidelines for exercise prescription in persons with CP are limited, there is no apparent reason to expect this group to respond differently than others do. See the next page for some basic guidelines and precautions for exercise testing and training in persons with CP.

Basic Guidelines and Precautions for Exercise Training of Persons With Cerebral Palsy

- Because of the limitations of persons with CP, the personal trainer needs to be creative and often needs to modify equipment and exercises.
- Most persons with CP will benefit most from a balanced approach addressing flexibility, muscle strength and endurance, and cardiorespiratory fitness.
- As with other clients, standard guidelines for cardiorespiratory training can be applied; moderate to vigorous intensity of 50% to 85% of $\dot{V}O_2$ or HRR, 30 or more minutes per session, four or more days per week should be the goal. Gradual progression is recommended as with sedentary persons without the disorder; in very deconditioned persons with CP, the recommendation is to begin with 5 to 10 minutes, twice per day, four or more days per week; increasing physical activity in daily life should be a goal as well.
- People with CP can perform standard moderate resistance training of 8 to 12 exercises for one to three sets of 8 to 12 repetitions, two to three days per week at 40% to 60% of maximum, although some exercises will need to be modified. In general, maximal loads should not be used for most persons with CP.
- In many persons with CP, athetosis and spasticity make use of free weights inadvisable; if a client with CP does use free weights, extreme caution and careful spotting are necessary.
- All standard principles such as avoidance of breath-holding, 48 hours of rest between working the same muscle groups, full range of motion, and controlled movement should be carefully applied to persons with CP.
- It is important to give attention to muscle imbalances, with exercises chosen to improve any deficiencies.
- It is particularly important that persons with CP have a period of aerobic warm-up (10-15 minutes) and stretching before and cool-down with additional stretching after resistance training. This is because of significant risk of loss of joint ROM in persons with CP.
- Because of interference from spasticity, guidelines for flexibility training in this population include stretching all major muscle groups to point of tension and holding for 60 to 120 seconds each. Special attention should be given to areas of limited range of motion; assisted stretching may be useful if performed cautiously; daily stretching of muscles that are causing the most problems with activities of daily living should be performed.
- The personal trainer must be aware of and sensitive to the fact that many persons with CP have cognitive, visual, hearing, and speech difficulties.
- Because of balance and coordination problems, supervision is recommended with the use of modes such as the treadmill, elliptical trainer, and cross-country ski machine.
- The personal trainer should emphasize proper nutrition in persons with CP, and in particular among clients who are overweight.

CONCLUSION

The scope of practice of personal trainers is expanding rapidly. Accumulating evidence supports the application of exercise training to numerous special populations including persons with several neuromuscular disorders. Increasing and sustaining moderate to high levels of physical activity among persons with SCI, MS, CP, and epilepsy are strongly encouraged. The functional and health benefits of regular exercise for these populations are similar to those for other persons when the activities are performed safely and effectively. Many persons in these groups are at increased risk for chronic metabolic disorders, at least partially because of the high frequency of physical inactivity among these populations.

Personal trainers working under the guidance of health care professionals should make an effort to promote their services to populations with the disorders covered in this chapter. The intrinsic rewards of working with persons who have these neuromuscular disorders, as well as others such as Parkinson's disease, muscular dystrophy, and post-polio syndrome, are many and certainly as meaningful as those derived from working with other clients, both nonathletic and athletic. Finally, two key references that should become part of the library of any personal trainer working with special populations are *ACSM's Resources for Clinical Exercise Physiology* and *ACSM's Exercise Management for Persons with Chronic Diseases and Disabilities* [22, 49].

STUDY QUESTIONS

1. A client with a complete spinal cord injury at L1 has been having shoulder pain while using her wheelchair. The personal trainer suspects it is from overuse. Which of the following exercises target the muscles that will help to restore balance at the shoulder?
   A. incline dumbbell bench press
   B. front shoulder raise
   C. seated row
   D. internal rotation with tubing
2. A 40-year-old client diagnosed with multiple sclerosis complained of significant fatigue following the previous three training sessions. Those sessions included 40-45 minutes of stationary bicycling with a target heart rate of 90-100 bpm and resistance training performing one set of 10 repetitions using 50% of her 1RM for five different exercises. Which of the following should be decreased during the next training session?
   A. bicycling intensity
   B. bicycling duration
   C. resistance training repetition number
   D. resistance training load
3. At the beginning of a training session, a client with a history of seizures tells the personal trainer that he had a low-grade fever the previous night and, as a result, he had a sleepless night. Which of the following exercise modifications should be made for this training session?
   A. avoid exercise
   B. decrease aerobic exercise intensity
   C. give extra attention on avoiding the Valsalva maneuver
   D. decrease aerobic exercise duration
4. A client diagnosed with cerebral palsy has functional use of his legs. Which of the following modes of exercise requires the LEAST amount of supervision?
   A. treadmill walking
   B. stairstepper
   C. stationary bicycle
   D. elliptical trainer

APPLIED KNOWLEDGE QUESTION

Fill in the chart to describe the general exercise contraindications and safety concerns for clients with SCI, MS, epilepsy, and CP.

	Exercise contraindications	Safety concerns
SCI		
MS		
Epilepsy		
CP		

REFERENCES

1. Ascherio, A., K.L. Munger, E.T. Lennette, D. Spiegelman, M.A. Hernan, M.J. Olek, S.E. Hankinson, and D.J. Hunter. 2001. Epstein-Barr virus antibodies and risk of multiple sclerosis. *Journal of the American Medical Association* 286: 3083-3088.
2. Bauman, W.A., and A.M. Spungen. 2000. Metabolic changes in persons after spinal cord injury. *Physical Medicine and Rehabilitation Clinics of North America* 11: 109-140.
3. Birk, T.J., E. Nieshoff, G. Gray, J. Steeby, and K. Jablonski. 2001. Metabolic and cardiopulmonary responses to acute progressive resistive exercise in a person with C4 spinal cord injury. *Spinal Cord* 39: 336-339.
4. Bradley-Popovich, G.E., K.R. Abshire, C.M. Crookston, and G.G. Frounfelter. 2000. Resistance training in paraplegia: Rationale and recommendations. *Strength and Conditioning Journal* 22: 31-34.
5. Burkett, L.N., J. Chisum, W. Stone, and B. Fernhall. 1990. Exercise capacity of untrained spinal cord injured individuals and the relationship of peak oxygen uptake and level of injury. *Paraplegia* 28: 512-521.
6. Burnham R.S., and R.D. Steadrand. 1994. Nerve entrapment in wheelchair athletes. *Archives of Physical Medicine and Rehabilitation* 75: 519-524.
7. Cerebral Palsy International Sports and Recreation Association. 1991. *Classification and Sports Rules Manual,* 5th ed. Nottingham, England: CPISRA.
8. Chad, K.E., D.A. Bailey, H.A. McKay, G.A. Zello, and R.E. Snyder. 1999. The effect of a weight-bearing physical activity program on bone mineral content and estimated volumetric density in children with spastic cerebral palsy. *Journal of Pediatrics* 135: 115-117.
9. Comi, G., L. Leocani, P. Rossi, and B. Columbo. 2001. Physiopathology and treatment of fatigue in multiple sclerosis. *Journal of Neurology* 248: 174-179.
10. Commission on Classification and Terminology of the International League Against Epilepsy. 1981. Proposal for revised classification of epilepsies and epileptic seizures. *Epilepsia* 22: 389-399.
11. Commission on Classification and Terminology of the International League Against Epilepsy. 1989. Proposal for revised clinical and electroencephalopathic classification of epileptic seizures. *Epilepsia* 22: 489-501.
12. Curtis, K.A., T.M. Tyner, L. Zachary, G. Lentell, D. Brink, T. Didyk, K. Gean, J. Hall, M. Hooper, J. Klos, S. Lesina, and B. Pacillas. 1999. Effect of a standard exercise protocol on shoulder pain in long-term wheelchair users. *Spinal Cord* 37: 421-429.
13. Damiano, D.L., and M.F. Abel. 1998. Functional outcomes of strength training in spastic cerebral palsy. *Archives of Physical Medicine and Rehabilitation* 79: 119-125.
14. Damiano, D.L., C.L. Vaughn, and M.F. Abel. 1995. Muscle response to heavy resistance training in spastic cerebral palsy. *Developmental Medicine and Child Neurology* 75: 658-671.
15. Davis, G.M. 1993. Exercise capacity of individuals with paraplegia. *Medicine and Science in Sports and Exercise* 25: 423-432.
16. Davis, G.M., and R.M. Glaser. 1990. Cardiorespiratory fitness following spinal cord injury. In: *Key Issues in Neurological Physiotherapy,* L. Ada and C. Canning, eds. Sydney: Butterworth-Heinemann, pp. 155-196.
17. Davis, G.M., and R.J. Shepard. 1988. Cardiorespiratory fitness in highly active versus less active paraplegics. *Medicine and Science in Sports and Exercise* 20: 963-968.
18. Davis, G.M., R.J. Shepard, and F.H.H. Leenen. 1987. Cardiac effects of short-term arm crank training in paraplegics: Echocardiographic evidence. *European Journal of Applied Physiology* 56: 90-96.
19. Davis, G.M., R.J. Shepard, and R.W. Jackson. 1981. Cardiorespiratory fitness and muscular strength in lower-limb disabled. *Canadian Journal of Applied Sport Sciences* 6: 159-165.
20. Davis, G.M., R.J. Shepard, and R.W. Jackson. 1991. Exercise capacity following spinal cord injury. In: *Cardiovascular and Respiratory Responses to Exercise in Health and Disease,* J.R. Sutton and R. Balnave, eds. Sydney: University of Sydney, pp. 179-192.
21. Davis, G.M., S.J. Tupling, and R.J. Shepard. 1986. Dynamic strength and physical activity in wheelchair users. In: *1984 Olympic Scientific Congress—Sports and Disabled Athletes,* C. Sherrill, ed. Champaign, IL: Human Kinetics, pp. 139-148.
22. Durstine, J.L. 2002. *ACSM's Exercise Management for Persons with Chronic Diseases and Disabilities,* 2nd ed. Champaign, IL: Human Kinetics.

23. Ferrara, M.S., W.E. Buelly, B.C. McCann, T.S. Limbird, J.W. Powell, and R. Robl. 1992. The injury experience of the competitive athlete with a disability: Prevention implications. *Medicine and Science in Sports and Exercise* 24: 184-188.

24. Ferrara, M., and J. Laskin. 1997. Cerebral palsy. In: *ACSM's Exercise Management of Persons with Chronic Diseases and Disabilities,* J.L. Durstine, ed. Champaign, IL: Human Kinetics, pp. 206-211.

25. Figoni, S.F. 1986. Circulorespiratory effects of arm training and detraining in one C5-6 quadriplegic man. *Physical Therapy* 66: 779.

26. Figoni, S.F. 1993. Exercise responses and quadriplegia. *Medicine and Science in Sports and Exercise* 25: 433-441.

27. Figoni, S.F. 1997. Spinal cord injury. In: *ACSM's Exercise Management for Persons with Chronic Diseases and Disabilities,* 1st ed., J.L. Durstine, ed. Champaign, IL: Human Kinetics, pp. 175-179.

28. Figoni, S.T., R.A. Boileau, B.H. Massey, and J.R. Larsen. 1988. Physiological responses of quadriplegics and able-bodied men during exercise at the same oxygen uptake. *Adapted Physical Activity Quarterly* 5: 130-139.

29. Figoni, S.F., C.G. Gupta, and R.M. Glaser. 1999. Effects of posture on arm exercise performance of adults with tetraplegia. *Clinical Exercise Physiology* 1: 74-85.

30. Franklin, B.A., K.I. Swentek, K. Grais, K.S. Johnston, S. Gordon, and G.C. Timmis. 1990. Field test of maximum oxygen consumption in wheelchair users. *Archives of Physical Medicine and Rehabilitation* 71: 574-578.

31. Gates, J.R., and R.H. Spiegel. 1993. Epilepsy, sports, and exercise. *Sports Medicine* 15: 1-5.

32. Hjentnes, N. 1977. Oxygen uptake and cardiac output in graded arm exercise in paraplegics with low level spinal lesions. *Scandinavian Journal of Rehabilitation Medicine* 9: 107-113.

33. Hjentnes, N. 1984. Control of medical rehabilitation of para and tetraplegics by repeated evaluation of endurance capacity. *International Journal of Sports Medicine* 5: 171-174.

34. Hutzler, Y.A., A. Chacham, U. Bergman, and I. Reches. 1998. Effects of a movement and swimming program on water orientation skills and self-concept of kindergarten children with cerebral palsy. *Perceptual and Motor Skills* 86: 111-118.

35. Hutzler, Y., A. Chacham, U. Bergman, and A. Szeinberg. 1998. Effects of a movement and swimming program on vital capacity and water orientation skills of children with cerebral palsy. *Developmental Medicine and Child Neurology* 40: 176-178.

36. Jackson, R.W., G.M. Davis, P.R. Kofsky, R.J. Shepard, and G.C.R. Keene. 1981. Fitness levels in lower limb disabled. *Transactions of the 27th Annual Meeting of the Orthopedic Society* 6: 12-14.

37. Kammerman, S., and L. Wasserman. 2001. Seizure diagnosis: Part 1. Classification and diagnosis. *Western Journal of Medicine* 175: 99-103.

38. Kammerman, S., and L. Wasserman. 2001. Seizure disorders: Part 2. Treatment. *Western Journal of Medicine* 175: 184-188.

39. Kofsky, P.R., G.M. Davis, G.C. Jackson, C.R. Keene, and R.J. Shepard. 1983. Field testing: Assessment of physically disabled adults. *European Journal of Applied Physiology* 15: 109-120.

40. Kofsky, P.R., R.J. Shepard, G.M. Davis, and R.W. Jackson. 1986. Classification of aerobic power and muscular strength for disabled individuals with differing patterns of habitual physical activity. In: *1984 Olympic Scientific Congress—Sports and Disabled Athletes.* Champaign, IL: Human Kinetics, pp. 147-156.

41. Korczya, A.D. 1979. Participation of epileptic patients in sports. *Journal of Sports Medicine* 19: 195-198.

42. Laskowski, E.R. 1994. Strength training in the physically challenged population. *Strength and Conditioning* 16: 66-69.

43. Liaw, M.Y., A.C. Lin, P.T. Cheng, M.K. Wong, and F.T. Tang. 2000. Resistive inspiratory muscle training: Its effectiveness in patients with acute complete cervical cord injury. *Archives of Physical Medicine and Rehabilitation* 81: 752-756.

44. Linn, W.S., A.M. Spungen, H. Gong Jr., R.H. Adkins, W.A. Bauman, and R.L. Waters. 2001. Forced vital capacity in two large outpatient populations with chronic spinal cord injury. *Spinal Cord* 39: 263-268.

45. McLean, K.P., P.P. Jones, and J.S. Skinner. 1995. Exercise prescription for sitting and supine exercise in individuals with tetraplegia. *Medicine and Science in Sports and Exercise* 27: 15-21.

46. McLean, K.P., and J.S. Skinner. 1995. Effect of training position on outcomes of an aerobic training study on individuals with quadriplegia. *Archives of Physical Medicine and Rehabilitation* 76: 139-150.

47. Mellett, C.J., A.C. Johnson, P.J. Thompson, and D.R. Fish. 2001. The relationship between participation in common leisure activities and seizure occurrence. *Acta Neurological Scandinavica* 103: 300-303.

48. Mulcare, J.A. 1997. Multiple sclerosis. In: *ACSM's Exercise Management for Persons with Chronic Diseases and Disabilities,* J.L. Durstine, ed. Champaign, IL: Human Kinetics, pp. 189-193.

49. Myers, J., W. Herbert, and R. Humphrey, eds. 2002. *ACSM's Resource for Clinical Exercise Physiology: Musculoskeletal, Neuromuscular, Neoplastic, Immunologic, and Hematologic Conditions,* 1st ed. Baltimore: Lippincott Williams & Wilkins.

50. Nakken, K.O. 1999. Physical exercise in outpatients with epilepsy. *Epilepsia* 40: 643-651.

51. Nakken, K.O., P.G. Bjorholt, S.L. Johannssen, T.Loyning, and E. Lind. 1990. Effect of physical training on aerobic capacity, seizure occurrence, and serum level of antiepileptic drugs in adults with epilepsy. *Epilepsia* 31: 88-94.

52. Nakken, K.O., and R. Lossius. 1993. Seizure-related injuries in multihandicapped patients with therapy-resistant epilepsy. *Epilepsia* 34: 846-850.

53. Nash, M.S., S. Bilsker, and A.E. Marcillo. 1991. Reversal of adaptive left ventricular atrophy following electrically stimulated exercise training in human tetraplegics. *Paraplegia* 29: 590-599.

54. Noseworthy, J.H., C. Lucchinetti, M. Rodriguez, and B.G. Weinshenker. 2000. Multiple sclerosis. *New England Journal of Medicine* 343: 938-952.

55. Ogyniemi, A.O., M.R. Gomez, and D.K. Klass. 1988. Seizures induced by exercise. *Neurology* 38: 633-634.

56. Oligati, R., J.M. Burgunder, and M. Mumenthaler. 1988. Increased energy cost of walking in multiple sclerosis: Effect of spasticity, ataxia, and weakness. *Archives of Physical Medicine and Rehabilitation* 69: 846-849.

57. Oligati, R., J. Jacquet, and P.E. Di Prampero. 1986. Energy cost of walking and exertional dyspnea in multiple sclerosis. *The American Review of Respiratory Disease* 134: 1005-1010.

58. Peck, D.M., and D.B. McKeag. 1994. Athletes with disabilities: Removing barriers. *The Physician and Sportsmedicine* 24: 59-62.

59. Petajan, J.H., E. Gappmaier, A.T. White, M.K. Spencer, I. Mino, and R.W. Hicks. 1996. Impact of aerobic training on fitness and quality of life in multiple sclerosis. *Annals of Neurology* 39: 432-441.

60. Petajan, J.H., and A.T. White. 1999. Recommendations for physical activity in patients with multiple sclerosis. *Sports Medicine* 27: 179-191.
61. Peterson, C. 2001. Exercise in 94 degrees F water for a patient with multiple sclerosis. *Physical Therapy* 81: 1049-1058.
62. Phillips, W.T., B.J. Kiratli, M. Sarkarati, G. Weraarchakul, J. Myers, B.A. Franklin, I. Parkash, and V. Froelicher. 1998. Effect of spinal cord injury on the heart and cardiovascular fitness. *Current Problems in Cardiology* 23: 649-704.
63. Ponichtera-Mulcare, J.A. 1993. Exercise and multiple sclerosis. *Medicine and Science in Sports and Exercise* 25: 451-465.
64. Poser, C.M., D.W. Paty, and L. Scheinberg. 1983. New diagnostic criteria for multiple sclerosis: Guidelines for research protocols. *Annals of Neurology* 13: 227-231.
65. Sadovnick, A.D., P.A. Baird, and R.H. Ward. 1988. Multiple sclerosis: Updated risks for relatives. *American Journal of Medical Genetics* 29: 533-541.
66. Schmitt, B., L. Thun-Hohenstein, L. Vontobel, and E. Boltshauser. 1994. Seizures induced by physical exercise: Report of two cases. *Neuropediatrics* 25: 51-53.
67. Sopka, C. 1998. Sports medical concerns for conditioning athletes with disabilities. *Strength and Conditioning* 20: 24-31.
68. Spiegel, R.H., and J.R. Gates. 1997. Epilepsy. In: *ACSM's Exercise Management for Persons with Chronic Diseases and Disabilities,* J.L. Durstine, ed. Champaign, IL: Human Kinetics, pp. 185-188.
69. Sutherland, G.J., and M.B. Anderson. 2001. Exercise and multiple sclerosis: Physiological, psychological, and quality of life issues. *Journal of Sports Medicine and Physical Fitness* 41: 421-432.
70. Svenson, B., B. Gerdle, and J. Elert. 1994. Endurance training in patients with multiple sclerosis: Five case studies. *Physical Therapy* 74: 1017-1026.
71. Tantucci, C., M. Massucci, R. Piperno, V. Grassi, and C.A. Sorbini. 1996. Energy cost of exercise in multiple sclerosis patients with low degree of disability. *Multiple Sclerosis* 2: 161-167.
72. Turk, M.A., C.A. Geremski, P.F. Rosenbaum, and R.J. Weber. 1997. The health status of women with cerebral palsy. *Archives of Physical Medicine and Rehabilitation* 78: S10-17.
73. United Cerebral Palsy, UCP Net. Cerebral palsy—facts and figures. Retrieved January 2001 from http://www.ucp.org/ucp_generaldoc.cfm/1/3/43/43-43/447.
74. White, A.T., T.E. Wilson, S.L. Davis, and J.H. Petajen. 2000. Effect of precooling on physical performance in multiple sclerosis. *Multiple Sclerosis* 6: 176-180.
75. Winnich, J.P., and F.X. Short. 1984. The physical fitness of youngsters with spinal neuromuscular conditions. *Adapted Physical Activity Quarterly* 1: 37-51.
76. Wise, J.B. 1996. Weight training for those with physical disabilities at Idaho State University. *Strength and Conditioning* 18: 67-71.
77. Yamasaki, M., K.T. Kim, S.W. Choi, S. Muraki, M. Shiokawa, and T. Kurokawa. 2001. Characteristics of body heat balance of paraplegics during exercise in a hot environment. *Journal of Physiological Anthropology in Applied Human Sciences* 20: 227-232.

CHAPTER 23

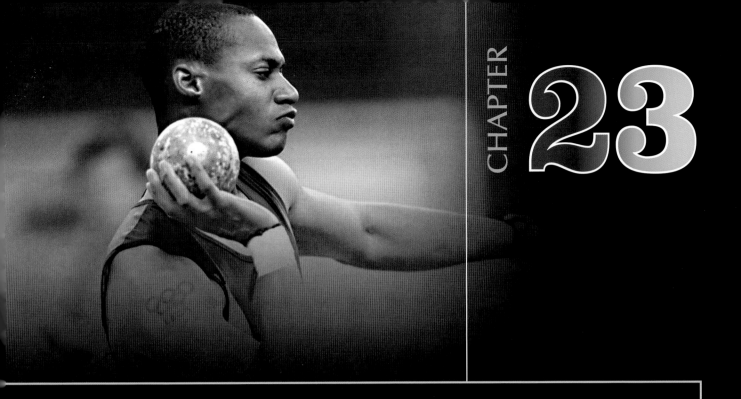

Resistance Training for Clients Who Are Athletes

David Pearson | John F. Graham

After completing this chapter, you will be able to

- understand how to apply overload and specificity to a resistance training program for a client who is training for a sport;
- understand the value, role, and application of a periodized training program;
- describe the cycles and phases of a periodized training program;
- understand how load and repetitions are manipulated in a linear and a nonlinear periodization model; and
- design a linear and nonlinear periodization program.

Personal trainers have the opportunity to work with a large variety of client types. Commonly, a client has a sedentary lifestyle with limited recreational pursuits, sometimes to the extent that he or she is very deconditioned or symptomatic of a cardiovascular or metabolic medical condition or confirmed disease. Alternatively, some clients are on the opposite end of the wellness continuum; they are very physically active, possibly both in their job and in personal time, with competition-laced goals and aspirations. Clients who are athletes have training needs that are much different from those of the general population. Following the application of the basic resistance training program design variables detailed in chapter 15, this chapter describes how to develop a more advanced periodized program that will help clients—labeled as athletes in this chapter—meet their competitive goals.

Factors in Program Design

Resistance training programs have been used for many years as an integral part of a total exercise program to enhance athletic performance. During the past two decades, the effectiveness of carefully planned resistance training programs as a method of improving body development and sport performance has been accepted on the basis of the scientific literature [1, 2, 21, 22, 30, 35, 36]. Significant benefits can be gained from the systematic and proper application of the overload and specificity principles, the two primary tenets of resistance training. Combined with the principles of periodization needed to optimize the exercise stimulus, resistance training provides one of the most potent and effective methods to increase muscular performance capabilities, improve sport performance, and help to prevent injury [9, 13, 35].

Overload Principle

The overload principle is based on the concept that the athlete must adapt to the demands of greater physiological challenges to the neuromuscular system. Thus, the training stress or loads placed on the muscles must be progressively increased for gains to occur [13, 30, 35]. As explained in chapter 15, the personal trainer can apply overload by increasing the amount of weight lifted in an exercise, incorporating more workouts in a week, including more (or more difficult) exercises, or adding sets to one or more exercises in a workout.

Specificity of Training

Specificity refers to the personal trainer's developing a program that trains an athlete in a specific way to produce a specific change or result. The more similar the training activity is to the actual sport movement, the greater the likelihood that there will be a positive transfer to that sport [3, 8, 14, 17, 18, 24, 34]. Although an athlete may enhance his or her speed and power with a nonsport-specific program [27], the most effective program will match the metabolic and biomechanical characteristics of the training program to the sport activity. This level of specificity will train the appropriate metabolic systems by including exercises that duplicate the joint velocities and angular movements of the sport. Therefore, the personal trainer should design the resistance training program to include at least one exercise that mimics the movement pattern of each primary skill of the athlete's sport (see table 23.1 for examples).

> The more similar the training activity is to the actual sport movement, the greater the likelihood that there will be a positive transfer to that sport.

> The personal trainer should design the resistance training program to include at least one exercise that mimics the movement pattern of each primary skill of the athlete's sport.

Although an increase in 1-repetition maximum (1RM) strength is a common outcome of all programs that involve lifting heavy loads, improving an athlete's ability to generate force at very rapid speeds requires training at high velocities [16]. Thus, improving a 1RM by conventional slow-velocity heavy resistance training does not assure the improvement of force development in ballistic sport movements (e.g., basketball jump shot, baseball pitch, volleyball spike). Instead, the personal trainer should select power exercises and assign moderate loads to allow the athlete to perform the movements explosively [3].

> Improving an athlete's ability to generate force at very rapid speeds requires the personal trainer to select power exercises and assign moderate loads to allow the athlete to perform those exercises explosively.

The text for this chapter has been edited from D. Pearson, A. Faigenbaum, M. Conley, and W.J. Kraemer, 2000, "National Strength and Conditioning Association's basic guidelines for the resistance training of athletes," *Strength and Conditioning Journal* 22 (4): 14-27 and J.F. Graham, 2002, "Periodization research and an example application," *Strength and Conditioning Journal* 24 (6): 62-70.

TABLE 23.1

Examples of Sport-Specific Exercises

Sport skill	Related sport-specific exercises*
Ball dribbling and passing	Close-grip bench press, reverse curl, triceps push-down
Ball kicking	Unilateral hip adduction/abduction, leg (knee) extension, leg raise
Freestyle swimming	Lat pulldown, lateral raise, lunge
Jumping	Power clean, push jerk, back squat
Racket stroke	Dumbbell fly, bent-over lateral raise, wrist curl/extension
Rowing	Bent-over row, seated row, hip sled
Running/Sprinting	Lunge, step-up, toe raise (dorsiflexion)
Throwing/Pitching	Pullover, overhead triceps extension, shoulder internal/external rotation

*This list is not exhaustive; many more sport-specific exercises can be included.

Adapted from Baechle and Earle 2000.

Periodization of Resistance Training

One of the most important developments in the technology of sport training has been the advancement of concepts related to periodization. **Periodization** is the systematic process of planned variations in a resistance training program over a training cycle [12, 13, 30, 35]. The primary goals of periodization are met by appropriately manipulating volume and intensity and by effectively selecting exercises. A significant amount of research has been performed that shows that this concept optimizes training adaptations [10, 20]. One of the primary advantages of this training approach is the reduced risk of overtraining due to the purposeful time devoted to physical and mental recovery [13, 23, 30]. Typically only core exercises are periodized, but all exercises can be varied for intensity and volume [13, 29, 30, 35].

Periodization is the systematic process of planned variations in a resistance training program over a training cycle.

Cycles and Phases

Periodized programs are typically divided into three distinct cycles. The **macrocycle** is the largest division, which typically constitutes an entire training year but may also be a period of many months up to four years (e.g., for an Olympic athlete). Macrocycles typically comprise two or more **mesocycles** divided into several weeks to a few months. The number of mesocycles is dependent on the goals of the athlete and, if applicable, the number of sport competitions contained within the period. Each mesocycle is divided into **microcycles** that can range from one week to four weeks, which include daily and weekly training variations [5, 6, 7, 11, 13, 30, 32].

In 1981, Stone and colleagues [31] in the United States developed an American model for strength and power sports by modifying the periodization program that had been created by the former Soviet Union and Eastern European countries [35, 36]. This approach divides a resistance training program into five mesocycles, each with a primary goal or focus:

- **Hypertrophy phase:** to develop a muscular and metabolic base for more intense future training using a resistance training program that includes sport-specific or nonsport-specific exercises performed at a high volume and a low intensity
- **Strength phase:** to increase maximal muscle force by following a resistance training program that focuses on sport-specific exercises of moderate volume and intensity
- **Strength/Power phase:** to increase the speed of force development and power by integrating sport-specific power/explosive exercises of low volume and high intensity

- **Competition or peaking phase:** to attain peak strength and power by performing a very high intensity and very low volume sport-specific resistance training program
- **Active rest phase:** to allow physiological and mental recovery through limited low-volume and low-intensity resistance training or by having the athlete perform physical activities unrelated to his or her sport

It has been found that greater strength and power gains can be achieved by repeating this set of five mesocycles more than once per year [13, 30]. The concept of variation is a vital factor that explains the advantage of performing the entire set of training phases *three* times in a single year instead of only once [13, 30].

Variation in Exercise Selection

Empirical evidence suggests that variations in exercise selection for the same muscle group result in greater increases in strength and power than a program with no variation in exercises. This does not mean that the personal trainer needs to vary the exercises performed in every training session or that all exercises must be changed when one change is made. However, changes in exercises may be made every two to three weeks, or some exercises can be varied on an every-other training session basis (i.e., with two somewhat different training sessions performed alternately). Still, certain core exercises need to be maintained through the training program so that progress in the major exercises can be continuously made [25].

Variations in exercise selection for the same muscle group result in greater increases in strength and power than a program with no variation in exercises.

Linear and Nonlinear Models of Periodized Resistance Training

The classic periodization model is generally a linear program; that is, training intensity gradually and continually increases and training volume gradually and continually decreases from one mesocycle to the next. If there is variation in the loading within the week or microcycle, the number of sets and repetitions for a given exercise does not change across the workouts. A variation on the linear model involves within-the-week or microcycle vacillations in both the assigned training load and the training volume for most (or all) core exercises. This type of periodization model is referred to as **undulating** or nonlinear [4, 13, 28].

Linear Periodization Model

For the linear model, weekly fluctuations in the core exercises occur such that the repetition maximum-level (RM) training (i.e., 100% of the assigned training load) is performed on one day (referred to as the "heavy" day), and subsequent training in the same week for the same exercise is performed at a "light" level (10-30% lighter loads than on the RM day), a "moderate" or "medium" level (5-10% lighter loads than the RM day), or both (depending on whether there are two or three workouts in a week)—all with the same set and repetition assignments. (Refer to the section "Within-the-Week Variation" on page 382 for further explanation.) An example of a linear program (although it shows only one week) is the "Sample Muscular Strength Program" in chapter 15. The "light" day loads are only 80% of the full "heavy day" RM loads, but the number of sets and repetitions (i.e., volume) remains the same across the workouts.

Advancing a linearly periodized program involves a gradual increase in intensity over multiple weeks (or microcycles) of training. Usually the length of time devoted to a particular intensity load ranges from two to four weeks. The program ends with an active rest phase prior to the start of another complete training cycle or an in-season (competitive) period.

A linear periodization program involves gradual and continual increases in training intensity and gradual and continual decreases in training volume from one mesocycle to the next, but no variation in the assigned number of sets and repetitions within each mesocycle.

Sample Linear Periodization Program

Before starting the periodized program, the personal trainer should recommend that the athlete complete a lower-intensity four- to six-week base training program. This introductory program will allow the athlete to learn exercise technique, gain an initial adaptation to resistance exercise stress, and prepare for the first training cycle. Loads are typically very light (e.g., 15-20RMs). This base program is especially important for beginners and may or may not be used with experienced, trained athletes.

A summary of the parameters of the linear periodization phases is included in table 23.2, and a sample program is shown in table 23.3.

TABLE 23.2

Summary of the Program Design of a Linear Periodization Program (Core Exercises)

Phase	Length (weeks)	Sets	Goal repetitions	Rest period length	Assigned load
Hypertrophy/ Endurance	2-4	3-5	8-12	1-2 minutes	~75%1RM
Strength	2-4	3-5	5-6	3-5 minutes	~85%1RM
Strength/Power	2-4	3-5	3-4	2-3 minutes*	90-93%1RM**
Competition	2-3	3-4	1-2	3-5 minutes	≥95%1RM**
Active rest	1-3	No resistance training			

*Some exercises or situations may require up to a 5-minute rest.

**The loads for power exercises (e.g., push press, power clean) need to be somewhat lighter to permit rapid and explosive movements (consult reference 3 for details about assigning loads for power exercises).

Adapted from Pearson, Faigenbaum, Conley, and Kraemer 2000.

- **Hypertrophy/Endurance phase.** This two- to four-week phase formally starts a periodized program. The personal trainer should direct the athlete to perform three to five sets of each exercise at an intensity that allows 8 to 12 repetitions (about 75%1RM) per set with a one- to two-minute rest period between sets and exercises. This will create a higher-volume, lower-intensity stimulus.
- **Strength phase.** Using the same length cycle of two to four weeks, the athlete performs three to five sets of five to six repetitions per exercise with an intensity of about 85%1RM. A three- to five-minute rest period is allowed between sets and exercises.
- **Strength/Power phase.** For the next two to four weeks, the athlete performs exercises that allow only three to four repetitions for three to five sets at 90% to 93%1RM. The personal trainer also includes power exercises (e.g., push press, power clean) with somewhat lighter loads [3] to permit rapid and explosive movements. A longer rest period between sets is recommended for adequate recovery.
- **Competition phase.** During a two- to three-week time period, the personal trainer further increases the load so that it allows only one to two repetitions at ≥95%1RM (slighter lighter loads for power exercises [3]). The athlete performs three to four sets of each exercise with a three- to five-minute rest period between sets and exercises. This phase allows for the peaking of strength and power abilities, which is especially important for sports that require maximal strength and rapid force development.
- **Active rest phase.** At this point, the athlete moves into the competitive season after a week of active rest or formally completes a one- to three-week active rest period before returning to the hypertrophy phase to repeat the periodized program.

Nonlinear Periodization Model

A nonlinear periodization model varies the intensity (load) and volume of the core exercises throughout the week. This is in contrast to the linear periodization model that modulates the load but keeps the volume intact. For example, the intensity of a four-day program could be Monday, "heavy"; Tuesday, "light"; Thursday, "power"; and Friday, "moderate." (The remaining days of the week are rest days.) This continues for a given time period before the athlete begins a competition period or a one- to two-week active rest phase.

A nonlinear or undulating periodization program involves within-the-week or microcycle vacillations in the assigned training load and volume.

Sample Nonlinear Periodization Program

As recommended prior to the start of the linear periodization program, the athlete may need to complete a four- to six-week base training program that incorporates many repetitions with light loads (e.g.,

TABLE 23.3

Sample Three-Day Linear Periodization Program

Phase	Week	Sets	Goal reps+	Rest period length (minutes)+	Monday "Heavy" day+ 100% of the assigned training load	Wednesday "Light" day+ 80% of the assigned training load++	Friday "Medium" day+ 90% of the assigned training load++
Hypertrophy/ Endurance	1	3	12	1	67%1RM	54%1RM	60%1RM
	2	4	10	1.5	75%1RM	60%1RM	68%1RM
	3	4	10	1.5	75%1RM	60%1RM	68%1RM
	4	5	8	2	80%1RM	64%1RM	72%1RM
Strength	5	3	6	3*	85%1RM	68%1RM	77%1RM
	6	4	6	3*	85%1RM	68%1RM	77%1RM
	7	5	5	3*	87%1RM	70%1RM	78%1RM
	8	5	5	3*	87%1RM	70%1RM	78%1RM
Strength/ Power	9	3	4	3*	90%1RM**	72%1RM	81%1RM
	10	4	4	3*	90%1RM**	72%1RM	81%1RM
	11	5	3	3*	93%1RM**	74%1RM	84%1RM
	12	5	3	3*	93%1RM**	74%1RM	84%1RM
Competition	13	3	2	5	95%1RM**	76%1RM	86%1RM
	14	4	2	5	95%1RM**	76%1RM	86%1RM
	15	4	1	5	100%1RM**	80%1RM	90%1RM
Active rest	16	No resistance training					

+These guidelines apply to core exercises only. For the load assignments, refer to chapter 15 for an explanation of the relationship between a percent of a 1RM and the number of repetitions that typically can be performed. ++The athlete should complete the same number of goal repetitions—not more simply because the loads are lighter. This applies also to the power exercises whose loads were lightened from the "heavy" day assignments. The %1RMs shown for the "light" and "medium" days were calculated by multiplying the %1RMs of the "heavy" day by 0.80 and 0.90 (respectively). *Some exercises or situations may require up to a 5-minute rest. **The loads for power exercises (e.g., push press, power clean) need to be somewhat lighter to permit rapid and explosive movements (see reference 3).

Adapted from Pearson, Faigenbaum, Conley, and Kraemer 2000.

15-20RMs) to reinforce proper exercise technique and provide a foundation for later phases. A nonlinear program can use the same time period as a linear periodization model (i.e., 12-16 weeks). The different training sessions are sequenced or rotated within a seven-day (or longer) microcycle.

The characteristics of nonlinear periodization workouts are listed in table 23.4, and a sample program is shown in table 23.5.

- **Monday ("heavy" day).** This workout emphasizes muscular strength by assigning three to four sets of each exercise with a 3- to 6RM load. To promote recovery, the personal trainer should allow a three- to five-minute rest period.
- **Tuesday ("light" day).** The lighter loads of this workout permit more repetitions, but they are still repetition maximums (e.g., 10-

TABLE 23.4

Summary of the Program Design of a Nonlinear Periodization Program (Core Exercises)

Training day	Sets	Goal repetitions	Rest period length	Assigned load
"Heavy"	3-4	3-6	3-5 minutes	85-93%1RM
"Light"	2-4	10-15	1-2 minutes	65-75%1RM
"Power"	3-4	2-4	2-3 minutes*	Power exercises: 30-60%1RM** Other core exercises: 90-95%1RM**
"Moderate"	2-4	8-10	1-2 minutes	75-80%1RM***

*Some exercises or situations may require up to a 5-minute rest. **For power exercises, the personal trainer should assign loads at 30-60%1RM to allow the athlete to perform them explosively. (For further information about determining loads for power exercises, refer to reference 3). Other core exercises should be assigned 2-4RM loads. ***Or loads 5-10% less than the "heavy" day loads.

Adapted from Pearson, Faigenbaum, Conley, and Kraemer 2000.

15RMs). The athlete performs two to four sets of each exercise with a one- to two-minute rest period between sets and exercises.

- **Thursday ("power" day).** There are two load and repetition schemes for this workout, depending on the exercise. For power exercises, the athlete performs three to four sets of two to four repetitions with 30% to 60%1RM to allow higher movement velocities; all other core exercises are assigned the same number of sets but at 2- to 4RMs. In addition, the personal trainer can include plyometric power exercises (e.g., with a medicine ball) to develop the power component in the training program of trained and experienced athletes. A two- to three-minute rest period between sets is recommended to allow adequate rest for the power exercises, but the 2- to 4RM sets may require additional recovery time.
- **Friday ("moderate" day).** This session uses loads 5% to 10% lighter than on the "heavy" day, or at least a sufficiently reduced intensity that allows 8 to 10 repetitions for two to four sets of each exercise. A one- to two-minute rest period is recommended between sets and exercises.

An example of a three-day nonlinear periodization program is to perform five sets with a 3RM load on the first training day of the week (i.e., the "heavy" day), three sets with a 10RM load on the next training day (the "light" day), and four sets with a 6RM load on the last training day (the "moderate" day). Again, both the load and volume are modified throughout the week.

Effectiveness of Linear and Nonlinear Periodized Programs

The effectiveness of a periodized program is attributed to the systematic variation that allows the athlete to adequately recover from the assigned loads and repetitions. Often the nonlinear method of periodization is used so that training can continue through the season. This is especially important for sports with long seasons (e.g., tennis, wrestling, basketball, hockey). Typically, during the in-season program, the frequency of training is reduced and the volume of exercise is modulated in relationship to the amount of competition and volume of sport practice. The key element of this type of training is the variation and ability to allow rest after a training or competition period [25].

During the in-season, training frequency is reduced and the volume of exercise is modulated in relationship to the number of competitive events and the volume of sport practice.

Further, although some sources suggest that there is no difference [4], it appears that the nonlinear model is more effective at promoting muscular strength gains than the linear model [20, 28, 33]. A probable reason is that the athlete is not exposed to continually greater training intensities. Instead, a nonlinear periodized program applies a training stress that contributes less to accumulated neural

TABLE 23.5

Sample Four-Day Nonlinear Periodization Program

Week	Monday				Tuesday				Thursday				Friday			
	"Heavy" day+				"Light" day+				"Power" day+				"Moderate" day+			
	Sets	Goal reps	Rest period length (min)	Load	Sets	Goal reps	Rest period length (min)	Load	Sets	Goal reps	Rest ++ period length (min)	Load	Sets	Goal reps	Rest period length (min)	Load**
1	3	6	4	85%1RM	2	15	1	65%1RM	3	4	3	P*: 30%1RM O*: 90%1RM	2	10	1.5	75%1RM
2	3	6	4	85%1RM	3	15	1	65%1RM	3	4	3	P: 32.5%1RM O: 90%1RM	3	10	1.5	75%1RM
3	4	6	4	85%1RM	3	15	1	65%1RM	4	4	3	P: 35%1RM O: 90%1RM	3	10	1.5	75%1RM
4	3	5	5	87%1RM	4	15	1	65%1RM	4	4	3	P: 37.5%1RM O: 90%1RM	4	10	1.5	75%1RM
5	3	5	5	87%1RM	4	15	1	65%1RM	4	4	3	P: 40%1RM O: 90%1RM	4	10	1.5	75%1RM
6	4	5	5	87%1RM	2	12	1.5	67%1RM	3	3	3	P: 45%1RM O: 93%1RM	2	9	2	85%1RM
7	4	5	5	87%1RM	3	12	1.5	67%1RM	3	3	3	P: 47.5%1RM O: 93%1RM	3	9	2	77%1RM

8	3	4	5	90%1RM	3	12	1.5	67%1RM	4	3	3	P: 50%1RM O: 93%1RM	3	9	2	77%1RM
9	3	4	5	90%1RM	4	12	1.5	67%1RM	4	3	3	P: 52.5%1RM O: 93%1RM	4	9	2	77%1RM
10	4	4	5	90%1RM	4	12	1.5	67%1RM	4	3	3	P: 55%1RM O: 93%1RM	4	9	2	77%1RM
11	4	4	5	90%1RM	2	10	1.5	75%1RM	3	2	3	P: 50%1RM O: 95%1RM	2	8	2	80%1RM
12	3	3	5	93%1RM	3	10	1.5	75%1RM	3	2	3	P: 52.5%1RM O: 95%1RM	3	8	2	80%1RM
13	3	3	5	93%1RM	3	10	1.5	75%1RM	4	2	3	P: 55%1RM O: 95%1RM	3	8	2	80%1RM
14	4	3	5	93%1RM	4	10	1.5	75%1RM	4	2	3	P: 57.5%1RM O: 95%1RM	4	8	2	80%1RM
15	4	3	5	93%1RM	4	10	1.5	75%1RM	4	2	3	P: 60%1RM O: 95%1RM	4	8	2	80%1RM
16	Active rest: no resistance training															

+These guidelines apply to core exercises only. For the load assignments, refer to chapter 15 for an explanation of the relationship between a percent of a 1RM and the number of repetitions that typically can be performed. ++Some exercises or situations may require up to a 5-minute rest. *For power exercises (P), the personal trainer should assign loads at 30-60%1RM to allow the athlete to perform them explosively. (For further information about determining loads for power exercises, refer to reference 3). Other core exercises (O) should be assigned 2-4RM loads. **Or loads 5-10% less than the "heavy" day loads.

fatigue [19]. Alternatively, the personal trainer will need to monitor a well-trained athlete who is following a nonlinear program because of the high relative loading; for example, even the "light" day involves RM loads [3].

CONCLUSION

Since one type of workout will not benefit every athlete in the same way, a training program should blend existing exercise science knowledge (e.g., adhering to the specificity and overload principles) with the practical requirements of administering an individualized exercise program. To this end, a personal trainer can design a periodized resistance training program that meets the needs of the athlete and attends to the specific demands of his or her sport.

STUDY QUESTIONS

1. Which of the following is the most sport-specific resistance training exercise for a volleyball player?
   A. push press
   B. lateral shoulder raise
   C. seated shoulder press
   D. leg press
2. Which of the following is the correct order of the divisions of a periodized program (from shortest to longest)?
   I. mesocycle
   II. microcycle
   III. macrocycle

   A. I, II, III
   B. III, II, I
   C. II, I, III
   D. II, III, I
3. Which of the following is the correct sequence of the phases of a periodized program?
   I. strength/power
   II. hypertrophy
   III. active rest
   IV. competition
   V. strength

   A. I, II, III, V, IV
   B. IV, III, II, I, V
   C. III, II, V, I, IV
   D. II, V, I, IV, III
4. A personal trainer includes the back squat exercise in an athlete's linearly periodized resistance training program. What is the load for a "medium" training day if the athlete's 1RM is 400 pounds (182 kilograms) and the number of goal repetitions is 4 per set?
   A. 360 pounds (164 kg)
   B. 325 pounds (148 kg)
   C. 285 pounds (130 kg)
   D. 255 pounds (116 kg)

APPLIED KNOWLEDGE QUESTION

Use table 23.3 as a guide to fill in the chart with the assigned loads for the bench press exercise for a well-trained athlete's linearly periodized resistance training program. His 1RM is 195 pounds. (Remember to round *down*.) Assume there are no increases in the athlete's strength across all of the training phases, despite that the athlete's 1RM would certainly improve over time. Also, refer to table 15.4 to determine the relationship between a percent of a 1RM and the number of repetitions that typically can be performed.

Phase	Week	Goal reps	*Tuesday* "Heavy" day	*Thursday* "Light" day	*Saturday* "Medium" day
Hypertrophy/ Endurance	1	12			
	2	10			
	3	8			
Strength	4	6			
	5	6			
	6	5			
Strength/Power	7	4			
	8	4			
	9	3			
Competition	10	2			
	11	2			
	12	1			

REFERENCES

1. American College of Sports Medicine. 1998. Position stand: The recommended quantity and quality of exercise for developing and maintaining cardiorespiratory and muscular fitness, and flexibility in healthy adults. *Medicine and Science in Sports and Exercise* 30 (6): 975-991.
2. Atha, J. 1981. Strengthening muscle. *Exercise and Sport Science Reviews* 9: 1-73.
3. Baechle, T.R., R.W. Earle, and D. Wathen. 2000. Resistance training. In: *Essentials of Strength Training and Conditioning,* 2nd ed., T.R. Baechle and R.W. Earle, eds. Champaign, IL: Human Kinetics.
4. Baker, D., G. Wilson, and R. Carlyon. 1994. Periodization: The effect on strength of manipulating volume and intensity. *Journal of Strength and Conditioning Research* 8: 235-242.
5. Chargina, A., M.S. Stone, J. Piedmonte, H.S. O'Bryant, W.J. Kraemer, V. Gambetta, H. Newton, G. Palmeri, and D. Pfoff. 1986. Periodization roundtable. *NSCA Journal* 8 (5): 12-23.
6. Chargina, A., M.S. Stone, J. Piedmonte, H.S. O'Bryant, W.J. Kraemer, V. Gambetta, H. Newton, G. Palmeri, and D. Pfoff. 1987. Periodization roundtable. *NSCA Journal* 8 (6): 17-25.
7. Chargina, A., M.S. Stone, J. Piedmonte, H.S. O'Bryant, W.J. Kraemer, V. Gambetta, H. Newton, G. Palmeri, and D. Pfoff. 1987. Periodization roundtable. *NSCA Journal* 9 (1): 16-27.
8. Coyle, E.F., D.C. Feiring, T.C. Rotkis, R.W. Cote, F.B Roby, W. Lee, and J.H. Wilmore. 1981. Specificity of power improvements through slow and fast isokinetic training. *Journal of Applied Physiology* 51: 1437-1442.
9. DeLorme, P. 1945. Restoration of muscle power by heavy resistance exercises. *Journal of Bone and Joint Surgery* 27: 645-667.
10. Fleck, S.J. 1999. Periodized strength training: A critical review. *Journal of Strength and Conditioning Research* 13 (1): 82-89.
11. Fleck, S.J., and W.J. Kraemer. 1988. Resistance training: Exercise prescription. *Physician and Sportsmedicine* 16: 69-81.
12. Fleck, S.J., and W.J. Kraemer. 1996. *Periodization Breakthrough!* Ronkonkoma, NY: Advanced Research Press.

13. Fleck, S.J., and W.J. Kraemer. 1997. *Designing Resistance Training Programs,* 2nd ed. Champaign, IL: Human Kinetics.
14. Gardner, G. 1963. Specificity of strength changes of the exercised and nonexercised limb following isometric training. *Research Quarterly* 34: 98-101.
15. Graham, J.F. 2002. Periodization research and an example application. *Strength and Conditioning Journal* 24 (6): 62-70.
16. Häkkinen, K., P.V. Komi, M. Alen, and H. Kauhanen. 1987. EMG, muscle fibre and force production characteristics during a 1 year training period in elite weightlifters. *European Journal of Applied Physiology* 56: 419-427.
17. Kanehisa, H., and M. Miyashita. 1983. Specificity of velocity in strength training. *European Journal of Applied Physiology* 52: 104-106.
18. Knapik, J.J., R.H. Mawdsley, and M.U. Ramos. 1983. Angular specificity and test mode specificity of isometric and isokinetic strength training. *Journal of Orthopedic Sports Physical Therapy* 5: 58-65.
19. Komi, P.V. 1986. Training of muscle strength and power: Interaction of neuromotoric, hypertrophic, and mechanical factors. *International Journal of Sports Medicine* 7 (Suppl): 101-105.
20. Kraemer, W.J. 1997. A series of studies: The physiological basis for strength training in American football: Fact over philosophy. *Journal of Strength and Conditioning Research* 11 (3): 131-142.
21. Kraemer, W.J., M.R. Deschenes, and S.J. Fleck. 1988. Physiological adaptations to resistance exercise: Implications for athletic conditioning. *Sports Medicine* 6: 246-256.
22. Kraemer, W.J., S.J. Fleck, and W.J. Evans. 1996. Strength and power: Physiological mechanisms of adaptation. *Exercise and Sport Science Reviews* 24: 363-397.
23. Kraemer, W.J., and B.A. Nindl. 1998. Factors involved with overtraining for strength and power. In: *Overtraining in Athletic Conditioning.* Champaign, IL: Human Kinetics.
24. Moffroid, M.T., and R.H. Whipple. 1970. Specificity of speed of exercise. *Physical Therapy* 50: 1693-1699.
25. Pearson, D. 1997. Weight training. In: *Physical Education Handbook,* 9th ed., N. Schmottlach and J. McManama, eds. New York: Prentice Hall.
26. Pearson, D., A. Faigenbaum, M. Conley, and W.J. Kraemer. 2000. National Strength and Conditioning Association's basic guidelines for the resistance training of athletes. *Strength and Conditioning Journal* 22 (4): 14-27.
27. Pearson, D., and G. Gehlsen. 1998. Athletic performance enhancement: A study with college football players. *Strength and Conditioning* 20 (3): 70-73.
28. Poliquin, C. 1988. Five steps to increasing the effectiveness of your strength training program. *NSCA Journal* 10 (3): 34-39.
29. Sale, D.G., J.D. MacDougall, A.R.M. Upton, and A.J. McComas. 1983. Effects of strength training upon motor neuron excitability in man. *Medicine and Science in Sports and Exercise* 15: 57-62.
30. Stone, M.H., and H.S. O'Bryant. 1987. *Weight training: A scientific approach.* Minneapolis: Burgess.
31. Stone, M.H., H.S. O'Bryant, and J. Garhammer. 1981. A hypothetical model for strength training. *Journal of Sports Medicine and Physical Fitness* 21: 342-351.
32. Stone, M.H., H.S. O'Bryant, J. Garhammer, J. McMillan, and R. Rozenek. 1982. A theoretical model of strength training. *National Strength Coaches Association Journal* 4 (4): 36-40.
33. Stone, M.H., J. Potteiger, K.C. Pierce, C.M. Proulx, H.S. O'Bryant, and R.L. Johnson. 1997. Comparison of the effects of three different weight training programs on the 1RM squat: A preliminary study. Presentation at the National Strength and Conditioning Association Conference, Las Vegas, NV, June.
34. Thepaut-Mathieu, C., J. Van Hoecke, and B. Maton. 1988. Myoelectrical and mechanical changes linked to length specificity during isometric training. *Journal of Applied Physiology* 64: 1500-1505.
35. Wathen, D., T.R. Baechle, and R.W. Earle. 2000. Training variation: Periodization. In: *Essentials of Strength Training and Conditioning,* 2nd ed., T.R. Baechle and R.W. Earle, eds. Champaign, IL: Human Kinetics.
36. Zatsiorsky, V. 1995. *Science and Practice of Strength Training.* Champaign, IL: Human Kinetics.

PART VI

Safety and Legal Issues

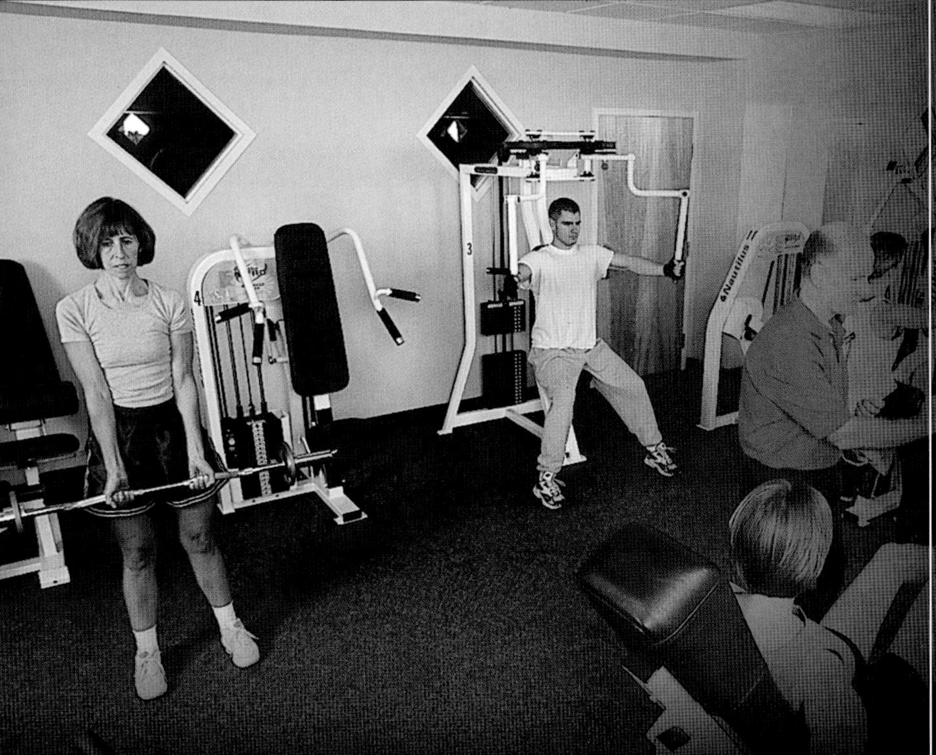

CHAPTER 24

Facility and Equipment Layout and Maintenance

Mike Greenwood

After completing this chapter, you will be able to

- assess equipment organization, placement, and spacing requirements of an exercise facility;
- understand the unique layout and maintenance needs of a home exercise facility; and
- identify facility and equipment maintenance and cleaning duties that promote a safe

Although personal trainers have numerous responsibilities regarding facility maintenance, no responsibility is greater than providing a safe training environment for every client. In fact, many of the personal trainer's responsibilities have the element of safety as a common denominator. Specifically, a safe exercise environment is the result of personal trainers putting into practice

- proper supervision, program design, and exercise instruction;
- relevant facility rules and policies;
- efficient facility design and equipment placement; and
- an effective maintenance plan that consists of facility and equipment cleaning and repair schedules.

This chapter focuses on the last two responsibilities and provides further guidelines for implementing facility and equipment maintenance in an exercise facility located in a client's home.

Facility and Equipment Layout

When determining the layout of an exercise facility, the personal trainer must organize and position the equipment to allow sufficient space for the client to get in and out of the area and for the personal trainer to supervise and interact with the client. Often, the most desirable layout is not possible because space is limited, especially in a home facility. Drawing a floor plan can enable one to visualize the present and potential locations of all equipment. Whatever the outcome, safety should always be the top priority when the personal trainer is determining facility and equipment layout [1, 2, 9].

Equipment Organization

There are three general types of equipment in an exercise facility—equipment used for resistance training, aerobic training, and stretching and body weight exercise. One of two methods can be used for organizing equipment in an exercise facility:

1. Cluster the resistance training equipment in separate locations in the facility based on the body part they target (e.g., chest, shoulders, back, arms, legs, abdomen) while also designating areas for aerobic exercise machines, stretching, and body weight exercise.
2. Divide the facility into separate training areas according to equipment type (e.g., free weights, resistance training machines, aerobic exercise machines, mats for stretching and calisthenics).

Organizing the training areas according to equipment type creates an efficient use of space but depends on the facility's size and clientele [7]. Larger facilities that service more clients have more equipment and a greater variety of equipment, so clustering equipment based on the body part targeted improves functionality and accessibility.

Safety should always be the top priority when the personal trainer is determining facility and equipment layout.

Equipment Placement

The following are general guidelines for equipment placement in an exercise facility.

- Equipment for exercises that require spotters (see chapter 13) should be located away from windows, mirrors, and doors to avoid distraction or collision with other clients; instead, they should be placed in areas that are easily supervised and accessible.
- The tallest machines or pieces of equipment (e.g., squat racks, power racks) should be placed along the walls. Also, they may need to be bolted to the walls or floors for increased stability and safety.
- Dumbbell racks are also typically placed against the walls and shorter, smaller pieces of equipment placed in the middle of the room to improve visibility and maximize use of space.
- Resistance training machines within a circuit are commonly placed in an order such that large muscle groups are trained first and small muscle groups last [9].
- An area separate from all exercise machines should be designated for stretching.
- Aerobic machines that require clients to be upright (e.g., treadmills, stair climbers, elliptical trainers) should be placed behind the aerobic exercise machines that require clients to be lower to the ground (e.g., rowing machines, stationary bikes, semi-recumbent cycles), so that the taller machines are closer to the wall and do not impair the visual field (e.g., for television watching) of clients using machines that are lower to the ground.

- All equipment should be placed at least six inches (15 centimeters) from mirrors.
- A separate room for group instruction classes is recommended.

Equipment Spacing

Safety and functionality are the main considerations when one is spacing exercise equipment. Proper spacing of equipment improves the personal trainer's supervisory ability and provides adequate room for clients to perform each exercise safely (called the **user space**). Spacing should also facilitate access between each piece of equipment (called the **safety space cushion**) and enhance traffic flow in, out of, and around the exercise facility. Table 24.1 shows the total space requirements (i.e., the user space plus a safety space cushion) of various types of exercise equipment [7, 10]. The following are guidelines suggested by the National Strength and Conditioning Association regarding equipment spacing [5].

Equipment should be spaced to allow clients to safely perform each exercise, facilitate access between each piece, enhance traffic flow, and improve the personal trainer's ability to interact with clients.

TABLE 24.1

Guidelines for Equipment User Space and Safety Cushion

Type of exercise or equipment	Needed user space and safety cushion for stand-alone pieces of equipment
Supine and prone exercises (e.g., bench press, lying triceps extension)	**Formula:** [Actual weight bench length (a user space length of 6 to 8 feet) + a safety space cushion of 3 feet on each side*] *multiplied by* [Actual bar length (a user space "width" of 4 to 7 feet) + a safety space cushion of 3 feet on each side*] **Example:** If a client is using a 6-foot-long weight bench for the bench press exercise with an Olympic bar: [6 feet + 3 feet + 3 feet] × [7 feet + 3 feet + 3 feet] = 156 square feet
Standing exercises (e.g., biceps curl, upright row)	**Formula:** [User space "length" for a standing exercise of 4 feet + a safety space cushion of 3 feet on each side*] *multiplied by* [Actual bar length (a user space "width" of 4 to 7 feet) + a safety space cushion of 3 feet on each side*] **Example:** If a client is performing the (standing) biceps curl using a 4-foot-long bar: [4 feet + 3 feet + 3 feet] × [4 feet + 3 feet + 3 feet] = 100 square feet
Standing exercises from or in a rack (e.g., back squat, shoulder press)	**Formula:** [User space "length" for a standing exercise (in a rack) of 4 to 6 feet + a safety space cushion of 3 feet on each side*] *multiplied by* [Olympic bar length (a user space "width" of 7 feet) + a safety space cushion of 3 feet on each side*] **Example:** If a client is performing the back squat exercise in a 4-foot-square power rack using an Olympic bar: (4 feet + 3 feet + 3 feet) × (7 feet + 3 feet + 3 feet) = 130 square feet
Olympic lifting area (e.g., power clean, lunge**; step-up**)	**Formula:** [Lifting platform length (a user space length of typically 8 feet) + a safety space cushion of 3-4 feet on each side*] *multiplied by* [Lifting platform width (a user space width of typically 8 feet)] + a safety space cushion of 3-4 feet on each side*] **Example:** If a client is performing the power clean exercise on an Olympic lifting platform with a 4-foot safety space cushion: [8 feet + 4 feet + 4 feet] × [8 feet + 4 feet + 4 feet]= 256 square feet

(continued)

TABLE 24.1 *(continued)*

Guidelines for Equipment User Space and Safety Cushion

Type of exercise or equipment	Needed user space and safety cushion for stand-alone pieces of equipment
Stretching and warm-up activities	**Formula:** [A user space length of 7 feet] *multiplied by* [A user space width of 7 feet] **Example:** If a client is performing a modified Hurdler's stretch: [7 feet] × [7 feet] = 49 square feet
Aerobic and resistance training exercise machines	**Formula** (see page 597 for generic guidelines for aerobic equipment): [The length of the actual machine (a user space length of 3 to 8 feet) + a safety space cushion of 3 feet on each side*] *multiplied by* [The width of the actual machine (a user space length of 1 1/2 to 6 feet) + a safety space cushion of 3 feet on each side*] **Examples:** If a client is running on a treadmill: [7 feet + 3 feet + 3 feet] × [3 feet + 3 feet + 3 feet] = 117 square feet If a client is performing the machine seated chest press exercise: [5 feet + 3 feet + 3 feet] × [4 feet + 3 feet + 3 feet] = 110 square feet
In a home exercise facility: Aerobic dance, kickboxing, calisthenics, body weight exercises	**Formula:** [A user space length of 5 to 7 feet] *multiplied by* [A user space width of 5 to 7 feet] **Example:** If a client is exercising to an aerobic dance videotape in a home facility: [6 feet] × [6 feet] = 36 square feet

*If this exercise or piece of equipment was placed in a group of similar equipment, then the safety space cushion would be only 3 feet on *one* side because the adjacent piece of equipment would provide the safety space cushion on the *other* side. Therefore, the space calculations would be [User space length + 3 feet] *multiplied by* [User space width + 3 feet].

**Although the lunge and step-up are not explosive or power exercises and therefore do not have to be performed on a platform, the "moving" or "traveling" nature of these exercises and others like them would benefit from the segregation provided by an Olympic platform. Thus, from a safety standpoint they are included in this row.

Adapted from Baechle and Earle 2000.

Facility Traffic Flow

- Traffic flow should be around the perimeter of resistance training and aerobic exercise machine areas. Different colors of flooring or carpet can be used to identify walkways through the facility.
- There should be at least one walkway that bisects the room to provide quick and easy access in and out of the facility in an emergency.
- An unobstructed pathway three feet (91 centimeters) wide should be maintained in the facility at all times as stipulated by federal, state, and local laws. Resistance training machines and equipment and aerobic exercise machines must not block or hinder traffic flow.
- Although ceiling height does not affect traffic flow on the floor, the ceiling should be free of low-hanging apparatus (beams, pipes, lighting, signs, etc.) and high enough to allow clients to perform overhead and jumping exercises. A minimum of 12 feet (3.7 meters) is recommended.

Stretching and Body Weight Exercise Area

- A 49-square-foot (4.6-square-meter) area (7 feet by 7 feet, or 2.1 meters by 2.1 meters) for each client should be allotted for stretching and warm-up activities.
- A larger area may be needed if the personal trainer performs partner stretching (e.g., PNF exercises) with the client.

Resistance Training Machine Area

- All resistance training machines and equipment must be spaced at least two feet (61 centimeters), preferably three feet (91 centimeters), apart. To effectively serve clients who use wheelchairs, more than three feet (91 centimeters) may be needed.

- If a free weight exercise is performed in a resistance training machine area (e.g., a circuit training workout area, a three-foot (91-centimeter) safety space cushion is needed between the ends of the barbell and all adjacent stations [7].
- Multistation machines can also be used for resistance training, but they require more space than single-station machines. If possible, more than the three-foot (91-centimeter) spacing is recommended between multistation machines and single-station machines.

Resistance Training Free Weight Area

- The ends of all Olympic bars should be spaced three feet (91 centimeters) apart.
- The area designated for a free weight station should be able to accommodate three to four people.
- Racks holding fixed-weight barbells should have a minimum of three feet (91 centimeters) between the ends of the bars.
- Weight trees should be placed in close proximity to plate-loaded equipment and benches, but not closer than three feet (91 centimeters).

Olympic Lifting Area

- The square footage for an Olympic lifting area should accommodate three to four people.
- The walkway around an Olympic lifting platform should be three to four feet (91-122 centimeters) wide.

Aerobic Exercise Area

- Ideally, a space cushion of three feet (91 centimeters) should be provided on all sides of aerobic exercise machines (placement too close to walls should be avoided) for safety and to allow clients and supervising personal trainers easy access.
- Table 24.1 gives precise space guidelines, but generic recommendations suggest 24 square feet (2.2 square meters) for stationary bikes and stair machines, 6 square feet (0.6 square meters) for skiing machines, 40 square feet (3.7 square meters) for rowing machines, and 45 square feet (4.2 square meters) for treadmills [5]. These recommendations include the needed space between the machines.

Ideally, a safety space cushion of three feet (91 centimeters) should be provided on all sides of exercise equipment.

Special Considerations for a Home Facility

Many of the considerations that exist for the commercial setting apply to the home exercise facility, but typically on a smaller scale with respect to available space and equipment. For example, it is still vital to consider equipment layout and placement according to available space. In fact, the client may look to the personal trainer for advice on purchasing home equipment. In addition, clients and personal trainers may need to address various aspects such as environmental issues and safety of children and pets.

Home Equipment Purchases

The purchase of appropriate home exercise equipment is one of the greatest challenges the personal trainer and client have to face. Once the amount of available exercise space is determined, the personal trainer and client can begin examining the abundance of home exercise equipment from reputable companies that provide attractive warranties to their customers. While it is vital to select exercise equipment based on the exercise goals and activity interests of the client, it is also imperative to purchase exercise equipment that will fit into the home (i.e., ceiling height, door width).

Obviously cost is always an important factor, but variety, diversity, portability, and space efficiency are also necessary considerations. Some personal trainers warn against the purchase of exercise equipment that can be dismantled and stored out of sight because this practice can become a barrier to reaching a client's exercise goals. Home exercise equipment that is stored out of sight can lead to exercise sessions that are out of mind!

Home Environment Issues

A home exercise facility presents additional safety concerns that revolve around access of children and pets to the exercise area. This aspect comes into play both when the facility is in use and when it is not. During use, the personal trainer and client/homeowner should keep children and pets a safe distance away from electrical outlets, bike pedals, treadmill belts, free weights, and so on to avoid serious injury. A see-through gate placed in the accessing door frames can help promote a safer home exercise environment.

When the equipment is not in use, all doors and windows that access the home facility should be locked. If this level of security is not possible (e.g., if there is no door to the exercise area), the personal trainer and client/homeowner should move the equipment to another location. If it is impossible to move all pieces of existing equipment, it may be necessary to disable various apparatus (i.e., unplug cords to treadmills, remove weight pins from machines, remove weight plates from bars, place bars out of the flow of traffic) to ensure that the living environment is safe—for example, that children will not be able to inadvertently turn equipment on.

The client and personal trainer should also make certain that the home exercise facility has sufficient electrical supply and access [5, 9]:

- All electrical outlets should be grounded (three-wire/pronged) with, preferably, 110- and 220-voltage capabilities.
- Additional electrical outlets should be available (or at least within nearby access) for vacuum cleaners and electric tools.
- Aerobic exercise machines should not exceed the electrical capabilities of home circuitry.
- When possible, outlets should be ground-fault circuit interruption (GFCI) protected so that power is automatically shut down in the event of an electrical overload [9].

Other important environmental issues that are often considered in the design of the home exercise facility include adequate lighting, air circulation, mirrors, and protective flooring. If a home exercise area is well lit and has proper air circulation, exercising becomes more enticing. Natural light from windows or skylights is an effective source of additional lighting [3]. Ceiling fans and portable variable-speed fans can be used to enhance air circulation in exercise areas. Mirrors can be a valuable tool for evaluating a client's exercise technique, but they also can add to the appearance and sense of spaciousness especially of a small home facility.

Rubberized flooring large enough for equipment to rest on is a wise choice to provide good traction and reduce noise levels [4]. A less expensive alternative is short-pile indoor/outdoor carpet, but it needs to be glued or anchored to the floor to prevent slippage [3]. With this type of floor covering, the client should use a padded mat for floor exercises to help reduce perspiration accumulation on the permanent carpeted surface.

Home Equipment Layout

Because a home exercise facility is smaller, has less equipment, and services fewer clients than a commercial facility, all fixed equipment (e.g., aerobic exercise machines and dumbbell racks) is typically arranged along the perimeter of the room fairly close to the walls. Also, the space cushion around equipment is often reduced (e.g., 18 inches [46 centimeters] instead of three feet [91 centimeters]).

An additional consideration for the home exercise facility is to provide 25 to 49 square feet (2.4-4.6 square meters) for activities such as aerobic dance, kickboxing, calisthenics, and body weight exercises [10]. It is also an advantage to allow enough space for items like television, VCR, DVD, radio, or CD player in the exercise area so the client may view exercise tapes and listen to music or news. Often, entertainment equipment can be mounted to a wall or the ceiling. Figure 24.1 shows an example of a home exercise facility.

A home exercise facility that has good lighting, proper air circulation, and enjoyable entertainment equipment is more enticing to exercise in.

Facility and Equipment Maintenance

Personal trainers must implement consistent inspection, maintenance, and cleaning schedules to ensure safety and a functional exercise environment for every client. Regular maintenance and cleaning schedules also contribute to the life expectancy of exercise equipment. If a personal trainer is knowledgeable about the function, proper use, maintenance, and cleaning of equipment, there is a greater likelihood that these tasks will be conducted thoroughly and correctly. In addition, personal trainers must be familiar with these tasks to safeguard their clients against injury and avoid litigation (refer to chapter 25 for more information).

Regular maintenance and cleaning schedules contribute to a safe and functional exercise environment and help to extend the life expectancy of equipment.

Facility Maintenance

Maintaining and cleaning exercise facilities begins with assessment of the types of surfaces that are present and the maintenance difficulties that could arise relative to each area. Personal trainers should frequently assess the condition of walls, floors, and ceilings, as well as the accessibility and safe placement of equipment. Cleaning the commercial exer-

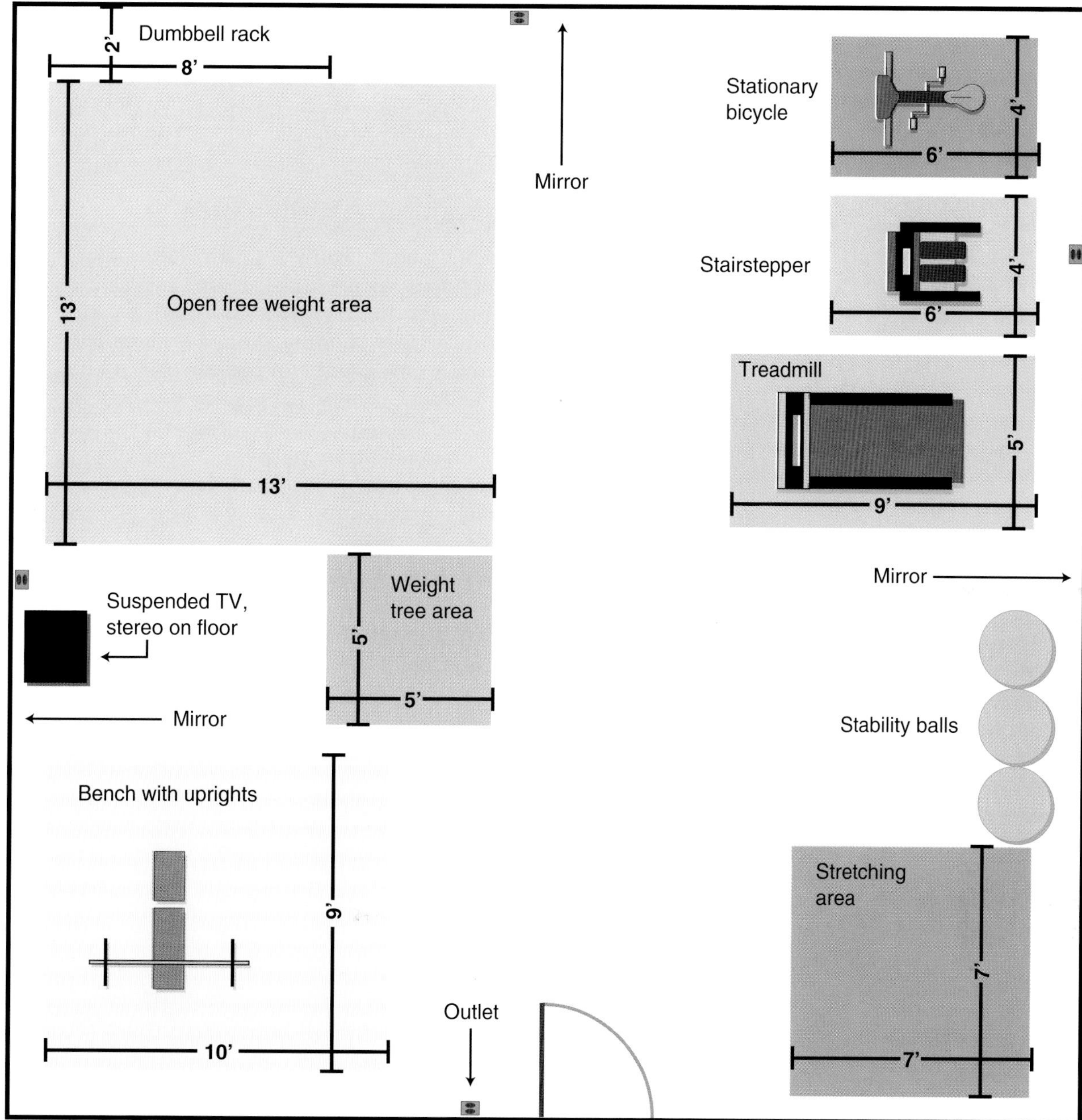

Figure 24.1 Example of a home exercise facility floor plan.

cise facility is handled not only by a custodial staff but often also by the personal training staff. Cleaning the home facility is commonly considered part of keeping up the home and therefore is done by the client. Alternatively, the personal trainer may be assigned (hired) to maintain and clean the home facility; either way, it is important to discuss such details during the personal trainer's initial interview with a new client.

Refer to the National Strength and Conditioning Association's (NSCA's) *Safety Checklist for Exercise Facility and Equipment Maintenance* for an inventory of facility maintenance tasks and cleaning schedule (page 604).

Floor

Flooring can be composed of such materials as wood, brushed cement, tile, rubber, interlocking mats, or carpet. The personal trainer needs to inspect, maintain, and clean the floor regularly. Wooden flooring must be kept free of splinters, holes, protruding nails, uneven boards, and loose screws. Inspection of these potential problem areas should occur daily during cleaning. Tile flooring should be treated with antifungal and antibacterial agents, especially in the aerobic exercise area. Tile floors should also be resistant to slipping and moisture and free from chalk and dirt buildup.

Resilient rubber flooring in the free weight and machine areas should be treated with antifungal and antibacterial agents in the same manner as the flooring in the aerobic exercise area. It must be kept free of large gaps, cuts, and worn spots. Interlocking mats must be secure, free from protruding tabs, and arranged so as not to pull apart or become wrinkled. The stretching area must be kept free of accumulated dust. Mats or carpets should be nonabsorbent (without odor or moisture) and should contain antifungal and antibacterial agents.

Carpeting must be kept free of tears, and walkways and high-traffic areas should be protected with additional mats. All areas must be swept and vacuumed or mopped according to designated cleaning schedules. Finally, flooring must be kept glued and fastened down properly, and all fixed equipment must be attached (bolted) securely to the floor.

Walls

Wall surfaces include mirrors, windows, exits, storage areas, and shelves. Wall surfaces should be cleaned two to three times a week or as needed. The personal trainer needs to inspect, maintain, and clean walls regularly. Walls in high-activity areas must be kept free of protruding apparatus (e.g., extended bars and lighting fixtures); and mirrors, shelves, and other fixtures must be attached securely to the walls.

Mirrors and windows must be cleaned most often in high-activity areas (e.g., near drinking fountains and doorways) and any cracked or broken sections replaced immediately. Further, mirrors present in any area must be attached (glued) to the wall at least 20 inches (51 centimeters) off the floor so they are not broken by equipment rolling or leaning against them. For example, the diameter of a 45-pound (20-kilogram) weight plate is 18 inches (46 centimeters); a mirror placed 20 inches (51 centimeters) off the floor provides a two-inch (five-centimeter) safety margin [6, 7].

Ceiling

Maintenance and cleaning of ceilings in the exercise facility are often overlooked. The personal trainer needs to inspect, maintain, and clean the ceiling. This practice also includes ceiling fixtures and attachments such as lights, air conditioning units, heating units, and ceiling fans. Tiled ceilings must be kept clean, and any damaged or missing tiles should be replaced as needed. Open ceilings with exposed pipes and ducts do not require regular dust removal but should be cleaned as needed.

Equipment Maintenance

Maintaining a facility also involves making sure equipment is functional, clean, and safe to use. Equipment that is constantly used and not consistently cleaned or maintained is potentially dangerous to the client and the personal trainer. In a commercial exercise facility, the personal training staff and local equipment representatives will clean and maintain the exercise equipment. Cleaning the equipment in a home facility can be handled by the client, but it is a responsibility of the personal trainer to properly maintain the equipment.

Refer to the NSCA's *Safety Checklist for Exercise Facility and Equipment Maintenance* for an inventory of equipment maintenance tasks and cleaning schedule (page 604).

Cleaning the equipment in a home facility can be handled by the client, but it is a responsibility of the personal trainer to properly maintain the equipment.

Stretching and Body Weight Exercise Area

Equipment commonly used for stretching includes padded mats, stretching sticks, elastic cords, and wall ladders. Mats in stretching areas should be cleaned and disinfected daily and should be free of cracks and tears. Areas between mats should be swept or vacuumed regularly to avoid dust and dirt buildup. The area should be free of benches, dumbbells, and other equipment that may create clutter and may tear mat surfaces. All equipment should be stored after use, and elastic cords should be secured to a base, checked for wear, and replaced when necessary.

Body-weight exercises typically involve the use of padded mats, utility benches, hyperextension benches, plyometric boxes, medicine balls, climbing ropes and wall panels, jump ropes, core stabilization equipment (stability balls and balance boards), and so on. All mats and bench upholstery should be disinfected daily and free of cracks and tears. The flooring below plyometric boxes and jumping equipment should be padded to protect the client from impact with a hard surface. The tops and bottoms of boxes should have nonslip surfaces for safe use and should be inspected monthly for excessive wear. Other equipment and accessories should be inspected regularly for functional safety and should be cleaned on a regular basis to extend their life span.

Resistance Training Machine Area

A large variety of resistance training machines (e.g., cam, pulley, cable, chain, plate-loaded, selectorized, pneumatic, isokinetic) are designed as a single station or a multistation. Bench upholstery and machine surfaces that come into contact with skin should be cleaned and disinfected daily and should be free of cracks and tears. Guide rods on selectorized machines should be cleaned and lubricated two to three times per week. No machine should have loose bolts, screws, cables, chains, or protruding or worn parts that need replacement or removal. Weight plates on resistance training machines should be inspected weekly for cracks. Extra L- or T-shaped pins designed for the selectorized machines and belts should be kept in stock so that clients do not try to improvise with unsafe substitutes. Chains, cables, and pulleys should be adjusted for proper alignment, tension, and smooth function on a weekly basis, as even minor misalignments can cause premature wearing and damage to belts and cables.

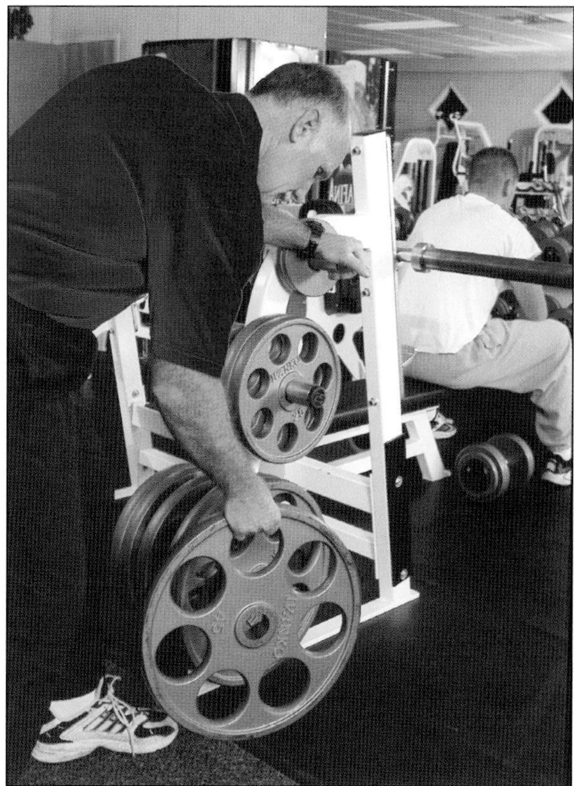

Figure 24.2 Weight plates must be removed from the bars and picked up off the floor and returned to the weight trees after use.

Resistance Training Free Weight Area

Free weight resistance training exercises involve the use of various types of bars, benches (with and without uprights or racks), squat or power racks, barbells, dumbbells, and trees for standard- or Olympic-sized weight plates. All equipment, including safety equipment (belts, locks, safety bars), should be returned to proper storage areas after use to avoid pathway obstruction. All bench and rack welds should be inspected monthly or as needed. In and around squat and power racks, the floor should be nonslip and should be cleaned regularly. Dumbbells should be checked frequently for loose hex nuts or broken welds. "Out of order" signs should be posted on nonfunctional or broken equipment (even in a home facility); or, more desirably, such equipment should be removed from the area or locked out of service. All protective padding and upholstery should be free of cracks and tears and cleaned and disinfected daily.

Olympic Lifting Area

Not all facilities have an Olympic lifting area, but those that do commonly have a segregated wooden lifting platform, Olympic bars, bumper plates, racks, locks, and chalk bins. Maintenance and cleaning of this area should occur regularly. Olympic bars should be properly lubricated and tightened to maintain the rotating bar ends. Bent Olympic bars should be replaced. The knurling (rough area) on Olympic bars should be kept free of debris and chalk buildup by means of occasional cleaning and brushing of these areas. All locks should be functioning, and rubber plates, wrist straps, knee wraps, and belts should be stored properly. The platform should be inspected for gaps, cuts, slits, and splinters (depending on the type of surface) and properly swept or mopped to remove chalk. The platform area should be free of benches, boxes, and other clutter to give the client sufficient room to safely perform power and explosive exercises (see chapter 13).

Aerobic Exercise Area

As with resistance training machines, there is a great assortment of aerobic exercise machines, including stationary bikes, treadmills, rowing machines, semi-recumbent bikes, sprint machines, stair climbers, elliptical trainers, skiing machines, and so on. In this area, equipment surfaces that come into contact with skin should be cleaned and disinfected frequently. This is particularly true during and after periods of heavy use. Cleaning and disinfecting not only protects clients from unsanitary conditions, but also extends the life of equipment surfaces and maintains their appearance. All moving parts (e.g., belts, chains, joints, flywheels) should be properly lubricated and cleaned two to three times weekly or when needed. During the cleaning process, straps, belts, connective bolts, and screws need to be checked for tightness or wear and replaced if necessary. Measurement devices such as rpm meters should be properly maintained; the manufacturer usually does this, but one can extend the life span of the equipment by wiping off sweat and dirt regularly. Equipment parts such as seats and benches should be easy to adjust.

CONCLUSION

In the design of an exercise facility, safety is the first priority when one is organizing, placing, and spacing the equipment regardless of its purpose or how it will be used. Equipment should be spaced to allow clients to safely perform each exercise, facilitate access between each piece, enhance traffic flow, and improve the personal trainer's ability to interact with clients. A home exercise facility has many of the same layout and maintenance requirements for the personal trainer, but environmental issues and the safety of children and pets may be jointly handled by the client/homeowner and the personal trainer. Further, the personal trainer has to develop an effective plan that focuses on maintaining and cleaning the facility and all equipment on a scheduled basis.

STUDY QUESTIONS

1. Which of the following are appropriate guidelines for the use of mirrors in a fitness facility?
   - I. 6 inches (15 centimeters) away from equipment
   - II. 20 inches (51 centimeters) away from equipment
   - III. 6 inches (15 centimeters) above the floor
   - IV. 20 inches (51 centimeters) above the floor

   - A. I and III only
   - B. I and IV only
   - C. II and III only
   - D. II and IV only
2. A client asked her personal trainer to design a home fitness facility in the client's basement. In addition to free weights and aerobic machines, she would like an area dedicated to stretching. Which of the following guidelines should the personal trainer follow?
   - I. Place it in the middle of the room between the weight trees, bench press station, and the treadmill to improve visibility.
   - II. Place it in an area separate from the exercise machines.
   - III. Plan for a minimum of 64 square feet.
   - IV. Plan for a minimum of a five-foot user space length and width.

   - A. I and III only
   - B. I and IV only
   - C. II and III only
   - D. II and IV only
3. An area of the fitness facility has two squat racks with Olympic bars, one hip sled, and three weight trees. Which of the following describes correct equipment spacing?
   - A. 20 inches (51 centimeters) between each weight tree
   - B. 24 inches (61 centimeters) between the squat racks and hip sled
   - C. 36 inches (91 centimeters) between the ends of the Olympic bars

D. 48 inches (122 centimeters) between the frame of each squat rack

4. How often should the guide rods on selectorized machines be cleaned and lubricated?
   A. daily
   B. twice a week
   C. once a week
   D. once a month

APPLIED KNOWLEDGE QUESTION

Assuming stand-alone stations, calculate the recommended total needed area (in square feet) for these pieces of equipment or exercise areas:

a. A client is performing the seated shoulder press exercise (length: 4 feet; width: 3 feet).
b. A client is performing the upright row exercise using a 5-foot long bar.
c. A client is using a 5-foot long weight bench for the lying triceps extension exercise with a 4-foot "EZ-curl" bar.
d. A client is performing the step-up exercise on an 8-foot Olympic lifting platform with a 3-foot safety space cushion.
e. A client is performing the front squat exercise in a 4 1/2-foot square power rack using an Olympic bar.
f. A client is exercising on a stair machine (length: 5 feet; width: 3 feet).
g. A client is performing a seated toe touch stretch.

REFERENCES

1. Adams, S., M. Adrian, and M. Bayless. 1984. *Catastrophic Injuries in Sports: Avoidance Strategies.* Salinas, CA: Coyote Press.
2. Armitage-Johnson, S. 1994. Providing a safe training environment, Part II. *Strength and Conditioning* 16 (2): 34.
3. Brooks, D.B. 1999. *Your Personal Trainer.* Champaign, IL: Human Kinetics.
4. Coker, E. 1989. Weightroom flooring. *NSCA Journal* 11 (1): 26-27.
5. Greenwood, M. 2000. Facility maintenance and risk management. In: *Essentials of Strength Training and Conditioning,* 2nd ed., T.R. Baechle and R.W. Earle, eds. Champaign, IL: Human Kinetics.
6. Kroll, W. 1990. Selecting strength training equipment. *NSCA Journal* 12 (5): 65-70.
7. Kroll, W. 1991. Structural and functional considerations in designing the facility, Part I. *NSCA Journal* 13 (1): 51-58.
8. National Strength and Conditioning Association. 2001. *Strength and Conditioning Professional Standards and Guidelines.* Colorado Springs, CO: National Strength and Conditioning Association.
9. Polson, G. 1995. Weight room safety strategic planning—Part IV. *Strength and Conditioning* 17 (1): 35-37.
10. Tharrett, S.J. and J.A. Peterson, eds. 1997. *ACSM's Health/Fitness Facility Standards and Guidelines,* 2nd ed. Champaign, IL: Human Kinetics.

NSCA's Safety Checklist for Exercise Facility and Equipment Maintenance

Exercise Facility

Floor

- ❑ Inspected and cleaned daily
- ❑ Wooden flooring free of splinters, holes, protruding nails, and loose screws
- ❑ Tile flooring resistant to slipping; no moisture or chalk accumulation
- ❑ Rubber flooring free of cuts, slits, and large gaps between pieces
- ❑ Interlocking mats secure and arranged with no protruding tabs
- ❑ Carpet free of tears; wear areas protected by throw mats
- ❑ Area swept and vacuumed or mopped on a regular basis
- ❑ Flooring glued or fastened down properly

Walls

- ❑ Wall surfaces cleaned two to three times a week (or more often if needed)
- ❑ Walls in high-activity areas free of protruding appliances, equipment, or wall hangings
- ❑ Mirrors and shelves securely fixed to walls
- ❑ Mirrors and windows cleaned regularly
- ❑ Mirrors placed a minimum of 20 inches (51 centimeters) off the floor in all areas
- ❑ Mirrors not cracked or distorted

Ceiling

- ❑ All ceiling fixtures and attachments dusted regularly
- ❑ Ceiling tile kept clean
- ❑ Damaged or missing ceiling tile replaced as needed
- ❑ Open ceilings with exposed pipes and ducts cleaned as needed

Exercise Equipment

Stretching and Body Weight Exercise Area

- ❑ Mat area free of weight benches and equipment
- ❑ Mats and bench upholstery free of cracks and tears
- ❑ No large gaps between stretching mats
- ❑ Area swept and disinfected daily
- ❑ Equipment properly stored after use
- ❑ Elastic cords secured to base with safety knot and checked for wear
- ❑ Surfaces that contact skin cleaned and disinfected daily
- ❑ Nonslip material on the top surface and bottom or base of plyometric boxes
- ❑ Ceiling height sufficient for overhead exercises (12 feet [3.7 meters] minimum) and free of low-hanging apparatus (beams, pipes, lighting, signs, etc.)

Resistance Training Machine Area

- ❑ Easy access to each station (a minimum of two feet [61 centimeters] between machines; three feet [91 centimeters] is optimal)
- ❑ Area free of loose bolts, screws, cables, and chains
- ❑ Proper selectorized pins used
- ❑ Securing straps functional

- ❏ Parts and surfaces properly lubricated and cleaned
- ❏ Protective padding free of cracks and tears
- ❏ Surfaces that contact skin cleaned and disinfected daily
- ❏ No protruding screws or parts that need tightening or removal
- ❏ Belts, chains, and cables aligned with machine parts
- ❏ No worn parts (frayed cable, loose chains, worn bolts, cracked joints, etc.)

Resistance Training Free Weight Area

- ❏ Easy access to each bench or area (a minimum of two feet [61 centimeters] between machines; three feet [91 centimeters] is optimal)
- ❏ Olympic bars properly spaced (three feet [91 centimeters]) between ends
- ❏ All equipment returned after use to avoid obstruction of pathway
- ❏ Safety equipment (belts, collars, safety bars) used and returned
- ❏ Protective padding free of cracks and tears
- ❏ Surfaces that contact skin cleaned and disinfected daily
- ❏ Securing bolts and apparatus parts (collars, curl bars) tightly fastened
- ❏ Nonslip mats on squat rack floor area
- ❏ Olympic bars turn properly and are properly lubricated and tightened
- ❏ Benches, weight racks, standards, and the like secured to the floor or wall
- ❏ Nonfunctional or broken equipment removed from area or locked out of service
- ❏ Ceiling height sufficient for overhead exercises (12 feet [3.7 meters] minimum) and free of low-hanging apparatus (beams, pipes, lighting, signs, etc.)

Olympic Lifting Area

- ❏ Olympic bars properly spaced (three feet [91 centimeters]) between ends
- ❏ All equipment returned after use to avoid obstruction of lifting area
- ❏ Olympic bar rotates properly and is properly lubricated and tightened
- ❏ Bent Olympic bars replaced; knurling clear of debris
- ❏ Collars functioning
- ❏ Sufficient chalk available
- ❏ Wrist straps, belts, and knee wraps available, functioning, and stored properly
- ❏ Benches, chairs, boxes kept at a distance from lifting area
- ❏ No gaps, cuts, slits, splinters in mat
- ❏ Area properly swept and mopped to remove splinters, and chalk
- ❏ Ceiling height sufficient for overhead exercises (12 feet [3.7 meters] minimum) and free of low-hanging apparatus (beams, pipes, lighting, signs, etc.)

Aerobic Exercise Area

- ❏ Easy access to each station (minimum of two feet [61 centimeters] between machines; three feet [91 centimeters] is optimal)
- ❏ Bolts and screws tight
- ❏ Functioning parts easily adjustable
- ❏ Parts and surfaces properly lubricated and cleaned
- ❏ Foot and body straps secure and not ripped
- ❏ Measurement devices for tension, time, and rpms properly functioning
- ❏ Surfaces that contact skin cleaned and disinfected daily

(continued)

Frequency of Cleaning and Maintenance Tasks

Daily

- ❑ Inspect all flooring for damage or wear.
- ❑ Clean (sweep, vacuum, or mop and disinfect) all flooring.
- ❑ Clean and disinfect upholstery.
- ❑ Clean and disinfect drinking fountain.
- ❑ Inspect fixed equipment's connection with floor.
- ❑ Clean and disinfect equipment surfaces that contact skin.
- ❑ Clean mirrors.
- ❑ Clean windows.
- ❑ Inspect mirrors for damage.
- ❑ Inspect all equipment for damage; wear; loose or protruding belts, screws, cables, or chains; insecure or nonfunctioning foot and body straps; improper functioning or improper use of attachments, pins, or other devices.
- ❑ Clean and lubricate moving parts of equipment.
- ❑ Inspect all protective padding for cracks and tears.
- ❑ Inspect nonslip material and mats for proper placement, damage, and wear.
- ❑ Remove trash and garbage.
- ❑ Clean light covers, fans, air vents, clocks, and speakers.
- ❑ Ensure that equipment is returned and stored properly after use.

Two to Three Times per Week

- ❑ Clean and lubricate guide rods on selectorized machines.

Once per Week

- ❑ Clean (dust) ceiling fixtures and attachments.
- ❑ Clean ceiling tile.

As Needed

- ❑ Replace light bulbs.
- ❑ Clean walls.
- ❑ Replace damaged or missing ceiling tiles.
- ❑ Clean open ceilings with exposed pipes or ducts.
- ❑ Remove (or place sign on) broken equipment.
- ❑ Fill chalk boxes.
- ❑ Clean bar knurling.
- ❑ Clean rust from floor, plates, bars, and equipment with a rust-removing solution.

From *NSCA's Essentials of Personal Training* by Roger W. Earle and Thomas R. Baechle, 2004, Champaign, IL: Human Kinetics. Adapted from Baechle and Earle 2000 and National Strength Training and Conditioning 2001.

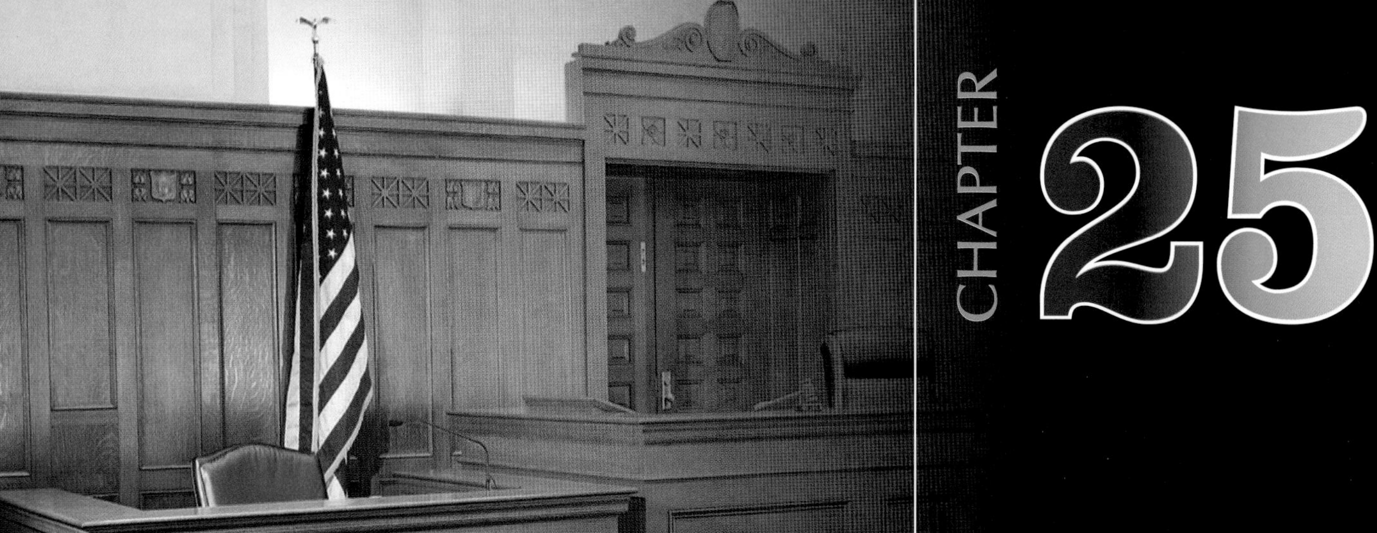

CHAPTER 25

Legal Issues in Personal Training

Anthony A. Abbott | JoAnn Eickhoff-Shemek

After completing this chapter, you will be able to

- explain basic aspects of the law and the legal system;
- define negligence and the four elements that an injured client must prove in a negligence lawsuit against the personal trainer;
- identify professional and legal responsibilities of the personal trainer; and
- develop and implement risk management strategies to minimize the possibility of litigation.

This chapter addresses the relevance of understanding the legal aspects of personal training in light of professional competency and risk management. Personal trainers are apprised of the "standard of care" as promulgated by the industry leaders. This chapter focuses on those essential services and protective actions that not only help insulate the personal trainer against litigation but also promote an air of professionalism while, even more importantly, providing safe and effective programming for the personal trainer's clientele.

As we analyze the legal system, we introduce basic concepts of law and accompanying terminology to provide the personal trainer with insights into issues affecting his or her business. The chapter reviews various divisions of the law and presents examples of such law. In the field of civil law, contracts and torts are emphasized, as this is the area within which the personal trainer is most likely to become legally embroiled. The anatomy of a lawsuit is examined to provide an understanding of the sequence of legal proceedings.

Understanding negligence is the personal trainer's primary concern as it relates to a failure to act or, more likely, a substandard performance. Elements of a negligence claim are analyzed in light of the duty owed to a client and whether the personal trainer demonstrated an appropriate "standard of care" in service provided.

Once the personal trainer understands the concept of negligence and its consequences, he or she must become aware of those specific situations in which one may create a risk of insult, injury, or possibly even death. Personal trainers have numerous physical settings or areas to consider when analyzing their susceptibility to a potential lawsuit, and this chapter addresses these areas of vulnerability.

Finally, this chapter addresses "lines of defense" for the personal trainer, or strategies for minimizing liability exposure. We view risk management first from the perspective of assessing potential areas of vulnerability, and then from the perspective of developing plans to address these issues. We discuss methods of implementing these plans along with the importance of follow-up procedures to evaluate effectiveness. Knowledge of protective legal documents is an obvious highlight of any strategy to minimize liability, and the chapter presents an analysis of such documents in the light of inherent injuries, negligence injuries, and extreme forms of conduct. Lastly, the authors appeal to the common sense and ethical concern of personal trainers to secure liability insurance if they have not already done so, and then explain the difference between general liability insurance and professional liability insurance.

We begin with a sample court case and a discussion of the perils of litigation.

Bailiff: "Here ye, here ye, the Circuit Court for Anywhere, U.S.A., is now in session, the Honorable Justus Wright presiding."

Judge Wright: "Mr. Bailiff, please call the first case."

Bailiff: "The first case on the docket, Your Honor, is Ima Dees Grundle vs. Sue Mee Traynor in the matter of a negligence lawsuit."

Judge Wright: "Counselors, please enter your appearance for the record for your respective clients."

Plaintiff's lawyer: "For the record, my name is Lye Belle Proffet, of the law firm Goodman, Goldman and Gotchyal, and I represent Ima Dees Grundle in her claim against Sue Mee Traynor and the Ms Fit Factory, a personal training studio for women."

Defendant's lawyer: "For the record my name is Stan Bye Yurman, of the law firm Schyster, Schuckster and Schwindler, and I represent Sue Mee Traynor, owner and operator of the Ms Fit Factory, in her defense of this claim."

Judge Wright: "Very well counselors, are there any preliminary matters?"

Ms. Proffet: "No, Your Honor."

Mr. Yurman: "No, Your Honor."

Judge Wright: "All right, Ms. Proffet, you may begin with a brief opening statement followed by Mr. Yurman's opening statement, and then Ms. Proffet, please call your first witness."

Ms. Proffet: "Your Honor, ladies and gentlemen of the jury, the plaintiff will prove that on Friday, January 3, 2004, Ima Dees Grundle suffered an unnecessary and severe injury that has left her permanently disabled, an injury that resulted from inappropriate and unsafe exercise instruction provided by the defendant, Sue Mee Traynor. At approximately 10 A.M. on this day, Ms. Grundle, not having been properly screened and tested regarding her capacity for exercise, was instructed to perform an exercise called a 'lunge' with weights or dumbbells in her hands. The defendant demonstrated a perfunctory example of this exercise without sufficient cautionary instructions or guidance relating to exercise progression. When Ms. Grundle lost her balance, the defendant was not in a position to assist or 'spot' her; and therefore, Ms. Grundle, dropping her weights, fell to the tile surface, at which time she tried to break her fall with her right hand, thereby leading to a compound fracture of the wrist. After numerous surgeries, lost time on the job, and great inconvenience to her family, not to mention the pain and suffering, Ms. Grundle continues to be burdened by a limited range of motion with her wrist as well as fingers and therefore has received a medical disability regarding her capacity to effectively perform many activities of daily living to include an inability to carry out some very basic hygienic tasks."

The Perils of Litigation

Hopefully, the personal trainer will never be named as a defendant in such a lawsuit for the costs are far more than monetary, as psychological stress, additionally, exacts a lasting toll. Moreover, lawsuits also lead to negative publicity that in turn can cause a loss of business and consequent income. Movies and television may lead one to believe that litigation is an exciting event, but this is a media myth. The reality is that for plaintiffs and defendants alike, lawsuits are time-consuming, expensive, and emotionally traumatic.

In a society that is becoming more litigious with every passing year, the personal trainer must recognize the reality of a potential lawsuit. Unfortunately, many personal trainers, like the proverbial ostrich hiding its head in the sand, do choose to ignore this possibility—a fact evidenced by the large percentage who fail to carry liability insurance. This "ignorance is bliss" attitude is also reflected in the low attendance at legal issues and risk management presentations often conducted for personal trainers at national conferences by professional fitness associations.

Increased Litigation

It would appear that the current escalation of litigation reflects a serious industry problem regarding client expectations versus service delivery. We will now examine how this problem arose.

Over the past 20 years, the fitness boom has come of age; and with it, facilities such as clubs, gyms, and spas have advertised the availability of "professional" fitness instruction, which implies safe and effective exercise programming. In reality, few fitness facilities, including personal training studios, have stringent education, experience, and **certification** requirements for their instructors and personal trainers. This is both unfortunate and unnecessary, for professional standards and rigorous certification programs are available through fitness industry leaders such as NSCA (National Strength and Conditioning Association) and ACSM (American College of Sports Medicine). This absence of professional training for fitness instructors and personal trainers often results in a lack of basic knowledge about screening, testing, planning, organizing, leading, and supervising groups, as well as teaching individuals, safely and effectively [26]. However, it would seem reasonable, from the standpoint of public safety, to expect some level of competence before fitness instructors and personal trainers are permitted to work with the public.

Competent personal trainers must become familiar with and practice the application of professional standards.

The significance of the problem centers on the public's right to be protected from unsafe practices, particularly in an area associated with the health promotion industry. Speaking to this point, John Dietrich, past president of American International Health Industries, stated as far back as 1983: "There are no **licensure** requirements or mandated training programs for health club fitness instructors (as well as personal trainers), yet who can deny the grave responsibility of an individual whose job it is to assist people in vigorous exercise [health promotion behavior] and the use of powerful machines" [11 p. 257]. Twenty years later, the problem still endures.

Lack of screening and inappropriate exercise programming may set the stage for an injury that can range from a temporary inconvenience such as a muscle strain to a permanent disability. More importantly, lack of comprehensive assessments, appropriate fitness tests, thorough evaluations, suitable program design, attentive supervision, and ability to respond rapidly to emergency situations may even lead to death. Additionally, the lack of safe and progressive exercise programming can lead to a client's inability to achieve desired training effects or the benefits of exercise. Failure to achieve positive and timely results causes discouragement and the inevitable abandonment of an exercise program.

Many health care professionals and fitness authorities are deeply concerned about the qualifications, or rather lack of qualifications, of exercise instructors and personal trainers. Understandably, college and university educators contend that the physical education/exercise science profession has been bypassed in the growth of the fitness industry; as a result, quality instruction and training have been generally absent. In an effort to keep their overhead down, facility owners or managers frequently hire minimum wage instructor/trainer staff while dismissing college-educated physical education or exercise science majors as "overqualified."

Seemingly, many fitness facility entrepreneurs have jumped on the fitness bandwagon for financial gain at the expense of their clientele's health and safety. Unfortunately, the same entrepreneurial fever and greed that have led to the hiring of untrained staff within the fitness industry have also led to disappointment within the arena of fitness instructor/personal trainer certification. It has been estimated that there are over 300 certification programs, most conducted by self-appointed fitness authorities who have no formal or very limited training in exercise science themselves. One must remember that a certificate is no more valuable than the training behind it and the standards used for awarding such a credential.

Training and Certification

Becoming a competent personal trainer requires an in-depth knowledge of human anatomy, physiology, kinesiology, and exercise science combined with practical training and experience [25]. This cannot be achieved through weekend cram courses and certification programs during which students are typically primed for specific questions to which they regurgitate the answers on examination. There is never sufficient time for practical training and thorough testing to ensure that candidates are capable of safe and effective exercise programming for the public.

To develop the knowledge, skills, and abilities of a competent personal trainer, one must undergo formal instruction in exercise science through an accredited university or a credible vocational school that provides comprehensive theoretical education and extensive practical training taught by qualified exercise physiologists. Upon completion of academic instruction coupled with substantial practical training in the areas of health assessment, fitness testing, performance evaluation, program design, and client supervision, serious and knowledgeable students seek **certification** through truly nonprofit professional associations such as the NSCA and the ACSM. Graduates of an athletic training program from an accredited university usually seek certification through the NATA (National Athletic Trainers' Association).

When personal trainers were administered a nationally validated survey test examining their knowledge base in exercise science, instructors with ACSM certification scored significantly higher than those who possessed other personal training certifications, not including the NSCA-Certified Personal Trainer® certification, which did not exist at the time [1]. This study also reflected that formal education, not experience, was the most significant factor correlating with a sound knowledge base including an understanding of exercise safety. In fact, this study demonstrated that the knowledge base of commercial fitness instructors within the state of Florida was no greater than that of members in the facilities where instructors were employed. More recent research has supported this observation by concluding that formal education in exercise science coupled with certification from either NSCA or ACSM, versus other certifications, was a strong predictor of a personal trainer's exercise knowledge base, whereas years of experience was not related to such knowledge [21].

In years past, individuals injured at fitness facilities would accept the blame themselves and rarely hold others responsible. Injured persons would attribute their strained muscles and tendons, sprained ligaments, or shoulder and low back pain to just being out of shape, and therefore would feel embarrassed to bring their injuries to anyone's attention other than their physicians [2]. Today, however, the public is beginning to hold health facilities, fitness instructors, and personal trainers accountable for unsafe instruction and inadequate supervision.

Relevance of Understanding Legal Aspects

With recent acceptance of personal training as a viable form of fitness instruction, and the concomitant growth of personal trainers within the fitness industry, it is predictable that more lawsuits will be filed against these individuals. Because many personal trainers operate out of their own studios as well as providing service within their clients' homes, injured parties have no recourse other than to bring legal action against the individual personal trainer. True, the personal trainer operating out of a fitness facility often finds that an injured party pursues a claim against the facility rather than the personal trainer since the facility is viewed as having deeper pockets. However, claims for which judgments have been rendered have been filed jointly against facilities and personal trainers alike.

Therefore, it should be obvious to personal trainers that it is incumbent upon them to be aware of the basic structure and function of our legal system.

Knowledge that this system may be an asset or a liability to the personal trainer's operation enables the personal trainer to take advantage of potentially protective mechanisms while avoiding those pitfalls that can undermine one's business.

Knowledge of and respect for the legal system enables one to become a more competent personal trainer and lessens the chances of becoming embroiled in litigation.

The Legal System

The American system of jurisprudence has foundations dating back to biblical times as well as heavy influences from our English ancestry. In fact, an abundance of our current laws arose from British common law [20]. Therefore, the sources of law within our legal system are derived not only from governmental mandates (statutory law) but also from common law (case law). Additionally, the legal system is divided into the two domains of civil law and criminal law.

Law Divisions

Common law is that collection of unwritten laws that is based upon customs, general usages, and court decisions. Most people are familiar with the concept of "common law marriage" that is the basis for highly publicized "palimony" cases. Common law is more frequently referred to as **"case law"** since it is typically arrived at through judicial decisions of past cases to which lawyers refer or which they cite when attempting to bolster their arguments. **Statutory law,** on the other hand, is enacted and authorized by statutes, ordinances, and codes. Consequently, it is often referred to as **codified law,** for it is written into law by acts of local, state, and federal governmental bodies. Codified or statutory laws typically impose duties or restrictions upon individuals; but sometimes such laws may even grant immunity, as does the "Good Samaritan" law [18].

Civil law is the system that applies to one's private rights and therefore to personal responsibilities or obligations that individuals must recognize and observe when dealing with others. Hence, this division of law addresses expressed grievances between individuals as well as with groups, corporations, and other entities and attempts to resolve such differences, often via monetary solutions. Civil law also comprises a system of remedies for violations of one's rights or the rights of a collective body. With respect to the personal trainer, the realm of civil law dealing with contracts and torts is the problematic area to be covered more extensively in this chapter.

Criminal law, in contrast, governs an individual's or group's conduct to society as a whole, rather than to individuals per se or to collective bodies. When individuals violate societal prohibitions or deviate from these laws, they are subject to governmental punishment including fines, imprisonment, or both. Although the personal trainer is less likely to become embroiled in a criminal violation, there always exists the possibility of the unauthorized practice of medicine or some allied health profession, as in attempting to diagnose and prescribe medicine or rehabilitative exercise. This unauthorized practice of an allied health profession may even include going beyond one's scope of practice by providing dietary counseling to clients.

Contract Law

The law of contracts governs the legal rights and obligations between individuals as well as between collective bodies that assent to an enforceable agreement. This agreement (contract) or promise (contract) generates a legal obligation to perform or not to perform some undertaking or some thing. Basically, there is an offer proposed by one party, and an acceptance of that offer by the other party. This agreement or contract reflects a promised exchange, which in personal training usually amounts to a service (exercise instruction) for money (financial remuneration).

Ideally, a **personal services contract** is agreed upon and spelled out between the personal trainer and client (see the contract on p. 182); and for this contract to be valid, certain requirements must be met. Contractual requirements are established when it is documented that a written agreement existed, that consensual words were articulated, or that implied conduct was expressed. There are many other contract types to be found within the fitness industry, contracts utilized not only by exercise facilities but also by personal trainers. Other client contracts include releases, waivers, express assumptions of risk, informed consents, and generally any type of exculpatory agreement. Additionally, contracts are often generated between business partners or associate personal trainers, as well as between personal trainers and independent contractors who work for them. Frequently, personal trainers work as independent contractors for fitness facilities with whom they have such contracts. The many contracts about which a personal trainer should be knowledgeable are covered more extensively in the section "Protective Legal Documents."

Tort Law

The law of torts governs the legal rights and obligations between individuals as well as between collective bodies in relationship to civil wrongs or injuries. By definition a **tort** is any wrongful act that does not involve a breach of contract and therefore may be cause for a civil suit for which a court of law can adjudicate compensation in the form of damages. The basic elements of a successful tort are fivefold, in that once a legal duty (#1) has been established and this reality is coupled with the fact that a documented breach (#2) of that duty was the actual or **proximate cause** (#3) of the verified insult, injury, or death (#4), then compensation or damages (#5) can be awarded.

Tortuous acts are primarily subdivided into two major categories, intentional and negligent conduct. As the name implies, an intentional tort reflects conduct that purposely brought about a given consequence such as a physical injury or a damaged reputation. However, unless the contrary is positively proven, courts give the benefit of the doubt to the defendant and presume that torts are of the negligent type.

People have a negligent tort brought against them for a failure to conform their conduct to a generally accepted standard or duty. When a duty has been confirmed, a court of law will judge a personal trainer's performance in relationship to established standards and guidelines published by peer professional associations such as NSCA and ACSM. Then, if this omission or commission is determined to be the proximate cause of a validated insult or injury, damages can be assessed.

Personal trainers are most likely to be sued under tort law as a result of negligence due to substandard performance.

Additionally, a third tortuous act is referred to as **strict liability,** which is the concept of "liability regardless of fault." Imposition of liability without fault is based on an ideology of social justice that demands compensation to the injured. The rationale for strict liability is that even if there is no negligence, "public policy demands that responsibility be fixed wherever it will most effectively reduce the hazards to life and health inherent in defective products that reach the market" [10 p. 176]. As relates to the personal trainer, documented defective equipment responsible for an injury or death will lead to a judgment against the manufacturer rather than the personal trainer who provides instruction on such equipment.

Anatomy of a Lawsuit

One can understand the anatomy of a lawsuit by considering the sequence of events that occurs during a typical personal injury claim [15]. If an individual feels that he or she has been injured due to the negligence of a personal trainer, that person may retain counsel who will attempt to negotiate a settlement or initiate a lawsuit against the personal trainer. In legal terminology, the injured party is then designated as the **plaintiff**. The personal trainer, who now becomes the **defendant,** will notify his or her insurance carrier, who in turn will instruct the personal trainer to retain counsel. Frequently the insurance company assists the personal trainer in locating and securing counsel. At this point, the insurance provider for the defendant may begin an investigation in hopes of preventing the suit from going forward or possibly concluding an early settlement, thereby limiting or minimizing the payout.

If an early termination to the suit cannot be achieved, then the lengthy process of **discovery** ensues. During discovery, all paperwork pertaining to the client–personal trainer relationship is inspected and analyzed. Papers such as personal services contract, medical history, lifestyle questionnaire, physical exam reports, physician clearance forms, informed consents, waivers, releases, express assumption of risk forms, fitness profiles, program design, workout logs, personal notes, and any other documents must be made available for scrutiny by both lawyers. During this pretrial phase, **interrogatories** and **depositions** of plaintiff and defendant are taken along with those of other parties who have any knowledge of or involvement with the incident in question. During deposition of the personal trainer, opposing counsel will query the personal trainer not only about the specific events leading to the injury, but also about the personal trainer's formal education in exercise science, certifications, practical experience, continuing education, and anything relating to the defendant's qualifications as a competent personal trainer.

During deposition, personal trainers must document their qualifications and competency.

Normally, courts insist that the opposing parties arrange an **arbitration** hearing in hopes of settling the matter out of court and thereby avoiding any further legal expenses to the parties involved, as well as the governmental entity having jurisdiction. When arbitration is unsuccessful, a jury trial is scheduled in order that the parties may present their cases and an **adjudication** be executed.

Negligence

Negligence should be a primary concern for all personal trainers and employers (e.g., managers or owners of fitness facilities) of personal trainers. Employers can be found vicariously liable for the negligent acts of their personal trainers through a legal doctrine called *respondeat superior.* Under this doctrine, if a client is injured due to the conduct of his or her personal trainer, the client can (and often does) sue both the personal trainer and the personal trainer's employer for negligence. Therefore, it is essential for personal trainers and their employers to understand negligence and know what steps they can take to help minimize liability associated with negligence. If the personal trainer is not an actual employee but is considered an independent contractor, the employer can still be vicariously liable. See the later section titled "Fitness Facilities and Independent Contractors."

Not all injuries are caused by the negligence (or "ordinary" negligence) of a personal trainer or his or her employer. Other causes include (a) "inherent" injuries, which are due to accidents that are not preventable and are no one's fault; and (b) "extreme forms of negligence," which are due to the gross negligence, willful and wanton, or reckless conduct of the defendant [9]. Injured individuals can also contribute to their own injury through their own negligence. Negligence as discussed in this chapter is often referred to by the law as "ordinary" negligence, distinguishing it from extreme forms of negligence.

Definitions

Negligence is the failure to conform one's conduct to a generally accepted standard or the failure to act as a reasonably prudent person would act under like circumstances [6]. Negligence can occur by omission, or failure to perform when performance is due (e.g., the personal trainer does not have the client complete a preparticipation screening form), or by commission, that is, performance in a negligent manner (e.g., the personal trainer teaches an exercise incorrectly or in an unsafe manner).

Negligence is the failure to conform one's conduct to a generally accepted standard.

In a negligence lawsuit, the plaintiff (e.g., the injured client who filed the lawsuit against his or her personal trainer, the defendant) has the burden of proof. The plaintiff must prove by the preponderance of the evidence (that degree of proof which is more probable than not) all of the following four elements:

- Duty—an obligation recognized by the law requiring the defendant (e.g., the personal trainer) to conform to a certain conduct that reflects the standard of care
- Breach of duty—the conduct of the personal trainer that was not consistent with the standard of care
- Causation—the connection between the breach of duty and the injury; the breach of duty must be the true cause of the injury.
- Damages—the loss due to the injury, which can include both economic damages (e.g., medical costs, lost wages) and noneconomic damages (e.g., pain and suffering)

Economic and noneconomic damages are considered **compensatory damages**—those that compensate the plaintiff for his or her actual loss or injury. For example, compensatory damages can be awarded to the plaintiff for ordinary negligence. Courts can also award the plaintiff **punitive damages**—those over and above the compensatory damages—to punish the defendant for acting willfully, maliciously, or fraudulently or to set an example for similar wrongdoers. For example, punitive damages could be awarded for extreme forms of negligence on the part of the defendant.

Also regarding damages, most states now have **comparative negligence** statutes that have replaced **contributory negligence.** Under contributory negligence, a plaintiff would be barred from recovering any damages if he or she contributed at all to his or her own injury; that is, the plaintiff would not receive any compensation. Under comparative negligence, negligence is measured in terms of percentages, and damages allowed are diminished in proportion to the amount of negligence attributable to the person for whose injury recovery is sought [6]. For example, if the damages totaled $100,000, the plaintiff's contribution to his or her injury was 50%, and defendant's contribution was 50%, the plaintiff would receive $50,000 instead of $100,000.

Duty and the Personal Trainer

Courts determine duty (or the **standard of care**) in various ways. Two ways applicable to personal trainers are through examination of (1) the standards of practice developed and published by professional organizations and (2) the special relationship that exists between the personal trainer and the client.

Standards of Practice

Standards of practice published by professional organizations are commonly referred to as standards, guidelines, position statements, and recommendations. Many organizations in the fitness field have published standards of practice to provide benchmarks of desirable practices for professionals. Two sets of standards of practice that have been peer reviewed and have achieved industry-wide consensus include

1. NSCA's *Strength and Conditioning Standards and Guidelines* [7]
2. *ACSM's Health/Fitness Facility Standards and Guidelines* [27]

These publications define standards and guidelines in a similar fashion. Standards are required procedures that reflect the standard of care, whereas guidelines are recommended procedures that are not intended to reflect the standard of care but are designed to further enhance the quality and safety of services provided. The National Strength and Conditioning Association published 11 standards and 13 guidelines within the following nine areas of potential **liability exposures** (situations that can create a risk of injury):

1. Preparticipation screening and clearance
2. Personnel qualifications
3. Program supervision and instruction
4. Facility and equipment setup, inspection, maintenance, repair, and signage
5. Emergency planning and response
6. Records and record keeping
7. Equal opportunity and access
8. Participation in strength and conditioning activities by children
9. Supplements, ergogenic aids, and drugs

The American College of Sports Medicine published six standards and over 500 guidelines. The six standards address the following:

1. Emergency plan
2. Pre-activity screening
3. Staff qualifications
4. Facility signage
5. Supervision of youth services and programs
6. Compliance to all relevant laws, regulations, and published standards

It is essential that all fitness professionals, including personal trainers, familiarize themselves with these published standards of practice and implement them within the daily operations of fitness facilities and programs or services. Published standards of practice can serve as a shield (minimize liability associated with negligence) for the personal trainer who adheres to them. However, they can also serve as a sword (increase liability associated with negligence) for the personal trainer who does not adhere to them.

Published standards of practice can be introduced as evidence (via expert witness testimony) in determining the duty of the personal trainer. Testimony by expert witnesses often helps the court determine whether or not the defendant's conduct reflected the current standard of care or duty owed toward the plaintiff. For example, in *Mandel v. Canyon Ranch, Inc.* [22], the expert witness for the defendant, Canyon Ranch, testified that Canyon Ranch did fulfill its duty (followed ACSM standards for pre-activity screening and emergency procedures) when Mandel died from an apparent cardiac arrest during a wallyball game. In this case, the court concluded that the conduct of the staff at Canyon Ranch was consistent with published standards of practice, and therefore it was difficult for the decedent's family to prove there was a breach of duty even though Mandel died. If there is no breach of duty, there can be no negligence. However, if one's conduct is inconsistent with published standards of practice, it can result in a breach of duty that can then lead to negligence. Because it is almost impossible to know which standards of practice will be introduced into a court of law, it is best to adhere to those that are the most stringent.

In addition to standards of practice, professional organizations have published ethical standards. These ethical standards may also be introduced into a court of law as evidence of duty, but probably would not carry the same weight as the standards listed earlier. The National Strength and Conditioning Association established the following Code of Ethics for those who hold the CSCS® or NSCA-CPT® certification [7]:

1. Respect the rights, welfare, and dignity of all individuals.
2. Strive to provide equal and fair treatment to all individuals and not discriminate against anyone.
3. Provide and maintain a safe and effective training environment.
4. Comply with all general laws of the land including, but not limited to, applicable business, employment, and copyright laws.
5. Accept responsibility for the use of sound judgment when working with their clientele.
6. Respect the confidentiality of their clientele while remaining accountable.
7. Refer their clientele to more qualified fitness, medical, or health professionals when appropriate.
8. Remain current on practical and theoretical foundations through continuing education activities.
9. Avoid engaging in any behavior or form of conduct that would constitute a conflict of interest or actions that adversely reflect on the profession or the National Strength and Conditioning Association, and the NSCA Certification Commission.
10. Strive to safeguard the public by reporting violations of this Code of Ethics.

Special Relationship

Another way courts can determine the legal duties of personal trainers is by examining the special relationship that exists between the personal trainer and the client. Courts may classify this special relationship as a fiduciary relationship. **Fiduciary relationships** exist when one person trusts in and relies upon another, for example, a lawyer and client, or a health care provider and patient. In a personal trainer-client relationship, the client trusts and relies upon the personal trainer's fitness expertise. In this type of special relationship, the personal trainer has additional duties involving good faith, trust, special confidence, and candor toward clients [6]. A breach of these duties could make the personal trainer liable. Because of these fiduciary responsibilities, the personal trainer could be held to a higher standard of care than other fitness professionals such as group exercise leaders. Also, given the extra training, education, and certification that many personal trainers have and the extra or higher fees paid by the client, personal trainers are likely to be held to a higher standard of care than other fitness professionals [20].

The trust and bond between client and personal trainer help define legal responsibilities.

Legal Duties of Personal Trainers

In a negligence lawsuit, the court will determine the duty of the defendant (e.g., the personal trainer) owed to the plaintiff (e.g., the personal trainer's client). Personal trainers should consider the issues in the following sections as potential **legal duties.** Many of these relate to standards of practice published by professional organizations such as NSCA and ACSM. By no means do these duties comprise all potential legal duties, but they do reflect the most common issues that arise in negligence lawsuits in the fitness field.

Qualifications

The competence of a personal trainer will be judged in a negligence lawsuit. The qualifications (or lack of qualifications) of the personal trainer could be used in determining negligence. Therefore, it is wise for personal trainers to obtain the appropriate qualifications. However, there are no state or national laws requiring any specific qualifications such as a degree, certification, or licensure in personal training. Education, whether it is a degree in exercise science (or a related field), adequate work experience, or both, is an important factor in determining the competence of the personal trainer.

Even if a personal trainer has a high level of qualifications, this does not mean that he or she could never be liable for negligence. A personal trainer's conduct could fall below the standard of care despite the number of degrees, experience, and certifications in the field the person has. However, when personal trainers obtain and apply in their practice the proper knowledge, skills, and abilities that education, experience, and certifications help provide, it should become less likely that their conduct will fall below the standard of care.

Preparticipation Screening and Medical Clearance

Both NSCA [7] and ACSM [27] require participants to undergo preparticipation screening before engaging in an exercise program. The major purpose of screening is to determine whether the client should have a medical exam (and perhaps a clinical graded exercise test) and whether or not medical clearance is needed prior to participation in fitness testing and an exercise program. See the sample screening forms in chapter 9, pages 183 and 184. Additional examples can be found in various books [18, 20, 27].

If personal trainers opt for developing their own screening form, they should use published standards and guidelines to serve as a guide in developing the form and selecting the criteria for requiring medical clearance. For example, preactivity screening typically requires screening of primary coronary risk factors (high blood pressure, high cholesterol, smoking, and sedentary lifestyle) and serious medical conditions such as diabetes, arthritis, and orthopedic restrictions [27]. After reviewing the data obtained in the health screening process, the personal trainer must determine if medical clearance is needed. Chapter 9 further explains this process and the resulting recommendations.

In addition to properly carrying out the preactivity screening process, it is essential that personal trainers not make medical diagnoses or prescribe treatment from the data collected on health history forms in order to avoid potential legal claims related to the unauthorized practice of medicine. All states have statutes that authorize certain licensed health care professionals to diagnose and treat. A violation of these statutes by "unauthorized" professionals such as personal trainers could result in criminal prosecution. It is imperative for a personal trainer to remember that he or she is only a "suspectician," not a "diagnostician."

Personal trainers are "suspecticians," not "diagnosticians"; that is, although they may feel that a particular diagnosis is likely, they may not make medical diagnoses or prescribe treatment.

Another potential legal problem regarding health history forms may arise when a personal trainer obtains this information and then either (1) does not have the knowledge or background needed to decipher it or realize what it may require, or (2) does not use it properly. This type of conduct could be used against the personal trainer to demonstrate foreseeability in a negligence lawsuit. Foreseeability is the ability to see or know in advance that harm or injury is a likely result from certain acts or omissions [6]. For example, if the personal trainer does nothing or does not know what to do when a client indicates on the health history form that he or she has diabetes, it is foreseeable that possible harm or injury could occur to the client. Therefore, it is important for personal trainers to have adequate knowledge and experience to understand, interpret, and use health history data appropriately.

If a medical clearance is warranted, a proper form should be utilized. See chapter 9, page 192, for a sample medical clearance form. One form can be used both for fitness testing and for the exercise program. If the physician states any restrictions or contraindications on this form, it is important for the personal trainer to properly implement these restrictions in the client's testing and exercise program and to document these actions. Failure to screen, obtain medical clearance when needed, and follow a physician's recommendations could constitute a breach of duty.

Fitness Testing

Before the personal trainer conducts a battery of fitness tests (e.g., cardiovascular, muscle strength/endurance, flexibility, and body composition), it is important to administer an informed consent. The **informed consent** is a protective legal document (see "Protective Legal Documents" further on) that informs the client of any inherent risks associated with fitness testing and participation in an exercise program. It can provide an **assumption of risk** defense for the personal trainer, meaning that the client was informed of the risks, understood and appreciated the risks, and voluntarily assumed them. See chapter 9, page 190, for an example of an informed consent form. It is critical that the informed consent be written and administered properly in order for it to be valid.

When determining which protocols to use for fitness testing, it is important to select those that would be appropriate for the client, given his or her health and exercise history. See chapter 10 for details on this issue. For example, it may not be appropriate to use a step test or treadmill test to obtain an estimate of cardiovascular endurance for a sedentary, overweight person with arthritis. It is also important for personal trainers to follow published guidelines for exercise testing: for example, to know the absolute and relative contraindications to fitness testing; monitor heart rate, blood pressure, and perceived exertion during the test; and know when to stop an exercise test [15]. Personal trainers who conduct exercise tests in nonclinical settings should also have the following recommended credentials [27]:

- A college degree in health/fitness or a related exercise science field or substantial vocational training in fitness testing, evaluation, program design, and exercise supervision
- Current professional certification from a nationally recognized organization in the

health/fitness industry that promulgates high standards

- Current CPR certification

Exercise Program Design and Scope of Practice

When developing the exercise program for the client, it is essential that the personal trainer design the program within his or her **scope of practice.** According to the NSCA Certification Commission, a personal trainer can assess, motivate, educate, and train clients and should refer clients to other health care professionals when appropriate [24]. Personal trainers should never diagnose, treat, or prescribe. If a personal trainer attempts to "diagnose" medical conditions, for example, from the data obtained from the health history, or to "treat" a medical condition through an exercise program for a client, he or she will likely be violating unauthorized practice of medicine statutes. It is very important to not say something like "This exercise will help treat your osteoporosis or high blood pressure" because that would be outside the scope of practice of the personal trainer or any fitness professional. A personal trainer can tell clients that the individualized exercise program designed for them will help them to achieve their fitness and health goals. Koeberle [20] recommends avoiding the use of the term "exercise prescription," which may have medical connotations, and using the term "exercise program" instead. Though this may be a good idea, the term "exercise prescription" is widely accepted and used throughout the fitness field. It is likely that, if ever addressed in a court of law, the intent behind the "exercise prescription" or "individualized exercise program" may be more the issue than what it is called.

Many Americans have major coronary risk factors and chronic conditions such as diabetes, arthritis, and orthopedic problems. It is a well-known fact that regular physical activity helps reduce coronary risks and is essential in preventing and controlling many chronic health problems [23]. Often, physicians refer their patients to a personal trainer or to a fitness facility so that patients can begin an exercise program that will not only improve their fitness level but also in turn improve their health. When setting up an exercise program with clients who have coronary risks and medical conditions (and perhaps even for those clients without risks or medical conditions), it is best for the personal trainer to establish an ongoing partnership with the client's physician. This can be done through two-way consultation, with the personal trainer reporting to the physician on the client's progress in the exercise program and the physician updating the personal trainer on the client's present state of health or regarding recommended modifications to the exercise program [20]. This two-way consultation is in the best interest of the patient/client and may prevent the personal trainer from incurring any potential legal problems with the unauthorized practice of medicine.

In addition to clients' relying on their personal trainers for their expertise in designing exercise programs, clients often want nutrition advice or want their personal trainer to put them on a special diet. Again, to avoid problems with the unauthorized practice of medicine or the unauthorized practice of an allied health profession (e.g., a registered, licensed dietitian), personal trainers should refrain from recommending any diet or specific supplements [20]. It would be best to limit any nutrition education or advice to general information on healthy eating as outlined in university textbooks on nutrition or to refer clients to a licensed, registered dietitian for any specific diet or nutritional questions.

Because of the special relationship created between the personal trainer and the client, clients may share personal problems, such as financial or relationship difficulties, with their personal trainers. Again, in this situation the personal trainer should not attempt to "counsel" clients, which could be considered outside the scope of practice. In these situations, it is best for the personal trainer to refer clients to a qualified counselor or therapist. The general rule is that any time the interests or needs of the client exceed the expertise or qualifications of the personal trainer, the personal trainer should refer the client to the appropriate health care provider.

> The proper scope of practice for personal trainers includes assessing, motivating, educating, and training clients to help them achieve their fitness and health goals; it does not entail diagnosing, treating, or counseling, which are responsibilities of licensed health care providers.

Supervision and Instruction

The failure to properly supervise and instruct clients is a significant liability exposure for the personal trainer. Injured clients have sued their personal trainers (and the personal trainers' employers) for negligence due to improper supervision and instruction on the part of personal trainers.

In fact, lack of supervision or inadequate supervision is the most common allegation of negligence [28]. The type of supervision provided by personal trainers can be considered "specific" because the personal trainer is directly interacting with an individual client [28]. Specific supervision requires the personal trainer to be with the client continuously throughout the training session. It also entails monitoring

- signs/symptoms of overexertion,
- intensity levels (heart rate and perceived exertion), and
- proper form and execution of each exercise (including spotting).

Personal trainers provide instruction to their clients on how to properly use exercise equipment (e.g., aerobic, free weight, fixed-weight, and functional training equipment) as well as in many other forms of exercise that are often taught, such as swimming, calisthenics, and stretching. All exercises must be taught correctly with proper form and execution. Personal trainers should also teach their clients general principles of safe and effective exercise, such as warm-up, cool-down, progression, monitoring intensity (heart rate and perceived exertion), signs/symptoms of overexertion, and ways to minimize risks associated with exercise. If a client gets hurt and sues the personal trainer for failure to provide adequate or proper instruction, most likely it will be a peer of the personal trainer (via expert testimony) who will help determine for the court whether or not the instruction was adequate and proper.

Another factor in determining if instruction was proper and adequate could be whether or not the instruction was appropriate given the client's health status and any medical conditions. (This is another reason to establish a two-way consultation with the client's physician.) For example, if a client is pregnant, it is essential for the personal trainer to follow the recommendations for exercise activity published by the American College of Obstetricians and Gynecologists (see chapter 18). If the personal trainer is unfamiliar with these guidelines or does not know how to apply them, he or she should refer the client to a personal trainer who is experienced and knowledgeable in this area. Again, any time the needs or interests of the client exceed the experience, expertise, or qualifications of the personal trainer, it is best to refer the client to a professional with the proper qualifications.

Supervision and Instruction Duties

- Remain with the client continuously throughout the training session.
- Devote complete attention to client and his or her activities.
- Instruct clients in proper exercise execution and safe use of equipment.
- Monitor for signs and symptoms of overexertion, intensity levels, and proper form and execution.
- Follow published recommendations regarding safe and effective exercise for clients with medical or health conditions (pregnancy, diabetes, arthritis, etc.).

Equipment and Facility Safety

The law classifies members and clients of fitness facilities as **business invitees** because of the mutual benefit that exists between them and the land owner/occupier (e.g., owner/manager of the facility). For example, the owner receives a monetary benefit, and the member/client receives all the programs and services provided with the fees paid. Land owners/occupiers have a duty to act reasonably toward invitees regarding the activities and conditions on their land. This involves reasonable inspection of the property for danger and reasonably repairing and/or warning of dangers. Eickhoff-Shemek [14] lists the following responsibilities to meet this duty:

1. Regularly inspect the premises and equipment to determine whether any condition exists that might be considered dangerous.
2. Document that the inspections have taken place, and file the document in a secure place.
3. If a condition could be considered "dangerous" by an invitee, it is necessary to (a) correct the condition (e.g., repair or remove the condition) and/or (b) warn the invitee of the possible danger (e.g., post proper signage that an invitee will see and understand).

Though this is a primary duty of the owner/manager of a fitness facility, a personal trainer who is self-employed and an independent contractor might be said to have stepped into the shoes of the owner/manager [20]. In this situation, it is the freelance personal trainer who owes a duty to act reasonably toward his or her business invitee client and needs to carry out the responsibilities just listed. The same responsibilities would apply if a personal trainer works with clients in their homes, even though the client in this case would not be classified as an invitee.

Numerous lawsuits have resulted from injury to individuals using exercise equipment. Clients injured on exercise equipment can sue their personal trainer, the equipment manufacturer, the facility, or all three. If the injury was due to a manufacturing, design, or marketing defect in the equipment, the client would sue the manufacturer for product liability. However, if the injury is due to the fault of the personal trainer, the client can sue the personal trainer (and the personal trainer's employer) for negligence [13].

One can minimize equipment-related negligence by implementing the many standards and guidelines published by NSCA [5, 7] and ACSM [15, 27]. These standards and guidelines reflect issues that often arise in equipment-related lawsuits, such as (1) not properly instructing or supervising participants who use the equipment; (2) not properly inspecting and maintaining the equipment according to the manufacturer's specifications; and (3) not properly warning individuals of risks when using equipment, for example, not ensuring that warning labels have been properly placed on the equipment.

It is worth noting that the American Society for Testing and Materials (ASTM) has developed standards for fitness facility safety and equipment labeling; and although currently they have published specific equipment standards only for stationary exercycles, they have plans in the near future for similar treadmill standards, as well as new standards for other types of exercise equipment [18]. Personal trainers are well advised to become familiar with this organization and its efforts to improve fitness facility operational safety through the implementation of new equipment standards.

The personal trainer is responsible for numerous legal duties, and each duty represents an area of vulnerability and possible exposure to liability. If personal trainers can remember the acronym "STEPS" (figure 25.1), they will go a long way toward avoiding the distressing experience of litigation. When a personal trainer is continually attentive to applying the "standard of care" to each of these five steps, then successful navigation through these potentially litigious waters is more than likely—it is almost assured.

Emergency Plan

Professional associations commonly recognize that a comprehensive **emergency plan** is of paramount importance and therefore a standard to which all facilities must adhere. As stated in the NSCA executive summary concerning professional standards and guidelines, "strength and conditioning professionals must develop a written, venue-specific emergency response plan to deal with injuries and reasonably foreseeable untoward events within each facility" [7]. Similar to this NSCA standard is a standard shared by ACSM and IHRSA, which states, "A club/facility must be able to respond in a timely manner to any reasonably foreseeable emergency event that threatens the health and safety of club/facility users. Toward this end, a club/facility must have an appropriate emergency plan that can be executed by qualified personnel in a timely manner" [19 p. 5, 27 p. 5].

By its very nature, a comprehensive emergency action plan consists of numerous strategies that are

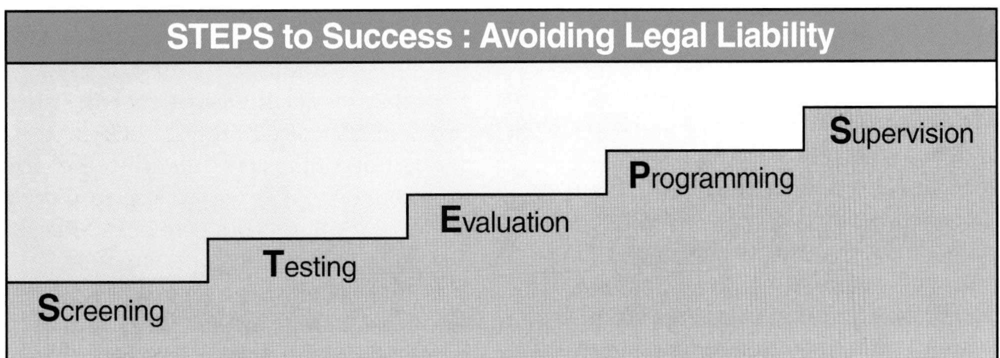

Figure 25.1 Applying the standard of care to each of these five steps will help in avoiding litigation.

concisely stated in order to handle untoward events that occur without warning [5]. The plan must be written, and all personnel involved should sign off on the fact that they have read, understood, and agree to comply with all actions outlined. This plan should include an emergency procedures sheet that highlights the sequence of events to follow and lists important emergency agencies and their phone numbers [27]. This sheet can be posted at convenient and strategic locations throughout a facility, thereby permitting periodic review by staff. Knowledge of agencies and numbers is worthless if phones are not readily available and rapidly operable. Whether the setting is a large health and fitness facility or a small personal training studio, these requirements of an emergency action plan remain the same.

Emergency plans must guarantee the fastest available access to emergency medical personnel and facilities. To this end, a good plan outlines specific roles for staff members, specifying, for example, who should recognize an untoward event, activate the emergency medical system (often by phoning 911), alert staff to the incident, attend to the person involved, secure first aid equipment, assist the principal caregiver(s), verify that responders are en route, take charge of crowd control, guide emergency responders to the scene, and, most importantly, take responsibility for the coordination of the overall effort. Additionally, other duties to be assigned are for staff who will notify the individual's family, record the incident, write up the after-action report, and follow through with corrective actions for those tasks that were not handled expeditiously and correctly.

From the initial recognition of the emergency to the final corrective actions report, numerous steps must be followed to maximize the health and safety of clientele. Each step needs to be analyzed with regard to the uniqueness of the facility, qualifications of the personnel, and the physical and financial resources available.

The proper handling of untoward events often requires the use of special emergency equipment; therefore, a first aid kit or multiple kits, depending upon the size of the facility, must be available. It is crucial that kits be properly marked, identifiable, accessible, and easily transportable, as well as stocked according to foreseeable events and the skills of responders. Consequently, kits must be periodically checked—at least once a month—to verify that contents match the enclosed recommended list of supplies. Equipment and supplies must be used according to manufacturer and recognized professional guidelines; and when people are using these materials, it is imperative that they follow precautions for preventing disease transmission as outlined by the Center for Disease Control and Prevention (CDCP) and the Occupational Safety and Health Administration (OSHA).

Emergencies entail not only the accidents and injuries one might anticipate but also crises such as fires, floods, tornadoes, earthquakes, hurricanes, severe storms, bomb threats, and even terrorist activities. Crises could also include sexual harassment, intoxicated clients, hazardous spills, thievery, unruly behavior, parking lot accidents, and health concerns or life-threatening events that may be peculiar to a given site. Fire evacuation plans, severe weather contingencies, and even procedures for handling and ejecting disruptive patrons are important considerations with which the professional personal trainer may have to deal.

Emergency and crisis plans must be practiced and rehearsed with regularity. Ideally, mock emergencies or crises should take place at least on a quarterly basis if not more often; and some of these rehearsals should occur unannounced. Responsible critiques and corrective actions from such rehearsals will only improve the plan. The emergency response plan, including rehearsals, should be evaluated by facility risk managers, legal advisors, and medical providers to ensure that timely and effective procedures are being followed as well as modified when needed [7]. It is recommended that facilities enlist a medical liaison to keep the emergency plan updated and to periodically evaluate the skills and ability of personnel, including personal trainers [27].

Emergency plans should be rehearsed (announced and unannounced) on a regular basis and followed up with timely critiques and corrective actions.

Ideally, professional personal trainers should be certified in both first aid and CPR, including use of an **automated external defibrillator (AED)**. Informal surveys reflect that although personal trainers are typically certified in CPR, most do not have certification in first aid. Of those with CPR, most are certified only in adult CPR, and this without training in AEDs. It would appear that the average personal trainer's commitment to the safety of his or her clients is lacking.

For personal trainers operating out of small studios or servicing clients within their homes, the responsibility of an emergency response falls solely upon their shoulders. Therefore, it is even more incumbent upon these individuals to be highly trained and extremely competent in delivering CPR and first aid.

Personal Trainer's Response to Cardiovascular Complications Cardiovascular complications within the fitness facility typically take the form of a **myocardial infarction (MI)** or **sudden cardiac arrest (SCA).** In either case, the facility or personal trainer must respond with emergency cardiac care. Such care requires appropriate training and equipment.

When a mild to moderate MI is suspected (tightness of the chest, radiating pain, etc.), activation of the emergency medical services (EMS) system is essential. In addition to making the member or client as comfortable as possible and keeping the person as calm as possible, the personal trainer (if properly qualified by, for example, the American Red Cross) should immediately administer emergency oxygen.

Emergency oxygen (O_2) is so vitally important because low oxygen levels to the heart are likely to lead to cardiac arrest, in which blood circulation ceases. In addition to activation of EMS, supplemental oxygen is probably the most important step that one can take in treating the suspected MI. The fact is that any victim of a potentially life-threatening illness or injury should receive emergency medical oxygen [4]. It has been determined that the administration of O_2 will only enhance or improve the likelihood of a positive outcome; in fact, it has been estimated that O_2 administration may double a person's chances of survival [4].

Although it is true that O_2 is a drug when given in concentrations beyond that found in the air we breathe, the Food and Drug Administration (FDA) has exempted the prescriptive requirement for emergency O_2. As stated by the FDA, anyone properly trained in O_2 administration can provide this emergency drug.

When an SCA occurs within the fitness facility, personal trainer's studio, or client's home, the prognosis is poor unless an AED is available. In the United States, SCA strikes approximately 350,000 people each year outside of the hospital environment, and more than 95% die. Rapid defibrillation is the only definitive treatment.

Because of the unavoidable response time of paramedics, defibrillation by EMS personnel is usually too late to provide successful resuscitation. Once blood stops circulating, every minute without defibrillation decreases the chances of survival by 10%. The only solution to this dilemma is the availability of an AED on the premises—an AED that can be immediately applied (figure 25.2).

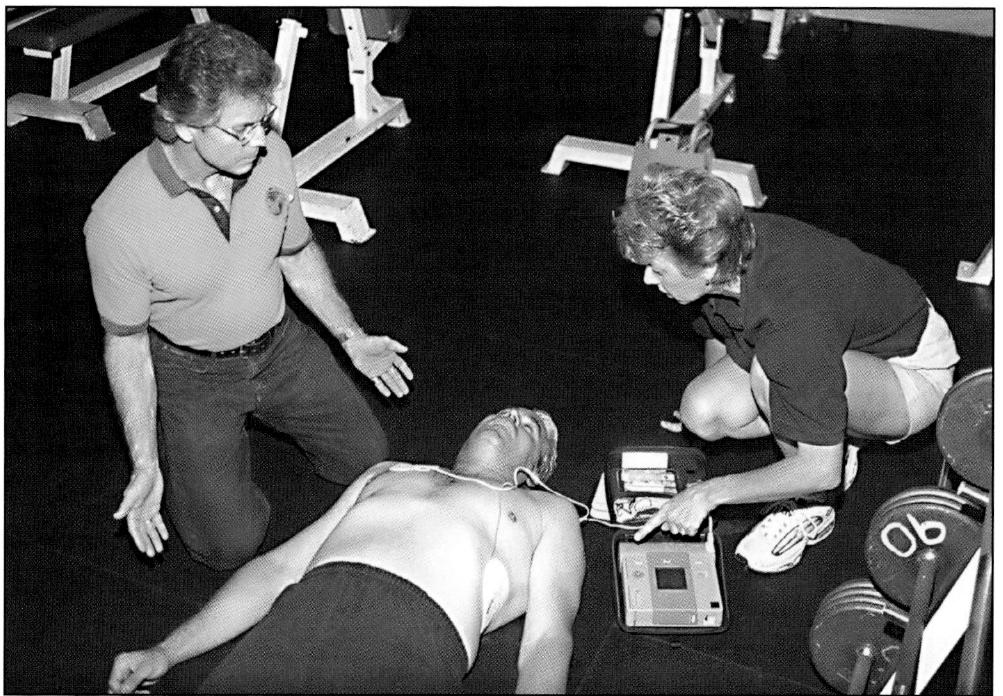

Figure 25.2 Client receiving defibrillation with an automated external defibrillator (AED).

AEDs have been effectively used for over 10 years and are credited with having saved hundreds of lives. As a result of their proven success, the House of Representatives passed the Cardiac Arrest Survival Act, which directs the Department of Health and Human Services to develop guidelines for placing AEDs in federal buildings nationwide. This legislative bill also establishes a "Good Samaritan" provision that will protect individuals from liability issues in those states that have not already enacted such laws regarding AEDs [3].

AEDs, Oxygen, and Litigation Some lawyers will argue that the use of AEDs and oxygen may increase fitness facilities' exposure to litigation by having them held to a higher standard of care. There is little merit to this argument, especially when one considers recent position stands by professional associations like AHA and ACSM. In early 2002, these associations published the AHA/ACSM Scientific Statement titled "Automated External Defibrillators in Health/Fitness Facilities," a supplement to their previous recommendations for emergency policies at facilities. In this statement, a public access defibrillation plan with AED is "encouraged" in fitness centers servicing a general membership and even "strongly encouraged" in centers with memberships over 2,500, as well as in those with programs for clinical populations [3].

In order to provide the gift of life as well as health to members and individual clients, facilities and personal trainers should have AEDs and oxygen readily available. This emergency equipment is essential if we are to give the people who incur MIs and SCAs a fighting chance. It stands to reason that personal trainers should encourage training for and use of such equipment within their respective fitness facilities; and if personal trainers are operating out of their own studios or within clients' homes, then it would seem prudent that they invest in this equipment and the concomitant training.

Having emergency oxygen and AEDs available reflects a professional commitment to an emergency response.

Record Keeping and Confidentiality

Record keeping is an integral part of any successful business. Written documentation of the operations of a fitness facility, a personal training studio, or an individual personal trainer's business not only is important to the financial success of that enterprise but also may be critical to the defense of a potential lawsuit. Notwithstanding the significance of typical business records, this section deals only with those records likely to be subpoenaed in a lawsuit.

Client Records Client records encompass a large variety of documents. Initial interview notes can substantiate the type of arrangement the personal trainer and the client anticipate and upon which they agree. During the initial interview or at a later meeting, a personal services contract may be drafted or finalized, further legitimizing the responsibilities of both parties. See chapter 9, page 182, for an example of such an agreement. If there are any addendums to this contract, they should be attached to the initial agreement.

After the contractual arrangement has been finalized, the personal trainer normally provides the client with a self-administered **medical history** form to be filled out by the client at home and later reviewed with the personal trainer (see p. 184 for a sample medical history form). After going through the medical history form with the client, the personal trainer must have the client sign off on the form, stating that the information provided is true and correct to the best of the individual's knowledge. It is crucial for someone—preferably someone other than the personal trainer—to witness the client's signature. Ideally, the client is required to complete a comprehensive medical history form; however, as a bare minimum, the personal trainer may just require the Physical Activity Readiness Questionnaire (PAR-Q) (see p. 183) [15]. It is advisable to review, update, and initial the PAR-Q and any medical history forms on a yearly basis and to advise clients in writing that they are responsible to report any significant changes in their medical or health history to the personal trainer.

To assist with this health appraisal, it is also recommended that the personal trainer walk the client through a lifestyle questionnaire that will provide a more comprehensive picture of the client's health status. Questions should be limited to those that provide pertinent information but do not create embarrassment or invade one's privacy.

Depending upon the client's health status as well as age and goals, the personal trainer may or may not require that the client be medically examined and that a physician clearance form be completed and returned to the personal trainer (see p. 192). Additionally, it is helpful for the personal trainer to have any physical exam reports inclusive of stress test results along with laboratory results (e.g., blood profiles). For this information to be released to the personal trainer, the personal trainer must provide the client with a **medical release** form. If the personal trainer is relying on information received from a phone contact with a physician or the physician's medical staff, then the personal trainer should document this communication by means of medical notes reflecting the date, the person spoken to, and the exact nature of the conversation.

If the client is to be scheduled for fitness testing, then this is noted in the personal trainer's appointment book or log, and the client is given an appointment letter that includes preparation directions for testing. Prior to testing, the client reads an informed consent (p. 190) and the personal trainer explains the form to the client. After ascertaining that any questions have been answered to the complete satisfaction of the client, the personal trainer ensures that the consent form is dated, signed, and witnessed. After testing, the client should receive a **fitness profile,** and the personal trainer should maintain an individual assessment recording form (see p. 211). With the information garnered from the health appraisal and fitness testing, the personal trainer is ready to write the exercise program.

In addition to the written exercise program, the personal trainer ought to record any educational materials provided to the client and educational sessions attended by the client. The personal trainer should keep a training log on each client to document workouts and reflect client progress. From the observation of training logs and the examination of follow-up fitness tests, the personal trainer may write progress notes that should be shared with the client as well as recorded in the client's file. Any congratulatory letters or motivational messages need to be photocopied and placed within the client's file. Any written correspondence to the personal trainer from the client should also be retained and filed appropriately.

Should an untoward event occur, it is necessary to complete and file an accident form or **incident report.** Any corrective action should be noted, as well as follow-up journaling of the client's prognosis and progress. This can also be an opportune time for a risk management evaluation.

Facility Records Fitness facilities as well as personal training studios are required to maintain suitable signage for locker rooms, wet areas (steam room, whirlpool), sauna baths, racquetball courts, pools, cardiovascular areas, weight rooms, and so on. It is mandatory that the signage (instructions or directives) exhibited on equipment be permanent and observable at all times. When equipment is defective or broken, it should be removed from the floor, or appropriate signs should be placed on the equipment to alert clients that it is not to be used. Records of manufacturer operational manuals, equipment instructions, and "out of order" signs may be helpful in the event of an incident related to an equipment injury. It can also be advantageous to have staff sign off on an agreement to comply form that states that they have read, understood, and will comply with manufacturer's instructions for the operation of specific equipment.

Regarding liability concerns with exercise equipment, it is important to document that equipment has been installed (installation record) according to the manufacturer's directives and, of particular importance, that unstable equipment has been secured to the floor in order to avoid its falling on clients. Every facility or studio needs to possess and make use of a preventive maintenance schedule for equipment; and this schedule must be verifiable through inspection logs along with corrective maintenance forms.

In line with the earlier discussion of untoward events, emergencies, or crises that could occur, it is mandatory that facilities and studios have a written emergency plan, which includes a risk management plan that allows for inspections and corrective action. Emergency plans provide for rehearsals, which are followed up with critique sheets and, again, corrective action forms. Also, as mentioned earlier, emergency procedures sheets are to be placed at convenient and strategic locations throughout the facility or studio to assist in emergency response as well as to permit periodic review by staff.

Confidentiality It is appropriate to briefly address the subject of confidentiality, particularly in light of the numerous records just discussed. Obviously, the personal trainer is going to have very personal information about clients, so the personal trainer must be very sensitive to how this information and data are handled. Additionally, when talking with the client, the personal trainer should not encourage the sharing of personal details other than those relating to medical, fitness, motivational, and business concerns but rather make every effort to avoid such sharing of unessential information.

If the personal trainer wishes to use a client's name, as in the case of referrals, for example, or any "before and after" pictures, it is important to obtain a signed and witnessed release form from that client. If the personal trainer wishes to use data from a client's fitness profiles (baseline and follow-up measurements) for statistical or marketing purposes, the informed consent that the client signs before fitness testing should include a statement to this effect.

Finally, it is not uncommon for personal trainers to work with underage clients, not only teens but also preteens. Personal trainers need to recognize that the maturity level of these clients is such that they often see events in a very different light than the personal trainer does, and therefore tremendous potential for misunderstanding exists. Personal trainers must be overly cautious when working with these young clients; and because of issues surrounding the "age of consent," personal trainers would do well to schedule sessions in open areas and public environments where training can be observed by other adults. Additionally, training young clients in small groups may lessen the chance of false accusations, especially when one is working with the opposite sex.

Strategies for Minimizing Legal Liability Associated With Negligence

Personal trainers may use three major risk management strategies to minimize legal liability associated with negligence:

1. Implement procedures that reflect the duties discussed in the preceding section.
2. Implement the use of waivers.
3. Purchase appropriate liability insurance.

Risk management is a proactive administrative process, meaning that one should address all three of these strategies before starting a personal training practice.

By implementing procedures that reflect legal duties, personal trainers provide themselves with a first line of defense if they are ever sued for negligence. Remember, the plaintiff will have to first prove that the personal trainer had a particular duty and that the personal trainer breached that duty. It will be quite easy for a plaintiff to prove that certain duties exist through the standards and guidelines published in the field. However, if the personal trainer can show that he or she did indeed implement the proper procedures (has evidence through records, etc.) within his or her practice, it will be more difficult for the plaintiff to prove that there was any breach of duty even though the plaintiff was injured. If there is no breach of duty, there cannot be any negligence, and the case will typically be dismissed.

A second line of defense for personal trainers is to have all clients sign a prospective release (**waiver**) prior to participation in the training program. Though a waiver should never be used as a substitute for implementing procedures that reflect legal duties, it can be used to protect personal trainers for their own negligence, for instance, failing to implement procedures that courts could determine as legal duties. There are numerous factors to consider before implementing a waiver, as discussed in the next section, "Protective Legal Documents."

A third and final line of defense is to have liability insurance. If a court rules that a defendant was negligent, the insurance company (as opposed to the defendant) will pay the damages up to the limits established in the policy. Personal trainers who are employees of a fitness facility will probably be included under the **general liability insurance** covering the facility and its employees for general acts of negligence. Personal trainers who are employees of a business, as well as those who are self-employed, can purchase professional liability insurance, often available at relatively inexpensive group rates. When purchasing liability insurance, it is important to consult with legal and insurance experts to help ensure that the insurance purchased will cover all activities conducted during personal training. For example, if training sessions are held outdoors, typical general liability and professional liability insurance may not cover these activities.

Protective Legal Documents

Several different types of protective legal documents exist, but the following three are commonly used in the fitness field:

- Informed consent
- Agreement to participate
- Prospective release (waiver)

Before discussion of the type of legal protection each of these provides, it will be helpful to review the three major causes of injury associated with physical activity:

- Inherent—injuries due to accidents that are not preventable and are no one's fault
- Negligence—injuries due to the fault of the defendant (and sometimes the plaintiff)

- Extreme forms of negligence—injuries due to the gross negligence, willful and wanton, or reckless conduct of the defendant [9]

For lawsuits arising from injuries caused by inherent injuries, an informed consent or an **agreement to participate** provides the best legal protection through what is called an assumption of risk defense [12]. Within each of these documents is a section informing the participant of the potential risks associated with the activity (e.g., type of injuries that can occur). This section helps serve as evidence of the assumption of risk defense, meaning that the client knew and fully understood the risks, appreciated those risks, and voluntarily assumed them. Generally, the law does not allow individuals to recover for injuries they have assumed.

For lawsuits arising from the negligence of the personal trainer, a prospective release or waiver provides the best protection. Within the waiver is a key section that includes an **exculpatory clause**—that clause explicitly stating that the client releases the personal trainer from any liability associated with negligence on part of the personal trainer [12]. This clause will provide evidence that the client gave up (waived) his or her right to pursue a successful negligence lawsuit against the personal trainer, but it must be written and administered carefully to be enforceable. The exculpatory clause does not provide protection for lawsuits due to inherent injuries. Therefore, an "assumption of risk" section is often added to provide this protection.

There are generally no legal documents to protect personal trainers for lawsuits arising from extreme forms of negligence. A few states may allow the use of a waiver to protect from such conduct, but most do not [9]. Extreme forms of negligence can occur when a defendant had prior knowledge that a danger or risk existed but took no corrective action to prevent the danger or risk; for example, a personal trainer has prior knowledge that a certain exercise can put a client at risk for injury, but has the client perform that exercise anyway. It is important to realize that this type of conduct could subject the personal trainer to punitive damages, which are very rarely, if ever, covered by liability insurance [20].

Making the Protective Documents Enforceable

Protective legal documents signed by the client prior to participation in the training program can provide important "evidence" in a court of law that strengthens the defense of the personal trainer. For example, if the personal trainer had a client sign a properly written and administered waiver, this document would serve as evidence that the injured client waived his or her right to sue for negligence. The personal trainer would then seek summary judgment—a pretrial motion in which the judge can dismiss the case because, as a matter of law, there is no issue to be tried in a court of law.

The law involving protective legal documents is quite complex and varies from state to state. Eickhoff-Shemek [12] provides the following factors to consider:

1. "A lawyer who is knowledgeable about the law regarding protective documents must review your protective legal documents to help ensure they are written properly and that they reflect the law in your state.
2. Informed consents and waivers are contracts and therefore can only be signed by adults. Only adults can enter into a contract. Agreements to participate are not contracts and therefore can be signed by minors.
3. Exculpatory clauses used in waivers are not enforceable in medical or research settings and in certain states (e.g., Virginia, Montana, and Louisiana [at the time of publication]) where they are against public policy. Regarding school settings such as colleges and universities, the general rule is that waivers are against public policy for required activities but may be enforceable for voluntary activities [9].
4. The exculpatory clause used in waivers is not allowed in informed consents or in agreements to participate. If an exculpatory clause is added to an agreement to participate for adults it then becomes a waiver.
5. Informed consents used in medical settings must be administered prior to a patient having any kind of medical procedure. If the informed consent is not written or administered properly, the health care provider (and the medical facility) could be found negligent for not informing the patient of particular risks [18]. This also applies to subjects in research settings who must also be properly informed of risks through informed consent.
6. All documents must be administered properly, for example, participants should have ample time to read them and a well-trained employee should orally explain the document to each participant.

7. Protective documents must be stored in a secure place for an amount of time consistent with the statute of limitations, which in some states may be up to four years" (p. 29).

It is recommended that personal trainers familiarize themselves with protective legal documents before consulting with a lawyer. For more information (and examples) on waivers and agreements to participate, see *Legal Aspects of Waivers in Sport, Recreation, and Fitness Activities,* reference [9]. For more information (and examples) on informed consents, see *Legal Aspects of Preventive, Rehabilitative and Recreational Exercise Programs,* reference [18].

Fitness Facilities and Independent Contractors

Fitness facilities often establish independent contracts with personal trainers. These contracts cover a variety of issues including those related to liability. For a sample independent contractor agreement (and an employment agreement) written for personal trainers, see *Legal Aspects of Personal Fitness Training,* reference [20]. Before a personal trainer signs an independent contractor agreement, he or she should have it reviewed by a knowledgeable lawyer. As previously mentioned, personal trainers who are self-employed **independent contractors** must purchase their own liability insurance, which will probably be a requirement in the contract.

The general belief is that a fitness facility would not be liable for acts or omissions of their independent contractors. However, this is not necessarily true. Herbert [17] states that fitness "facilities must be cognizant of the fact that they can be held liable for the negligent acts or omissions of those contractors where principles of ostensible agency or agency by estoppel are applied to a particular case" (p. 36). This can occur when clients of personal trainers have no notice or knowledge of the true relationship between the facility and the independent contractor (e.g., the personal trainer). Unless notified, a client could assume that his or her personal trainer is an employee as opposed to an independent contractor. To minimize liability associated with agency by estoppel, it is recommended that fitness facilities post notices stating that independent contractors provide certain services.

Because of *respondeat superior,* the legal duties of personal trainers are also the legal duties of employers who hire them as employees (as opposed to independent contractors). Employers must be aware of their many legal duties, develop and implement policies and procedures that reflect their legal duties, and conduct regular in-service training so that their personal trainers know how and why it is essential for them to properly carry out the policies and procedures. Employers and the personal trainers they hire as employees have a joint responsibility to ensure a safe program and facility for all clients, whereas independent contractors generally have the sole responsibility to ensure a safe program and facility for their own clients.

CONCLUSION

When personal trainers become thoroughly prepared and truly committed to providing the most effective exercise programs and the safest training environments, then this vocational pursuit will deserve the recognition of an allied health care profession. However, to become acknowledged as professionals, personal trainers must be willing to undergo formal instruction in exercise science through accredited university programs or credible vocational schools in order to receive not only comprehensive theoretical education but also extensive practical training taught by qualified exercise physiologists. As a result of developing the appropriate knowledge, skills, and abilities of an exercise professional, coupled with a sincere concern for clients, one can ascend the "STEPS to Success" and enjoy not only a personally rewarding and financially profitable career as a personal trainer, but also a bright and sunny future free from the ominous clouds of litigation.

STUDY QUESTIONS

1. While instructing a 55-year-old client on the forward lunge exercise, the personal trainer observes the client fall to the floor. Though an AED is available, the personal trainer "freezes" and does nothing. Which of the following is true regarding the personal trainer's handling of this situation?
   A. There was a breach of duty.
   B. The personal trainer was negligent by commission.
   C. Any injuries the client suffers are inherent, therefore the personal trainer was not required to assist the client.
   D. Because the client had high blood pressure and a history of heart disease, contributory negligence statutes would hold harmless the personal trainer's actions.
2. Telling a client which of the following falls OUTSIDE a personal trainer's scope of practice?
   A. "Performing the squat exercise will make your thigh muscles stronger and will help you walk up stairs more easily."
   B. "Walking on a treadmill five days a week will help treat your heart disease."
   C. "This shoulder press machine should be avoided until a physician evaluates the pain in your shoulder."
   D. "Holding your breath during the bench press exercise is not good for your high blood pressure."
3. Which of the following should be included in a facility's emergency plan?
   I. emergency procedures sheet
   II. staff roles and duties
   III. severe weather contingencies
   IV. critical confidentiality strategies

   A. I and III only
   B. II and IV only
   C. I, II, and III only
   D. II, III, and IV only
4. Which of the following documents offers the best type of legal protection in lawsuits stemming from inherent injuries?
   A. exculpatory clause form
   B. agreement to participate
   C. prospective release
   D. waiver

APPLIED KNOWLEDGE QUESTION

Based on the NSCA's *Strength and Conditioning Professional Standards and Guidelines* [7] document, describe specific situations that can create a risk of injury to a new client who has never exercised at a commercial fitness facility and has no experience with using exercise equipment.

REFERENCES

1. Abbott, A. 1989. Exercise science knowledge base of commercial fitness instructors in the state of Florida. Research study presented at the ACSM annual conference, Orlando, FL, 1991.
2. Alter, J. 1983. *Surviving Exercise.* Boston: Houghton Mifflin.
3. American Heart Association. 2002. Automated external defibrillators in health/fitness facilities, AHA/ACSM Scientific Statement. *Circulation* 105: 1147-1150.
4. American Red Cross. 1993. *Oxygen Administration.* St. Louis: Mosby Lifeline.
5. Baechle, T., and R. Earle, eds. 2000. *Essentials of Strength Training and Conditioning*, 2nd ed. Champaign, IL: Human Kinetics.
6. Black, H. 1991. *Black's Law Dictionary*, 6th ed. St. Paul, MN: West.
7. Brass, M., J. Eickhoff-Shemek, B. Epley, D. Herbert, J. Owens, D. Pearson, S. Plisk, and D. Wathen. 2001. *Strength and conditioning standards and guidelines.* National Strength and Conditioning Association Web site. Retrieved from www.nsca-lift.org/publications/standards.shtml.
8. *Chai v. Sports & Fitness Clubs of America, Inc.*, Case No. 98-16053 (Cir. Ct., 17th Jud. Cir., Brwd. Cnty., FL, 2000).
9. Cotten, D., and M. Cotten. 1997. *Legal Aspects of Waivers in Sport, Recreation, and Fitness Activities.* Canton, OH: PRC.
10. Cotten, D., J.T. Wolohan, and T.J. Wilde, eds. 2001. *Law for Recreation and Sport Managers*, 2nd ed. Dubuque, IA: Kendall/Hunt.

11. Dietrich, J., and S. Waggoner. 1983. *The Complete Health Club Handbook.* New York: Simon and Schuster.
12. Eickhoff-Shemek, J. 2001. Distinguishing protective legal documents. *ACSM's Health and Fitness Journal* 5: 27-29.
13. Eickhoff-Shemek, J. 2002. Exercise equipment injuries: Who's at fault? *ACSM's Health and Fitness Journal* 6: 27-30.
14. Eickhoff-Shemek, J. 2002. Legal duties toward trespassers, licensees and invitees. *ACSM's Health and Fitness Journal* 6: 30-32.
15. Franklin, B., ed. 2000. *ACSM's Guidelines for Exercise Testing and Prescription,* 6th ed. Philadelphia: Lippincott Williams & Wilkins.
16. Herbert, D. 1992. Use of health assessments/questionnaires. *Exercise Standards and Malpractice Reporter* 6: 6.
17. Herbert, D. 1994. Avoiding liability for independent contractors. *Exercise Standards and Malpractice Reporter* 8: 33, 36-37.
18. Herbert, D., and W. Herbert. 2002. *Legal Aspects of Preventive, Rehabilitative and Recreational Exercise Programs,* 4th ed. Canton, OH: PRC.
19. International Health, Racquet & Sportsclub Association. 1998. *Standards Facilitation Guide,* 2nd ed. Boston: IHRSA.
20. Koeberle, B., and D. Herbert. 1998. *Legal Aspects of Personal Fitness Training,* 2nd ed. Canton, OH: PRC.
21. Malek, M.H., D.P. Nalbone, D.E. Berger, and J.W. Coburn. 2002. Importance of health science education for personal fitness trainers. *Journal of Strength and Conditioning Research* 16 (1): 19-24.
22. *Mandel v. Canyon Ranch, Inc.,* Case No. 31277 (Super. Ct. of Ariz., Pima, County, 1998).
23. Nieman, D. 1998. *The Exercise-Health Connection.* Champaign, IL: Human Kinetics.
24. NSCA Certification Commission. 2002. *A National Study of the NSCA-Certified Personal Trainer.* Lenexa, KS: Applied Measurement Professionals.
25. Roberts, S. 1996. *The Business of Personal Training.* Champaign, IL: Human Kinetics.
26. Sharkey, B. 2002. *Fitness and Health,* 5th ed. Champaign, IL: Human Kinetics.
27. Tharrett, S., and J. Peterson, eds. 1997. *ACSM's Health/Fitness Facility Standards and Guidelines,* 2nd ed. Champaign, IL: Human Kinetics.
28. van der Smissen, B. 1990. Supervision. In: *Legal Liability and Risk Management for Public and Private Entities.* Cincinnati: Anderson.

APPENDIX

Business Management for the Personal Trainer

Patrick S. Hagerman

Personal training is a service business that follows the same format as many other businesses. Whether you work as an employee of a health club, or own the business, personal training requires the development of a framework that supports your career. This framework consists of the decisions you make regarding how your business is set up and run. The following guidelines are meant to provide an outline for making decisions and building the framework of a successful business, and to help you make personal training a profitable career.

Location

Personal training primarily takes place in one of three locations: at the client's home or workplace, in a health club or gym facility, or in a private personal training studio. Additionally, condominium developments in large cities or retirement communities may welcome personal training on-site. Personal training can really be done anywhere that you and the client can get together. Every location has some advantages and disadvantages that must be explored.

Personal training outdoors serves the needs of clients who are working toward events such as 10K races or cycling rides, but not those who want to ride the recumbent bike in front of the TV. Outdoor training allows for some variety because of the increased space available and is a good change of routine to help break up the monotony of always being inside. Outdoor venues are limited by the cooperation of the environment. If the weather (temperature, humidity, rain, snow, wind) is not conducive to a safe training session, it is best to arrange a suitable indoor location.

Commercial health clubs, fitness centers, hospital wellness centers, and YMCAs are abundant in most cities. Additionally, many apartment complexes, businesses, and hotels have fitness centers available for their residents or patrons. The main benefit of these types of facilities is the abundance and variety of equipment and the controlled atmosphere. A downside is that equipment has to be shared with others, and your work hours are limited to the operating hours of the facility.

Training clients in their home has the advantage of being very convenient for the client. The trade-off is the inconvenience that the personal trainer must endure in traveling from client to client. You may also have to provide any equipment that is needed if the client does not have home exercise equipment. This will limit you to what you can carry and requires more creative training techniques.

Private personal training studios are becoming more popular as personal trainers seek to combine the benefits of a commercial fitness center with the privacy of in-home training. Private studios allow personal trainers to control all aspects of the training environment, including the equipment, the hours of operation, and the number of personal trainers and clients who are using the facility at any one time.

Selecting the location that suits your particular style of training may sometimes require finding a combination of locations. There are clients who prefer in-home training, or who cannot travel to a club or studio, along with clients who prefer the atmosphere of a large club. Alternating locations could increase your ability to serve different types of clients. In addition, seasonal variations may require changes from outdoor to indoor activities throughout the year. Ultimately, you will find a location that suits both your clients and your style of training.

The difference between locations often relates to more than just the amount and type of equipment available. You may move between locations during a career in personal training, so it is important to know that all locations are not the same. Table A.1 lists some of the main factors that will influence your choice of a location.

TABLE A.1

Factors to Consider When Choosing a Personal Training Location

	Client's home	Health club	Private studio
Overhead	Low	Low	High
Travel time	High	Low	Low
Equipment variety	Small	Large	Moderate
Distractions	Telephone Other family members	Noise Other members	Minimal
Income	Retain all	Share with club	Need to pay the bills first
Exposure to other prospective clients	Low	High	Low
Competition with other personal trainers	Minimal or none	High	Low
Privacy	High	Low	High

Business Structure

The legal structure of the business is one of the most important decisions that must be made at the very outset of your planning. If you will be working as an employee of a health club or training company, you typically are not involved with decisions about business structure. However, if you are planning to work for yourself, the structure of the business will affect decision making throughout the life of the business, so some care in choosing the right structure is necessary. As your business grows and changes, you should periodically rethink your business structure to determine if it is still the best form for you. The three types of business structures described next are seen in all industries. Highlights of each one are provided here. For additional information, visit your local chamber of commerce or Small Business Administration office (www.sba.gov).

Sole Proprietorship

A sole proprietorship is basically a one-person business in which the owner and worker are the same person. Anyone can start a sole proprietorship simply by stating that he or she is "in business." Sole proprietorships are usually established in the name of the person doing business, or through the use of an assumed name (e.g., Joe's Personal Training). Assumed names can be established by filing the proper forms (usually with the local county clerk) and can be used on bank accounts and advertising.

If you create a sole proprietorship, you own all the assets of the business and control all aspects of the business. There is no separate legal entity, and therefore you will be individually responsible for the business's liabilities. For example, if you purchase equipment for the business but fail to make your payments, the creditor can sue both the business and you personally. Creditors can go after the business assets, as well as your personal assets such as your house, car, and bank account. Additionally, a sole proprietorship can have employees, in which case the owner is also legally responsible for all business decisions made by the employees.

Preparing taxes for a sole proprietorship is easy. All profits from the business are added to your personal income, allowable business expenses are deducted, and what is left is taxed at the applicable individual tax rate. The business does not file any additional federal tax forms. The downside is that the owner must pay self-employment tax on the business income.

Ending a sole proprietorship is as simple as ceasing business operations. A sole proprietorship exists as long as the owner does business, or until the business, including all assets, is sold to someone else.

Partnership

Beginning a partnership requires a lot of trust and cooperation, so choosing the right person or persons to be in business with is crucial. A general partnership begins when two or more individuals agree to create a business whose assets, profits, and losses each will equally own. A partnership can be established with an oral agreement, but it is advisable to draw up a written agreement that addresses the major issues related to doing business. This agreement can cover who the partners are, how new partners will be added, how partners can leave, and how profits and losses are divided. Every decision made in a partnership requires agreement among all the partners.

A partnership may use the names of the partners (Tom, Dick, and Harry) or establish an assumed name. A partnership should keep bank accounts and financial records that are separate from the personal accounts and records of the individual partners involved in the partnership. This way, all the partners will have access to the accounts and the ability to audit the accounts at any time. Unless otherwise agreed upon, each partner generally owns an equal portion of the business, has an equal say in business decisions, gets an equal portion of the profits, and is liable for an equal portion of the losses and bills.

Additionally, general partners are liable both together as the business, and individually as owners, for any debts. A creditor can demand that an individual partner pay any money owed to the creditor, which would require that partner to get reimbursement from the other partners. You should make sure that the persons you decide to form a partnership with can individually afford to share any debt or losses.

Taxes for a partnership are a bit more complicated than for sole proprietors. A partnership tax return is filed, but the partnership does not pay taxes. The profits and expenses are divided among the partners, who then individually pay taxes on their share. Partners must also pay the self-employment tax on their share of the profits.

Partnerships are valid as long as the partners remain in business. Partners may be added or leave the partnership in accordance with the partnership agreement. Partnerships can also be sold if all of the partners agree.

Corporation

Establishing a corporation takes considerably more time and money initially, but the benefits may outweigh the costs in the long term. Incorporation leads to a higher level of perceived professionalism from the public and an improved ability to borrow funds from financial institutions, as well as reducing personal liability for corporation debts. Several types of corporations can be formed, so obtaining legal counsel during the start-up process is advised.

A corporation is a separate legal entity, with the owners as shareholders. A corporation can have one or many shareholders. Each state has different requirements for creating a corporation. Your state corporation commission or secretary of state's office can provide you with the necessary paperwork and instructions. In most cases you will be required to prepare and file articles of incorporation or a certificate of incorporation, as well as pay a filing fee. You will have to decide on a name for your corporation, which will be used in all business transactions. The name cannot be the same as that of any other corporation in your state, regardless of whether or not you are operating in the same town, and should not be so similar to that of another corporation that misidentification is possible (e.g., Joe's Personal Training vs. Joe's Personnel Training).

Since a corporation is a legal entity separate from its owners, the corporation must have a separate bank account and financial records. When a corporation is set up this way, in accordance with individual state laws, any liabilities of the corporation belong to the corporation only. Creditors seeking payment may look to the assets of the corporation only, not the individual owners. Likewise, the assets and money earned by the corporation are the property of the corporation, not the individual owners.

The individual owners have ultimate control over the operation of the corporation. The owners are usually organized as officers, including a president, vice president, secretary, and treasurer. One person may hold all of these positions if that person is operating the corporation as the sole owner.

Since the corporation is a separate entity, the owner(s) or officers are paid either a wage or a salary by the corporation. They may also receive an equal share of the company profits in the form of dividends. How often a corporation pays dividends is determined by that corporation. You can decide that your corporation will pay dividends every month, quarter, year, or on any other basis you choose.

The corporation must file its own tax forms each year, separately from the individual owners. The corporation pays taxes on its profits before dividends are paid, and the individual owners must pay taxes on the dividends they receive. This is known as double taxation. To avoid double taxation, a corporation may elect to form as a subchapter S corporation. This requires the filing of additional forms with the Internal Revenue Service at the time the corporation is established. An S corporation does not pay taxes on business profits, but instead directly passes those profits or losses on to the owners, who then pay the taxes at the applicable individual tax rate. The assistance of a certified public accountant is advised when one is filing corporation taxes.

A corporation is generally considered to exist forever. A corporation can be dissolved only through filing with the appropriate state offices. A corporation can be sold with the agreement of all owners or shareholders and the transfer of all assets.

Table A.2 highlights the major differences between a sole proprietorship, partnership, and corporation.

Employee or Independent Contractor

The line between an employee and an independent contractor can be fuzzy and hard to define. A person is an employee if he or she is held to any behavioral or financial controls. Behavioral control involves direction and control regarding how you train your clients. If a club owner or manager instructs you as to how you should design specific workout programs, provides training regarding how their members or clients should be trained, or intervenes in your training program in any way, they are exerting behavioral control. Financial control includes setting limits on how much you can charge clients, on how much you are allowed to work (limiting how much you can make), and on your ability to work for others in a similar capacity. Finally, if any taxes are withheld from your paycheck, you are an employee. If there are no behavioral or financial controls or withholdings from your paycheck, you are an independent contractor. The one exception to these rules is the situation in which you work within a club owned by other parties as an independent contractor and must conduct your business within the operating hours of the club. In this instance, the club is allowed to exert control over your work schedule because of when it is open to the public, but you are still an independent contractor.

Sometimes these situations are more complicated, and the distinction is not clear. In the first two of the following examples, the difference between an employee and independent contractor is clear. The third example is more complicated.

Example 1

You are hired by Club Fitness to do personal training. Club Fitness instructs you in how you are to train your clients. Club Fitness decides that you can charge only $35 per session and can work only up to 40 hours per week. Additionally, you are not allowed to personal train at any other club while you work at Club Fitness. You are an employee because Club Fitness exerts both behavioral and financial controls.

Example 2

You are hired by Club Fitness to provide personal training to its members. Club Fitness has no say in how you train your clients. You charge your clients whatever you want, and work as many or as few hours per week as you want. You are not limited to personal training just

TABLE A.2

Comparison of Business Structures

	Sole proprietorship	Partnership	Corporation
Difficulty to form	Low	Moderate	High
Cost to form	Low	Moderate	High
Owner liability	High	High	Low
Difficulty of tax preparation	Low	Moderate	High
Difficulty of record keeping	Low	Moderate	High
Cost to terminate	Low	Moderate	Moderate

at Club Fitness, but can train anywhere you want. You are an independent contractor because Club Fitness exerts neither behavioral nor financial controls.

Example 3

You are hired by Club Fitness to do personal training. Club Fitness does not give instruction on how you should train your clients, but it specifies that you must charge $35 per session so that all the trainers in the club are charging the same. You can work as many hours as you like, and you can work anywhere you like. You are an employee because Club Fitness exerts financial control over how much you can charge. You have behavioral control and some financial control, but not total financial control. If Club Fitness has any behavioral or financial control in any capacity, no matter how small, you are an employee.

A final point concerning independent contractors working in a fitness facility is the need for written agreements between the two parties. Having written documentation of the relationship between the facility where you will work and your business is the only way to make sure that your arrangement will not be altered by the facility's management. This agreement should describe the relationship of the two parties, the length of the agreement and conditions under which the agreement can be canceled, any exclusive rights you have to the personal training business within the facility, what access you have to the facility, what kind of marketing you can do within the facility, and how much the facility will receive for rent or use of equipment. It is advisable to have an attorney assist you in writing this agreement, or consult with you before you sign an agreement provided by a facility.

Financial Decisions

The financial decisions you make in your business will determine whether you thrive or flounder. Many small businesses fail within the first year because of poor financial planning and decision making. Financial decisions need to be made before you open your doors. You should decide on how you will do your bookkeeping, how you will choose your price, and how you will raise the capital needed to start or expand your business.

Bookkeeping

Regardless of the business model you decide to use, you should always establish a business checking account and record-keeping system separate from your personal finances. Having separate records allows you to chart your business from month to month, recognize income and expense patterns, and keep track of your cost of doing business. There are several computer programs that can make day-to-day accounting simple, such as *Quicken*® or *Quickbooks*®.

Day-to-day accounting should include detailed accounts of both income and expenses. Each time a client makes a payment for services or products, that income should be recorded in a category that describes the source of the income. For instance, you will want to keep track of how much you make from training sessions, selling products, consultations, and any other income sources. Tracking income in separate categories allows you to identify trends over time and to make decisions on how profitable your services and products are. Business-related expenses should be carefully tracked because you may be able to reduce your taxable income at the end of the year by filing an itemized tax return. You should consult a certified public accountant regarding what expenses are tax deductible in your specific situation. Normally, tax-deductible expenses include equipment, rent and utilities, wages paid to other trainers or for professional services such as accounting, automobile expenses such as mileage and insurance if you travel to clients' homes, business-related travel to conferences and workshops, and dues paid to professional organizations. Each expense should be documented, and receipts should always be kept for several years.

When it comes time to file tax forms, unless you are a certified public accountant, hire one. Filing inaccurate or inappropriate tax forms is a problem that is easily avoided by using a certified public accountant. Spend some time talking with a certified public accountant at the start-up of your business to determine what accounting methods are suitable for your business, what expenses are eligible as tax deductions, and how to forecast your financial needs and prepare budgets that will keep you in business. The advice of a professional accountant will also be invaluable in preparing your financial data should you decide to borrow money or acquire loans.

Choosing Your Price

In order to stay in business, a business must make money. You must decide how much you are going to charge for your services. Typically, the law of supply and demand will dictate your price within a certain range. For instance, if personal trainers in your area, working in the same environment, are charging between $35 and $45 per hour, your price should be somewhere within this range. In certain instances you may be able to charge more than your competitors if you can justify doing so because of the services you provide, the location you work at, or your educational level.

Another approach to determining your fee, rather than just picking a fee that seems reasonable and competitive, is to calculate what fee is necessary based on your income goals and business expenses. First decide how much you want to make after expenses (net income). Next, determine what expenses you will have—both recurring (monthly rent/loan payments) and one-time (equipment purchases). Add these two totals together to find what your gross income needs to be. It is a smart idea to add in a 10% contingency to cover any unforeseen expenses or drops in income (sick days, canceled appointments, etc.).

To determine your hourly fee based on this calculated gross income, you now need to decide how many hours a week you want to work. While it may be tempting to say that you will work 40 to 50 hours a week, you must consider any travel time to and from work or clients' homes; time spent doing administrative tasks such as accounting, marketing, advertising, and returning phone calls; and maintaining equipment or cleaning your studio. Any business-related task that takes up part of your time should be included. Generally, you can assume that 10 to 15 hours a week will be spent on these tasks during your first year of business, and 5 to 10 hours a week after you have established yourself.

Deduct the time spent on administrative tasks from the total time you want to work, and that will be the total number of hours you have left to train clients.

The final calculation involves dividing your estimated gross income by the number of weeks you plan on working each year, then by the number of hours you have available to train. The result is what your hourly fee needs to be to meet your goals. Figure A.1 shows that a trainer who wishes to make $50,000 a year in profit, has $10,000 in expenses, and wants to take two weeks off this year will need to charge $44 per hour over a 30-hour work week to meet his or her goals. The form on page 635 is a worksheet that you can use to determine your hourly rate. (Note that these calculations do not factor in applicable local, state, and federal income taxes.)

Raising Capital

The cost of starting a new personal training business depends largely on where you are going to be training. If you choose to work within a health club, in a gym, or in clients' homes, your main expenses will be taxes, uniforms, insurance, and office supplies (business cards, letterhead, etc.). If you will be opening a private studio, your expenses will increase as you add equipment, rent and utilities, advertising, and additional insurance.

Two options exist for raising capital: spending money only as you make it, and borrowing money from friends, family, investors, or financial institutions. Financial institutions prefer to loan money to corporations and often require that any assets of the business (e.g., fitness equipment that is purchased) be held as collateral. In the case of a start-up business, financial institutions may also require a personal guarantee or personal assets as collateral.

When approaching a financial institution to borrow money, you must prepare a business plan that includes marketing, advertising, and operating plans; a description of the market and the share of the market the business will acquire; and financial

Hourly Rate Calculation

A. Personal net income	$50,000.00
B. Annual operating expenses	$10,000.00
C. Subtotal (A + B)	$60,000.00
D. Contingency (10% of C)	$6,000.00
E. Necessary gross income (C + D)	$66,000.00
F. Necessary income per week (E ÷ 50)	$1,320.00
G. One-hour training session fee (F ÷ 30)	$44.00*

*Consult a financial planner to determine the impact of income taxes; your necessary gross income may need to be adjusted to accurately calculate your hourly rate.

Figure A.1 Example of an hourly rate calculation.

Hourly Rate Calculation Worksheet

A. Personal net income goal $________

B. Annual operating expenses

1. Rent ________
2. Utilities ________
3. Marketing ________
4. Insurance ________
5. Equipment ________
6. Office supplies ________
7. Conferences ________
8. Affiliation dues ________
9. Automobile ________
10. Banking fees ________
11. Income tax ________
12. Other ________

Total expenses $________

C. Subtotal (A + B) $________

D. Contingency fee (10% of C) $________

E. Necessary gross income (C + D) $________

F. Necessary income per week (E ÷ number of weeks you wish to work per year) $________

G. One-hour training session fee (F ÷ number of hours you wish to train clients per week) $________

From *NSCA's Essentials of Personal Training* by Roger W. Earle and Thomas R. Baechle, 2004, Champaign, IL: Human Kinetics.

data. Your Small Business Administration office can help you prepare this document.

Marketing

Before you can start an advertising or marketing program, you must determine your business goals. Goals will include how much you want to spend on marketing, what segment of the population you want to reach, and how fast you want your business to grow. The last item, growth of the business, must be approached realistically. It would be great to do some advertising, gain enough clients to keep you busy, and start a waiting list; but what do you do with the overflow? Can you handle a fast increase in business? Are your facilities capable of handling the number of people you may potentially reach? Do you have the resources to handle a certain amount of growth at this time? Determine both the immediate and long-term goals of your business, and make your marketing decisions with the goals in mind.

The segment of the population you wish to serve is called the target market. This is the group of people your marketing should be designed to reach. If your business will concentrate on aiding the 50-plus age group, then target your marketing to reach this population. Most broad forms of marketing (print, radio, TV) will access large segments of the market that you may not want to reach. Therefore, both your marketing approach and delivery must be tailored to the particular segment. It is also a good idea to determine the target market of your competition in order to make sure that this market is not overly saturated with personal trainers. If everyone in your area is going after the 50-plus age market, then the adolescent marketplace may be a more open one.

The actual marketing and advertising strategies you employ will depend on your target market, budget, and the amount of time you want to personally spend on this task. The following list includes the most common types of marketing and the respective cost levels.

Marketing Devices and Costs

- **Word of mouth/Referrals [free]:** Encourage current clients to send their friends to you.
- **Print advertising [$$-$$$]*:** Purchase ads in newspapers, magazines, and local events calendars.
- **Television and radio [$$$]:** Purchase 15- to 30-second ads.
- **Personal appearances/Presentations to local groups [$]:** Give short talks on general fitness concepts; follow up with question and answer sessions.
- **Writing for local papers [$]:** Write weekly columns with your contact info at the end.
- **Yellow pages [$$-$$$]:** This is undoubtedly the first place someone will look (big ads cost more).
- **Flyers [$]:** Hand-deliver flyers that you make on your home computer.
- **Direct mail [$$]:** Professionally designed flyers are delivered to particular ZIP codes.
- **Product ads (T-shirts, pens) [$-$$$]:** Give products to clients and at health fairs—a T-shirt is a walking billboard.
- **Charity gift certificates [$$]:** Donate certificates for free consultations or one free session; these are usually bought by someone who can afford your services.
- **Volunteering at health fairs [$]:** Get your name in circulation; offer drawings for sessions.
- **Brochures and business cards [$-$$]:** Always have business cards handy; brochures can sell your services for you—design your own brochure or have it professionally done.
- **Joining local chamber of commerce [$]:** Network with other business owners and persons likely to be able to afford your services.

*$ = cheap; $$ = moderate; $$$ = expensive.

What you choose to say through your various marketing efforts should be a reflection of your target market's goals. In order for your marketing to do its job, your message must convey what your target market wants to hear. For instance, if you are targeting the 20 to 35 age group, it is not a good idea to tout the benefits of exercise as "preventing osteoporosis and improving balance and cardiovascular endurance"; this message will not appeal to this group's goals. A better approach would include wording such as "exercise for definition and muscle tone" or "prevent increased body fat." Likewise, if you are marketing toward young athletes, programs for weight loss are probably not going to be a big seller. Establish what the goals of your target market are through some simple research at your local library. Many studies have been done on what certain age-specific demographics perceive as necessary health/fitness-related goals.

Your marketing efforts should also communicate the benefits of your services in terms of your experience, education, location, and what you can offer the client that is different from what other personal trainers offer. What makes you special is what you need to communicate in your marketing.

Insurance

Having proper insurance coverage is a requirement, not a decision. Any business that desires to stay in business will cover all liabilities with insurance; the same goes for personal training. There are several types of insurance you should be aware of. While each is appropriate for all types of business structures, which ones you need depends on your location. Consult an insurance agent who works with the fitness field to determine the types of coverage you need.

Liability

Liability insurance policies generally pay for any damages that are awarded by the courts, and sometimes cover any legal fees incurred during a defense. All personal trainers, regardless of the location they work in, should have personal injury and professional liability insurance. Personal injury liability insurance helps to protect against libel, slander, or wrongful invasion of privacy. Professional liability insurance helps to protect against bodily injury arising from services provided or negligence.

General commercial liability covers individuals or businesses against accidents and injuries that happen on the business premises (in the gym, on the sidewalk up to the gym, slip and falls, etc.). If you own a private training studio, you will need this (even if you are renting space). If you work as an employee, your employer should provide this type of insurance.

Personal Health

If you work as an employee of a fitness center, you may be entitled to health benefits from your employer. If you are an independent contractor or own your own business, you should investigate personal health insurance for yourself. Most major insurance companies have plans for small businesses that are based on the number of full-time employees, or plans that add you to a group of similar businesses to give you a discounted rate. Health insurance should be investigated at the beginning of your business planning, because the typically high monthly rates ($200 and up) will need to be figured into your regular expenses.

Property Insurance

If you own the business and either rent or own the location, and have any assets such as equipment, you need property insurance. Similar to homeowners' insurance, property insurance protects against fire, theft, vandalism, and other incidents that can affect your business negatively.

Closing Thoughts

The success of a personal training business depends on the foundation upon which it is built. The process of establishing a new business and then nurturing that business requires continuous attention to the details of each topic discussed in this appendix. While each personal trainer may approach his or her business from a different perspective, we all have the same goal: to develop our business into a profitable career. Use this information as a starting point and take the initiative to read more about business management, marketing, and development. Your business will thrive.

Answers to Study Questions

Chapter 1
1.B, 2.C, 3.A, 4.A

Chapter 2
1.A, 2.C, 3.D, 4.C

Chapter 3
1.C, 2.A, 3.D, 4.A

Chapter 4
1.D, 2.A, 3.B, 4.C

Chapter 5
1.A, 2.D, 3.A, 4.A

Chapter 6
1.C, 2.C, 3.B, 4.A

Chapter 7
1.B, 2.C, 3.D, 4.B

Chapter 8
1.B, 2.C, 3.A, 4.B

Chapter 9
1.B, 2.B, 3.C, 4.D

Chapter 10
1.D, 2.B, 3.C, 4.D

Chapter 11
1.B, 2.B, 3.B, 4.A

Chapter 12
1.A, 2.A, 3.B, 4.B

Chapter 13
1.C, 2.C, 3.A, 4.B

Chapter 14
1.B, 2.B, 3.D, 4.B

Chapter 15
1.B, 2.D, 3.D, 4.C

Chapter 16
1.C, 2.C, 3.B, 4.A

Chapter 17
1.A, 2.C, 3.D, 4.C

Chapter 18
1.D, 2.A, 3.A, 4.C

Chapter 19
1.C, 2.D, 3.B, 4.C

Chapter 20
1.D, 2.B, 3.C, 4.B

Chapter 21
1.C, 2.C, 3.C, 4.A

Chapter 22
1.C, 2.B, 3.A, 4.C

Chapter 23
1.A, 2.C, 3.D, 4.B

Chapter 24
1.B, 2.D, 3.C, 4.B

Chapter 25
1.A, 2.B, 3.C, 4.B

Suggested Solutions for Applied Knowledge Questions

Chapter 1

Structure/Substance	Role during a muscle action
Myosin cross-bridges	• Bind to sites on the actin, then rotate (swivel in an arc) to cause the actin to slide over the myosin
ATP	• Splits to provide energy for movement (e.g., for the dissociation of actin and myosin after the power stroke)
Calcium	• Is released into the sarcoplasm by the sarcoplasmic reticulum when the motor neuron receives an action potential • Binds with troponin
Troponin	• Lies on top of the tropomyosin • Binds with the released calcium • Shifts the tropomyosin off of the actin's binding sites to allow the myosin cross-bridges to attach to the binding sites
Tropomyosin	• Covers the binding sites on the actin when at rest • Binds with troponin once the calcium is released
Acetylcholine	• Carries the action potential across the synapse from the axon terminal of one axon to receptor sites on the second neuron (to continue the electrical impulse)

Chapter 2

$\dot{V}O_2$ = 140 beats/min × 100 ml blood/beat × 11 ml O_2/100 ml blood = 1,540 ml O_2/min

= 1,540 ml O_2/min divided by (132 pounds divided by 2.2 kilograms per pound)

= 1,540 ml O_2/min divided by 60 kilograms

= 25.7 ml $O_2 \cdot kg^{-1} \cdot min^{-1}$ divided by 3.5 ml $O_2 \cdot kg^{-1} \cdot min^{-1}$

$\dot{V}O_2$ = 7.3 METs

Chapter 3

Activity	Carbohydrate	Fat
Client is sitting in a chair listening to the personal trainer	Least	Most
During the first few seconds of the treadmill test	Most	Least
During a stage in which the client has reached steady state	Least	Most (a shift toward fats)
At the end of the test as the client reaches maximum	Most (a shift toward carbohydrates)	Least

Chapter 4

Source of external resistance	Resistance training exercises
Gravity	Many exist, for example, standing shoulder press, free weight bench press, lat pulldown, angled leg press
Inertia	Power clean, snatch
Fluid	Pneumatic (compressed air) resistance exercises
Elasticity	Rubber tubing exercises
Electronically controlled	Isokinetic-based rehabilitation machines

Chapter 5

System	Two adaptations *(more listed in the text; e.g., table 5.2)*
Nervous	• Increased EMG amplitude • Increased skill • Increased motor unit recruitment • Increased motor unit firing rate • Decreased co-contraction • Increased motor unit synchronization
Muscular	• Increased cross-sectional area • Increased size and number of myofibrils • Fiber subtype shift from Type IIb to Type IIa
Skeletal	• Increased bone formation/mass
Metabolic	• Possibly increased concentration of ATP and CP • Possibly increased concentration of creatine kinase and myokinase
Hormonal	• Increased concentration of testosterone • Altered epinephrine response • Increased sensitivity of receptor sites
Cardiovascular	• Augmentation of the development of endurance and running efficiency • Increased capillarization • Decreased myoglobin and mitochondrial density

Chapter 6

System	Two adaptations *(more listed in the text; e.g., tables 6.1 and 6.2)*
Nervous	• Morphological change in the neuromuscular junction • More negative resting membrane potential • Increased density of membrane ion channels • Changes in the motor endplate
Energy	• Increased storage of glycogen and intramuscular triglycerides • Increased time to exhaustion • Increased availability of free-fatty acids • Shift in lactate threshold • Increase in mitochondrial density
Skeletal	• Increased thickness of the meniscus • Increased hydroxyproline and calcium concentrations • Increased site-specific bone mineral density
Cardiovascular (blood vessels)	• Increased cross-section of coronary blood vessels • Increased capillary density • Increased a-$\bar{v}O_2$ difference
Endocrine	• Increased insulin sensitivity • Increased parasympathetic stimulation • Decreased release of epinephrine and norepinephrine
Cardiovascular (heart)	• Increased $\dot{V}O_2$max • Increased stroke volume • Increased cardiac output • Increased size of the heart chambers • Decreased resting heart rate • Decreased submaximal exercise heart rate • Increased blood volume

Chapter 7

Nutrient	General daily requirements
Kilocalories	• Based on table 7.2: 154 lb × 16 kcal/lb = 2,464 kcal • Based on table 7.3: REE = (8.7 × weight in kilograms) + 829 REE = (8.7 × 70) + 829 REE = 609 + 829 REE = 1,438 kcal Activity factor for "light" activity level: 1.5-1.6 (use 1.55) Total calorie needs = REE × 1.55 Total calorie needs = 1,438 × 1.55 Total calorie needs = 2,229 kcal
Protein (grams)	Minimum of 0.8 grams per kilogram of body weight: 70 × 0.8 = 56 g
Carbohydrate (grams)	Probably about 5 grams per kilogram of body weight: 70 × 5 = 350 grams
Fat (percent of total kilocalories)	≤30% of total calories consumed

Nutrient	General daily requirements
Monounsaturated fat (% of total fat intake)	33% of total fat intake
Polyunsaturated fat (% of total fat intake)	33% of total fat intake
Saturated fat (% of total fat intake)	33% of total fat intake
Vitamin A	700 micrograms
Vitamin E	15 milligrams
Calcium	1,000 milligrams
Iron	18 milligrams
Fluid	1.5 to 2.7 quarts (1.4-2.6 liters) or more

Chapter 8

1. Make goals specific, measurable, and observable:
   - The client provided a *specific* goal of a 90-pound increase in his 1RM.
   - The goal increase is *measurable* (i.e., it is a certain load).
   - The goal is *observable* in that the client and the personal trainer can visually see that the leg press is loaded with the goal weight and a 1RM attempt is either successful or not successful; there is no "in between."
2. Clearly identify the time constraints:
   - The client stated a six-month time frame.
3. Use moderately difficult goals:
   - A 90-pound increase is very large and may have to be modified (although the client's training status is not mentioned; a relatively untrained healthy male client can probably attain this goal, but other client types may have difficulty).
4. Record goals and monitor progress:
   - The client can be retested every four to eight weeks to monitor progress.
   - A workout card or wall poster can be a valuable visual motivator.
5. Diversify process, performance, and outcomes:
   - If the client can tolerate it, a periodized resistance training program (see chapters 15 and 23) will be the most effective method.
6. Set short-range goals to achieve long-range goals:
   - If the client will be retested every eight weeks (two months), his short-term goals could be to reach a 1RM of 255 pounds in two months, 285 pounds in four months, then 315 pounds in six months.
7. Make sure goals are internalized:
   - Since the client provided his own goal, it is likely that he has internalized it.
   - The personal trainer should discuss the goal with the client to find out why the client provided that particular goal; this will help the personal trainer determine what type of feedback or motivation is appropriate for the client (e.g., if the client's friend has a 1RM of 310 pounds, the client's stated goal of 315 pounds may indicate an ego-involved goal orientation).

Chapter 9

Based on comparisons to the coronary artery disease risk factor thresholds (table 9.1):

- Family history: no risk—his father's heart attack occurred after age 55 (his grandmother's heart attack is not a factor).
- Cigarette smoking: no risk—he is a nonsmoker.
- Hypertension: no risk—blood pressure is below the 140/90 mmHg reading.
- Hypercholesterolemia: at risk—his cholesterol is over the 200 mg/dL recommendation and his HDL level is at the 35 mg/dL cutoff
- Fasting glucose: no risk—his reading is below the 110 mg/dL recommendation.
- Obesity: no risk—his BMI is less than 30 kg/m^2.
- Sedentary lifestyle: at risk—client is sedentary.

Based on the risk stratification categories (table 9.2), the client is at a "moderate" risk.

Chapter 10

Client	Description	Fitness component to be tested	Test One	Test Two
Male 27 years old	Has been participating in 5-km runs for 3 years	Cardiovascular endurance	1.5-mile run	12-minute run
Female 33 years old	Has been resistance training consistently for 10 years	Muscular strength	1RM bench press	1RM back squat
Female 41 years old	Has been diagnosed as obese by her physician	Body composition	Girth measurements	BMI *or* waist-to-hip ratio
Male 11 years old	Has no exercise experience or training	Muscular endurance	1-minute sit-up test	Push-up test

Chapter 11

- Age-predicted maximal HR: 220 – 36 = 184 beats/min
- 85% age-predicted maximal HR: 184 × 0.85 = 156 beats/min
- 50% age-predicted maximal HR: 184 × 0.50 = 92 beats/min
- 90% age-predicted maximal HR: 184 × 0.90 = 166 beats/min
- Step 1: Plot all of the average HR measurements that are between 50% and 90% of age-predicted maximal HR (Y-axis) versus the corresponding work rates (X-axis) on a graph (if desired, use the graph seen in figure 11.5). Note that the stage 1 HR and work rate are not plotted.
- Step 2: Construct a horizontal line at 184 beats/min (the age-predicted maximal HR).
- Step 3: Construct a line of best fit for the plotted data points (from step 1) and extend the line beyond the horizontal line at 184 beats/min. In this case, the line passes through the two plotted points of (600, 130) and (750, 158).
- Step 4: Drop a vertical (perpendicular) line *from* the point where the horizontal line (at 184 beats/min) intersects the line of best fit *to* the X-axis.
- Step 5: Identify the X-axis value that corresponds with the vertical line. This X value is the predicted maximal work rate that will be used to calculate the estimated $\dot{V}O_2$max. In this applied knowledge problem, this vertical line reveals a predicted maximal work rate of about 890 kg · m^{-1} · min^{-1}.
- Step 6: Use equation 11.5 to convert the kg · m^{-1} · min^{-1} value to watts:
  - --Equation 11.5: Work rate (in watts) = work rate (in kg · m^{-1} · min^{-1}) ÷ 6.12
  - --Predicted maximal work rate (in kg · m^{-1} · min^{-1}) from step 5 is 890 kg · m^{-1} · min^{-1}
  - --Predicted maximal work rate (in watts) = 890 kg · m^{-1} · min^{-1} ÷ 6.12
  - --Predicted maximal work rate (in watts) = 145 watts
- Step 7: The client's body weight in kilograms is already provided: 76 kilograms
- Step 8: Use equation 11.6 to determine the predicted $\dot{V}O_2$max score in ml · kg^{-1} · min^{-1}:
  - -- Equation 11.6: $\dot{V}O_2$max (ml · kg^{-1} · min^{-1}) = [(10.8 × watts) ÷ body weight] + 7
  - -- The predicted maximal work rate (in watts) from step 6 is 145 watts
  - -- Body weight (kg) = 76 kg
  - -- $\dot{V}O_2$max (ml · kg^{-1} · min^{-1}) = [(10.8 × 145) ÷ 76] + 7
  - -- $\dot{V}O_2$max (ml · kg^{-1} · min^{-1}) = 27.6 ml · kg^{-1} · min^{-1}
- Step 9: Use table 11.17 to compare the predicted $\dot{V}O_2$max of 27.6 ml · kg^{-1} · min^{-1} to normative values:

-- 27.6 ml · kg^{-1} · min^{-1} for a 36-year-old male ranks at less than the 10th percentile.

Chapter 12

a. What static flexibility exercises focus on the hip extensors?
   - Forward lunge: gluteus maximus, hamstrings (also: iliopsoas, rectus femoris)
   - Lying knee to chest: gluteus maximus, hamstrings (also: erector spinae)
   - Semistraddle (modified hurdler's stretch): hamstrings (also: erector spinae, gastrocnemius)

b. What dynamic flexibility exercises involve the hip extensors?
   - Lunge walk: gluteus maximus, hamstrings (also: iliopsoas, rectus femoris)
   - Reverse lunge walk: gluteus maximus, hamstrings (also: iliopsoas, rectus femoris)
   - Hockey lunge walk: gluteus maximus, hamstrings (also: iliopsoas, rectus femoris, hip adductors)
   - Walking side lunge: gluteus maximus, hamstrings (also: rectus femoris, hip adductors)
   - Walking knee tuck: gluteus maximus, hamstrings

c. What body-weight exercises strengthen the hip extensors?
   - Several resistance training exercises shown in chapter 13 can be performed with only the client's body weight that will train the hip extensors (e.g., squat, forward lunge).

d. What stability ball exercises actively (concentrically, not isometrically) train the hip extensors?
   - Supine leg curl: gluteus maximus, hamstrings (also: erector spinae)
   - Supine hip lift: gluteus maximus, hamstrings (also: erector spinae)
   - Reverse back hyperextension: gluteus maximus, hamstrings (also: erector spinae)

Chapter 13

1. Bench press: common errors
   - Bouncing the bar on the chest during the upward movement phase to help raise the bar past the sticking point
   - Arching the back to raise the chest to meet the bar during the downward movement phase
   - Raising the hips or the head off the bench during the movement
2. Back squat: common errors
   - Allowing the heels to lift off the floor, the torso to flex further forward, or the upper back to round during the upward movement phase
   - Allowing the knees to move in (via hip adduction) or out (hip abduction) during the movement
   - Allowing the arms to relax or the elbows to drop down and forward
3. Front squat: common errors
   - Allowing the heels to lift off the floor, the torso to flex forward, or the upper back to round during the upward movement phase
   - Allowing the knees to move in (via hip adduction) or out (hip abduction) during the movement
   - Allowing the arms to relax or the elbows to drop down and backward
4. Shoulder press: common errors
   - Pushing with the legs or rising off the seat to help raise the bar upward
   - Excessively arching the back during the upward movement phase
5. Power clean: common errors
   - Allowing the upper back to round (i.e., losing the flat-back position), especially during the first pull
   - Extending the knees faster than (and/or before) the hips
   - Allowing the bar to travel upward too far away from the body
   - Using a "reverse curl" movement to move the bar into the catch position

Chapter 14

	Walking	Running
Body position	• The head should be held upright with the eyes looking straight ahead. • The shoulders should be relaxed but not rounded. • The upper body should be positioned directly over the hips. • Body should be upright with the torso positioned directly over the hips.	Same as walking (see left column), plus: • The lower back should not be arched.

(continued)

(continued)

	Walking	Running
Foot strike	• Heel strikes the ground and then the weight is immediately spread over the foot by a gentle rolling heel-to-ball action. • Primarily this heel-to-ball roll starts near the outer side of the heel and continues forward and slightly inward toward the middle of the ball of the foot at push-off.	Same as walking (see left column), plus: • Bouncing with each step should be avoided. Different from walking in this way: • Some elite runners run primarily ball-to-heel.
Arm action	• The left arm swings forward when the right foot strides forward. • The right arm swings forward when the left foot strides forward. • The arms swing naturally from relaxed shoulders. • The arms are held bent at the elbow at 90 degrees. • The elbows pass fairly close to the sides. • The arms and hands swing primarily in a forward and backward motion. • The hands should not cross the midline of the body. • On the forward swing the hands come to the level of the chest at the nipple line. • On the backward swing the hands reach the hipbone at the side of the body. • The hands are cupped loosely.	Same as walking (see left column). Different from walking in these ways: • Only some arm action occurs from the shoulders. • Much of the arm movement comes from the lower arm. • The elbow is unlocked. • The angle at the elbow opens during the arm downswing and closes during the upswing. • The forearms are carried between the waist and chest.

Chapter 15

10RM loads and their estimated 1RMs for these selected exercises:

Exercise (all cam machines)	10RM (pounds)	Estimated 1RM (pounds)
Vertical chest press	60	80
Seated row	50	65
Shoulder press	45	60
Biceps curl	35	45
Triceps extension	30	40
Leg (knee) extension	70	95
Leg (knee) curl	60	80

Assigning loads:
Repetition range to match training goal: 6 to 12 per set
Goal repetitions: 8
Loading (%1RM) range to match the training goal: 67 % to 85 %1RM
%1RM associated with 8 goal repetitions: 80 %1RM

* Calculate training loads from the estimated 1RM:

Exercise (all cam machines)	Estimated 1RM (pounds)	×	%1RM associated with 8 goal repetitions (in decimal form)	=	Calculated trial load	Assigned training load (rounded down)
Vertical chest press	80	×	0.80	=	64	60
Seated row	65	×	0.80	=	52	50
Shoulder press	60	×	0.80	=	48	45
Biceps curl	45	×	0.80	=	36	35
Triceps extension	40	×	0.80	=	32	30
Leg (knee) extension	100	×	0.80	=	80	80
Leg (knee) curl	80	×	0.80	=	64	60

Chapter 16

Type	Intensity	Duration	Frequency	Goals
LSD	Lower than normal; 50% to 85% HRR	Longer than normal; 30 minutes to 2 hours	No more than twice a week	Improve anaerobic threshold; develop endurance in the involved muscles; promote fat use; improve glycogen sparing
Pace/Tempo: intermittent	At lactate threshold; RPE of 13 to 14 (or 4-5, depending on the scale)	Repeated work intervals of 3 to 5 minutes alternated with rest intervals of 30 to 90 seconds	1 to 2 times per week	Improve $\dot{V}O_2$max
Pace/Tempo: steady	At lactate threshold; RPE of 13 to 14 (or 4-5, depending on the scale)	One session of 20 to 30 minutes	1 to 2 times per week	Improve $\dot{V}O_2$max
Interval	At or above lactate threshold and $\dot{V}O_2$ max; 90% to 100% of HRR	Repeated work intervals of 3 to 5 minutes alternated with rest intervals at 1:1 to 1:3 work:rest ratio	1 to 2 times per week *(not mentioned in chapter)*	Complete more work at a higher level of intensity than in a continuous exercise session; enhance the body's ability to clear lactate from the blood

Chapter 17

Mode	• Since her 1RM squat is 1.5 times her body weight, she can perform lower body plyometric drills • Without knowing her 1RM bench press, one cannot be certain whether she can safely perform upper body plyometric drills

(continued)

(continued)

Activity-specific drills and their intensity *(table 17.2 and the technique checklists)*	Choose from these lower body drills: • Two-foot ankle hop (intensity level: low) • Double-leg vertical jump (intensity level: low) • Skip (intensity level: low) • Single-leg push-off (intensity level: low) • Jump to box (intensity level: low) • Double-leg tuck jump (intensity level: medium) • Split squat jump (intensity level: medium) • Double-leg hop (intensity level: medium) • Jump from box (intensity level: medium) • Depth jump (intensity level: high) • Depth jump to second box (intensity level: high) If she is able to qualify to perform upper body plyometrics, she could include these exercises: • Depth push-up (intensity level: medium) • Power drop (intensity level: high)
Frequency	2 × a week (as long as this does not result in overtraining due to the frequency of teaching aerobic classes)
Volume *(table 17.4)*	100-120 total (foot) contacts (since she is resistance trained and performs plyometric drills now during a class she teaches)

Chapter 18

	***Minimum* exercise program**	***Optimal* exercise program**
Number of activity sessions per day	3	3
Intensity of the activity sessions *(described by words)*	Moderate, alternated with rest	Moderate to vigorous, alternated with rest
Intensity of the activity sessions *(described by number of* $kcal \cdot kg^{-1} \cdot day^{-1}$*)*	3-4	6-8
Intensity of the activity sessions *(described by number of kilocalories per day)*	Using 3 $kcal \cdot kg^{-1} \cdot day^{-1}$: 90 kcal	Using 7 $kcal \cdot kg^{-1} \cdot day^{-1}$: 210 kcal
Approximate total duration of the activity sessions	30 minutes	60 minutes
Examples of the activity sessions	Recess *(more listed in the text)*	Circuit exercises *(more listed in the text)*

Chapter 19

Dietary modifications:

- Refer to a registered dietician.
- Select foods that are aligned with the client's cultural and ethnic background.
- Select foods that help to decrease risk of CVD risk factors (e.g., follow the TLC diet).
- Create a deficit of 500 to 1,000 kilocalories per day.
- Women: not less than 1,000 to 1,200 kilocalories per day (1,200-1,600 for women who weigh more than 165 pounds [75 kilograms] or for women who exercise regularly).
- Set a weight loss goal of 10% of body weight over the first six months, then set new goals.
- Aim for a 1- to 2-pound (0.45- to 0.9-kilogram) weight loss per week.

- Change food choices to lower caloric and fat intake.

Exercise program guidelines:

- Increase expenditure to help contribute to the reduced food intake (deficit) of 500 to 1,000 kilocalories per day.
- Aim for a mode, intensity, and duration of activity that will expend at least 150 kilocalories per day (1,000 kilocalories per week); progress toward 300 kilocalories per day (2,000 kilocalories per week).
- Start all exercise at a low level.
- Aerobic conditioning:
  - -- Mode: use low-impact activities.
  - -- Frequency: five days per week (or daily).
  - -- Duration: can begin with two daily sessions of 20 to 30 minutes each; eventual goal: 40 to 60 minutes per day.
  - -- Intensity: 40% or 50% to 70% $\dot{V}O_2$max.
- Resistance training:
  - -- Begin with body-weight exercises.
  - -- Intersperse with aerobic exercise.
- Flexibility training:
  - -- Frequency: daily (or at least five days per week).

Lifestyle change support suggestions:

- Self-monitoring:
  - -- Record activity and dietary behaviors, habits, and attitudes (e.g., use the "Small Steps . . . Big Changes® Diet and Activity Diary" form).
  - -- Identify the obstacles to regular exercise.
- Rewards:
  - -- Provide big or small, tangible or intangible rewards (from the personal trainer, the client, or the client's family or support group).
  - -- Small rewards are for reaching small goals; big rewards are for reaching big goals.
- Goal setting:
  - -- Set realistic, stepwise short-term goals to reach larger, long-term goals.
  - -- Fill out and sign an activity/exercise self-contract.
- Stimulus control:
  - -- Identify social or environmental cues that trigger undesired responses.
  - -- Modify those cues and determine ways to manage the situation.
- Food consumption behavior changes:
  - -- Eat more slowly.
  - -- Use smaller plates.
  - -- Do not skip meals.
  - -- Develop techniques over time that work well for a specific client.

Chapter 20

	Beginning exercise program				Exercise concerns
	Mode	Intensity	Frequency	Duration	
Hypertension	Aerobic exercise: • Walking • Jogging • Swimming Resistance exercise (multijoint exercises): • Weight machines • Elastic bands • Circuit training	Aerobic exercise: • 40% $\dot{V}O_2$max • 8 RPE on 6-20 scale • Expenditure of 700 kcal per week Resistance exercise: • 16 to 20 reps • 50%1RM • 1 set	Aerobic exercise: • 3 days per week Resistance exercise: • 2 days per week	Aerobic exercise: • 15 minutes Resistance exercise: • 30 minutes	• If the blood pressure is Stage 1, cancel the exercise session and advise the client to speak with the doctor • Avoid the Valsalva maneuver

(continued)

(continued)

<table>
<tr><th rowspan="2"></th><th colspan="4">Beginning exercise program</th><th rowspan="2">Exercise concerns</th></tr>
<tr><th>Mode</th><th>Intensity</th><th>Frequency</th><th>Duration</th></tr>
<tr><td>MI</td><td>Aerobic exercise:
• Not limited, but include treadmill walking when possible</td><td>Aerobic exercise:
• 40% $\dot{V}O_2$max
• 9 RPE on 6-20 scale
Resistance exercise:
• 20 reps
• 1 set</td><td>Aerobic exercise:
• 3 days per week
Resistance exercise:
• 2 days per week</td><td>Aerobic exercise:
• 15 minutes</td><td>• Monitor client for angina, palpitations, shortness of breath, diaphoresis, nausea, neck pain, arm pain, back pain, or a sense of impending doom
• Avoid the Valsalva maneuver</td></tr>
<tr><td>Stroke</td><td>Aerobic exercise:
• Ergometer
Resistance exercises
Flexibility exercises
Coordination and balance exercises</td><td>Aerobic exercise:
• 30% $\dot{V}O_2$ peak (not *max*)
• 9 RPE on 6-20 scale
Resistance exercise:
• Eventually strive for 3 sets of 8-12 reps</td><td>Aerobic exercise:
• 3 days per week
Resistance exercise:
• 2 days per week</td><td>Aerobic exercise:
• 5 minutes
Flexibility exercise:
• Before and after each session (as little as 5 minutes)</td><td>• Balance and strength are affected
• A 1RM cannot be determined; start with very light resistance training loads</td></tr>
<tr><td>PVD</td><td>Aerobic exercise:
• Walking
Resistance exercise:
• Same as for hypertensive clients</td><td>Aerobic exercise:
• Walk until it hurts, stop, then do it again, and so on</td><td>Aerobic exercise:
• Near daily</td><td>Aerobic exercise:
• 10 minutes</td><td>• PVD clients cannot walk for more than 2 to 5 minutes without having to stop and rest due to calf pain</td></tr>
<tr><td>Asthma</td><td>Aerobic exercise:
• Walking
• Jogging
• Swimming
Resistance exercise:
• General resistance training</td><td>Aerobic exercise:
• 11 RPE on 6-20 scale
Resistance exercise:
• 16-24 reps</td><td>Aerobic exercise:
• 3 days per week
Resistance exercise:
• 2 days per week</td><td>Aerobic exercise:
• 5 minutes</td><td>• Monitor intensity via RPE and the sense of shortness of breath
• Avoid temperature extremes</td></tr>
</table>

Chapter 21

Describe an appropriate beginning exercise program for this client.

- Most likely, this client will be able to tolerate any type of beginning resistance training program (see chapter 15 for details on designing a muscular endurance training program).
- The important exception is that all resistance exercises that over stress the neck and shoulder joints should be avoided (e.g., upright row and shoulder press).
- This client will be able follow nearly any type of aerobic exercise program and, preferably, will eventually progress to performing vigorous aerobic activity.

How should her present program be modified?

- This client should regress the resistance training program to perform isometric muscle actions only.
- Also, the personal trainer can increase the diameter (e.g., with tape, felt, or foam) of the bars and handles of the resistance machines to allow the client to more effectively grasp and hold them.
- While the wrists are sore and inflamed, rest may be the best decision.

Chapter 22

	Exercise contraindications	Safety concerns
SCI	• Exercising within 2-3 hours after a meal • Exercising while ill	• Overuse injuries at the shoulders, wrists, and elbows • Heat- and cold-related injuries • Poor venous return • Spasticity • Exercise-induced hypotension • Extra padding on equipment
MS	• Possibly muscular strength testing • Rapidly advancing resistance training loads • Vigorous/High aerobic exercise intensities (i.e., exercise to exhaustion) • Complex skill-oriented exercises • Exercising through an exacerbation	• Heat sensitivity and intolerance • Fatigue • Dehydration • Hip abductor/adductor spasticity • Sensory loss/Poor balance • Muscle imbalance across joints (agonist vs. antagonist) • Depression
Epilepsy	• Possibly vigorous exercise	• Effects of weight loss on the side effects of medication • Seizures
CP	• Short or nonexistent aerobic warm-up and stretching	• Seizures • Contractures • Poor coordination/balance • Joint pain • Spasticity

Chapter 23

Phase	Week	Goal reps	*Tuesday* "Heavy" day	*Thursday* "Light" day	*Saturday* "Medium" day
Hypertrophy/ Endurance	1	12	130 pounds	100 pounds	115 pounds
	2	10	145 pounds	115 pounds	130 pounds
	3	8	155 pounds	120 pounds	140 pounds
Strength	4	6	165 pounds	130 pounds	145 pounds
	5	6	165 pounds	130 pounds	145 pounds
	6	5	170 pounds	135 pounds	150 pounds
Strength/ Power	7	4	175 pounds	140 pounds	155 pounds
	8	4	175 pounds	140 pounds	155 pounds
	9	3	180 pounds	140 pounds	160 pounds
Competition	10	2	185 pounds	145 pounds	165 pounds
	11	2	185 pounds	145 pounds	165 pounds
	12	1	195 pounds	155 pounds	175 pounds

Chapter 24

a. (4 feet + 3 feet + 3 feet) × (3 feet + 3 feet + 3 feet) = 90 square feet

b. (4 feet + 3 feet + 3 feet) × (5 feet + 3 feet + 3 feet) = 110 square feet

c. (5 feet + 3 feet + 3 feet) × (4 feet + 3 feet + 3 feet) = 110 square feet

d. (8 feet + 3 feet + 3 feet) × (8 feet + 3 feet + 3 feet) = 196 square feet

e. (4.5 feet + 3 feet + 3 feet) × (7 feet + 3 feet + 3 feet) = 136.5 square feet

f. (5 feet + 3 feet + 3 feet) × (3 feet + 3 feet + 3 feet) = 99 square feet

g. (7 feet) × (7 feet) = 49 square feet

Chapter 25

Many examples exist; here are a variety of situations based on the nine areas of potential liability exposures listed in the NSCA's *Strength and Conditioning Professional Standards and Guidelines* document:

1. Preparticipation screening and clearance:
   - The client has a preexisting condition that increases injury risk.
2. Personnel qualifications:
   - The client is trained by someone who is not professionally certified.
3. Program supervision and instruction:
   - The client is left to perform new or unfamiliar exercises without supervision.
   - The client receives instruction, but is not corrected when he or she cannot perform the exercise properly.
4. Facility and equipment setup, inspection, maintenance, repair, and signage:
   - The equipment is not frequently inspected for wear.
   - The equipment is not properly maintained according to the manufacturer's specifications.

- Standard warning labels are not properly placed on the equipment.

5. Emergency planning and response:
   - The facility does not have an emergency plan.
   - The staff of the facility have not been trained to know and follow the emergency plan.
6. Records and record keeping:
   - Medical history forms and informed consent forms are not kept on file.
   - Modifications made to existing equipment are not kept on file.
   - The client does not have a workout card.
7. Equal opportunity and access:
   - The facility does not meet ADA guidelines.
8. Participation in strength and conditioning activities by children:
   - The exercise program is not modified for a child's capacities.
   - A child client is made to use adult-sized equipment.
9. Supplements, ergogenic aids, and drugs:
   - A client is pressured to purchase and use supplements sold by the facility.
   - A client is provided false information about supplements.

Glossary

Compiled by Torrey Smith

This glossary includes those terms that are bolded red in the text.

2-for-2 rule—A guideline that can be used to increase the load when two or more repetitions above the repetition goal are completed in the final set of an exercise for two consecutive training sessions.

acceleration—An increase in velocity.

actin—One of the two primary myofilaments that bind with myosin to cause a muscle action.

adenosine triphosphate (ATP)—The universal energy-carrying molecule manufactured in all living cells as a means of capturing and storing energy.

age-predicted maximal heart rate (APMHR)—The estimated maximum heart rate as influenced by age (i.e., 220 – age).

agonist—A muscle that is shortening to perform a concentric action.

all-or-none principle—Principle that describes when a muscle cell membrane reaches or exceeds its electrical threshold to result in a muscle action.

alpha-blocker—A drug that opposes the excitatory effects of norepinephrine released from sympathetic nerve endings at alpha-receptors and that causes vasodilation and a decrease in blood pressure.

alternated grip—A grip in which one hand is pronated and the other hand is supinated.

amenorrhea—Loss of menses for at least three consecutive menstrual cycles.

amortization phase—The time between the eccentric and concentric phases.

anabolic—Referring to the synthesis of larger molecules from smaller molecules.

anatomical position—Position in which a person stands erect with arms down at the sides and palms forward.

angina—A pain in the chest related to reduced coronary circulation that may or may not involve heart or artery disease.

angular velocity—An object's rotational speed.

antagonist—A muscle, typically anatomically opposite to the agonist, that can stop or slow down a muscle action caused by the agonist.

appendicular skeleton—Skeletal subdivision that consists of the shoulder girdle, arms, legs, and pelvis.

arteriovenous oxygen difference (a-$\bar{v}O_2$ difference)—The difference in the oxygen content of arterial blood versus venous blood expressed in milliliters of oxygen per 100 milliliters of blood.

assistance exercise—Exercises that involve movement at only one primary joint and recruit a smaller muscle group or only one large muscle group or area.

assumption of risk—A defense for the personal trainer whereby the client knows that there are inherent risks with participation in an activity but still voluntarily decides to participate.

atherosclerosis—A progressive degenerative process through which the interior lining of the arterial walls becomes hardened and inelastic.

atrium—An upper chamber of the heart that functions to pump blood to the lower chamber of the heart (i.e., ventricle).

auscultate—To listen to the sounds of the body by using a stethoscope.

automated external defibrillator (AED)—A portable device that identifies heart rhythms; uses audio or visual prompts, or both, to direct the correct response; and delivers the appropriate shock only when needed.

autonomic dysreflexia—Manifestation of a spinal cord injury that disrupts normal regulation of arterial blood pressure.

axial skeleton—Skeletal subdivision that consists of the skull, vertebral column, and thorax (rib cage).

ballistic stretching—A type of stretching that involves active muscular effort and uses a bouncing-type movement in which the end position is not held.

beta oxidation—A series of reactions in which free fatty acids are metabolized for energy for aerobic activity.

beta-blocker—A drug that opposes the excitatory effects of norepinephrine released from sympathetic nerve endings at beta-receptors; used for the treatment of angina, hypertension, arrhythmia, and migraine.

bioelectrical impedance analysis (BIA)—A body composition test that measures the amount of impedance or resistance to a small, painless electrical current.

bioenergetics—The energy pathways of metabolism.

bracketing—A type of training in which an exercise or sport movement is performed with a lighter-than-normal or a heavier-than-normal resistance.

bradycardia—A resting heart rate of less than 60 beats per minute.

breach of duty—Conduct of a personal trainer that is not consistent with the standard of care.

calcium channel blocker—Calcium antagonist that acts directly on the smooth muscle cells of blood vessels to cause vasodilation for the treatment of angina and hypertension.

cardiac output ($\dot{Q}$)—The quantity of blood pumped by the heart per minute expressed in liters or milliliters (i.e., SV × HR).

catabolic—Referring to the breakdown of larger molecules into smaller molecules.

cerebral palsy—A group of chronic musculoskeletal deficits causing impaired body movement and muscle coordination.

chronic obstructive pulmonary disease (COPD)—A condition or dysfunction of the pulmonary system (e.g., chronic bronchitis, emphysema, asthma).

civil law—The system that applies to one's private rights and therefore to personal responsibilities or obligations that individuals must recognize and observe when dealing with others.

closed grip—A grip in which the thumb is wrapped around the bar so that the bar is fully held in the palm of the hand.

closed kinetic chain—A movement during which the most distal body part's motion is significantly restricted or fixed; often occurs with lower (or upper) body movements with the feet (or hands) on the floor.

complex training—A combination of resistance and plyometric training.

compound set—Two different exercises for the same primary muscle group that are completed in succession without an intervening rest period.

concentric action—Action that occurs when a muscle overcomes a load and shortens.

construct—A neural process that cannot be directly observed but must be indirectly inferred through the observation of behavior.

contraindication—An activity or practice that is inadvisable or prohibited because of a given injury.

contusion—Condition in which tissue below the skin (e.g., muscle) is damaged but the skin is not broken; typically caused by excessive external impact.

core exercise—Exercises that involve movement at two or more primary joints and recruit one or more large muscle groups or areas.

Cori cycle—A gluconeogenic process, taking place in the liver, in which lactate is converted to glucose.

coronary artery disease (CAD)—A condition or dysfunction of the cardiovascular system (e.g., atherosclerosis, myocardial infarction, angina).

coronary risk factor—A characteristic, trait, or behavior that affects the probability of developing cardiovascular disease.

criterion-referenced standard—A method to compare data that involves a combination of normative data and experts' judgment to identify a specific level of achievement.

cross-training—A method of combining several exercise modes within one exercise program.

damages—Economic or noneconomic losses due to an injury.

deceleration—A decrease in velocity.

defendant—The person being sued or accused in a court of law.

diastolic blood pressure—The pressure exerted against the arterial walls between beats when no blood is ejected from the heart or through the vessels (diastole).

Dietary Reference Intakes (DRIs)—Current recommendations for the intake of vitamins and minerals; replaced the *Recommended Dietary Allowances*.

dislocation—Complete displacement of the joint surfaces.

duration—Measure of the length of time an exercise session lasts.

duty—Obligation to demonstrate an appropriate standard of care.

dynamic stretching—A type of stretching that utilizes speed of movement and is specific to a sport or movement pattern.

dyslipidemia—Abnormal lipid (fat) levels in the blood, lipoprotein composition, or both.

dyspnea—Shortness of breath.

dystonic spasm—Brief recurring muscle contractions that result in twisting and repetitive movements or abnormal posture.

eccentric action—Action that occurs when a muscle cannot develop sufficient tension and is overcome by an external load, and thus progressively lengthens.

edema—The escape of fluid into the surrounding tissues, resulting in swelling.

elasticity—The ability of a muscle fiber to return to original resting length after a passive stretch.

electron transport chain (ETC)—A series of oxidative reactions that rephosphorylate ADP to ATP.

end-diastolic volume—The volume of blood from the left atrium that is available to be pumped by the left ventricle.

endomysium—The connective tissue encasing individual muscle fibers.

epilepsy—Two or more unprovoked, recurring seizures.

epimysium—The connective tissue encasing the entire muscle body.

excess postexercise oxygen consumption (EPOC)—The oxygen uptake above resting values used to restore the body to the pre-exercise condition; also termed "oxygen debt."

exculpatory clause—An agreement explicitly stating that the client releases the personal trainer from any liability associated with negligence on the part of the personal trainer.

exercise arrangement—The specific sequence of exercises within a resistance training workout.

exercise choice—The exercises selected for inclusion in a resistance training program.

exercise order—*See* exercise arrangement.

exercise selection—*See* exercise choice.

false grip—A grip in which the thumb is not wrapped around the bar but instead is placed next to the index finger.

fascia—A fibrous tissue that envelops muscles, groups of muscles, and other soft tissue.

fascicles—Bundles of muscle fibers. Also referred to as fasciculi or fasciculus (singular).

fast-twitch (Type II)—A type of motor unit (and muscle fiber type) that is recruited for anaerobic activity.

feedback—The knowledge of results or awareness of success or failure.

Fick equation—$\dot{Q} = \dot{V}O_2 \div a\text{-}\bar{v}O_2$ difference.

fiduciary relationship—A rapport that occurs when one person trusts in and relies on another (e.g., personal trainer and client).

field test—An assessment that is performed away from the laboratory and does not require extensive training or expensive equipment.

first-class lever—A lever for which the applied and resistive forces act on opposite sides of the fulcrum.

five-point body contact position—Proper body positioning to maximize stability and spinal support in supine and seated exercises.

flexibility—The ability of a joint to move through an optimum range of motion (ROM).

fluid ball—The abdominal fluids and tissue that are kept under pressure by the diaphragm and abdominal muscles to support the vertebral column from the inside out.

force arm—A line starting from and perpendicular to the line of action of the force, extending to the fulcrum.

forced repetition—Repetitions that are successfully completed with assistance from a spotter.

forced vital capacity—The volume of air moved that results from maximal inspiration and maximal expiration.

freestyle (front crawl)—A swimming stroke with a straight and prone body position, an overhand arm motion, and a flutter kick.

frequency—The number of workouts performed in a given time period (typically one week).

friction—The resistance to motion of two objects or surfaces that touch.

frontal plane—A vertical plane that divides the body or organs into front and back portions.

fulcrum—The point about which a lever pivots.

functional capacity—The highest rate of oxygen transport and utilization that is reached at maximal physical exertion; also referred to as $\dot{V}O_2$max.

general warm-up—A type of warm-up that involves performing basic activities requiring movement of the major muscle groups (e.g., jogging, cycling, or jumping rope).

gestational diabetes—The onset of a diabetic condition that occurs only during pregnancy.

gluconeogenesis—The formation of glucose from lactate and non-carbohydrate sources.

glycogenolysis—The breakdown of glycogen.

glycogen—The stored form of glucose.

glycolysis—The breakdown of carbohydrates (either glycogen stored in the muscle or glucose delivered in the blood) to produce ATP.

goal repetitions—The number repetitions a client is assigned to perform for an exercise.

goal setting—A strategy for increasing the level of participation or causing a behavioral change.

Golgi tendon organ—Sensory organ lying within the tendons of the musculotendinous region that recognizes changes in tension in the muscle.

grip width—The distance between the hands when placed on a bar.

health appraisal—Process to screen a client for risk factors and symptoms of chronic cardiovascular, pulmonary, metabolic, and orthopedic diseases in order to optimize safety during exercise testing and participation.

heart rate reserve (HRR)—The difference between a client's maximal heart rate and his or her resting heart rate (i.e., APMHR – RHR).

high-density lipoproteins (HDLs)—Proteins produced in the liver that contain the largest amount of protein and the smallest amount of cholesterol; when elevated, these contribute to a decreased incidence of coronary artery disease.

hyperinsulinemia—High levels of insulin in the blood.

hyperlipidemia—Elevated concentrations of cholesterol, triglycerides, lipoproteins, or a combination of these.

hyperplasia—An increase in the number of muscle fibers.

hypertension—Traditionally, high blood pressure at rest that is defined as ≥140/90 mmHg (either or both numbers).

hyperthermia—Elevated body temperature.

hypertrophy—An increase in cross-sectional area of the muscle fiber.

hypoglycemia—Blood glucose level of ≤65 mg/dL.

independent contractor—A self-employed professional who works within the confines of, but is not controlled by, another business or facility.

informed consent—A protective legal document that informs the client of any inherent risks associated with fitness testing and participation in an exercise program.

innervation—Stimulation of a muscle cell by a motor nerve.

intensity—The demand or difficulty of an exercise session that determines exercise duration and training frequency.

intermittent exercise—Several shorter bouts of exercise interspersed with rest periods.

isokinetic—Referring to dynamic muscle activity in which a joint moves through a range of motion at a constant velocity.

isometric action—Action that occurs when a muscle generates a force against a resistance but does not overcome it, so that no movement takes place.

Karvonen formula—A method to determine exercise heart rate that takes into consideration a client's age and resting heart rate.

ketosis—High levels of ketones in the bloodstream caused by incomplete breakdown of fatty acids.

Korotkoff sounds—Vibrations that are heard, through the use of a stethoscope, as a result of blood flow through a constricted artery.

Krebs cycle—A series of reactions that continues the oxidation of glucose, glycogen, or pyruvate to create ATP.

lactate threshold (LT)—The exercise intensity at which blood lactate begins an abrupt increase above the baseline concentration.

lactate—An end-product of glycolysis; most common marker to identify lactic acid accumulation.

lactic acid—An end-product of glycolysis.

legal duty—An obligation recognized by the law requiring a person to conform to certain conduct that reflects the standard of care.

licensure—The legal authority or formal permission from authorities to carry on certain activities that by law or regulation require such permission.

liftoff—The movement of the bar from the supports of a bench or rack to a position in which the client can begin the exercise.

line of action of a force—The line along which the force acts, passing through the force's point of application.

load—The amount of weight assigned to an exercise set.

long-term goal—A strategy of sequencing and combining short-term goals to reach the client's primary outcome.

low-calorie diet (LCD)—A calorie-reduced yet nutrient-dense diet to achieve a caloric deficit.

low-density lipoproteins (LDLs)—Proteins that transport primarily cholesterol; when elevated, these contribute to an increased incidence of coronary artery disease.

macrocycle—The largest periodization division, typically composed of two or more mesocycles.

maximal heart rate (MHR)—The actual maximum heart rate.

maximal oxygen uptake ($\dot{V}O_2max$)—The greatest amount of oxygen that can be utilized at the cellular level for the entire body.

mean arterial pressure—The average blood pressure throughout the cardiac cycle (i.e., [(SBp – DBp) ÷ 3] + DBp).

mechanical advantage—The ratio of the length of the moment arm through which a muscular force acts to the length of a moment arm through which a resistive force acts.

medical clearance—Approval by a physician indicating that the client is fit for exercise.

mesocycle—A division of a periodized program that lasts several weeks to a few months.

metabolic equivalent (MET)—Resting oxygen uptake that is generally estimated to be 3.5 ml $O_2 \cdot kg^{-1} \cdot min^{-1}$.

metabolic syndrome—Any combination of three or more of the following unhealthy conditions: abdominal obesity, high triglycerides, low HDLs, hypertension, and high fasting glucose.

microcycle—A division of a periodized program that lasts from one to four weeks and can include daily and weekly training variations.

mitochondria—Specialized cellular organelles where the reactions of aerobic metabolism occur.

mode—The specific type of exercise or activity that will be performed during an exercise session.

moment arm—*See* force arm.

motivation—A psychological construct that influences behavior, commitment, attitude, and the desire to exercise.

motor unit—A motor nerve and all the muscle fibers it innervates.

multijoint exercise—An exercise that involves movement at two or more primary joints.

multiple sclerosis—An immune-mediated (autoimmune) disorder that is characterized by inflammation and progressive degeneration of nervous tissue.

muscle fiber—The structural unit of muscle. Also referred to as a muscle cell.

muscle spindle—Sensory organ within muscle fibers that relays sensory information about length and speed of stretch to the central nervous system.

myocardial infarction—A result of the death of heart tissue due to an occluded blood supply; also referred to as a heart attack.

myofibrils—The elements of a muscle fiber that primarily consist of actin and myosin.

myofilaments—The two primary proteins in a myofibril (i.e., actin and myosin).

myopathy—Any disease of a muscle.

myosin—One of the two primary myofilaments that bind with actin to cause a muscle action.

near-infrared interactance (NIR)—A body composition test that measures changes in the absorption of light at various anatomical sites; sometimes referred to as "near-infrared reactance."

negligence—The failure to conform one's conduct to a generally accepted standard or the failure to act as a reasonably prudent person would act under the circumstances.

neutral grip—A grip in which the palm faces in and the knuckles point out to the side, as in a handshake.

normotensive—Referring to normal blood pressure.

norm-referenced standard—A method to compare data that involves comparing the performance of a client against the performance of others in the same category (e.g., percentile scores).

one-repetition maximum (1RM)—The greatest amount of weight that can be lifted with proper technique for only one repetition.

onset of blood lactate accumulation (OBLA)—The exercise intensity at which blood lactate accumulates faster than it is removed.

open grip—*See* false grip.

open kinetic chain—A movement during which the most distal body part is free to move; often occurs with lower (or upper) body movements with the feet (or hands) off the floor and typically involves pushing or pulling against a machine.

osteoporosis—A disorder characterized by the demineralization of bone tissue that results in a decreased bone mineral density.

outcome goal—A goal that is gauged by social comparison (e.g., the desire to beat an opponent).

overhand grip—A grip in which the hand grasps the bar with the palm down and the knuckles up.

overload—A training stress or intensity greater than what a client is used to.

overstriding—A walking or running gait in which the foot hits too far in front of the body's center of gravity, causing a braking effect.

overtraining—A condition in which a client trains too much or rests too little, or both, resulting in diminished exercise capacity, injury, or illness.

oxidative system—The primary source of ATP at rest and during aerobic activities.

oxygen debt—*See* excess postexercise oxygen consumption (EPOC).

oxygen deficit—The difference between the amount of oxygen required for exercise and the amount of oxygen actually consumed during exercise.

pace/tempo training—A type of training program that involves an exercise intensity at the lactate threshold.

paraplegia—Injury to thoracic segments T-2 to T-12 causing impairment in the trunk, legs, pelvic organs, or a combination of these.

parasympathetic nervous system—A part of the nervous system that, when stimulated, slows down various systems of the body (decreases heart rate).

PAR-Q (Physical Activity Readiness Questionnaire)—An assessment tool to initially screen apparently healthy clients who want to engage in low-intensity exercise and identify clients who require additional medical screening.

passive warm-up—A type of warm-up that involves receiving external warmth or tissue manipulation (e.g., hot shower, heating pad, or massage).

pennation angle—The angle between the direction of the muscle fibers and an imaginary line between the muscle's origin and its insertion.

percent of 1RM-repetition relationship—The inverse correlation between an assigned load and the number of repetitions a client can perform with that load.

percent of APMHR method—A method to determine exercise heart rate that takes into consideration a client's age.

percentile—Percentage of scorers at or below the client's score.

performance goal—A goal that is gauged by a self-referenced personal performance standard (e.g., client's desire to beat his or her own record).

perimysium—The connective tissue encasing groups of muscle fibers (fascicles).

periodization—The systematic process of planned variations in a resistance training program over a training cycle.

phosphagen system—The primary source of ATP for short-term, high-intensity activities.

plaintiff—The "injured" person who brings a suit or complaint into a court of law.

plasticity—The tendency of a muscle to assume a new and greater length after a passive stretch even after the load is removed.

post-ictal state—The period immediately following a seizure.

postural alignment—The proper body position in which the head is upright, the shoulders are relaxed but not rounded, and the pelvis is slightly tilted posteriorly to align the torso over the pelvis.

potentiation—The increase in the activity of the agonist muscle caused by the reflexive response of the muscle spindles and the release of the storage of elastic energy.

power (or explosive) exercise—A structural core exercise that is purposely performed very quickly.

power—The rate of performing work; force × velocity.

preadolescence—Period of time before the development of secondary sex characteristics, corresponding roughly to the ages 6 to 11 years in girls and 6 to 13 years in boys.

process goal—A goal that is gauged by the amount or quality of effort during an activity (e.g., the desire to demonstrate perfect exercise technique).

program design variable—An aspect of an exercise program that, when manipulated properly, creates a safe, effective, and goal-specific outcome.

progression—The gradual and consistent increase in the intensity of an exercise program.

pronated grip—*See* overhand grip.

prone—Lying facedown.

proprioceptive neuromuscular facilitation (PNF)—A type of stretching that involves a partner and both passive movement and active (concentric and isometric) muscle actions.

proprioceptor—Specialized receptors in muscles, joints, and tendons that relay messages to the central nervous system about body and limb movements.

proximate cause—A cause that immediately precedes and produces an effect.

punishment—Any act, object, or event that *decreases* the likelihood of future target behavior (when the punishment follows that behavior).

pyramid training—A type of training variation in which the load is progressively increased in sequential sets with a corresponding decrease in the number of goal repetitions.

pyruvate—A precursor of lactic acid during the final steps of glycolysis.

quadriplegia—Injury between the highest thoracic (T-1) and highest cervical (C-1) segments of the spine resulting in impairment of the arms, trunk, legs, and pelvic organs.

rate coding—The control of the motor unit firing rate (i.e., the number of action potentials per unit of time).

rate-limiting step—The slowest reaction in a series of reactions.

rate-pressure product—An estimation of the work of the heart (i.e., double product; HR × SBp).

rating of perceived exertion (RPE)—A self-rating system that accounts for all of the body's responses to a particular exercise intensity.

recruitment—The process in which tasks that require more force involve the activation of more motor units.

reinforcement—Any act, object, or event that *increases* the likelihood of future target behavior (when the reinforcement follows the target behavior).

reliability—An expression of the repeatability of a test or the consistency of repeated tests.

repetition maximum (RM)—The greatest amount of weight that can be lifted with proper technique for a specific number of repetitions.

repetitions (or reps)—The number of times a movement of an exercise is completed.

resisted sprinting—A method to increase stride length and speed-strength by increasing the client's ground force production during the support phase.

respondeat superior—A legal doctrine by which employers can be found vicariously liable for the negligent acts of their employees (e.g., personal trainers).

rest period—The time interval between two sets.

resting heart rate (RHR)—The heart rate associated with the client's resting metabolic rate. *See also* resting metabolic rate.

resting metabolic rate (RMR)—A measure of the calories required for maintaining normal metabolism.

risk management—A facet of the emergency plan designed to decrease and control the risk of injury from client participation and, therefore, the risk of liability exposure.

risk stratification—A method to initially classify clients as being at low, moderate, or high risk for coronary, peripheral vascular, or metabolic disease.

rotational work—The product of the force exerted on an object and the distance the object rotates.

safety space cushion—The recommended area between each piece of equipment that enhances traffic flow in, out of, and around the exercise facility.

sagittal plane—A vertical plane that divides the body or organs into left and right portions.

sarcomere—The segment of a myofibril between two adjacent Z lines (bands), representing the functional unit of skeletal muscle.

sarcopenia—Muscle loss due to aging.

sarcoplasmic reticulum—Highly specialized network system in a muscle fiber that stores calcium ions.

scope of practice—Legal boundaries that determine the extent of a personal trainer's professional duties.

second-class lever—A lever in which the applied and resistive forces act on the same side of the fulcrum, but with the applied force acting through a moment arm that is longer than that of the resistive force.

seizure—An uncontrolled electrical discharge within any part of the brain, causing physical or mental symptoms that may or may not be associated with convulsions.

self-determination—A desire to participate in an activity for self-fulfillment as opposed to trying to meet the expectations of others.

self-efficacy—A perceived self-confidence in one's own ability to perform specific actions (e.g., reach a short-term goal) that lead to a successful outcome.

self-talk—A client's "internal voice."

series elastic component (SEC)—The structures that, when stretched, have the ability to store energy that may be released upon an immediate concentric muscle action.

set—A group of repetitions that are performed consecutively.

short-term goal—A strategy of establishing an attainable step that brings the client closer to reaching the long-term goal.

single-joint exercise—An exercise that involves movement at only one primary joint.

size principle—The recruitment of larger and more motor units as a response to an increased force requirement.

slow-twitch (Type I)—A type of motor unit (and muscle fiber type) that is recruited for aerobic activity.

spasticity—A state of increased tonus of a muscle characterized by heightened deep tendon reflexes.

specific warm-up—A type of warm-up that involves performing movements that mimic the sport or activity (e.g., slow jogging before running or lifting light loads on the bench press before lifting training loads).

specificity—A strategy to train a client in a certain way to produce a particular change or result.

speed-endurance—The ability to maintain running speed over an extended duration (typically longer than six seconds).

speed-strength—The application or development of maximum force at high velocities.

sphygmomanometry—Measurement of blood pressure using an inflatable air bladder-containing cuff and a stethoscope to auscultate the Korotkoff sounds.

split routine—An exercise routine in which different muscle groups are trained on different days or training sessions.

sprain—Injury to a ligament.

sprint-assisted training—A method to increase stride frequency by having the client run at speeds greater than he or she is able to independently achieve.

stage of readiness—The degree or extent to which a client is ready to begin an exercise program.

standard error of measurement—The difference between a person's observed score—what the result was—and that person's true score, a theoretically errorless score.

standard of care—A set of criteria for the appropriate duties of a personal trainer. *See also* scope of practice.

state anxiety—The actual experience of anxiety, characterized by feelings of apprehension or nervousness, that is accompanied by an increased physiological arousal.

static stretching—A type of stretching performed at a slow constant speed, with a stationary endpoint.

status epilepticus—A seizure lasting more than 30 minutes or a seizure that occurs so frequently that consciousness is not restored.

sticking point—The most difficult part of the exercise that typically occurs soon after the transition from the eccentric to the concentric phase.

strain—Injury to a muscle.

stretch reflex—The immediate contraction of a muscle caused by a rapid stretch of that muscle.

stretch-shortening cycle (SSC)—The series of three phases that explains the mechanical and neurophysiological reactions to a plyometric movement.

stride frequency—The number of steps per minute.

stride length—The distance covered with each step.

stroke volume—The quantity of blood ejected by the left ventricle expressed in milliliters of blood per beat.

structural exercise—An exercise that loads the trunk (vertebral column) and places stress on the lower back.

subluxation—Partial displacement of the joint surfaces.

superset—Two different exercises for opposing or antagonistic muscle groups that are completed in succession without an intervening rest period.

supinated grip—A grip in which the hand grasps the bar with the palm up and the knuckles down.

supine—Lying down on the back, facing up.

sympathetic nervous system—A part of the nervous system that, when stimulated, speeds up various systems of the body (increases heart rate).

systolic blood pressure—The pressure exerted against the arterial walls as blood is forcefully ejected during ventricular contraction (systole).

tachycardia—A resting heart rate of more than 100 beats per minute.

target behavior—A behavior that is the focus for change or improvement; also called an operant.

target heart rate range (THRR)—The minimum and maximum heart rates per unit of time that are assigned for an aerobic exercise session.

tendinitis—Inflammation of a tendon.

test protocol—Procedures required for administering a reliable test.

test-retest method—A strategy to promote reliability by repeating a test with the same individual or group.

tetraplegia—*See* quadriplegia.

therapeutic lifestyle change (TLC)—A lifestyle modification that includes diet, physical activity, and weight loss.

thermic effect of food—An increase in energy expenditure above resting metabolic rate, caused by the digestion and assimilation of food.

third-class lever—A lever in which the applied and resistive forces act on the same side of the fulcrum, but with the resistive force acting through a moment arm that is longer than that of the applied force.

tidal volume—The amount of air moved during inhalation or exhalation with each breath.

torque—The tendency of a force to rotate an object about a fulcrum.

tort—A breach of legal duty other than a breach of contract that results in a civil wrong or injury; may be the foundation for a civil suit to collect damages.

total peripheral resistance—The impedance of blood flow caused by exercise, nervous stimulation, metabolism, and environmental stress.

trait anxiety—The potential perception or probability that a certain situation will cause anxiety.

transverse plane—A horizontal plane that divides the body or organs into upper and lower portions.

trial load—An estimated load that is based on a percent of the client's body weight.

triglycerides—A group of fatty compounds that circulate in the bloodstream; the predominate storage form of fat.

tropomyosin—A protein, attached to actin, that prevents actin from binding to the myosin cross-bridges.

troponin—A protein, attached to tropomyosin, that when activated shifts the tropomyosin to allow the actin to bind to the myosin cross-bridges.

type 1 diabetes mellitus—A disease in which the pancreatic beta cells are destroyed by an autoimmune process leading to absolute insulin deficiency; formerly known as "insulin-dependent diabetes mellitus" (IDDM).

type 2 diabetes mellitus—A disease resulting in insulin resistance in peripheral tissues and an insulin production deficit of the pancreatic beta cells; formerly referred to as non-insulin-dependent diabetes mellitus (NIDDM).

underhand grip—*See* supinated grip.

understriding—A walking or running gait in which the foot takes too short a stride, causing wasted energy.

undulating—Referring to a type of periodized training program that involves within-the-week or microcycle vacillations of training load and volume.

user space—The recommended area that a client needs to perform an exercise safely.

validity—The degree to which a test or test item measures what it is supposed to measure.

Valsalva maneuver—The act of breath-holding that contributes to maintaining intra-abdominal pressure; the client tries to exhale against a "closed throat."

variation—A purposeful change of the program design variable assignments to expose a client to new or different training stressors.

venous return—The return of the blood to the right atrium from the body (periphery).

ventricle—A lower chamber of the heart that functions to pump blood from the heart (right ventricle pumps to the lungs, left ventricle pumps to the body).

very low density lipoproteins (VLDLs)—Proteins that transport primarily triglycerides; when elevated, these contribute to an increased incidence of coronary artery disease.

visualization—The ability of the brain to draw and recall mental images that can create positive emotional responses and improve motivation.

volume—The total amount of weight lifted in a training session (i.e., total repetitions × the weight lifted per repetition) *or* the total number of repetitions completed in a training session (i.e., the number of repetitions performed in each set × the number of sets).

waiver—A contract that serves as evidence that the injured client waived his or her right to sue for negligence.

Wolff's law—The deposition of bone tissue (i.e., an increase in bone density) as a response to mechanical stress.

work—The product of the force exerted on an object and the distance the object moves (i.e., force × distance).

work-to-rest ratio—The relationship between the duration of the exercise interval and that of the recovery interval.

Credits

Figures

Figures 1.1, 1.2, 1.3, 1.4, 1.5, 1.6, 1.7, 1.8, 1.9, 6.1, 6.2, 6.4, 6.5 a-b, 6.9, 6.10, 16.2 Reprinted, by permission, from J.H. Wilmore and D.L. Costill, 1999, *Physiology of sport and exercise*, 2nd ed. (Champaign, IL: Human Kinetics), 29, 30, 32, 33, 35, 36, 55, 55, 58, 61, 282, 284, 199, 190, 261, 552, 621.

Figure 1.10 Fig. 18.1 p. 479 from EXERCISE PHYSIOLOGY 2nd, by Sharon A. Plowman and Denise L. Smith. Copyright © by Pearson Education, Inc. Reprinted by permission.

Figures 2.1, 2.3, 2.4, 2.5, 2.8, 2.10, 2.11, 3.1, 3.2, 3.3, 3.4, 3.5, 3.6, 3.7, 3.9, 3.10, 4.1, 4.2, 4.3, 4.4, 4.5, 4.8, 4.9, 4.10, 4.11, 5.1, 5.3 Reprinted, by permission, from T.R. Baechle and R.W. Earle, 2000, *Essentials of strength training and conditioning*, 2nd ed. (Champaign, IL: Human Kinetics), 116, 117, 119, 119, 120, 121, 122, 74, 77, 78, 79, 80, 81, 82, 86, 87, 30, 31, 31, 33, 34, 38, 39, 43, 44, 145, 152.

Figure 2.6 Reprinted from *Textbook of Medical Physiology*, 9th ed., A.C. Guyton and J.E. Hall, Copyright 1996, with permission from Elsevier Science.

Figures 2.7, 2.9 Reprinted, by permission, from W.D. McArdle, R.I. Katch, and V.L. Katch, 1996, *Exercise physiology: Energy, nutrition, and human performance*, 4th ed. (Philadelphia, PA: Lippincott, Williams, and Wilkins), 241, 230.

Figure 4.12 Adapted, by permission, from E.A. Harman, M. Johnson, and P.N. Frykman, 1992, "A movement oriented approach to exercise prescription," *NSCA Journal* 14(1): 47-54.

Figure 6.3 Reprinted, by permission, from J.H. Wilmore and D.L. Costill, 1999, *Physiology of sport and exercise*, 2nd ed. (Champaign, IL: Human Kinetics), 190. Originally adapted, by permission, from G.A. Brooks and J. Mercier, 1994, "Balance of carbohydrate and lipid utilization during exercise: The 'crossover' concept," *Journal of Applied Physiology* 76: 2253-2261.

Figure 6.6: From HANDBOOK OF PHYSIOLOGY: SECTION 12: EXERCISE: REGULATION AND INTEGRATION OF MULTIPLE SYSTEMS, edited by Loring B. Rowell and John T. Shepherd, copyright © 1996 by The American Psychological Society. Used by permission of Oxford University Press, Inc.

Figure 6.7 Reprinted from C. Snow-Harter, 1992, "Exercise, calcium and estrogen: Primary regulators of bone mass," *Contemporary Nutrition* 17(4). By permission of author.

Figure 8.1 Adapted, by permission, D.E. Sherwood and D.J. Selder, 1979, "Cardiorespiratory health, reaction time and aging," *Medicine and Science in Sports* 11: 186-189.

Figure 8.2 Reprinted from *Neurobiology of Aging*, Vol. 11, R.E. Dustman et al., "Age and fitness effects on EEG, ERPs, visual sensitivity, and cognition," pp 193-200, Copyright 1990, with permission from Elsevier Science.

Figure 9.1 Physical Activity Readiness Questionnaire (Par-Q) © 2002. Reprinted with permission from the Canadian Society for Exercise Physiology. http://www.csep.ca/forms.asp

Figure 9.2 Reprinted, by permission, from T. Olds and K. Norton, 1999, *Pre-exercise and health screening guide* (Champaign, IL: Human Kinetics), 29.

Figure 14.1 Adapted, by permission, from G. Town and T. Kearney, 1994, *Swim, bike, run* (Champaign, IL: Human Kinetics), 44.

Figure 14.2 Adapted from: *Sports and fitness equipment design*, Kreighbaum E. and M.A. Smith (eds.) Human Kinetics Publishers, (1996). By permission of author.

Figure 14.6 Adapted, by permission, from M. Evans, 1997, *Endurance athletes edge* (Champaign, IL: Human Kinetics), 76.

Figure 14.12 Adapted, by permission, from American Red Cross, 1992, *Swimming and diving* (Washington, DC: American Red Cross), 116.

Figure 16.3 Reprinted, by permission, from G. Borg, 1998, *Borg's perceived exertion and pain scales* (Champaign, IL: Human Kinetics), 47, 50.

Figure 17.1 Reprinted from *Eccentric muscle training in sports and orthopaedics*, M. Albert, Copyright 1995, with permission from Elsevier.

Figure 18.5 Reprinted, by permission, from W. Westcott, 1996, *Building strength and stamina: New nautilus training for total fitness* (Champaign, IL: Human Kinetics), 15.

Figure 18.6 Reprinted, by permission, from W. Westcott and T. Baechle, 1999, *Strength training for seniors: An instructor guide for developing safe and effective programs* (Champaign, IL: Human Kinetics), 22.

Figure 19.1 Reprinted, by permission, from C.W. Baker and K.D. Brownwell, 2000, Physical activity and maintenance of weight loss. In *Physical activity and obesity*, edited by C. Bouchard (Champaign, IL: Human Kinetics), 315.

Figures 20.2, 20.3 Reprinted, by permission, from A.S. Fauci et al., 1998, *Harrison's principles of internal medicine*, 14th ed. (New York: McGraw-Hill Companies), 1345-1352.

Figure 21.2 Reprinted from *Mechanical low back pain*, 2nd ed., J.A. Porterfield and C. DeRosa, p.138, Copyright 1998, with permission from Elsevier.

Tables

Tables 6.1, 10.2 Reprinted, by permission, from American College Sports Medicine, 1998, *ACSM's resource manual for guidelines for exercise testing and prescription*, 4th ed. (Philadelphia, PA: Lippincott, Williams, and Wilkins), 161, 631.

Tables 6.2, 6.3 Adapted, by permission, from J.H. Wilmore et al., 2001, "Heart rate and blood pressure changes with endurance training: The Heritage Family Study," *Medicine and Science in Sports and Exercise* 33(1): 107-116.

Table 6.4 Reprinted from *Textbook of medical physiology*, 10th ed., A.C. Guyton and J.E. Hall, p. 976, Copyright 2000, with permission from Elsevier Science.

Table 6.5 Reprinted, by permission, from J.H. Wilmore and D.L. Costill, 1999, *Physiology of sport and exercise*, 2nd ed. (Champaign, IL: Human Kinetics), 45.

Table 7.3 Adapted, by permission, from National Research Council, 1989, Recommended dietary allowances. Courtesy of the National Academies Press, Washington, D.C.

Table 7.4 From www.nap.edu.

Table 9.1 Reprinted, by permission, from American College of Sports Medicine, 2000, *ACSM's guidelines for exercise testing and prescription*, 6th edition (Philadelphia, PA: Lippincott, Williams, and Wilkins), 24. Originally adapted, from Summary of the second report of the National Cholesterol Education Program (NCEP) expert panel on detection, evaluation, and treatment of high blood cholesterol in adults (Adult Treatment Panel II), 1993, *Journal of the American Medical Association* 269: 6015-3023.

Table 9.2 Adapted, by permission, from American College of Sports Medicine, 2000, *ACSM's guidelines for exercise testing and prescription*, 6th edition (Lippincott, Williams, and Wilkins), 26.

Tables 9.3, 10.4 Reprinted, by permission, from American College of Sports Medicine, 2000, *ACSM's guidelines for exercise testing and prescription*, 6th edition (Lippincott, Williams, and Wilkins), 27, 80.

Table 10.1 Adapted, by permission, from American College of Sports Medicine, 2000, *ACSM's guidelines for exercise testing and prescription*, 6th edition (Lippincott, Williams, and Wilkins), 77. Data from Institute for Aerobics Research 1994.

Table 10.2 Reprinted, by permission, from American College of Sports Medicine, 1998, *ACSM's resource manual for guidelines for exercise testing and prescription*, 3rd edition (Lippincott, Williams, and Wilkins), 631.

Tables 10.3, 11.17, 11.28 Adapted, by permission, from American College of Sports Medicine, 2000, *ACSM's guidelines for exercise testing and prescription*, 6th edition (Lippincott, Williams, and Wilkins), 80, 77, 86.

Table 11.1 Reprinted, by permission, from V.H. Heyward, 2002, *Advanced fitness assessment and exercise prescription*, 4th ed. (Champaign, IL: Human Kinetics), 27.

Tables 11.2, 11.5, 11.6, 11.18, 11.19, 11.21 Reprinted, by permission, from G.M. Adams, 2002, *Exercise physiology laboratory manual*, 4th ed. (New York: McGraw-Hill Companies), 250, 224-225, 178-179, 149.

Tables 11.8, 11.9 Reprinted, by permission, from A.R. Frisancho, 1990, *Anthropometric standards for the assessment of growth and nutritional status* (Ann Arbor, MI: University of Michigan Press).

Table 11.7 Reprinted from National Institutes of Health, National Heart, Lung, and Blood Institute, 1998, *Clinical Guidelines on the Identification, Evaluation and Treatment of Overweight and Obesity in Adults (Executive Summary)*. NIH Publication 98-4083. Available online at www.nhlbi.nih.gov. Accessed January 13, 2003.

Tables 11.10, 11.11 Reprinted from S. Abraham, C.L. Johnson, and M.R. Najjar, 1979, *Weight by height and age for adults 18-74 years* (Hyattsville, MD: U.S. Department of Health, Education, and Welfare). Publication (PHS) 79-1656.

Table 11.12 Reprinted, by permission, from V.H. Heyward, 2002, *Advanced fitness assessment and exercise prescription*, 4th ed. (Champaign, IL: Human Kinetics), 171.

Table 11.13 Adapted, by permission, from V.H. Heyward and L.M. Stolarczyk, 1996, *Applied body composition assessment* (Champaign, IL: Human Kinetics), 12.

Table 11.14 Adapted, by permission, from L.A. Golding, C.R. Myers, and W.E. Sinning, 1989, *Y's way to physical fitness*, 3rd ed. (Champaign, IL: Human Kinetics), 125-136.

Table 11.15 Adapted, by permission, from G.A. Bray and D.S. Gray, 1988, "Obesity Part I–Pathogenesis," *Western Journal of Medicine* 149: 432.

Table 11.16 Reprinted, by permission, from American College of Sports Medicine, 1998, *ACSM's resource manual for guidelines for exercise testing and prescription*, 3rd edition (Lippincott, Williams, and Wilkins), 75.

Table 11.16 Reprinted, by permission, from American College of Sports Medicine, 1998, *ACSM's resource manual for guidelines for exercise testing and prescription*, 3rd edition (Lippincott, Williams, and Wilkins), 77.

Tables 11.18, 11.19, 11.21 Reprinted, from G.M. Adams, 2002, *Exercise physiology laboratory manual*, 4th ed. (New York: McGraw-Hill Companies), 178, 179, 149. Reproduced with permission of The McGraw-Hill Companies.

Table 11.20 Adapted, by permission, from P.O. Åstrand, 1960, "Aerobic capacity in men and women with special reference to age," *Acta Physiologica Scandinavica* 49(Suppl. 169): 45-60.

Tables 11.22, 11.23 Reprinted, by permission, from J.R. Morrow et al., 2000, *Measurement and evaluation in human performance*, 2nd ed. (Champaign, IL: Human Kinetics), 234, 235.

Table 11.24 Reprinted from the U.S. Department of Health and Human Services and the President's Council on Physical Fitness and Sports, 2002, *The 2002-2003 President's Challenge: Physical Activity and Fitness Awards Program*, p. 20. Available online at www.fitness.gov. Accessed December 31, 2002.

Tables 11.25, 11.26 Reprinted, by permission, from V.H. Heyward, 2002, *Advanced fitness assessment and exercise prescription* (Champaign, IL: Human Kinetics), 119-120.

Table 11.27 Adapted, by permission, from YMCA, 2000, *YMCA Fitness testing and assessment manual*, 4th ed., edited by L.A. Golding, C.R. Myers, and W.E. Sinning (Champaign, IL: Human Kinetics), 200-211.

Table 11.28 Reprinted, by permission, from American College of Sports Medicine, 2000, *ACSM's guidelines for exercise testing and prescription*, 6th ed. (Philadelphia, PA: Lippincott, Williams, and Wilkins), 86.

Table 11.29 Adapted, by permission, from YMCA, 2000, *YMCA Fitness testing and assessment manual*, 4th ed., edited by L.A. Golding, C.R. Myers, and W.E. Sinning (Champaign, IL: Human Kinetics), 113-124.

Table 11.30 a-b a. Reprinted, by permission, from Health Canada, 1986, "Age-gender norms for push-up test and percentiles by age groups for trunk forward flexion using a sit-and-reach box," *Canadian Standardized Test of Fitness Operations Manual*, 3rd ed., (Canada: Health Canada), and V. Heyward, 2002, *Advanced fitness assessment and exercise prescription*, 4th ed. (Champaign, IL: Human Kinetics), 125.

Table 11.31 Adapted, by permission, from YMCA, 2000, *YMCA Fitness testing and assessment manual*, 4th ed., edited by L.A. Golding, C.R. Myers, and W.E. Sinning (Champaign, IL: Human Kinetics), 200-211.

Table 11.32 Reprinted, by permission, from Health Canada, 1986, "Age-gender norms for push-up test and percentiles by age groups for trunk forward flexion using a sit-and-reach box," *Canadian Standardized Test of Fitness Operations Manual*, 3rd ed., (Canada: Health Canada).

Table 15.1 Adapted from T.R. Baechle and R.W. Earle, 2000, *Essentials of strength training and conditioning*, 2nd ed. (Champaign, IL: Human Kinetics).

Table 15.5 Adapted from T.R. Baechle and B.R Groves, 1998, *Weight training: Steps to success*, 2nd ed, (Champaign, IL: Human Kinetics), 112-113, and T.R. Baechle, and R.W. Earle, 1995, *Fitness weight training* (Champaign, IL: Human Kinetics).

Table 15.7 Adapted, by permission, from T.R. Baechle and R.W. Earle, 1995, *Fitness weight training* (Champaign, IL: Human Kinetics), 121.

Table 15.10 Adapted from T.R. Baechle and R.W. Earle, 2000, *Essentials of strength training and conditioning*, 2nd ed. (Champaign, IL: Human Kinetics), and R.W. Earle, 1999, Weight training exercise prescription. In *Essentials of personal training symposium workbook* (Lincoln, NE: NSCA Certification Commission).

Table 16.3 Adapted, by permission, from American College of Medicine, 2000, *ACSM's guidelines for exercise testing and* *prescription,* 6th edition (Lippincott, Williams, and Wilkins), 152-153, and adapted, by permission, from B.E. Ainsworth et al., 2000, "Compendium of physical activities: An update of activity codes and MET intensities," *Medicine and Science in Sports and Exercise* 32(9) Suppl: 186-189.

Table 18.1 Reprinted from C. Corbin, R. Pangrazi, and G. Welk, 1994, "Toward an understanding of appropriate physical activity levels of youth," *Physical Activity and Fitness Research Digest* 1(8): 1-8.

Table 19.2 Reprinted from National Institute of Health, and National Heart, Lung, and Blood Institute, 1998, *Clinical Guidelines on the Identification, Evaluation, And Treatment of Overweight and Obesity in Adults (Executive Summary).* NIH Publication 98-4083. Available online at www.nhlbi.nih.gov. Accessed January 13, 2003.

Tables 19.4, 19.5 Reprinted from National Institute, and National Heart, Lung, and Blood Institute, 2000, *The Practical Guide, Identification, Evaluation, and Treatment of Overweight and Obesity in Adults.* NIH Publication 00-4084. Available online at www.nhlbi.nih.gov. Accessed November 21, 2002.

Tables 19.6, 19.12, 19.16 Adapted, by permission, from American College of Sports Medicine, 2003, *ACSM exercise management for persons with chronic diseases and disabilities,* 2nd ed. (Champaign, IL: Human Kinetics), 138, 151, 145.

Tables 19.7, 19.8 Reprinted, by permission, from C. Otis and R. Goldingay, 2000, *The athletic women's survival guide* (Champaign, IL: Human Kinetics), 74.

Tables 19.9, 19.11 Reprinted from National Institute, and National Heart, Lung, and Blood Institute, 2001, *The Third Report of the National Cholesterol Education Program (NCEP) Expert Panel on Detection, Evaluation and Treatment of High Blood Cholesterol in Adults (Adult Treatment Panel III) Executive Summary.* NIH Publication 01-3670. Available online at www.nhlbi.nih.gov. Accessed November 21, 2002.

Table 20.1 Adapted from *The Sixth Report of the Joint National Committee on Prevention, Detection, Evaluation, and Treatment of High Blood Pressure (JNC VI), Archives of Internal Medicine* 157: 2413-2446, 1997. NIH Publication 98-4080.

Table 23.1 Adapted, by permission, from T.R. Baechle and R.W. Earle, 2000, *Essentials of strength training and conditioning,* 2nd ed. (Champaign, IL: Human Kinetics), 400.

Tables 23.2, 23.2, 23.4 Adapted, by permission, from D. Pearson et al., 2000, "National Strength and Conditioning Association's basic guidelines for the resistance training of athletes," *Strength and Conditioning Journal* 22(4): 14-27.

Table 24.1 Adapted, by permission, from T.R. Baechle and R.W. Earle, 2000, *Essentials of strength training and conditioning,* 2nd ed. (Champaign, IL: Human Kinetics), 560.

Forms and Text

Chapter 9 form Health Risk Analysis Adapted, by permission, from B.J. Sharkey, *Fitness and health,* 5th ed. (Champaign, IL: Human Kinetics), 63-67.

Chapter 24 form NSCA's Safety Checklist for Exercise Facility and Equipment Maintenance Reprinted, by permission, from T.R. Baechle and R.W. Earle, 2000, *Essentials of strength training and conditioning,* 2nd ed. (Champaign, IL: Human Kinetics), 596-601. Adapted in part from NSCA, 2001, *Strength & Conditioning Professional Standards and Guidelines* (Colorado Springs, CO: National Strength and Conditioning Association).

Chapter 6 text, page 115 Adapted, by permission, from T.R. Baechle and R.W. Earle, 2000, *Essentials of strength training and conditioning,* 2nd ed. (Champaign, IL: Human Kinetics), 166.

Chapter 9 text, page 180 Reprinted, by permission, from American College of Medicine, 2000, *ACSM's guidelines for exercise testing and prescription,* 6th edition (Lippincott, Williams, and Wilkins), 24.

Chapter 11 text, page 236 Adapted, by permission, from American College of Medicine, 2000, *ACSM's guidelines for exercise testing and prescription,* 6th edition (Lippincott, Williams, and Wilkins), 84.

Chapter 18 text, pages 462, 466 Reprinted, by permission, from American College of Medicine, 2000, *ACSM's guidelines for exercise testing and prescription,* 6th edition (Lippincott, Williams, and Wilkins), 232-233.

Chapter 18 text, pages 465, 466 Adapted from *International Journal of Gynecology and Obstetrics,* 77 "Exercise during pregnancy and the postpartum period," pgs. 79-81, Copyright 2002, with permission from Elsevier.

Chapter 18 text, page 466 Adapted, by permission, from A.F. Cowlin, *Women's fitness program development* (Champaign, IL: Human Kinetics), 133.

Chapter 19 text, page 492 Adapted, by permission, from C. Vega, 2001, Nutrition. In *Aquatic Fitness instructor manual: A resource for aquatic fitness professionals* (Nokomis, FL: Aquatic Exercise Association).

Photos

Chapter 1 opener ©Kristiane Vey/Jump
Chapter 2 opener ©Digital Vision
Figures 2.2a and b ©Human Kinetics
Chapter 3 opener ©Kristiane Vey/Jump
Figure 3.8 ©Kristiane Vey/Jump
Chapter 4 opener ©Human Kinetics
Figure 4.6 ©Digital Vision
Chapter 5 opener ©Digital Vision
Figure 5.2 ©Stuart Hamby/Human Impact Photography
Chapter 6 opener ©Martina Sandkuhler/Jump
Figure 6.8 ©Digital Vision
Chapter 7 opener ©Empics
Figure 8.3 ©Digital Vision
Figure 9.1 ©Martina Sandkuhler/Jump
Chapter 14 opener ©Digital Vision
Chapter 15 opener ©Digital Vision
Chapter 16 opener ©Digital Vision
Figure 16.1 © Kristiane Vey/Jump
Chapter 17 opener ©Sporting Pictures
Chapter 18 opener ©Sport The Library/Brian Drake
Figure 18.7 ©Human Kinetics
Chapter 19 opener ©Digital Vision
Chapter 20 opener ©Marco Grundt/Jump
Figure 20.1 ©Getty Images
Figure 20.4 ©Catherine Ledner/Getty Images
Chapter 22 opener ©Sporting Pictures
Figure 22.1 ©Human Kinetics
Figure 22.2 ©Digital Vision
Chapter 23 opener ©Empics
Chapter 25 opener ©Corbis
Figure 25.2 Photo courtesy of Anthony A. Abbott

Index

Note: Page numbers followed by an italicized *f* or *t* refer to the figure or table on that page, respectively.

About the Editors

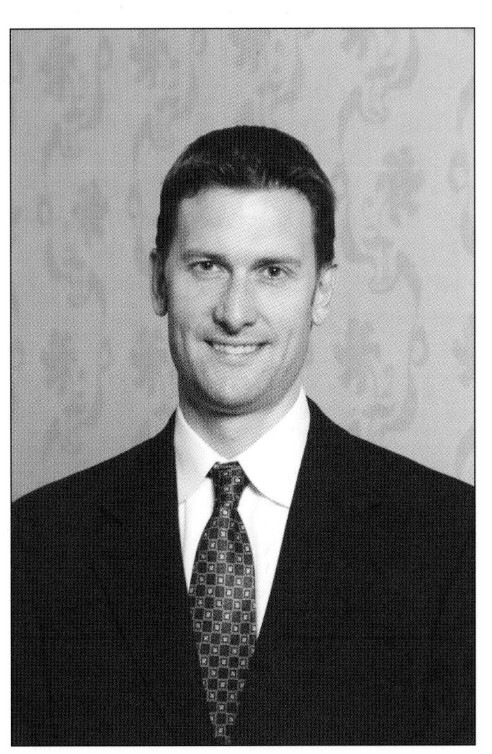

Roger W. Earle, MA, is the associate executive director and director of exam development for the NSCA Certification Commission. As an NSCA-Certified Personal Trainer and Certified Strength and Conditioning Specialist, he has been a practicing professional for more than 15 years.

Earle received his bachelor's degree in exercise science (magna cum laude) from Creighton University and his master's degree in exercise science (summa cum laude) from the University of Nebraska. He is coeditor of *Essentials of Strength Training and Conditioning, Second Edition.*

Before his work with the NSCA Certification Commission, Earle was a Division I strength coach and an exercise science faculty member at Creighton University for nine years.

Earle makes his home with his wife and children in Glendale, Arizona.

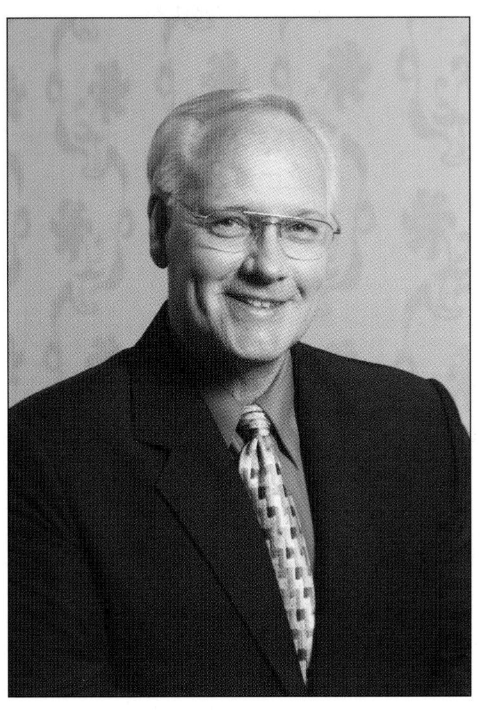

Thomas R. Baechle, EdD, is executive director of the NSCA Certification Commission and professor and chair of the department of exercise science and athletic training at Creighton University in Omaha, Nebraska.

In his notable career covering more than 30 years as a fitness professional and academician, Baechle has earned numerous certifications, taught at respected universities, held a variety of professional and civic offices, and volunteered for many national and international associations and organizations related to fitness and personal health. He also is widely published and lectures frequently on topics relating to his area of expertise.

Among his recent honors are the 2002 Distinguished Faculty Service Award from Creighton University, the Lifetime Achievement Award from the NSCA in 1998, and the Award of Merit for Excellence in Education and Development of Professional Standards from the International Fitness Institute in 1996. Baechle makes his home in Omaha.

About the NSCA

As the worldwide authority on strength and conditioning, the National Strength and Conditioning Association (NSCA) supports and disseminates research-based knowledge and its practical application to improve athletic performance and fitness.

The NSCA is a 26,000-member nonprofit educational association with members in 56 countries. Membership in the NSCA provides professionals with access to high-quality strength and conditioning publications, first-rate educational conferences and clinics, and a multitude of educational services in addition to networking and job opportunities for its members.

The NSCA Certification Commission offers two nationally accredited fitness-related certifications—the Certified Strength and Conditioning Specialist® and the NSCA-Certified Personal Trainer®. Both of these certifications meet the accreditation guidelines of the National Commission for Certifying Agencies and are recognized by the National Skills Standards Board.